The Organisation of Mind

The Organisation of Mind

Tim Shallice
Institute of Cognitive Neuroscience,
University College London
and
Cognitive Neuroscience Sector
SISSA Trieste

Richard P. Cooper
Department of Psychological Sciences,
Birkbeck, University of London

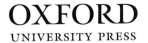

OXFORD
UNIVERSITY PRESS

OXFORD
UNIVERSITY PRESS

Great Clarendon Street, Oxford OX2 6DP

Oxford University Press is a department of the University of Oxford.
It furthers the University's objective of excellence in research, scholarship,
and education by publishing worldwide in

Oxford New York

Athens Auckland Bangkok Bogotá Buenos Aires Calcutta
Cape-Town Chennai Dar-es-Salaam Delhi Florence Hong-Kong Istanbul
Karachi Kuala-Lumpur Madrid Melbourne Mexico-City Mumbai
Nairobi Paris São-Paulo Singapore Taipei Tokyo Toronto Warsaw

with associated companies in Berlin Ibadan

Oxford is a registered trade mark of Oxford University Press
in the UK and in certain other countries

Published in the United States
by Oxford University Press Inc., New York

British Library Cataloguing in Publication Data

Data available

Library of Congress Cataloguing in Publication Data

Library of Congress Control Number: 2010942078

ISBN 978-0-19-957924-2

10 9 8 7 6 5 4 3 2 1

Typeset in Swift
by Glyph International, Bangalore, India
Printed in Italy
on acid-free paper by
L.E.G.O. S.p.A. Lavis TN

Whilst every effort has been made to ensure that the contents of this book are as complete,
accurate and up-to-date as possible at the date of writing, Oxford University
Press is not able to give any guarantee or assurance that such is the case. Readers are
urged to take appropriately qualified medical advice in all cases. The information in this
book is intended to be useful to the general reader, but should not be used as a means
of self-diagnosis or for the prescription of medication.

Preface

Neuroscience research relevant to cognitive processes has grown dramatically in the past two decades, largely due to the increasing availability of sophisticated technologies such as those used in neuroimaging. This growth has led to great advances in our understanding of the brain bases of cognitive processes, but in our view this progress is being undermined by a stance that tends to ignore or consider as irrelevant the cognitive level of analysis. This threat comes in two forms. From below, there is a reductionist view, which suggests that explanation can proceed without cognitive-level concepts, and moreover that such concepts are in themselves misleading. From above, there is a view that central cognition is non-modular or non-decomposable, and that brain-based approaches are irrelevant.

Our aim in this book is to refute the philosophical positions implicit in both of these views. Thus, the title *The Organisation of Mind* deliberately echoes Hebb's (1949) groundbreaking monograph *The Organization of Behavior*. We do not presume that our book will have the longevity of Hebb's, or that it resolves the mysteries of mind, but it does aim to embody a position on the state and future direction of cognitive neuroscience, together with a hypothesis concerning mind and its organisation.

This book is not intended to be a standard cognitive neuroscience text. It certainly does not cover all areas that would be relevant in such a text. Thus, our concern is primarily with higher-level aspects of mind and not with 'early' perceptual processes or 'late' motor processes. Similarly we do not consider emotion, motivation, development, social cognition, or the cognitive functions of neurotransmitter systems or the many interactions between each of these and cognitive processing. Even on the topics and methods that we do cover we are selective. Instead we aim to address in some detail the basic theoretical and methodological disputes on the topics we treat. At a more basic level, we assume a working knowledge of brain anatomy and how it can be visualised. Readers unsure of details in this area are advised to consult other sources, such as are available on the net.

Our intended audience is academics and graduate research students in cognitive neuroscience and related disciplines, such as cognitive psychology, cognitive science, neuropsychology, systems and behavioural neuroscience, and philosophy of mind. Conceptually the book consists of three sections. The opening chapters present the historical and methodological foundations of cognitive neuroscience. The emphasis throughout is on the relation between the computational methods of cognitive science, the patient-based methods of cognitive neuropsychology, and the brain-imaging methods of contemporary neuroscience. At issue is the question of how these sets of methods may advance our understanding of mind. It is argued that both sets of empirical methods have substantial limitations, but also that these limitations may be ameliorated if theoretical inferences are supported by evidence grounded in both neuropsychology and neuroimaging. This argument is illustrated in the central and closing chapters. In the second part, we discuss three distinct fundamental concepts arising from a computational view of mind, namely representation, buffers or short-term stores, and operations on representations. It is argued that together these provide the foundations for routine or automatised processing. The final chapters are then concerned with systems that may bias such routine processing in non-routine situations and additional systems required by such biasing, such as episodic memory and the systems involved in consciousness and thinking.

We are grateful to many people for their assistance during the many years that this project has taken to complete, particularly Fabio Campanella and Rosalyn Lawrence. Versions of individual chapters were read by Fergus Craik, Cristiano Crescentini, Karalyn Patterson, Alessandro Treves, Antonio Vallesi and Elizabeth Warrington. Their criticisms have helped to greatly improve the text. We have also benefitted greatly from interactions with our colleagues in the institutions in which we have worked—University College London (TS), Birkbeck, University of London (RC) and SISSA Trieste (TS). We much appreciated too the most helpful assistance of the OUP team. Most of all we are grateful to Maria and Tracy to whom the book is dedicated. Without their encouragement, support and tolerance of the inordinate time taken, the project would have never reached fruition.

Contents

Cognitive Neuroscience: The Seeds are Sown

1.1 The Origins of Cognitive Neuroscience

It has been known since Hippocrates in 400BC that 'from the brain and from the brain only ... we think, see, hear, ... distinguish the ugly from the beautiful, the bad from the good, the pleasant from the unpleasant' (Jones, 1923). Today every first-year student in the life sciences is aware that different regions of the cerebral cortex carry out different types of process. We have all seen, even in reports in newspapers, that a particular part of the temporal lobe of the cerebral cortex is activated when a face is recognised (Kanwisher, McDermott & Chun, 1997) or that lesions involving a part of frontal cortex can cause one to lose one's sense of humour (Shammi & Stuss, 1999). Such examples suggest that the mind has a complex structure. Uncovering the mind's organisation, and how any part of it operates, may then seem a technically complex but conceptually straightforward process, given the power of modern brain-imaging procedures. However, beneath the technologically brilliant surface, lies a hidden intellectual crevasse. Our knowledge of brains is mainly derived from the types of empirical procedures and conceptual frameworks that are characteristic of reductionist materialist approaches in biology, in general. Yet brains have two other aspects. They are the vehicles of intelligent action and thought, and scientifically, since Babbage, such processes have been a province of engineering and, later, computer science. They are also the physical basis of mind, whose properties we know from philosophy and psychology. Yet our exponentially increasing knowledge about brain function does not allow one to directly answer questions about intelligence and mind.

Many bridges exist between the realm of biomedicine on the one hand and on the other hand those of engineering, computer science, psychology and philosophy—collectively that of cognitive science. The bridges are somewhat fragile, but they need to be crossed. The empirical methods available to the cognitive sciences internally have proved inadequate over the last fifty years to resolve the theoretical questions the sciences pose. Yet to ignore the cognitive sciences and to attempt to build an understanding of cognition, just from the brain sciences, would lead to a thicket of information without structure or perspective. One needs to link the empirical power of the one approach to the theoretical insights of the other. The interface is the discipline of cognitive neuroscience.

In science, as we all know, 'history is bunk'. We know that the author of a journal article may genuflect by means of referencing to discoverers of a finding or proposers of theory. In reality we also know that this is just part of the intellectual property relations of the social structure of science, not something that is directly intellectually useful. In cognitive neuroscience, though, this standard view is wrong. To understand how and why the intellectual crevasse exists in the field requires an understanding of its history, which is complex, as cognitive neuroscience arises from many different fields.[1]

Sixty years ago, virtually nothing scientific was known about the general organisation of the mind. The most influential psychologists who were interested in discovering basic laws about its workings—although they refused to call it 'mind'—were concerned with the principles of how it changed over time. They were trying to establish laws of learning (for a definitive account, see Hilgard, 1948). Most of the principal theorists did not understand that the mind had a structure. Indeed some of the leading figures of the period explicitly rejected the attempt to uncover specific mechanisms for carrying out cognitive operations—'hypothetical constructs'—as they called them. Instead they had the naïve belief that behaviour could be predicted through applying a set of simple equations with stimuli and motivations as input—the so-called intervening variable approach of Clark Hull (1943). Some, such as Burrhus Skinner, stridently argued that one could dispense even with this level of theorising.[2]

At that time, as befits what Thomas Kuhn would call a pre-paradigm science, how one conceived of the mind as an object of scientific study depended critically on where one studied it. Behaviourism, exemplified by theorists such as Hull and Skinner, was essentially an American phenomenon. Yet their main European contemporaries left little general legacy. The Gestalt psychologists, mainly German and mainly Jewish, had withered in exile (see Mandler & Mandler, 1969). They made important experimental findings on many aspects of cognition (see Koffka, 1935; Duncker, 1945). However their conceptual frameworks were dominated by generalisations from their discoveries on the lower levels of perception. Their theoretical extrapolations from perception to thought were in general not fruitful.[3] In Switzerland, Jean Piaget had discovered many important empirical phenomena concerning cognitive development, but his Hegelian theoretical edifice too

---

[1] We assume those reading this book will come from many types of intellectual background. Those familiar with the history of the relevant fields can skip to Chapter 2. Others should pick and choose according to their areas of knowledge. Some knowledge of the gross brain anatomy and physiology is assumed.

[2] One major behaviourist, Edward Tolman (1932), had a much more sophisticated view and indeed greatly influenced the cognitive map theorists of hippocampal function to be discussed in Chapter 2.

[3] See Humphrey (1951) for a benign assessment.

was to go completely out of fashion. In Britain, Frederic Bartlett (1932) had shown how the concept of 'schema', derived from the ideas of the neurologist Henry Head, could be applied fruitfully to memory but otherwise his theoretical approach had little impact.

But what of the brain sciences? Surely they were more advanced. Indeed, from the work of the Cambridge neurophysiologists, Alan Hodgkin, Andrew Huxley and Roger Keynes, how the neuron worked had become well understood. Yet how neurons operated collectively, in different regions of the cortex, remained obscure. With the partial exception of the speech areas, all parts of the cortex outside the sensory and motor areas were labelled 'association cortex'. This term was a conceptual fig-leaf; the referent masquerading as the neural underpinning of the only interesting process then attributed to mind—the forming of associations. In practice it meant 'terra incognita'. If asked to specify how 'association cortex' might operate, brain scientists would characterise it by 'equipotentiality' or 'mass action'. This was the hypothesis developed by the animal psychologist, Karl Lashley: that it is just the number of neurons and connections operative in the cortex that matters for its computational functioning. On this view, where in association cortex the neurons are and how they are organised were considered essentially irrelevant for understanding higher cognitive processes.

Or consider neuropsychology, the study of the cognitive disorders observed in neurological patients. By the 1950s, a large range of different types of disorder were known to clinical neurology.[4] However the disorders were mainly characterised by loose and vague descriptions, and not by experimental results. Few of those interested in the scientific understanding of the mind thought these clinical syndromes of much theoretical relevance. Even within the field, potentially interesting phenomena seen in individual patients were frequently dismissed as artefacts.[5] Instead as an antidote to the looseness and variety of the clinical descriptions of individual patients that filled the literature, progress was held to depend on the use of *group studies*. These involved comparing the averages of quantitative measures of the performance of groups of patients, with each group having lesions in a different part of the brain. The results too seemed of little theoretical interest. A major reason was that the measures were normally derived from performance of clinical tests (e.g. Hécaen & Albert, 1978). Performance of theseé tests tended to

involve many different computational processes, as they were pragmatically developed and not designed from a theoretical perspective.

With the benefit of hindsight, one can see that before 1950 there were many islands of progress in the sea of ignorance. For instance, in the study of thinking, the Wurzberg school in Germany and their successors, such as Selz (1922), had made important advances.[6] In phenomenology—broadly the use of introspection to characterise one's own thought processes—there had been splendid nineteenth-century work, peaking in the masterpiece of William James (1890). However, the dominance of the ideology of behaviourism as *the* supposed method for studying what had previously been 'the mind' meant that both James and the Wurzberg school, who relied on reflection and descriptions of mental states, were generally ignored in later psychology.

Similarly in neuropsychology great advances had been made in the last thirty years of the nineteenth century by the so-called 'Diagram-Makers', another mainly German school, who tried to develop general models of cognitive processes, in particular those involved in the comprehension or production of words. Their theoretical innovations were based on the behaviour of what they termed 'pure cases', i.e. neurological patients held to have highly selective and theoretically relevant disorders, who we would now describe as having damage to only a single process or subsystem. Their models (see Figure 1.1 from Lichtheim, 1885) involved centres for attaining particular types of representation, such as 'motor word representations' and where 'concepts are elaborated', together with the connections between them. Apart from the labels these models look much like the information-processing diagrams of one hundred years later. However, a generation or two later they, too, became 'ripe for ruthless destruction' as 'false gods' (Head, 1926, pp. 65–66).[7] Essentially the dominant view in which students were trained in the mid 20th century was that the Wurzbergers, James, the Diagram Makers and their like were curiosities from a prescientific era. In actuality what passed for science at the time in, say, psychology was intellectually arid.

---

[4] See, for example, the book of Macdonald Critchley (1953) on parietal lobe syndromes.

[5] See the critique of Bay (1953) on the existence of agnosia and of Schuell & Jenkins (1959) on the existence of different types of aphasia.

[6] For a fascinating account of the Wurzberg School see Humphrey (1951).

[7] The present book is in many respects complementary to an earlier book of one of us *From Neuropsychology to Mental Structure* (Shallice, 1988) (referred to as FNMS). Where an issue or neuropsychological syndrome has been extensively discussed there, reference will be made rather than the material being repeated. For extended discussion of the early history of neuropsychology see FNMS Chapter 1.

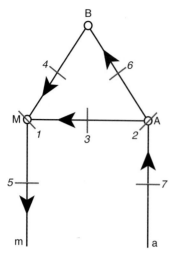

Fig. 1.1 Lichtheim's diagram showing his putative organisation of language processing. A is the centre for auditory word-representations; M the centre for motor word-representations; and B where concepts are elaborated. a and m are auditory input and speech motor output, respectively. The numbers 1 to 7 correspond to interruption points. Different forms of aphasia where held to result from damage to the different points. M was held to be localised within Broca's area (within left inferior frontal gyrus), while A was held to be localised in Wernicke's area (within the left posterior superior temporal gyrus).

1.2 The Seeds are Sown: the Period 1950–70 (Biomedical Sciences: Systems Neuroscience)

It was in the period 1950–70 that the first major developments occurred for what was to become modern cognitive neuroscience. However, in these developments lay the origins of a future problem. For the seeds came from two different species of plant, and it has remained very difficult to graft one on to the other. The first involved applying the standard approaches of the biomedical sciences more systematically to the cortex. They were rooted in the reductionist methods of experimental biology. The second came from conceiving of the mind as analogous to the operation of a computer program or, more generally, by analogy with how artefacts work. In addition to these differences of intellectual background, the two communities were sociologically very different. Moreover, the latter group of disciplines—the ones that became cognitive science—were riven by intellectual disputes within individual fields and, just as critically, by a lack of effective interaction between them.

Within the first type of approach the most basic method to be effectively used was to study the behavioural consequences of creating lesions in specific parts of the brains of animals. This had been applied successfully in the nineteenth century, but had stalled after

the characterising of the functions of the sensory and motor cortices. In the first half of the twentieth century the method had begun to be successfully applied to elucidate the function of subcortical structures, such as nuclei of the hypothalamus. The potential for applying the approach to the cortex had, though, been held back ideologically by Lashley's concept of mass action. However, in the 1950s and 1960s, the method became increasingly widely used to study cortical function. It became apparent that damage to different lobes of the cortex had very different effects. Thus, lesions to the temporal cortex were observed to lead to difficulties in previously acquired visual discriminations (Mishkin & Pribram, 1954). To give a more complex example, lesions to frontal cortex were found to produce what was later known as a problem in 'working memory'. For instance, a monkey is placed in a testing apparatus. It can see but not reach two food wells. One is baited with some attractive food; 30 seconds later, say, the animal has to choose which food well to approach when allowed to reach for the food, which it has not been able to see since the baiting. When an animal that has had a lesion in its frontal lobe has to select between the two food wells, it has major problems. It becomes unable to go consistently to the one that was baited on that trial.[8]

Positively, what these phenomena implied for how the animal's mind worked was not readily apparent. Thus the 'working memory' idea was not applied to frontal cortex until the work of Fuster & Alexander (1971) to be discussed shortly. However, negatively, support for Lashley's concept of 'mass action' rapidly waned. It was realised that impairments depended critically on the area of the cortex involved, as well as how large the lesion was.

More dramatic were the findings using a second method, that of *single cell recording*. In the 1950s, following earlier work on the eye of the horseshoe crab by H. Keffer Hartline in the 1920s, an American sensory physiologist, Steven Kuffler (1953), working on cats at Johns Hopkins, had used electrodes to record from the peripheral visual systems. He found that the cells had highly specific properties. For instance, the ganglion cells in the third layer of the retina, responded to a circular area in a particular part of the visual field—its receptive field—but their firing was inhibited by stimulation of any part of a circular surround.

Some years later, the method was applied to investigating the main relay between the retina and the cortex,

---

[8] We have somewhat compressed history. The initial discovery that frontal monkeys have such a problem occurred somewhat earlier, by Jacobsen, Wolfe & Jackson (1935). However, intensive work on the phenomenon did not occur until the 1960s (see e.g. Warren & Akert, 1964).

the lateral geniculate nucleus (LGN) (Hubel & Wiesel, 1961). Then in a remarkable piece of serendipity, the neurophysiologists David Hubel and Thorsten Wiesel (1962), working at Harvard, moved on to investigate the primary receiving area of visual cortex itself, so-called V1. They demonstrated that cells there have highly specific properties. They discovered that in certain layers of V1, in particular in its layer 4, which receives its input from earlier systems, there are many so-called 'simple' cells, which are optimally activated by a bar of light in a particular orientation. Hubel and Wiesel also observed cells with more complex properties. For instance, they found cells that respond to edges with a particular orientation anywhere in a certain area of the visual field; others require edges that stop. These were 'complex' cells.

The animals studied by Hubel and Wiesel were lightly anaesthetised. The technical advance soon followed of employing microelectrodes to record from cells in the brains of awake, behaving animals. With this it was shown that cells in other regions of cortex could have much more abstract properties. Thus cells with so-called 'place fields' were found in the hippocampus by the American emigré to London, John O'Keefe, working with Jonathan Dostrovsky (1971). These were cells that fired whenever the animal moved into a particular part of its environment (see Figure 1.2). In the same year, 'working memory' cells were discovered in prefrontal cortex by the Catalan psychiatrist turned neurobiologist working in Los Angeles, Joaquin Fuster, with Garrett Alexander (1971). They had placed microelectrodes in the so-called dorsolateral part of the prefrontal cortex (DLPFC) while an intact animal was carrying out the type of delayed response task, discussed above with respect to the effects of lesions. Neurons in this region responded very actively over the 30-second interval (see Figure 1.3). A year later, Charlie Gross working with Rocha-Miranda and Bender (1972) discovered a cell in inferotemporal cortex that responded to a stimulus as specific as a hand. An effective method for obtaining findings on more complex functions of the cortex had been born.

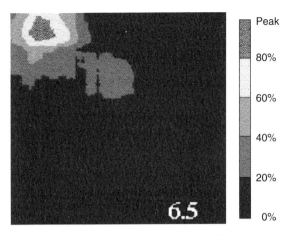

Fig. 1.2 Firing map of a place cell from region CA1 of the rat hippocampus. The map shows the firing rate of one cell as the rat moved around a square box (1.22m x 1.22m). Only when the rat was near the top left corner of the box did the cell fire at near to its peak rate, which in this instance was 6.5 Hz as shown in the bottom right corner. Adapted by permission from Macmillan Publishers Ltd: Nature (J. O'Keefe and N. Burgess (1996) Geometric determinants of the place fields of hippocampal neurons. Nature, 381, 425–428), copyright (1996).

Turning to humans, scanning procedures of the gross electrical activity of the brain, the *electroencephalogram* (or EEG) (for continuous recording) or *the evoked response* (for recording of stimulus induced activity), were beginning. Recording of the gross electrical activity of the cortex in animals goes back to the ninieteenth century but initiation of recording of the EEG in humans is generally credited to the German physiologist Hans Berger (Swartz & Goldensohn, 1998). The linking of evoked responses to cognitive phenomena began in the 1960s. Two related examples were the discovery of contingent negative variation (CNV) by Walter et al. (1964) and the *Bereitschaftspotential* by Kornhuber and Deeke (1965). In the CNV, when a stimulus is preceded by a warning signal, an electrical response can be detected over much of the frontal cortex for 1 s or more prior to the occurrence of the signal. The amplitude of this response

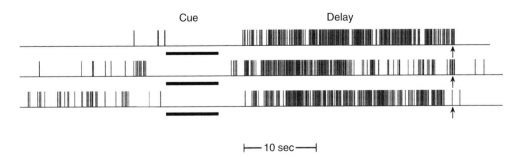

Fig. 1.3 Firing activity of a cell from monkey dorsolateral prefrontal cortex (DLPFC) during three consecutive trials of a delayed response task. The delay was 32 secs. From J.M. Fuster & G.E. Alexander, 1971, Neuron activity related to short-term memory, Science, 173(3997), 652–654. Reprinted with permission from AAAS.

decreases with repeated presentation, reflecting habituation. That the frontal response declines with habituation suggests that frontal processes are responsive to novelty, as we will see in Chapter 9. The *Bereitschaftspotential* is a closely related wave that occurs in the second preceding voluntary movement; its relation to awareness is discussed in Chapter 11. More types of evoked response will be discussed later in the book. However, the mapping between them and cognitive processes has always been more complex than for the effects of lesions on cognition.

1.3 The Seeds are Sown: the Period 1950–70 (Biomedical Sciences: Neuropsychology)

Over this twenty-year period, advances were also beginning to occur in human neuropsychology—the investigation of the effects on cognitive processes of lesions occurring as a result of neurological disease in patients. As we have just seen, at this time it was being shown in animals that lesions to different parts of the cortex have different effects. Similar phenomena were also beginning to be studied again experimentally in patients. The standard method at the time was the *neuropsychological group study* procedure. On this approach, the *average* performance of patients with lesions affecting one part of the brain on a given test or experiment is compared with the average performance of those with lesions in another part of the brain. During this period the method was beginning to produce intellectually challenging results, if the regions were appropriately chosen and the tasks well selected. Thus, the Manchester-born neuropsychologist, Brenda Milner (1963), working in Montreal, showed that patients with dorsolateral prefrontal lesions could not change their mental 'set'. They were presented with a pack of cards, each of which had a number of shapes all in the same colour. The shapes themselves, their colour and number changed from one card to the next. The patient was required to sort the pack of cards according to a rule they had to discover by trial-and-error. For instance, this might be to sort by the colour of the cards. When, however, they got a run of cards right, indicating they had discovered the rule, it was changed to, say, sorting based on the number of stimuli on the card. The patient had to discover this rule too and then move to a third rule and so on. Patients with dorsolateral prefrontal lesions tended to perseverate on an early discovered rule. They could not shift to following a new rule. Patients with lesions elsewhere in the brain did not show this effect.[9]

Or consider perception. Damage early in the visual system—say in Brodmann area 17, the site of V1—causes visual sensory difficulties in part of the so-called *visual field*. The Italian neurologists, Ennio De Renzi, Giuseppe Scotti and Hans Spinnler (1969), worked with patients who had a difficulty in recognising objects, which arose from an impairment at a higher level of the perceptual process. Technically this is called a *visual agnosia*. It is not just a problem attributable to visual sensory problems, such as a so-called *field defect*. De Renzi and his colleagues showed that the form the agnosia took differed according to the hemisphere of the lesion. Patients with lesions to the posterior part of the right hemisphere were impaired when the task was made visually difficult, for instance by their having to name each of an overlapping set of outline drawings. By contrast some patients with lesions to the posterior part of the left hemisphere had difficulty deciding whether two percepts, which were visually very different—say a real doll and the photograph of a visually quite different doll—represent the same sort of thing. They had a difficulty processing the 'meaning' of the object.[10]

More surprisingly, however, a very different type of method from that of lesion-based group studies was returning to favour, having been essentially ignored as unscientific for fifty years. This was the detailed characterisation of the cognitive difficulties of individual patients whose disorders had a particular theoretically interest. This method was conceptually much further from the animal lesion work, seen as the scientific standard in the area, than was the group-study approach, since the individual case method rapidly began to lose much of its links with localisation. In the mid-1960s, Norman Geschwind (1965), a neurologist at the Harvard Medical School, started the intellectual rehabilitation of forgotten neuropsychology from the nineteenth century. He resurrected the work of the 'diagram-makers', discussed in Section 1.1, on pure cases of language disorder, which had been derided by influential commentators of a generation or two before. This work of scholarship was empirically in tune with work using the group-study approach being carried out by the neuropsychologist Harold Goodglass and his colleagues, also in Boston, on different types of aphasia syndromes, i.e. different types of language difficulty resulting from neurological disease. They showed that patients with more posterior lesions within the so-called 'language areas' of the left hemisphere tended to have fluent, if semantically empty, speech—they manifested so-called Wernicke's aphasia. By contrast, those with more anterior lesions in the region had less fluent speech, with a loss of verbs and also of words with

---

[9] See Section 12.6 and FNMS Chapter 14 for more information on this test—the so-called Wisconsin Card-Sorting Test.

[10] See FNMS Chapter 8 for more details.

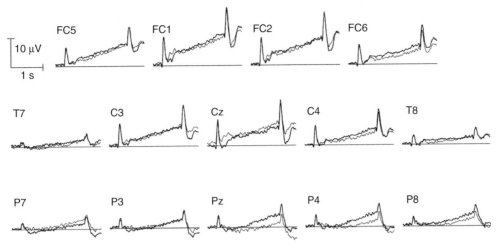

Fig. 1.4 Mean CNV trace recorded from 10 healthy subjects over two sessions at 14 standard electrode sites, including frontal (FC5, FC1, FC2, FC6), temporal (T7, T8), central (C3, Cz, C4) and parietal (P7, P3, Pz, P4, P8) scalp locations. Potentials were obtained from 200 trials per subject in a task in which a warning tone was presented followed 2 second later by a stimulus tone (high pitch or medium pitch). Subjects had to ignore high pitch stimuli but make a key-press response to medium pitch stimuli. Each trace shows a 2.8 sec interval from 200 msec before the warning tone to 600 msec after the stimulus. Reprinted from W. Gerschlager, F. Alesch, R. Cunnington, L. Deecke, G. Dirnberger, W. Endl, G. Lindinger and W. Lang, Bilateral subthalamic nucleus stimulation improves frontal cortex function in Parkinson's disease, Brain, 1999, 122(12), 2365–2373, by permission of Oxford University Press.

more purely syntactical roles, so called 'function words' such as prepositions, pronouns and conjunctions; this was Broca's aphasia (Goodglass, Quadfasel & Timberlake, 1964; Benson, 1967).[11]

It was not just nineteenth-century theorising, but also a nineteenth-century method—the *single-case study*—that then began to resurface as an empirical procedure. However it was carried out in a much more quantitative empirical fashion than it had been a century before. Impairments of high-level processes in particular individual patients with striking disorders of apparently great interest were increasingly frequently described. The paradigmatic example that revitalised the approach was a study by the neuropsychologist, Brenda Milner, whose work on frontal lobe function we just discussed, together with the neurosurgeon William Scoville (Scoville & Milner, 1957) in Montreal. They showed how a lesion involving the hippocampi—structures on the medial surface of the temporal lobes—and anatomically nearby structures could produce a dramatically dense amnesia, a loss of the patient's knowledge of their own past. Other examples were the analyse of Marcel Kinsbourne and Elizabeth Warrington (1962) in London on simultanagnosia, an inability to recognise more than one object at the same time, and by John Marshall and Freda Newcombe (1966) in Oxford on a novel reading disorder, deep dyslexia. The earliest of these single-case studies were carried

out within a theoretical framework derived from physiological psychology and clinical neurology, although using experimental techniques derived from human experimental psychology. The last of these papers, and shortly thereafter studies on memory disorders by the American Wayne Wickelgren (1968) and by Warrington and Shallice (1969), were strongly influenced theoretically by a second, quite different, type of conceptual framework alluded to earlier. This was the 'information-processing' framework from the cognitive sciences, which ultimately derived from the machine perspectives on mind that came from research stimulated by the Second World War.

1.4 The Seeds are Sown: the Period 1950–70 (The Cognitive Sciences: Information-Processing Psychology)

The 1950s saw the beginning of a second cluster of approaches, which 25 years later were collectively to become cognitive science. Unlike the biomedical sciences, they had few close working links with each other. However, they had two things in common. The first was a negative characteristic: they were little, if at all, influenced by biomedical work on brain function. Their second, more positive aspect was that they were all affected, to varying degrees, by conceptions of mind deriving from an engineering framework that developed in the late 1940s and 1950s stimulated by the invention of computers.

---

[11] See FNMS Chapter 7.

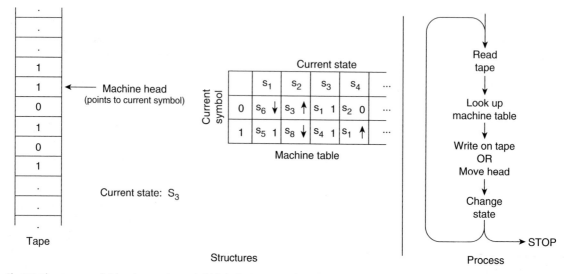

Fig. 1.5 The structures (left) and processing cycle (right) of a Turing Machine. The machine's tape consists of a sequence of cells, each containing a symbol. The machine's head points to one of those cells. On each processing cycle the machine changes the current cell (by moving the machine head up or down, or by writing to the tape) and the current state. The details of the operations are specified in a machine table, which lists the operations for all state/symbol pairs. Arrows indicate the direction of movement of the tape head.

In the biomedical work we have been discussing, the difficulties faced by the pioneers were the standard scientific ones of conceiving of the experiment and, for neuropsychology, of hypothesising a novel clinical condition that would make the experiment relevant. Then there was the standard scientific problem of the time of carrying out empirical work with what would now be considered primitive equipment. With the exception of work such as that of Hodgkin and Huxley, which is not central to the history of the cognitive neurosciences, the advances were not very abstract or mathematical. The approach was rooted conceptually in experimental biology and medicine.

The critical developments that led to the cognitive sciences differed from those in the biomedical sciences, both in their fields of origin and in their intellectual style. Cognitive science has a variety of precursors. Possibly the most important intellectual influences came from mathematical logic. About one hundred years ago, Bertrand Russell and Alfred Whitehead attempted to develop a programme by which all of mathematics could be derived logically from very basic axioms. In 1931, in a classic paper, the Austrian Kurt Gödel showed formally that any such programme must be inherently internally contradictory or incomplete in the sense that there would be certain true theorems that could never be proved; no procedure could ever establish their truth. This situation led the Cambridge logician, Alan Turing, in a paper in 1936 to attempt to characterise what types of functions—in the mathematical sense—are capable of being computed. In the process, he invented the most basic conceptual computing engine—the Turing machine.

The Turing machine (see Figure 1.5) involves four components. There is a tape, which holds an infinite number of cells—each of which contains one of a finite number of symbols (e.g. a 0 or a 1). Then there is a machine head. It can read a cell on the tape, write a symbol on to the current cell or move to a different cell. Thirdly, the machine has a state. There are only a finite number of possible states that the machine may be in, and the state may change during the machine's operation, as specified by the fourth component of the Turing machine, namely its 'machine table'. This specifies what the machine must do when it is in a particular state and reads a given symbol. It specifies the state that the machine goes to next (which may be the special *Stop* state). In addition it specifies whether the machine head should either move up or down one cell on the tape or write a symbol to the current cell of the tape.[12] A computable function is a function for which

---

[12] The design of Turing's machine was in part motivated by the idea of a person carrying out a mathematical operation with pencil and paper. Thus, in the original conception of the Turing machine, the machine's head corresponds to a perceptual process, its state transition table corresponds to its long-term memory, its current state represents its short-term memory, and writing to the machine's tape corresponds to a motor process. This conception has been largely forgotten with the widespread use of computers in which the machine's tape is seen as a kind of (internal) working memory. Curiously, the logician Emil Post, working in New York, also produced a model of computation in 1936. The model was developed independently of Turing's, but bares strong similarities. The common influences were the work of Kurt Gödel and Alonzo Church.

an appropriate machine table exists that allows it to be computed.

Turing's paper acted as a pivot between a rarefied academic endeavour of no apparent practical benefit and the development of the machine that most revolutionized our material life in the second-half of the twentieth century—the computer.[13] However, important as were these intellectual factors, equally important were the applied pressures operating in various branches of electrical engineering to conceive of human 'operators' as analogous to the machines they controlled. Then the overall behaviour of the system of human plus machine could be better understood and controlled.

Around the time of the Second World War, the gradual development of increasingly complex calculating machines—of which the most sophisticated up until then had tended to be analogue—was given a great fillip by the pressure to produce a variety of military applications. The ideas of three men working with these types of application, in addition to Turing, left a deep legacy. A little after Turing's classic paper, the Hungarian Norbert Wiener (1948) produced a major mathematical treatise on the operation of man-made systems, which sense aspects of the environment and use this information to 'act' upon it, for instance, in the operation of servo-controlled guns; this book was the origin of what he called *cybernetics*. The second of these seminal figures was the Bell Labs scientist, Claude Shannon, who conceived of how one could measure the capacity of information channels such as those used in telephone communications. The fundamental unit he developed with Warren Weaver was the *bit* of information. This corresponds to a reduction by a factor of 2 in the degree of uncertainty the recipient of a message has about the state of affairs being described by the sender (Shannon, 1948). Most of all, there was the development of the computer and with it—particularly important at the theoretical level—were the ideas of the Hungarian mathematician Johannes von Neumann (1958) on the basic concepts underlying programming.

This epoch of practical and theoretical work on the beginning of intelligent machines spawned many fields, which would later coalesce—up to a point—into cognitive science. A key strand was the development of information-processing psychology in the early 1950s by the groups of George Miller in Boston, Donald Broadbent in Cambridge and Paul Fitts in Michigan. This started with

the attempt to characterise the speed of mental processing in terms of Shannon and Weaver's measures of information capacity, which had just been developed. The study of how rapidly people could carry out simple mental operations had begun in the first great period of the investigation of mind in the last-third of the nineteenth century by the Dutchman, Franciscus Donders (1868). However, the question was of little interest to the Behaviourists or the Gestalt School. The need to apply psychology in the Second World War, however, led the Scottish psychologist Kenneth Craik (1943), in his book *The Nature of Explanation*, to put the missing mental components back into the human mind. Partially echoing Turing, he specified that there are three critical types of steps required for a knowledge-based system to operate. The first is that the stimulus must be translated into an *internal representation*. The second is that a set of cognitive operations should transform one internal representation into a series of others. In turn, in a third type of step, one of these representations can be translated into action.[14] In a later work, Craik made his model more concrete and predated Wiener by viewing the human operator as an intermittent servomechanism.[15] This way of viewing the thought process revived interest in the duration of basic cognitive operations, investigated nearly a century before by Donders, of how long a simple cognitive operation would take.[16]

Stimulated by Craik's ideas, Bill Hick (1952) in Cambridge and, a little later, Ray Hyman (1953) in Baltimore applied Shannon's ideas to their 'human operators'. They considered one of the simplest possible situations—choice reaction time—when a subject has to respond as rapidly as possible in selecting one from n possible responses, say by pressing one of n response keys when the appropriate one of n stimuli, say lights, occurs. Hick found that reaction time (RT) is proportional to $log(n+1)$, where n is the number of alternatives. In other words it could be characterised as closely related to the amount of information measured in Shannon's 'bits' that is being transmitted from the perceptual to the response part of the 'human operator'. However, if one makes a slight variation to this basic situation, such as making the subject much more practiced (Leonard, 1959), then the speed at which behaviour depending on mental processes takes place is not generally characterisable as obeying the $log(n+1)$ law. Thus the attempt to quantify the amount of information being transmitted in

---

[13] Turing's life is a remarkable refutation of the claim of the pure mathematician, G.A. Hardy—produced in the same place and time as the Turing machine—for the positive value of advanced pure mathematics in *The Mathematician's Apology*, that it had no practical applications. For an account of Turing's life—intellectual, practical, personal and political—leading to his suicide, see the splendid biography of Hodges, 1983.

---

[14] This must be one of the first, if not the first, use of the concept of internal representation.

[15] Craik was killed in 1945 in a bicycle accident when he was only 31.

[16] See Sanders (1998) for more detailed discussion.

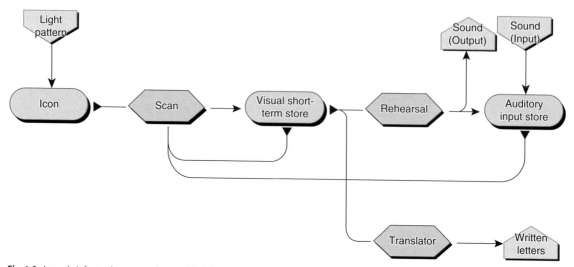

Fig. 1.6 An early information-processing model of short-term memory for visual verbal input used by Sperling to explain the findings of his 1960 paper on stimuli such as arrays of letters (see Sperling, 1967, Figure 4). The Icon was actually called the visual input store. The Visual Short-Term Store was actually called the recognition buffer. The diagram uses the conventions of the COGENT modelling environment described in Section 3.6.

cognitive operations in terms of information theory ground to a halt rather rapidly.[17]

Conceiving of a person carrying out a simple task as a system transmitting information could, however, be productively applied in a less quantitative fashion. The behavioural procedures available in human experimental psychology allow one to give plausible characterisations of the 'human operator' as a set of specific processors and memory stores with particular types of information being transmitted between them. One of the earliest such models is Sperling's (1960) model of short-term retention of visual verbal material, illustrated in Figure 1.6, which is to be discussed shortly. This approach was a more qualitative product of conceiving of the human mind from an engineering perspective. Experiments on groups of normal adult subjects thus began to be carried out with the aim of specifying what the functions of the individual processors were and how they were connected. This type of theorising, that of 'information-processing', or more derogatorily 'box-and-arrow' models, rapidly became popular following a classic analysis of attention by Donald Broadbent (1958) of the Applied Psychology Unit, Cambridge (see, e.g. Neisser, 1967; Norman, 1968). In addition Miller, Galanter and Pribram (1960) showed how the routine–subroutine structure of programmes could be used as a fruitful analogy for the control of action.

The main experimental methods that were used involved giving normal 'subjects'—i.e. volunteers[18]—sets of very simple tasks, which differed on one or more critical variables. The measures used were the time taken by subjects to carry out the tasks in the different experimental conditions (the reaction times) or the relative rates at which they made errors.

Stable data, which have sufficient precision for effective theoretical use, can indeed be obtained by human experimental psychological methods, if the experimental procedures adopted are skilfully refined. A good example came from a now classic memory paradigm involving the retrieval of lists of unrelated words.[19] Many lists of different words, randomly selected from a large pool, are presented to each subject, one word at a time at a fixed rate. After each list has finished, the subject attempts to recall as many words as they can from it. From the correct recall performance of each subject, so-called 'serial position curves' can be derived. The serial position of a remembered word is its ordinal position in the list when presented. An example of the summed results is given in Figure 1.7.

---

[17] Whether the logarithmic relation between RT and number of alternatives is indeed linked to amount of information being transmitted in the information theory sense remains an open question.

[18] The term 'subject' is now often considered to be politically incorrect. However, it is a technical term implying *appropriately* that the participant has voluntarily agreed to follow in detail the instructions of the experimenter. The experiment is useless unless the subject accepts to do so. The feeble term 'participant' misses the Gricean point.

[19] Another good example from this period was the methodology invented by the American psychologist Saul Sternberg (1969)—the so-called 'additive factors' procedure. This will be discussed in more detail in Chapter 3.

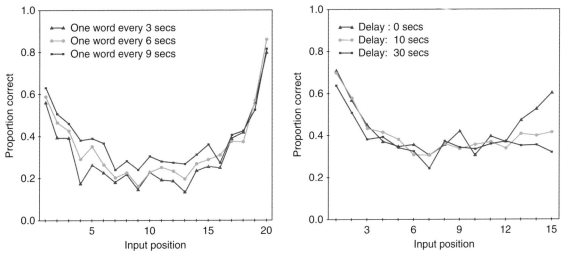

Fig. 1.7 'Serial position curves' showing the proportion of words correctly recalled from each serial position for (a) three different presentation rates and (b) three different filled delay conditions (data from Glanzer & Cunitz, 1966). In a filled delay condition the subject counted upwards from a presented number. Note that the curves are qualitatively similar for different presentation rates, with each showing a 'primacy effect', with better recall for words near the start of the list, a flatter middle section and a 'recency effect', with better recall for words near the end of the list. Redrawn from Journal of Verbal Learning and Verbal Behavior, 5(4), M. Glanzer & A.R. Cunitz, Two storage mechanisms in free recall, pp 351–360, Copyright (1966), with permission from Elsevier.

Using this method, it was shown by Murray Glanzer of New York University working with Anita Cunitz (Glanzer & Cunitz, 1966) that the recall of words presented in the last few serial positions of a list has very different characteristics from that of words retrieved from earlier positions. First, performance on the words retrieved from near the end of the list improves very rapidly as one moves towards the final position (the so-called 'recency effect'). Second, this increase is essentially unaffected by a variable like how slowly the words are presented, unlike the flat, middle part of the list or the good performance on the first few words—the so-called 'primacy effect'. Third, the 'recency' effect disappears if the subject has to carry out a 30-second period of distracting activity before attempting to recall the words in the list. This distraction has no effect on recall of the earlier part of the list. Glanzer and Cunitz, therefore, argued that the recency part of the curve appeared to be based principally on the subject recalling words from a store different from that involved in retrieval from the earlier part of the list. The two types of store were originally characterised as *primary* and *secondary* memory by the Harvard pair of Nancy Waugh and Don Norman (1965).

This theoretical framework was doubly productive. First, it linked naturally with models of visual short-term storage developed a little earlier using a different experimental paradigm by George Sperling (1960), also at Harvard. Sperling's paper, which involved a more complex type of reasoning analogous to that employed by Glanzer and Cunitz, is the first really powerful use of human experimental psychological methods to

derive theoretical conclusions, which essentially remain valid today. He distinguished two different types of visual short-term store—one very short-lasting and taking in information in parallel from the visual array—often called the *icon*—and the other depending on serial processing of information from the icon to what we will call the *visual short-term store*. The model is illustrated in Figure 1.6.

Second, 'Con' Conrad (1964) and Alan Baddeley (1966a) in Cambridge had shown that words or letters retained for intervals of a few seconds or so are particularly susceptible to *acoustic*—actually *phonological* confusion—or interference. Thus, when a list of letters is recalled the stimuli '... PD ...' may be retrieved as '... BT ...'. However, if information is held for longer, say a few minutes, the confusions that occur are between semantically related items. So *bull* might be recalled as *cow*. Moreover, Gus Craik (1968)[20] in London, predicted that when subjects make substantive errors in the free recall of word lists, the type of error should differ according to the word's position in the list. Indeed, the recency part of the serial position curve is subject to phonological confusions, while items recalled from the earlier part of the list are subject to semantic confusions.

A typical model of the time had the conceptual structure illustrated in Figure 1.8. The support that the behavioural evidence provides for the model is based

---

[20] No relation to Kenneth Craik referred to earlier.

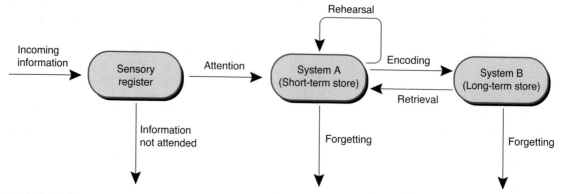

Fig. 1.8 The Modal Model of memory. To make quantitative predictions, the model may be elaborated by specifying equations for, e.g., the probability of an item being forgotten from the Short-Term Store within a time window, or the probability of an item in the Long-Term Store being rehearsed within a time window. See Waugh and Norman (1965) or Atkinson and Shiffrin (1968). For visual input the Sensory Register would correspond to the Icon of Figure 1.6. At the time a plethora of names were given to an essentially similar set of concepts.

on two types of characterisation of the components of the model:

1 The way that systems A and B are affected by any variable X, depends on the relation between X and the hypothetical functions of A and B.

2 A property of a system can be characterised in terms of some mathematical function.

An example of this second property is that the amount of information stored in system A (i.e. short-term storage) decreases as a monotonic function of the number of different semantically unrelated words to which attention is directed which immediately follow it. In Waugh and Norman (1965), the function was exponential decline. By contrast, such interference has no—or at least an order-of-magnitude less—effect on the contents of a second hypothetical subsystem B (long-term storage).[21]

Principle 2, if one ignores the qualifying clause about attending to subsequent words, and considers only the function relating interference and amount of information stored, is of a type standard in many areas of science. Principle 1, however, is interesting in two respects. First, it depends on a system-level property—the function of the hypothetical subsystem. Second, it is an intuitive, not a formal, property. Thus if one was to assume, as was frequently done in the 1960s following the ideas of Hebb to be discussed shortly, that the function of a hypothetical short-term store is to hold information in labile form while it is laid down in long-term storage, then why a particular mathematical function occurs in principle 2 becomes understandable.

That rapid exponential decay of information should be the underlying basis of the recency effect as held by Waugh and Norman is explained through its being a plausible way for a short-term storage system to operate. However, the contrasting effects of the phonological and semantic dimensions—both on interference and on errors—do not follow in any obvious fashion from this perspective. Rather, these latter properties follow if store A is viewed as having a different type of function, namely that of being a holding short-term store specifically for speech operations, as for instance suggested by Shallice and Warrington (1970) and compatible with the working memory model of Baddeley and Hitch (1974). This function too is in turn compatible with an exponentially decaying trace.[22] This example is typical of the relation in human information-processing psychology between empirical findings and hypothetical functions of components of an information-processing system referred to as principle 1; usually it is partly based on unimplemented and inherently intuitive ideas about how a hypothetical mechanism might work computationally. However, when a prediction such as the one about error type and list position is corroborated, *both* the model and the intuitive way the model has been developed are supported; this process is known as bootstrapping.

This type of methodology has, however, an Achilles' heel. As already pointed out, the models to which the empirical findings were related, were frequently not precise. Nor could they be, given the partly intuitive nature of the link between evidence and model. To test a specific mathematical function—principle 2—was the exception, not the norm. Take the concept of the words

---

[21] The need to add a qualification arises as long-term storage is also affected by so-called *retroactive interference* but with a much slower and qualitatively different interference effect to short-term storage (Underwood, 1957).

[22] However, it also explains why the effects of experimental decay can be much reduced if 'semantic support' is available. See Chapter 7 for further discussion.

being 'attended' to, which qualifies the example given of principle 2; this relates to hypothetical processes that are not themselves modelled. Moreover, the results of any particular paradigm are often affected by many factors. So, seemingly subsidiary aspects, both of the task—such as the familiarity or precise meaning of the stimuli, the time for which they are presented or over which they have to be retained—and also of the subjects—their age, experience of the task and so on—can alter the pattern of results in unexpected ways.

Take the free recall experimental paradigm again. New variants were introduced later in the 1970s. One, for instance, was when subjects were presented with a list of words but had to count for 20 seconds after each word. This idea was to remove any short-term trace of the words, which has just been held to be responsible for the recency effect. This, however, led to an apparently rather similar recency effect to that just discussed (e.g. Tzeng, 1973). In other experiments, Baddeley and Hitch (1977) showed that you could obtain a recency effect if you asked rugby players to recall the matches they had played in a season. It was then argued by many, incorrectly as it now appears, that as these forms of recency effect were unlikely to result from retrieval from a short-term store, so the more classical free recall recency effect did not either (but see Brown, Neath & Chater, 2007, for a contemporary unitary account of recency effects over different time scales). The alternative view differentiated two types of recency effect with different underlying processes, and the model shown in Figure 1.8 was held to be directly relevant to paradigms with the same temporal characteristics as the classical free recall one.

On the basis of experimental psychology methods alone as used at the time, this latter conclusion was *ad hoc*. The methods were often not powerful enough to discriminate effectively between the alternative accounts of a given experimental paradigm that were put forward. Nor was the problem limited to a single paradigm. Quite often, a new paradigm would be introduced that seemed to provide a clear and simple choice between rival theories of a function. Soon, though, the experimental paradigm itself would become an object of study as it began to be realised that a complex set of processes were involved when the cognitive system implemented the paradigm. This was the sociological process described by Tulving and Madigan (1970, p. 442) as the 'functional autonomy of methods' in which 'yesterday's methods have become today's objects of study.'

Some of the empirical paradigms developed did have theoretically transparent results, which have stood the test of time. The free-recall paradigm was one, as we will see. Others, however, led to apparently never-ending disputes, as the paradigm's progeny became more and more complex. This somewhat disappointing state-of-affairs even led some of the leading practitioners of the information-processing approach to abandon it for a strange set of beliefs derived from the Cornell psychologist, James Gibson. This was that if one characterises the perceptual environment well enough, then the behaviour produced will be transparent and over-determined. Even scientists previously very influential in the information-processing field (Neisser, 1976; Turvey, 1973) abandoned that approach for the Gibsonian perspective. As the determination of the internal structure of the mind using human experimental methods had proved to be harder than initially hoped, in response the Gibsonians held it to be unnecessary! Most of the practitioners held fast. But overall progress was slow.

1.5 The Seeds are Sown: the Period 1950–70 (The Cognitive Sciences: Linguistics)

Before the 1950s, in the intellectual climate of behaviourism, what went on inside the organism was a taboo issue. Linguistics at the time was essentially descriptive. In the early 1950s, the American theoretician, Noam Chomsky of MIT, took ideas from the logician, Emil Post (1943), and applied them to completely redirect linguistics. Chomsky attempted to specify the operations involved in producing or comprehending a sentence. Of the three strands of cognitive science, in this area the theorists of the human operator as a machine had their most abstract influence.[23]

Linguists distinguish between phonology—how words are realised as sounds, morphology—how words are constructed out of more elementary components, such as inflections, semantics—the meanings of words, pragmatics—how sentences are constrained by the context in which they are uttered, and syntax—grammar. Chomsky was primarily concerned with syntax. He argued that what is critical is to articulate a system of rules, which comprise the knowledge that underlies our ability to comprehend and produce language. Syntax, as he redefined it, is the determination of the most efficient grammar of a language, where a grammar is a system of rules for specifying all, and only all, of the possible sentences of the language.

---

[23] Chomsky has been, undoubtedly, the most remarkable intellectual of the second-half of the twentieth century. In addition to dominating his discipline for over 50 years, which is itself unparalleled in this period, he has remained a real intellectual instead of just retreating into his speciality, producing a whole stream of tightly argued and empirically detailed political works (e.g. Chomsky, 1969).

TABLE 1.1 Context-free grammar rules for a simple fragment of English.

Non-Terminal Rules	Terminal Rules
S → NP VP	Det → the
NP → Det Noun	Noun → lion
VP → IV	Noun → tiger
VP → TV NP	Noun → leopard
	IV → roars
	TV → hates
	TV → sees

Chomsky argued, in the tradition of Turing and Post, that an appropriate way to represent grammars is as a series of *rewrite rules*. A rewrite rule takes the form:

$A → B$, or if A then B,

where *A* and *B* are each strings of symbols.[24] If there are no further rules that can apply to a string of type *B*, then its symbols are part of the *terminal vocabulary*, i.e. the actual words of the language. Those of type *A* are the *non-terminal vocabulary*, which involve more abstract concepts such as 'noun' or 'verb phrase' (VP) from traditional grammar. A very simple example is shown in Table 1.1.

Grammars come in different types, such as:

1 *Finite-state grammars*, where every rule has one of two forms (i) $A_1 → B A_2$ or (ii) $A_1 → B$, where each *A* is a single non-terminal item and *B* is a string (or sequence) of terminal items.[25]

2 *Context-free grammars*, where every rule is of the form $A → B$, where *A* is a non-terminal item and *B* is a string of terminal and/or non-terminal items.

3 *Context-sensitive grammars*, where every rule is of the form $X A Y → X Z Y$, where *A* is a non-terminal item and *X*, *Y*, *Z* are all strings of non-terminals and terminals and *Z* is non-empty.

The set of rules given in Table 1.1 are for a context-free grammar.[26] They enable one to say that sentences in this grammar are composed of strings such as: (i) *The lion roars*, (ii) *The tiger hates the lion,* and (iii) *The leopard sees the tiger.*

In his early work Chomsky (1959a) showed the inadequacy of finite-state grammars as grammars of natural language;[27] they were shown not to be able to realise particular types of syntactic structure. Thus finite-state grammars cannot deal with the syntactic structure of so-called centre embedding. As an example, the following valid English sentence contains as elements the meanings of the three sentences from above:

The lion the tiger the leopard sees hates roars.

In principle, if not in practice, such a process of adding an additional clause in the centre of a sentence can be carried out infinitely. Now in a finite-state grammar, two separate parts of a string cannot both come from the same re-write rule if there is an 'alien' element between them. The relation between such an embedded sentence and the sentence components on either side cannot, therefore, be derived from a finite-state grammar. In order to derive the above sentence, one would need to add a context-free rule, such as $NP → NP S$. Chomsky therefore argued that the grammars of natural language must be at least of the context-free type.[28]

Chomsky also argued that a special type of *rewrite rule*, called a *transformation*, is required to capture the similarity in meaning between sentences with different surface forms, such as *The tiger hates the lion* and *The lion is hated by the tiger*. This is captured by the transformation rule:

$$NP_1 + V + NP_2 → NP_2 + auxiliary \text{ (i.e. is)} + V^* + by + NP_1$$

The overall approach developed by Chomsky provides a valuable formalisation for capturing many of the empirical regularities of syntax, and a wide range of domains of syntax have been investigated using his approach. The empirical phenomena are basically the judgement by linguists of what are legitimate or illegitimate usages in a language. The task of the theoretician is to find the most effective formalisation within the overall constraints of the approach.

Early on, attempts were made to link information-processing approaches with transformational linguistics. The idea was to measure the processing characteristics of each hypothetical transformation, such as the time it takes (e.g. Mehler & Miller, 1964; Clifton & Odom, 1966). However these attempts failed (Fodor, Bever & Garrett, 1974). In response, the dogma was developed that linguistics is not required to make predictions about

---

[24] Multiple application of such rules give rise to hierarchically-structured trees, with the two sides of each rule corresponding to neighbouring levels.

[25] In such representations order is critical. Thus in (i) *B* comes before A_2 in the string.

[26] Note that inclusion of the rule $S → NP VP$ ensures that this is not a finite-state grammar, as that rule involves two non-terminal items on the right hand side.

[27] And also context-free grammars.

[28] In fact, Chomsky argued that even context-free grammars were insufficiently powerful to capture natural language. The arguments against context-free grammars were later undermined by Gazdar, Klein, Pullum and Sag (1985) assuming that more complex syntactic categories than those traditionally used are incorporated into the grammar.

experimentally obtained measures, such as reaction time. Chomsky (1965) therefore argued that it is critical to distinguish between *linguistic competence*, which linguistic theory must explain, and *linguistic performance*, which is influenced by a host of factors, such as short-term memory capacity, with which linguistics is not essentially concerned.[29]

Transformational grammar and its descendents remain a major intellectual achievement and a valuable way of representing language. It is, though, essentially concerned empirically with a very abstract characterisation of language—what linguists think is proper usage—rather than with how people behave when using language in specific situations. Overall, the ideology of the competence/performance distinction essentially immunised linguistics from any serious consideration of psycholinguistic (cognitive psychological) results. There has continued to be no major intellectual rapprochement with information-processing psychology, either in its methods or its contents.[30] This doctrine, and the even more rigid rejection by the majority of the field of the computational approach of connectionism 20 years later, helped to create a fragmented, rather than a unified, cognitive science.

1.6 The Seeds are Sown: the Period 1950–70 (The Cognitive Sciences: Computer Simulations of Mind)

The most direct attempt to realise the ideas of Alan Turing and Johannes von Neumann lay in the field of computer modelling of mental and brain processes. In the 1950s, the decade after the computer was invented, two rather different strands began to develop in this field: those of symbolic artificial intelligence (or AI) and of connectionism or neural networks.

One strand took as its basis the developing logic of the computer program and tried to mimic different types of cognitive process in terms of complex programs. Terms like 'representation' and 'operation', from the early approach of Kenneth Craik, fit naturally within this conceptual framework of symbolic AI. The prototypic cognitive process to be modelled was problem-solving, but symbolic AI simulations were also made of

many other types of cognitive process, including language, perception and memory.[31]

The other strand instead took the operation of the neuron as its basic element and attempted to show how basic cognitive operations could be realised in terms of circuits built of elements, each of which operated in a simplified fashion like a neuron. Here the referents of terms like 'representation' and 'operation' are much more complex beasts than for symbolic AI, so this strand maps much less easily on to other symbolic approaches in cognitive science.

Within the symbolic AI strand, critical early attempts were the so-called Logic Theorist of Allen Newell, Clifford Shaw and Herb Simon (1958) and the General Problem Solver (GPS) of Newell and Simon (1961) that followed it.[32] GPS and later developments, such as the programs of Newell and Simon (1972), planned how a system should behave when presented with a pencil-and-paper problem to solve, such as *cryptarithmetic* ones, which we will illustrate in Section 1.7, or the well-known missionaries-and-cannibals problem. Its main approach was to use so-called 'backward chaining' from the goal, often called *means-ends analysis*. Newell and Simon (1972) illustrated it by the following example: I want to take my son to nursery school. What is the difference between what I have and what I want? One of distance. What changes distance? My automobile. My automobile won't work. What is needed to make it work? A new battery. What has new batteries? An 'auto-engineer' shop ... and so on.

To make such a procedure work, GPS needed three types of thought element. Two are analogous to key elements of the Turing machine. Thus it needs knowledge in some form of *representation* of the state of the relevant part of the world. In addition, it needs *goals*, representations of the problem to be solved. Finally, it needs *operations*, which it can use so as to move in steps from the current state of the world to that of the goal. It then selects, principally by means-ends analysis, a series of such steps.

GPS at the time seemed to open up the possibility of artificial thinking machines. Indeed, in 1958 Herb Simon predicted that it would be only 10 years before a computer would be able to beat chess champions and be capable of posing new mathematical theorems (Russell & Norvig, 1995). However, there turned out to be many difficulties. The major problem was that GPS and its immediate successors obtained a solution to their problem by searching through a so-called state-space

---

[29] In retrospect the competence-performance ideology was especially inappropriate, as the empirical observations did not fit the theory related to transformations, such as the passive, which had a theoretical status that was changed in later versions of Chomsky's approach.

[30] The desire for intellectual separation from the other field was reciprocated by much of information-processing psychology at the time transformational grammars were first articulated (see e.g. Broadbent, 1968).

[31] Boden (1977) remains an excellent history of the early development of the field.

[32] Before his highly influential collaboration with Newell and Shaw, Simon had carried out work in economics for which he was later to obtain a Nobel Prize!

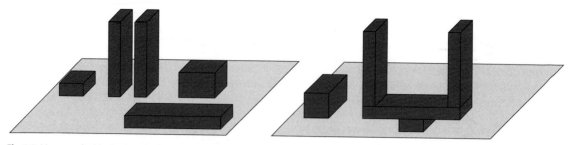

Fig. 1.9 How can the blocks given in the state on the left be assembled to produce the state on the right, given that you can only use one hand? This problem is too difficult for HACKER, but BUILD is able to "think" of using the large block as a stabilising weight during the construction process and later remove it.

where all the possible states that the system can be in are explicitly specified. Such an approach does not deal well with many human problem-solving methods. These include the use of analogies and the use of perceptual features of the representation, as in work with diagrams (see Boden, 1988). Progress would turn out to be far less fast than Simon thought.

GPS was the start of what later became known as the *production-systems approach* to the simulation of the thought processes, to be discussed further in the next section. More generally it and the Logic Theorist started the research programme of *symbolic AI*. In the 1970s, symbolic AI was to ride high, as a potential approach for understanding mind, being influential in areas as far from problem-solving as language (e.g. Winograd, 1972) and vision (Winston, 1975).[33] In the domains of problem-solving and planning themselves, for instance, programs like Sussman's (1975) HACKER and Fahlman's (1974) BUILD were able to use procedures developed from GPS to solve quite complex planning problems. For instance, in the control of robots that were stacking objects as in warehouses (see Figure 1.9), they would order the sequence of actions appropriately. By the 1970s, the standing of symbolic AI was very high.

Symbolic AI is currently much less influential in cognitive neuroscience than the second strand of work on computer simulation of mind—now called connectionism—which began from somewhat related roots but rapidly diverged. Connectionism was much influenced by very early discussions on the conceptual relation between the logic circuitry of computers and the behaviour of neural networks. These arose from a collaboration between the physiologist and psychiatrist, Warren McCulloch, and a mathematician, Walter Pitts, in 1943. Their paper showed how networks with particular arrangements of neuron-like elements could mimic the making of logical inferences. The elements had thresholds; they fired if, and only if, the sum of the inputs arriving in the preceding time slice exceeded

the threshold. For instance, a network with two input neurons connected to one output neuron could behave either like an AND-gate or an OR-gate (see Figure 1.10). And more complex networks could compute more complex logical expressions.

This work influenced the Canadian neuropsychologist, Donald Hebb (1949). Hebb speculated that a network of neurons having strong excitatory interconnections with each other—a *cell assembly*—could act as a device for categorising whether a perceptual input to the brain was an example of a certain discrete type of representation, say an *elephant*. Hebb also produced a theory of how such a network might be formed by learning. Assume that when a neuron fires, this is followed shortly thereafter by the firing of a second neuron on to which it synapsed. Then Hebb speculated that what we now call the *weight* of the synaptic connection between the neurons is strengthened. In other words, at any later time, the second neuron would receive a stronger input from the first and so, if the first fires again, the second becomes more likely to fire than it did before. Repeated application of this process will tend to produce a group of neurons with the property that, if more than a certain number begin to fire, then the firing rate in the whole assembly will rise to maximum.[34]

There are now a variety of forms of the 'Hebb rule' which are derived from Hebb's original somewhat vaguely specified verbal account (see Dayan & Abbott, 2001, Chapter 8). The simplest form is:

$$a\frac{d\vec{w}}{dt} = \vec{v}.\vec{u},$$

where a is a time constant that modulates how fast weights can change, $\vec{w}$ is the vector of the 'weights' for

---

[33] For its standing then see, for instance, the most intellectually challenging of the cognitive psychology textbooks of the time, that of Lindsay and Norman (1977).

[34] It was pointed out by the Canadian psychologist Peter Milner (1957) that without a complementary inhibitory process or other means of reducing weights, the continued application of Hebb's rule could lead to all active neurons tending to fire at maximum whenever an input occurred—the *kindling* problem—so no discriminative behaviour could occur. This means that Hebb's rule needed modifications.

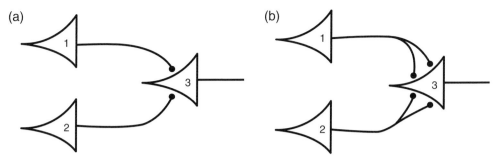

Fig. 1.10 Two simple networks consisting of two input neurons and one output neuron. Inputs are on the left and outputs are on the right. The network on the left (a) functions as an AND-gate as both input neurons must be activated to activate the output neuron. The network on the right (b) functions as an OR-gate. Only one input need be activated to activate the output neuron. Reproduced with kind permission from Springer Science+Business Media: Bulletin of Mathematical Biophysics, A logical calculus of the ideas immanent in nervous activity, 5(4), 1943, p. 130, W.S. McCulloch and W. Pitts, figure 1c, 1b.

the connections from all the input cells synapsing with a given neuron, v is the output activity of the neuron and $\vec{u}$ is the vector of activations of the input cells (see Figure 1.11).[35]

Hebbian learning is one of the most widely used learning rules for artificial neural networks. Hebb therefore produced both a plausible neural analogue for a representation—the 'cell assembly'—and a plausible speculation about learning—'Hebbian learning'. Hebb certainly did not give his ideas an adequate empirical test, at any level. His ideas on learning were not unique to him. His model in its original form could not work. However, his overall conception made the idea of a cognitive neuroscience that was theoretically rich and empirically investigable concrete for the first time. It was his greatest achievement.[36]

Hebb's speculations stimulated actual computer simulations of hypothetical neural networks, particularly in the work of the New York engineer Frank Rosenblatt (1958) on *perceptrons*. A perceptron is a highly simplified network that was designed to permit the study of lawful relationships between how a nerve net is organised, how its environment is structured and the 'psychological performances of which it (the network) is capable' (Rosenblatt, 1962). More concretely, a perceptron is a series of sets of units that are connected with each other only using feed-forward connections. There is no

looping. Each of these connections has a weight that can be altered by a learning algorithm (see Figure 1.12).[37]

Perceptrons appeared to provide an effective start to understanding how a real neural network could simulate cognitive operations. However, the approach suffered a major setback in the late 1960s. In a striking parallel to what we have seen happened in information-processing psychology at much the same time, one of the original proponents of the overall approach published a key work, which, twenty years after he started it, seemed to undermine the approach. The Brutus of the new field of connectionism was MIT computer scientist, Marvin Minsky, who with Dean Edwards had produced the first ever neural network computer in 1951 (see Russell & Norvig, 1995).

Perceptrons can have different numbers of layers. Consider simple perceptrons, which have only an input and an output layer. In 1962 Rosenblatt proved for them his *perceptron convergence theorem*. This theorem showed that, if a solution exists, then such an elementary two-layer perceptron would always learn in finite time any given input–output mapping. The problem lay in the initial premise. Minsky, working with the intellectually versatile South African emigré, Seymour Papert (1969), proved that there were certain input–output mappings thath could not be learned by a simple perceptron. An example is the so-called exclusive-or (XOR) mapping (see Figure 1.13). With two input and one output unit, the rule to be learned is that the output

---

[35] A very interesting development of the Hebb rule is an alterative plasticity rule proposed by Bienenstock, Cooper and Munro (1982), where the right-hand side of the Hebb rule equation is multiplied by $(v - T)$, where T is a threshold that determines whether synapses are strengthened or weakened. It fits better with experimental neurophysiological evidence.

[36] Hebb's contributions were not all positive. In a theoretical analysis in 1945 he held that the frontal lobes are essentially valuable only during development, which indirectly legitimised prefrontal leucotomy. Moreover, he initiated the field of sensory deprivation research, which led to refinements of psychological torture techniques.

[37] A 'learning algorithm' is a method of gradually adjusting the weights on the connections between neurons in an artificial neural network that depends upon the pattern of firing of the network on each trial or on how satisfactory is the network's output on the trial. It is the motor of the network's learning. There are many types of learning algorithm (see Chapter 3). An excellent example is Hebbian learning, which, however, was not used in perceptrons. The one most usually applied for perceptrons was the delta-rule (see Section 1.7).

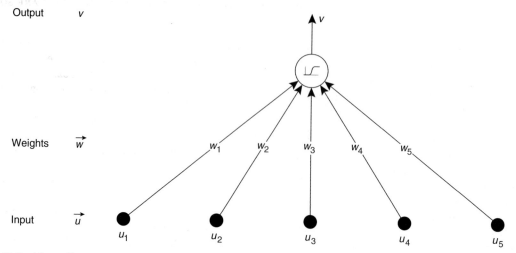

Output v

Weights $\vec{w}$ w_1 w_2 w_3 w_4 w_5

Input $\vec{u}$ u_1 u_2 u_3 u_4 u_5

Fig. 1.11 Feed-forward inputs to a single neuron. Inputs and weights are given by vectors. Weights may be adjusted by a learning rule such as that of Hebb. (See text, Figure 1.19 and Dayan & Abbott, 2001, for additional details.)

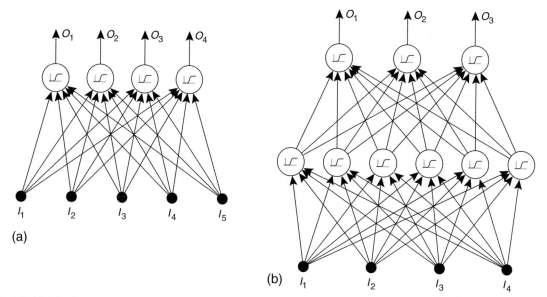

(a)

(b) I_1 I_2 I_3 I_4

Fig. 1.12 (a) A simple perceptron consisting only of a layer of input units and a layer of output units. (b) A perceptron which adds a layer of hidden units.

I_1	I_2	O
0	0	0
0	1	1
1	0	1
1	1	0

(a)   (b)   (c)

Fig. 1.13 Three depictions of the exclusive or (XOR) function. (a) The required output (O) of the XOR function for each pair of inputs (I). (b) A Venn-Diagram representation of the function. (c) A graphical representation of the required output of XOR as a function of its two inputs. Hollow red circles represent inactive (zero) outputs. Filled red circles represent active (one) outputs. The function is not linearly separable as it is not possible to draw a single straight line on the graph which separates inactive from active outputs, as illustrated by the four dashed grey lines.

unit must be activated, *if, and only if*, either one *but not both* of the input units is on; otherwise the output unit is to remain inactivate.[38]

Minsky and Papert's proof essentially stopped research on connectionist approaches to understanding the system-level operation of the brain for more than ten years. As will be discussed, symbolic AI was to undergo a similar retrenchment ten years later. In information-processing psychology the blow was somewhat less severe, as the rejectionist position advocated by Neisser and Turvey was adopted by only a minority in the field; but confidence in the field was still shaken. By 1970 then, there were the beginnings of the cognitive sciences. However, of the four approaches we have considered, at least one was in internal turmoil, in another such turmoil was to occur within ten years, and for the other two there were major internal critics. The approaches all also tended to be intellectually isolated with little contact with each other and, as discussed in Section 1.5, often hostile to the other.[39] When the neuroscience set of disciplines began to roll, the cognitive science ones were ill-equipped to match them.

1.7 The Blossoming Disciplines 1970–95: the Cognitive Sciences: Computer Modelling of Mind and Linguistics

For the fields that were becoming the cognitive sciences, the period 1970–95 saw progress that was real but generally fairly slow by comparison with the related disciplines in neuroscience.[40] In most fields of cognitive science, the traumas following 1970 were overcome. One can see a clear relation between the position dominant in the 1990s and that dominant in the field in the 1960s or 1970s. There has been no general rejection of the previously dominant positions, as happened, for instance, in the history of 'hard-core' psychology before 1960. However, 'normal science' in the sense of Kuhn, where the vast majority of the experts accept a common set of positions and methods, had yet to be achieved, and in most of the fields there remain sizeable groups of expert sceptics.

In the 1970s, as we have just seen, connectionism was ignored as fatally flawed by the many carriers of the symbolic AI banner. It was in self-destruct mode. In the 1980s, however, it had a spectacular rise in influence. The major breakthrough came in 1982. The Princeton bio-physicist John Hopfield drew an analogy between how networks of highly idealised neurons might work and processes involved in magnetic interactions between atoms within solid materials, in particular so-called *spin-glasses*, where the interaction is disordered.

In the previous section we introduced artificial neuron-like units of the type proposed by McCulloch and Pitts (1943) in their initial analysis of neural nets (see Figure 1.10). Hopfield considered how networks of such units behave (see Figure 1.14). With time held to occur in discrete steps, he assumed that each 'neuron' is either fully on or off at each time-slice. By analogy with statistical physics, he introduced the idea that the network had an overall energy. In the analogy, a unit in the network corresponds to a molecule that is in one of two states. The molecule is influenced by its neighbours to switch states or remain in the same state. When all units are on, the system has maximum energy. Using this analogy, Hopfield showed that if the units in a network are symmetrically connected, and if they are each updated at random, then a function corresponding to the (potential) energy of the physical system decreases or remains constant at each update. In other words, in the updating procedure, the energy of the neural net moves towards a minimum. How the system's state changes over time, given the updating process, can be thought of as a trajectory in a *state space*.

Hopfield's key idea was that the different potential minima, termed *(point) attractors* (see Figure 1.15), could each represent individual memories. Given the updating law, that meant that if the system in the physics example is anywhere within the so-called *basin of attraction*, then, over time, the state will move to its point attractor. Again there is an analogy with memory. Accessing a memory, given a cue, would be equivalent to the state of the system moving from somewhere in the memory's basin of attraction to its point attractor (the energy minimum). If the unit represents a complex object, say, then when it responds to elements of a sensory input, the procedure corresponds to *pattern completion*.

The Hopfield net was a highly schematised model of memory retrieval. Moreover, it did not learn. Hopfield had only shown that such a system could represent the analogues both of storing a number of different memories and of retrieval, which would depend on the initial state of the system (including its input). From this very simple beginning, the field moved in two directions. Within the theoretical physics community, the theory of such systems progressed very rapidly by developing the analogies with solid-state physics (see Amit, 1989). For instance, there is a major theoretical problem for Hopfield nets of the trajectories landing in irrelevant

[38] See Hertz, Krogh and Palmer (1991, Chapter 5), for extended discussion of this issue.

[39] The lack of cross-talk at the time between artificial intelligence, cognitive psychology and linguistics was very well demonstrated quantitatively by Pylyshyn (1983) using citation counts.

[40] To lessen the memory load for the reader unfamiliar with them, the fields for 1970–95 are considered in the reverse order to those for 1950–70.

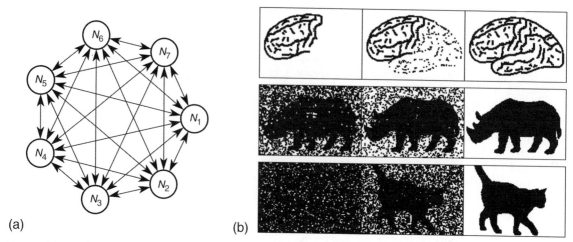

Fig. 1.14 (a) A Hopfield network consisting of seven units. All units are interconnected with symmetric weights and all units may serve as input and output units. (b) States of a Hopfield network consisting of 150 × 100 binary units which encodes three stored images. The panels on the left show three images presented to the network. The middle panels show a state of the network part-way through the settling process for each case. The right panels show the final stable states of the network when the settling process has converged. The top-most example shows how, given a partial image, the network is able to fill-in or recall a complete image. The second example shows how given a corrupted image the network is able to produce a "'cleaned-up" version. The third shows that given a completely random initial state the network will settle to one if its known states.

local minima—into which the so-called *gradient-descent* process of moving to a lower energy level can easily fall (see Figure 1.15). This problem was overcome by making the process noisy. Using methods derived from this approach, it became possible, for instance, to measure how many memories could be stored in a system. This was then applied to estimating the capacities of particular neural systems, such as the hippocampus (e.g. Treves & Rolls, 1994).

The other prong of the development of the field involved learning. Consider a stochastic (i.e. noisy) Hopfield net in which some of the units are so-called 'visible' ones: they are the input and output interfaces the network has with the environment. It is assumed that on each trial the environment fixes the state of some of these units; it 'clamps' them (see Figure 1.16). Then, as was discussed above, given the current values of the weights of the connections, the net will move to a certain energy minimum. Assume, however, that in addition a learning process is taking place and that it is early in this process. Then in the settling process that occurs in a Hopfield net, the minimum state initially reached—the point attractor—is likely to be far from what would have occurred if the net had been allowed

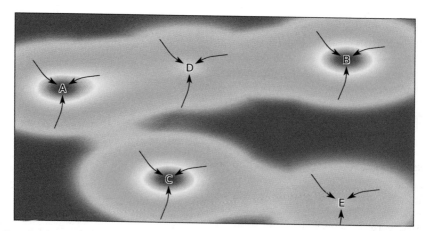

Fig. 1.15 A two dimensional representation of the energy surface of a Hopfield network. The network is put into its initial state based on a given set of cues. The state is then updated so that the network's energy moves towards a point attractor (points A, B and C in the figure). If the update process involves only adjusting single units at each step so as to minimise energy, i.e. a process of gradient descent, then the network may settle into a local minimum (points D or E). Adding noise appropriately to the update process avoids this problem.

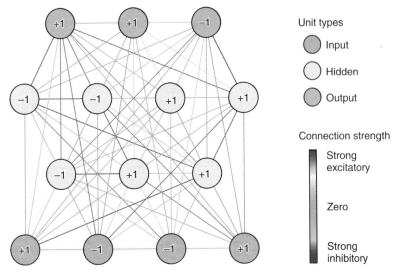

Fig. 1.16 A Hopfield network with input and output units (i.e. a Boltzmann machine). Units are of three types: input units, output units and hidden units. Units are either clamped to +1 or −1, or are stochastic. Stochastic units take the value S = +1 with probability g(h$_i$) and S = −1 with probability 1−g(h$_i$), where h$_i$ = $\sum_j w_{ij} \cdot s_j$ and g(h$_i$) = $\frac{1}{1+e^{(\alpha_i - \frac{2h_i}{T})}}$. The parameter *T* is known as the temperature while α$_i$ is a threshold.

to run free, i.e. to settle to a minimum without any of the units being clamped.

In a British–American collaboration, Geoff Hinton and Terry Sejnowski in 1983 showed that such a 'Boltzmann machine' network would improve its ability to reproduce the appropriate state of the output units (i.e. to categorise its inputs) if a complex learning procedure is applied to the weights (see Figure 1.17) (Hinton, Sejnowski & Ackley, 1984). The procedure involves two phases. In the first, the *positive phase*, the system has its input and output units clamped, as discussed above. The system is then allowed to settle. This produces for each pair of nodes *i* and *j*, and hence for each connection w_{ij}, a probability p^+_{ij} that the nodes are

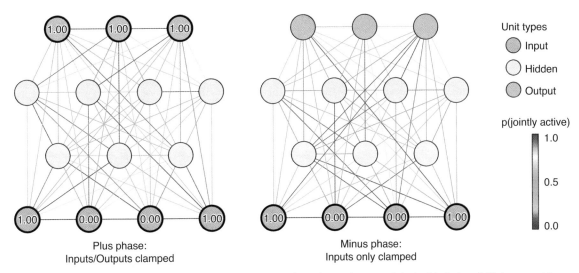

Plus phase:
Inputs/Outputs clamped

Minus phase:
Inputs only clamped

Fig. 1.17 Learning in the Boltzmann Machine proceeds in two phases for each input/output pair. In the "plus" phase (left) the network is allowed to settle with both input and output units clamped to the desired pattern. For each pair of units, i and j, the probability that they are both "on" is determined. This is referred to as p$^+_{ij}$. (This probability is not necessarily zero or one as the network is stochastic, so even when it has settled units will spontaneously change state with some finite probability.) In the "minus" phase (right) the network is allowed to settle with just the input units clamped. Again, for each pair of units, I and j, the probability that they are both "on" is determined. This is referred to as p$^-_{ij}$. If multiple input/output patterns are to be learnt, this process is repeated for all patterns, yielding average values for p$^+_{ij}$ and p$^-_{ij}$. Weights are then adjusted, with the weight between units i and j being adjusted in proportion to the difference between p$^+_{ij}$ and p$^-_{ij}$. Note that in this figure the lines between units represent probabilities, not connection strengths.

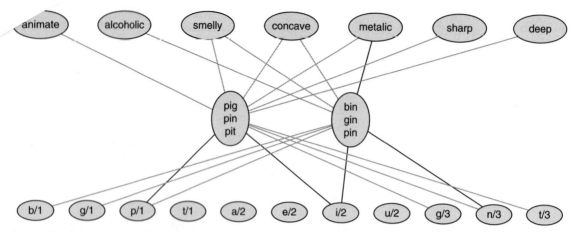

Fig. 1.18 The abstract structure of Hinton and Sejnowski's (1986) Boltzmann machine mapping orthographic representations (bottom) to semantic representations (top).

both active at the same time in the positive phase. This is referred to as a Hebbian term. In the second phase, the *negative phase*, the network is allowed to run with its inputs clamped but its outputs can now vary freely. Again, the network is allowed to settle. This produces for each connection an 'anti-Hebbian' term p^-_{ij}, corresponding to the probability that the nodes joined by the connection are simultaneously active in the negative phase. Weights between nodes i and j are then adjusted by an amount proportional to the difference between the Hebbian and anti-Hebbian terms. Early in learning the two settlings will lead to very different end-points. So the overall weight change of a positive phase minus a negative phase is considerable. Late in learning there is little overall alteration in the weights. With a set of input vectors to be categorised, different inputs can be sampled on different positive phases of the learning algorithm.

The complex learning process developed by Hinton and Sejnowski in order to learn to categorise inputs, therefore alternates between a positive phase and a negative phase. The model had an interesting link with a speculation put forward by Crick and Mitchison (1983), at about the same time, that dream sleep has the function of *unlearning* inappropriate tendencies when the brain's neural network is unconstrained by input or output. The phases are, therefore, sometimes referred to as 'wake' and 'sleep' phases.[41]

The Boltzmann machine was a beautiful idea. Its learning procedure—Hebbian learning—was biologically plausible. Its 'wake' and 'sleep' phases were biologically suggestive. However, it has one great drawback: it is

terribly slow. Running it involves four nested loops. So in practice it was rarely used for simulations of any empirically plausible cognitive or brain process.[42] One case where it was used was in an early simulation of the reading of words, a topic to be much discussed empirically in Chapters 4 and 5. Marshall and Newcombe (1973), using neuropsychological methods, had argued that reading aloud and reading-to-meaning were fundamentally distinct processes based on anatomically distinct routes. Their evidence was derived from two types of acquired dyslexia they had described—surface dyslexia and deep dyslexia—each having one or other route preserved (Marshall & Newcombe, 1966, 1973).[43] Hinton and Sejnowski (1986) modelled the reading-to-meaning process using a Boltzmann machine with three 'layers' (see Figure 1.18). The output of their net corresponds to one type of representation, say, that of the meanings of each word. Its input is clamped with the visual form of that word; in this early model this consists of a representation of each of the letters in their ordinal position within the word, e.g. H in position 1, A in position 2, T in position 3. With that input, the network has to learn to produce each word's meaning, again represented as a list of semantic features; in the original one they are mimicked by random vectors! Hinton and Sejnowski showed that their Boltzmann machine could learn the mapping. Moreover they demonstrated that the trained network was resistant to minor damage. Thus, when one of the 20 intermediate units was removed, the network's accuracy remained high (98.6%).

---

[41] The learning rule in the sleep phase is often called the 'anti-Hebbian' modification rule. It is not biologically implausible. According to Dayan and Abbott (2001) it corresponds to synaptic modification in cerebellar Purkinje cells.

[42] A deterministic version of the Boltzmann machine (Peterson and Anderson, 1987) works much faster and has been used in simulations (see e.g. Plaut & Shallice, 1993a; discussed in Chapter 4).

[43] These syndromes are described in more detail in Chapter 4; see also Figure 1.30.

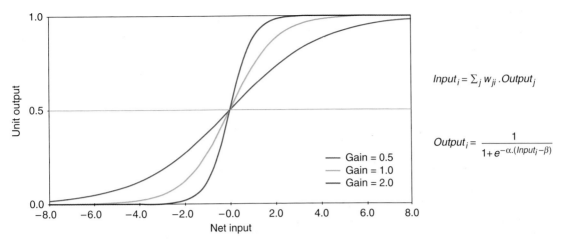

Fig. 1.19 The so-called sigmoid activation function typically used to calculate the output of a unit in a connectionist network given its input. In general, the input to unit i is the weighted sum of outputs from units which feed into unit i. If that weighted sum exceeds a threshold (zero in the graph, β in the equation) the unit's output will be between 0.5 and one. Otherwise it will be between 0.5 and zero. When the gain (α in the equation) is high the function is steep and values near the threshold will map to values near zero or one (blue line in the graph). When the gain is low the function rises gently and values near the threshold map to values nearer to 0.5 (red line in the graph).

We have described Boltzmann machine learning in some detail as this elegant and biologically plausible, but ultimately prohibitively slow, algorithm paved the way for a quick-but-dirty way of enabling networks to learn—*back-propagation*—which has since been the stock-in-trade of connectionist modellers at the cognitive level. Back-propagation has been independently invented several times, initially by Bryson and Ho (1969). It was, however, the rediscovery by Rumelhart, Hinton and Williams (1986) that led to it becoming extremely popular when the field had been primed by Hopfield nets, Boltzmann machines and simpler interactive activation models (McClelland & Rumelhart, 1981), which do not represent individual neurons—to be discussed in Chapter 3.

Back-propagation is a learning algorithm used in a multi-layer network in which activation flows through the system in one direction only from input to output—a *feed-forward* system.[44] The network is required to learn to produce a given output. Consider again the example of reading words discussed above. In a feed-forward implementation, at a particular stage of learning, the weights of the connections will have reached certain values. When a given word is presented to the network, this results in a wave of activation passing through the layers, which in turn leads to a pattern of activations in the output units.

Naturally, before learning is complete, the output representation (the meaning) activated differs from what it should be. The back-propagation algorithm alters the weights, so that with the same word as input the output will be less different than it was from the target value (i.e. the best representation of the word's meaning). This is done for each word in turn and the algorithm then recycles for another *epoch* of learning trials, one for each word and so on.[45]

Back-propagation generalises the so-called delta rule applied in the study of perceptrons, discussed in Section 1.6. For any one output unit, i, the change in the weight of the connection from a hidden unit, j, is be given by:

$$\Delta w_{ij} = a \cdot \sum_p [\text{error in unit } i] \cdot f'(\text{input to unit } i) \cdot [\text{output of unit } j]$$

where the summation is over all training patterns, p, a is a constant (the learning rate), and f' is the derivative of the activation function for the unit (see Figure 1.19). For earlier connections too—those involving the layers of the network other than input and output—the 'hidden units'—the error signal is computed by a backward pass through the network; first the weights of the last set of connections are updated, then those of the ones before them and so on by a recursive process. The formula employed is closely related to the delta rule, just discussed, which applies for the output units.

The initial discussion of back-propagation—Rumelhart et al. (1986)—gives a very clear and detailed account.

---

[44] While Hinton and Sejnowski's Boltzmann machine account of reading was layered, it was not feed-forward. As in all Boltzmann machines, all connections were bi-directional, so activation could circulate from the output units back to the intermediate units.

[45] In fact updating the weights typically occurs at the end of each epoch.

basic learning rule has subsequently been developed in a variety of ways (see Hinton, 1989; Hertz et al., 1991; Chapter 6). One development that has been particularly influential was the formulation of *back-propagation through time*, an extension of back-propagation for networks with feedback or *recurrent* connections and where the network's behaviour is a function of its input or processing history. Such networks are able to capture temporal structure, as occurs in domains such as language and action to be discussed in Chapters 4 and 8. In some situations, standard back-propagation is sufficient for learning temporal structure within a recurrent network.[46] In others, particularly where a recurrent network is required to reproduce a specific sequence of known length (as in the Botvinick and Plaut model of action selection to be discussed in Section 8.3) or where its input is fixed while activation circulates through the network until it reaches a stable state (as in the Plaut and Shallice (1993a) model to be discussed in Section 4.11), back-propagation through time is needed.

Networks that learn by back-propagation were endlessly criticised later as being inadequate for modelling the mind on the grounds that they are biologically unrealistic (e.g. Crick, 1989; Douglas & Martin, 1991). However, they have two great virtues. Theoretically, as Minsky and Papert had shown, simple perceptrons had had the problem that they could not learn many simply describable types of input–output mapping, such as giving one output if a pattern is symmetrical and another if it is not. Empirically, it was found that multi-layer back-propagation nets can learn such mappings. Secondly, they learn much faster than say, Boltzmann machines. They can therefore be used in practice to simulate the operation of a system that is composed of units that very abstractly behave like neurons and which carries out a particular function.[47] They have, for instance, been used to simulate processes in the other main reading procedure: spelling-to-sound (e.g. Seidenberg & McClelland, 1989), semantic memory (knowledge) operations (e.g. Farah & McClelland, 1991), face recognition (e.g. Farah, O'Reilly, Vecera, 1993), and aspects of speech perception (e.g. McClelland & Elman, 1986), amongst many other examples. Thus they helped to provide a framework of models of how different specific higher-level processes might operate, which are made more plausible by using units that compute in parallel in a broadly analogous way to neurons. The objection that they are biologically unrealistic can be countered by pointing out that all models are abstract simplifications, and for that reason cannot be completely faithful to reality. This issue is discussed more extensively in Section 3.7.

By comparison with the more empirical methods to be discussed in the next section, the application of these models to the domain of cognition has been highly controversial, not only with respect to the particular learning algorithms used. The best known models were subject to able but highly polemical attacks that were much broader in their targets. These attacks came from two sources. One was from those favouring non-distributed connectionist models, so called *localist nets* to be discussed in Section 3.7 (e.g. Page, 2000). More critically, the attacks have come from those in fields with a more formal structuralist tradition, like that in linguistics, who have viewed any attempt to grapple with the microstructure of cognition in a neurally more plausible fashion as a return to the intellectually barren perspectives of the behaviourists. Connectionism was seen by Chomsky and his followers as just a new manifestation of behaviourism. In a famous polemic against his fellow-Bostonian Skinner's (1957) book, *Verbal Behaviour*, Chomsky (1959b) had himself extended his analyses of context-free grammars to attempt to show that behaviourism was intellectually inadequate as an account of language behaviour. His followers attempted to make analogous critiques of connectionism (e.g. Fodor & Pylyshyn, 1988; Pinker & Prince, 1988). This attitude still continues (Fodor, 2000).[48]

The analogy between behaviourism and connectionism is in fact quite inappropriate. Behaviourist approaches to syntax had been shown formally by Chomsky to be incapable of capturing the complexity of the grammatical regularities found in language. There is *no* demonstration—and as we will see later there cannot be—that the much more complex formalisms that connectionism can provide, when compared with a typical set of rewrite rules, are incapable of capturing the essence of syntax. It will be a theme of this book that this criticism is essentially retrogressive. Connectionist theoreticians themselves have not been so hostile to other cognitive science approaches as the followers of Chomsky have been to them. However, they have generally been dismissive of what they consider the box-and-arrow theorising characteristic of earlier information-processing psychology, which they consider unduly primitive.

Symbolic artificial intelligence, by contrast, suffered the complementary trajectory to connectionism. By the 1980s it was clear that programs that planned in advance for all contingencies that might occur—they used so-called *conditional (or contingency) planning*—ran

---

[46] See, for example, Elman (1990).

[47] We will use the term *function* to characterise the input–output mapping of a subsystem that can be separately characterisable.

[48] Chomsky in conversation even once described connectionism to one of us as an intellectual fraud.

into severe problems. In real life situations they proved very fragile. For instance, it may be too complex to enumerate exhaustively all the possible contingencies or unexpected events that may occur, there may be random elements, motor execution may be faulty or the situation may be such that a short-cut solution is available (see Russell & Norvig, 1995). In the 1980s, a new approach, *reactive planning*, therefore became popular and was seen as a replacement for the symbolic AI approach. In a series of papers in the 1980s, the MIT computer scientist Rodney Brooks (1991) argued for the effectiveness of robots that have fairly minimal internal states. He rejected explicitly trying to determine as the *answer* to a problem a set of long strings of moves, with each string being conditional on a particular state of the world that might develop. Instead, he argued that the robot's behaviour should be based on a large repertoire of *behavioural models*, each of which can control a particular sort of behaviour, such as wall-following, obstacle-checking or exploration.[49] However, the development of such robots tended to move further towards solutions to particular practical problems; they lost contact with cognitive science more generally.[50]

There has, however, been one type of symbolic AI system that survived the general unpopularity of symbolic models, and also left a strong legacy in the rest of cognitive science—*production systems*. Production systems take us back, both conceptually and historically, to a system close to the basic Turing machines. In the 1940s, the logician Post, who influenced Chomsky, considered a type of computational system in which the operators—termed *productions*—were so-called *condition–action* pairs. These pairs are like a more cognitive version of the old stimulus–response elements of behaviourist theories. A condition can be satisfied either by the perceptual input or by the contents of a *working memory*. If it is so satisfied, then, other things being equal, an action is produced. *Actions* in turn are not just behaviours; they can involve putting tokens of representations into the working memory.

Production systems were initially developed for simulations of cognition by Allen Newell and Herb Simon, who had already introduced the first two AI programs—Logic Theorist and GPS. In their 1972 book, they showed that a sequence of the firings of production rules, each of which involves putting information into working memory, can, over a series of time-cycles, be seen as an analogue of the flow of the thought process. Moreover the

D = 5	G = ?	D O N A L D +
O = ?	E = ?	G E R A L D
N = ?	R = ?	R O B E R T
A = ?	B = ?	
L = ?	T = ?	

Fig. 1.20 A standard cryptarithmetic problem. The 'sum' is valid arithmetic, where each letter stands for a different digit. Given that the letter D stands for 5, what digits do each of the other letters stand for?

sequence is determined by the goals set up, which are also represented as elements in working memory. Productions act as a potentially parallel set of operators, each being both at a local level *modular* and yet given a working memory they can be applied together. Such systems can become the basis of a plausible model of thought. To test their model, Newell and Simon used *protocols*, namely the product of the subject *thinking aloud* as they are solving the problem. They demonstrated that in a situation like that of solving cryptarithmetic problems (see Figure 1.20), there was a very reasonable qualitative fit between the operation of the program and the protocol of a typical subject.

Newell and Simon applied production systems to a variety of cognitive domains with varying degrees of success.[51] However, over the next few years, other more complex production systems were developed, which culminated in the 1980s in two different but related strands, each of which had considerable empirical success. One strand consisted of *Soar* (Newell, 1990), shown in Figure 1.21. Above we said that 'other things being equal', an action is produced when a condition is satisfied. However, normally other things are not equal! The conceptual problem that Soar tackled is the way that, in a production system, the conditions of two or more productions may be satisfied on a particular time-cycle. Yet their *actions* may potentially be in conflict in some way. For instance, the results of effecting one production may remove the pre-conditions for selecting the other. In the 1970s, production systems avoided this problem by a variety of conflict-resolution procedures, so that typically only one production fired on a cycle (see e.g. McDermott & Forgy, 1978). Conflict-resolution procedures could, for instance, favour productions whose conditions matched against those working memory elements that had been most recently added or changed; they could favour more specific ones requiring many constraints to be satisfied over more general ones, which are elicited more frequently. They could simply order the conditions and operate by random selection with replacement. The designers of Soar

---

[49] These behavioural models can have a hierarchical structure with high-level ones being able to modify the lower-level ones or override their outputs.

[50] The reactive-planning approach was itself subject to strong criticism in the following decade—see Section 9.1.

---

[51] See Boden (1988) for an effective critique of Newell and Simon's early work.

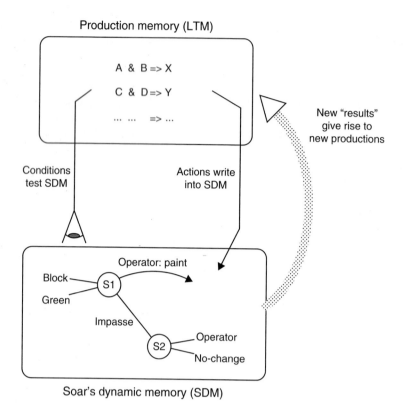

Fig. 1.21 A schematic illustration of Soar. Rules in Production Memory match against and modify elements in Soar's Dynamic Memory, which is structured in terms of goals (S1) and subgoals (S2). Reproduced with permission from R.M. Young and R.L. Lewis, 1999, The Soar cognitive architecture and human working memory. In A. Miyake and P. Shah (eds.) Models of Working Memory. Cambridge University Press.

viewed all such procedures as *ad hoc*. So they instituted a software version of Rodin's Thinker. When multiple productions are satisfied, Soar creates a so-called *impasse*. A new problem is posed to the system, namely, which of the potentially competing productions to select. Only when that is solved, either putatively or definitively, does the program continue with its original problem.

Soar developed from two strands of Newell's previous research—the General Problem Solver discussed in Section 1.6 and the *Model Human Processor* (MHP), which was developed in collaboration with Stu Card and Tom Moran (Card et al.,1983). The MHP was a *box-and-arrow diagram* of the hypothesised information-processing components relevant to a human computer operator. It specified different representational codes for different components and different processing times for different kinds of operation. In association with the GOMS (Goals, Operators, Methods and Selection Rules) methodology for task decomposition, it allowed one to predict how long a subject would take for different tasks, such as text editing using different interfaces or recalling computer commands using different abbreviation schemes (see e.g. John & Newell, 1987). In the limited

domain for which it was developed, it fitted relevant findings well. Newell, however, viewed Soar as a unified theory of the mind. So he tried to apply Soar to empirical phenomena in a wide variety of cognitive domains. The attempt was too ambitious. Soar is too cerebral a system to work well in domains, involving, say, spatial operations or the retrieval of one's autobiographical memory of the past, so-called *episodic memory*, to be discussed in Chapter 10. Moreover, both the cortex and the cognitive system contain too many special-purpose computations, which made it premature to attempt a unified theory of cognition at that stage of cognitive science's development (see Cooper & Shallice, 1995). Soar has, therefore, become an AI system mainly oriented to applied problems such as command-and-control, and now has relatively little influence in cognitive science (but see Young & Lewis, 1999, for an alternative view).[52]

---

[52] This remains true despite recent modifications to Soar which have involved the addition of distinct semantic and episodic memory components, and long-term and short-term visual stores (Laird, 2008). Thus, cognitive science has had substantial

The other strand is a system with similarities to Soar but where a much greater sustained effort has been made to incorporate psychological concepts. This much modified theory is the so-called *ACT* (for Adaptive Control of Thought) set of models developed by the Carnegie-Mellon psychologist John Anderson, initially with Gordon Bower as the program HAM (Anderson & Bower, 1973) but then developed through ACT-E and ACT* to ACT-R (Anderson, 1993). ACT-R is a hybrid system with both symbolic and subsymbolic aspects. It has been tested in much more detail than Soar in a variety of cognitive domains. Moreover its mechanisms and operation are much more influenced by concepts of modern cognitive psychology than is Soar. For instance, it contains separable declarative and procedural memory components, cognitive processes to be discussed in Chapter 10. Moreover in its latest version (J. Anderson, 2007) it is much influenced by cognitive neuroscience. We will, therefore, discuss it further, later in the book, rather than here (see Sections 3.8, 7.9 and 12.9).

ACT-R is currently the most influential symbolic AI system in cognitive science. However, by comparison with connectionism, symbolic AI now has relatively little influence. In part, this is because symbolic approaches are most suited to modelling complex tasks where behaviour is often best understood in terms of application of a strategy, and where different individuals may adopt different strategies. Strategic knowledge then becomes essentially a free parameter of the models, making them difficult to falsify. Even so, in Chapters 9 and 12 we will argue that the influence of symbolic AI deserves to be greater!

A second area where symbolic models might have been adopted, and one which does not appear to be subject to individual differences in strategy, is in comprehending and producing language. Given the rejection by Chomskyan linguists of connectionist approaches, and the structural elements of modern linguistic theories exemplified by phrase structure grammars (see Table 1.1), one might anticipate that the development of symbolic systems during the 1980s and 1990s would have led to significant cross-fertilization with linguistics. This has not been the case. Chomskyan linguistics instead developed as a distinctly separate endeavour, led primarily by a series of key texts by Chomsky himself.

One of the primary influences behind developments in linguistics during this period was a move towards

perceived parsimony. This was apparent in the development of theories covering different aspects of language. These included *X-bar theory*, *case theory* and θ-*theory* (Chomsky, 1981). Take, for example, X-bar theory, a general theory of the structure of phrases. Here, all phrase structure rules take one of three forms:

$$\overline{\overline{X}} \rightarrow \text{Spec}_x\ \overline{X}$$

$$\overline{\overline{X}} \rightarrow \text{Adj}_x\ \overline{X}$$

$$\overline{X} \rightarrow \text{Comp}_{x1}\ ...\ \text{Comp}_{xn}$$

In such rules, X is a variable that ranges over syntactic categories, such as noun (N) and verb (V). The rules permit structures such as those shown in Figure 1.22. For example, the first rule captures the generalisation that in English a noun phrase ($\overline{\overline{N}}$) consists of nominal *specifier* (e.g. a determiner, such as *the*, or a genitive phrase, such as *the footballer's*) followed by something of category $\overline{N}$ (e.g. a noun followed by zero or more complements (comp), (such as *boots*), while a sentence ($\overline{\overline{V}}$) consists of a verbal specifier (e.g. a noun phrase such as *the footballer's boots*) followed by something of category $\overline{V}$ (i.e. a standard verb phrase, such as *kicked the ball*).

Of course, even in English, many grammatically correct sentences do not fit the basic phrase structure rules of X-bar theory. Sentences involving so-called *raising* or *control* verbs, and non-standard constructions, such as *topicalisation* and *cleft sentences*[53] were allowed by the grammar by the use of empty slots in the surface form, technically a *trace*, and *move* operations. Move operations allowed a syntactic element to be realised in the surface form in a non-standard position, while a phonologically empty item—the trace—was held to be left in place of the moved element. The primary obsession then became one of specifying, in concrete terms, conditions under which movement was, or was not, possible (see, e.g. Chomsky, 1981, 1986). Why, for example, should one of the following be grammatical and the other not?[54]

Who did you speak to before you met?

* Who spoke to you before you met?

---

recent influence, but the influence has been one-way. In our view this is unfortunate. Some aspects of Soar as traditionally conceived, particularly related to impasses and subgoaling, fit well with neuroscience evidence on the processing of novelty; see Section 9.4.

[53] Raising and control verbs are those such as *try*, as in *John tried to help Mary*, where the semantic subject (*John*) of the embedded clause (*help Mary*) is realised in the surface form as the subject of the sentence. Topicalised constructions are those where the topic of the sentence is realised in the surface form as the sentence initial phrase as in *Mary, John tried to help*. Cleft sentence begin with *it or that* as in *It was Maradona who handled the ball*.

[54] In these examples we use the linguistic convention of an asterisk to indicate an ungrammatical sentence.

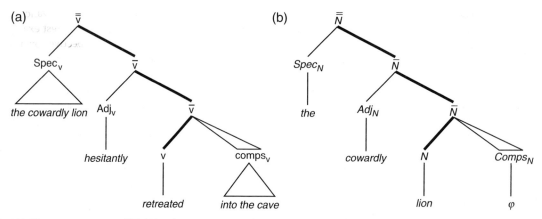

Fig. 1.22 Phrase structure trees within X-bar theory. A common abstract structure underlies both (a) sentences (the maximal projection from the category V) and (b) noun phrases (the maximal projection from the category N). The symbol φ represents a null constituent.

The proposed solution involved specifying barriers to movement in terms of abstract constraints based on structural notions, such as *C-command* and *government*. These notions are defined in terms of the position of nodes within syntactic tree structures (see Figure 1.22).

A further stimulus for developments in linguistic theory following Chomsky's initial work was the logical problem of learning a language. The question was how a language, which can have a potentially infinite number of strings of words, could be learned when the child hears only a finite set of valid sentences. Chomsky had long argued that this problem was solved by what he called *universal grammar*—general 'conditions on the form and organisation of any human language' (Chomsky, 1968, p. 71). These conditions were held to be essentially psychological constraints that followed from innate computational or neural processes involved in language comprehension and production. In the 1980s, universal grammar was made more concrete through the *principles and parameters* approach (Chomsky, 1981; Chomsky & Lasnik, 1993). The idea was that universal grammar specified a set of parameterised constraints concerned with issues such as the order of items on the right-hand side of phrase structure rules in X-bar theory, of whether pronouns have to be present in the surface form (as in English) or are optional (as in Italian and many other Romance languages). Languages were held to differ in their *parameter settings* (as well, of course, as in their lexical items). Given this, learning a language would be a matter of learning the parameter settings (and the lexical items)—something that might reasonably be inferred from exposure to a small set of grammatically correct sentences.

A major shift occurred in the mid-1990s with the rise of the *minimalist programme* (Chomsky, 1995). Minimalism refocused mainstream linguistic theory by viewing language as linking two hypothesised cognitive systems: the conceptual/semantic system and the phonetic/ articulatory system. Language is therefore understood as a 'perfect' mapping between the interfaces of these systems—between logical form and phonetic form. The two systems are held to impose constraints on the interface representations. For instance, logical form must be interpretable, so it cannot contain the equivalent of unbound variables, such as *chases(Fido, x)*, where *x* is not specified.

The mapping specified by the language module, between logical form and phonetic form, is also held to be 'optimal' and subject to two 'economy' principles: the principle of *economy of derivation* and the principle of *economy of representation*. The details of the economy principles are not important to the current discussion. What is critical is that minimalism is a radical departure from earlier versions of Chomskyan theory. It does away with established conceptual frameworks, such as that involved in X-bar theory. Additionally, it limits phrase structure to binary rules (i.e. rules with exactly two elements on the right hand side) and reduces the number of operations on phrase structure to just two, *merge* and *move*.

In some ways, the minimalist approach would appear compatible with a cognitive neuroscience view of mind, particularly in view of the assumptions concerning the relation of language to the conceptual/ semantic system and the phonetic/articulatory system. However, there is no cognitive neuroscience evidence that relates to these systems within the minimalist programme. Moreover there are many difficulties within the approach as it currently stands. As Lappin, Levine & Johnson (2000) argue, the notions of *perfection* and *optimality* are poorly specified. Somewhat sweepingly, they argue that minimalism 'rests upon an obscure metaphor rather than a precise claim with clear empirical content' (p. 666), and that it represents a sociological but unscientific revolution in linguistic theorising.

Linguistics, even that part which is concerned with syntax, is far from just the movement identified with Chomsky. A number of different types of theorising remain popular amongst major practitioners (e.g. Gazdar et al., 1985; Pollard & Sag, 1994; Steedman, 2000; Bresnan, 2001). None of these approaches has been refuted, and many are much more naturally implemented as a program within an information-processing approach. However, these types of theorising have never commanded the linguistic mainstream. So the intellectual wall between cognitive psychology and linguistics has remained fairly impermeable in the psychology to linguistics direction.

1.8 The Blossoming Disciplines 1970–95: the Slow but Steady Advance of Human Experimental Psychology

The history of human experimental psychology has been less dramatic than those of linguistics, symbolic AI and connectionism. Despite its main theoretical tool—the information-processing model—being treated dismissively by connectionists, the field has produced steady empirical advances. In many respects it has shown a type of development somewhat similar to those occurring in single-cell recording, neuropsychology and functional imaging, to be discussed in the next section. More important, the field has reached what Kuhn would describe as 'normal science'. However, this has not occurred in the way Kuhn held to be prototypic of the advanced sciences. In the classic Kuhnian model, empirical anomalies build up in the existing theoretical framework.

They are resolved by a major theoretical advance, such as Newton's or Darwin's, to take the greatest examples. This in turn restructures basic perspectives over large areas of the field. Instead, in human experimental psychology, outstanding theoretical disputes became resolved more by developing knowledge of the conditions under which each of the competing theories is appropriate, rather than by any single all-purpose theoretical reorganisation of the field. At the same time, a variety of new, more subtle questions became posed and novel experimental procedures were developed to tackle them. In addition, as occurred for the neuroscience methods to be considered shortly too, there was a rapid colonising of new topic areas.

Take, as an example, the field of attention. The modern approach to the area began with practical questions in ergonomics being posed at the end of World War II. How many channels of communication can be maintained with a pilot? Colin Cherry (1953), an Englishman at MIT, discovered that when two passages are played to a pilot simultaneously, one to each ear, then if the pilot understands the gist of one—on the so-called primary channel—he (as it was in those days!) extracted little information from the other—the secondary channel. He would even fail to detect a switch in the language of the message (see also Treisman, 1964).

As mentioned earlier, the so-called *early selection* theory of attention was proposed by Donald Broadbent (1958) (see Figure 1.23) in order to explain why capacity is so highly limited. Attention was assumed to operate like a filter to allow information from one and only one message to reach higher centres. This theory was soon realised to be too stark. Anne Treisman in her DPhil

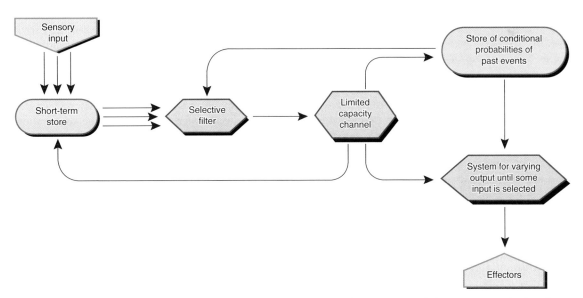

Fig. 1.23 The early selection model of attention (see Broadbent, 1958, Figure 7, p 299). Selection occurs before processing, with selected information passing through a limited capacity channel. The Short-Term Store would correspond to the Icon of Figure 1.6.

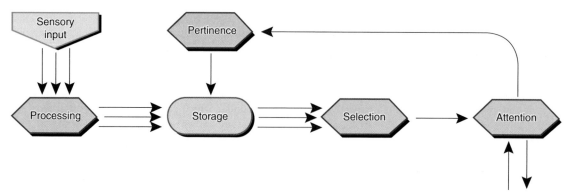

Fig. 1.24 The late selection model of attention (see Norman, 1968, Figure 1, p 526). Selection occurs after processing and storage of the sensory input.

dissertation at Oxford (see Treisman, 1964) suggested that the all-or-none filter should be replaced by an attenuating filter. On this account, some information reaches higher centres from channels other than the primary one. But on all channels except the first, the input is greatly reduced. However, within a couple of years a rival 'theory' had been put forward by Deutsch & Deutsch (1963) (see also Norman, 1968 and Duncan, 1980). This was the *late selection* theory (see Figure 1.24). On this approach, a choice between messages was made only after each had been reasonably fully analysed semantically. Only then is one selected to control action or to reach consciousness.

A key result, held to support this second position, was obtained by Moray (1959). The subject has the task of continuously echoing back speech heard on the primary channel—*shadowing*. Moray showed that a person's own name is detected more frequently than a control name on a secondary channel. On the late selection theory, the content of the message on the secondary channel affects whether it is detected, and so one's own name—being semantically highly important—becomes selected.

For many years the field was split between these two rival camps of theorists. Forty years later, the conditions under which each of these two formulations of attention is the more appropriate are known. First, if one assumes that there is an attenuating filter, rather than an all-or-none filter—as all proponents of early selection have argued since Anne Treisman's initial proposal—then on early selection theory there must be some form of later selection too, so the contrast between the theories is not so great as was initially assumed. Second, it is generally accepted that if two conditions hold, then early selection theory is valid (see Cowan, 1995; Pashler, 1998; for reviews). The first condition is that both input channels involved are in the same sense modality, as in the early shadowing experiments. The second is that the task involves demanding

operations at the stages that follow the purely perceptual ones.

Both of the qualifications are necessary. As far as the first condition is concerned, when structurally unrelated inputs are presented on different processing channels, then effective processing can occur in parallel across input systems. This is so even when the demands on later stages of the system by the primary task are quite heavy. Thus Allport, Antonis and Reynolds (1972) had subjects shadowing prose and sight-reading difficult pieces on the piano with relatively little interference between them (for tighter but less dramatic supporting evidence, see also Treisman & Davis, 1973, and Gipson, 1986).

The second qualification is also relevant. Thus, if all that is required is that the subject just monitors for particular targets, then a number of input streams can be checked simultaneously (Duncan, 1980). This type of finding can be generalised to the following 'law': the degree to which late selection, rather than early selection, operates depends upon the *cognitive load* of the primary task (Lavie, 1995). With low loads, late selection tends to hold; with high loads, early selection is the rule.

That early selection effects are primarily found within a single modality made the loci of selection likely to be modality-specific. Indeed strong human experimental evidence was obtained by Duncan (1984) that the unit of selection in vision was the segmented object, as previously suggested by Neisser (1967). The basic principle is that the selection process operates on the perceptual input at a processing stage *after* one in which the scene is segmented *pre-semantically* into different objects in parallel (Driver & Baylis, 1998). There are many demonstrations supporting this principle. Thus, similarly to Duncan (1984), Egly, Driver and Rafal (1994) found that, if attention is orientated towards one position in space, one is faster to move attention to the position if it is within the same object, than to an equidistant position in another object.

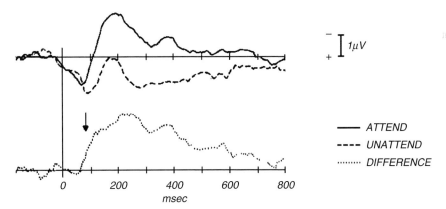

Fig. 1.25 Event-related potentials (ERPs) as measured at the medial frontal site (Fz) for short auditory stimuli of high or low pitch presented through stereo headphones and with an apparent location either to the left or the right of the subject. A subject had to attend to either the high or the low pitch tones and was required to indicate the locations of the attended tones. The lower panel shows the difference between 'attended' and 'unattended' waves. Each wave represents the mean of approximately 500 stimulus presentations over 8 subjects (4000 stimuli). Copyright © 1983 by the American Psychological Association. Reproduced with permission. J.C. Hansen and S.A. Hillyard, 1983, Selective attention to multidimensional auditory stimuli, Journal of Experimental Psychology: Human Perception and Performance, 9(1), 1–19. The use of APA information does not imply endorsement by APA.

In the last example we conflated work on a slightly different topic—how attention is shifted (Posner & Cohen, 1984)—with that of the selection of an object to be attended. One of the characteristics of the development of research on attention, using experimental psychological methods, has been the very variety of different aspects that have been studied in the last couple of decades. Shifting attention itself can be so-called *endogenous* (i.e. voluntarily self-initiated) or *exogenous* (i.e. semi-involuntarily driven by a stimulus). Attention can be divided or shared. And many further aspects have been addressed, such as alertness and vigilance (Broadbent, 1971), and attention-to-action (Norman & Shallice, 1986; Posner & Petersen, 1990), which will be discussed in later chapters. Thus, as resolutions have been obtained on the more basic aspects of the field, so new debates have opened up. The process is much more similar to geographical exploration than the prototypical Kuhnian model of the history of an advanced science.

The resolution so obtained of the early versus later selection debate could have been carried out by human experimental methods alone. Other aspects of attention work have been adequately addressed by these methods too. However, the sense of resolution of the earlier debates and the progress on the later issues have been greatly helped by a broadening of the methods used. Attention has become the subject of a wide panoply of cognitive neuroscience methods, not just those of human experimental psychology. Thus, very early in the modern history of the field, Hillyard, Hink, Schwent and Picton (1973) used electrophysiological-evoked response techniques to be discussed in the next section. They showed that an early component of the so-called evoked response, recorded at scalp electrodes, was reduced if attention was directed away from a stimulus, compared with when it was directed towards it. Moreover, the divergence occurred a mere 60–80 msec after stimulus presentation (Hillyard & Picton, 1987) (see Figure 1.25). This is hard to reconcile with a solely late-selection position. Moreover, Lavie's load theory, too, has been beautifully supported by functional imaging results (see Figure 1.26).

The issue of early or late selection is just one of the many aspects of attention that have been investigated by cognitive neuroscience methods. Thus, Corbetta and Shulman (2002) produced strong evidence from functional imaging that anatomically separate systems are involved in so-called *exogenous* (bottom-up) and *endogenous* (top-down) forms of the capture of attention (see Section 9.3). Moreover, a wide set of cognitive neuroscience techniques has been used. Even single-cell studies of attention have been a growth area (see e.g. Desimone & Duncan, 1995). So have neuropsychological analyses of the syndrome, unilateral neglect, in which the patient cannot orient attention to one part of the world, typically the left (e.g. Driver & Mattingley, 1998). Thus studies using the procedures of human experimental psychology now combine with many other cognitive neuroscience methodologies, and the combination tends to produce results that are more dramatic than the use of human experimental psychology procedures alone. Attention is no longer just a psychological area of study. Instead it is a field of cognitive neuroscience.

For instance, take the idea that visual attention operates on segmented objects. This was supported by experiments on normal subjects by Duncan (1984).

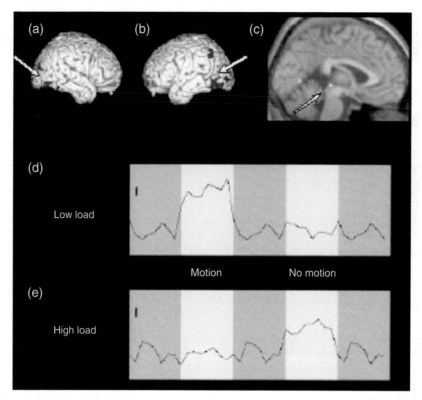

Fig. 1.26 Interaction effects of visual motion and linguistic-processing load. Subjects were presented with a word surrounded by white dots. In the low linguistic-load condition subjects were required to indicate whether a word was presented in upper or lower case. In the high linguistic-load condition they were required to indicate whether the word was bi-syllabic. In both conditions they were told to ignore the white dots, which may or may not have been moving. In the low-load condition activity was seen in area MT V5 with moving dots, suggesting that the motion of the dots was processed (consistent with a late-selection model), but in the high-load condition it was not (consistent with an early-selection model). (a) and (b) The interaction effect in V5. (c) Modulation of attention-related activity is also seen in the superior colliculus. (d) and (e) Mean activity over all subjects in V5 for low and high load conditions. From G. Rees, C.D. Frith and N. Lavie, 1997, Modulating irrelevant motion perception by varying attentional load in an unrelated task, Science, 278(5343), 1616–1619. Reprinted with permission from AAAS.

Driver, Baylis and Rafal (1992) used a left neglect patient, CC, to produce a much more dramatic phenomenon supporting the same position. Subjects viewed figures, such as those shown in Figure 1.27. They were asked to report the form of the central line by indicating whether it matched the line shown in the bottom of the display. Normal subjects have no difficulty on the task, but report the figure in yellow as appearing in the foreground on a striped, shapeless blue background. CC also performed well when the yellow figure appeared on the left (as in Figure 1.27a), and hence when the border was to the right of the foreground figure. This was true regardless of whether the border fell to the left or the right of fixation. However, when the yellow portion of the diagram was on the right (as in Figure 1.27b), and hence the line was to the left of the figure, CC performed at chance. Again, this was true whether the boundary line was to the left or right of fixation. The results suggest that object segmentation occurs

pre-attentively, with neglect relating to the left side of segmented objects, rather than just occurring in the left visual field.

There are other areas of human experimental psychology where major progress has been made, such as object or face recognition, word processing, short-term memory and so on. However, the empirical methods internal to human experimental psychology itself remain weak by comparison with the harder sciences. Take Frost (1998), discussing models of the different means by which words are read, itself a field opened up by the neuropsychological advances briefly refereed to in the last section. 'The process of recognising printed words has been studied for many years and has been a very active field of scientific inquiry. It has provided researchers not only with novel and ingenious experimental techniques, but also with rich and comprehensive sets of data that describe almost every aspect of reading. Yet despite the abundance of accumulated

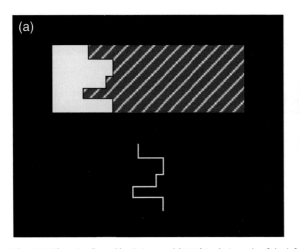 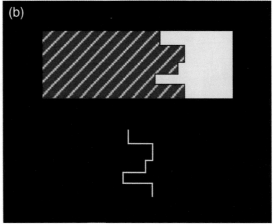

Fig. 1.27 The stimuli used by Driver et al (1992) in their study of the left-neglect patient CC. Subjects were required to indicate whether the line within the top rectangle matched that below it. Controls performed equally well when the foreground was on the left (a) or the right (b). Patient CC was selectively impaired with stimuli of type (b), where the dividing line was on the left of the yellow figure, seen as the foreground. Reprinted by permission from Macmillan Publishers Ltd: Nature Neuroscience (J. Driver and J.B. Mattingley (1998) Parietal neglect and visual awareness, Nature Neuroscience, 1(1), 17–22), Copyright (1998).

data, the major controversies that have dominated the field for so many years seem to be as lively as ever. Experiments are being run each year by the hundreds, yet their results fail to convince the unconvinced' (p.71). This is because Frost's 'novel and ingenious experimental techniques' typically means new experimental paradigms. The data they produce are fairly coarse, such as manipulation X leads to a slower response to stimulus type Y than type Z. Moreover, if one takes any particular new paradigm, then Tulving and Madigan's lament, discussed in Section 1.4, still applies; how the paradigm should be realised, even for a simple model, can itself require extensive investigation. At the same time there are a rapidly growing number of models of increasing complexity.

Thus the situation in an area such as reading is that there are a large number of experimental paradigms, which each provide evidence that needs explaining in terms of a range of models. More powerful forms of data tend to be required to differentiate adequately in such domains between the escalating number of possible theoretical accounts and paradigm-specific interpretations. The situation in an area requiring more complex processes, such as problem-solving, where cognitive neuroscience methods have had, until recently, relatively little influence, has been even more static theoretically. Broad theoretical frameworks, such as the *mental models* approach (Johnson-Laird, 1983) and a *mental logic* one (e.g. Braine, 1978), were still confronting each other in much the same way as they did 20 years before (e.g. Braine & O'Brien, 1998; Goodwin & Johnson-Laird, 2005; Reverberi et al, 2007).

A broad generalisation is that, the more successful human experimental psychology research has been in an area, the more there has been a widening of the approaches that have been used. So from the original studies, which used only experimental psychology techniques on adult human subjects, studies in successfully developing areas tend now to encompass a wide variety of other cognitive neuroscience approaches. Indeed, the development of successful experimental paradigms internal to cognitive psychology now almost inevitably leads to their adoption in a wider cognitive neuroscience context. A consequence is that the contributions of human experimental psychology methods themselves can easily be overlooked. Yet, as we will see, all these other methods are dependent upon the appropriate selection of a task for the subject to carry out. Which tasks are useful and which are not and how they are tackled by subjects, is, *par excellence*, the domain of human experimental psychology. Moreover, it will be argued later that the classic type of theoretical framework derived from human experimental psychology—the information-processing one—remains critical for cognitive neuroscience.

If one considers the approaches comprising cognitive science as a whole, there has then been real progress within each individual discipline, but in none of them has it been as dramatic as within the more neuroscience-based fields, shortly to be discussed. Within each field there remain sceptics about most theoretical perspectives. Most critically, exponents of different approaches often remain in conflict with each other and, even where there is no conflict, aficionados of the different approaches often remain well separated intellectually from each other. Thus, the leading proponents of the neural network modelling tend to be reductionists and, with a few exceptions like Jay McClelland

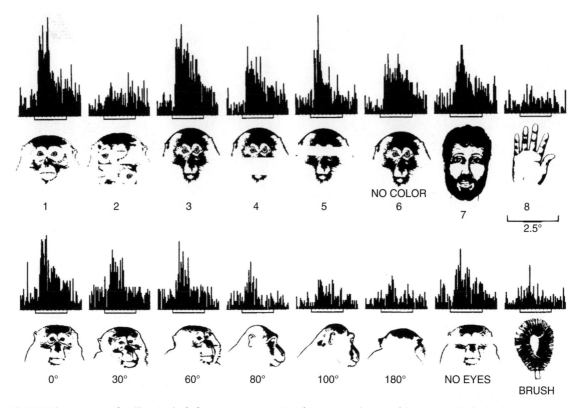

Fig. 1.28 The response to face-like stimuli of a face-receptive neuron in inferior temporal cortex of the macaque. Each stimulus was presented for 2.5 secs, as indicated by the bar underneath each histogram. Reproduced with permission from Desimone et al (1984) Stimulus selective properties of inferior temporal neurons in the macaque, Journal of Neuroscience, 4, 2051–2062. Figure 6A, 6B, p 2057.

and David Plaut, consider cognition too flaky to be tractable. Those from the symbolic tradition influenced by Chomsky in turn tend to regard connectionism as quasi-behaviourist. Symbolic AI is shunned by virtually all, and human experimental psychology considered mundane. So cognitive science remains highly fragmented.

1.9 The Blossoming Disciplines 1970–95: the Macro-level Neurosciences

The period 1970–95 may have seen steady but slow advance in the cognitive sciences. By contrast, it saw rapid progress for the neurosciences. For the systems and cognitive areas of neuroscience with which we are concerned in this book, all of the approaches discussed in the earlier sections developed both extensively by colonising all areas of the cortex and intensively by the introduction of new methods.

The speed of advance has been rapid in both single-cell recording and neuropsychology. Using single-cell recording the initial work on visual cortex by Hubel and Wiesel was followed soon after by key discoveries by Dubner and Zeki (1971) and Zeki (1974) on so-called V4, a structure very responsive to the colour of the

stimulus and V5, one responsive to its movement.[55] After that there was an explosion in the number of visual regions investigated. By 1995, 32 different visual regions had been identified (Van Essen & Deyoe, 1995). This does not mean, however, that each of the different regions has been unambiguously worked out. Thus, even now, the extent to which colour is particularly relevant to the processing being carried out in V4 remains a matter of controversy (e.g. Hadjikhani et al, 1998; Heywood & Cowey, 1998; Moutoussis & Zeki, 2002).

Over the period, many tasks were developed in a somewhat analogous fashion to what was occurring in human experimental psychology. These though were tasks that produced activation in particular regions of the brain. To give just two examples, Perrett, Rolls and Caan (1982) found that cells in the superior temporal sulcus are activated when a monkey looks at a face. Shortly after, Desimone et al. (1984) found cells with similar properties in the inferior temporal cortex (see Figure 1.28). A more complex example is the so-called

---

[55] This was originally known as MT (medial temporal lobe) and this is still the usage in the USA. The V-labelling is logical as it indicates that *anatomically* the relevant regions form a network derived initially from V1 (Brodmann area 17).

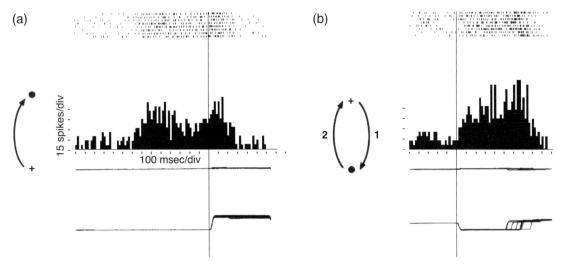

Fig. 1.29 Firing properties of a sustained-response cell in the posterior parietal cortex of a macaque during the double-saccade task. (a) A single saccade from the fixation point vertically up. (b) A double saccade, first vertically down and then back up to the original fixation point. Each panel shows the raster trace of firing over 8 trials, the corresponding histogram, and the vertical eye position. Reproduced with kind permission from Springer Science+Business Media: Experimental Brain Research, Memory related motor planning activity in posterior parietal cortex of macaque, 70(1), 1988, p. 218, J.W. Gnadt and R.A. Andersen, figure 3.

double-saccade task of Sparks and Mays (1980). Two lights—A and B—come on very briefly. The animal must saccade (make an eye movement) to look first to where A is and then to where B is. Using this task, Gnadt and Andersen (1988) (see Figure 1.29) found that when the animal looks at A, there are cells in a part of the posterior parietal cortex—the lateral intra-parietal sulcus (LIP, discussed in Section 3.4)—that code where the position of B is in the visual field with respect to fixation at A. A response occurs in these neurons when the eyes reach A, even though there is no longer a stimulus at B. In this paradigm, LIP appears to be concerned with a process of remapping the spatial frame-of-reference to guide the second saccade.

Using tasks such as these, many properties of cells in particular subregions of the parietal, temporal and frontal, both premotor and prefrontal, cortices have been established. Or to be more accurate, tasks were developed that activated in a fairly specific fashion a certain proportion of cells in particular subregions. Such tasks were also developed for many other structures, such as the hippocampus, amygdala and basal ganglia. However, just as in neuropsychology, the approach remained a craft. If a new task was developed, there was no method, other than the semi-intuitive skill of the investigator, to know what parts of cortex would be appropriate to investigate.

Cognitive neuropsychology too advanced on a wide front. First, the single-case study methodology became highly productive. It is striking, however, that the types of processes that were studied tended initially to be

very different from those investigated by single-cell recording. They reflected processes that were often noted by clinicians to be affected by cortical lesions in humans. Thus one of the first systems to be explored was the reading system, a type of system that is never, for obvious reasons, investigated using single-cell recording. Marshall and Newcombe's initial two-route approach—a product of the 1960s and early 1970s and referred to in Section 1.7—was developed in various ways. The critical subsystems involved, and in particular, the range of syndromes produced when particular subsystems were damaged, were worked out in the 1970s and early 1980s (see e.g. Coltheart, Patterson & Marshall, 1980; Patterson, Coltheart & Marshall, 1985). The types of model that were produced and how they map on to syndromes are illustrated in Figure 1.30 and Table 1.2. Analogous advances were made slightly later for the writing systems.[56]

The structure of many other systems too began to be uncovered by neuropsychological methods. For instance, following the early pioneering work of the Italian neurologist, Ennio De Renzi, and his collaborators discussed in Section 1.3, the different levels of

---

[56] For detailed discussion see FNMS Chapters 4 to 6. The reader will note that this figure follows the standard information-processing convention that inputs are from the top and outputs are from the bottom. This is opposite to the convention for connectionist models; see e.g. Figures 1.11 and 1.12. Geoff Hinton claims responsibility for the latter on the grounds of implementing bottom-up and top-down processing iconically.

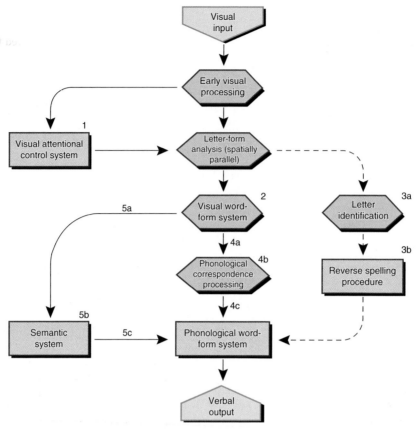

Fig. 1.30 A standard two-route model of the processes believed to be involved in reading of normal subjects (circa 1980s) based on figures of FNMS. Table 1.2 gives the correspondences to the putative functional locus of acquired dyslexic syndromes. The two normal reading routes are indicated by labels 4abc and 5abc. In addition the model contains a route (indicated by 3ab) which is held to be used when patients with damage to the visual word-form system read by the very slow and error prone compensatory strategy of explicitly identifying the individual letters of the word and using reversed spelling (see Warrington & Langdon, 2002) (shown in figure) or explicit visual combining (see Kay & Hanley, 1991) in order to read. It is available to normal adult readers but rarely used by them.

process involved in object recognition and how they can break down were established by neuropsychological methods in the 1970s (see e.g. Warrington & Taylor, 1978). This was followed by analogous work in the 1980s on face recognition (Bruce & Young, 1986; Ellis & Young, 1988).[57]

Or, to take another example, the 1970s and 1980s saw the isolation of systems involved in many different forms of memory. These included (i) episodic memory (i.e. autobiographical memory), (ii) semantic memory (knowledge), (iii) verbal short-term memory, (iv) visual short-term memory and (v) so-called priming, i.e. unconscious facilitation of a specific cognitive process. These forms of memory will be discussed extensively in Chapters 7 and 10. That these different systems could be separated was shown as early as the mid-1970s by the way they could be selectively impaired or selectively

spared in particular disorders, such as (i) amnesia, which selectively involves episodic memory, but not semantic memory (Kinsbourne & Wood, 1975) or priming (Warrington & Weiskrantz, 1968); (ii) 'semantic dementia', which complementarily impairs semantic but not episodic memory (Warrington, 1975); and two short-term memory syndromes, which do not involve episodic long-term memory or semantic memory: (iii) verbal (Warrington & Shallice, 1969) and (iv) visual (De Renzi & Nichelli, 1975).[58]

A key aspect of the success of the field has been the cross-talk between the information-processing models derived from human experimental psychology investigations and ones derived from neuropsychological studies. As discussed in Section 1.6, McCulloch and Pitts, and then Hebb, made the first metatheoretical link between the cognitive science and the neuroscience disciplines.

---

[57] See FNMS Chapter 8.

[58] See FNMS Chapters 3, 13 and 15 for extended accounts.

TABLE 1.2 Mapping of of dyslexia syndromes onto damaged components of a standard two-route reading model of the 1980s (Figure 1.30). For justification of the mappings see FNMS Chapters 4, 5 and 13. The final column gives sections where the syndrome is most discussed.

Peripheral Acquired Dyslexias:

Attentional Dyslexia	1	FNMS
Neglect Dyslexia	1 (but to one hemispace only)	FNMS
Visual Dyslexia	2 (without relative preservation of 3)	FNMS
Pure Alexia	2 (with relative preservation of 3)	4.12, 5.10

Central Acquired Dyslexias:

Deep Dyslexia	4 and partial 5	4.6, 4.11
Phonological Dyslexia	4 or 5 plus 4c	4.7, 4.9, 5.10
Surface dyslexia	5	4.6–4.9
Reading without semantics	5	4.6, 4.8, 4.9

However, the first major concrete linkage was provided by cognitive neuropsychology. One way the link was manifest was that experimental procedures that had been developed for use with normal subjects were now applied to patients. Striking dissociations were discovered. As a simple example, Figure 1.31 shows the performance of PV an 'auditory-verbal short-term memory patient', on the memory task of free recall of auditorily presented stimuli, which was discussed in Section 1.4 (Vallar & Papagno, 1986).[59] It can be seen that the recency effect, which was discussed in Section 1.4 with respect to normal subjects (see Figure 1.7), *and only that part of the serial position curve*, is selectively impaired in this patient for stimuli that are presented auditorily. This fits with many other findings that this group of patients have a selective impairment of the auditory-verbal short-term store or in the terminology of the later versions of the Baddeley and Hitch (1974) working memory model the 'input phonological buffer'.[60] Moreover, the complementary pattern is found in classical amnesia, the syndrome discussed in Section 1.3 (Baddeley & Warrington, 1970).

A second concrete way in which the disciplines became linked was that it began to be required that information-processing theories derived from either of the two empirical domains—human experimental psychology and neuropsychology—should explain the results of both. This meant they could be refuted by findings from either empirical domain. Current models of the reading system provide an excellent example of this. The link will be discussed in Chapter 4.

1.10 The Blossoming Disciplines: the Development of Imaging Procedures

Within the macro-neurosciences, progress has, however, been most dramatic using the new techniques of functional imaging (brain scanning). Functional imaging has its origins in electroencephalography, discussed in Section 1.2. However, the major advances came with the application of positron emission tomography (PET) to studying cognitive processes in the 1980s. This allowed processes to be localized much more effectively than was possible with EEG. PET became a viable technique with the work of Ter-Pogossian et al. (1975) and was first extensively applied to the study of cognitive processes by Ingvar, Roland and their co-workers in Scandinavia (e.g. Roland, Skinhøj & Lassen, 1981). This was followed 10 or so years later by the development in the USA of a technique with much greater spatial and temporal resolution, that of functional magnetic resonance (fMRI) by Ogawa, Lee, Kay and Tank (1990) and Kwong et al. (1992). This second technique only began to be applied widely in experimental investigations concerning functional localisation in the mid-1990s.

The success of functional imaging as a powerful empirical tool for cognitive neuroscience depended critically on two key methodological advances. One was the introduction of methodologies for isolating components involved in the task. This initially involved so-called 'subtraction' procedures and was developed by explicit analogy with methods used in information-processing psychology. Cognitive subtraction was an analogue of the chronometric methods for decomposing a task into stages, referred to briefly in Section 1.4. It was based on a procedure for decomposing response times originally proposed by Donders in the nineteenth century and much developed by Saul Sternberg at Bell Labs in the 1960s. This isolates the individual stages involved in the time to respond correctly to a stimulus. Indeed, one of the initial St. Louis team of innovators in functional imaging methodology was Mike Posner, who together with Saul Sternberg, had been the prime exponent of the chronometric approach in early modern human information-processing psychology (see Posner, 1978).

The basic idea that Donders had was to develop a general method for studying how long thought processes

---

[59] Related findings on other such patients had been obtained by Shallice and Warrington (1970) and Warrington, Logue and Pratt (1971).

[60] This syndrome will be discussed in more detail in Chapter 7. See also FNMS Chapter 3 and Vallar and Shallice (1990) for detailed discussions.

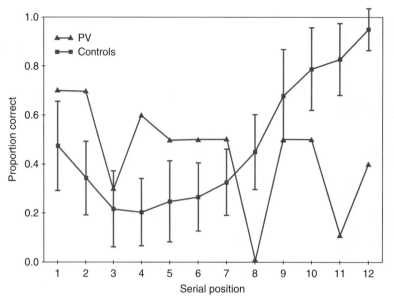

Fig. 1.31 Serial position curves for PV (red line) and control subjects (blue line with error bars). Lists consisted of 12 items presented auditorily. Control data is from 16 subjects matched to PV on age and education level. (See also Figure 1.7.) Redrawn from Brain and Cognition, 5(4), G. Vallar and C. Papagno, Phonological short-term store and the nature of the recency effect: Evidence from Neuropsychology, 428–442, Copyright 1986, with permission from Elsevier.

took. He assumed that the total time to respond was the sum of the time to complete each of a number of stages, which operated in series. He then compared two tasks, which appeared to require the same component processes except that one specific stage was required for one task but not for the other. For instance, if subjects must respond to one of two lights, then if only one light is illuminated the decision can be based on whichever one of the two comes on. Alternatively, if they both come on but in different colours, the decision can be based on the colour. Donders used the procedure of subtracting the first RT from the second to obtain an estimate of 50 msec to discriminate colours (see Sanders, 1998).

The study, which showed that, with the introduction of a more rigorous methodology, functional imaging could be turned into an effective method, was that of Petersen, Fox, Posner, Minton & Raichle (1988, 1989). In a somewhat analogous fashion to the history of cognitive neuropsychology, subtraction was first applied in functional imaging to the processes underlying reading and auditory word processing. This time, however, the study involved an investigation of the normal reading process, instead of how it malfunctions following neurological disease, as discussed in the previous section.

Subjects had five tasks. In the first they did nothing and their eyes were closed. In the second they again did nothing but their eyes were open. In the third they viewed nouns silently. In the fourth they read nouns aloud. In the fifth they had to generate a verb given a

corresponding noun, such as *eat* given *cake*. Using a Donders-type approach, the different processes involved in the task could be localised by subtracting the activation produced when task *n-1* was carried out from that when task *n* was done. Thus the activation produced in the naming nouns task minus that involved in the silent reading of nouns was held to correspond to the set of processes involved in name retrieval and production. The most famous contrast was probably that of verb generation minus reading or repeating, held to be involved in producing semantic associates and producing a localisation in the left anterior inferior frontal gyrus (see Figure 1.32).[61] This initial study was followed shortly later by isolation of regions of the human cortex critically involved in colour and movement processing (Lueck et al, 1989), in vigilance (Pardo, Fox & Raichle, 1991) and in willed action (Frith et al., 1991).

The dramatic success of these early studies led to a flood of further papers. However, the development of a real science depends upon a technique for producing results that are clearly reliable, so that proper replication becomes possible. The second breakthrough, which allowed this, again came from the developing of a method by analogy with ones used in the less exact sciences.

---

[61] The localisations for the functional anatomy of reading claimed in this paper are probably not completely correct; see e.g. Cohen et al, 2003, and Chapter 5 where problems with the subtraction method are also discussed.

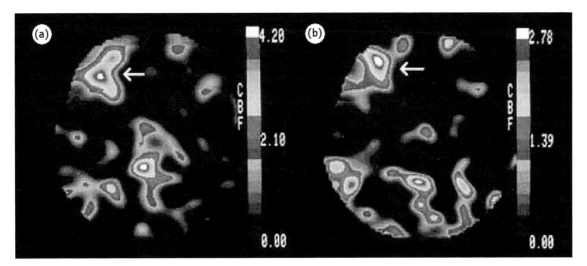

Fig. 1.32 Activation in the left inferior frontal gyrus arising when a verb had to be generated from a noun with that occurring from (a) repeating or (b) reading aloud a noun subtracted from it. Reprinted by permission from Macmillan Publishers Ltd: Nature (S.E. Petersen, P.E. Fox, M.I. Posner, M. Mintun and M.E. Raichle (1988) Positron emission tomographic studies of the cortical anatomy of single-word processing. Nature, 331, 585–589), copyright (1988).

This was the introduction of a highly sophisticated procedure for analysing functional imaging results—statistical parametric mapping (SPM) by Karl Friston and his colleagues (Friston, Frith, Frackowiak & Turner, 1995). This allowed the investigator to compare the activation produced by different but related tasks, and to distinguish probably real (i.e. statistically significant) effects from potentially random changes.[62] This meant that observed effects became clearly replicable. Thus the stream of results that were beginning to be produced with cognitive tasks by the use of PET methodology and later fMRI could become part of a proper scientific database.

1.11 The Current Situation: Social Aspects

We now have a many-faceted set of methods, both experimental and theoretical, for determining the nature of mind. We have four primarily empirical neuroscience-based methods concerned with (i) the use of single and multiple cellular recordings, (ii) the behavioural effects of lesions in animals, (iii) human neuropsychology and (iv) functional imaging. In addition there are four main relevant areas of cognitive science—with, overall, a more theoretical stance—(v) information-processing/human experimental psychology, (vi) neural network modelling, (vii) symbolic artificial intelligence

and (viii) linguistics. Some of these methods, particularly the more neuroscience-based ones, are developing very fast. Others are doing so rather more sedately, but all are advancing.

It might seem then that we have reached the stage in science where progress is incremental and straightforward: Kuhnian normal science. All that would appear to be required is 'micro-science' working on highly specific issues, such as, say, the operation of short-term memory or the functions of ventrolateral prefrontal cortex. Each such topic could be approached with the set of methods now known to be effective and which have been increasingly refined since the 1960s. This could also be done relatively independently of what else is known about other aspects/areas of the brain/mind. In the social organisation of the field, this would be reflected in the production of the specific paper and the textbook. General discursive analyses of the field, such as this, would be redundant.

However, the smooth trajectory of the field towards an advanced science is hindered by major intellectual and social obstacles. The intellectual obstacles are two-fold. One derives from the differing histories of the two sets of fields that comprise cognitive neuroscience. This has been a theme of this chapter and is also the subject of the next two chapters. The second is the weakness of the behavioural paradigms to produce results that convincingly select between different plausible theories, whether supported by brain-based evidence or not. This is especially the case in experimental paradigms where trials last more than a second or two.

The difficulties of intellectual interaction between the two approaches are deeply embedded in two somewhat

---

[62] Critically, the method took account of the way that change can potentially be detected at many different loci in the brain using statistical procedures related to so-called Bonferonni corrections. For more detailed discussion see Chapter 5.

overlapping social discontinuities that stem from the varied origins of the range of disciplines required. First, there is the division that occurs across science between theoreticians and experimentalists. This is more grave, in contrast to a field, say, like physics, as there have not been centuries of co-existence and mutual respect. This division is compounded by a second that relates to the different social origins and practices of modern cognitive science and modern neuroscience.

At the empirical level, an investigation in the cognitive sciences virtually always involves one person or at most a small team of two or three people, cheap technology and possibly a few well-selected patients or a patient population.[63] A single study can consist of a whole series of experiments or other type of investigations or analyses, each carried out to test theoretical inferences about the findings of previous ones. Also, each can be carried out fairly quickly, as the resources required are minimal and so the team is not so dependent on major grant support.

Neuroscience research, by contrast, is part of biomedical science. Most of the research recruits to the field come from a biomedical, not a cognitive science, background and know little of cognitive science. Moreover, parts of the biomedical sciences, in particular functional imaging and cellular neuroscience, are much closer to 'big science' in their social organization than are the cognitive sciences. The teams of researchers tend to be larger and need much technical support. Use of the equipment, for instance, in functional imaging, is highly expensive. Again, especially in functional imaging, the varieties of advanced technical expertise required means that collaborators are often drawn from different disciplines with each expert having a somewhat limited knowledge of the specialities of the other. The experiment is, therefore, of necessity more of a political act, in that it is more dependent on large-scale funding and negotiation between investigators than is cognitive science.[64] Also, in functional imaging, more than in cognitive science, publications in high-status journals are urgently needed to provide the intellectual seed corn to justify receiving sizeable research grants in the next round, and these are essential for research to proceed. As each experiment requires access to scarce and expensive resources there is normally neither time nor money to run a whole series of experiments, with each successive experiment dealing with

problems thrown up by the earlier ones, before a paper is submitted.

Thus in functional imaging one now frequently comes across studies where the experimental procedure has been developed *de novo* apparently without any attempt to link it with existing cognitive paradigms or cognitive theorising and where the patterns of activation resulting are 'explained' in an *ad hoc* fashion using everyday language concepts. High-status journals collude by facilitating publication of studies that can easily be described, so as to catch the lay public eye. This state of affairs has allowed the engineer turned psychologist Uttal (2001) to mount a scathing and plausible, but in our view essentially incorrect, attack on the interpretation of functional imaging results in terms of a set of mental *components* or *isolable systems* to employ the terminology used so far. Uttal supports his case by considering the cognitive concepts used in functional imaging. He lists explanatory cognitive concepts employed and domains of study in 22 imaging experiments to support the following claim: 'There are a large number of more or less inadequately defined mental components and activities that have been associated with particular regions of the brain by PET and MRI techniques and the list is growing rapidly. I contend that the recent wave of research using imaging techniques has led to proliferation of hypothetical psychological, cognitive or mental components without a proper foundation of clear-cut answers to the questions of accessibility and analysability.' He further argues, 'It is possible that we are being led astray from a true more valid and more realistic conceptualisation of the unified nature of mental processes based on widely distributed brain mechanisms.'

This book as a whole will, we trust, provide an answer to Uttal's basic critique and a riposte to his rejection of localisation-of-function. However, that the critique could have been produced at all by a competent scientist cannot just be attributed to the social structure of cognitive neuroscience. It stems as much from the way that cognitive scientists have failed to provide neuroscientists with appropriate conceptual tools to make the link to imaging studies. This is not, however, in our view because the concepts do not exist. Instead it is because each set of conceptual frameworks in cognitive science tend to be contested explicitly or implicitly by another set of theoreticians. This derives from the intellectual style of the cognitive sciences, contrasting as it does with that of the biomedical sciences. Much of cognitive science, such as the disciplines of linguistics, cognitive psychology and the more cognitive aspects of neuropsychology too, have an internal style that has echoes of the philosophical origins of the issues it addresses. The theoreticians frequently indulge in major gladiatorial combat over frameworks, as in the

---

[63] For the sociological aspects certain parts of neuropsychology, in particular much of cognitive neuropsychology, is better considered within the cognitive science domain than within the biomedical domain.

[64] This social division is not all-or-none. Thus traditionally, systems neuroscience was a small science area, although it is less so now.

battles connectionists and symbolic theorists have fought over implicitly agreed terrain (to be discussed in Chapter 3), such as models of how the past tense is produced in language (see Section 8.7). There is a love of polemic, which frequently verges on the deliberately arcane. Neither side in a polemic is willing to allow any validity to the ideas of the other. So the theoreticians do not bother to consolidate. This means that, overall, the field gives the impression to outsiders that it has no solid substance. In particular, it fails to provide a clear set of concepts to which someone trained as a neuroscientist can relate. Instead, cognitive science theoreticians have articulated a mass of concepts, many of which are held to be in conflict as explanations of mental processes with another group of concepts.

To take one example, information-processing models or *box-and-arrow* models based on the *isolable systems* approach are often seen in the field as *passé*. They are not considered 'wrong' but they are ignored. To the more neuroscience-orientated cognitive scientist they are forgotten in favour of direct explanation in terms of neurophysiology. By the more computer-science orientated they are disdained for connectionist models. By those orientated towards linguistic theory they are vague performance-related notions, not relevant for understanding the interesting processing structures involved in language.

In their adoption of these types of confrontational and dismissive attitudes, cognitive scientists forget the utility of multiple models with different grains and different functions within the same domain. This unwillingness of cognitive scientists to consolidate has contributed greatly to the relative neglect by neuroscientists of the products of cognitive science research. As critically, the different social styles of the two domains exacerbate the intellectual divisions that exist.

In the next two chapters, however, we will argue that, intellectually, a strong link between the two types of discipline is essential if we are to understand cognition, but that the relation between the two is necessarily complex. Within this setting, the sociological divisions we have discussed make the intellectual problems more difficult to confront. For only one pair of subdisciplines have the interrelations been worked out fairly well, that of human neuropsychology and information-processing cognitive psychology (see, e.g. Caramazza, 1986; Shallice, 1988). In most other cases, transfer of information between the fields exists. However it is done intuitively, not within an overall theoretical framework. This book aims to provide an introduction to the basic conceptual structures required.

Why *Cognitive* Neuroscience?

2.1 Introduction: the Reductionist Approach

At the end of the last chapter we discussed the sociological differences between research in neuroscience and that in cognitive science, and the difficulties this created for relating brain-related evidence to cognitive-level theorising. But maybe this is all unnecessary. In the 1980s, Patricia Churchland, a philosopher-of-science very knowledgeable about neuroscience (see e.g. Churchland & Sejnowski, 1992), argued that the concepts we currently have at the cognitive level, are essentially pre-scientific and compared them to phlogiston (Churchland, 1986). She was referring, very explicitly, to the everyday concepts we apply to mind—*belief*, *desire*, *hear*, etc.—but also argued that it was 'boneheaded' (p. 373) to treat the concepts of information-processing psychology and linguistics autonomously and as if separated from any neuroscientific basis. Should one, then, just not bother with the current concepts of cognitive science and build new and better ones from a neuroscience base?

From the opposite perspective it has been argued by the philosopher-of-mind, Jerry Fodor, that information derived from brain-based investigations has so far told us little of importance of how the mind functions and, by implication, was unlikely to be informative in the future.[1] An inference from both these arguments is

---

[1] This line of argument is presented informally in the *London Review of Books*, where Fodor (1999) recalls a post-talk dinner at which a group of 'neuroscientists' were unable to explain to

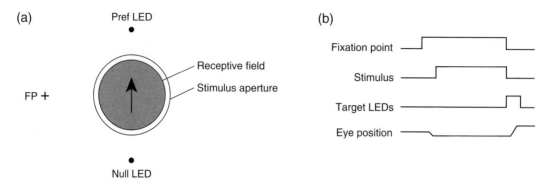

Fig. 2.1 The psychophysical paradigm of Britten et al (1992). (a) The spatial layout of the task. FP is the fixation point. Once the monkey established fixation, a moving random dot pattern appeared in the stimulus aperture. (The arrow indicates the direction of movement for this trial.) After 2 secs the stimulus was removed and two LEDs, corresponding to two possible directions of motion, appeared. The monkey was required to indicate the direction of perceived movement by making a saccade in the direction of the appropriate LED. (b) The temporal sequence of events during a trial. Redrawn with permission from K.H. Britten, M.N. Shadlen, W.T. Newsome and J.A. Movshon, 1992, The analysis of visual motion: A comparison of neuronal and psychophysical performance. The Journal of Neuroscience, 12(12), 4745–4765. Figure 2, p 4748.

that the attempt to link brain-based experimental findings with the theoretical frameworks of cognitive science is pointless.

Consider first the reductionist perspective, which essentially eliminates as irrelevant current cognitive science ideas. How might it work? Consider a beautiful example from Movshon and Newcombe and their colleagues on the systems underlying movement perception. The key initial step in this field was a discovery made on monkey vision in the period following Hubel and Wiesel's breakthrough. As mentioned in Section 1.9, Dubner and Zeki (1971) found that in MT/V5, an area in the posterior part of the superior temporal sulcus, neurons showed great sensitivity to movement (see also Zeki, 1974). About 90% of the cells responded strongly to one direction of movement through the cell's receptive field—their preferred direction—and much less, or not at all, to movement in the opposite direction.

Ten years later, a syndrome was discovered in humans in which the patient becomes insensitive to moving stimuli. The first patient described with this disorder (LM) had a threshold duration for detecting movement (999 msec) four times longer than that of control subjects (275 msec) and yet had completely normal performance on, say, colour or shape discriminations (Zihl et al., 1983). These psychophysical results corresponded to her perceptual experiences. LM said that when she poured coffee into a cup, the fluid appeared frozen 'like a glacier' (p. 315). If a lesion is made in MT/V5, monkeys

too have an impairment in detecting movement (e.g. Newsome & Paré, 1988; Marcar & Cowey, 1992).

In a series of experiments, Movshon, Newsome and their colleagues followed up these findings by a much more complex study. They correlated the firing patterns of many neurons in MT/V5 with the results of psychological experiments with the monkeys—one for each neuron. For a particular neuron, the psychological experiment required the monkey to detect whether there was a stimulus moving in the preferred direction of the neuron. When the stimulus is presented in the receptive field of the neuron, the activity of the neuron is measured (e.g. Britten et al., 1992) (see Figure 2.1). The team was able to develop a computational model (see Figure 2.2) in which the behavioural response of the monkey corresponded well to the pooled activity of at least 50–100 neurons (with the same preferred direction) in MT/V5. The output of the units standing for V5 neurons is fed to a 'central decision mechanism' (Shadlen et al., 1996). This applies *signal detection theory*, a procedure used in psychophysics (Green & Swets, 1966). In a physical system, detection depends upon the signal being discriminable from intrinsic noise of the system on some dimension. So in signal detection theory, noise sampled from a normal distribution is assumed to be added to the signal: the decision is made as to whether the signal (plus noise) has occurred against the alternative of another sample of noise alone. To do this a criterion is set and whether the observed value on the dimension is greater than the criterion is checked. In Shadlen et al.'s model, the dimension reflected the summed output of MT/V5 units.[2]

him why investigations of brain processes could tell us anything interesting about the mind. One of us was one of those enjoying the food and the argument. This book is in part stimulated by, and a response to, Fodor's sceptical line of argument.

---

[2] Computational models of movement detection have developed considerably further than this simple model (see, e.g. Rust

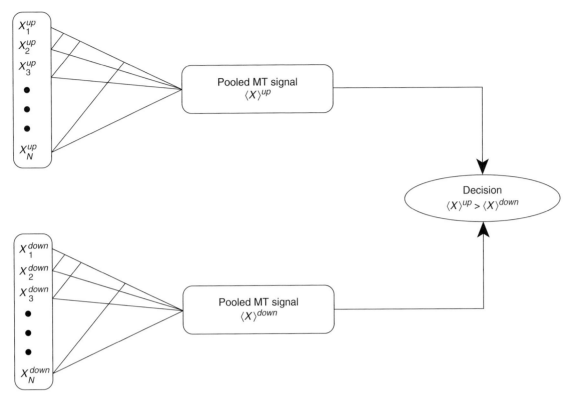

Fig. 2.2 The model of Shadlen et al (1996). Psychophysical judgments were modelled as the comparison of two signals, one being based on the average response of neurons preferring the up motion and the other from the average response of neurons preferring the down motion. Redrawn with permission from M.N. Shadlen, K.H. Britten, W.T. Newsome and J.A. Movshon, 1996, A computational basis of the relationship between neuronal and behavioral responses to visual motion. The Journal of Neuroscience, 16(4), 1486–1510. Figure 2, p 1489.

Consider schematically how the cognitive neuroscience of movement perception might be viewed as developing. It starts with initial observations of empirical correspondences between aspects of stimuli being presented to an animal—say dots moving in a particular direction—and neuronal activity in the animal's brain. Then there are more detailed investigations of the properties of individual neurons in relation to the characteristics of the stimuli. Finally, a model is produced of the relationship between the neural activity and behaviour. The stimuli in the experiments represent a very simple physical property of the environment. The behaviour of each neuron is assumed just to represent this property. The behaviour of neurons is weakly correlated prior to pooling, but all are held to be qualitatively equivalent.

The other parts of the history of work on the topic can be considered less important. More detailed characterisation of the function of the system by behavioural studies and work on the effects of lesions in humans or functional imaging studies were essentially of only

secondary relevance to its development. The main line of research could proceed apparently independently of more complex characterisations of the function of the region, or of any analysis of human behaviour; neither, for instance, played any role in the development of Shadlen et al.'s computational model.

One could abstractly characterise the stages in the investigation as follows:

(1a) Find a task (or tasks) that activates a particular region of the brain well; it is not important how this occurs.

(1b) Carry out detailed studies on the microanatomy of the region.

(2) Examine how the cells in the region are activated by the task (or tasks).

(3) Build a computational model of how the cells are functioning in the task (or tasks).

(4) Modify (1a) and do further studies of type (1b) and (2) to test the model. If they do not fit, return to stage (3).

The reductionist programme outlined above may not even depend on any concept of the function of region V5. Without any such conception, one can treat

et al., 2006). In addition, motion perception involves other areas as well as MT/V5 (Giese & Poggio, 2003).

the paired observations of stimulus presentations and neuron firings as given and build a model like that of Shadlen et al. to explain them. However that ignores the problem of selecting the tasks and inputs with which to test a region and, more particularly, how one can be confident that the sets of tasks and inputs so far used are a sufficient set to characterise the operation of the region adequately. Moreover, it ignores the motivation for the model. In this case, the way that particular stimuli were used to investigate the region by Movshon, Newcombe and their collaborators occurred historically in a situation where the probable function of the region was clear, following the early work of Semir Zeki and his collaborators. More generally, a set of neurons with multiple inputs and outputs could, on a connectionist approach, be conceived to be subject to many learning processes and not be characterisable by any simple function.

Even ignoring this last possibility, can one assume that the ascription of a function to a region is typically a fairly straightforward early step in the research process? Thus, before Hubel and Wiesel's breakthrough it was very difficult to conceive that a cortical cell might code for a property of the stimulus like movement (see Hubel's Nobel address quoted by Nicholls et al., 2001, p. 410). After their work, it became easier to believe that a cortical region might code for a particular dimension of the stimulus, and to use relevant stimuli for experimental investigations. The later work, though, depended on Zeki's earlier functional characterisation of V5 to know that the tasks and range of stimuli used were appropriate. More critically, no biologist would find it surprising that a highly developed organism contained a system specifically sensitive to moving stimuli and its environment (see e.g. Lettvin et al., 1959). The idea that regions of the brain have functions and that the function of region MT/V5 is that of detecting and characterising moving stimuli hardly rests on any cognitive science concepts.

An investigation of this type can be seen as basically a bottom-up or reductionist research programme. Is it likely to be effective for investigating all forms of mental process? Clearly, for some processes in humans—but we do not know how many—there is no correspondence in animals. Thus, with the exception of the possibility of work with patients who have had certain types of operation for epilepsy (see e.g. Quiroga et al., 2005), single-cell recording cannot be carried out. But maybe an analogous procedure could use fMRI or that plus EEG or MEG.[3]

2.2 A Reductionist Program for Investigating More Central Processes?: the Case of the Hippocampus

The approach sketched above is implicitly localisationist. It depends upon the concept of a brain region. The first requirement for the approach to work in an analogous fashion in more central systems must then be that there are higher-level subsystems that are as specific in their localisation as regions like V5. Empirically, if one assumes that the prefrontal cortex is the seat of the cortical processes furthest from the perceptual input and so most protypically central, and one looks at how it is activated in high-level cognitive tasks, then disconcertingly specific activation sites are indeed seen. Take, for example, a study by Paul Burgess, Angela Quayle and Chris Frith (2001) on holding an intention on-line, while carrying out another task. The study requires that at any time later, if a particular type of stimulus occurs, the subject must return and complete the primary task. The relevant process—maintaining an intention in an active state—is about as far from an input process as one could reasonably hope to investigate, given that the key processes in such cognitive activities as composing sonnets still remain rather difficult to capture experimentally! Again, however, for the process of retaining an intention active, we have regions activated that appear to be of the same sort of anatomical specificity as the human equivalent of V5 (see Figure 2.3).

One could raise many technical objections to this type of comparison of size between regions isolated in different functional imaging studies. However, for holding and realising intentions, just as for work on movement perception, neuropsychological investigations—including both ones using single case designs and ones using group-study methodology—also fit with the assumption that an automatically relatively specific high-level subsystem can be damaged selectively (see Shallice & Burgess, 1991; Burgess et al., 2000). Moreover, the idea that the setting up or realising of intentions is dependent on such a subsystem is also compatible with the specific difficulties these patients have. Thus, evidence from both functional imaging and neuropsychology points to the idea that there is a specific system in anterior medial prefrontal cortex that is involved in the regulation of intentions.[4]

---

[3] Magnetoencephalography (MEG), pioneered by Cohen (1972), is an imaging technique that measures magnetic fields produced by the same electrical activity that is measured in EEG.

Because of the mechanisms underlying the electrical aspects of neural activity and differences in the properties of electrical and magnetic fields, MEG is more sensitive than EEG to cortical activity from structures relatively near to the skull.

[4] The methodology of this study will be discussed in Chapter 5 and the cognitive aspects in Chapter 9.

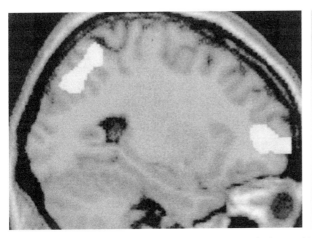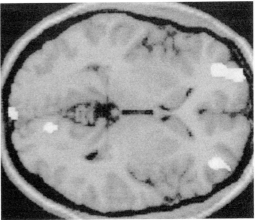

Fig. 2.3 Regions activated in the study of P. Burgess et al (2001) when a subject, in addition to an on-line task, maintains an intention but does not have to realise it. The regions include right parietal and bilateral frontopolar cortices (given in so-called sagittal and axial views of the activated region). Reprinted from Neuropsychologia, 39(6), P.W. Burgess, A. Quayle and C.D. Frith, Brain regions involved in prospective memory as determined by positron emission tomography, 545–555, Copyright (2001), with permission from Elsevier.

The existence of specific high-level systems does not, though, mean that a reductionist programme like that used in the research programme on movement perception would work in the same way for more complex processes. When one examines the investigation and analysis of central systems more directly, it is soon apparent that there are many difficult problems in the attempt to transfer directly to more central systems, the approach so successful in movement perception.

That specifying the processes being investigated at a rough functional level, as in the 'regulation of intentions' example just considered, is an absolutely key step in cognitive neuroscience research on complex processing, and moreover not one that is simply carried out in one brief initial historical step, will be a major theme of the book.[5] It can be illustrated by the example of work on the hippocampus, where the critical work on the functions of the structure were the results of brilliant serendipitous observations. However, there was not one such set of observations but two, and each pointed to a different function.

The hippocampus receives input from virtually all parts of cortex through relays, principally first in the perirhinal and parahippocampal cortices, and then the entorhinal cortex and, in return, again through the entorhinal cortex, it projects back to the cortex (see Figure 2.4). It became a widely studied structure as a result of the observations of Milner and Scoville, discussed in Section 1.3, that selective severe amnesia could occur following lesions to it and related structures. This condition had resulted as a devastating

unanticipated side-effect of operations for reducing the frequency of intractable epileptic seizures. Large bilateral lesions of the medial temporal lobe had been made in the patient's brain to remove epileptic foci and so lessen the incidence of seizures. The hippocampus, as it lies on the medial surface of the temporal lobes, was also removed and was held to be the principal structure which when damaged produced an amnesic state.

For the present, assume that sceptics, such as Gaffan (2002), about the role of the hippocampus in memory are greater in number and in influence than they actually are. Also travel back to the late 1960s. Stimulated by Milner's work, a former McGill student, John O'Keefe, was investigating a possible role for the hippocampus in memory. His team made a most surprising finding. This was the serendipitous discovery of so-called *place cells* in the hippocampus of the rat (O'Keefe & Dostrovsky, 1971; O'Keefe, 1979). These are cells that respond when the animal is in a particular place in a known environment (see Section 1.2). From these and similar observations, O'Keefe and Lynn Nadel (1978) put forward the theory that the hippocampus acts as a *cognitive map*, which enables the animal to find its way around in familiar surroundings. The utility of the notion that the hippocampus holds a representation of the known environment of the animal was strongly supported by the invention of the so-called Morris water-maze (Morris, 1984). In this procedure, the rat is placed in a circular pool from which it cannot escape. There is, however, a hidden platform. A normal rat will rapidly learn where the platform is, even though it cannot be seen, and when placed again in the maze will swim immediately to its position. A lesion to the hippocampus makes learning of the location by the rat extremely slow.

---

[5] There is no requirement that this specification should be able to be made in everyday language, as has been done for MT/V5.

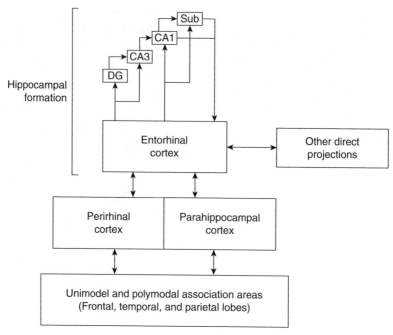

Fig. 2.4 Connectivity of the hippocampal formation (consisting of the entorhinal cortex and the hippocampus proper - the dentate gyrus, CA3, CA1 and subiculum) and its connections to the medial temporal cortex. Redrawn with permission from L.R. Squire and S.M. Zola, 1996, Structure and function of declarative and nondeclarative memory systems, Proceedings of the National Academy of Sciences of the United States of America, 93(24), 13515–13522. Figure 7, p. 13518. Copyright (1996) National Academy of Sciences, U.S.A.

Moreover, as in the outline of a reductionist approach to cognitive neuroscience discussed earlier, an effective computational model has been developed to explain the way the cells behave in different environments. Input to the hippocampus from the cortex is funnelled through the entorhinal cortex from which it passes to the dentate granule cells, then to the so-called CA3 pyramidal cells and to CA1 cells and then to the subiculum, from where there are outputs back to entorhinal cortex, as well as to other parts of cortex and subcortical structures (e.g. via a fibre tract called the fornix). Figure 2.5 shows both the global anatomy and internal structure. On the Neil Burgess–John O'Keefe model (1996) (see Figure 2.6), the critical CA3 and CA1 regions, which are the locus of the place cells, are functionally conflated. Each place cell receives input from a large number of so-called *boundary vector cells* (Hartley et al., 2000), which each respond maximally to the animal's distance from a perceptual boundary in the environment. The firing rate of the place cells is proportional to the amount by which a simple sum of the inputs it receives from the boundary vector cells is greater than a threshold. The model is a simple feed-forward system.[6] It gives a good account of empirical properties of the fields of place cells and how they are altered by clever experiments that restructure, in a systematic

way, the animal's learned environment. Thus when the rat is trained in an environment of a given shape, say a square, and the shape is changed by moving the borders of the enclosure, the places where particular cells respond are necessarily changed. The most interesting changes are where the place fields actually split into two. The model fits well with the characteristics of the cells (see Figure 2.7).[7]

The parts of the model can also be treated as elements in a more complex overall model of how the rat moves in the environment (see Figure 2.8). In the more complex model, the roles of particular areas of the hippocampus and a number of areas of cortex are specified (see Byrne, Becker & Burgess, 2007). These proposals fit with properties of cells in other systems.

That the hippocampus of the rat is actually involved in enabling the animal to find its way around a familiar environment has been amply supported by later findings. Thus, if the animal is to use visual cues to work out where it is and to 'navigate' from there to its eventual goal, it is vital to know in what direction it is looking. This is achieved by so-called *head direction* cells, which only fire when the animal's head is pointed in a certain direction and which are remarkably independent

---

[6] Certain levels include competitive learning.

[7] Many other models also adopt cognitive map functions for the hippocampus (e.g. Zipser, 1985; Sharp, 1991; Redish & Touretsky, 1998; Hartley et al., 2000).

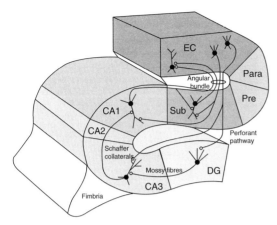

Fig. 2.5 Anatomy of the hippocampus. From D. Amarel and P. Lavenex, 2007, Hippocampal neuroanatomy. In P. Andersen, R. Morris, D. Amaral, T. Bliss and J. O'Keefe (eds.), The Hippocampus Book. Oxford University Press. Figure 3.1, p 38. Reprinted by permission of Oxford University Press, Inc.

frame of reference that is body-centred (egocentric) to one that is independent of the particular orientation of the animal in the environment (allocentric). Moreover, yet another type of cell that fits with the model has recently been found in entorhinal cortex. These are the boundary vector cells of Hartley et al. (2000). They fire when the animal is close to the borders of the environment (Solstad et al., 2008).

Thus one seems to have an example of the ascription of a function to a region—the hippocampus—which occurred early in the history of the investigation of the structures, which then guided the research aimed at understanding the behaviour of its neurons and, as we will discuss, aimed at relating their behaviour to a computational model. The history of research on the hippocampus seems to fit the reductionist approach of cognitive neuroscience as well as that on movement perception did. The tasks used were derived initially from the ascribed function but later were derived by extrapolation from the computational model.

However, there is one complication in this account. The hippocampus became a fashionable structure to investigate with Milner's work, not because of its role in navigation but because it was held to have another function—that of being the source of autobiographical memory.

of the animal's actual position (Taube et al., 1990); in different positions in the environment the preferred directions for such a cell are parallel; they are not simply converging on a distant salient stimulus. Their role in the model is to support the transformation between a

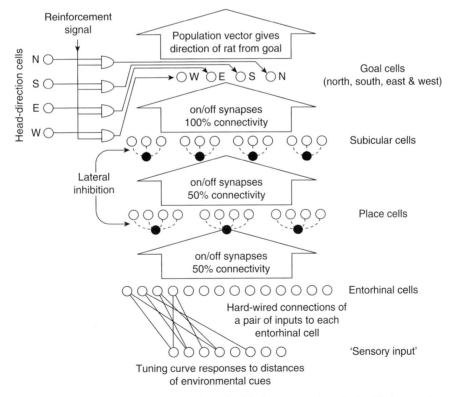

Fig. 2.6 The population vector model of Burgess et al (1994) of the role of the hippocampus in navigation. The input to the network is the position of the rat relative to the cues in the environment. The network's output specifies the direction the rat should move to reach the goal. Redrawn from Neural Networks, 7(6–7), N. Burgess, M. Recce and J. O'Keefe, A model of hippocampal function, 1065–1081, Copyright (1994), with permission from Elsevier.

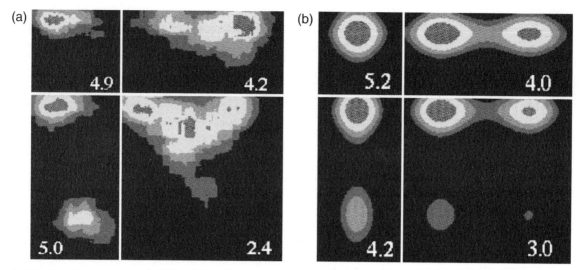

Fig. 2.7 Firing rates of a hippocampal place cell from (a) CA1 and (b) an equivalent cell in the model of O'Keefe and Burgess (1996). The rat was placed in a rectangular o square enclosure and allowed to explore while firing activity was recorded. The geometry of the box was then changed to one of the other three rectangles as discussed in the text. The figure in the lower corner of each cell indicates the peak firing rate in Hertz. See also Figure 1.2. Adapted by permission from Macmillan Publishers Ltd: Nature (J. O'Keefe and N. Burgess (1996) Geometric determinants of the place fields of hippocampal neurons. Nature, 381, 425–428), copyright (1996).

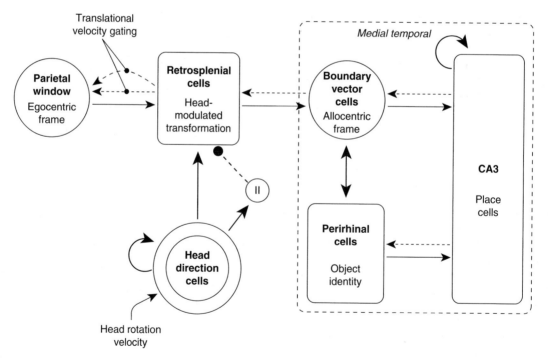

Fig. 2.8 The rat navigation model of Byrne et al (2007), which includes the components of the population vector model (Figure 2.6). Perirhinal cells respond to known landmarks. Place cells encode location within a Cartesian grid. Boundary vector cells encode landmark locations on a polar grid in allocentric space (i.e. environmental organised), while cells in parietal window encode landmark locations in egocentric space (i.e. relative to the subject). Transformation between the two is achieved by the retrosplenial transformation layer. Head direction cells encode the direction of the head. II are inhibitory interneurons. Copyright © 2007 by the American Psychological Association. Adapted with permission. P. Byrne, S. Becker and N. Burgess (2007) Remembering the past and imagining the future: A neural model of spatial memory and imagery, Psychological Review, 114(2), 340–375. The use of APA information does not imply endorsement by APA.

And that supposed function did not die in 1971 with the discovery of place cells. Instead it also led to a rich line of research. The lesions created by Scoville were very large and so many have since argued that the hippocampus was not the critical structure that when removed led to amnesia occurring (see e.g. Horel, 1978; Gaffan, 2002). That the hippocampus was the critical structure in producing the devastating memory impairments observed following the early experiments into epilepsy by Scoville was, however, suggested by behavioural experiments carried out somewhat later by Milner and her colleagues in groups of epileptic patients. In order to reduce their seizures, the patients had had parts of the temporal lobe in one hemisphere removed in operations that were more conservative than Scoville's earlier ones. The patients were tested on a variety of tasks involving memory, such as the retention of a short story over a 40-minute period and maze learning (see Milner & Teuber, 1968). Deficits were much more severe when the hippocampus was involved.

As an example, one of Milner's students, Corsi (1972) (reported in Hécaen & Albert, 1978) used two verbal and two non-verbal memory tasks and compared four groups of patients with lobectomies of the left temporal lobe and four with analogous right temporal lobectomies. For each hemisphere, the four groups differed in whether the hippocampus was lesioned and, if so, by how much. In all the memory tasks, the deficit was proportional to the degree of hippocampal removal.[8]

About the same time in 1972, the Canadian psychologist Endel Tulving, working with Wayne Donaldson, put forward the concept of an *episodic memory* to characterise a system which they held to underlie our everyday life experiences of the retrieval of autobiographical memories. They contrasted episodic memory with *semantic memory*, the systems underlying knowledge. Semantic memory itself was a concept that the AI theorist Ross Quillian (1968) had just begun to investigate within computer science. After the idea of episodic memory was introduced to clinical neuropsychological research by Kinsbourne and Wood (1975), it became a standard view that the hippocampus was critically involved in some aspect of the episodic memory system and that lesions to it thereby give rise to organic amnesia. This view remains a standard one in human neuropsychological research, see e.g. Nadal and Moscovitch (1997), although some authors consider that, with respect to memory, the hippocampus is part of a more extensive system also involving medial temporal cortex which acts as an undifferentiated whole (e.g. Squire & Zola, 1996).[9]

Even earlier than for the navigation account, what was essentially the episodic-memory approach to hippocampal functions led to the development of a computational model, in this case by the Cambridge theoretician, David Marr (1971). In Marr's model, the cerebral cortex stores much of what would now be known as episodic memory. However, he conjectured that representations of events in the cortex would be somewhat limited, as he held the cortex to be essentially built to retain categorical information, i.e. semantic memory, as we would now call it. Marr therefore postulated an additional system. He assumed that the different aspects of an event would be coded as different elements (in different groups of neurons). These, he believed, would be rapidly associated with each other in the hippocampus. The model used the neuroanatomy of the hippocampus as a guide and employed *Hebbian learning*, discussed in Section 1.6, and orthogonal coding of input dimensions.[10] The model remained virtually unique until the late 1980s. Since then many related models, based on the idea that the hippocampus supports episodic memory, have been developed (e.g. Gluck & Myers, 1993; McClelland et al., 1995; Alvarez & Squire, 1994; Meeter & Murre, 2005).

Some of the memory models (e.g. that of Gluck & Myers) are not greatly concerned with the details of the anatomy and physiology of the hippocampus. For the current argument we will take the memory model of Treves and Rolls (1992, 1994) and compare it to the Burgess–O'Keefe cognitive map model that we discussed earlier with respect to how they characterise the processing being carried out by particular types of cells in the hippocampus.

Treves and Rolls took a different tack for their modelling than did Neil Burgess and his collaborators. Instead of trying to fit detailed empirical results of particular behavioural experiments, they were concerned with how the detailed microanatomy of the hippocampus and its connections to the cortex could affect storage and retrieval of episodic memories. Thus they argue that the CA3 and CA1 regions have somewhat different functions and, moreover, that the relation between them is held to be represented by attractor networks in the Hopfield sense, as discussed in Section 1.7, rather than by simple feed-forward systems. An episodic memory, of say, this moment in your life, could contain many elements, sights and sounds from your current surroundings, your comprehension of the meaning of this sentence, your approval or otherwise of the

---

[8] For similar later findings see Kilpatrick et al. (1997).

[9] The term *declarative* memory is often used to cover both episodic and semantic memory. Its use though lessens the clarity

with which hippocampal functions can be discussed; see Chapter 10 for further discussion.

[10] It also used inhibitory normalisation to avoid the kindling phenomena to which a purely Hebbian mechanism is subject.

argument it carries, other thoughts about this book, your thoughts about the coming evening and so on. CA3 cells are seen by Treves and Rolls as holding representations of such elements of episodic memories. Each attractor basin comprises the representation of each single, full episodic memory. It is formed by the pattern of activity of the CA1 cells, which are receiving input from the CA3 cells, which in turn are coding the elements.

The theory also provides an account of other aspects of the anatomy that do not figure prominently in the Burgess–O'Keefe theory. Thus the CA3 cells receive two sets of input—one from dentate granule cells involving the so-called mossy fibres and another that by-passes them, coming direct from the entorhinal cortex (see Figure 2.4). It is shown in simulations that if CA3 cells receive only this second input, then learning would not occur. The mossy fibres are viewed by Treves and Rolls as a 'sort of unsupervised teacher' that strongly influences which CA3 neurons can fire. Moreover, it is held that this pathway has the properties necessary to carry the signals that switch the hippocampus from encoding into initiating recall. Thus Treves and Rolls predicted that the direct pathway on to the CA3 neurons should be associatively modifiable, and indeed this has been found to be the case (Berger et al., 1996). Moreover, if the dentate gyrus inputs are eliminated, learning is impaired (Lassalle et al., 2000; Lee & Kesner, 2004).

Finally, Treves and Rolls argue that the difference in number between hippocampal pyramidal cells and neocortical cells is such that monosynaptic mapping of the CA3 cells onto the neocortex could not work for capacity reasons. Instead they argue that a series of unpackings of the memory trace through intermediary systems is necessary before the cortex is reached. And indeed the subiculum, the entorhinal cortex and the parahippocampal/perirhinal cortex provide these intermediary representations.

The Burgess–O'Keefe and Treves–Rolls models appear to be unrelated. One is concerned with giving an explanation of the empirical properties of CA1 and CA3 cells in certain experiments, the other with justifying the details of the microanatomy and by capacity constraints. The models are each completely dependent on the functions they are trying to simulate.[11] Yet they are functional models of the same set of neurons—the CA3 and CA1 pyramidal neurons—in the same structure, the hippocampus.

There are then two different conceptions of the function of the hippocampus. One is that it is the seat of the knowledge an animal uses to find its way around in a familiar environment. The other is that it is critical for episodic memory, the system required for our experience of remembering past events. The former was an extrapolation from the behaviour of hippocampal cells in the context of the geography of the animal's immediate environment. The latter characterisation, which admittedly is the more disputed one, arises from neuropsychology and from a conceptual framework derived from cognitive psychology. What is striking about these characterisations of the function of the hippocampus is that they are still—over forty years later—spawning computational models of hippocampal function, which are held to be rooted in the anatomy and physiology of the hippocampus and also acting as conceptual frameworks to guide empirical investigations.

How are the two perspectives to be reconciled? First, it is still just about possible that the hippocampus only realises one of these functions; that the apparent properties of the hippocampus, which lead to one of the claimed functions, produce a conceptual illusion. This could have been because a property apparently concerned with space was actually just a manifestation of memory. This possibility was made implausible by the discovery of head-direction cells. It was made virtually inconceivable by a more recent and dramatic discovery of a completely unexpected type of cell that has been found in the entorhinal cortex. These are the so-called *grid cells* (Hafting et al., 2005). They respond when the animal is in one of a number of positions on a hexagonal grid in the environment (see Figure 2.9).[12] Moreover, as one passes through the entorhinal cortex in the ventral direction, the size of the grid increases. It appears that hippocampus place cells can be seen as the sum of the effects of grids of all the different grains superimposed on the place field site, in a rather Fourier-like arrangement (see Solstad et al., 2006). While direct recording of grid cells in human entorhinal cortex has—for obvious reasons—not yet been carried out, recent elegant fMRI experiments have shown that the human entorhinal cortex appears to have the properties one would expect if it too contained grid cells (Doeller et al., 2010).

The discovery of grid cells makes virtually certain the assumption that place fields really do functionally represent environmental places and are not some complex epiphenomenon of the task and some different function of the hippocampus CA1 and CA3 cells. We are clearly dealing with an integrated spatial navigation system.

---

[11] Computationally, the Burgess–O'Keefe model initially used feed-forward nets, the other is built on attractors. However, later versions of the Burgess–O'Keefe model, e.g. N. Burgess et al. (2001), also use attractors.

[12] This is true for a roughly square field; it is not, though, for instance, if the environment is made into a tortuously maze-like structure (see Sargolini et al., 2006).

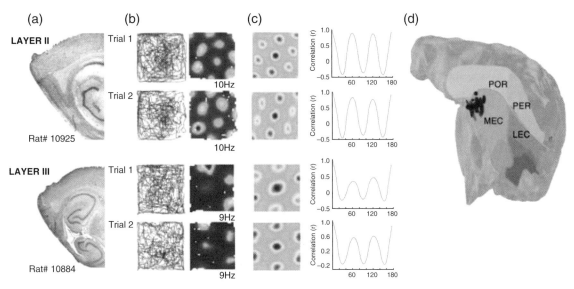

Fig. 2.9 Grid cells in rat medial entorhinal cortex (MEC). (a) Sections of layers II and III of the cortex, showing recording sites (red dots). (b) Trajectory of moving rat plus colour-coded locations of where spikes occurred (left) and firing fields of representative grid cells from the locations in (a) (right). (c) Autocorrelation map and periodicity over space for the rate maps from (b). (d) The region of the medial temporal lobe in which recordings were made. (LEC=Lateral Entorhinal Cortex; PER=Perirhinal Cortex; POR=Postrhinal Cortex). From F. Sargolini, M. Fyhn, T. Hafting, B.L. McNaughton, M.P. Witter, M.-B. Moser, E.I. Moser, 2006, Conjunctive representation of position, direction, and velocity in entorhinal cortex, Science, 312(5774), 758–762. Reprinted with permission from AAAS.

The alternative 'function artefact' possibility is that the apparent episodic memory properties of the hippocampus may derive from regions of temporal cortex other than the hippocampus. Yet hippocampal rats are held to show impairments of non-spatial memory, such as learning a sequence of odours (Kesner et al., 2002). And even such a strong advocate of the 'spatial' position as O'Keefe (2007) accepts that non-spatial information is held in the hippocampus, although he argues that proportionally fewer cells are involved than for spatial processing. Moreover, ascribing episodic memory as a function of the hippocampus explains many related phenomena. For instance, cholinergic input to the hippocampus from a structure, the basal forebrain, lying beneath the prefrontal cortex, appears to have a memory-control function; presence or absence of cholinergic input seems to switch hippocampal operation from a memory-encoding to a memory-retrieval mode (Hasselmo & Wyble, 1997).[13] Most critically, patients with selective problems in episodic memory and lesions apparently restricted to the hippocampus have been described (see e.g. Warrington & Duchen, 1992; Kartsounis, Rudge & Stevens, 1995; Vargha-Khadem et al., 1997;[14] Cipolotti et al., 2001). The issue will be addressed in more detail in Section 10.8.

From a modelling perspective, attractors, used by Treves and Rolls to characterise the memory-carrying function of the hippocampus, turn out to describe properties of place cells. Thus Wills et al. (2005) adapted the Burgess–O'Keefe (1996) procedure of altering the spatial structure of the rat's box. This time, however, they altered it more gradually and smoothly from one form, say a square, to another, a circle. They found that hippocampal place cells had attractor properties, they switched fairly sharply from responding to place X in one environment to responding to place Y in the changed one. It is as though the rat's brain, at a certain point in the transformation, decides that it must be in a qualitatively different place.

It is almost certain that the hippocampus has both functions. If so, how can they be reconciled? One possibility is that, anatomically, the hippocampus has two partially separate functions. The perirhinal/postrhinal cortices and the entorhinal cortex both have a division between two regions: one where cells related to navigational processes are common and one where they are not found. The hippocampus could well contain such an anatomical subdivision.

Another possibility is that the spatial function may be more basic as in the Nadel–Moscovitch theory to be discussed in Section 10.3. Alternatively, the memory function might still be the more basic. Thus Redish

---

[13] These memory control functions will be discussed further in Section 10.10.

[14] This is a developmental case that complicates interpretation

(see e.g. Thomas & Karmiloff-Smith, 2002).

(1999) argues that the role of the hippocampus in navigation is primarily to enable the animal to self-localise on re-entering a familiar environment. On this theory, once the animal is oriented in a familiar environment, it does not require the hippocampus. This context-switch function, on his view, could be easily extrapolated to the memory function. However, it is in conflict with the on-line navigation function of many implementations of the cognitive map theory, such as the Burgess–O'Keefe position.

Or take the view of Eichenbaum and Cohen (2001). They argue that three 'guiding principles' explain how hippocampal cells operate. '(a) discrete subsets of cues and actions are encoded by hippocampal cells in terms of appropriate relations between the items; (b) the contents of these representations overlap to generate a higher order framework on 'memory space' and (c) animals can conceptually 'navigate' this memory space by stepping across learned associations to make indirect novel associations or other inferential judgements among items in the memory space' (p.303). On this perspective, the cognitive map is a vague analogy of how the hippocampus might work when carrying out an episodic-memory function. However, even on this view there is a clash with the Burgess–O'Keefe formulation, as on that position

spatial organisation of the environment is viewed as innately specified in the hippocampal circuitry and the discovery of grid cells makes this entirely plausible. The function of the hippocampus is not *just* then that of forming associations between environmental cues; it has a real spatial basis.

Maybe the spatial function is specific to lower animals. In fact, London taxi drivers need to pass 'the knowledge', a test of their detailed navigational knowledge of an enormously complex city, which is not based on a grid (!). They have a larger posterior right hippocampus than controls, and the longer they have been a taxi driver, the larger it is (Maguire et al., 2000; see also Maguire, Woollett & Spiers, 2006) (see Figure 2.10). And when they performed taxi-driving route-finding in a virtual environment, their hippocampus is activated (Maguire et al., 1998). So this is not a plausible possibility.

The position that seems most plausible to us is that the *computational tasks* posed by navigation are rather similar to those posed by episodic memory. A rat must know thousands of qualitatively different places. The attractor properties of place cells indicate that places are not necessarily psychologically continuous. Some may grade smoothly into others; but for some,

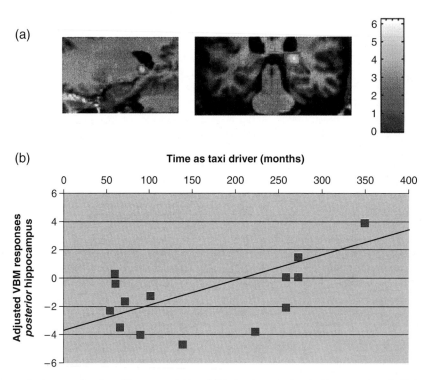

Fig. 2.10 Hippocampal volume as a function of time as a taxi driver. (a) Regions larger in size; the hippocampi are the C-shaped areas in the coronal view (right). (b) The volume of grey matter in the right posterior hippocampus correlated positively with time as a taxi driver. Reprinted with permission from E.N. Maguire, D.G. Gadian, I.S. Johnsrude, C.D. Good, J. Ashburner, R.S.J. Frackowiak and C.D. Frith, 2000, Navigation related structural change in the hippocampi of taxi drivers, Proceedings of the National Academy of Sciences of the United States of America, 97(8), 4398–4403. Copyright (2000) National Academy of Sciences, U.S.A.

the transition is abrupt, as when the rat, relying on its whisker sensory system, moves from one texture of ground, say rock, to another, grass. In an analogous way, two neighbouring episodes in memory can be sharply psychologically distinct or can blend into each other. Both have a core structural element—space and time, respectively—and both also require the binding of many different elements as cues. Moreover, when the information is later retrieved, only a subset of the cues is likely to be the same as when the complex was learned or encoded. To us it is most likely that this is an example of exaptation in evolution, where organs or structures that were prepared by natural selection for a different function are used for a new one; the later episodic-memory function would utilize the architecture that initially evolved for navigation (see O'Keefe & Nadel, 1978). That this could happen would be because of the similarities in the two computational tasks.

What is clear, however, is that for this complex structure deep in the system—and the cerebral cortex is an even more complex structure than the hippocampus—the more detailed research programme of knowledge of the microanatomy and of the physiological properties of the neurons involved in specific experimental situations has been driven by its perceived function(s). And after nearly 40 years we still do not know how its two candidate functions relate. This overall functional relation has not in practice been transparent from knowing the properties of how the components of the hippocampus behave, even though many variants on a range of tasks have been employed to study it. A reductionist bottom-up research strategy would have failed. In a highly complex system it is, therefore, vital to understand the overall computational tasks of a region! Moreover, one of its candidate functions—episodic memory—derived conceptually from cognitive psychology; it is not a characterisation that would arise straightforwardly in a reductionist framework.

An additional point, to which we will return in the next chapter, is that if either of these theories is on the right lines, then a particular computational task requires a specific microanatomy and a specific electrophysiology to implement it. In this case, the hippocampus may even be implementing two very different functions, if it is the case that one evolved from the other. The components themselves are not merely 'hidden units' in a large undifferentiated connectionist net in which the properties of one part are just a consequence of learning influences propagating through many layers of processes, they need to be honed to perform specific computational tasks.

The two examples considered so far, of V5/MT and the hippocampus, differ in a variety of ways. First, the internal structure of the system is far more complex in the latter case than the former. Thus in the Shadlen et al. model, all the units behave in qualitatively the same fashion. Second, on either of the accounts of the function of the systems we have considered, that of the hippocampus is the more abstract, as it is less simply related to any particular physical characteristic of a stimulus or response. Third, the tasks used are much more complex in the hippocampal case. This example then illustrates that there are likely to be much more severe methodological problems in investigating more central processes than those involved in low-level processes like movement perception.

If one wishes to generalize the example of the hippocampus to more central cortical functions, one needs to add two caveats. The first is that the term 'region', held to be the material basis of a function, may be very clearly defined, as we will see in Chapter 3, for parts of parietal cortex, or less precisely so, as will be discussed for regions of lateral frontal cortex in Chapter 9. More critically, the term 'computational task' is not necessarily to be understood in everyday language terms. More abstractly it means that the processes carried out in this region are ones that need to be characterised *as a whole* in relation to the processes occurring in other parts of the brain. These may include the characterisation of the processes by analogy with a mechanism that has a function for the whole system that contains it, such as a *buffer*. However, the relation between the part and the whole may be more abstract; for example, as a set of *hidden* units involved in translating one type of representation to another or as a vehicle for holding basis functions. Examples of the models of Zipser and Andersen (1988) and of Pouget and Sejnowski (1997) will be given in the next chapter. However, in both cases, the properties of the region are being abstractly characterised as a whole in relation to an analogous level of characterisations of other interacting parts of the global system. This requires a different type of conceptual framework from the more straightforwardly reductionist ones that characterise the operation of a region in terms of how the processing subcomponents work; that is, its internal neural operation.

2.3 Further Conceptual Problems in Investigating More Central Systems

Instead of arguing that characterisations at the cognitive level of how a system functions are irrelevant because a reductionist bottom-up programme will work, the more real worry is that Fodor is right and that even both sources of knowledge may be insufficient to cope with the overall complexity of the systems under investigation and the lack of power of our sources of empirical evidence. For in addition to the need to investigate the role a region plays in the overall system, there are a host of other differences between investigating simpler low-level processes and complex central ones.

1. An obvious point, but one with great practical significance, is that for many processes, e.g. ones involved in language, skilled action or the higher thought processes, there are no animal analogues, so the most directly reductionist approach cannot even be considered. Even a methodology like fMRI provides only a much grosser type of information in humans than does single-cell recording in animals. Thus there are currently no human equivalents to the methods that continually provided the main empirical motor for research on the cognitive neuroscience of movement perception.[15]

2. A second problem relates to a key component of the process of obtaining empirical findings in human cognitive neuroscience. Consider a typical scientific experiment such as the X-ray diffraction study of Wilkins et al. (1951) of the A form of DNA, which provided the critical evidence that DNA had a helical structure. The process of obtaining data may be separated into three stages:

(i) Select an appropriate object of study; in this case it was the DNA sample (or part of it).

(ii) Use an appropriate investigation procedure (X-ray diffraction).

(iii) Obtain measures which can be used in theory building (X-ray diffraction pattern images).

As far as the first stage was concerned, there were many subtle and complex questions concerning whether the form of DNA being used was pure, or whether, say, it was an inappropriately dry laboratory sample (see Arnott et al., 2006). However, given that the DNA form was pure—and all scientific investigations, including ones in cognitive neuroscience, have analogous qualitatively but investigable aspects[16]—the procedure by which quantitative data was obtained from it can be rigorously characterised. Thus, in stage (iii) how measures constrain theoretical inferences about the nature of the stage (i) object is completely well-defined. The method of X-ray diffraction had been well understood, both as a procedure and theoretically since 1912. Even though the model building process was complex and indeed initially faulty, as it was historically in the case

of DNA (see Wilkins, 1963), the process by which one maps the output of the stage (ii) procedures into deductions concerning the theoretical possibilities for a model of the underlying structure is virtually completely determined prior to the investigation. The inference procedure in going from the observed data to theoretical models is constrained by the mental equivalent of a fixed rigid structure.

Some aspects of cognitive neuroscience have similar characteristics. Consider for instance the inference from locations of photon absorptions at the detectors to activation levels in the cortex when using PET. However, the situation in general in cognitive neuroscience is completely different. Ever since single-cell recording was released in the 1960s from the constraint of being applied in the anaesthetised animal to being applied in the behaving animal, stage (ii) has involved the result of a task being carried out by the animal. When we move to humans, an enormous range of tasks have been used and new ones are being invented at an increasing rate. Moreover, we have no way of constructing a task for higher level processes, such that it reflects the operation of certain processes and no others. The paradigms used have been intuitively generated by some experimenter and how subjects will behave in them is unknown before they are tried.

Historically, as we discussed in Section 1.4, experimental tasks are developed because they are assumed to reflect some hypothetical key process fairly directly, but often they turn out rather rapidly to be very complex. A classic example was the so-called Sternberg (1966) serial-search short-term memory paradigm, which was enormously widely used in the early 1970s and then became much less popular. The basic assumption driving its use was that the linear fit of reaction times to number of items to be remembered reflected an underlying high-speed serial scanning process (see Figure 2.11). Only when, ten years later, results from cleverly designed experiments (see Monsell, 1978) made this assumption much less plausible, did the task drop out of fashion; instead the results began to seem to reflect a complex combination of different processes. New tasks continue to have complicated evolutions. A recent example is that of task-switching (Allport et al., 1994; Rogers & Monsell, 1995) which also rapidly escalated in popularity and only then did its underlying complexity become apparent (see Chapter 9).

The lack of transparency of the available tasks means that the analysis of the system and of the tasks that use it must be developed together. When assessing models in the light of the experimental results, one cannot conceptually treat the task as though it is a completely constrained measurement procedure, as, say, X-ray diffraction in the earlier example or the experimental

---

[15] There is one exception. This is recording from electrodes in patients who have had them implanted to detect the onset and source of epileptic seizures (e.g. Quiroga et al., 2005). This method, however, is relatively little used. Moreover it is currently essentially limited to investigations of medial temporal cortex.

[16] Analogous examples in cognitive neuroscience will be given in Chapter 4.

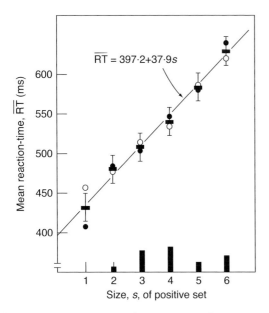

$$\overline{RT} = 397 \cdot 2 + 37 \cdot 9s$$

Fig. 2.11 Mean reaction time and percentage error from item-recognition experiments in which a subject is required to indicate if a given digit occurred in a just-presented set of digits. Filled circles represent positive responses. Open circles represent negative responses. The results are suggestive of a sequential process of memory scanning. From Memory scanning: New findings and current controversies, S. Sternberg, 1975, The Quarterly Journal of Experimental Psychology 27(1), 1–32, Psychology Press, reprinted by permission of the publisher (Taylor & Francis Group, http://www.informaworld.com).

apparatus in classical physics. The whole investigation process is an order of magnitude more complex.

3. If the inferential indeterminacy of the task itself was not sufficient of a problem, a related problem concerns the nature of a task. For lower-level processes the tasks are often very simple, as in the movement perception experiments discussed above. Task performance can then be plausibly modelled in terms of the mapping of a small number of variables relating to the physics of the environment on to responses as in say responding only to whether or not a stimulus can be detected to be moving in one direction or another. Moreover, if the model of movement perception fits the findings, this supports the characterisation of the task as well as the model itself.

Cognitive tasks, even apparently simple ones, are in fact highly complex. To start with, in adult humans, carrying out the task typically involves obeying instructions—a process we cannot currently scientifically characterise. And even tasks that seem fairly straightforward to explain to a subject can have hidden complexities. Take one of the most common and simple experimental procedures used in research on word processing in language—the *lexical decision* task—where letter strings are presented on a monitor and the

subject must decide as quickly as possible whether they form a word or not. The system must first attempt to remove the effects of the word and the response that occurred on the previous trial. It must prepare for the precise time of occurrence of the stimulus and attention must be given to the appropriate part of the screen. If the letter string is at all long, an eye movement must be prepared and executed. General visual perceptual processes related to form and possibly space perception will be involved, as well as ones specifically related to orthographic analysis. Phonological and semantic representations are likely to be involved.[17] A potentially complex decision may then be required, which can involve consideration of the visual form of the letter string, its realised sound and possibly its meanings. Moreover, the decision process will often take into account the type of non-word stimulus that has occurred in the experiment so far. Finally, the decision must be realised either as a key press or verbally.

Each of these processing domains, as we will call them, is itself internally complex. In Chapter 3 we will discuss the complex processes underlying word production, which would be involved if a verbal response has to be produced. Moreover, the processes can interact in a complex fashion. For instance, the size of the spatial attentional window that is responsible for determining what set of letters will be processed simultaneously at the orthographic level is influenced by whether semantic or phonological transformations will follow in the more central part of the reading process (Làdavas et al., 1997b). Yet lexical decision is simplicity personified compared, say, to tasks involving judgements of whether recollection or knowledge underlies a recognition response in episodic memory, which we are about to discuss.

4. The problem is not just one of the variety of different processes involved. It can also relate to the very nature of the processes. Take, for instance, the fMRI studies of Henson et al. (1999a) (see Figure 2.12) and Eldridge et al. (2000), which use the so-called *remember–know* experimental paradigm developed by Tulving (1985) and Gardiner and Java (1990). The experiment has *Study* phases and *Test* phases. In the Test phase the subject must decide whether a word shown had been presented just beforehand in the previous study list. However, if the answer is 'Yes' s/he has to refine the response by making an additional decision. This is whether s/he explicitly recollected the word being presented or just knew that it had occurred, because it was familiar but without any conscious memory of it actually being presented. The contrast between the 'Remember' and the 'Know'

---

[17] At least in some subjects how much stress is placed on each is partially under voluntary control; see Monsell et al. (1992).

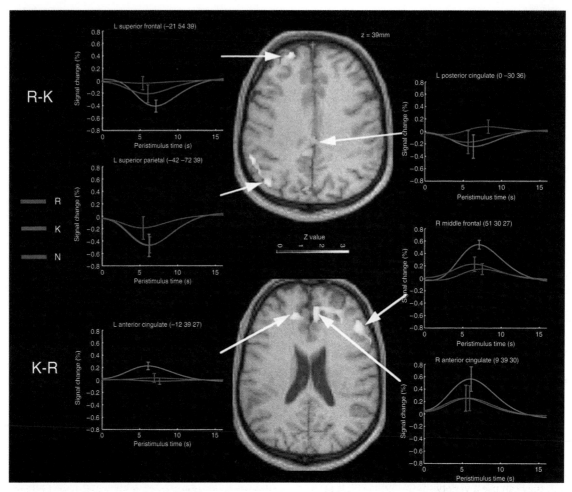

Fig. 2.12 Regions found by Henson et al (1999) to show enhanced responses to correct remember versus correct know judgements (top: R - K) and correct know versus correct remember judgements (bottom: K - R) using the remember-know paradigm of Tulving (1985) and event-related fMRI. (See text; N is a 'No' response.) Reprinted from Henson et al, 1999, Recollection and familiarity in recognition memory: An event-related functional magnetic imaging study. The Journal of Neuroscience, 19, 3963–3972. Figure 3, p 3969.

condition gave theoretically interesting results, which will be discussed in Section 10.8. However, in the functional imaging analysis one is dividing trials into different types—using what are called event-related fMRI procedures—by how the subject virtually instantaneously reflects on their experience of remembering. To give a complete account of the results it would be necessary to explain how subjects can provide a characterisation of their own mental states, one of the deepest issues in the philosophy-of-mind. Even for the results to be theoretically useful at all, the experimental contrast must be valid experientially; that is, it must correspond to a division that fits with the natural history of mental life (see Section 11.6). It is, therefore, a very major matter indeed even to decide whether the experimental data has any scientific meaning at all.

We are here far from the domain of detecting the movements of a spot of light. Surely, it can be argued,

cognitive neuroscience does not need to depend upon tasks where the degree of reflection required of the subject is so complex. However, for very many tasks that are extensively used, one cannot describe what the subject is doing in terms of simple physical properties of the environment. Take the lexical decision task. A letter string is presented to the subject and s/he must determine whether it is a word or not. But what is a word? Maybe following what an extreme follower of Patricia Churchland's attack on the phlogiston-like nature of everyday language folk psychological terms might claim, a word might eventually be characterised by certain types of firing in structures in the perisylvian cortex. However, even if true, as the only or main criterion for what a word is, this would be a mystification. It is clearly to be *primarily* defined in terms of the practices of the speakers of a certain language. As a concept, it relates to concepts in phonology, morphology and semantics. To attempt to explain behaviour in this task independently of this level of conceptual framework would clearly be absurd.[18]

But are there not simple tasks where the requirements of the task can be directly characterised in terms of the physics of the environment? Even here when one moves to humans, at least, there can be considerable complexities. Consider so-called visual pattern masking, where a word is presented for 30 msec or so and is followed by a complex meaningless pattern, often made up of components of letters—loops, straight lines, junctions of the two and the like. This following mask makes the word presented 20 or so msec earlier very difficult to see. Yet if the word is presented slightly later in a different case, facilitation of word processing (i.e. *priming*) occurs. Priming of semantic associates can probably also occur (e.g. Marcel, 1983b) or at least of an item's semantic characteristics (Kouider et al., 2007).[19]

A control condition that is often used is to present the stimulus for a duration that is so short it cannot be detected above chance. But what does this mean? A subject going through a series of trials will use all sorts of cues to try to detect whether a stimulus occurred before the mask. Take the situation of so-called *metacontrast masking* where a small stimulus, such as a bar, is very briefly presented but followed very shortly after—such as by 40–80 msec—by two other spatially very close bars, which do not quite overlap it. Phenomenally, the first bar is not seen. But if subjects are asked to guess whether the initial bar was actually present or not, they can use a variety of cues—the apparent duration of the whole stimulus combination, whether there is any appearance of movement or expansion in the seen bars or whether there was an after-image of the first bar, which they infer correctly or otherwise to imply that the bar was presented (see Held, 1996, for review). In other words, what seems an almost automatic low-level perceptual report—whether the first bar was or was not seen—is, in practice, a complicated and idiosyncratic mixture of inferences and other aspects of perception. The typical subject is behaving in a much more complex way than the 'central decision mechanism' of the Shadlen et al. model, which merely sums the output of V5 neurons and determines whether they exceed a threshold. The person in the metacontrast experiment is selecting what type of cue to use, and is guessing, making use of knowledge about the task structure. Yet the pattern of activation obtained in any imaging experiment, for instance, which uses such paradigms, must reflect such processes, too, unless they are explicitly controlled for. To ignore such factors can potentially lead the theorist into doubtful conclusions as we will see in Section 11.12.

5. These problems are exacerbated as task performance for higher-level processes can often be non-static. Learning occurs and therefore the state of the subject changes during the course of the task. This greatly complicates interpretation of many scanning experiments. Moreover it can make what used to be considered the most powerful neuropsychological method—the single case study—very difficult to apply for higher-level cognition.[20]

These points entail that, to account for an experimental finding, one needs two different types of theories/models/accounts to explain the performance of a subject in a given task, namely:

(i) a model of how the relevant parts of the cognitive system are organised *and*

(ii) an account of what programs—more specifically strategies or control processes—are being run to execute this particular type of task.[21] More formally, it will be argued in Chapter 9 that the set of schemas in operation in execution of the task need to be specified.

We refer, in point (ii), to *type of task*, since in principle any change in stimuli, responses, instructions or a host of variables, such as time-of-day, can change the control processes in operation (see Chapter 9). Yet unless one assumes that control processes are generally essentially unchanged across otherwise similar tasks, no progress could be made in developing satisfactory models relating to the on-line operation of the systems controlled, those of point (i). Modelling would not be sufficiently constrained by the data. The development of theories requires that many sets of input–output results are explained by the same model. However, to account for particular results, this assumption of identical control processes across similar tasks may need to be relaxed. To do this of course reduces the falsifiablity of the model of the on-line processes under consideration.

Quite frequently behavioural studies aim to account for particular parts of the natural history of task performance

---

[18] Typically connectionist models of the domain include representations of words as nodes or attractors (see Section 1.7) in the model; they too must be parasitic on concepts coming from linguistics.

[19] The claim was disputed for many years (see e.g. Holender, 1986), but is now generally accepted (see e.g. Abrams et al., 2002). For further discussion see Section 11.4.

[20] For discussion see FNMS Chapter 14.

[21] The contrast between an on-line process and a control process, which is methodologically very important, was first made in a paper on short-term or working memory—that of Atkinson and Shiffrin (1968).

in terms of somewhat loosely characterised processes not tied down to any specific model. The very complexity of the processes underlying task performance make such studies important, because using an extensively studied task one can have more confidence than with a novel one that any abstraction of what are held to be key processes involved in task performance will not overlook the effects of processes in cognitive levels or domains other than those with which the investigator is concerned. They facilitate process (ii) above.

Typically it is assumed implicitly that the model is behaving optimally, given an abstract characterisation of the task, and that this is transparently reflected in the subject's behaviour. However, we will find many situations discussed in later sections where that is not so, as in a number of cases discussed above. Tulving and Madigan's caveats, referred to in Section 1.4, are as necessary today as in 1970.

Moreover, if to account for performance in any given task one requires two different types of assumption—one concerning the model (i), and the other (the type (ii) one) specific to the individual task, and even to sub-varieties of it—then it is clear that there are many theoretical degrees of freedom in accounting for the experimental evidence. To make matters worse, the data our empirical procedures provide are not that powerful for theoretical purposes. The results are essentially highly limited in their grain. We cannot effectively assess any variable on better than ordinal scales, with a few exceptions, such as the additive factors methodology to be discussed in the next chapter. Thus, even with fMRI, using a standard analysis procedure e.g. SPM (statistical parametric mapping—see Chapter 5), the most usual type of theoretical conclusion is that an area is significantly more activated in condition A than in condition B. With a few exceptions, such as linear effects or ones related to additive factors methodology, we do not concern ourselves with quantitatively *how much* more the region is activated in condition A than condition B. This gives our data limited power to differentiate between theories.

These difficulties mean that to attempt to understand central processes, we need to use every type of empirical and theoretical assistance we can obtain. A major theme of the book is that for this purpose we need brain-based evidence, as well as purely behavioural support. The necessary complexity of the theoretical environment and the relative weakness of the data available mean that evidence that puts stronger constraints on possible theories, which the brain-based data do, cannot be ignored. Complementarily though, we require cognitive conceptual frameworks, as without them we will be theoretically blind. Using the combined approaches of *cognitive* neuroscience is vital.

2.4 The Theoretical Problems of Investigating Central Systems

The discussion of the methodological difficulties in the previous section used implicitly the assumption that the mind/brain is composed of, and *entirely* composed of, isolable systems each with a different micro-function. Theoretically the idea that the mind is composed of a set of 'isolable' processing systems (and memory stores) each with its own specialised function was common early in the development of information-processing psychology (e.g. Posner, 1978; Morton, 1981). The approach fitted well with the dissociations being described by cognitive neuropsychologists (see Shallice, 1981). So in that field too, the same type of position was supported together with the natural idea that the isolable systems were each located physically in different parts of the cortex.

For the more reductionist cognitive neuroscientists this approach is an almost unquestioned perspective (see e.g. Ochsner & Kosslyn, 1999). Indeed the idea that the mind is 'massively modular' and that it has no essentially non-modular parts has become a standard view in modern sociobiological speculations (consider Cosmides & Tooby, 1994; Pinker, 1997). Theoretical arguments have, though, been presented against this position, at least as being applicable to all cognitive processes. If these arguments hold then the difficulties of inferring from findings to the theoretical structure of the mind will become even more complex. Consider the line of argument developed by Fodor (1983) when he was popularising the term 'cognitive module' and formalising, and extending the concept of isolable (or functional) subsystems, which was already well-accepted in information-processing psychology (see e.g. Posner, 1978; Morton, 1981). Fodor used the term in a much more detailed sense than did Marr, but he also limited its application only to some cognitive processes.

Modules, Fodor claimed, have many characteristics.[22] Apparently, following Chomsky (1980), he assumed that humans have different domains of knowledge, such as of language, of space, of physical objects, of persons, of numbers and so on. Modules, he claimed, operate within only one domain (Chomskyan modularity). In addition, he argued that they are innately specified, and are *not* assembled from more basic elements by learning (Darwinian modularity). Considering how they are implemented in the brain, he held them to be hardwired (anatomical modularity), and to have characteristic breakdown patterns—the specific impairments

---

[22] The way we label some of these characteristics follows an exhaustive review article on modularity (Seok, 2006).

known from neuropsychology (neuropsychological modularity). They are held *not* to be implemented by relatively equipotential neural mechanisms. Turning to their computational role, a module is informationally encapsulated (computational modularity), by which he means that it receives input from, and sends output to, only a very limited set of other systems. In addition, he considered them to be *computationally autonomous*, in that they do not share any general resource, such as attention or memory, with other modules. Finally, modules have a characteristic pattern of development (developmental modularity).

This is a long and abstract set of properties. At least one is highly implausible—that of *computational autonomy*. That attentional processes, for instance, do not affect otherwise modular processes is clearly false. Evidence for top-down attentional influences at very early stages of the perceptual system can be obtained from a variety of methods—functional imaging experiments (Macaluso & Driver, 2005), electrophysiological ones, as discussed in the Section 1.8, and single-cell recording (Moran & Desimone, 1985). Moreover sets of neurotransmitter systems, such as dopamine, serotonin, acetylcholine and noradrenaline, each activate a wide swathe of cortex, probably implementing different computational functions (see Yu & Dayan, 2005; Dayan & Huys, 2009).[23] One can, however, modify Fodor's position by allowing a module to satisfy most or nearly all of the properties that he outlined. It is probably this implicit modification of his theory that has led to notions related to it becoming highly popular in developmental psychology (e.g. Leslie & Frith, 1988), as well as in cognitive neuropsychology (Caramazza & Shelton, 1998—see Chapter 6). Moreover, the idea that cognition is domain-specific fits with ideas derived from single-cell recording for separable dorsal and ventral systems to be discussed in Chapter 3, which were originally related to functions of the temporal and parietal cortices but which have been extended even into prefrontal cortex (e.g. Goldman-Rakic, 1987).

There are many other problems with Fodor's position. The most obvious ones concerns how learning occurs. Humans have an enormous range of cognitive and motor skills and knowledge. How do they acquire it? The pure structuralists (including Fodor) using syntax as their model say 'parameter setting'. There is a set of choices available innately and when a child learns a given language, 'choices' are made by the combination of environment and child, in the sense that one of the a

priori possible values of the parameters becomes selected and fixed. The child's language system makes the 'choice'. This account has a certain plausibility for the acquisition of syntax or morphology. Consider instead skilled operations in thought or action. When a child learns to tie a shoe-lace or to use the single-transferable-vote procedure in elections, or to play a French defence type of position in chess, what parameters are being set? The whole issue of learning cannot be finessed so crudely. Whatever the ancillary problems with Fodor's position, his arguments, however, put firmly on the intellectual agenda the idea that the mind may contain a set of modules, each in a specific cognitive domain.

However, Fodor's own position was more complex and actually at odds with the massively modular position. The title of Fodor's book—*The Modularity of Mind*—alliterative and elegant as it is, was misleading. Fodor in fact argues that informationally encapsulated systems, each within a specific cognitive domain—his modules—cannot create cross-domain analogies. Yet analogy, he argued, was central to many higher-level thought processes. He used the example of scientific discovery. 'What is known about the flow of water gets borrowed to model the structure of the atom; what is known abut the behaviour of the market gets borrowed to model the shaping of operant responses. And so forth' (Fodor, 2000). The point is that 'analogical reasoning' would seem to be a process that depends upon the transfer of information between cognitive domains previously assumed to be mutually independent. By definition, according to him, systems that only contain informationally encapsulated subsystems cannot reason analogically (Fodor, 1983, p. 107). According to Fodor—and he still holds this view (see Fodor, 2000)—half the mind, the input systems, is modular. The other half of the mind, however, is *not* modular; it is equipotential. Even more starkly, he argues it will never be understood by scientific methods.

Fodor supported his philosophical argument with two quasi-empirical ones. The first was that artificial intelligence had yet to devise an effective modular theory of thought. This is, in fact, pragmatically a stronger argument now than when it was produced in 1983! The second was that there was nothing known on the neuropsychology of thought. This was clearly untrue at the time.[24] However, there are still major claims that there may be structures underlying 'general intelligence', which are internally equipotential (see e.g. Duncan et al., 2000). So Fodor's position cannot be immediately rejected on empirical grounds.

---

[23] A second property—that they are 'hard-wired'—is also difficult to hold, given the evidence on the word-form system in reading; see Sections 4.12 and 5.10.

[24] See FNMS Chapter 14.

One possibility is that Fodor's view on the intrinsic complexity of the processes underlying thought may be too extreme, but not completely wrong. For instance, it is possible that higher-level systems are not completely equipotential, but that they are in some sense more weakly encapsulated than lower-level ones. This position has some similarity with the perspective that derives from a source that Fodor would excorciate as a vehicle for understanding higher-level cognition, namely connectionism. Thus Rumelhart and McClelland (1986) argued 'it seems fairly clear that there is not some single neuron whose functioning is essential for the operation of any particular cognitive process. While reasonably circumscribed *regions* of the brain may play fairly specific roles, *particularly at lower levels of processing* [italics added], it seems fairly clear that within regions, performance is characterised by a kind of graceful degradation in which the system's performance gradually deteriorates as more and more neural units are destroyed. [...] Again this is quite different from many serial symbolic processing models in which the disruption of a single step in a huge program can catastrophically impact the overall performance of the whole system.' (p. 134). They continue 'Neuropsychological investigation of patients with brain damage indicates that there is no part of the cortex on whose operation all other parts depend. Rather it seems all parts work together, influencing one another and each contributes to the overall parts of the task and to the interpretation into it of certain kinds of constraints or sources of information. To be sure brain mechanisms control vital bodily functions and the overall states of the system, and certain parts of the cortex are critical for receiving information in particular modalities, but higher level functions seem to be characterised by distributed, rather than central control' (Rumelhart & McClelland, 1986, pp. 134–135). Rumelhart and McClelland qualify this slightly, but do not materially alter their position, by discussing and endorsing Luria's (1966) somewhat vague views on brain function and the role of frontal cortex. However, they do this by referring to concepts like *subsystem* and *strategy*, which float in an undefined fashion above their dense set of connectionist concepts.

Their position—which we will term that of 'early connectionism'—is less strong than Fodor's and more surrounded by caveats. However, consider a large multi-layer connectionist net that has a set of specific and separate input-processing domains and that carries out many different input–output tasks. In addition, include a constraint such that units on a higher level receive most of their inputs from 'nearby' units on 'lower' levels. Then units at higher levels would tend to be less specialised.[25]

Thus again one would expect higher-level systems to be internally less separable into subsystems than lower-level ones.

Rumelhart and McClelland's position therefore reinforces that of Fodor in suggesting that a qualitatively different type of system may underlie higher levels of processing when contrasted with the more modular lower-level systems. Modularity then cannot be assumed from a general argument; it must be empirically supported.

What then are we to make of findings similar to those of Henson et al. (1999) and P. Burgess et al. (2001) discussed earlier in the chapter, which suggest that quite tightly localised systems with abstract higher-level functions exist? If the general positions of Fodor and of early Rumelhart and McClelland were correct, then to presuppose that the localised regions of statistically significant differences in activation arise from differential activation of different localised subsystems would be incorrect. Some other explanation for the pattern of results would need to be sought. We will return to this issue in Section 5.7.

Thus in the course of such considerations, very broad issues about the organisation of cognition interact with highly specific points of imaging methodology concerned with, say, the creation of the so-called BOLD signal in fMRI (see Chapter 5). One cannot assume from the limited arguments concerning functional imaging presented so far that the operation of higher-level processes is necessarily based on isolable subsystems. Assume, however, that the localized activation in higher-level systems, observed when subjects carry out tasks involving more complex cognitive operations, is derived from anatomically restricted isolable subsystems. One can still take a position in some way more in the spirit of Fodor's than of the 'massive modularity' view on the relation between input and central processing. It may be that there is a qualitative difference in the organisation of cognition between higher-level central processes and lower-level input ones and that the difference in organisation is not merely a matter of degree.

2.5 The Overall Structure of the Cognitive System

Overall this leaves three types of positions, which accept that there is some qualitative difference between lower- and higher-level processes, which loosely can be called the domains of on-line perceptual-motor performance

---

[25] For an algorithm that realises the 'nearby' constraint rigorously, see Plaut (2003). Technically, one also needs to add to this argument the constraint that the settling-time of the system is relatively short.

and of thought, respectively. All three positions assume that the lower-level systems are in some sense modular.

A1. This position assumes that there is a change in the *degree of specialisation* of systems, as one moves from lower- to higher-level processes. However, this change can be all-or-none (A1a), as in Fodor's perspective, or it can be partial, as in the early Rumelhart and McClelland perspective (A1b). Moreover, if 'central processes' do differ qualitatively from input processes, one has the second issue—which we will call a type B one—of where the line is drawn. Newell (1990), as will be discussed shortly, drew the line at a relatively high level—the tackling of a novel problem. For Fodor, however, the line is much lower. Take word meaning. Fodor (1983) argues that 'input processing for language provides no semantic analysis "under" lexical items'. He holds that the output of the perceptual input systems are what Rosch et al. (1976) called *basic categories*. A basic category is the concept that is psychologically salient in the hierarchy when one moves from the most specific to the most general concept that refers to an entity. Thus in the hierarchy *poodle*, *dog*, *mammal*, *animal*, *physical object*, *thing*, the basic category is *dog*. Thus for Fodor semantic decomposition of a word—that a dog is an animal—is in that part of the cognitive system—the central system—of which to paraphrase Wittgenstein—one cannot speak.

A2. One can argue instead that both Fodor and early Rumelhart and McClelland were essentially wrong, and that the principle of modularity applies at all levels. For instance, take the program Soar (Newell, 1990), discussed in Section 1.7, which is one of the two culminations of the AI work in production systems. The development of Soar depended critically on the argument that qualitatively different types of process need to occur when the system is attempting to cope with a problem which is novel for it by comparison with one which is routine for it. In Soar, when the system does not know the answer to some problem, it sets up a so-called *impasse*. This creates what is called a new *problem-space* and the system continues to operate in this new problem-space, only returning to its original problem when it has solved the new problem (see Figure 2.13). One impasse may of course lead to another and so on in potentially infinite regress.

In this aspect of his work with Soar, Newell was adapting to production systems, a fundamental symbolic AI idea, first implemented by Sussman (1975) in his program HACKER, of a separation between the routine processing part of the system and that for confronting novelty.[26] To implement such a system in the mind/brain would require only one additional system. This would need to detect an impasse—which is

computationally fairly easy—and set up a new problem-space to temporarily override the previously active problem space and to confront the impasse. Finally, the system would need to hand over control to the new problem space. Control would be passed back when the impasse was solved. Intuitively, anatomically this could be materially a fairly small simple system but one that controls all other systems in a particular way. This could then be a qualitatively different system from the other modules but computationally no more complex than any other of the modular systems. Thus the qualitative conceptual distinction between a central system that is conceptually non-modular because it is not domain specific and modular non-central systems would be compatible with overall anatomical modularity.

A3. A related possibility, discussed extensively later in the book, particularly in Chapters 9 and 12, is that there are separate systems which deal with novelty, abstraction, analogy and the like. This would be different from the Newell-type of position in that, on this approach, there is a separate domain of processing with its own set of subsystems for dealing with different aspects of higher-level thought processes. Such subsystems would be modular in the anatomical sense, but not in Fodor's sense, as they would be modulating many different domains of processing. Thus Fodor's distinction between central and input processes remains appropriate. However central systems are no longer assumed to be equipotential.

Whichever of these alternatives is accepted, there is a further issue that needs consideration. Humans are conscious. Indeed people are necessarily conscious of some aspect of what they are doing, whenever many key central processes are carried out. This will be discussed in Chapter 11. This is not just an optional additional philosophical question. In the discussion earlier in the chapter of the detection of stimuli in a pattern-masking paradigm, the subject's behaviour was dependent upon which aspect of the situation they were *conscious* of, and so upon which they *chose* to base their action (see Weiskrantz, 1997, for related discussion). In, say, the remember–know paradigm they must even reflect on their conscious states.

Yet we have absolutely no agreement about how, even in principle, one can understand the brain bases of conscious processing. However, it is plausible that this involves some qualitative difference from processes unrelated to consciousness. It would, therefore, be rash to assume that an answer to this question will not greatly influence many other questions concerning central processes. One might be able to study V1, as Crick and Koch (1995) pointed out, and ignore consciousness.[27] It would seem unwise to study cognitive

---

[26] See FNMS Chapter 14.

[27] But see Silvanto et al. (2005), for a counter-argument.

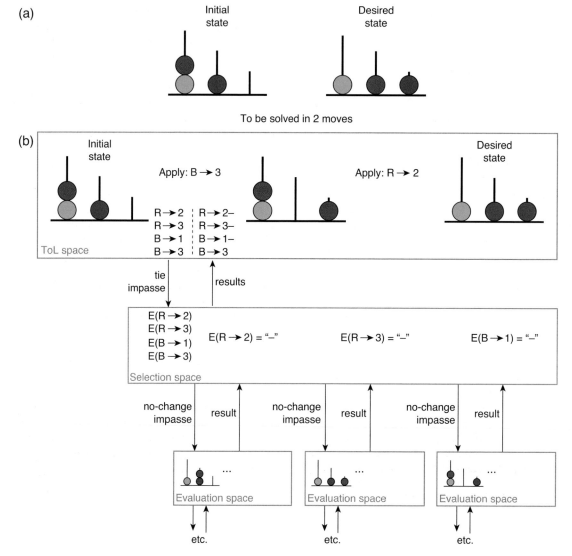

Fig. 2.13   Problem solving and impasses in the Soar production system. (a) A simple 2-move Tower of London problem (see Section 12.5). The coloured circles represent balls on sticks of different heights. The goal is to move one ball at a time so as to transform the initial state into the desired state. (b) A partial trace of Soar solving the problem using a look-ahead strategy. Given the initial state, four moves are possible. Each move is initially considered to be equally viable. This creates a tie impasse, which is resolved by moving to a selection space and then to a series of evaluation spaces in which possible moves are evaluated. In this case, three of the four possible moves receive a negative evaluation. This resolves the initial subgoal as a tie no longer exists. The remaining move is then selected and applied. The process then repeats until the goal is achieved.

systems located further forward in the brain, such as those located in the anterior cingulate or dorsolateral prefrontal cortex, with that assumption.

We are therefore left with three very broad possibilities (issue A) on how the mind/brain is organised. One (A1) is that it has an informationally encapsulated modular (input) system and a second central system, which is more equipotential and less informationally encapsulated. The second (A2) is that it is essentially entirely modular with one special impasse-resolving subsystem. The third (A3) is that it is entirely modular but with two

very broad classes of subsystems, one informationally encapsulated and rather concrete in its functions and the second not so, but *not* equipotential, as it has a set of subsystems each having highly abstract functions. Two of these possibilities produce questions (issue B) about where the line between the two types of system should be drawn. Finally, all give rise to a third type of question. Whatever answers one gives to issues A and B, how could a system that is operating in this way give rise to consciousness (issue C)? This question, though, in turn, may throw light on issues A and B!

One may summarise the argument so far in two ways. The first is that the process of determining how the higher-level systems in the mind/brain operate depends on characterising what approximately their functions are and how they are connected to other such systems. Such questions are inextricably bound up with general questions about the organisation of the mind. These questions are extremely complex, both methodologically and theoretically. And this complexity is not a mere quantitative matter. The data we need to use for theory-building are not derived from a scientifically solid, well-understood empirical procedure, as in the harder sciences, but depend upon high-level processes like interpretation of instructions, strategies and reflections which are far from easy to characterise.

A second set of issues arises if we provisionally isolate a system or set of systems. One would naturally want to develop a more detailed model of how the system operates. However, to do this we must face two additional types of problem. First, in conflict with the position advocated by Kosslyn (1992), it will be argued that it is possible to isolate systems even if we do not know exactly where they are in the brain. Cognitive neuropsychology has indeed demonstrated this. Obviously if we do not know exactly where a system is in the brain, we cannot have any idea of its underlying anatomical microstructure or physiology. Second, and in practice more critically, even if we do have a reasonably accurate localisation of the region, we may be dealing with a process that is found only in humans. In this case, too, we are not likely to have much knowledge of the anatomical microstructure of the region and even

less of its specific cellular physiology. One cannot therefore develop models by using the approaches adopted in the type of work discussed earlier in the chapter of Shadlen et al., N. Burgess et al. and Treves and Rolls, where the elements of the model are derived from specific neurobiological information. Therefore one cannot rely on the standard reductionist approach of building up from simpler elements.

How is one to proceed? One possible approach is to forget about any evidence related to neuroscience when attempting to understand such complex processes. However, the purely internal development of cognitive science fields has not been promising. Human experimental psychology by itself, for instance, does not have powerful enough methods to be really effective in isolation. It has been most successful where it attempts to make use of cognitive neuroscience evidence, as was illustrated in the discussion of attention in Section 1.8. Symbolic artificial intelligence is also under a cloud. The Chomskian linguistics approach, even on its own terms, offers only a very partial view of language performance as opposed to its core domain of language competence, and says nothing about all the other forms of higher cognitive processes. Its new minimalist version almost accepts that its methods cannot lead to a definitive theory. We therefore argue that it is vital to bite the bullet and attempt to integrate brain-based empirical evidence with a cognitive science characterisation of the observed behaviour, using a full range of cognitive theories. How this might be done is discussed in the next chapter.

CHAPTER 3

Bridging the Theoretical Gap: from the Brain to Cognitive Theory

3.1 **Introduction: Return to Marr**

Why is there a term *cognitive* in cognitive neuroscience? Does it represent merely the aspirations of neuroscientists, the goal of what their subject should achieve? Or does it also represent a type of theorising, which is necessary for understanding the brain/mind? In the last chapter we argued that one should choose the second alternative.

In Section 2.3 we referred to the *functions* of particular systems, a term that straddles engineering and biology, phenomenological concepts like *awareness, strategy, recollection* and *task*, linguistic concepts like *word* and *semantics*. How can we relate such cognitive concepts to concepts we use to characterise the operation of a material object like the brain? More concretely, the empirical methods derived globally from the neurosciences that we mainly discuss in this book are those from functional imaging and from neuropsychology. The former involves direct measurements of brain function. The latter obtains its theoretical interest because the observed effects reflect physical damage to the brain. It therefore seems necessary to consider how cognitive-level theories can be related to empirical findings of such types linked to brain processes and to neurobiological levels of explanation.

As we saw in the last chapter some critics have argued that theorising in the two domains—that of cognitive science and neuroscience—cannot be effectively linked. However, this is a minority view. For the majority, what are the theoretical domains being held to be linkable and what type of bridges are to be built between them? Many theorists have discussed the matter. Amongst these theorists one can differentiate between (i) an approach from the brain sciences, such as that of Marr (1982), (ii) an approach from philosophy-of-mind, such as that of Cummins (1983), (iii) approaches from computer science, such as those of Pylyshyn (1984) or Newell (1990) and (iv) an approach from information-processing and developmental psychology (Morton, 2004).[1] In addition, there are connectionist approaches (e.g. Smolensky, 1988).

The theorist who is still, after 20 years, generally the most quoted on this topic is the mathematician turned theoretical neurophysiologist, David Marr, based in Cambridge and then MIT, who died very young, shortly after producing his best known work, his 1982 book on Vision.[2] Marr is often thought of as a brilliant meteor, a theorist who left the research field with a research programme that, while apparently specifically concerned

with vision, was in fact a more general manifesto on how to conceive of a brain that implements cognitive processes. But, it is generally believed, the programme never materialised. We will give a more positive assessment of his legacy.

Marr himself had worked on models of the cerebellum and hippocampus before turning to cortex. His 1982 book followed McCulloch and Pitts, who were discussed in Section 1.6, in seeing the nervous system as essentially an information-processing device. In a development of work initially with Poggio (Marr & Poggio, 1976), Marr specified three different levels of theory of how cognitive processes are implemented in the brain (Marr, 1982). The most abstract level on which the device can be analysed is what he calls the *computational theory* level. To Marr the computational theory of the device is concerned with the goal of the computation, and the logic of the strategy by which it is carried out. Sejnowski and Churchland (1989), referring concretely to object perception, gave a clearer characterisation of this second part by calling it 'the computational level of *abstract problem analysis*, decomposing the task (for example determining structure from motion) into its main constituents' (p. 302).

Marr considers this to be the critical level from an information-processing perspective in the context of perception, but as discussed in the previous chapter, the position would apply even more strongly for more central processes. For him 'an algorithm is likely to be understood more readily by understanding the nature of the problem being solved than by examining the mechanism (and the hardware) in which it is embodied'. In a similar vein he argues that 'trying to understand perception by studying neurons is like trying to understand a bird's flight by studying only feathers. It just cannot be done. In order to understand bird flight, we have to understand aerodynamics; only then does the structure of feathers and the different shapes of bird's wings make sense' (Marr, 1982, p. 27). Marr held the perspective in a strong form. He even extended this belief to the study of processes early in vision, namely to questions such as why retinal ganglion cells and lateral geniculate cells have the receptive fields they do.

Marr's main example of why the computational level is critical was derived from 1970s AI vision and neuropsychology. In the early 1970s, programs such as those of Freuder (1974) and Tenenbaum and Barrow (1976) used their knowledge about what scenes can contain to segment the image. Thus the knowledge that desks have telephones on them was used to segment out a black blob half-way up the image of an office scene and 'recognise' it as a telephone. Marr does not deny that such processes are used in perception. However, he argues that they cannot be critical. His evidence was

---

[1] Morton's approach is more general than the others and compatible with them.

[2] Marr died of leukaemia in 1980. The book was published posthumously.

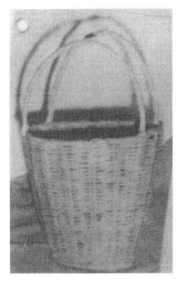 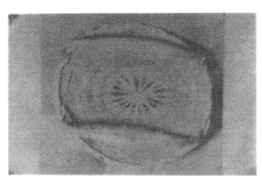

Fig. 3.1 The 'unusual views' matching test of Warrington and Taylor (1973). Patients have to name or identify unusual views of an object (right) and later the usual views (left). In the different views matching test patients must select from a choice of two which is the 'usual view' that goes with a particular 'unusual' one. Reproduced with permission from Shallice (1988) From Neuropsychology to Mental Structure, Cambridge University Press. (Figure 8.2, p189.) Copyright © 1988, Cambridge University Press.

derived from a neuropsychological study of Warrington and Taylor (1978).

This study concerned patients with left posterior lesions who were 'associatively agnosic' in Warrington's sense. When objects are presented to such patients they do not know what they are. They can neither name them nor know how to use them. Yet their visual systems can carry out the complex and difficult operations required to match correctly two pictures of these same objects, when they are viewed from two quite different directions.[3] Such a different-views matching test clearly makes extensive use of image segmentation operations. Yet the patient can carry these out without knowing what the object is. This led Marr to reject the idea that the accessing of the 3D form of an object typically makes extensive use of top-down information from semantic representations. Marr therefore argued for a computational model of visual processing in which there is a processing stage that produces a 3D model of the scene prior to the one in which meaning and significance were assigned.

Farah (1990) in fact presents strong arguments against some of Marr's interpretations of Warrington and Taylor's findings. However, Marr has two arguments that depend upon two complementary sets of findings of Warrington and Taylor (in right and left posterior

patients, respectively). The other argument concerns right parietal patients who present with a so-called *apperceptive agnosia*;[4] they cannot identify objects from photographs taken from non-canonical perspectives or colloquially 'unusual views' (see Figure 3.1). Farah's arguments undermine Marr's claims that the findings from right parietal patients support the existence of a pre-semantic representation which is *viewpoint-independent*. They do not undermine his argument that top-down information is not generally critical for attaining an adequate pre-semantic representation, such as a structural description.

Thus at his level of computational theory we may specify that a complex function (object recognition) is the result of sub-functions. We therefore have something like:

$$y = h(g(f(x))),$$

where x is a representation of the visual input,

f is a function that segments the visual input,

g is a function that uses knowledge of the visual structure of objects to categorise them visually,

h is a function that applies knowledge other than of visual structure and form to the visually categorised structure and

y is a representation of the recognised object.

Once we have a function broken down in this way, we effectively have a recipe for carrying out the computation: take the input, apply function f to that input, then

---

[3] In an influential book, Farah (1990) uses the term 'associative agnosia' in a different sense. We will adopt Warrington's usage that it refers to patients who do not know what objects signify—what they are—but in whom processes prior to semantic ones are intact. See FNMS Chapter 8 for more detailed discussion.

[4] See FNMS Chapter 8.

apply function g to the result and h to that result. The procedure is very coarse, but in principle we can apply the same technique to decompose functions f and g into subfunctions, and thereby specify the procedure at a lower 'level' (or at a finer conceptual grain).[5] Of course, this approach can also be used when two or more subfunctions are suspected of operating in parallel:

$$y = g(f_1(x), f_2(x)).$$

Here there is no requirement that f_1 and f_2 be evaluated in sequence.

Concentrating on the first two only of these three visual stages, Marr claimed that 'the quintessential fact of human vision' is that its computational task is to 'tell about shape and space and spatial arrangement.'[6] By *task* Marr did not just refer to a human or animal subject tackling a real problem situation. Instead he referred to the function of a subset of the processes the animal is carrying out, which can be considered a computationally separable part of the whole. For instance, Marr talks of the task of extracting structure (i.e. form) from motion as a functional subpart of visual perception.

Marr's next level—that of the algorithm—specified the abstract series of steps that are carried out in order to implement each of the constituent computational subtasks determined by the previous level. They correspond to a computer program.[7] The lowest of Marr's levels is that of the hardware implementation. This is how the nervous system realises the algorithm. Dawson (1998) characterises Marr's position as the *tri-level hypothesis* namely by 'What information-processing problem is the system solving? What information-processing steps are being used to solve the problem? How are these information-processing steps actually carried out by a physical device? These three questions define the tri-level hypothesis.' (Dawson, 1998, p. 9).

At about the same time as Marr was analysing the computations carried out in the brain, a second relevant concept was developed by the philosopher Cummins (1983) in an attempt to understand psychological levels of explanation. His term is *functional analysis*. Here we have a similar label to a term used by Marr but instead of an attempt at a rigorous specification of some necessarily small component of the cognitive system we have a top-down procedure. Cummins phrased his idea in philosophical language. 'Functional analysis consists in analysing a disposition into a number of less problematic dispositions such that the programmed manifestation of these analysing dispositions amounts to a manifestation of the analysed disposition' (p28). In simpler terms functional analysis is top-down decomposition of a complex process into a program involving simpler operations, just of the type Marr conceived. The information-processing level of theorising discussed in Section 1.4 is an example of the approach, while a programming language in which one can build standard types of information-processing models and examine how they would behave is considered in Section 3.6.

While Marr came to the problem from physiology and mathematics, and Cummins from philosophy, the third overlapping approach derives from computer science. This uses the concept of *architecture* or *functional architecture*. Early computers had a standard four-box architecture (see Figure 3.2) (Ware, 1963). Newell (1990) gives a closely related, but somewhat more fine-grained, characterisation of the functions that all classical computer architectures perform (see Table 3.1).[8]

Some discussions of the concept *functional architecture* tend to provide a low-level referent for the term. Thus Pylyshyn (1984) argues 'Specifying the functional architecture of a system is like providing a manual that defines some programming language. Indeed defining a programming language is equivalent to specifying the functional architecture of a virtual machine.' Here the emphasis is on the type of micro-functions that can be computed which is close to the capacities required by what Marr would include in the algorithmic level. However, Pylyshyn says, again referring to the *functional*

---

[5] The issue of the extent to which recognition depends upon top-down as well as bottom-up processes was far from settled by the Warrington and Taylor findings (see, for example, Dayan et al., 1995, and Silvanto et al., 2005, for modelling and empirical findings for the alternative perspective.) What Warrington and Taylor's findings do suggest is that top-down information is not critical across the broad processing domains of semantic and structural description characterisations.

[6] In Section 6.3 it will be argued that Marr's separation of levels in object recognition was essentially correct.

[7] There is another direct link between Marr's kind of hierarchical functional decomposition and the conception of an algorithm— the LISP programming language. LISP programs are sets of function definitions, bottoming out in low-level functions, such as *read, write, sum, log,* etc. So a LISP program can provide a hierarchical decomposition of a function into subfunctions, and an algorithm for calculating or applying the function. In fact, parts of the algorithm depend on the LISP interpreter. Thus, the above functional decomposition is actually agnostic about the order, if any, in which f_1 and f_2 are evaluated. However, there are logics of computation (e.g. Girard, 1987) that allow such commitments to be specified.

---

[8] This classical architecture, sometimes referred to as the von Neumann architecture or stored-programme computer, is based on von Neumann's (1945) work on the EDVAC machine, and Mauchly and Eckert's earlier work on the first programmable computer, ENIAC.

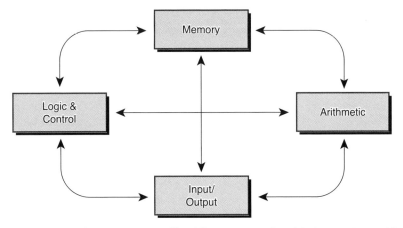

Fig. 3.2 An early standard computer architecture consisting of four fully-interconnected modules (see, e.g., Ware, 1963).

architecture of the system, 'It includes the basic operations provided by the biological substrate, say for storing and retrieving symbols, comparing items, treating them differently as a function of how they are stored and so on, as well as such basic resources and constraints on the system, as a limited memory. It also includes what computer scientists refer to as 'the control structure' which selects which rules to apply at various times.' (p. 30). One can read this as meaning that certain types of operation are available rather than that each of the individual commands are specified.

We will follow Newell (1990) and assume that the concept *human functional architecture* involves more than one level of grain of concept. This too fits well with the way Cummins thinks about functional analysis. He uses the idea of *causal subsumption*. In *causal subsumption* you work down from a high-level function by decomposing it into a set of somewhat lower-level functions and then by iteration down to a fixed 'bottom set' of basic functions. In fact, Marr's own use of the term *level* is rather confused. On the surface, he can be viewed as in Dawson's characterisation of his position as referring just to this *domain*

sense of level, in terms of the contrast between conceiving of abstract problem analysis, of algorithms and of hardware. However, the examples of the hardware *level* that Marr gives, such as 'synaptic mechanisms, action potentials, inhibitory interactions and so forth' (Marr, 1982, p. 26), make it clear that this sense is not well separated in his formulation from the Cummins–Newell *grain* sense of level. To avoid confusion we will not use the term *level* in the sense of *conceptual grain*, the first sense of level, that of Cummins and Newell. We will restrict it to the *conceptual domain* sense, that which corresponds to Dawson's tri-level approach. *Level* in the sense of *conceptual domain* then refers to the scientific conceptual framework in which the concepts and arguments are derived. The three relevant conceptual domains are:

(1) *computational task* where the concepts and arguments are derived from logic or branches of mathematics;

(2) *functional architecture* where the concepts come from computer science;

(3) *brain hardware* where the concepts come from the brain sciences.

TABLE 3.1 Functions of classical computer architectures (see Newell, 1990) and how they relate to the standard four-box architecture shown in Figure 3.2. Newell also includes a generic category of components added for increased speed and reliability (parallel processing, memory caches, etc.)

Primitive operations (e.g., increment counter, add operands) (Arithmetic + Logic & Control)

The fetch–execute cycle:
- Get the current operation pointed to by the program counter (Logic & Control).
- Apply the operation to its arguments (Logic & Control + Arithmetic).
- Store the result (Logic & Control + Memory).
- Update the program counter to point to the next operation (Logic & Control).

Enable construction of and access to data structures (Logic & Control + Memory).

Enable input and output processes (Input/Output).

Enable interrupts, dynamic resource allocation, memory protection (Logic & Control + Memory).

3.2 **The Rejection of the Marrian Approach**

Many readers may think that this positive discussion of Marr's arguments and concepts, which essentially come from the 1970s and 1980s, is out-of-date. It is often believed that the assumption that the way of describing the human mind as analogous to a computer program operating like a poor man's Turing machine is not useful. As discussed in Section 1.7, so-called 'Old-fashioned Strong AI'—the most direct realisation of this approach—was held by many to have burnt out in the 1980s, as its grand program was realised to be impossible (see e.g. Brooks, 1991). Gibsonian psychologists, such as Turvey (1974) and Neisser (1976), held that to do justice to the high number of degrees of freedom of the action system and the high-dimensional way that the perceptual world guides action requires that one develop a dynamical model and not a mono-causal abstraction of a series of discrete stages or operations; this view is supported by a school of philosophy (Port & van Gelder, 1995; van Gelder, 1998). Indeed, at the most abstract level, many philosophers-of-mind rejected functionalism—the view that consciousness is to be understood as a product of certain computational operations of the human cognitive system (e.g. Searle, 1980).

Most of all, however, the rejection of the utility of concepts linked to functional architectures comes from the success of connectionism (see Section 1.7). To the connectionists, the aspects of the conscious human mind that seem most like the products of the operation of the serial computer—reasoning and the like—are seen as the epiphenomenal froth thrown up in the wake of the motor of brain processing. Much more critical, it is felt, is to use concepts abstracted from the operation of the motor itself.[9]

Instead of rejecting the concept of *functional architecture*, we will broaden it and include classes of connectionist concepts discussed in Section 1.7, such as Boltzmann machines and Hopfield nets, as types of functional architectures. We take this approach rather than the dismissal of the three conceptual domain (tri-level) perspective for three reasons. The first is that the connectionist approach to cognitive processes has never eliminated the need for representing the domain of abstract problem analysis distinctly from that of the domains of the algorithms that implement it and more particularly of hardware. Thus a connectionist model of a cognitive process is typically couched as a model of X, where X specifies in an abstract form what input–output

mapping is required of the system being modelled. Take the seminal reading models of Seidenberg and McClelland (1989) and Plaut et al. (1996) that map from the written form of a word to its spoken form (see Figure 3.3). Hypothetically the mapping from the sensory input (not shown) to the input to the computational problem domain, that is in the above example—the orthographic representation[10] of letters and their positions within a word—and the corresponding mapping for outputs, could be realised so that the now many-layered model could represent input–output processing without any explicit representation of concepts like *grapheme*[11] and *phoneme*.[12]

However, as suggested by the arguments in Chapter 2, such a reductionist strategy entails a major intellectual cost. There are questions that are naturally posed if one sees the mapping as one from a set of graphemes to a set of phonemes, which would be far from natural to pose if one viewed the mapping as between certain types of visual squiggles and movements of the articulators. Thus within phonetics there are held to be a hierarchy of units in which speech production is organised: *distinctive features*, *phonemes*, *syllable onsets*, *rimes*, *syllables*, *feet*. One could argue that the existence of such units might be inferred bottom-up from the physiology of the speech production system, although 'might' is very much the operative term, as it would be very difficult to produce. However this could hardly be the case for the existence of units in the orthographic system analogous to those at higher levels of the speech production system, but this has been suspected since the 1970s (see Mewhort & Beal, 1977). One possibility from a reductionist perspective is that higher-level units in the orthographic system correspond to letters that frequently occur together—that form strong sequential dependencies. However, Prinzmetal et al. (1991) showed this was not an adequate account. They used a so-called conjunction error paradigm, where subjects were presented very briefly with words composed of coloured letters. They found that the colour of a letter tended to be misreported as the colour of a neighbouring letter if the two letters were in the same syllable more than if the two letters were in different syllables. Thus within the cognitive, as opposed to reductionist, framework appropriate questions naturally arise such as, for instance, do syllables have orthographic representations as well as speech output ones, or do subsyllabic units such as syllable onset (e.g. *pa* for *pan*) or rhyme (*an* for *pan*) exist

---

[9] For a connectionist criticism of Marr's tri-level framework see Sejnowski and Churchland (1989). Indeed the article can be viewed as an implicit polemic against the utility of cognitive models.

[10] Units relating to written words.

[11] This term is most often used to refer to the written form of a letter but sometimes to the letter cluster that corresponds to a phoneme, e.g. *ch*.

[12] This refers to the smallest linguistically distinctive unit of speech of which one can be aware, e.g. /s/ (in English).

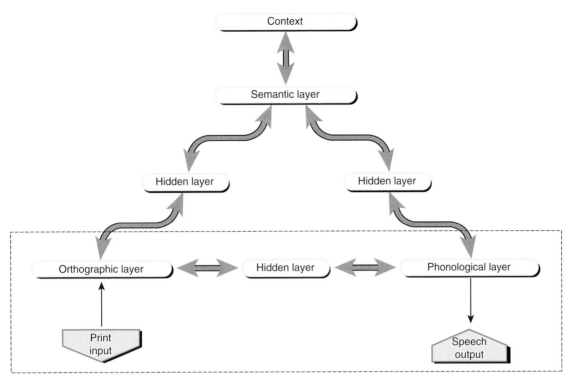

Fig. 3.3 The "triangle" model of reading of Plaut et al (1996). Only the lower section included in the rectangle is implemented.

within the orthographic system, as well as within the speech output one? (But, for somewhat contrasting perspectives in Spanish, see: Álvarez et al., 2004; Conrad et al., 2008) Seeing the mapping in a reductionist fashion as from visual squiggles to movements of the articulators would mean that one would not consider such questions. They demand a different conceptual framework—a cognitive one.

Secondly, connectionist models are often based on earlier information-processing models of the functional architecture. Take again the connectionist models of reading discussed above. As described in Section 1.9, early models based on neuropsychological evidence (e.g. Marshall & Newcombe, 1973) differentiated a semantic route from a phonological route. This differentiation is accepted in virtually all connectionist models of reading, such as that of Plaut et al. (1996), to be discussed extensively in the next chapter. Indeed the only aspect of standard information-processing models of reading not accepted in the Plaut et al. connectionist model framework is the distinction between a lexical and a non-lexical phonological route (compare Figure 3.3 and Figure 3.4, which gives the *Dual-Route Cascaded*, DRC, model of Coltheart et al., 2001).[13] This, however, was never unequivocally accepted by earlier information-processing

theorists attempting to explain neuropsychological evidence (see Shallice et al., 1983; Shallice & McCarthy, 1985; Norris, 1994). Moreover a separation between the two routes has been implemented within connectionist models (see Zorzi et al., 1998; Perry et al., 2007). In this domain, connectionist models are in some respects more detailed implementations of information-processing ones.

There is a third broader reason why a concept like functional architecture must almost certainly be useful. Once you have a set of functions with well-defined interface specifications that can be informally thought of in terms of the box-and-arrow diagrams of cognitive neuropsychology,[14] you can mix and match functions subject to the interface requirements. So a system that is functionally modular has a certain 'generative capacity' where new functions can be assembled out of existing subfunctions. This type of re-use is more efficient from an engineering perspective than engineering each global function from scratch.

The most critical point is that any specific connectionist model is necessarily grossly simplified by comparison with the system that it is held to represent. While it is rarely done, the model—or occasionally the models—actually implemented is (or are) treated as one

---

[13] The Dual-Route Cascaded model is in fact a 3-route model, as we will see later.

[14] For a formal characterisation see the signature conceptual framework of Fox et al. (2006).

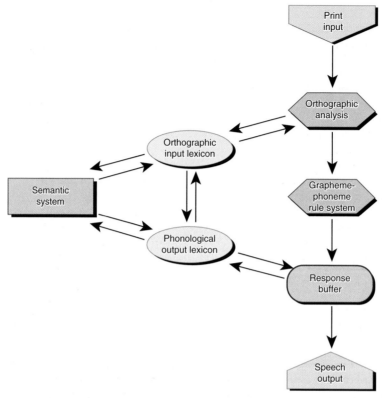

Fig. 3.4 The so-called 'Dual-Route' Cascaded (DRC) model of reading of Coltheart et al (2001).

(or more) example(s) of a broad class of models which have a set of common properties. One of the broad class of models is presupposed to correspond to the relevant subsystems in the brain itself. Just occasionally, as in the models of deep dyslexia to be discussed in Section 4.10, the theory of the models is made explicit. It is held that models with a certain set of abstract properties will, if damaged, give rise to certain sorts of behaviours. Then the theory corresponds more to the *computational task* domain of Marr, with the actual implementations being in the functional architecture domain.

3.3 Modules, Isolable Subsystems and Functional Specialisation

As far as cognition is concerned, the arguments discussed in the last section are negative ones for not dismissing as part of the intellectual flotsam of a past century the concepts of the tri-level approach and more specifically *functional architecture*. However, they do not provide a strong positive argument that any doubters need to confront concretely. One should also consider why the concept is scientifically useful for understanding cognitive processes.

It is impossible in a book of this size to consider all the functional architectures that have been proposed. Thus Dawson (1998), for instance, lists 24 examples and

many more could be considered. Leaving aside the extension to connectionist models in the preceding section, functional architectures have components and so componentiality needs to be justified. A prerequisite for the concept of functional architecture to be valuable comes from the utility of the concepts of *isolable subsystem* and of *modularity* discussed in Chapter 2.

Moreover, given the discussions, in Sections 3 and 4 of the last chapter, of the complexity and lack of empirical power of cognitive tasks, it may well be that the only tractable way to decompose, even a simple and rapid piece of cognitive processing, is by starting with a modular theory. Subsequent discussion in later chapters will suggest that the strategy, apparently similar to that of the drunk looking under the street light for his lost wallet, may actually work! However, we are used to mechanisms having components. We find it easy, possibly too easy, to use modularity as a conceptual approach.[15] As discussed in the last chapter (Section 2.4),

---

[15] In the next chapter we will discuss a critique of the use of modularity for explaining neuropsychological dissociations, that of van Orden, Pennington and Stone (2001). On looking it up in Google Scholar we noted that the first listed citation quoted it as justifying inferences to modularity from double dissociations, so ingrained is the conceptual framework!

the philosopher Jerry Fodor (1983) made the concept of modularity explicit in a way that made little reference to the earlier information-processing literature which had made extensive, and mainly implicit, use of the related but looser notion of *isolable subsystem*. However, as we also discussed, for Fodor for a system to be a module it had to pass 11 (!) criteria and at least one of the eleven is clearly invalid. We cannot, therefore, be as constraining about the properties of modules as Fodor wanted to be. Yet Fodor showed that the idea needs some flesh. We will list properties of what we will generally call *isolable subsystems*, or *systems* for short, to distinguish the current conceptual framework from that of Fodor.[16]

The simplest notion accepted by many information-processing psychologists such as Posner (1978), Tulving (1985) and one of us (FNMS Chapter 2) is well articulated by Sternberg (2001) whose characterisation of modularity is:

M1: '*Two parts (sub-processes)* ***A*** *and* ***B*** *of a complex (mental) process are defined as modules, if and only if, they are separately modifiable.*' (p. 151)

This is an operational criterion. However, it may be considered to be too broad. It depends on what one means by a mental process. Thus one can damage independently two different regions of a continuum of a processing space such as that realised in area V1 (see Shallice, 1988). One would not want to call them 'isolable subsystems'. Or consider layers in a multi-layer connectionist net. One would hardly want to call them each a subsystem.

To partly deal with these issues and to relate the concept of modularity to that of functional architecture, we will add:

M2: *The process carried out in the subsystem, so modifiable, computes a particular type of input–output mapping—which at the finest grain we will call a basic cognitive operation. This can be characterised as having a discrete subfunction within the system as a whole.*

This criterion is of course far from being operationalisable. It depends on theory. Moreover, again one can view a given layer of hidden units as transducing between domain A and domain B and so having a discrete subfunction. So, it is unclear how useful it is to consider a system which satisfies just M1 and M2 as modular. A system that satisfies them need have only *weak modularity*.[17]

For *strong modularity* in addition one needs additional criteria. One possibility is:

M?: *There exists a decomposition of the system such that the computational interactions within subsystems are much more complex than those between subsystems.*

This reflects a very common view. However, one should bear in mind the comments of Mumford (1994), namely 'In the cortex, roughly 65% of all cells are pyramidal cells which send their output to distant cortical areas, as well as locally via their axon collaterals. This means that there is *no hiding of local information*, no 'local variables' or protected data. [...] Instead of black boxes with opaque walls, we have apartments in a cheap housing complex with very thin walls! All your neighbours hear everything which is going on in your home. Instead of 'hiding local variables', a device central to all modular programming, every little whimsy that occurs to you goes out instantly to all and sundry.' (p. 135). We therefore favour a very different type of constraint, namely:

M3: *The output of the system is characterisable as a representation.*

This implies that the system computes a function in a low-dimensional space with each dimension being either discrete (categorical) or continuous.[18] Where there are multiple recipient systems, M3 would be compatible with Newell's (1990) characterisation of a 'symbol', namely a pattern that provides the same one-to-one mapping onto patterns in *more than one* distal system within the overall cognitive system. Again this is a theoretically dependent criterion.

If the Marrian framework is to be useful in cognitive neuroscience, there needs to be a brain basis to the concept, so in addition we assume:

M4: *The subsystem needs to be relatively spatially localised in the brain.*[19]

---

[16] There is no material difference between a *system* and a *subsystem*. The difference depends purely on the context in which the system/subsystem is considered.

[17] We will see in the next chapter, in the discussion of the connectionist model of reading-to-meaning of Plaut and Shallice (1993a), that one can obtain *partially* separable *non-transparent* modifiability, in the sense that lesions to one part of a complex system can affect processing more related to one stimulus set and those to another part affect processing more related to a different stimulus set. Yet the functions separately damaged are only highly indirectly related to the measures which operationalise the double dissociation.

[18] The lowness of the dimensionality needs to be at least 3. Consider either the position of an object in 3D space (continuous) or the maximum number of arguments of a verb (discrete). In linguistics a verb like *pour* takes three arguments concerning the source, theme—i.e. the liquid—and the destination.

[19] The issue of how and why modules evolved is complex. We refer the reader to Bullinaria (2007, 2009), for a computational analysis of the issue (see also Section 3.7.).

Can one obtain purely behavioural evidence for the existence of modularity for cognitive processes? The classic arguments stemming from Chomskyan linguistics for the computational modularity of syntactic processing are undermined in psycholinguistic experiments by, for instance, the demonstration of the many ways by which semantic factors influence parsing.[20] Thus, Tannenhaus et al. (1995) presented subjects, who were looking at a scene, with a sentence and monitored their eye movements to objects in the scene referred to by the sentence, as they heard it. Analysis of the eye movements did not produce what one would expect given a purely syntactic parsing account of how the sentence would be understood. For instance, when the sentence *Put the apple on the towel in the box* occurred and there was only one towel present, they supported the assumption that subjects interpret *the towel* as the destination of the movement. When, however, two towels are present, the interpretation appears to be that *on the towel* refers to the initial location of the apple. Thus parsing is influenced by the semantics of the scene.

Turning to information-processing psychology, behavioural methods *alone* rarely provide strong evidence for a particular modular structure and hence for modularity itself. Take the Baddeley–Hitch working memory model discussed in Chapter 1 as a paradigmatic model of the later part of the early development of information-processing psychology. We will see in Section 7.5 that in a somewhat modified form, namely that of Baddeley (1986), it accounts very well for both neuropsychological findings and functional imaging findings. However, as we will again see in Section 7.7, it has had its hegemony challenged by a host of competitors. Moreover it has spawned a number of more detailed implementations which are at best only weakly modular. Behavioural evidence does not clearly distinguish between them.

The clearest purely behavioural examples that apply property M1 are the use of chronometric procedures, particularly those of Sternberg (1969, 2001). This is because, unlike most psychological theorising, the approach does not rely on balancing the relative strengths of evidential support across a wide set of different experimental paradigms. Sternberg (2001) gives a most detailed analysis of his concept of modularity (assumption M1) and provides many relevant empirical examples. He differentiates two basic ways by which one may provide support for the existence of a modular system. Basic to both is the idea of whether one can find two factors *F* and *G* which influence the two hypothetical processes **A** and **B** selectively, in the sense that *F* should influence **A** but not **B** and *G* should have the

complementary effect of influencing **B** but not **A**.[21] However, Sternberg points out that we cannot observe the effects of *F* on **A** and of *G* on **B** directly, but only on measures that reflect these effects. Where Sternberg's two methods differ is in how these influences are manifested in measures of behaviour or brain states. It should be appreciated that, as Sternberg points out, just as for neuropsychological double dissociations (see FNMS Chapter 11), the finding of two factors *F* and *G* with such selective effects, does not *prove* the underlying system is modular. The degree to which that hypothesis is supported depends on the plausibility of any alternative hypotheses which make the same prediction.

When *pure measures*—M_A and M_B—are available, then a variation in factor *F* needs to influence M_A but not M_B, with variation in factor *G* having the complementary effect. Sternberg gives three examples. The most clear-cut support for such separability of process is provided by an example from the operation of a timing subsystem in the rat. Using a Skinner Box, Roberts (1981) found that the *peak rate* of lever pressing and the *peak time* at which lever pressing occurs are influenced by different factors. Unfortunately this is an example from a paradigm far from cognition. However, relatively pure measures do occur in cognition. Thus, the Glanzer and Cunitz study of the effect of different factors in serial position curves, discussed in Section 1.4, is one such. Certain factors, such as interfering material presented at the end of the list, affect only the recency part of a serial position curve in a free recall of word lists experiment. Other factors, such as rate of presentation, affect the amount retrieved in the early part.[22]

Sternberg's own major innovation (in Sternberg, 1969) was to introduce a critical procedure in the second situation, when only *composite measures* M_{AB} are available; that is, where each measure reflects the operation of more than one process. Combining them requires a *composite rule*. This was his *additive factors* procedure for combining different levels of the two factors *F* and *G*. The *composite measure* originally used by Sternberg was reaction time, as briefly discussed in Section 1.10. The *composite rule* was the sum, it being required that:

$$RT = K + T_A + T_B,$$

where T_A is the time to carry out process **A**, influenced by factor *F* but not factor *G*,

T_B is the time to carry out process **B** influenced by factor *G* but not factor *F*,

and *K* is a constant.

---

[20] See Harley (2008) for an excellent review.

[21] This was called the critical variable methodology in cognitive neuropsychology; see FNMS Chapter 10.

[22] In fact the second set of factors also affects the last few serial positions. So the example is not completely clean.

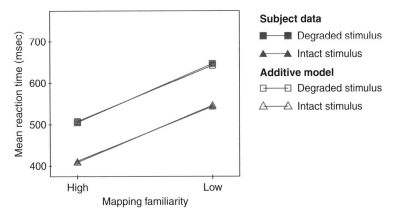

Fig. 3.5 Results of the study of Sanders, Wijnen and van Arkel (1982). Subjects viewed dot-patterns of digits which were either intact or degraded, and responded either with the digit's name or the name of the successor digit. The human data (in red) matches well with an additive model (in blue). (Data from A.F. Sanders, J.L.C. Wijnen and A.E. van Arkel, 1982, An additive factor analysis of the effects of sleep loss on reaction processes, Acta Psychologica, 51, 41–59.)

These give rise to another possible criterion for a subsystem using Sternberg's (2001) ideas on stages of processing:

> M?: *Subsystems are the seats of 'functionally distinct operations that occur during non-overlapping epochs, and such that responses occur when both[23] operations have been completed'* (Sternberg, 2001, pp. 159–160).

This presupposes that the transmission of information from one subsystem to the next essentially occurs as a packet, short in time compared with that of the operation of the subsystem. Each subsystem is then responsible for a discrete processing stage. An example is where one factor affects visual operations and a second affects language ones. Take, for instance, the study of Sanders (1998), which Sternberg gives. Subjects saw on a screen one of the digits 2, 3, 4, 5 depicted in dot patterns, and had to respond with a name 'two', 'three', 'four' and 'five'. The visual factor varied was perceptual difficulty, produced by degrading the stimulus with yet further dots. The language factor varied was the conceptual difficulty, by having the subject respond in one set of conditions by the next digit name, i.e. 'three' for 2 instead of by its own name 'two'. The results, which fit with a modular decomposition approach, are shown in Figure 3.5.

However, there are two major problems for the Sternberg method. One is that models with quite different underlying principles—in particular, ones that do not fit this criterion—can produce a similar pattern of results. Thus Sternberg gives the examples of McClelland's (1979) cascade model of reading, an activation-based model, which is a precursor to the interactive-activation model of McClelland and Rumelhart (1981) to be discussed

later in Section 3.7. It has been shown by Ashby (1982) that it can produce close approximations to that given by additive factors for the predictions on observed means. And Miller, van der Ham and Sanders (1995) show that other types of cascade model can give roughly additive effects on means and in some cases on variances. Roberts and Sternberg (1993) argue that these alternatives can be distinguished from the modular model by more refined aspects of the RT distributions, but this is a rather outré response. Indeed Ashby (1982), commenting on differences between a purely additive stages model and nonadditivities produced by McClelland's cascade model, concludes that 'only a remarkable empirical effort would succeed in detecting these nonadditivities' (p. 605). In this respect the Sternberg approach using behavioural evidence is subject to a very general problem for purely behavioural evidence—that it is often possible to build a number of plausible models of a process and it is unclear from purely behavioural data which is to be preferred.[24]

There are few theorists who would deny the existence of some qualitative functional step at some point within the cognitive system between the analysis of perceptual input and the preparing of the response output, which are what the Sanders (1998) study aims to differentiate. The second major problem for the additive-factors approach is that it is much more critical to specify the internal organisation within each of the systems and within other high-level systems. We know of only one case where methods such as these have been used to analyse the functional architecture of a tightly organised system with many hypothetical subsystems such as those involved in, say, reading (e.g. Coltheart et al., 2001) or

---

[23] For generality, 'all' would be preferable to 'both'.

[24] The alternative models of the reading process are an obvious example of this point—see Section 1.8 and Chapter 4.

speech production (e.g. Levelt, 1989).[25] Yet within these grosser processing domains it is much more probable that the relation between successive subsystems is non-linear than linear (Harrison et al., 2007).

The existence of these two unresolved problems is discouraging for purely behavioural experiments. However, it should be noted that behavioural measures are not alone in under-determining the possible models that can explain them. We will see a similar problem occurring in one aspect of neuropsychology in the next chapter. Moreover, it is not clear that single-cell recordings, say, also sufficiently constrain the possible plausible models of how neural systems operate. Thus, radically different approaches to the computational function of V1 are beginning to be produced, claiming it is involved in many levels of visual analysis on the basis of single-cell recording. Deco and Lee (2004) argue that V1 neurons are involved in multiple visual routines including higher-level visual processing. We do not have a view on these ideas. However they suggest that any single level analysis of brain processing may well be insufficient.

Can we provide stronger evidence for modular structure? We will argue in the next two chapters that to combine evidence from neuropsychology and functional imaging with the purely behavioural evidence is the way forward.[26] However, if modularity is to be in any way plausible in cognitive neuroscience, then it must have an anatomical basis.

3.4 The Anatomical Bases of Modularity

Two contrasting principles can be seen to apply in the anatomy of the cerebral cortex. The first is a basic similarity of structure throughout the cortex. The local organisation of the cortex is grossly the same wherever it is examined (Rockel et al., 1980; Braitenberg & Schuz, 1991). Thus it typically has a 6-layer structure with bottom-up input arriving at layer 4 and top-down input in layers 1 and 2. Moreover it has been argued (Douglas & Martin, 1991) that there is a basic neural circuit which is reproduced across different regions of cortex.

At the same time, if one looks in more detail, there are many differences between regions, more minor but consistently occurring across different members of a species. In the first decade of the twentieth century, the study of these differences—cytoarchitectonics—led the German anatomists Korbinian Brodmann and Oskar Vogt, and an Australian one, Alfred Walter Campbell, to divide the cortex into regions according to its local structure. The divisions were based on the number and structure of individual layers in particular areas, the density of cells and cell sizes—both overall and within given layers—the total thickness of cortex and the relative thickness of different layers. To these can be added the connectivity, which for instance delimits area V5/MT, discussed in the previous chapter.[27] Yet other divisions can be made using more complex measures—immunological, histological or physiological (Douglas & Martin, 1991). To complicate matters still further, some of the divisions are sharp, while others are more gradual.

The anatomical differences were originally codified in a series of papers and were summarised by Brodmann in his 1909 book. Each hemisphere was divided into about 50 areas.[28] Minor anatomical differences exist between most areas, but the connectivity of a particular region is also specific and the functional responses of the cells tend to be different. This is also true of anterior regions; there is no gross evidence of less differentiation in more anterior systems as one might expect on the equipotential central system hypothesis of Fodor discussed in the previous chapter. For instance, Figure 3.6 from Rempel-Clower and Barbas (2000), shows the nature of connectivity between different parts of frontal cortices (lateral: Brodmann area (BA) 8, 9, 10, 12 and 46; orbital: BA 11, 13, 14 and 25) and of temporal cortex (BA 28 and 36 and an area called TE). It can be seen that the connections are not only specific to parts of each lobe but also to different layers of cortex within those lobes. This clearly suggests functional differences. The connections shown in Figure 3.6 are from the rhesus monkey but it is implausible that the human brain is any less specific.[29]

---

[25] The exception is in the WEAVER implementation of part of Levelt's model by Roelofs (1997) discussed in Section 3.5.

[26] Sternberg (2001), himself, gives two possible lines which use cognitive neuroscience evidence.

[27] V5/MT was originally characterised both for anatomical and physiological reasons. It was a densely myelinated area of cortex, which physiologically contained a so-called *retinotopic map* of the contralateral visual field (Allman & Kaas, 1971). In other words, the part of V5/MT that is activated relates in a systematic way to the position on the retina of the stimulus.

[28] One problem with Brodmann's analysis is that it was based on a single human brain. Moreover, many neuroanatomists consider the Brodmann terminology misleading for particular areas of cortex. The alternative, however, is to use a wide range of different verbal labels for areas, each with its own anatomical implications. For simplicity and because of its widespread use, we will generally use Brodmann area labels.

[29] As far as Fodor's overall thesis is concerned, it should not, though, be assumed that anatomical differences necessarily refute the hypothesis of some form of decreasing functional specialisation with conceptual distance from sensory and motor systems. Indeed as one moves from primary cortical areas (such as BA 1, 2, 3, the primary somatosensory system) to supramodal ones, there is an increase in the total length of the dendrites of neurons of about one-third and in the number

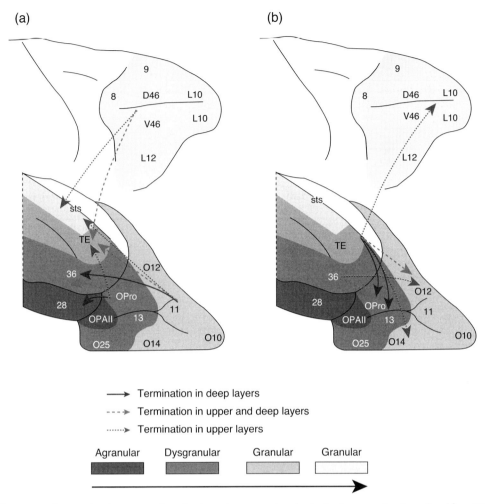

Fig. 3.6 The pattern of connections between prefrontal and anterior temporal cortices in the rhesus monkey. Reproduced from N.L. Rempel-Clower and H. Barbas, The laminar pattern of connections between prefrontal and anterior temporal cortices in the Rhesus monkey is related to cortical structure and function, Cerebral Cortex, 2000, 10(9), 851–865, by permission of Oxford University Press.

This anatomical and physiological type of differentiation of regions occurs on a number of different anatomical grains. In the visual brain—the part of the cortex where the activity of cells can be increased by visual stimuli—much more specific anatomical organisation is known based on the detailed neuroanatomy, on the responsiveness of cells to particular types of stimuli, and on connectivity. This has led to the use of Zeki's V-nomenclature for regions smaller than Brodmann

areas (see Figure 3.7), with V1 as the initial processing region for visual input at the cortical level. However, even those regions are being subdivided, especially the higher ones. For instance, region V6 in Brodmann area 19 has been subdivided into a more purely visual area V6 and a visuomotor one V6a (Galletti et al., 1996) (see Figure 3.8). This is based both on the pattern of connectivity to other regions and on the different conditions under which the firing of the cells can be driven.

It is not just the visual brain which is being divided more finely. Similarly the premotor area—Brodmann area 6—is now divided into a considerable set of subregions F1 to F7 (Matelli et al., 1985). Areas 20 and 21 of temporal cortex have been divided into four subregions (Morel & Bullier, 1990), and so on.

How do these subregions connect with other regions? The fronto-parietal connections are collectively known as the 'dorsal route' being involved in co-ordinating

---

of dendritic spines, the regions of neurons where most input synapses occur, of about two-thirds (Jacobs et al., 2001). This implies that regions of the brain with the more abstract functions have the highest connectivity. However this change is not an all-or-none one across critical regions, as a very crude anatomical realisation of Fodor's framework might suggest, but a graded one across types of cortical regions.

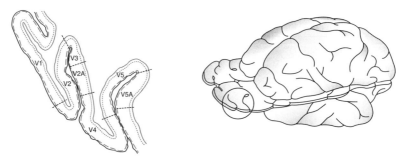

Fig. 3.7 A horizontal section through the occipital lobe of the macaque monkey brain, showing the anatomical organisation of Zeki's V nomenclature for regions of the visual cortex. Adapted with permission of Royal Society Publishing from S. Zeki, 2005, The Ferrier Lecture 1995. Behind the Seen: The functional specialization of the brain in space and time. Philosophical Transactions of the Royal Society B: Biological Sciences, 360(1458), 1145–1183 (Figure 4b, p. 1149).

visuo-motor interactions in the control of simple actions, and grossly contrasting with the 'ventral route' concerned with object identification (Ungerleider & Mishkin, 1982; Milner & Goodale, 1995). They have been mapped in great detail (see Figure 3.8) and involve a highly complex but specific set of connections. Any individual region receives its main input from a small set of other regions but also has a weaker input from a wide set of others. What do these regions do? They are collectively involved in sensorimotor integration between eye, hand and arm in reaching and grasping objects. This is more properly the role of the dorsal–dorsal route (Rizolatti & Matelli, 2003) involving more superior parietal regions. As we will see in Chapter 8, more inferior parietal regions—a complementary ventral-dorsal route—implement more complex activities which depend on eye-hand co-ordination. As far as lower-level motor control is concerned, the neurons, for instance, in VIP—the ventral intraparietal regions—are activated by both visual and somatosensory input in certain positions, and primarily by stimuli the animal can reach (Colby et al., 1993). They are particularly active during movements to the mouth. Those neurons in the medial intraparietal regions, MIP, are similar but the response of the neuron is dependent upon the position of the monkey's arm. They are critically involved in reaching (Snyder et al., 2000). The anterior intraparietal region (AIP) responds to moving stimuli in any modality. They elicit grasping (Murata et al., 2000). The neurons in the lateral intraparietal (LIP) region are triggered during eye movements (Andersen et al., 2004).

Most of these effects are described from the use of single cell recording in the monkey. However it has been shown by functional imaging that similar structures exist in the human (see Culham & Valyear, 2006). Thus Bremmer et al. (2001) extrapolated from the single-cell recording studies of AIP. They examined the regions which are activated by movement in different modalities using Price and Friston's cognitive conjunction methodology to be discussed in Section 5.7. Their results

are shown in Figure 3.9. One region in each hemisphere was activated by a moving stimulus, regardless of the modality in which it was presented. This was in the intraparietal sulcus, just as for the monkey.

We may now ask whether these subregions, which have different connectivity to other regions and have different cellular properties, could be the potential hardware basis of subsystems. They are certainly less informationally encapsulated than idealised Fodorian modules as they often receive input from quite a wide set of systems, but their *main* inputs come from a fairly limited set of other regions. More important, from a negative perspective as far as Fodorian modules are concerned, they have strong top-down inputs. Most critically, to see them as computationally modular is misleading as they are part of a complex system where their computations are being integrated on-line in real time with those of other subsystems in the operation of a more global process, the linking of vision with on-line action. When you use an object you typically first look at it, then move towards it, look at it again, reach and then grasp it (Land et al., 1999). Thus a notion of discrete modules à la Fodor is inappropriate. At the very least though they could be thought of as the anatomical basis for isolable processing subsystems with subsystem characteristics M1—concerned with separability—and M4—with spatial localisability. Without a more adequate computational account of the whole system, which we still do not have, it is impossible to decide about M2 and M3—whether the system computes a subfunction with outputs corresponding to representations. From the Marconi et al. depictions (Figure 3.8), it would appear that the same output is *not* generally being used by multiple subsequent subsystems, suggesting that M3 may not hold. However these subsystems also form many hierarchies with, say, the ventral intraparietal regions (VIP) being part of the dorsal visual system which is itself part of the higher visual system. We will call them collectively the *object use system*.

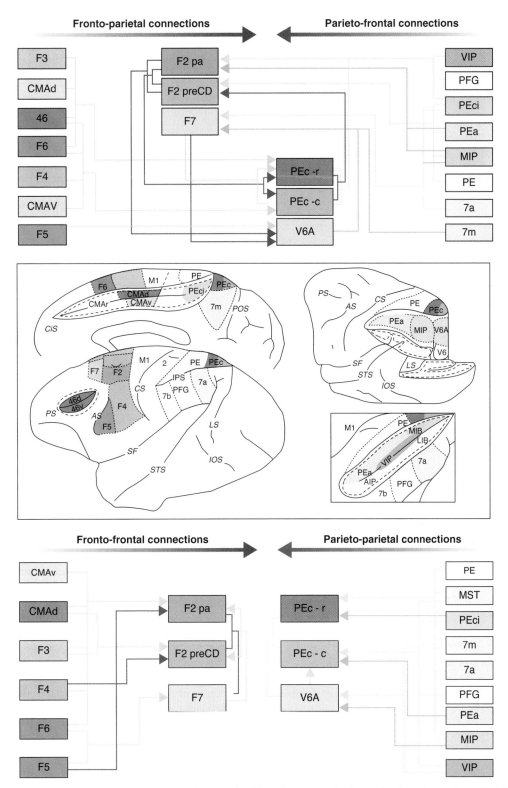

Fig. 3.8 Anatomical relationships between systems in the parietal and frontal cortices involved in eye-hand coordination in reaching for an object. Reproduced from B. Marconi, A. Genovesio, A. Battaglia-Mayer, S. Ferraina, S. Squatrito, M. Molinari, F. Lacquaniti and R. Caminiti, Eye-hand coordination during reaching. I. Anatomical relationships between parietal and frontal cortex, Cerebral Cortex, 2001, 11(6), 513–527, by permission of Oxford University Press.

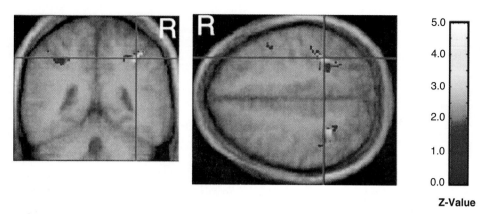

Fig. 3.9 Regions activated in posterior parietal and premotor cortex involved in multi-modal motion processing. Reprinted from Neuron, 29(1), F. Bremmer, A. Schlack, N.J. Shah, O. Zafiris, M. Kubischik, K.-P. Hoffmann, K. Zilles and G.R. Fink, Polymodal motion processing in posterior parietal and premotor cortex: A human fMRI study strongly implies equivalencies between humans and monkeys, pp 287–296, Copyright (2001), with permission from Elsevier.

But, the reader may well ask, why should one consider the system dealing with visuo-motor connections as having relevance for understanding the brain bases of cognition? Visuo-motor co-ordination is unconscious. Much of cognition is conscious. As we will see in Chapter 11 this is a treacherous basis on which to make a principled division between higher and lower-level processing. But visuo-motor co-ordination is also not symbolic. Cognition is typically symbolic.

This response though would be premature. As we will see in Chapters 6 and 8, the left inferior parietal lobe plays a key role in a key human accomplishment—tool use. And one can see the precursors of this in the monkey. In certain neurons on the anterior bank of the intraparietal sulcus, the size of the receptive field can expand when a tool is being used (Iriki et al., 1996) (see Figure 3.10). Moreover, consider a prototypically symbolic activity—the use of syntax—which incidentally is typically processed in an unconscious fashion. How did syntax evolve? Some authors (Hauser et al., 2002) argue that it just involved the evolution of recursion (see Jackendoff & Pinker, 2005, for a critique).[30] Alternatively others, e.g. Rizzolatti and Arbib (1998), have suggested language evolved from the systems necessary for the control of action. Consider a concept like argument-structure. As Schwartz et al. (1991) have shown, related concepts are required in understanding high-level

disorders of action (see Chapter 8) so the Rizzolatti–Arbib position is inherently plausible. Moreover consider the relation between semantics and syntax. Behavioural experiments, as we discussed in the last section, show that these syntactic choices are influenced by semantic ones and vice versa. A structure with some similarity to that of the interplay of the subsystems in visuo-motor control of action seems to be required.[31]

None of these, though, are compelling arguments. However, one domain, which even the most refined cognitive afficianado would accept as symbolic, is the domain of number—the basis of our deepest type of abstraction—mathematics. A critical region involved in certain aspects of the processing of number is the intraparietal sulcus, home to many of the types of visuo-motor transformations discussed above. Thus, Eger et al. (2003) presented numbers, letters and colours and had subjects respond to particular targets within each category. Numbers selectively activated the intraparietal sulcus bilaterally. As Simon et al. (2002) have shown, the regions involved in basic forms of number processing—particularly those involved in estimating small numerosities in the process called subitising—are in close proximity with the regions concerned with the object use system discussed above (see Figure 3.11). Why should this be? A promising proposal is the hypothesis of Feigenson and Carey (2003) that subitising develops from the system involved in keeping track of the paths of each of a small number of objects in order to act appropriately to individual ones. Pylyshyn and Storm (1988) have shown that we have this capacity for up to 5 objects when presented with 20 identical moving ones. On this hypothesis it is not surprising

---

[30] Hauser et al. never characterise what they mean by 'recursion', other than saying that it provides 'the capacity to generate an infinite range of expressions from a finite range of elements' (p 1569). Thus it allows the generation of structured expressions where the structure exceeds that allowed by a finite-state grammar—see Section 1.5. In computer science a recursive process is more restricted, namely to one that calls itself. Hauser et al. suggest that this potential for recursion is derived from hippocampal processing. This is grossly implausible.

---

[31] Except that the semantic processing would also involve the inferior temporal cortex; see Chapter 6.

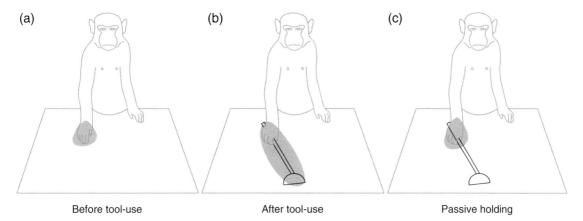

Fig. 3.10 Receptive fields of a cell in the intraparietal sulcus in three conditions of the Iriki et al study. Reprinted from Trends in Cognitive Sciences, 8(2), A. Maravita and A. Iriki, Tools for the body (schema), pp 79–86. Copyright (2007) with permission from Elsevier.

that the two processes are dependent upon anatomically related structures. Cognitive processing and non-cognitive (e.g. sensory-motor) processing are not hermetically sealed to each other. New functional subsystems may evolve in the human by evolutionary piggy-backing on systems carrying more primitive

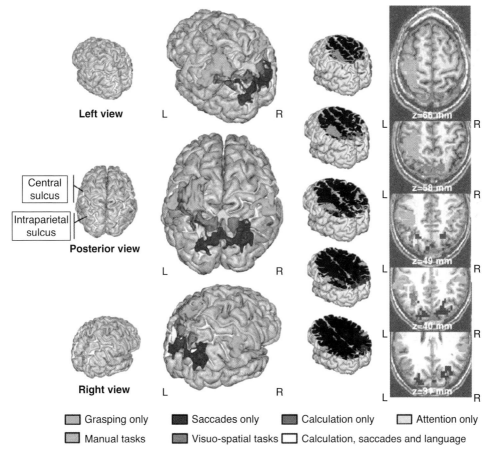

Fig. 3.11 Regions activated in and near the intraparietal sulcus in tasks requiring simple arithmetic operations and ones involved in hand-eye coordination in reaching or grasping. Reprinted from Neuron, 33(3), O. Simon, J.-F. Mangin, L. Cohen, D. Le Bihan and S. Dehaene, Topographical Layout of Hand, Eye, Calculation, and Language-Related Areas in the Human Parietal Lobe, 475–487, Copyright (2002), with permission from Elsevier.

functions with which they continue to co-exist, as we discussed for the hippocampus (see Section 2.2).

Leaving this issue aside, a weakened version of the *isolable subsystem* concept as a processing unit in the cognitive system is clearly compatible with what is known of the anatomy of the cerebral cortex. However it is not necessarily entailed by it.

This discussion can be summarised by outlining a set of additional properties of isolable subsystems which will be assessed later in the book. We therefore extend the properties listed in Section 3.3, beginning with Fodor's most basic property of a module:

M5: *Subsystems form into complex networks with other subsystems, so that each is carrying out only a particular subfunction of a much more complex overall function. Individual subsystems may enter into a variety of such networks each with a different overall function.*

M6: *Subsystems may have overlapping functions with other subsystems, in particular when the function of a higher-level process piggy-backs on that of a lower-level one.*

M7: *The functions of subsystems can be highly abstract.*[32]

M8: *The anatomical realisation of subsystems, specified in assumption M4, does not entail that they collectively 'tile' the cortex physically such that any neuron, hyper-column (or other anatomical unit) is a part of only one system; they could be part of more than one.*[33]

Indeed there are many claims that individual regions of cortex can subserve multiple functions. Thus Broca's area, traditionally the seat of key output speech functions (see Figure 1.1) has been held to be involved in recognition of bodily actions, syntax, musical syntax and harmonic sequence analysis, working memory, phonological-to-orthographic translation, inner speech and detecting embedded figures (Skoyles, personal communication). M.L. Anderson (2007) has indeed argued that individual brain regions are activated on average by over 9 types of task. In our view it is currently impossible to make any such estimate, since we have no inventory of I-O functions or of what size regions of cortex should count as a brain region. However we think it likely that extensive overlapping of the tiling of I-O functions onto the brain exists.

We require one final assumption:

M9: *Subsystems can be acquired by learning.*[34]

---

[32] This relates to the issue just discussed, but it will be considered in more detail in Chapters 9 and 12.

[33] This is the anatomical complement of assumption M6.

[34] See the discussion of the word-form system in Sections 4.12 and 5.10.

We will redefine a *non-brain based form of weak modularity* as the property of any system which satisfies assumptions M1, M2 (with *function* broadly characterised so as to include hidden units), M5, M6, M7 and M8. In its brain-based form we add M4 and M9. For *strong modularity* we add M3.

3.5 Information-processing models: the example of speech production

We have just seen that the concept of an isolable subsystem is compatible with the anatomy of the cortex but it is not entailed by it. From the computational perspective, in a Marrian fashion as discussed in Section 3.1, complex functions that need to be carried out by the cognitive system can often be divided naturally into different subfunctions, where each subfunction that is frequently employed can be realised by a very different type of computational transformation.[35] Moreover, this can be done from an information-processing perspective independently of knowledge of the brain basis.

Consider the production of speech. There is an enormous amount of knowledge and many theories about particular aspects of it: of syntactic aspects, as discussed in Sections 1.5 and 1.7; of how individual words are put together from their underlying components that have relevance at the semantic or syntactic level (*morphemes*) like *bigger* from *big* and *...er*; of the phonological structure of words and of phenomena like stress patterns both internal to the word and across a string of words. We have perhaps less secure knowledge of other aspects—of what can be spoken about, of the social organisation of conversation, of pragmatics—but even in these areas there is still much that is known. However, until the 1980s relatively little was known about the general organisation of the systems underlying it, how these different aspects interacted with each other, and especially how they interacted in real time when one produced speech. This situation began to change in the 1980s. Then the American, Merrill Garrett (1980, 1988), and in more detail the Dutchman, Pim Levelt (1989; Levelt et al., 1999), put forward theoretical frameworks, which appeared to capture many aspects of the whole underlying structure. The theoretical

---

[35] Consider two transformations $I_1 \rightarrow O_1$ and $I_2 \rightarrow O_2$ and assume that there is a similarity metric across all pairs (I_{1i}, I_{1j}), across all pairs (I_{2i}, I_{2j}), across all pairs (O_{1i}, O_{1j}) and across all pairs (O_{2i}, O_{2j}). Then the two transformations $I_1 \rightarrow O_1$ and $I_2 \rightarrow O_2$ would be of 'a very different type' if there is no pair of mappings such that if {I, O} maps input/output pairs of one transformation onto input/output pairs of the other transformation, then (i) I is similarity-preserving from I_1 to I_2, and (ii) O is similarity-preserving from O_1 to O_2.

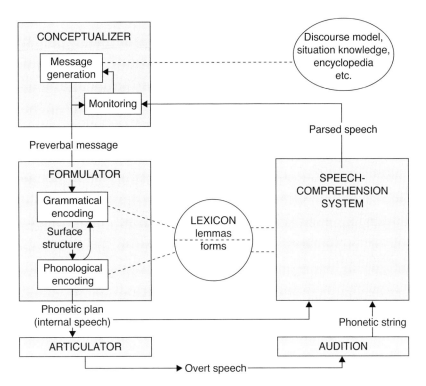

Fig. 3.12 Levelt's (1989) "blueprint" for the speaker as an information processing system. Boxes represent processing components while circles/ellipses represent knowledge stores. Reproduced from Levelt, W. J. M., Speaking: From Intention to Articulation, figure 1.1, page 9, © 1989 Massachusetts Institute of Technology, by permission of The MIT Press.

framework Levelt, in particular, articulated is far from completely accepted (for alternatives see e.g. Foygel & Dell, 2000; Caramazza, 1997). However, it represents the one that most broadly characterises the different types of computational tasks involved in speech production.

In Marrian fashion, Levelt's approach involves three grains of theorising. The coarsest grain is to subdivide the overall process of transforming thought into utterances into three broad component processes with apparently very different computational tasks, one process being subdivided into two parts; in addition, more controversially, it characterises the representations which are passed from one component process to the next. This is illustrated in Figure 3.12.

For instance, the *Conceptualiser* realises thought in what is termed a *preverbal message*. The preverbal message has many characteristics. It must specify the nature of the speech act, whether it is a question, directive or command, say, and the degree of politeness required. It must specify the time of what is referred to—past, present or future. It must contain a propositional structure that will involve function/argument relations of various degrees of complexity, as mentioned in Section 3.4. It also requires more subtle information, such as what is the focus of the utterance. The elements of this are held to be lexical concepts.

Essentially the existence of the *Conceptualiser* is inferred mainly by a priori means in Levelt's initial account of his theory. The representations in the core part of the speech production system, such as those involved in morphological, syntactic and phonological operations, are very different and obey different rules from those processes giving rise to what can be spoken about or those concerned with specifying the nature of the speech act, per se. Thus the *Formulator* deals with certain clearly language-related operations, such as compiling the syntax of an utterance, and the *Conceptualiser's* role is to produce an input on which the *Formulator's* operations can plausibly operate. However, although the concept of the *Conceptualiser* was initially put forward by Levelt principally for a priori reasons related to giving a complete account of the whole speech production process, since then, a disorder at the *Conceptualiser* stage of processing has proved to be a valuable characterisation of a neuropsychological syndrome—*dynamic aphasia* (Warren et al., 2003; Robinson et al., 2005)—to be discussed in Section 9.13. In this syndrome, the patient is able to produce what are syntactically and phonologically quite complex sentences, such as those used in describing a picture presented to them, but they have great problems in producing sentences in most other situations; for instance, they are grossly impaired in producing a

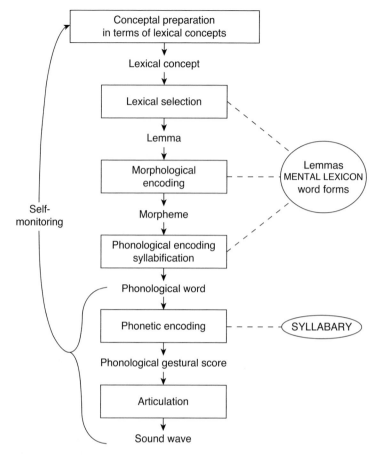

Fig. 3.13 Subprocesses held to be involved in the Formulator and Articulator components of Levelt's model. From W.J.M. Levelt, A. Roelofs and A.S. Meyer, A theory of lexical access in speech production, Behavioral and Brain Sciences, 22(1), 1–75, 1999, © Cambridge Journals, published by Cambridge University Press, reproduced with permission.

sentence if it has just to include a single concrete noun given to them.

Complementarily at the other end of the speech-production mechanism, the processes involved in lexical selection seem to be carrying out a computationally relatively distinct operation from those involved in realising on to the articulators the phonological structure of the words to be uttered. Moreover they can be separately impaired in aphasia (for a review see e.g. Nickels, 2001).

This coarsest grain of Levelt's theoretical framework is, however, mainly useful in allowing the Marr–Cummins type of causal subsumption; it provides a starting point for the more detailed breakdown of the three component processes into subprocesses. For instance, if one takes one vertical thread through the overall process—that involved in the selection and production of individual words—then Figure 3.13 illustrates how the *Formulator* component process is held to carry this out. Here, there are two critical concepts. The first is the *lemma*, which is held to represent the

potential syntactic role of a word (and in some way its semantics) but not its phonological form. The second is the *phonological word*, which corresponds on Levelt's account to a syllabified, metrically[36] and phonologically specified representation that is inaccessible in, say, the tip-of-the-tongue phenomenon, i.e. when one knows a word but cannot quite remember its phonological form.[37] Levelt's use of both these concepts as representations in an information-processing account of cognitive processes is controversial. His *lemma* concept has been particularly criticised (e.g. Caramazza, 1997;

---

[36] Metrical features of a word specify the relative stress to be placed on individual phonemes and hence provide the prosody of the sequence of phonemes that constitute the word.

[37] The division between the *Formulator* and the *Articulator* is held to be at the level of the phonetic plan, which includes specification of phonological words, as syllabification does not necessarily respect word boundaries; consider the sentence *He'll escort us*, where the last two words are normally syllabified *e-scor-tus* (Levelt et al., 1999).

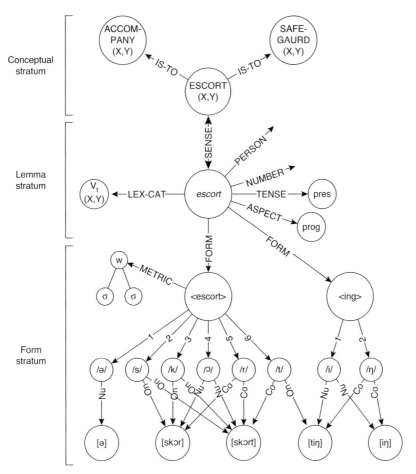

Fig. 3.14 Processes involved in transforming lexical concepts into phonemic forms within the WEAVER model. From W.J.M. Levelt, A. Roelofs and A.S. Meyer, A theory of lexical access in speech production, Behavioral and Brain Sciences, 22(1), 1–75, 1999, © Cambridge Journals, published by Cambridge University Press, reproduced with permission.

Harley, 2008). Levelt et al., however, point out that in speech errors, word exchanges such as *we completely forgot to add the list to the roof*, where *list* and *roof* are interchanged (from Garrett, 1980), typically concern elements in the same syntactic category in different phrases. They would involve inter-lemma switches. By contrast so-called segment exchanges such as *rack pat* for *pack rat* (from Garrett, 1988) do not respect syntactic category and typically concern elements from the same phrase. They would, therefore, be at the level of the phonological code, possibly in an output phonological buffer.[38]

The third stage of the deepening of the Levelt approach is to implement portions of this second grain

model of part of the overall process as a fully-specified computational model. For instance, the WEAVER model of Roelofs (1997) (see Figure 3.14) realises the subprocesses involved in transforming lexical concepts into phonological words (inputs to syllable-based articulatory programs) as a model with interactive-activation characteristics (see Section 3.7.3). This quantitatively compared with experimental data. The WEAVER model is, however, strongly modular in that it satisfies Sternberg's temporal property of processing stages discussed in Section 3.3. Its stages are temporally all-or-none, rather than cascaded. Activation does not flow to stage *n+1* until a selection is made at stage *n*. Levelt et al. (1999) review data from a variety of reaction time paradigms in normal subjects, which they hold to support the model, but this position has been much contested (see e.g. Stemberger, 1985; Dell, 1986; Harley, 1993; Caramazza, 1997) and indeed a cascade process is now considered more plausible (see e.g. Morsella & Miozzo, 2002; Harley, 2008).

---

[38] Theorising on the different types of short-term storage of representations involved in speech production is not a central part of the Levelt framework. It will be discussed further in Chapter 7. For functional imaging evidence broadly consistent with this grain of theorising see Indefrey and Levelt (2004).

We will discuss the alternative perspectives on issues related to the positions taken up by Levelt, Roelofs and their colleagues in later chapters, particularly 7 and 8. Our purpose in presenting the model here is to show how the different levels of the Marr–Cummins functional decomposition approach can exist at the cognitive level in one processing domain, without relying on evidence on its brain basis. What is critically important is that while the theory can be and indeed has been challenged, both at different grains and in different sub-domains, these challenges, even if successful, can be seen as part of an iterative processes for which the Levelt theory provides an essential starting-point. Furthermore, a theory of this general type provides a necessary unifying structure for scientific study in the area and more concretely for any theoretical interpretation of certain forms of cognitive neuroscience evidence.

Moreover, the ubiquity of language in the human species, its absence in other species and the constancy of the major subdivisions of the language process (i.e. syntax, semantics, morphology and phonology) as far as is known across cultures, make highly plausible the quasi-Chomskyan idea that the blueprint of at least the grosser domains of organisation of the speech production system are represented in some form in the human genotype.[39]

3.6 The COGENT Formalism

A major criticism of information-processing psychology is that the models that are produced are essentially a combination of diagrams and labels with no predictive power; *box-and-arrow models*, they are somewhat contemptuously called.[40] This criticism has often been met by the development of fully explicit computational implementations of specific information-processing models (e.g. the WEAVER model of Roelofs discussed

above). However, there is typically no transparent mapping between such explicit computational implementations and the original box-and-arrow diagrams on which they are based. COGENT (Cooper & Fox, 1998; Cooper, 2002) is a formalism that addresses this issue by providing a computational environment in which box-and-arrow diagrams may be first sketched and then fleshed out into computationally complete 'executable specifications'.[41]

The essential notion of COGENT is that box-and-arrow diagrams convey, by virtue of conventions for diagram interpretation, constraints on the subprocesses of a model and the information or communication channels between them. COGENT provides a set of types of component that may be assembled like Lego blocks into a model. A box-and-arrow diagram in COGENT therefore consists of a set of boxes of various types (processes, buffers or compounds) with communication links between those boxes. The components, their functions, and graphical representations are listed in Table 3.2.

To illustrate the notation, Figure 3.15 shows a COGENT rendering of Levelt's speech production model depicted in Figure 3.12. Most components of the diagram are compound boxes, reflecting the coarse grain of this level of theorising. Figure 3.16 illustrates the subprocesses of two of the components of Figure 3.15, the *Formulator* (see Figure 3.13), which consists of a series of rule-based processes, and the *Lexicon*, which comprises several interactive activation networks. Comparing these diagrams with those above (i.e. Figures 3.12, 3.13 and 3.14) clarifies the way in which the subprocesses of the *Formulator* operate through excitation of different strata within the *Lexicon*. Thus, the vertical arrows in Figure 3.13 depict the stage-wise operation of processes, rather than flow of information between them.

A COGENT box-and-arrow diagram may be fleshed out into a fully specified computational model by providing details of the internal functioning of each box (i.e., the rule set for each rule-based process, parameter values and initial states for all buffers and knowledge stores, and the box-and-arrow diagrams contained within each compound box). For non-compound boxes, this fleshing out requires a commitment to a representational language. The principal represented unit of COGENT is borrowed from the Prolog programming language. It is the *term*. Examples include *numbers*, *atoms* (i.e., symbols with no internal structure, which are represented by

---

[39] Within these areas some doubts have been raised about whether, for instance, all languages have a rule-governed syntax with hierarchical structure—grouping of words into phrases, before reaching up to the sentence level, e.g. in the Australian language Warlpiri (Hale, 1983); but see Legate (2002), and more generally Evans & Levinson (2009).

[40] Jacobs and Grainger (1994) in a very thoughtful review article proposed that there are three types of 'formats' for models, namely *verbal*, *mathematical* and *algorithmic*. We consider that box-and-arrow models should be considered a fourth type of format, since purely verbal models do not have their directed graph aspect (see Glymour, 1994). *Algorithmic* is also not an ideal term because it implies strict sequential processing. We will use the term *computational* for *algorithmic*. Our view is that verbal, box-and-arrow, and computational formats attempt to realise Marr's level 2 but with different degrees of detail. COGENT allows one to bridge the gap between the box-and-arrow and the computational formats.

---

[41] The COGENT cognitive modelling environment described here is unrelated to a second system developed within cognitive neuroscience that bears the same name—the COGENT system for the design of experimental stimuli for brain imaging and psychophysical studies—which was developed at University College London. For more details, see http://cogent.psyc.bbk.ac.uk/

TABLE 3.2 Components provided by the COGENT graphical cognitive modelling environment. There is a correspondence between many of the components and the chapters in this book, as indicated.

Icon	Name, Function and Properties
	Memory buffers allow the temporary storage of information. Parameters govern a buffer's storage capacity, decay rate, access characteristics, etc. (See Chapter 7.)
	Knowledge stores allow the long-term storage of knowledge, possibly in a structured form (e.g., with relations between individual elements). (See Chapter 6.)
	Processes carry out operations, generating outputs based either on their inputs or on the contents of buffers to which they have access. In COGENT their behaviour may be specified in terms of condition-action rules, where a rule's conditions may access a buffer's contents and/or carry out complex manipulations and translations of information and a rule's actions may alter buffer contents and/or send information to other model components. COGENT's rule language extends standard production system rule languages (see Section 1.7) by allowing conditions which involve complex logical operations in addition to matching against elements within a buffer. (See Chapter 8.)
	Networks consist of sets of nodes, where each node has an activation value. There are two types of network components: *layers*, where the nodes function independently, and *interactive activation networks*, where lateral inhibition operates between subsets of nodes. Parameters govern the response of nodes to net excitation and the nature of lateral inhibition. (See Chapter 1 and Section 3.7.3.)
	Data sources & data sinks provide input and output capabilities.
	Compounds are subsystems with internal structure which may be specified as an embedded box-and-arrow diagram.
	Communication links allow information to be transferred from one box to another. They are of three types: *read, send* and *recode*. The third is specifically for connectionist models where communication links can recode information through a matrix of weighted connections. Connection weights may be trainable through standard connectionist learning algorithms such as those discussed in Sections 1.6 and 1.7, namely Hebbian learning, delta-rule learning and back-propagation of error, and grey-scale shading of the arrow's tail indicates the density of connectivity.

character strings beginning with a lower-case letter), *variables* (represented by character strings beginning with an upper-case letter), *compound terms* such as *dribbles (maradona)*, which might represent the meaning of the proposition 'Maradona dribbles,' and *lists*.[42] The representation language is deliberately general, allowing models to be specified using either symbolic propositional representations or feature-based representations (which take the form of lists of atoms or numbers), or combinations of both.

To provide a concrete illustration of COGENT's representation and rule languages in information processing psychology, consider again the WEAVER account of speech production given by Roelofs and colleagues and described above. Figure 3.16b illustrates how the *Lexicon* might be implemented as a series of interactive activation networks. The node for the conceptual representation of *escort* might be represented in the *Conceptual Stratum* by a term such as:

concept(escort(x,y), [Condition1, Condition2, …])

where Condition1, Condition2, … is an unspecified set of conditions that must hold if the *escort(x,y)* node is to be selected (see Roelofs, 1997 and Levelt et al., 1999 for more details). Similarly, the node in the *Lemma Stratum* for the present progressive form of *escort* might be represented by a term such as:

lemma('escort', [tense=present, aspect = progressive], [concept=escort(x,y)])

Lemma selection may then be encoded by a suitable rule in *Lexical Selection*:

IF: node(concept(C, ConceptConditions), Activation) is in Lexicon: Conceptual Stratum *and* Activation is greater than T *and* preconditions_satisfied(Concept Conditions) *and* corresponding_sense(C, L)

THEN: send excite(lemma(L, Diacritics, Lemma-Conditions), E) to Lexicon: Lemma Stratum

where T and E are numerical parameters that correspond to the selection threshold and the amount of excitation passed to lower level nodes once a higher level node has been selected. This rule relies on two subsidiary functions, *preconditions_satisfied* and *corresponding_sense*. The former must implement WEAVER's verification process by checking, for all elements whose activation is above the selection threshold, that their selection preconditions

---

[42] In addition, the language includes a fixed set of predefined *operators*, such as + and –, which may also be used as terms in their own right.

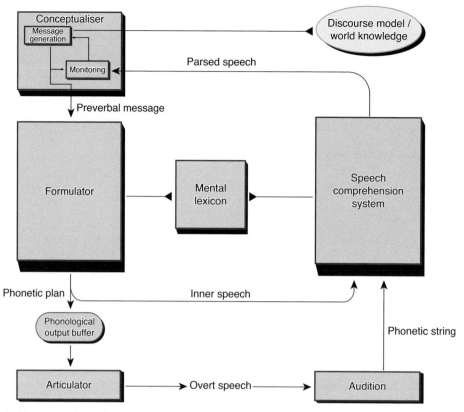

Fig. 3.15 Levelt's blueprint for the speaker drawn in COGENT (see Figure 3.12). Rectangular boxes correspond to compound processes with internal structure. The internal structure of the Formulator and Mental Lexicon components is further decomposed in Figure 3.16. For the Phonological Output Buffer addition, see Section 7.5.

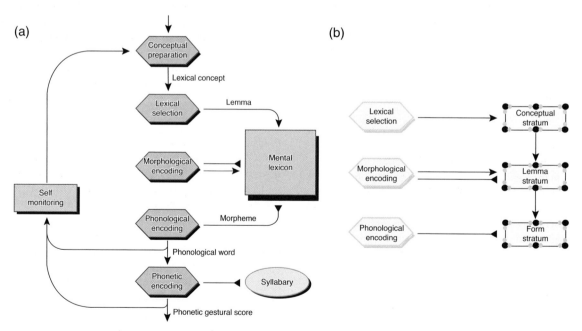

Fig. 3.16 COGENT renderings of (a) the Formulator and (b) the Mental Lexicon of the model of speech production of Levelt and colleagues (see Figures 3.12, 3.13, 3.14). Note that the Mental Lexicon is decomposed into three interactive activation networks, reflecting the decomposition of processing shown in Figure 3.14. The process boxes on the left of the Mental Lexicon diagram are shown in "faded" form to indicate that they represent inputs/outputs to the Mental Lexicon system, rather than components of the system itself.

are met. The latter must encode links between nodes in the *Conceptual Stratum* and the *Lemma Stratum*.

3.7 Complementarity: Connectionist Models Too

The intellectual appeal of the classic information-processing models rests on four types of metatheoretical support independent of the empirical support an individual model has. The first is the power of the computational metaphor. The second is that such models can represent the great differences in the computational tasks that the different parts of the mind must carry out. These two lines of support suggest a computational basis for modularity. The third expands that, as such models allow the interactions between these many different types of process to be rigorously specified. Finally, their components may map onto the anatomical and functional specificity of different brain regions.

However the distributed nature of neural networks and the gross anatomical similarity of different regions of the cortex suggest that modularity needs to be combined with its apparent opposite—distributed processing of a connectionist type—to give a more complete account of the neural bases of cognition. Cognitive neuroscience requires complementarity too.

Consider one of the parietal areas discussed in the previous section and illustrated in Figure 3.8, area 7a. Like other regions in the higher visual system the cells here respond to visual stimuli with their firing being affected by the position of the stimulus in the visual field, its so-called retinotopic location. However it is also affected by where the animal is fixating.[43] In a classic study, Richard Andersen, Greg Essick and Ralph Siegel (1985) recorded from area 7a for stimuli varying in their position in the visual field but with the fixation point also varying. They found that the response of the neurons was influenced in a complex way by both factors. In particular the response for a particular position in the visual field was modulated by the position at which the animal was fixating (see Figure 3.17).

How might this operate? In collaboration with the neural network modeller, David Zipser, Richard Andersen trained a single simple 3-layer feed-forward neural network (see Figure 3.18a) by back-propagation (see Section 1.7). It had two sets of input units—one set representing the position of the stimulus in the visual field and the other the position of the fixation point.

The net also had a single set of output units which represented the position in space of the stimulus (in head-centred co-ordinates). Examination of the activations of the hidden units in response to stimuli at different retinal locations revealed that the hidden units developed receptive fields qualitatively similar to those found by Andersen et al. (1985) for selected neurons in area 7a (see Figure 3.18b). Thus, some hidden units responded maximally when, for example, the stimulus was presented at specific retinal locations, while others showed more complex response functions sensitive to both retinal location and fixation point.

The approach of Zipser and Andersen has been formalised and greatly extended by Pouget and Sejnowski (1997, 2001). First, in the same style as Andersen et al. (1985), they argued that for a given perceptual input the outputs of certain neurons in inferior parietal cortex and area 7a could be modelled as a Gaussian function of input retinal location modulated by a sigmoidal function of eye position. They noted that functions of this general type (i.e. the product of a Gaussian and a sigmoid) form what is called mathematically a *basis*. Thus, in a fashion analogous to Fourier decomposition, any non-linear function may be approximated by a linear combination of elements from the basis. Pouget and Sejnowski (2001) therefore model neurons in area 7a as weighted sums of these basis functions.

As in the Zipser and Andersen model, the Pouget and Sejnowski model takes as inputs a representation of a position in the visual field and a representation of eye-position (see Figure 3.19). The model produces two outputs: one in retinocentric coordinates and one in head-centred coordinates. Several banks of hidden units—two representing the left hemisphere and two representing the right—implement the basis functions. Thus they assume that visual field input units respond as a Gaussian of the location of the input in the visual field. The eye-position input units respond as a sigmoidal function of the eye position. The hidden units then compute the product of these inputs. Weights from input to hidden units are fixed such that the hidden units maintain the retinotopic map present in the input visual field. However, at the same time the hidden units implement a bias to contralateral space, with more units in the left hemisphere being tuned to the right visual field and vice versa. This bias in receptive fields for neurons in area 7a has since been found in monkeys by Battaglia-Mayer et al. (2005). The output units of the model compute weighted sums (i.e. linear combinations) of the hidden units, with weights from hidden to output units learned through a standard gradient descent procedure (see Section 1.7).

Since the hidden units encode basis functions, the model is able to learn reliably the appropriate mapping from inputs to outputs. Pouget and Sejnowski therefore

---

[43] Points in the space near an animal may be represented in a variety of different ways. As discussed earlier, representations may be *retinotopic*, but in addition they may be *head-centred* (coded in terms of their positions with respect to the main anterior-posterior axis of the animal's head), *body-centred* (coded with respect to the main axis of the animal's body), and so on.

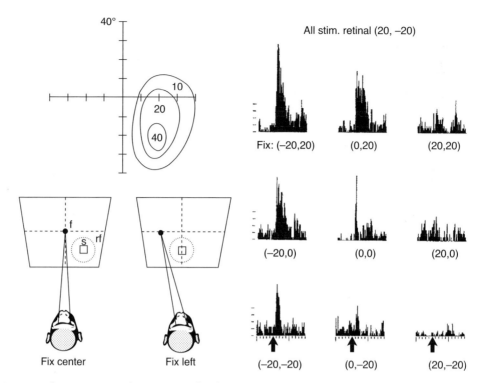

Fig. 3.17 Responses of a posterior parietal neuron to stimuli in the same spatial location when the animal fixates on different positions in space. From R.A. Andersen, G.K. Essick and R.M. Siegel, 1985, Encoding of spatial location by posterior parietal neurons. Science, 230(4724), 456–458. Reprinted with permission from AAAS.

evaluated their model by lesioning it and relating the effects to the unilateral neglect syndrome discussed in Section 1.8. This is appropriate because neglect is normally associated with damage to (typically right) parietal cortex. The fully-trained model was lesioned by removing the right hemisphere banks of hidden units. The resultant model was then used to simulate performance on a range of clinical tasks normally used to

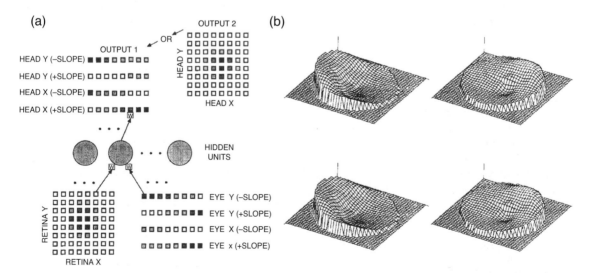

Fig. 3.18 (a) The three-layer feed-forward network of Zipser and Andersen (1988) trained to map from representations of the position of the stimulus in the visual field and the position of the fixation point to a representation of the position in space of the stimulus in head-centred co-ordinates. (b) Sample receptive fields of (top) neurons from area 7a and (bottom) model neurons. Adapted by permission from Macmillan Publishers Ltd: Nature (D. Zipser & R.A. Andersen, A back-propagation programmed network that simulates response properties of a subset of posterior parietal neurons. Nature, 1988, 331, 679–684), copyright (1988).

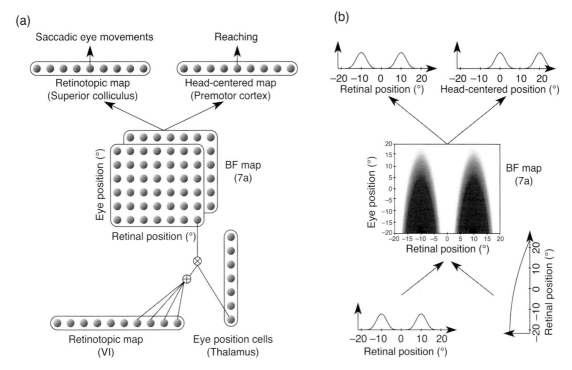

Fig. 3.19 (a) The architecture of Pouget and Sejnowski (2001) for simultaneously computing the positions of objects in several different reference frames using a set of basis functions. (b) The pattern of activity when two visual stimuli are presented at +10° and -10° on the retina and when the eye is pointing at 10°. Copyright © 2001 by the American Psychological Association. Reproduced with permission. A. Pouget & T.J. Sejnowski (2001) Simulating a lesion in a basis function model of spatial representations: Comparison with hemineglect. Psychological Review, 108(3), 653–673. The use of APA information does not imply endorsement by APA.

assess neglect such as *line cancellation* and *line bisection*.[44] On each of the tasks the model produces behaviour qualitatively similar to that of neglect patients. Here, then, we see how a process involving one of the subregions considered earlier from the perspective of modularity is well captured by the behaviour of a connectionist network.

As we argued above, connectionist nets can be seen as a type of functional architecture derived from a finer grain to that of isolable subsystems in the hierarchical structuring of units of the nervous system. In this case it would be the grain of *local networks* (to use the terminology of Sejnowski & Churchland, 1989). On this approach connectionist nets should not be seen as a functional architecture in conflict with that of the

subsystem-based information-processing level. Rather, they are a complementary functional architecture derived by extrapolation from the hardware domain at a finer conceptual grain.

The suspicious reader might be sceptical of such a Panglossian conclusion. Why, might she not ask, would a connectionist brain be organised into subsystems. The standard Panglossian answer, derived from such noteworthy figures as Herbert Simon and David Marr, is that it is the only way in which the evolution or development of a complex system carrying out multiple tasks can work. But their position is a mere assertion. When Bullinaria (2007) attempted to model such evolution using a three-layer feed-forward network, he found that the situation was much more complex. The network was trained on a task with two independent outputs—a 'what'/'where' task loosely based on the distinction between ventral and dorsal routes for processing visual information touched on in Section 3.4. The task was modelled with one set of input units, two sets of output units but overlapping hidden units. Bullinaria found that modularity emerged in some conditions but not others. Subtle changes in implementation details led to qualitatively different behaviour. For instance,

---

[44] In line cancellation subjects are presented with a page of short straight lines of random orientation and length. They are required to put a mark through every line. Neglect patients generally fail to mark some of the lines on the left of the page. In line bisection subjects are presented with a single horizontal line and asked to mark the centre of the line. Neglect patients tend to place their mark towards the right of the line, with the deviation from centre depending on the length of the line.

modularity emerged when the learning algorithm minimised sum-squared error across all outputs or when the network was sparsely connected, but not when the learning algorithm minimised what is called *cross-entropy* across all outputs and also the network was densely connected. Given that neural connectivity is relatively sparse, Bullinaria concludes that evolution is indeed likely to favour a modular neural organisation, regardless of the learning algorithm.

The modelling of the behaviour of specific neural circuits is not, however, the main way in which connectionism has been used in the study of cognition. Too little is generally known about the detailed neural architecture underlying most cognitive processes. Instead most of the connectionist models of cognitive processes to be considered are ones where the properties of the units and connections are derived from hypothetical generic neural circuits rather than ones where the specific architecture is based on good anatomical and physiological knowledge. Thus this second type of net has an underlying structure that only very abstractly resembles the nervous system, being composed of sets of units which each have a very general relation to that of a neuron and where the sets of units are linked according to one or other fairly standard general principle such as feed-forward, recurrent nets or attractor-based nets (see Figure 3.20). We will meet many examples of such models in this book. One is the model of reading referred to earlier in this chapter; see Figure 3.3.

Four types of objection to the use of connectionist (artificial neural net) models of cognitive functions need, however, to be considered.

3.7.1 Connectionist Networks are 'Mere Implementations'

Early in the development of connectionist nets it was argued that the relation between subsystems and neural nets is merely one in which the latter are used to implement the former (see Broadbent, 1985). This would mean that on the cognitive level they add little to an information-processing account as far as behaviour is concerned. If we take, for instance, connectionist models of reading, such as the Plaut et al. model, then this is far from accurate, as we will see in Chapter 4. They make many predictions which are not derived from the information-processing types of model with which they are related. This objection is no longer valid.

3.7.2 The Models are Biologically Implausible

As discussed in Section 1.7, it is often claimed that many aspects of connectionist networks are not biologically plausible. The use of the back-propagation learning

algorithm is perhaps the most extreme example (see Crick, 1989; Douglas & Martin, 1991; O'Reilly, 1996). Thus, back-propagation networks rely on a very slow learning process.[45] Moreover the error signal from the previous trial is fed back in each epoch of learning from the output layer to the preceding layer and then back one layer at a time to the first set of connections. This process is generally considered to have no plausible neural analogues.[46] Thus it is held that such connectionist models cannot be treated as an appropriate abstraction from local brain networks.

This argument misunderstands the functions of models. A model cannot represent all of reality. It contains an abstraction of only *some* aspects of a situation which, if the model is a good one, are key aspects. One makes simplifying assumptions that are false for greater mathematical or computational tractability. Thus Fabbri and Navarro-Salas (2005) in a recent book on the evaporation of matter/energy from black holes argue 'The history of research on black holes tells us that important physical insights have been gained through the study of simplified models of gravitational collapse. The paradigm is the Oppenheimer and Snyder model (1939). Despite its simplicity, forced by the difficulties of the technical treatment of more realistic situations, it turns out to produce a very accurate picture. ... The assumption of perfect spherical symmetry, the main criticism of black hole opponents, was not, in the end, a real drawback' (p. vii). Thus some aspects of a model may have no adequate correspondence at all in the real situation. They are required in order to make the model formally tractable, either by mathematical or computational means. Philosophers-of-science (e.g. McMullin, 1985) call such models containing false assumptions *Galilean models*. What is sauce for the physicist should be sauce for cognitive neuroscientist too.

Therefore to use this approach it is important, as discussed earlier, to distinguish between the scientific theory—those aspects of models which are held to represent reality—and the implementation details. Thus Cooper et al. (1996) argue for distinguishing between the 'essential theory'—what they refer to as the A, or above-the-line, content of a model—and implementation details—what they refer to as the B, or below-the-line, content of a model. Implementation details are usually necessary for a simulation to be run, but a model is much more powerful if the critical aspects of its behaviour are independent of such details. Unfortunately frequently in practice in neural network modelling of cognitive processes no attempt is made to

---

[45] Learning becomes unstable if the learning rate parameter is too high.

[46] But see Hinton (2010).

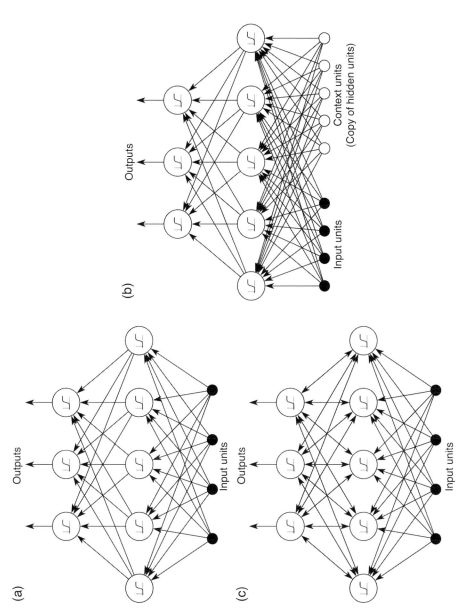

Fig. 3.20 Three network architectures each with three input units, five hidden units and three output units. (a) A three-layer feed-forward network; (b) A simple recurrent network; and (c) an attractor network. The simple recurrent network adds context units to the basic three-layer network, which copy the state of the hidden units on the previous cycle (see Elman, 1990). The attractor network adds bidirectionality. Attractor networks can also be formed by the addition of clean-up units – see e.g. Figures 4.11 and 4.21.

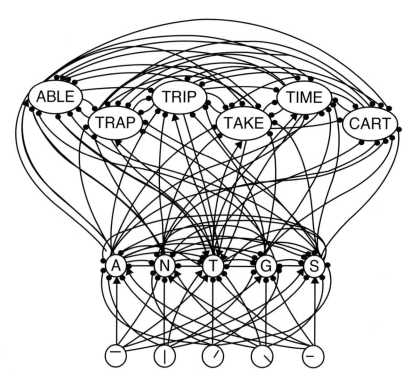

Fig. 3.21 A part of the interactive activation network model of word recognition of McClelland and Rumelhart (1981). The figure shows some of the neighbours of the letter T in the first position in a word, together with their interconnections. Copyright © 1981 by the American Psychological Association. Reproduced with permission. J.L. McClelland and D.E. Rumelhart (1981). An interactive activation model of context effects in letter perception: Part 1. An account of basic findings. Psychological Review, 88(5), 375–407. The use of APA information does not imply endorsement by APA.

vary the implementation details and thereby demonstrate such independence. However this is merely sloppiness on the part of the modellers. It need not be the case, as we will see in Chapter 4. Thus unrealistic assumptions can be parts of individual models without being an aspect of the general theory.

3.7.3 **Distributed Connectionist Models are Unnecessarily Complicated**

The third objection to connectionist models argues that the most common form of the approach—use of distributed representations—is unnecessarily complex. It is held that all that is required to capture what distributed connectionist models purport to explain are the properties of much simpler models, so-called 'localist' ones. Localist models are ones in which at the key conceptual level there are units that are fully activated by one and only one of the representations in the domain of the model. Also when transmission of information to other systems is required the output of these specific units stands for a particular representation. Thus these individual units in the critical part of the net have a privileged relation to one and only one representation.

The prototypic model of this type is the model of the lower levels of the word reading process proposed by

McClelland and Rumelhart (1981) and Rumelhart and McClelland (1982) (see Figure 3.21).[47] In this model there are single units that correspond to each level of processing. At the lowest level these are the strokes that represent parts of individual letters, e.g. — and /. The next layer consists of representations of the letters A, B, etc. Finally there are representations for each of the words in the set being considered, e.g. TRIP. When a word is presented to the net, activation flows through the system from the units corresponding to strokes to the units corresponding to letters to those corresponding to words. When a unit is excited, activation flows to the units to which it is connected in the neighbouring layers, so helping them to become activated more strongly. Each of the connections between units on the same level is inhibitory. This produces competition and limits the number of units that can be active.

In the initial interactive activation model of reading the weights of the connections were set by hand so as to make the system produce the appropriate output.

---

[47] This may be viewed as an alternative for the stages of the reading process modelled in the Plaut et al. model up to the first set of hidden units.

The interest of the model was in how well it matched behavioural studies of a variety of reading paradigms.

In each cycle of processing time the activation value a_i of each unit i is updated according to the following equations:

$$\Delta a_i = (max - a_i) . net_i - decay . (a_i - rest) \text{ [if } net_i \geq 0]$$

$$\Delta a_i = (a_i - min) . net_i - decay . (a_i - rest) \text{ [if } net_i \leq 0]$$

where $net_i = \sum a_j.w_{ji}$ is the net input to a unit, *decay* takes a fixed value between 0 and 1, and *a* ranges between *min* (–0.2) and *max* (+1.0).

Given strong activation in the input units—the units representing strokes—the activation of the output units will increase, with the output unit representing the most likely interpretation of the input increasing most quickly and suppressing, through inhibitory connections, alternative interpretations. After a number of time steps an identification is made by selecting probabilistically from the output units, with the probability of selecting each unit being proportional to the exponential of its activity (i.e., according to the so-called Luce (1959) selection rule). This is treated as identification of the item.

While many other connectionist models of reading now exist, the McClelland and Rumelhart model probably remains the model that provides, given appropriate updating, the best fit to relevant empirical results in normal subjects. These relevant empirical results involve visual aspects of the reading process, where one is concerned with the identification of individual words made difficult by being presented in brief exposures or masked or both (see Jacobs & Grainger, 1994; Grainger & Jacobs, 1996).

Many localist models, such as the McClelland and Rumelhart model of reading, do not learn. Values of the weights are set by hand. As this allows the modeller to set many variables, this makes the models potentially unconstrained and a priori difficult to falsify.[48] However, with the exception of the models of ordering of component actions to be discussed in Chapters 7 and 8, localist models have not been applied to neuropsychological or functional imaging data. By contrast distributed models are highly constrained by the task domain. The representations they build are ones that are structured by the learning process to capture the statistics of the input–output mapping or the input space they are modelling. Moreover units in the representations respond to a variety of stimuli much as higher-level neural representations typically do (see Chapter 6). These key features are not captured by localist models.

In an important article, Page (2000; see also Bowers, 2009; Plaut & McClelland, 2010), however, argues for the superiority of localist over distributed models for a number of reasons. His main argument is that standard connectionist models suffer from what is known as *catastrophic interference*. If the network has learned some mapping and then it is taught a new mapping, which interferes with the first (A–B A–C in the jargon of interference theory of verbal learning), then the learning of the first set of input–output relations is overwritten (Grossberg, 1987; McCloskey & Cohen, 1989; French, 1999). Page points out that this problem can be reduced but not eliminated by making distributed representations sparser, namely by having a lower density of units that are activated for any given input.

However, following Plaut and McClelland (2000), one can also see this characteristic as indicating that distributed representations are useful vehicles for capturing the slow learning of highly complex but fairly stable environments, which is what the higher organism is required to acquire in a very slow developmental process in many domains.[49] Dealing with rapid changes in the environment or in the input–output contingencies would, as Plaut and McClelland point out, require additional systems for coping with situations where rapid learning of the new contingencies is required. McClelland, McNaughton and O'Reilly (1995) have argued that this is an evolutionary function of the hippocampus (see Section 10.2). We will argue that the prefrontal cortex is essential for coping with novelty, and one can argue that certain neurotransmitter systems such as the cholinergic and noradrenaline systems have a related role (Yu & Dayan, 2005).

Page makes further criticisms of distributed networks. An important objection is that models with distributed representations are difficult to manipulate. Moreover they cannot easily represent operations such as holding sequences of items. The first part of this point is related to the objections of Fodor and Pylyshyn (1988), which will be addressed below, while we will return to the second of these points in Chapters 7 and 8. With the exceptions of these last two points, we do not find Page's arguments compelling.

3.7.4 Connectionist Models are Insufficient as Models of Symbolic Cognitive Processes

Connectionist models are often called 'subsymbolic' and seen as contrasting with symbolic models (e.g. Smolensky, 1986). A final objection is that a model like that of Andersen and Zipser may work well for an area of brain function related to low-level operations

---

[48] Some localist models do learn (see Page, 2000).

[49] See also O'Reilly and Munakata (2000).

and representations. However, the model contains nothing at all related to a symbolic representation, and the theoretical paradigm does not extrapolate effectively to deal with symbolic operations. This pre-theoretical objection has been captured most effectively by Fodor and Pylyshyn (1988). They argued that symbolic systems like language have two properties that are not well captured by connectionist systems. First, they respect general *systematic* relationships. Thus a conjunction like *and* specifies the relation between the two noun phrases it links and the complementary verb phrase in the sentence in an equivalent fashion whatever the noun phrases are. The associated property always applies to the referents of both noun phrases, not merely on 99% of occurrences. Or, to express the point in another way, if you can understand *Mary loves Tom* you can understand *Mary loves Jerry*. In addition Fodor and Pylyshyn argue that symbolic systems have a second property of *compositionality*, namely that the units of a sentence, words (or better morphemes), have similar nuggets of meaning whatever the rest of the sentence. These are important objections.

Consider first compositionality. Certain classes of connectionist models such as those derived from Hopfield nets discussed in Section 1.7 have a so-called attractor structure. The Plaut et al. (1996) word reading model is typical in this respect. The existence of feedback connections (between the phoneme units and 'hidden' units) means that when a state of the model occurs which is close to one of a certain number of learnt points, the internal dynamics of the model will result in its state moving over time towards the fixed point (see Figure 1.15). As a consequence, every time an output of that type occurs from that net other systems receive the very same input from it. This was Newell's definition of a symbol as discussed in Section 3.3. The finite set of attractors within the behaviour space of the system can be seen as satisfying the 'compositionality' requirement. Examples of such models will be given in the next chapter. At the neurophysiological level, evidence for the existence of attractors is surprisingly thin. However some exists. For instance, Akrami et al. (2009) recorded from inferotemporal neurons of monkeys while they were presented with a set of pictures, such as of objects, animals and people. For a given neuron two pictures were selected—one of which reliably activated the neuron (the + picture) and the other of which (the – picture) did not. They then presented the monkeys with morphs between the two pictures with differing percentage of each in different trials. For the more negative morphs the responses of the neuron varied according to the percent of the + picture. For the more positive morphs, instead, the responses became virtually identical about 600 msec after stimulus onset, as one would expect if an attractor had been accessed.

As far as systematicity is concerned, several authors have argued that Fodor and Pylyshyn have underrated the systematicity of connectionist models (e.g., Chalmers, 1996; Hadley, 1997).[50] In particular, connectionist models are well able to learn systematic relationships when trained within systematic domains. For example, take the Plaut et al. (1996) simulation again. The network trained on the mapping between structured representations of orthography and of phonology can develop what the authors refer to as 'componential' attractors—attractors with a substructure that reflects the common substructure (i.e., systematic relations) of the source and target domains.

More critically, Cain (2002) argues that Fodor and Pylyshyn have not shown that connectionist models of a thought operation cannot be systematic. They have shown merely that there is nothing in the connectionist paradigm per se that constrains such models to be systematic. However, this objection to Fodor and Pylyshyn can be turned on its head. What Fodor and Pylyshyn have argued is that there is nothing intrinsic in the connectionist architecture that explains systematicity, whereas it is the natural consequence of a symbolic computational theory of the organisation of mind.

We will therefore continue to consider distributed connectionist models. However they are optimal when the model has to produce a single learned representation as an output, or a set of learned representations one for each position slot, as in the Plaut et al. model. When a more complex output is required then localist models may in practice be easier to use.[51] However, given Fodor and Pylyshyn's general objections to connectionist models, particularly with respect to systematicity, it is also important to consider a generally less fashionable type of model: symbolic models and particularly ones based on production systems, which we introduced in Sections 1.6 and 1.7.

3.8 More Advanced Symbolic Architectures

The difficulties that connectionist models face with respect to compositionality and particularly systematicity stem from the use of feature-based approaches to representation by such models. Feature-based representational systems come initially from ideas on semantic memory (e.g. Smith & Medin, 1981). Moreover, in such models feature-based representations are naturally realised by arrays of neuron-like units which represent the inputs and outputs of a process. They are

---

[50] See Dawson (1998) for helpful discussion.
[51] We will consider alternative localist and distributed models for the same cognitive processes in a number of later chapters.

therefore designed to represent tokens of various types, but they cannot represent relations between arbitrary tokens in any direct way. The inability to represent relational information is a serious problem for connectionist models, as there is no obvious alternative representational scheme, beyond a feature-based one, which they may use.[52]

The alternative approach to representation typically adopted by symbolic models is based on symbolic propositions. These are structured representations consisting of a relation with one or more arguments. The arguments, in turn, may be atomic symbols or other symbolic propositions. Thus, one may represent the meaning of a sentence such as *John believes that Fido is a dog* by the proposition:

believe(john, isa(fido, dog))

Such propositional representations, are themselves rooted in symbolic logic, and so naturally support both systematicity and compositionality. Thus, a symbolic model which was able to generate the above proposition as a representation of the semantic content of the above sentence would, unless specifically engineered otherwise, generate the corresponding representation of the semantic content for an equivalent sentence with different referents. Of course, the inferential power of propositional representations comes at a large cost. It is far from clear how such representations could be coded in neural terms. Overall this means that feature-based and propositional representations represent alternatives with complimentary strengths and weaknesses, and as our argument about attractors shows they are potentially compatible.

In cognitive science, propositional representational systems have been most widely used in production system models which we introduced in Sections 1.6 and 1.7. It is within such models that the concept of functional architecture has seen its most extensive development, as discussed in Section 1.6. Newell (1990) generalised his earlier work on problem-solving with Simon (Newell & Simon, 1972) to all cognitive processes by arguing that all cognition (including reasoning and language, but also that involved in laboratory tasks such as serial recall and choice reaction time) can be viewed as a form of problem-solving. In support of this argument, Newell extended his Soar production system (Laird et al., 1987) by adding perceptual and motor subsystems to allow it to interact with the environment. The resultant functional architecture (see Figure 3.22) fits well with a modular view of the mind working in

discrete time steps. Input processes (*perceive* and *encode*) operate in a stage-wise fashion to deliver a representation of the environment to central cognition (the *attend*, *comprehend*, *task* and *intend* processes, all of which are performed by the central production system). When this completes its operations, it triggers stage-wise output processes (*decode* and *motor*).

There are many criticisms one can make of this particular functional architecture (e.g. there are no direct links from input processes to output processes, so even the simplest of behaviours must involve central cognition) (see Cooper & Shallice, 1995), and it has seen little development since Newell's death in 1992 (though see Laird, 2008, for some recent developments). The importance of the architecture is that it was the first explicit functional architecture for a relatively complete theory of mind.[53]

Several more recent functional architectures of the mind have developed the production system approach in different ways in an attempt to close the gap between the conceptual framework of production systems and empirical viability. We will briefly consider two— 4CAPS (Capacity Constrained Concurrent Cortical Activation-based Production System: Just & Varma, 2007) and EPIC (Executive Process Interactive Control: Meyer & Kieras, 1997a, 1997b)—before considering a third—ACT-R (Adaptive Control of Thought—Rational: Anderson et al., 2004a; Anderson, 2007)—in more detail. The functional architectures differ in their assumptions concerning central and peripheral systems, and in whether more than one production can fire at a time. Table 3.3 summarises key features of Soar and these three other functional architectures.

4CAPS grew out of work by Marcel Just and Patricia Carpenter (1992), who were concerned with individual differences in sentence comprehension tasks. It is based on the assumption that association cortex in any region of the brain functions as a production system. It is thus assumed that cognitive processing is the product of the operation of multiple production systems, with each specialised to operate on different types of representations. These systems are held to function in parallel and to be located in different cortical regions (see Figure 3.23). The various production systems are further assumed to be both *activation-based* and *capacity constrained*. The former means that the rule that fires in any production system at any time depends on the activation of elements in that production system's working memory. The latter means that there is an upper limit on the net activation of all working memory elements for each

---

[52] But see the model of semantic memory of Rogers et al. (2004), extensively discussed in Chapter 6, for a connectionist approach to such issues.

[53] There are certainly precursors to such explicit functional architectures, including Turing's original description of the Turing machine discussed in Section 1.4.

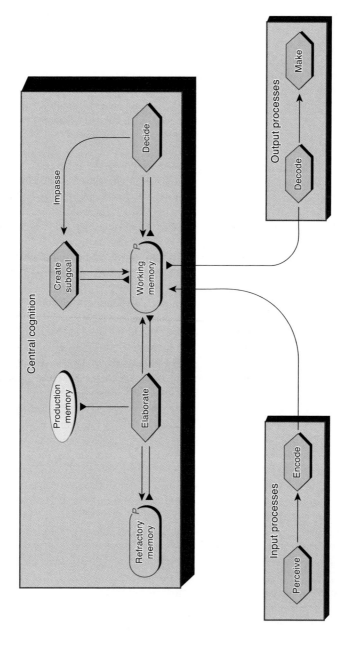

Fig. 3.22 The Soar architecture. The operation of Central Cognition consists of four stage-wise processes—*attend, comprehend, task* and *intend*—each of which involves the six processing systems operating in the same way but on different types of data. *Attend* focusses on one input. *Comprehend* analyses that input for significance. *Task* sets a specific task. Finally, *intend* determines and triggers the response. See Figure 1.21 for details on the Production and Working (their labelled 'Dynamic') Memories.

TABLE 3.3 A comparison of four production system cognitive architectures. Conflict resolution refers to the process of selecting one production to fire when many productions may match against the production system's working memory. In parallel production systems, all matching productions fire in parallel, and so conflict resolution is not necessary.

	Central system	Peripheral subsystems
Soar	Serial production system; Preference-based conflict resolution.	N/A
4CAPS	N/A	Multiple serial production systems; Activation-based conflict resolution.
EPIC	Parallel production system; no conflict resolution.	Serial processing is assumed but no algorithmic details are specified.
ACT-R	Serial production system; utility-based conflict resolution.	Serial processing is assumed but no algorithmic details are specified.

production system. This upper limit varies across individuals, and is held to account for individual differences in cognitive ability. If a task requires more activation than available then activation is scaled down within the subsystem as necessary. The net activation of a production system at a given cortical location is further assumed to be reflected by the BOLD signal of fMRI (see Chapter 5, and especially Section 5.3). 4CAPS has been applied with some success by Just and colleagues to model both behaviour and fMRI data on a range of tasks (e.g. Just & Varma, 2007), while its predecessor, 3CAPS, which did not attempt to map production systems to cortical regions, has been used to explore the deficits of frontal patients on certain goal-directed problem-solving tasks (Goel et al., 2001; see Section 12.5). However, 4CAPS does not specify a definitive set of production

systems or localisations. Thus, individual models developed in 4CAPS may use different production systems and different localisations. Until this problem is addressed, it is difficult to see how the 4CAPS research program can become cumulative.

EPIC has a much more bottom-up history. It was developed in an attempt to provide a detailed account of data of one particular experimental psychology paradigm concerning the *psychological refractory period*. These experiments involve the carrying out of two reaction time tasks with different stimulus–response characteristics at almost the same time; thus one task might be an auditory task and the other a visual one. Typically there is a delay in responding to the second of the stimuli (when compared with presenting the two tasks independently), referred to as the psychological refractory

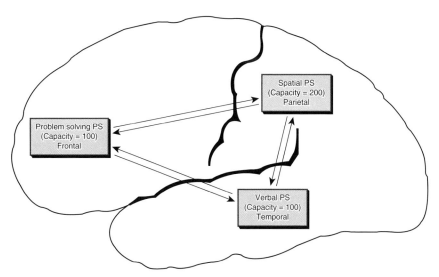

Fig. 3.23 The 4-CAPS architecture. It is assumed that distinct capacity-constrained production systems are localised in different regions of cortex. The capacity of each production system is assumed to be subject to individual variation, but the architecture does not specify the exact set of production systems or their locations. Three possible production systems are shown in the figure: problem solving, verbal and spatial.

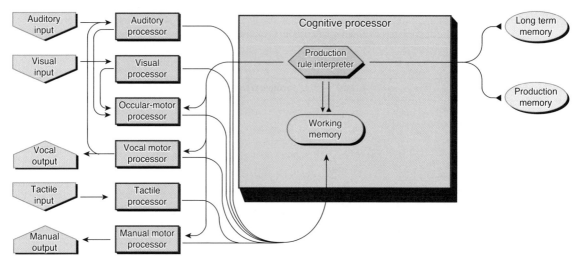

Fig. 3.24 The EPIC architecture. The cognitive processor is a simple production system without conflict resolution. This processor interacts with the world via a set of modality-specific peripheral modules. (See Meyer and Kieras, 1997a, 1997b.)

period (PRP). PRP effects had previously been accounted for by the assumption of serial central processing or of bottlenecks in response selection (see e.g. Pashler, 1998). Meyer and Keiras (1997b) presented an alternative account based on a functional architecture that fully adopted the Fodorian view of an equipotential central process with modular peripheral processes (see Figure 3.24). Thus, input and output processes for a variety of modalities were specified in terms of their response characteristics and timing behaviour. By contrast, central cognition was modelled by a simple production system in which multiple production rules could fire in parallel. Within the architecture, PRP type effects were shown to arise from the control strategies used by central cognition in order to avoid blocking or jamming of output subsystems that were simultaneously required by the separate tasks.

EPIC's subsystems (which are referred to as 'processors' by Meyer & Keiras, 1997a, 1997b) have at least characteristics M1–M3 of those discussed in Section 3.3. Thus, they are separately modifiable, may be characterised as having discrete subfunctions and have representations as outputs. EPIC makes no specific claims about neural localisation (M4), though given the peripheral functions assigned to subsystems, gross localisation is straightforward. For instance, EPIC's auditory processor would correspond to auditory cortex.

Byrne and Anderson (2001) challenged the EPIC account of PRP effects, and in particular the claim that central cognition can be modelled by a parallel production system. They demonstrated that PRP-like effects could be obtained in cognitive tasks, suggesting that as with peripheral processing, central cognitive processing too was serial. In support of this claim, Byrne and Anderson extended the ACT-R serial production system,

first discussed in Section 1.7. This production system model has its origins in very early work of John Anderson and Gordon Bower (1973). It has since been extensively developed by Anderson and his colleagues (e.g. Anderson, 1983; Anderson & Lebière, 1998; Anderson et al., 2004a; Anderson, 2007).[54] Byrne and Anderson added to ACT-R the perceptual and motor processes of EPIC and demonstrated that, unlike EPIC, the extended system could indeed account for their cognitive PRP effects. Subsequent developments have led to ACT-R embracing EPIC's modularisation of peripheral processes and extending it to some processes normally regarded as being part of central cognition, namely declarative memory, goal setting and short-term memory (Anderson et al., 2004a; Anderson, 2007; see Figure 3.25).

How is this degree of modularity justified? Essentially, Anderson and colleagues have extrapolated the abstract functional role of peripheral subsystems to other parts of the production system, as described below. At the same time they have bolstered their arguments by recruiting findings from neuroscience that support gross localisation, both of EPIC's original subsystems and of ACT-R's additional ones.[55]

To understand the extrapolation of functional roles it is necessary to consider in some detail the functioning of EPIC-like subsystems within ACT-R (see Figure 3.25).

---

[54] The developmental trajectory of ACT-R may be viewed as following the methodology of a Lakatosian research programme (Lakatos, 1970), with successive changes extending a *hard core* of theoretical assumptions. See Cooper (2006) for a detailed analysis of the evolution of the architecture.

[55] ACT-R subsystems therefore obey, in addition to criteria M1-M3, criterion M4.

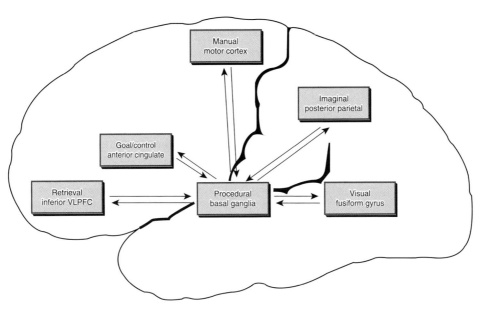

Fig. 3.25 The ACT-R architecture. Each box represents a module. The central module ("procedural") is a serial production system, held to be localised within the basal ganglia. Peripheral modules are distributed across the cortex and each includes a one-item buffer which acts as an interface between the module and the central production system. (See Anderson et al., 2008b.)

Such subsystems are explicitly referred to within ACT-R as modules. This reflects the fact that ACT-R modules share a precise information processing characterisation which differentiates them from the central production system processor. Thus, each ACT-R module interfaces with the central cognitive processor through its own limited capacity buffer, which is capable of storing one *chunk* of information.[56] This is true of both perceptual buffers (e.g., auditory and visual buffers) and motor buffers (e.g., manual and vocal buffers)[57] associated with the perceptual and motor modules. Given these perceptual and motor buffers, the conditions of a standard production rule[58] would match against the contents of any subset of buffers, or against any elements in the production system's working memory. Similarly, the actions of such a rule would alter either the contents of any buffer or working memory. ACT-R's extrapolation, then, is to treat working memory as just another module. This simplifies the structure of production rules because all production rule conditions are reduced to matching against the contents of module buffers, while all production rule actions are reduced to over-writing the contents of module buffers.[59]

More specifically, ACT-R breaks the critical working memory component of a production system into three: goal memory, short-term memory and declarative memory. It simultaneously adds three extra components. One is an intentional module, which sets and maintains goals in the goal buffer (held to be localised within dorsolateral PFC). The second is an 'imaginal' module, which allows storage of intervening results during performance of a task (held to be localised in the posterior parietal cortices). The third is a declarative module (consisting of the hippocampus and temporal lobe structures), which has the function of retrieving chunks from long-term memory that match cues in the retrieval buffer (held to be localised within ventrolateral PFC).

Since ACT-R assumes that only one production may fire on any cycle, a mechanism is needed to select between competing productions when more than one matches the contents of the various buffers. In such cases, the production with the greatest utility is selected. Utility is here determined via a learned cost–benefit trade-off.

[56] This scheme differs from that in EPIC, where input subsystems add their outputs directly to working memory, and output subsystems are triggered by signals from the central processor.

[57] See Chapter 7 for relevant discussion.

[58] See Section 1.7.

[59] Each ACT-R module therefore has a buffer that may be accessed or modified by the central processor. In addition, each module has an associated module-specific process that may also

access or modify the buffer. Thus, the central processor might set the focus of visual attention by writing an appropriate element in the so-called location subfield of the visual buffer. Subsequently, the vision module will elaborate the content of the visual buffer with a representation of the scene at the specified location. Similarly, the central processor might set cues in the working memory module's buffer, resulting in a recall process elaborating the content of the working memory buffer with the most active match to those cues.

Neither the ACT-R approach nor the EPIC one makes commitments to the algorithmic details of how their peripheral modules operate. Instead, modules are specified purely in terms of the outputs they generate given inputs and the time taken to generate these outputs. This is a very different approach from the connectionist one. They adopt the equivalent of Sternberg's temporal criterion for processing stages and, in the case of ACT-R, make declarative memory modular. These assumptions influence the timing predictions of the architecture.

To illustrate this, consider retrieval from declarative memory. In ACT-R this requires two production rules—one to initiate retrieval from the retrieval module and another to 'harvest' the results. The first would place retrieval cues in the retrieval buffer. This will result in processing within the declarative module, which will attempt to retrieve a chunk associated with those cues. As far as the time to carry out the overall operation is concerned, this depends on the time to retrieve a chunk. This in turn depends on the chunk's activation—a numerical quantity that increases whenever a chunk is retrieved but also decays over time.[60] The decay assumption gives rise to a recency effect, and the boost to activation on retrieval produces a frequency effect. If retrieval is successful, the declarative module places the retrieved chunk in the retrieval buffer. Only once the chunk has been retrieved can a second production apply, namely one whose conditions match the chunk in the retrieval buffer. It is assumed that the architecture takes 50 msec for each production to fire, whatever modules are involved. This means that the time for the complete retrieval process becomes 100 msec plus the time to retrieve the chunk.

Models of a range of tasks and cognitive functions have been developed within ACT-R, including models of attention tasks (Lovett, 2005), memory tasks (Anderson et al., 1998), skill acquisition (Lee & Anderson, 2001), problem-solving (Anderson & Douglass, 2001) and language processing (Lewis & Vasishth, 2005). Like all production system architectures, ACT-R draws a sharp distinction between knowledge and control (i.e. the way that the knowledge is used). The architecture specifies a general control regime but knowledge must be specified on a task-by-task basis. Thus, applying a production system architecture to a specific task, such as immediate serial recall of a list of items or playing chess, requires one to specify a theory of the knowledge and strategy believed to be used by subjects when performing that task.[61]

In addition, ACT-R has numerous parameters that affect its detailed behaviour. Thus, as mentioned above, whether a specific production fires depends on its utility, a numerical quantity derived from three factors: the expected probability of achieving the current goal given the production, the value of the current goal, and the anticipated cost in terms of time to achieve that goal if the production is fired. Similarly, whether a specific chunk is recalled given a retrieval cue depends on the chunk's activation, which is dependent upon the strength of associations between that chunk and other chunks, the rate of activation decay, and so on. All of these quantities have numerical parameters. Indeed, depending on how one counts, ACT-R has as many as 30 parameters, although not all of them will apply for any particular task and many have default values that apply across many tasks. When all of the parameters are assigned appropriate values, and task knowledge is given, ACT-R is able to produce quantitative 'predictions' for reaction times and error rates. Moreover, given additional assumptions about neural localisation of modules and the relationship between activity in those modules and the BOLD signal—assumptions to be discussed in Section 5.5—ACT-R also predicts neural activity as reflected in fMRI imaging studies.

The number of free parameters that may be adjusted *post hoc* in order to fit rather than predict existing data is of significant concern. Thus, Lovett (2002) produced an ACT-R model of the Stroop task to be discussed in Chapter 9. By varying 12 (!) parameters she was able to fit 92 data points arising from five experiments with an overall R^2 goodness-of-fit measure of 0.95 (see also Lovett, 2005). However, there are methodological problems with the data fitting approach. For example, a good fit says little about a model if the model could, with appropriate parameter settings, account for qualitatively different patterns of behaviour (Roberts & Pashler, 2000). Techniques such as cross-validation[62] and the use of default values across tasks have been proposed to improve the methodological limitations of data fitting, but use of the former approach remains rare, while the latter is still open to criticism since the production rules used for any task can be argued to be equivalent to free parameters (Howes et al., 2009). Data fitting, therefore, remains a significant methodological problem for the evaluation of models developed

---

[60] See Anderson et al. (2004a), for equations that give retrieval times in terms of these factors.

[61] Note that any computational model of a mental process that does not have an inbuilt learning component will need to make

similar assumptions. However, this aspect of production systems raises a danger—namely that they can be used as general purpose programming languages.

[62] Cross-validation involves adjusting a model's parameters to yield a good fit to one dataset and then using the model, with fixed parameters, to predict a second, independent, dataset.

within production system architectures such as ACT-R (Cooper, 2007a).

A further issue relates to the mapping of functions to neural structures within ACT-R, which is coarse, and extends to subprocesses of the central production system (see Figure 3.25). While it gains some support at a broad level, and this includes support from studies specifically testing predictions from the ACT-R account (Anderson et al., 2004b; Anderson et al., 2008a), there are many findings from imaging and patient studies with which it is not consistent. For example the retrieval module is held to be centred on left BA45/46, but this conflates retrieval from working memory, semantic memory and episodic memory. And as we will see in Chapter 10, this is just one of the many regions of prefrontal cortex involved in memory retrieval, and even its lateralisation is somewhat suspect, at least for episodic memory. Similarly, the anterior cingulate is held to be the location of the goal module, but, as we will discuss in Chapter 9, there are many theories of what its function is. We will discuss such issues in more detail in Chapters 9, 10 and 12. It is conceivable that these inconsistencies can be dealt with by refinement of the ACT-R functional architecture and the way it maps onto neural structures, but this remains to be demonstrated.

There is a more general concern with the relation between production system architectures and neuroscience. As noted above, such architectures distinguish between task knowledge and the control mechanism that uses that knowledge. While there have been few attempts to model neuropsychological disorders within production system architectures, those attempts that have been made have assumed that disorders affect the *use* of knowledge rather than task knowledge itself. Thus, Kimberg and Farah (1993) demonstrated that decreasing the degree of spreading activation within the declarative memory of an early (pre-modular) version of ACT-R led to behaviour similar to that of frontal patients on four standard clinical tasks when they were modelled.[63] The tasks were the Stroop task, the Wisconsin Card Sorting Test—both to be discussed in Chapter 9—a motor sequencing task, and a memory for context task. Significant changes have been made to the operation of spreading activation in recent versions of ACT-R, but there is no reason to believe that Kimberg and Farah's result would not hold in the current version. In a second relevant study, to be discussed in Section 12.5, Goel et al. (2001) demonstrated that increased decay of working memory elements within 3CAPS, the predecessor of 4CAPS, led to frontal-type behaviour on the Tower of Hanoi problem—a goal-directed block-moving problem discussed at length in Chapter 12. Both of these accounts imply that executive dysfunction following frontal brain lesions results from a generalised deficit in working memory, and hence that differences between patients with executive dysfunction must be attributed to selective deficits of different types of content within working memory (following Goldman-Rakic, 1996). This is a serious theoretical position that cannot be dismissed without substantial counterargument, but neither architecture (ACT-R or 3CAPS) provides any a priori reason for assuming that working memory aspects of prefrontal function should be structured according to types of content, and hence subject to the kind of content-specific deficits that Kimberg and Farah need to postulate in order to account for why individual frontal patients may perform well on some tasks but poorly on others.[64]

We have seen that production system architectures provide explicit, plausible, operationalisations of the concepts of functional architecture and modularity, including subsystem criteria M1 to M4. However the existing models have significant limitations. Thus, in both ACT-R and EPIC there is no mechanistic account of the functioning of subsystems—they are specified only in terms of their interface requirements and their timing parameters. This kind of specification is sufficient for a theoretical statement within the conceptual domain of a functional architecture, but insufficient for the conceptual domain of brain hardware, yet in providing localisations of subsystems, ACT-R and 4CAPS at least are concerned with this domain. Similarly, current attempts to account for neuropsychological disorders within production system architectures fail to explain why, for example, there are qualitatively different disorders of executive function.

3.9 Conclusions

The overall conclusion of the previous chapter was that we need cognitive-level theories for understanding the mind. Neuroscience alone would be insufficient. The overall conclusion of this chapter is much more eclectic. Four main types of model have been discussed—box-and-arrow diagrams, distributed connectionist models, localist connectionist models and production systems—and all have been held to be useful candidates for confrontation with brain-based evidence.

As the aim of this book is to address in some detail the relation between empirical areas of particular

---

[63] There have as yet been no attempts to relate lesion data to the localisation of function proposed in the current version of ACT-R.

[64] The limitations of relying on different types of working memory content and capacity as the sole factors for explaining executive dysfunctions following prefrontal lesions will be discussed in Chapters 7 and 9.

relevance for higher-level cognition and specific types of model rather than to be encyclopaedic in coverage, discussion will be restricted to these four types of architecture. They are only a smallish subset of those that could potentially be applied to cognitive neuroscience findings. Other computationally powerful approaches include reinforcement learning models (Sutton & Barto, 1998), Bayesian approaches (see Chater et al., 2006), including Bayes nets (Tenenbaum, 1999), and Deep Belief nets (Hinton et al., 2006). Some of these theoretical frameworks are now beginning to be extensively applied in certain areas of cognitive neuroscience such as in perception (Kersten et al., 2004), the role of certain neurotransmitters, including acetylcholine (Yu & Dayan, 2005), dopamine (Niv et al., 2007) and serotonin (Dayan & Huys, 2009), and the effects of reward and punishment (O'Doherty et al., 2004). However these are all topics which are not addressed in detail in this book.

The most basic type of models to be considered are isolable subsystem models. It has been argued that they are essential if we are to make progress. However such models come in families of types, depending upon which of the criteria M1-M9 are held to apply. Assumptions about modular systems will come up in all subsequent chapters. Unless otherwise specified the line of the book will generally be to view the cognitive system as composed of separable subsystems which compute distinct functions, many of them with the character of representations or combinations of representations. Internally, however, the subsystems may be well-characterised as connectionist systems. However the discussion of the anatomical differences between different regions of cortex entails that each connectionist systems should have specific additional characteristics which allow a particular type of input–output operation to be more easily performed. The favoured input–output operation is a function of the specific anatomy of the subsystem itself.

From a Marrian epistemological perspective, we will group the four main types of model into two as far as the cognitive level is concerned. The first type reflects the modular organisation of the mind; the organisation of the overall system is represented by a box-and-arrow diagram together with verbal specifications of the nature of computations implemented in each subsystem. The second type—which includes all three other types of model—corresponds to Marr's algorithmic level of description by providing a computational characterisation of the processes carried out in each subsystem.

The four main classes of models also involve two classes of representation—distributed and localist. The more detailed models will contain elements that should map onto representations in the more broad-ranging models. A key assumption is that these two types of representation can be linked by the concept of the *attractor*.[65] Of the models we consider, the more detailed distributed connectionist analyses will tend to be of particular simple domains with relatively simple outputs. They will be addressed particularly in Chapters 4 and 6. The broader information-processing localist connectionist or symbolic (production system) models will be of more complex domains. They will be discussed most in Chapters 7, 8 and 12.

Having specified in theoretical terms this set of possible ways of capturing cognitive processes, we can now turn to considering how empirical information in cognitive neuroscience relates to such models. We will argue that each of the empirical methods available presents complex problems for making inferences to the underlying structure of the cognitive system. For instance, for EEG and MEG one has the extremely thorny problem that the observed changes in potential at threshold does not adequately constrain which are the underlying pattern of possible sources—the so-called problem of source analysis (Scherg & Berg, 1991). For single- and multiple-cell recording, one has, particularly for higher level processes where extensive training is required, the question of what the relation is between the training and the properties of the cell(s) as studied.

We will therefore limit detailed consideration to two broad classes of methods. The first, to be discussed in Chapter 4, is where one observes behaviour in a subject in whom part of the brain is not functioning normally; this can be either—as in cognitive neuropsychology—because the person has suffered from a neurological disease or—as in transcranial magnetic stimulation (TMS)—because the brain region has been temporarily (and safely) made ineffective. The second class of methods, addressed in Chapter 5,—functional imaging—depend on using measures of brain activity in particular regions of cortex; we will concentrate on functional magnetic resonance imaging (fMRI) and positron emission tomography (PET). It will turn out that while these

---

[65] The relation between connectionist and production system models is more complex. In a purely theoretical exercise, Touretzky and Hinton (1988) showed that a production system architecture could be designed out of components obeying connectionist principles. A variety of specific assumptions had to be added to the connectionist principles with respect to the underlying operation of the components. Strangely this work has not been extensively developed since, though a connectionist implementation of an early version of ACT-R does exist (see Lebière and Anderson, 1993). It will be argued in later chapters that it is necessary to add specific additional assumptions to general connectionist ones for plausible models of particular functions with specific input–output characteristics.

two types of methods are very different, they are remarkably similar as far as the inferences they allow to models of the underlying cognitive processes. Moreover, at least for theories of the isolable system type, they are mutually supportive. Thus cognitive neuroscience will be seen to make progress because the theoretical conclusions that can be drawn are robust across very different types of sets of supporting assumptions and empirical methodologies.

CHAPTER 4

From Cognitive Impairment to Cognitive Models

4.1 The Empirical Methods of Cognitive Neuroscience

A continuing theme in the last three chapters has been that empirical results that combine brain-related methods with measures of behaviour afford a better opportunity for testing cognitive models than do investigations of normal subjects alone. In this and the next chapter we put more flesh on this claim. What are the critical types of findings and how do they relate to models?

Facts in science are frequently complex and typically depend upon a range of presuppositions. Within cognitive neuroscience, these divide into a number of broad classes:

1 Some derive from sciences 'harder' than ours, such as the physics of magnetic resonance imaging. We just assume they are correct theories and that the techniques are reliable and valid.

2 Some depend on rather gross simplifying assumptions about the brain as a physical and physiological object. One example is that of so-called source analysis using EEG, where assumptions have to be made that the source of the electromagnetic field measured by the EEG has certain physical properties.[1] In neuropsychology one typically assumes that the cognitive system investigated has not changed qualitatively during the process of recovery from a lesion.

3 We also need to make presuppositions similar to those that underlie psychological experimentation in normal subjects; that, for instance, any changes in underlying variables during the course of an experiment are roughly linear and that carry-over effects from one condition to another are equal over tasks. This then justifies the use of experimental designs such as Latin Squares in the construction of experiments.[2]

4 Finally, there are a group of simplifying presuppositions that are put forward to allow one to aim to make progress. These include, in addition to the type 2 ones discussed above, presuppositions such as that individuals who do not have a developmental cognitive disability are qualitatively similar in the organisation of their cognitive systems. If this were not true for a particular process, then the methodology of averaging across subjects to produce group means could easily lead to the mean being a pattern of performance that is qualitatively unlike that of any

member of the group.[3] But in complementary fashion, if this presupposition is false, inferences from the detailed study of individual members of the population, the methodology of choice in cognitive neuropsychology over the last 30 years, would not be appropriate for inferences to the organisation of cognition in the population as a whole. Considering basic perceptual processes, say, which appear to have a strong genetic link, this presupposition appears reasonable, but for the more complex processes of higher cognition with which this book is concerned, they are essentially articles of faith, necessary to make a possible start to the scientific enterprise.[4]

The first two types of presupposition are specific to each particular empirical methodology. In contrast, if inferences are to be made from findings from a cognitive neuroscience-type of empirical paradigm in humans to cognitive theorising, then the last two types of presupposition tend to be required whatever brain-related empirical methodology is being used. It is, therefore, important to make them explicit. If they do not hold—either generally or in particular cases—any theoretical conclusion will be worthless. Indeed without making the inference procedure explicit, the possible relevance—or lack of it—of data to theory is unlikely even to be addressed!

The empirical methods of cognitive neuroscience fall into two broad classes. In one, how the system malfunctions due to a permanent or temporary change to brain functioning is examined, or very occasionally, how it functions exceptionally well. It is argued that the pattern of performance that results provides insight into the operation of the undamaged system. In the other, physical measurements of some aspect of brain processes are made when normal subjects are carrying out tasks. As we will see in the next two chapters it is a complicated business to draw conclusions about cognition from any of the methods of cognitive neuroscience. In this and the following chapter we will therefore examine in detail one example of each type. In later chapters we will refer to results obtained with other methods; it is presupposed that analogous, but no doubt very different, inference procedures could be produced for them, but we are not aware of it having been done.

It is not, however, our aim to be comprehensive in our coverage. Rather, our aim in this chapter is to examine the assumptions underlying the cognitive neuropsychological approach in which cognitive structure is

---

[1] For instance Phillips et al. (2002), assume that sources lie in the grey matter, are orthogonal to the cortical sheet and their activity changes smoothly along the cortical sheet.

[2] But see Poulton (1973) for a fiercely sceptical view and Allport and Wylie (2000) for precautionary data.

[3] See the extensive discussion in FNMS Chapter 9.

[4] One possibility is that a large majority of the 'normal' population has one type of organisation of cognition in a given domain but a small group differs. This possibility would particularly undermine the single-case approach.

deduced from cognitive impairment. Specifically we will argue that, while a set of general assumptions can and should be set up, it may on occasions also be appropriate to consider whether one or more of those assumptions has been violated. The possibility of such violations will weaken the inferences that may be drawn from neuropsychological impairments to theories of normal cognitive structure, if those inferences are not supported by other lines of evidence. Similarly, in the next chapter we are principally concerned with the overall logic of the inferences from functional imaging. Again we do not aim to be comprehensive in our discussion of methods.

4.2 **The Methodology of Cognitive Neuropsychology**

The most traditional way to make inferences from cognitive neuroscience to theories of the organisation of the cognitive system has been through the findings of empirical studies of the cognitive effects of brain damage. In neuroscience, when lesions are made in animals they are typically created by surgery. In humans they arise from naturally occurring neurological disease. In the last two decades, these methods have been supplemented by the development of transcranial magnetic stimulation (TMS) for use in humans. In its most common application, TMS is a benign way of inducing what is typically a very short-lasting malfunction of a region of cortex by the application of a brief rapidly changing magnetic field across it (see Walsh & Pascual-Leone, 2003; Miniussi et al., 2010). In this book we will assume that the TMS findings we will discuss can be treated in an analogous fashion to a highly temporary naturally occurring lesion. Since the 1980s, more traditional methods have also been supplemented by the study of cognitive processes in children with developmental abnormalities. This approach has been most productive, as far as the study of the normal cognitive system is concerned, with respect to conditions like autism; the approach placed forcibly on the intellectual agenda the possibility that there could be a specialised cognitive system for holding representations of mental states (Baron-Cohen et al., 1985).[5] Interpretation of developmental disorders is, however, an order-of-magnitude more complex than that of acquired disorders. We will not consider them.

Methodologically we will concentrate on the cognitive effects of naturally occurring lesions in adult humans. Neuropsychological evidence is theoretically important because of the ubiquity of dissociations

following localised lesions. Neurological damage arises from many different aetiologies—tumours, both malignant (gliomas, astrocytomas, metastases) and benign (most meningiomas), vascular accidents (strokes)—both infarcts (blockage of an artery by an embolism) and haemorrhages—dementing conditions, traumatic head injury and many others. For the sufferer their effects range from that of a restricted form of disablement to the destruction of all life quality. Their effects on cognition depend to the first order on where in the brain the lesion is situated. Localised lesions produce, in many cases, what is scientifically the most relevant type of cognitive deficit—ones that are highly selective in what cognitive processes are impaired, or in rare cases are highly selective in what is spared (see Moscovitch & Umiltà, 1990).

The dissociations that are observed between a patient's gross inability to carry out certain cognitive tasks and his or her normal or near-normal performance on closely related ones are the type of dramatic observations that give neuropsychological evidence its special force for providing insight on normal function by comparison with observations of the behaviour of normal subjects in experiments. Many factors make the cognitive experiment on normal subjects a rather blunt instrument for testing theories of normal cognition. This is because these factors—the degree of practice, the precise nature of the material, individual differences, time-of-day and so on—can alter the qualitative pattern of the subject's performance. However the influence of such factors pales by comparison with the dramatic selective deficits that can result from brain damage. Moreover such dissociations occur for all domains of cognitive processing and typically there are a fair number in a given domain.

Dissociations can concern two different types of operations carried out on the same material or the same operation effected on two different types of material. As an example of the former type, patients can lose selectively the ability to be aware of a stimulus, especially when it is in a fairly crowded field (extinction or unilateral neglect, as discussed in Section 1.8) or the ability to point accurately to it when by itself (optic ataxia). The former tends to arise with right inferior parietal lesions (Vallar, 1993; Maguire & Ogden, 2002; Bjoertomt et al., 2002; Mort et al., 2003; but for a contrasting view see Karnath et al., 2001) and most typically affects stimuli in the left visual field. The latter arises with superior parietal lesions, particularly of the right hemisphere (Ratcliff & Davis-Jones, 1972; Perenin & Vighetto, 1988; Battaglia-Mayer & Caminiti; 2002; Pisella et al., 2009; but see also for a different position Karnath & Perenin, 2005). Thus lesions to the superior posterior medial parietal cortex can produce optic ataxia without neglect (Coulthard et al., 2006). The contrast

---

[5] A variety of developmental disorders were known and studied before the 1980. It was at this time, though, that the empirical phenomena under investigation impinged strongly on our understanding of normal cognition.

reflects the differential dependence of the two tasks of reaching and of attending on different subsystems of the parietal cortex.[6]

An example where there is a dissociation between different types of representation, when the same operation is used upon them, comes from the domain of semantics. When patients have to match a word to one of a number of pictures there is a double dissociation between identification of artefacts on the one hand and of living things and foods on the other (relatively preserved artefacts: Warrington & Shallice, 1984; relatively preserved living things and foods: Warrington & McCarthy, 1983, 1987; for reviews see Gainotti, 2000 and Capitani et al., 2003). This dissociation will be discussed extensively in Chapter 6.

That dissociations are often strongly counterintuitive is shown by the frequent and laudable attempts to explain them away in terms of already known factors when they are first described. Thus when the above semantic syndromes were first described—for instance, that of selective loss of living things and foods—the referees were highly sceptical. Over the following ten years a variety of attempts were made to explain away this selective loss in terms of some more basic variable, which was not related conceptually to the operational contrast between the semantic categories that dissociated. The variables used to explain the differences in performance between categories included item familiarity, the structural complexity of items and the density of category examples in the multi-dimensional 'space' of semantic representations (see e.g. Stewart et al., 1992; Funnell & De Mornay Davies, 1997; Gaffan & Heywood, 1993). This type of view is still present, most recently in the application of the concept of *relevance* to the disorder (Lombadi & Sartori, 2007).[7] The gravest problem faced by such attempts to explain away the phenomena is the existence of the complementary dissociations, where living things and foods are relatively preserved.

There is, though, a more basic issue, namely what counts as a dissociation. In the early days of cognitive neuropsychology it was common to use a simple statistical test, such as chi-squared, and a significant difference between the more intact and more impaired performance was considered to be evidence of a dissociation. However, such significant differences can easily occur when two individuals are drawn from the normal population too (see Laws et al., 2005). Somewhat later the idea of a dissociation was refined. In FNMS Chapter 9, the terminology was introduced of a *classical* dissociation, where the better performed task is carried out

completely normally but the impaired task is well below the normal range, a *strong* dissociation where the better performed task is not performed at the normal level but where there is still a large difference between how the two tasks are carried out and a *trend* dissociation where the difference is significant but performance is not qualitatively all that different between the two tasks. It was argued that the trend dissociation has no inferential value, a position substantiated by the later Laws et al. study.

A slightly more sophisticated method is to use z-scores and to consider that one has a classical dissociation if the value of z is less than the 0.05 level for one test and more than it for the other. This approach has numerous problems.[8] With the typical size of control group used in most cognitive neuropsychological studies, Crawford and Garthwaite (2005a) showed that the type I error rate could be as high as 10%. Crawford and Howell (1998) have introduced a modification of the t-test, which allows one to measure abnormality of performance on a single test more adequately. However, even the use of this procedure does not show that a difference in performance across the two tests is abnormal. To do this a revised standardised difference test has been proposed by Crawford and Garthwaite (2005b).[9] Even this procedure can be questioned as far as strong dissociations are concerned. The high error rate that occurs in patients showing putative strong dissociations compared with normal subjects could easily magnify absolute individual differences found in the normal control group. We will return to this issue in Chapter 6, when the topic of categorical specificity, based on strong dissociations, is considered.

Why should the behaviour of individual neurological patients be subject to such detailed questioning? The reason is that given certain assumptions, to be

---

[6] See Section 3.4 and Figure 1.27.

[7] See Chapter 6 for further discussion.

[8] Crawford and Garthwaite (2005a) argue that z-scores are legitimate for the purpose of establishing impairment if used with very large control samples as in most standardised tests. However they point out that in most cognitive neuropsychological single-case studies, a control group is employed which has a few subjects only.

[9] The test statistic proposed by Crawford and Garthwaite (2005b) is:

$$t_{n-1} = \frac{(X^* - \bar{X}) - (Y^* - \bar{Y})}{\sqrt{(s_x^2 + s_y^2 - 2s_x s_y r_{xy})\left(\dfrac{n+1}{n}\right)}},$$

where X^* and Y^* are the scores of the patient on tasks X and Y, n is the number of controls, $\bar{X}$ and $\bar{Y}$ are the means of the controls on the two tasks, s_x and s_y are the standard deviations of the controls on the two tasks, r_{xy} is the correlation between the tasks in controls. Crawford and Garthwaite show that this statistic is distributed according to t with $n-1$ degrees of freedom.

discussed shortly, the empirical domain of any cognitive model of normal function includes the relevant neuropsychological disorders. Furthermore, the ubiquity of dissociations in neuropsychology is most easily explained by 'multiple modularity' with each dissociation reflecting a line of cleavage in the functional architecture with the patient having an impairment of one or more than one of the isolable subsystems involved but preserved performance on the complementary tasks arising because apparently related subsystems are unimpaired.

Maybe, though, neuropsychological dissociations do not entail such a dramatic theoretical conclusion. Up until the 1970s a pre-cognitive human experimental psychologist could easily have justified his or her neglect of neuropsychological phenomena by arguing that they were a fairly random and unpredictable consequence of damage to a very complex neural network, and did not transparently reflect any simple structural property of the network.[10] Or could it not be the case that neuropsychological dissociations represent some complex consequences of the process by which the brain adapts to neurological insult rather than of the system as it existed prior to the acute onset of a disability?

We will consider now the first of these points just presented, as, if valid, it would undermine the theoretical relevance of many of the arguments based on neuropsychological evidence given in this book. The second is an example of a range of empirical possibilities about the brain which need to be treated in the context of the assumptions necessary in making inferences from neuropsychological data to cognitive theory.

4.3 Can Undifferentiated Neural Nets Give Rise to Dissociations when Damaged?

Can a dissociation arise without there being any line of cleavage in the functional architecture between two different subsystems? The answer is yes. Many possibilities exist.[11] The two core tasks may merely differ in difficulty or in the demands they make on a single system. The standard way of showing that this second possibility does not apply is to describe two complementary dissociations—a so-called *double dissociation* as in the two forms of category specific disorder considered above.[12] We will return to this issue shortly. Putting this task-difficulty possibility on one side, it is often loosely

assumed that this type of evidence entails an explanation in terms of isolable systems.[13] In fact there are a variety of other architectures that are compatible with the evidence (see Figure 4.1 for a few possibilities), if the appropriate assumption is made of where the functional lesion is in the model. Thus one of the simple possibilities, shown in Figure 4.1, is that the regions damaged may be better construed as a continuum of a processing space rather than two separable systems.

More critically, could it not be that neural networks when damaged can give rise to dissociations or better double dissociations? In the last chapter we based a discussion of how modularity might have evolved on the work of Bullinaria. Bullinaria, together with Chater (1995), has made the most detailed study of this related issue too. They examined the behaviour of a 3-layer back-propagation network (see Chapter 1 and Figure 4.2). The net was required to learn both 'mappings' between input and output that correspond to the system's obeying a rule and also mappings that correspond to 'exceptions' to the rule. This choice was made to see whether the network could produce complementary dissociations analogous to those found in particular pairs of syndromes. One example—to be discussed in Section 4.6—is the contrast between *surface dyslexia* (where pseudowords unambiguous in their spelling-to-sound mapping, e.g. *durn* or *stimp* can be pronounced correctly but exception words, e.g. *yacht* or *pint* cannot) and *phonological dyslexia* (which has the opposite characteristics).[14] The network's training involved the use of a supervised learning algorithm related to back-propagation, which effected a form of gradient descent (see Section 1.7 and Figure 1.15). It was carried out to a high level of accuracy. Part of the training set consisted of pairs that satisfied the identity relation (this corresponded to learning a rule); in this situation the output pattern of 0s and 1s must faithfully reproduce the input pattern. The other part of the training set consisted of a subrule. If the first units were 1111 or 0000, then the *subrule* was to 'flip' the last three output units. For instance, with the input 111110101 the net had to produce the output 111110010.[15] The former were called examples of the rule, the latter of the subrule.[16]

---

[13] See for discussion of this point van Orden et al. (2001).

[14] A second example is the contrast between the deficits in being able to produce regular forms of the past tense and irregular forms; this will be discussed in Section 8.7.

[15] In another simulation real exceptions were used but the results were similar.

[16] Subrules are analogous to the subregularities that are a characteristic property of many non-regular input–output mappings; consider the pronunciation of the words starting with *war...*, e.g. *war, warn, warp, warm*, etc, which differ consistently from the standard pronunciation of *ar* in English as in *car*.

---

[10] For arguments related to this see Gregory, 1961; Fodor et al., 1974.

[11] See FNMS Chapters 10 and 11 for extensive discussion.

[12] In fact there are considerable complications with respect to this response; see FNMS Chapter 10.

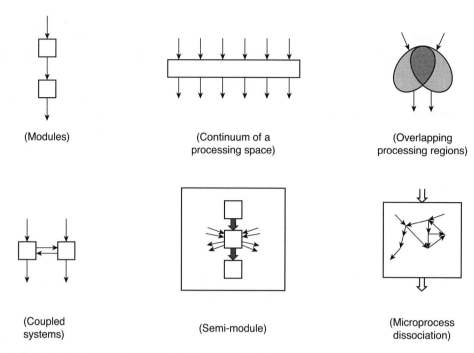

(Modules)

(Continuum of a
processing space)

(Overlapping
processing regions)

(Coupled
systems)

(Semi-module)

(Microprocess
dissociation)

Fig. 4.1 Some functional architectures that can produce dissociations when damaged. Reproduced with permission from Shallice (1988) *From Neuropsychology to Mental Structure*, Cambridge University Press; figure 11.2, p. 250. Copyright © 1988, Cambridge University Press.

Bullinaria and Chater wanted to see whether pairs of lesions within the network—either to the connections or to the hidden units—could produce double dissociations. Essentially they found that if the network was fairly small—9 input units, 100 hidden units and 9 output units—strong dissociations between the ability to use rules and to know exceptions could occur. Thus removing one set of hidden units could lead to as much as a 75% greater loss of the subrule than of the rule. Lesioning a different set could lead to a 48% greater loss of the rule than the subrule. However, when the number of hidden units was increased to 600, then lesions generally affected the subrule mapping more than the rule mapping. A greater preservation of subrules only very rarely occurred and even in those cases the mean subrule advantage was only 3%, with one example of 17%. Essentially the lesions had much more of a mass-action effect, with nearly all the lesions having a greater effect on the task which required the greater quantity of computational resources.[17] The larger the number of hidden units, the more the network behaved in a mass-action fashion, failing to show dissociations that could not simply be attributed to the quantitative differences in the resource requirement of the two tasks. When the network produced dissociations favouring the resource-rich task, it appeared to be because individual units or connections had significant importance in carrying out the mapping.[18] The conclusion follows that if we assume that the relevant networks in the brain are very large, then one would not expect double dissociations to arise by lesioning within a network that lacked structure and lacked internal architectural dimensions that reflected an input or output dimension.

To summarise, generalising from this example, a double dissociation appears not to be explicable in terms of some form of random damage within an otherwise equipotential network. Instead it would appear to require some type of functional specialisation of part of the cognitive system. However, functional specialisation need not necessarily take the form of isolable systems, as Figure 4.1 makes clear. Moreover, as we will see in Section 4.8, a double dissociation can exist with variation in only a single parameter in a network. Nevertheless, the isolable system is the most natural initial basis on which to build a more elaborate theory, as the next section will show.[19]

In this section we have presented an argument that neuropsychological findings are potentially relevant for

---

[17] The concept of 'resource' will be discussed further in Section 4.5.

[18] Similar conclusions were made in an unpublished paper of Medler et al., discussed in Dawson (1998).

[19] As Coltheart (2001) points out, any scientific data are, in principle, open to many possible interpretations. Unless, however, one can be provided, then an in principle objection to the obvious possible interpretation loses its force.

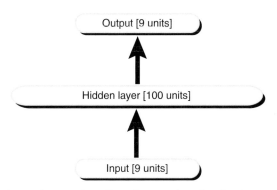

Fig. 4.2 The network used by Bullinaria & Chater (1995) in their explorations of the effects of lesions on the processing of regular (rule-governed) and irregular (exception) items.

understanding cognitive structure. In the next section we formalise the inferential procedure.

4.4 Basic Inference Assumptions

To make inferences from neuropsychological findings to models of normal function one needs a set of assumptions. An initial simple set of assumptions was put forward by Caramazza (1986). One of us shortly thereafter put forward a more complex set.[20] Somewhat related positions have been taken by Vallar (2000) and Coltheart (2000).

Caramazza begins with two initial assumptions. The first is that we have *a hypothesis (plus subsidiary hypotheses, initial conditions and so on) of how the task is carried out by a normal subject (he calls it M for model)*. For reasons that will become apparent shortly, we need to split this assumption into two; the second of which has a group of subsidiary assumptions.

(i) *That we have a model (plus subsidiary hypotheses, initial conditions and so on) of how the cognitive system is organised in a given processing domain.*[21] Examples would include the types of model considered in Chapter 3.

(ii) *A subject attempts to carry out a task, namely he or she attempts to produce outputs of type B, when inputs of type A occur. A subject is assumed to be able to understand what is specified by type A and type B and to be motivated to behave according to the task requirements, which are often given by the instructions. It is also assumed that we have a hypothesis about how the subject tackles the task.*[22] For a task like 'name this object', the realisation of the task in the model is intuitively straightforward. However a task involving, say spatial inferences

such as: *George is taller than Henry. Morris is taller than George. Who is the tallest?* may be tackled either by use of spatial imagery and visual spatial comparison or by a more algebraic approach (see Huttenlocher, 1968, and Section 12.2)[23]. There is a choice between the alternatives, which appears to be voluntary, at least in some subjects, and cannot simply be inferred from the overall functional architecture.

The next critical assumption of Caramazza's is:

(iii) *That a hypothesis is available about how the model is modified in this particular case by brain damage (his L for locus damage).*

Typically this is just assumed to be the failure of a part or parts of the model to operate—the subtraction assumption. In the case of one connectionist model, the deep dyslexia model of Hinton and Shallice (1991) and Plaut and Shallice (1993a), Plaut (1996) has made a more complex set of assumptions. The model is to be discussed further in Section 4.11. Plaut's approach was to 'lesion' the model and then retrain it to simulate a relearning process. However, such sophisticated attempts to realise assumption (iii) in a more complex fashion have unfortunately been extremely rare.

There is one further assumption that is generally assumed to be required in practice, in addition to the three above:

(iv) *The underlying cognitive systems are organised in the same fashion across all individuals in a particular reference group (i.e. members of the same culture).*

A key advance in neuropsychology lay in the appreciation at the advent of cognitive neuropsychology that the method of investigating in detail the pattern of behaviour shown by individual patients or a small group of highly similar patients could be very useful for understanding normal function, even though the behaviour of an individual case is traditionally seen in medicine as too insecure a datum to provide a basis for scientific generalisation. The methodological step forward, though, had a heel of the Achillean sort, in that it rested on the uncritical acceptance of assumption (iv).

It should be noted that on the standard approach of cognitive neuropsychology, patients are selected for study because they present to the clinician with a theoretically interesting disorder. They are not drawn from a population in any fashion that can be statistically justified, e.g. as by random selection. Thus, without an assumption of the above type, inferences cannot be drawn from the performance of a single patient, or even a small *selected series*, to the organisation of the

---

[20] See FNMS, in particular Chapter 10.

[21] The term 'domain' is used for convenience. In theory every hypothesis could apply to the cognitive system as a whole but this would be grossly unwieldy.

[22] See the discussion in Section 2.3.

[23] The former 'spatial paralogic' strategy is in fact complex—see Pylyshyn (2003)—but still very different from the direct rule-following manipulation of symbols.

normal system. With it, the performance of a single patient is in principle all that is necessary to provide support, or alternatively present difficulties, for a theoretical model of possible function. In practice, however, replication of the disorder—the demonstration of a functional syndrome—is critical.[24]

To assume qualitative similarity of cognitive organisation across all members of a culture who do not have a developmental abnormality may seem both a very strong and rather implausible assumption, as well as one suffering from the caveat that at best it is hard to determine whether it is true and at worst it may be untestable. However, as discussed in Chapter 3, group study that averages across group performance or uses standard statistics for group comparison implicitly makes the only slightly weaker assumption that the large majority of the 'normal' population have qualitatively equivalent processing systems.

When first enunciated the assumption was based only on faith together with the clinical intuition, that was essentially untested, that damage to a particular region of the brain had qualitatively the same effects across all patients with the same locus of lesion. Now, however, a possible test of the assumption is available using functional imaging. Somewhat amazingly, no study appears to have been carried out explicitly to test it.[25]

4.5 More Specific Inference Assumptions

In this book we will make more specific assumptions. Most of the more specific assumptions replace one of the more general ones. Thus assumption 1 incorporates assumption (i), 2 incorporates (ii) and 5_{NR} is a more specific version of 5_N which is more specific than (iii); if however a more specific assumption fails then one can move back to the more general one. In so doing we qualify two of the above assumptions in order to derive consequences from them or to cope with simple problems which arise from inferences based on the more basic versions. The first assumption is that:

1. One has a model (plus subsidiary hypotheses, initial conditions and so on) of how the cognitive system is organised in a given processing domain. The underlying system is weakly modular in the sense of assumptions M1, 2, 5, 6, 7 and 8 of Sections 3.3 and 3.4. Each module computes a basic I-O function.

This allows us to decompose execution of a task into separable stages.[26] The importance of this assumption is that the number of processes involved in a typical cognitive task is very large indeed as discussed in the last two chapters. We next assume that:

2. When a subject attempts to carry out a task, he or she attempts to produce outputs of type B, when inputs of type A occur. A subject is assumed to be able to understand what is specified by type A and type B and to be motivated to behave according to the task requirements which are often given by the instructions. Task performance requires, in addition to a model of the relevant on-line processes, the use of a procedure. The procedure specifies what subsystems and connections are relevant to the carrying out of the particular task.

If one takes any reasonably complicated cognitive domain, such as that of single word processing as shown in Figure 4.3, then the carrying out of any individual task involves only a subset of the systems and connections potentially available. For instance reading-to-meaning, reading aloud without paying attention to meaning, shadowing (echoing back speech), copying written words and transcribing speech to writing all involve different combinations of the same set of subsystems and connections to be achieved. In Chapter 9 it will be argued that the key process involved for selecting the particular set of on-line components and connections used for when a given task is being realised are one or more *action or thought schemas* depending upon whether one is in the domain of action or thought.

The concept of *action schema*, standing for one level of control unit for action, will be discussed in detail in Section 8.3. We will use the term *thought schema* as different from an *action schema* in that it involves qualitatively different types of representations (see Chapters 6, 8 and 12). Instead of *thought schema* the term *task-set* is often used (e.g. Allport et al., 1994). However the concept is typically undefined and, if interpreted literally, it would imply that to each task condition there is a single task-set, which would not be justified.[27] Abstractly having a satisfactory model of the procedure(s) employed for

---

[24] It should be noted that if assumption (iv) is made, topics of potential interest such as *synaesthesia* and *absolute pitch* must be excluded from study, since they are only found in a subset of the normal population.

[25] The test would need to be based on assumptions concerning individual differences in localisation of function—see the discussion of the fMRI experiment of Crescentini et al. (2009) in Section 5.3.

[26] As discussed in Section 3.2, even well-developed connectionist models, such as that of Plaut et al. (1996), only attempt to model a part of the overall process. They also can be conceived of as having separable subcomponents; we do not, however, presuppose that the state of the hidden units in such a model corresponds to a representation (assumption M3). This is why we use the characterisation of weak modularity.

[27] We will ignore for the present complications such as that some stimuli elicit their own procedure as in the so-called Stroop task, where subjects have difficulty in naming the colour in which a colour-word, e.g. *red* is written. These issues will be considered in Chapter 9.

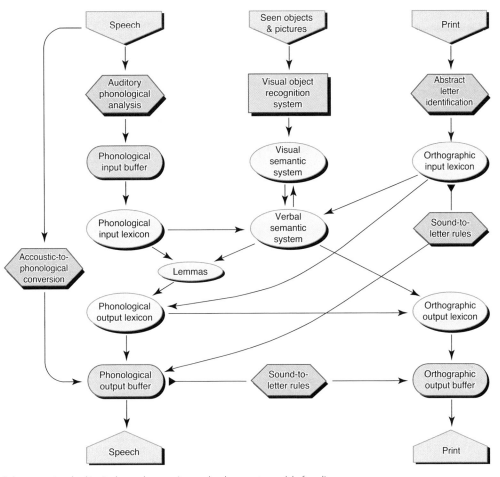

Fig. 4.3 Sub-systems involved in single word processing on the three route model of reading.

a given task is as important as the specification of the functional architecture.

The switching on of processing components and connections is not all that schemas control. They also have what we call *arguments* (following linguistic usage). These are the variables that specify which stimulus or remembered representation is to be operated upon. As we will discuss in Chapter 8, action schemas must have an internal structure since as stated above they need to satisfy multiple constraints. Schemas can also, for instance, set thresholds. A common experimental procedure is to instruct the subject to produce a response before a given temporal deadline, such as 500 msec after stimulus onset. This is presumably carried out by a learning process which involves varying the output thresholds for processing components.

A *procedure* corresponds to the operation of the implemented schemas involved in executing a task. The procedure is typically set up as a result of the subject's understanding the task instructions and voluntarily deciding to follow those instructions. However, as we will see shortly, the process can be far from transparent

to the investigator, especially when the subject is other than a normal adult of the same culture.

Theoretical explanations using box-and-arrow models normally just assume implicitly that for a particular task there is a specific procedure that is applied. Computational models, by contrast, need to make some of the assumptions about the procedure in operation more explicit. For instance, the so-called Dual Route Cascaded model of reading aloud, of Coltheart et al. (2001) shown in Figure 3.4 and which will be considered extensively later in the chapter, builds on proposals of Coltheart et al. (1977) and Grainger and Jacobs (1996) in assuming that the task of lexical decision involves three decision criteria.[28] Thus the theory requires assumptions about the procedure involved in each task discussed, in addition to the specification of the functional architecture.

---

[28] In Coltheart et al.'s modelling, there are two ways by which a YES response can occur—by activation in any one lexical unit exceeding a threshold or by the summed activation rapidly going high—and also a complicated time deadline for NO responses.

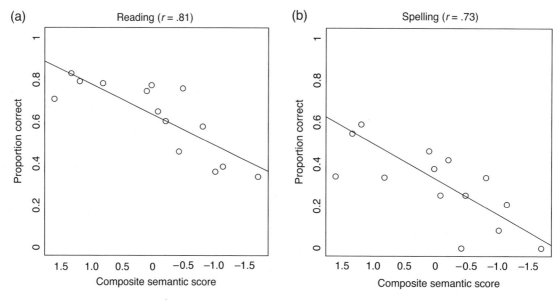

Fig. 4.4 Scatterplots showing the correlation between a measure of semantic impairment (composite semantic score) and the proportion correct for (a) reading aloud and (b) spelling words irregular in their spelling-to-sound correspondences for 14 semantic dementia patients. Adapted with permission from Patterson et al. (2006) 'Presemantic' cognition in semantic dementia: Six deficits in search of an explanation. *Journal of Cognitive Neuroscience, 18,* 169–183. Copyright © 2006, MIT Press Journals.

We will introduce here, as it will become relevant later, an assumption based on the brain-based aspects of weak modularity from Section 3.4 (assumptions M4 and M9), namely that:

> 3. *Specific computational operations depend upon individual I-O systems, which are anatomically relatively focally localised. In particular each of the I-O functional systems (F_i) is held to occupy a relatively restricted region of the brain (b_i), its base region. Within each hemisphere the base region can be viewed as a continuous sheet at a reasonably gross anatomical level.[29]*

This assumption is loosely specified with respect to what counts as a 'region' and how anatomically similar it needs to be in different individuals, or how all-or-none it needs to be. This vagueness is unavoidable given our present state of knowledge.

A further assumption is, however, critical for allowing inferences to be drawn to normal function from both single-case and group studies. This was one derived from Caramazza (1986); it is assumption (iv) of the previous section, namely that:

> 4. *The cognitive system is organised in the same fashion across all individuals in a particular reference group (i.e. members of the same culture).*

We now come to the main specific neuropsychological assumption, Caramazza's subtraction assumption—assumption (iii).[30] It becomes:

> 5_N. *The damaged system is a reduced but not reorganised version of the normal system*

At the end of the chapter a corollary of this assumption and assumption 3 becomes important, namely that:

> 3_N. *All patients who have selective loss of the base function should have lesions that anatomically affect the same region or the main input or output pathways to and from it. Moreover patients with lesions to the region should show loss of the base function.*

This assumption, however, played no role in traditional cognitive neuropsychology of the 1970s and 1980s, at least for 'ultra cognitive neuropsychologists' who rejected group studies. It will not be referred to for most of this chapter which is concerned with the methodology of 'single-case' cognitive neuropsychology.

Most simply one could assume that a subsystem is either working normally or it is not working at all. However this idea is a gross oversimplification. There are many situations where it is useful to consider varying degrees of impairment. For instance, as we will discuss later in this chapter, Patterson et al. (2006) drew major theoretical conclusions from the existence of a strong

---

[29] The last part of this assumption becomes relevant in the next chapter.

[30] For simulations suggesting that this assumption may be valid at best only at a gross level see Alstott et al. (2009).

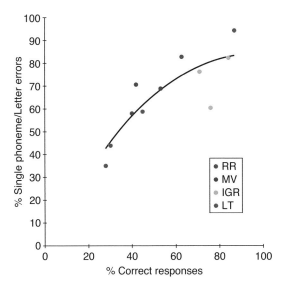

Fig. 4.5 Percentage of single phoneme/letter errors made by four patients plotted against their percentage of correct responses. The curve is the best-fitting quadratic passing through (0, 0). Adapted from T. Shallice, R.I. Rumiati & A. Zadini (2000) The selective impairment of the phonological output buffer. *Cognitive Neuropsychology*, 17(6), 517–546, reprinted by permission of the publisher (Taylor & Francis Group, http://www.informaworld.com).

correlation across patients all of whom presented with a particular functional syndrome—semantic dementia. This was between their performance on reading words and a composite score of semantic ability (see Figure 4.4, left). These conclusions assume that the effect of the output of the semantic system on other systems can be viewed as lying on a continuum between total impairment and normal operation. In a quite different context Shallice et al. (2000) were studying disorders of the output phonological buffer, to be discussed in Chapter 7. They showed that the relation between the percentage of errors involving only a single phoneme and overall per cent correct lay on the same curve for three different tasks—repeating, reading and writing non-words—in four different patients, their patient LT and also IGR (Caramazza et al., 1986), MV (Bub et al., 1987) and RR (Bisiacchi et al., 1989) (see Figure 4.5). Again one can represent effectively the capacity of the system in terms of a single variable. [31] This can be expressed as:

5_{NR}. *To a first approximation, the efficacy of a subsystem for carrying out the tasks for which it is required is given by a parameter r (for resource) lying between 0 and 1. The performance of any task is $f(r_1, r_2, r_3, ..., r_n)$ where $f=1$ when $r_1 = r_2... = r_n = 1$ and where $f(r_i)$ is a monotonic non-decreasing function of all the r_i including those lying between 0 and 1.*

The function $f(r_i)$ is a performance-resource function, first introduced for the analysis of divided attention dual-tasks in normal subjects (Norman & Bobrow, 1975; Navon & Gopher, 1979) (see Figure 4.6). As an increasing amount of the available resource of a subsystem, which is required by both tasks, is allocated to one of the two tasks, say, by altering the relative rewards for succeeding in the two tasks, so performance on that task increases. It reaches a maximum value when all the available resource is allocated to the task. By analogy the concept can be applied—in reverse—as the increasing loss of resource in a patient as a subsystem becomes progressively more impaired, say in a dementing process.[32]

On the assumption of single-valued monotonic resource functions, if two tasks rely critically on a single subsystem, then two patients can show a single dissociation, even if they both have damage to this subsystem merely due to differences in task difficulty. However the two patients cannot show a double dissociation, if this is appropriately defined as patient X performing better than patient Y on task A and with the reverse pattern on task B. This can be simply illustrated using the elegant notation developed by Newell and Dunn (2008) of the state-trace graph. This plots how two behavioural measures (dependent variables) relate to each other as the experimenter-controlled independent variables used in the experiment change. It is assumed that each behavioural measure has an upwardly monotonic relation with any system resources required. Then if both dependent variables are manifestations of the operation of a single common resource, the state-trace plot will be a single upwardly monotonic function (see Figure 4.7a).

This is simply proved. If $y = f(r)$ is upwardly monotonic in r then if $y_1 > y_2$ it follows that $r_1 > r_2$. If in addition $x = g(r)$ is upwardly monotonic in r then if $y_1 > y_2$ it follows that $x_1 > x_2$. Hence y is upwardly monotonic in x. Therefore a cross-over double-dissociation cannot be realised by a single resource (see Figure 4.7b).[33]

These assumptions—1–5—will need to be examined further. The first two may not apply in some cases. In

[31] This was also shown for another error characteristic, namely the rate of single substitution errors.

[32] If one averages over, say, 30% removals of artificial neurons in a simulation, then one is implicitly making this type of assumption.

[33] This is a simplification—see FNMS Chapter 10 for extensive discussion. Newell and Dunn make the well-known and correct criticism of inferences from single dissociations to multiple resources but completely mischaracterise the argument from FNMS in dismissing dissociations; the counter-example they give does not have cross-over characteristics (see e.g. FNMS Figure 10.5 for analogous cases). Glymour (1994), more substantively, has argued that this assumption of a potentially varying resource makes the theoretical methodology of cognitive neuropsychology inherently unfalsifiable and so non-progressive. For a response, see Shallice et al. (2000).

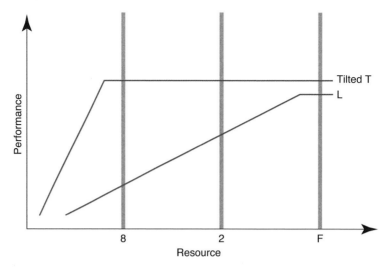

Fig. 4.6 Performance-resource functions for a target-detection task where targets are tilted Ts (red) or Ls (blue) in a background of upright Ts (see Beck & Ambler, 1973). Grey lines represent the resource allocated to the target in three conditions: focussed attention (F); when the target is in one of two positions (2); and when it is in one of eight positions (8). The graph demonstrates how performance when targets are tilted Ts can remain constant, while performance when targets are Ls increases from 8 to 2 to F. Redrawn from *Cognitive Psychology*, 7(1), D.A. Norman & D.G. Bobrow, On data-limited and resource-limited processes, 44–64, Copyright (1975), with permission from Elsevier.

certain situations, the third and fourth may well be found to be over-simple; there may, for instance, be qualitatively different types of damage to the same subsystem. There may also be problems in applying the fifth. However, before considering these problems, what do the assumptions bring us?

As far as cognitive neuropsychology is concerned—the drawing of inferences from neuropsychological findings on single patients to the organisation of the normal cognitive system, with assumptions 1, 2, 4 and 5—the functional architecture for implementing a procedure may be viewed as a directed graph with nodes for processing systems and directed connections, which enable an input to be transformed into an output (see Glymour, 1994). Normal performance entails that at least one intact path can be found between input and output. Moreover given a model of the on-line functional architecture (assumption 1), any given pattern of damaged components and connections will predict which of a set of input–output mappings should allow normal performance and for which it should be impaired. Given that the procedure used in each task involving the input-output mappings can be specified, the pattern of performance across tasks therefore strongly constrains the models of the functional architecture that are possible.

In addition to the assumptions underlying the processing models, this leaves three additional assumptions, namely 2, 4 and 5_{NR}. The first of these specifies that the functional architecture in a particular domain is at the service of the subject's motivation and intentions. We typically assume that the subject makes the most efficient use of the functional architecture available in

the domains relevant to the task.[34] However, the adopted procedure may be far from transparent in its consequences, as in *sotto voce* letter-by-letter reading, to be discussed in Section 4.12. Moreover, the payoff function is often ill-specified, as in the standard instruction: *be as fast as you can making as few errors as possible*. Assumption 5_{NR} has a similar status. It is necessary to check that tasks across which the performance of subjects is being compared are roughly of equivalent difficulty. If this is not done, misleading inferences can be drawn, as in the case of one-way dissociations. Finally, assumption 4 is standardly just assumed. It is the implicit creed on which cognitive neuropsychology was based. In Section 4.9 we will show that it cannot go unquestioned.

4.6 The Application of the Assumptions

To examine more concretely how these assumptions can be used, but also to see where they may be questioned, we will mainly use the domain of the acquired dyslexias, the area which saw the most dramatic early flowering of the use of the cognitive neuropsychology approach in the 1970s and 1980s. Between 1957 and 1979 seven new types of acquired dyslexia were discovered, to add to the one nineteenth century form that survived—pure

---

[34] The validity of this additional assumption is supported by its widespread use in the adaptive behaviour literature where subjects are assumed to maximise some payoff function (e.g. Anderson, 1990; Howes et al., 2009).

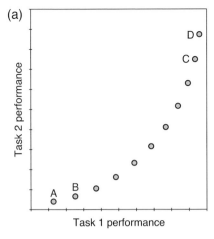
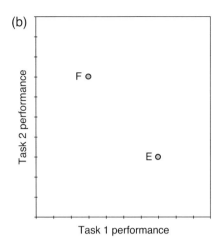

Fig. 4.7 (a) A state-trace plot showing performance on two tasks as a function of the resource required by the tasks. Points A and B demonstrate how two patients can show a single dissociation, with performance on task 2 being similar for A and B while performance on task 1 is better for B than for A. Points C and D demonstrate that the reverse dissociation can also arise from a deficit affecting a single resource. (See Newell & Dunn, 2008.) (b) Since the state-trace plot for single resource processes must be monotonically increasing, a deficit to a single resource cannot result in a double dissociation, defined as one patient (E) performing better on task 1 than another patient (F), but worse than that other patient on task 2.

alexia (Dejerine, 1892) (see Table 1.2). By the end of the 1980s a number of plausible box-and-arrow models had been developed to explain them.

The acquired dyslexias can be divided into two groups. In the first type—pure alexia, visual dyslexia, neglect dyslexia, and attentional dyslexia—the problem appears to lie in the attainment of an adequate internal orthographic representation of the letter string. We will consider them—the so-called *peripheral acquired dyslexias*—in more detail later. However this division itself suggests a functional separability between ortho-graphic and post-orthographic processes in reading. In the *central acquired dyslexias* the representation of the letter string which is passed from the orthographic to other systems, and which we will call its *word-form*, is assumed to be adequately attained. The problem lies later in processing—in the accessing of appropriate phonologi-cal or semantic representations.

In Chapter 1 we introduced two forms of central acquired dyslexia—deep and surface dyslexia—first described by Marshall and Newcombe (1966, 1973). Many more such patients of each type have now been described. Thus, when Plaut and Shallice (1993a) pro-duced their theoretical analysis of the syndrome, at least 35 patients had been described as examples of deep dyslexia. Surface dyslexia, in turn, has been found to be a common consequence of semantic dementia; Woollams et al. (2007) in a single paper describe the performance of about 50 such patients.

For each of these syndromes if one looks at the types of word that patients find easy or difficult to read and also at the errors they make, then the two types of evi-dence seem to point to a critical dimension accounting

for the syndrome. And the critical dimension is different for the two syndromes.

In the case of deep dyslexia, patients read concrete nouns far better than abstract nouns or other parts of speech. For instance, KF (Shallice & Warrington, 1975), the second deep dyslexic described in detail, read 73% of concrete nouns such as *tractor* correctly but only 14% of abstract nouns such as *faith*, 32% of adjectives such as *green,* and 10% or less for other parts of speech. Complementarily, when attempting to read words these patients typically make errors which are either semantically or visually related to the presented word, such as *bush → tree* or *sword → words*.[35] If we leave on one side the visual errors, which in some deep dyslexic patients can be a high proportion of all errors, it is clear that a semantic dimension is relevant for both differen-tiating words that can from those that cannot be read and for characterising errors.

By contrast, in surface dyslexic patients, the critical dimension relates to the regularity of the spelling-to-sound mapping. Thus a patient like MP (Bub et al., 1985) read words that use the most typical spelling-to-sound correspondences in the language given the ortho-graphic context such as (for English) *house, bricks, dinner, faith* at over 90% correct whatever their frequency in the language, and with a normal naming latency.[36]

---

[35] They also make morphological errors of producing inappro-priate affixes such as *card → cards*; they could be either seman-tic or visual or in a different class.

[36] Not all patients characterised as 'surface dyslexic' by these investigators in fact read so fluently; they do not read an

Words that used less standard spelling-to-sound correspondences, such as *tomb* (pronounced as *toom*) or *colonel* (pronounced as *kernel*), were read much worse. How badly they were read depended on their frequency of occurrence in the language. Very high frequency irregular words were read 80% correctly; ones occurring less than 25 times per million were read less than 40% correctly. The overwhelmingly most frequent type of error was a regularisation—that is, pronouncing the word as it is spelled.

At least two factors in spelling-to-sound translations are relevant to surface dyslexia. One is whether the pronunciation of the word corresponds to the spelling-to-sound 'rules' of the orthography of the language. The other is how consistently a string of letters larger than a single letter but smaller than a word is pronounced. Thus words ending ...*ind*, e.g. *hind, find, bind* are relatively consistently pronounced to rhyme with *mind*, where the *i* is technically pronounced in an irregular fashion (compare *bit*). A group of 12 semantic dementia patients who were 80% correct on reading regular consistent words showed increased errors of 18% for lack of regularity underlying a mapping and 12% for lack of consistency in the mapping; these being essentially orthogonal effects (Jefferies et al., 2004).

These two syndromes were ones that had initially provided the basic motivation for multiple-route models of reading, which are descendants of the two-route model of Marshall and Newcombe (1973). Such models all contain one or more systems concerned with the orthographic analysis and categorisation of letter strings, which we will discuss more extensively later in the chapter. They then have separate routes, one or more, giving rise respectively to phonological and semantic representations of the written word. The deep dyslexic patients are held to read by a 'semantic' route[37] and the surface dyslexic patients by a 'phonological' route. The simplest such model (see Figure 3.3) is now often called the 'triangle' model. In gross functional architecture, if not in its details, it resembles that of Marshall and Newcombe (1973).

If one restricts consideration to systems and connections prior to the phonological and semantic systems for the two routes, respectively, then the model predicts up to four different types of disorder:

1 A general deficit of visual processing (for a lesion prior to the orthographic system).

2 A deficit of orthographic processing that will affect the attaining of both phonological and semantic representations of the presented word; we will discuss this so-called *pure alexia* or better *word-form alexia* later in Section 4.12 of this chapter.

3 A condition in which reading aloud becomes dependent on the use of the mappings from orthography to phonology; this roughly corresponds to surface dyslexia.

4 A condition in which reading becomes solely dependent on the mappings from orthography to semantics and from semantics to output phonology. What this corresponds to is unclear without a better specified account of how the route operates. However, if one assumes an absolute loss of the phonological route and partial damage to the semantic route one has a plausible if intuitive account of deep dyslexia.[38]

The existence of surface and deep dyslexia does not logically entail a model including multiple reading routes. Yet only one group of theorists have rejected the multiple route framework—at least with respect to the existence of separable semantic and phonological routes. They are van Orden and colleagues (see e.g. van Orden et al., 2001). However—at least in some versions of their approach—even they presuppose separable orthographic, phonemic and semantic 'nodes' with separable interactions between each (see e.g. van Orden et al., 1997).[39]

Interpretations of other disorders in the domain are, however, far from straightforward. In 1979 two new syndromes were described, both of which seemed to require at least major modifications to the triangle model, if that is based directly on the Marshall and Newcombe account. During the 1980s and 1990s the theoretical choices made to explain the group of four syndromes diverged rapidly.

The first of the two new syndromes was *phonological alexia*, first described in two forms by the French neuropsychologists Beauvois and Derouesné (1979) (see also Derouesné & Beauvois, 1979). In phonological alexia the patient is able to read words very well but

orthographically regular non-word such as *frint* in the same fluent fashion with which a normal subject does. Some of these patients were probably using a non-standard compensatory procedure to cope with a pure alexia by explicitly sounding out the word phoneme-by-phoneme instead of using knowledge of the word's spelling; see FNMS Section 4.5. This type of patient provides an example of where a non-transparent procedure (assumption 2) masks the true nature of the patient's difficulty.

[37] An exception is that Coltheart (1980a) and Saffran et al. (1980) in fact do not consider that deep dyslexic patients read by the standard semantic route. Coltheart considers that they use a qualitatively different semantically-based route in the right hemisphere. See Section 4.11.

[38] Certain aspects of the syndrome are apparently not that well explained, such as, for instance, the visual errors. We will return to this point later.

[39] Where they essentially differ from other accounts is in holding that extensive reverberating interactions between the different nodes are taking place over most of the duration of the access process.

has great difficulty in reading pronounceable non-words. By now more than twenty such patients have been individually described (see e.g. Patterson, 2000; Caccappolo-van Vliet et al., 2004a, 2004b) and the syndrome occurs frequently after left parietal or prefrontal lesions (Rapcsak et al., 2009).

The second syndrome was preserved lexical reading—reading in the absence of comprehension or *reading without semantics*—first described briefly by Schwartz et al. (1980a) in patient WLP. Patient WLP could read virtually all words aloud but did not understand most of them. Thus she could only categorise 7/20 low-frequency animals names as animals but could read correctly 18/20 including words such as *hyena* irregular in their spelling-to-sound correspondences. Another such patient was reported a few years later by McCarthy and Warrington (1986a) and further ones by Cipolotti and Warrington (1995a), Lambon Ralph et al. (1995), Raymer and Berndt (1996), Lambon Ralph et al. (1998), Gerhand (2001) and by Blazely et al. (2005).

4.7 Computational Models and a More Complex Dataset

Does one need to modify the Marshall–Newcombe version of the triangle model to account for these two new syndromes, and if so how? Indeed one does. How, for instance, could reading without semantics be explained? There have been a variety of different approaches as to how this should be done. In addition, though, in the same period a major change occurred with regard to theory development, namely in how the models of normal function, which provide the 'flesh' for the functional architecture of assumption 1, are specified. Early in the history of cognitive neuropsychology, models were of the box-and-arrow type having only rough verbal specifications of component subsystems (see Section 3.6). However, although the theoretical problems posed by phonological alexia and reading-without-semantics had become apparent by 1980, and the first computational model in the area of the central dyslexias was not published until 1989, the choice between the rival successions to Marshall and Newcombe is now primarily viewed not as a selection between box-and-arrow models, but between computational models.

The simplest modification is to argue for three routes (see Figure 3.4),[40] a position initially put forward in box-and-arrow model form by Morton and Patterson (1980) (see also Coltheart, 1978) but developed computationally by Coltheart et al. (1993) and then in a somewhat modified form further by Coltheart et al. (2001). The model builds on the highly successful interactive activation model of McClelland and Rumelhart (1981), discussed in Section 3.7, but uses its principles for the operation not just of a single route but of three routes—a non-lexical grapheme-phoneme conversion route, a non-semantic lexical route and a semantic route.[41] On this account phonological alexia and reading-without-semantics represent the lexical non-semantic route operating without the non-lexical route or without the semantic route respectively.[42]

The lexical non-semantic route operates as an updated version of the McClelland and Rumelhart (1981) interactive-activation network as far as the orthographic word-forms are concerned. The corresponding phonological word-forms they activate then serially activate phoneme units. The non-lexical grapheme–phoneme conversion route operates in a strictly left–right fashion in which correspondences for longer sets of letters, e.g. *igh* are applied before those corresponding to any smaller set they contain e.g. *i*. When a rule is applied the corresponding phoneme unit is activated by the mean of the activation of its component letters. Fitting the model involves estimating its 31 parameters. We will consider the adequacy of the model in the next section.

However this has not been the only response to the existence of the two new syndromes. At least three alternative approaches were developed which maintained some version of a single phonological route position. One approach, that of Howard and Franklin (1988) and Hillis and Caramazza (1991), has been to hold to the basic Marshall and Newcombe model but to argue that reading-without-semantics occurs by a summation of the output of a non-lexical route and an impaired but not non-existent semantic route. It was already known, e.g. from AR (Warrington & Shallice, 1979) and ML (Shallice & Saffran, 1986), that patients not able to read a word aloud or unable to precisely access its meaning could still know its rough meaning. They could, for instance, very frequently know its superordinate category (see Section 6.3). Thus it was argued by Hillis and Caramazza that a patient might be able to read the *y* of *yacht* and know it was a water-going type of transport; so the system would induce by summation *yacht*.

A second, and much the best known alternative, was to make the phonological route a feed-forward 3-layer connectionist net mapping orthographic letter strings corresponding to whole words onto phonological representations. The initial version developed by Seidenberg and McClelland (1989) relied on clever but

---

[40] This model is often very confusing referred to as the 'dual-route' model, referring specifically to the two phonological routes.

[41] In fact the semantic route has not been simulated and so in the later versions of the model makes no contribution to reading aloud.

[42] This would also be the case for another computational model—that of Zorzi et al. (1998).

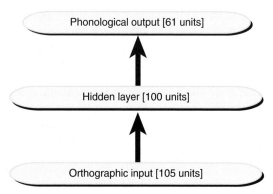

Fig. 4.8 The 3-layer feed-forward network used by Plaut et al (1996) for modelling the mapping from orthographic to phonological representations. This represents at a different conceptual grain the part shown in the rectangle of Figure 3.3.

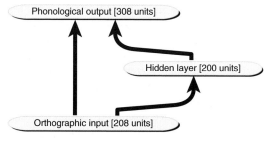

Fig. 4.9 The dual-route feed-forward model of Zorzi et al (1998) for mapping orthographic representations to phonological ones. Direct connections from the orthographic layer to the phonological layer learn regularities in the mapping while exceptions are acquired by the hidden layer route.

psychologically unrealistic orthographic and phonological representations. A version with much more plausible orthographic and phonological representations was therefore developed by Plaut, McClelland, Seidenberg & Patterson (1996) (see Figure 4.8). Like the Coltheart et al. DRC model, but unlike the Hillis–Caramazza one, this was computationally explicit. The net was trained on all the monosyllabic words in English. 30 units coded graphemes in syllable onsets; they represented either single letters, e.g. *I*, or letter pairs, e.g. *TH*, 27 units coded for vowel graphemes as either individual letters, e.g. *O* or letter pairs, e.g. *OO*, and 41 units coded for graphemes in the syllable coda, either single, double or triple letters, e.g. *T, TT* or *TCH*. Thus a word like THROUGH is represented by activation of syllable onset units *TH* and *R*, vowel unit *OU* and syllable coda unit *GH*. Similar principles were applied for the phonological output system. The weights of the orthographic-to-phonological pathway were then trained using back-propagation in a way that reflected the frequencies of words in the language.

A third possibility, put forward by Shallice et al. (1983) and Shallice and McCarthy (1985), and developed computationally by Norris (1994), was to argue that the phonological 'route' contained a number of levels of correspondence—graphemes, subsyllabic units such as initial consonant cluster (e.g. *str* of *straight*), rimes (i.e. vowels plus final consonant cluster e.g. *aight* of *straight*) and syllables as well as whole morphemes. What made this theory more constrained was the assumption that units and connections were differentially resistant to impairment— depending on their frequency in the language. Thus whole-word correspondences are assumed to be generally more fragile than grapheme-phoneme level ones. This was required to explain surface dyslexia, where the grapheme-phoneme level correspondences still operate even when word-level ones are no longer effective. In terms of assumption 5_{NR} the amount of resource needed depends upon the frequency with which the unit occurs in the language. Therefore generally the translations of morpheme-size units requires more resources and are therefore more liable to be lost than those operating on syllabic, sub-syllabic or grapheme-size units.

This is far from the complete set of theories that have been developed in this domain. In particular, the model of Zorzi et al. (1998) is empirically at least as solid as any of the ones discussed (see e.g. Zorzi, 2005). In this model the single phonological pathway of the Plaut et al. triangle model is expanded into two pathways, one without a set of hidden units and the other just like the hidden-unit pathway in the Plaut et al. model (see Figure 4.9). It therefore has in effect an architecture like a DRC model implemented in a Plaut et al.-like connectionist fashion. As a consequence it can mimic aspects of both more basic models (see also Perry et al., 2010 for an extension of the model to multi-syllabic words). Yet there is no clear a priori justification for the assumption of the two types of route.

How do the two most basic approaches deal with the set of four syndromes? One of them does it by rejecting some of the simple assumptions previously described. Consider, first, phonological alexia. As far as the DRC model is concerned, it is simply explained by the loss of efficiency of the non-lexical route (see Coltheart et al., 1996). For the other model, there are major complications. No attempt was made by Plaut et al. (1996) to simulate phonological alexia in the definitive version of the triangle model. However Harm and Seidenberg (2001) did do so with a closely related model. The phonological output units of the Plaut et al. model can be supported by *clean-up units* in order to build strong attractors at the output phonological-word level.[43]

---

[43] An improvement in the Harm and Seidenberg model is that the positional coding of orthography does not use the absolute position of letters in the input string. Instead this is carried out relative to the vowel. For clean-up units see Figures 1.14 and 4.11.

Harm and Seidenberg then added noise to the output units and obtained a behaviour pattern corresponding to phonological alexia. If the correspondence between orthography and phonology was stronger for graphemes and phonemes then the simplest way to explain phonological alexia on this approach was as a problem of the output phonological system.

This account corresponded to an important empirical theme for explaining phonological alexia. In 1985, Derouesné and Beauvois, the original discoverers of phonological alexia, had performed a very detailed analysis of one such patient, LB1. LB1, who was French, was 98% accurate in reading irregular words. He scored 68% in reading non-words which sounded like words (e.g. *kacé* sounding like *cassé*) or *ylau* sounding like *ilot*). However when the non-words, which were closely matched in other respects, did not sound like words (e.g. *tiko*, *aufo*) he was much worse (30%). It is clear that if the output phonological representation is based on an attractor, as in Harm and Seidenberg's simulation, and one is not available, performance would indeed be predicted to be worse.

More directly, Patterson and Marcel (1992) had tested a number of phonological alexic patients on a variety of purely phonological tasks such as blending phonemes to form a word as in /k/.../ae/..../t/ → cat and segmentation as in cat → /k/.../ae/..../t/. All were impaired. This too supported the idea that phonological alexia could be attributed to problems in the production of the non-words rather than in the transmission of information from the orthographic system.

However the beginning of a dent in this conclusion came from a study by Patterson (2000) on the phonological alexic CJ. She argued 'One could certainly not conclude that CJ's phonological skills were normal; but given that he *failed* to produce a correct response to about 80% of simple non-words in reading, his roughly 80% *correct* performance in both segmentation and blending even with non-word responses suggests that his non-word reading failures cannot be attributed entirely, or even primarily, to a general phonological weakness impeding the production of unfamiliar phonological forms.' (Patterson, 2000, p. 68). Later, Caccapolo-van Vliet et al. (2004a, 2004b) described three patients, MO, IB and RG2, with Alzheimer's disease, whose word reading was at the (i) 96%, (ii) 96%, (iii) 98% level, respectively. By contrast the reading of non-words was far worse, (i) 50%, (ii) 43%, (iii) 56%, respectively. However if one carried out tests that were specifically of the phonological system itself, such as blending or segmentation, then the patients behaved almost perfectly. Thus it appeared that the impairment could not be attributed to a problem in the

phonological output system, such as in the phonological output buffer (see Section 7.5).[44]

The Plaut et al. version of the triangle model, then, cannot use the Harm and Seidenberg explanation to account for the reading of these three patients. It also has difficulties with the other of the two newer syndromes—reading without semantics. It was shown by Patterson (1990) for the earlier connectionist implementation of a single phonological route—that of Seidenberg and McClelland (1989)—that the pattern of performance when the route is damaged does not correspond to surface dyslexia. The Plaut et al. model has a more subtle version of the same problem. When lesioned, the route gives rise to worse performance on exception words than on regular words, but the larger effect is a decline on regulars themselves with increased lesion severity (see Figure 4.10).

Some surface dyslexic patients, e.g. MP (Bub et al., 1985; Behrmann & Bub, 1992) fit the model well. MP was 98% correct with low frequency regular words, dropping to 73% with low frequency exception words. Others however, for instance KT (McCarthy & Warrington, 1986a), show a much more rapid decline, namely from 89% to 26%.

How is one to account for such differential effects of the regularity of a word's spelling-to-sound correspondence and in particular that it can be so great. On the DRC model it is easy. The non-lexical route remains intact but both the other routes are impaired to a greater or lesser degree. From the perspective of the connectionist triangle model, Plaut et al. make a most surprising two-step move. The first step is to argue, in a very consistent fashion given the triangle model, that reading words aloud will involve both of the two routes. However in the simulation, the semantic route was not in fact implemented. Instead it is assumed that the semantic pathway provides an additional contribution to the activation of the output phonemic units which depends on the word's frequency and the training *epoch*.[45] Thus an exception word such as *pint*, which has a pronunciation which is learned later, will have had a larger contribution to its eventually correct pronunciation from the semantic route than will a regular word

---

[44] Unfortunately no tests where non-words homophonic with words, e.g. *kwite*, like those carried out by Derouesné and Beauvois, appear to have been used with these patients. Thus one cannot completely rule out an explanation in terms of an impairment within the phonological output system.

[45] An epoch in a typical connectionist learning algorithm refers to one cycle of presentation of each of the stimuli, possibly with selection being probabilistic and depending on each word's frequency. The contribution of the semantic pathway assumed by Plaut et al. was upwardly concave asymptoting after about 1000 epochs for high frequency words.

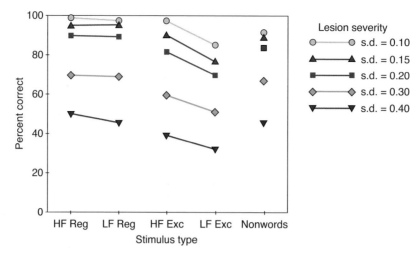

Fig. 4.10 Performance of Plaut et al's (1996) attractor network after lesions of various severities to the weights from hidden units to phoneme units. Lesions were effected by adding noise with mean zero and variable standard deviation to the weights. Performance is shown for high-frequency and low-frequency regular and exception words, and for nonwords. Copyright © 1996 by the American Psychological Association. Adapted with permission. D.C. Plaut, J.L. McClelland, M.S. Seidenberg & K. Patterson (1996), Understanding normal and impaired word reading: Computational principles in quasi-regular domains. *Psychological Review, 103(1)*, 56–115. The use of APA information does not imply endorsement by APA.

learned relatively quickly. However, as the semantic route gains in power in later epochs and contributes extensively to the pronunciation of exception words, so the weights of connections in the phonological route become increasingly specialised for regular words.

The second move made by Plaut et al. is to argue that there are individual differences in the degree of learning. They argue that MP's pattern of performance corresponds to a network which had had 400 epochs of practice, KT's to 2000 epochs. They then assume that surface dyslexia just corresponds to a loss of resource in the semantic system. This hypothetical contrast between MP and KT's degree of practice is a very surprising way to explain cognitive neuropsychological findings as it breaks one of the standard assumptions of cognitive neuropsychology; it violates assumption 4 above. However, before discussing this it should be pointed out that the other 'new' syndrome, reading without semantics, makes the problem even worse. If the semantic pathway is being used increasingly to support the reading of exception words, how can reading without semantics, in patients like WLP, arise? As the learning progresses Plaut et al.'s logic implies that exception words should be being acquired through an increasing use of the semantic route, but that is just the route that the patients are assumed to have lost.

The account of surface dyslexia given by Plaut et al. thus introduced two moves which were at the time relatively new, at least within the research programme of cognitive neuropsychology. The first is that apparently non-semantic processes may be computationally explained in terms of a combination of semantic and

non-semantic processes operating in parallel.[46] The second is that individual differences in the state of the cognitive system, prior to the lesion may need to be evoked to account for the distributions of patterns of performance that exist in a given domain. Adding this assumption of course greatly reduces the falsifiability of cognitive neuropsychology theorising. Does one gain anything from this apparently *ad hoc* extra complexity of adding an additional variable? The answer is that one does. The model makes additional predictions that can be tested, and they work. This makes it what the philosopher-of-science, Lakatos (1972), called a progressive scientific research programme. Thus one prediction is that the more damaged the semantic pathway, the more that irregular words will be read as regularisations, in other words they are read in terms of the most frequent grapheme-phoneme correspondences in the language.

The apparently implausible nature of the presuppositions that were forced on Plaut et al. (1996) in order to try to account for the characteristics of surface dyslexia, reading without semantics and phonological alexia might easily have led them to abandon the single phonological route approach and to accept multiple phonological routes as in the DRC model. Instead, however, Plaut with different sets of colleagues took two quite different ways to confront these difficulties.

---

[46] In this respect the model is in the spirit of the proposals of Howard and Franklin (1988) and Hillis and Caramazza (1991), discussed earlier in this section.

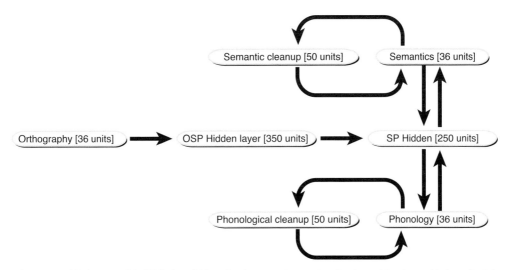

Fig. 4.11 The *Integrated Pathway* model of Kello (2003). Note that, in comparison to the triangle model, orthographic input feeds into nodes in the hidden layer between phonological and semantic representations. (See Kello & Plaut, 2003, Figure 8.)

4.8 **On the Adequacy of Models**

We will discuss in some detail the two approaches that Plaut with his colleagues took since they allow us to address a key metatheoretical issue: what makes a model a good account of empirical data. We will compare their two approaches using the four criteria suggested by Jacobs and Grainger (1994) (see also Chomsky, 1986) in their analytic view of models of reading of that period, namely:

1 *Descriptive Adequacy.* The degree of accuracy with which a model predicts or more typically post hoc explains a dataset.[47]

2 *Generality.* The breadth of the empirical studies for which the model provides an account.

3 *Simplicity and Falsifiability.* The fewer the number of assumptions it makes and the wider the area of conceivable results that are excluded by the model the better.[48]

4 *Explanatory Adequacy.* A model is to be preferred if its predictions derive directly from core assumptions rather than from *ad hoc* combinations of assumptions.

To return to the specific example, one approach Plaut and colleagues took was to abandon the complications of combining information from the semantic and phonological routes that had led to the need to postulate

individual differences and instead to provide the phonological route alone with the necessary computational flexibility. Thus Kello et al. (2005) have investigated another type of single-route model in which they examined in detail a proposal initially made by Kello (2003). This model, for reasons that are not directly relevant in the current context, maps orthographic representations into the hidden units which lie between phonological and semantic representations (see Figure 4.11). It is assumed, entirely appropriately, that such hidden units will be well developed before a child learns to read and that the output goal of the phonological pathway enables the child to access both phonological and semantic information very directly (see for relevant discussion Joanisse & Seidenberg, 1999; Kello & Plaut, 2003).

On the psychological level the argument of Kello et al. (2005) skates over many complications. One is the necessity of distinguishing between input and output phonological representations (see FNMS Chapter 7). A second is why the learning-to-read process for a child learning by phonics should not prioritise phonological 'targets' as opposed to hidden unit 'targets'. These can be viewed as negative aspects using the explanatory adequacy criterion.

Computationally, one critical variable that Kello et al. (2005) manipulate is input gain on the hidden units in a three-level feed-forward model. The input gain is a variable that changes the slope of the activation function used in connectionist simulations (see Figure 1.19). When the gain is high, the activation function comes to resemble a step function and competition effects are strong; processing of the target word is mainly affected only by very similar items. However, when the gain is low the activation function has a relatively gentle

---

[47] Very frequently explanations even for computational models involve *ad hoc* tweaking of the parameters to deal with some characteristic of the experiment which is held to be special.

[48] How to compute the number of assumptions of a connectionist model is a complex issue to which we will return in Section 4.11.

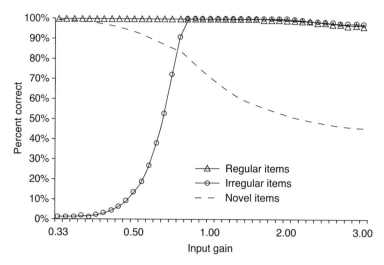

Fig. 4.12 Performance of the distributed connectionist model of Kello and colleagues as a function of input gain. At all levels of gain, performance on regular items is near perfect. However, when gain is high performance on irregular items is substantially better than performance on novel items. The reverse situation holds when gain is low. Thus manipulating a single parameter can give rise to a double dissociation in the network's performance. Reprinted from Dissociations in Performance on Novel Versus Irregular Items: Single-Route Demonstrations With Input Gain in Localist and Distributed Models, C.T. Kello, D.E. Sibley & D.C. Plaut (2005), *Cognitive Science*, 29(4), 627–654. Copyright © 2005, Cognitive Science Society, Inc., reprinted by permission of the publisher (Taylor & Francis Group, http://www. informaworld.com).

gradient, and the processing of any given input pattern is affected by a wider range of competitors.

Training is carried out with the input gain set to one. 'Lesioning' is held to affect only the input gain. The abilities of the net can be divided into three zones (see Figure 4.12). If the post-lesion gain is low, the regular items can be processed satisfactorily due to the influence of many items contributing. However, for the same reason, the net fails to respond appropriately with irregular items. The performance of the model mimics surface dyslexia. For high values of the gain, the net shows the opposite pattern, since very few critical mappings contribute to performance. Now, the performance of the model resembles phonological alexia. For values of the gain close to one, performance is generally quite good; thus the model mimics the normal subject.

How is one to assess such a model? We have discussed the four criteria of Jacobs and Grainger above. With regard to their third criterion, the model is not falsifiable. Every pattern of performance, at least for this aspect of reading, can be explained.[49] Second, there is no claim for any property of the net's behaviour being different from those of previous ones in the domain. It makes no special claims on Jacobs and Grainger's first criterion. The net has no clear 'signature' properties that distinguish it from earlier models. It does not make strong predictions about as yet

untested phenomena. Finally—and to us least important—only a very limited number of phenomena in the empirical domain of the net, are actually explained; it does not deal with most of the phenomena, say, discussed in the review of Zorzi (2005). The model is weak, then, on the second criterion of Jacobs and Grainger. In addition, the authors give no strong arguments about why lesions should lead to input gain being either greatly increased or decreased from one; it differs greatly in this respect from a model like Plaut et al. (1996). This uses the natural computational implementation of a lesion in terms of reducing the strength or number of connections of a pathway.[50] This is another aspect of explanatory adequacy. In this respect too it differs from other models which manipulate activation gain such as that of Cohen and Servan-Schreiber (1992). In this model, which aims to account for certain phenomena manifested by schizophrenic patients, the gain variable is manipulated in order to simulate the effect of changes in the level of a neurotransmitter, dopamine.

The way that the Kello et al. model attempts to account for both surface dyslexia and phonological alexia is most ingenious. It is conceivable that certain aspects of the model may turn out to be on the right lines. However, connectionist models have so many degrees of freedom that 'tweaking' them to produce the required results in the absence of clear intellectual

---

[49] Note in addition that performance could be degraded further by actually lesioning the route.

[50] They also add noise which is somewhat less intuitive.

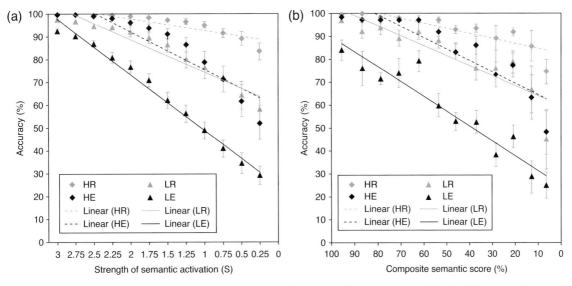

Fig. 4.13 The correlation between reading accuracy and a measure of the strength of the semantic contribution for high and low frequency regular and exception words for (a) the triangle model, and (b) a group of 51 semantic dementia patients. H stands for high frequency and L for low. R stands for regular spelling-to-sound mapping and E for an exceptional one. See Section 4.5 for the composite semantic score. Copyright © 2007 by the American Psychological Association. Reproduced with permission. Woollams et al, 2007, SD-squared: On the association between semantic dementia and surface dyslexia. *Psychological Review, 114*(2), 316–339. The use of APA information does not imply endorsement by APA.

motivation for the tweaking or when they do not make strong additional predictions is dangerous. Overall, the model does poorly on the criteria of Jacobs and Grainger, in particular with respect to explanatory adequacy and to generality.

The other approach taken by Plaut, this time in collaboration with Patterson, Woollams, Lambon Ralph and other colleagues, was to withdraw from some of the most extreme speculations about individual differences made in the Plaut et al. (1996) study but to develop a research programme combining both empirical and computational methods to see if evidence could be obtained for the basic approach taken in that paper—that is, to attempt to explain surface dyslexia and reading without semantics. The critical step the group took was to abandon the individual case method of examining single patients showing striking dissociations. Instead they took as their empirical base semantic dementia—the disease process that has given rise to the largest number of surface dyslexic patients examined and to all the patients showing reading without semantics.[51] For present purposes, the critical point is that such patients can have a progressive degradation of their semantic representations with relatively little effect on systems other than semantics, at least in the

earlier stages of the disease process. One can then consider what happens to reading aloud in a larger sample of such patients. The so-called case-series approach was used, where each patient's results are considered individually and not pooled in an overall average, as they would be in a more standard group study. Computationally essentially the same simulation was run as before but broadened in its semantic aspects.

The largest empirical study carried out was that of Woollams, Lambon Ralph, Plaut and Patterson (2007), in which they examine predictions concerning the relation between semantic impairment and surface dyslexia in a very detailed way. As mentioned earlier, they examined the performance of 51 semantic dementia patients! Many of the patients were tested in more than one time period in the progression of their semantic dementia, giving rise to 100 separate sets of observations. Woollams et al. then compared the performance of these patients with a modification of the Plaut et al. (1996) model in which the contribution of the semantic route, S, was allowed to vary over quasi-subjects over a range of 3 to 7 instead of being fixed at 5 which gave rise to the results shown in Figure 4.10.[52] Figure 4.13 shows the performance of the model and the patients grouped by severity on four sets of words—high-frequency regulars (HR), low-frequency

---

[51] Semantic dementia will be discussed more extensively in Chapter 6. See FNMS Chapter 12 for detailed discussion of classic early cases of Warrington (1975).

[52] They provide no independent test of the S = 3 to 7 range or of the number of epochs assumed in the learning process.

Nonreal > Real   Real > Nonreal

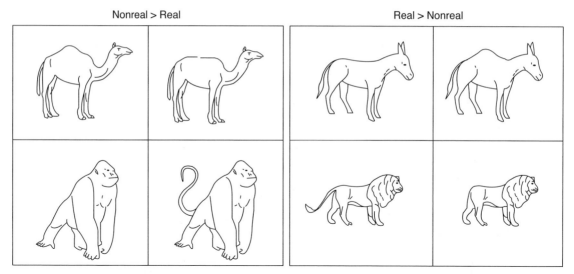

Fig. 4.14 Example stimuli used to test object decision in semantic dementia patients and controls by Rogers et al (2003). Nonreal > real (and vice versa) refers to the performance of the semantic dementia patients. From Object recognition under semantic impairment: The effects of conceptual regularities on perceptual decisions. T.T. Rogers, J.R. Hodges, M.A. Lambon Ralph & K. Patterson, *Language and Cognitive Processes*, 2003, *18*(5/6), 625–662, reprinted by permission of the publisher (Taylor & Francis Group, http://www.informaworld.com).

regulars (LR), high-frequency exceptions/irregulars (HE) and low-frequency exceptions/irregulars (LE). The fit is clearly good, although not perfect. Another important supporting finding for the interpretation in terms of the Plaut et al. triangle model is that non-word performance should not be influenced by the fate of the semantic system; and it does not show the same type of decline with increasing semantic impairment as does word reading. Over four increasing levels of semantic impairment non-word reading was correct on 82%, 70%, 85% and 74% of occasions.

The Woollams et al. findings provide impressive support for the Plaut et al. triangle model approach to surface dyslexia.[53] However, it should be noted that the pattern of performance shown by the surface dyslexic patient KT (McCarthy & Warrington, 1986a) (discussed above), with a drop of 89% for low-frequency regular words to 26% for low-frequency irregular words, would not be reproduced by their network.[54]

Predictions about reading are not the only type of predictions the group has tested. And as this chapter is about neuropsychological methodology in general and not just the acquired dyslexias, it is satisfying that predictions can also be made from the group's position in four other cognitive domains where semantic support is theoretically of potential assistance for item production. Patterson et al. (2006) looked at the performance of 14 semantic dementia patients on six different tasks. Two involved reading, namely reading aloud and lexical decision. However, the other four did not and ranged widely over cognitive domains. One involved the analogue of lexical decision with respect to objects in that subjects must choose which of two line drawings represents a real object and which does not (see Figure 4.14). A second required the subject to copy a line drawing of an object presented roughly 10 sec beforehand. A third was the generation of the past tense of a verb, just given in the present tense in a simple sentence.[55] Finally, the subject was asked to spell a spoken word. Performance on all these tests showed the equivalent of a regularity effect; thus Figure 4.15 shows how the errors on the low-frequency irregular items are typically characterisable as 'Legitimate Alternative Rendering of Components', i.e. regular forms. Figure 4.16 illustrates this in the delayed copying of a rhinoceros.

[53] The authors argue that a theoretical consequence of their position is that surface dyslexia should not exist except in the presence of impairments to the semantic route. In fact a very few exceptional cases do exist in the literature, for instance patient NW of Weekes and Coltheart (1996). Relatively preserved reading of regular over irregular words can occur for other reasons, for instance, as a compensatory strategy in pure alexia (see FNMS Chapter 4 for discussion of this compensatory strategy). NW was in fact slower at reading than normal subjects so this account remains possible for him. However it would not account for his similar problems in spelling.

[54] The closest version for an initial semantic contribution of 7 units would be a drop from roughly 90% → 60%. Whether any

individual case in their series showed a drop equivalent to KT is not discussed.

[55] This experimental paradigm—which has been bitterly fought over—will be discussed in Chapter 8.

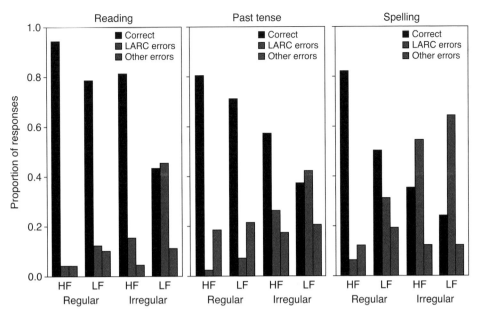

Fig. 4.15 Effects of regularity on reading, past tense formation and spelling, for a group of 14 semantic dementia patients. LARC errors are responses formed from legitimate alternative rendering of components (see text). Adapted with permission from Patterson et al (2006) 'Presemantic' cognition in semantic dementia: Six deficits in search of an explanation. *Journal of Cognitive Neuroscience, 18,* 169–183. Copyright © 2006, MIT Press Journals.

An assessment was also carried out of the semantic comprehension of the patients based on their performance on three semantic tests. Figure 4.17 shows the relation between the impairment on the semantic test and their performance on two of the six tests just discussed. In all cases there was a strong correlation between the semantic score and performance on the test.[56]

Given that all the subjects were patients with semantic dementia, which is a progressive disease that begins in a relatively localised fashion in the anterior inferior temporal lobe (see Chapter 6) but then becomes more widespread, could the correlations just arise from so-called associated deficits, and so reflect a more generalised degree of atrophy in the more severely affected patients? The results would then have no theoretical significance as far as the functional organisation of cognition is concerned. At present the odds seem to be against this interpretation. To assess this possibility, three other tests, which do not involve representations of familiar objects but require visuo-spatial thinking, were used. These were (i) the well-known intelligence

test, Progressive Matrices, (ii) the neuropsychological test of copying of a complex figure, the so-called Rey Figure and (iii) the Cube Analysis subtest of the VOSP (Visual Object and Space Perception) battery of Warrington and James (1991) (see Figure 4.18). In all these cases the patients showed no correlation at all between the semantic score and performance on the test (0.01, –0.09, –0.11). If the degree of generalised atrophy is the critical variable affecting performance, a correlation would have been expected here too. This supports the finding of Woollams et al., discussed earlier, on nonword reading.

The issue is far from closed and indeed we will return to it later. In addition to the issue of whether the theoretically critical findings of Patterson et al. and Woollams et al. can be dismissed as arising from associated deficits, Perry, Ziegler and Zorzi (2007) have produced the counter-argument that the semantic route is not important in the reading aloud of normal subjects. Indeed the evidence is mixed but mainly supports the existence of an effect (Strain et al., 1995; Shibahara et al., 2003 and other studies; for review see Woollams et al., 2007, versus Baayen et al., 2006). Thus the extra complication arising from incorporating a semantic route into the simulation is therefore productive in that it leads to principles which are held to characterise many aspects of cognition, not merely reading. The gain in descriptive adequacy, generality and, in particular, explanatory adequacy more than make up for the decrease in simplicity and falsifiability.

---

[56] In certain cases, however, the correlations were only significant if outliers were removed; as outliers are cases where the result was going in the opposite direction to the hypothesis, rather than cases where the results were discordant on some theoretically irrelevant dimension, this procedure does not seem justifiable. However, we will make the assumption that the results are valid.

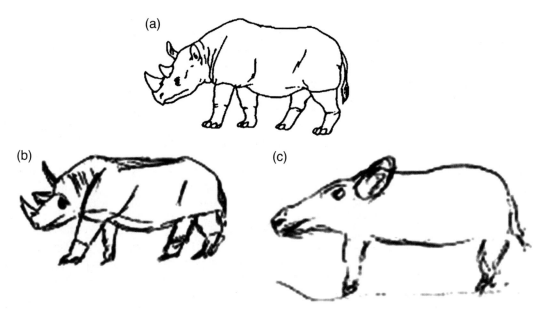

Fig. 4.16 Drawings by a semantic dementia patient of a rhinoceros. (a) The stimulus drawing to be copied. (b) The copy made by the patient while the stimulus drawing was in view. (c) The drawing made from memory 10 sec after the stimulus drawing was removed from view. Reprinted with permission of Royal Society Publishing from K. Patterson, 2007, The reign of typicality in semantic memory. *Philosophical Transactions of the Royal Society B: Biological Sciences*, 362(1481), 813–821; figure 3, p. 819.

We have contrasted the two models of Plaut and colleagues with respect to the neuropsychological data. To a reader familiar with the literature on the normal reading process the current stress on the neuropsychological aspects of the evidence may well appear somewhat one-sided. For instance, Zorzi (2005), in an excellent overview of computational models of the more central parts of the reading process, considers six phenomena that have

been described in the normal reader and only two neuropsychological syndromes as the empirical data base to use to compare rival models. Indeed it should be pointed out that the emphasis we have given to brain-based findings over ones using human experimental psychological methods with normal adult subjects is probably most appropriate when making earlier broad brush specifications of the functional architecture. Here, by contrast

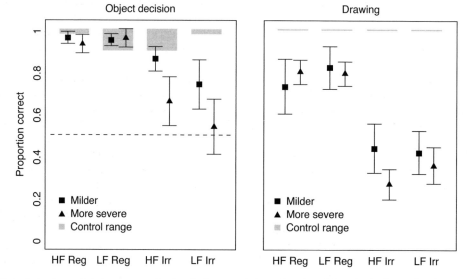

Fig. 4.17 Effects of stimulus regularity in two processing domains in semantic dementia patients (of two levels of severity) and controls. HF = High Frequency; LF = Low Frequency; Reg = Regular words; Irr = Irregular (i.e. Exception) words. Reproduced with permission from Patterson et al (2006) 'Presemantic' cognition in semantic dementia: Six deficits in search of an explanation. *Journal of Cognitive Neuroscience, 18*, 169–183. Copyright © 2006, MIT Press Journals.

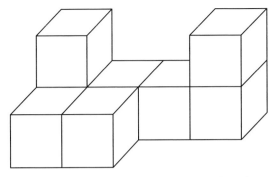

Fig. 4.18 A block figure similar to those used in the cube analysis subtest of the Visual Object and Space Perception (VOSP) battery. Subjects are required to count the number of cubes in each figure.

one is dealing with rival detailed computational models with many assumptions.

Zorzi et al. examine in detail the DRC model, the Plaut et al. triangle model and the Zorzi–Houghton–Butterworth model. The Z–H–B model succeeds with all six of the 'normal' reading phenomena and the other two models on five of the six. The problem for the Plaut et al. triangle model arises in a paradigm called the *position of irregularity* effect; the slowing produced by an irregular letter-sound correspondence becomes smaller the later it occurs in the word (e.g. *gnat* versus *lamb*) (Coltheart & Rastle, 1994). As we will see later, the triangle model at least needs to be updated to deal with a related phenomenon.

We have not paid as detailed attention to the DRC model as to the Plaut et al. one. This may seem surprising. The DRC model has much less contorted explanations of the three syndromes just considered—surface dyslexia, phonological alexia and reading without semantics—than does the Plaut et al. model. There is, however, a problem when models of the complexity of the DRC model confront findings of experiments on normal subjects. The model contains 31 different parameters which need to be set. This means that although it scores fairly high on descriptive adequacy on the Jacobs and Grainger criteria, it comes very low on simplicity. It is very difficult indeed to examine the properties of a 31-dimensional parameter space, which is what is required to properly assess its goodness of fit to the data. Instead Coltheart et al. chose a single set of values for the 31 parameters by a pragmatically sensible but otherwise arbitrary procedure and then examined how the model behaved with this single set of parameters. The model generally does very well, but one has no idea of how robust the model's performance is to variations in the parameters. Zorzi (2005) also makes a variety of criticisms of the intricate special-purpose assumptions necessary to get the model to work as well as it does. So it is unclear how to assess the generally excellent fit of the model with this particular

parameter set to data. In addition it should be noted that the apparently excellent fits of a computational model of this complexity to quantitative data can be somewhat misleading. Take reaction times, which can be derived directly from the models by using the number of cycles required to reach thresholds. To obtain fits concerning the position of irregularity effect Coltheart et al. alter parameters in an *ad hoc* fashion. In justification they point out that reaction time involves processes other than those covered by the reading model so that precise fits should not be expected. However this makes the quantitative fits they obtain much less impressive.

Just as critically, if the arguments presented by Plaut and his colleagues on surface dyslexia are correct and the semantic route contributes to reading aloud, then the good fits of the other models to normal data must be seriously questioned. This is because they do *not* incorporate any simulation of the semantic route. Neuropsychological findings would then undercut the excellent fits of the other models to normal data.

To summarise, it would be premature to decide which of the three main models of the phonological reading process is to be preferred. On the Jacobs–Grainger criteria for assessing models they are relatively strong in different areas. Thus, for instance, the DRC model and the Zorzi–Houghton–Butterworth model are probably strongest in predictive adequacy but weak on simplicity, especially the DRC model, while the Plaut et al. triangle model is very strong on explanatory adequacy.

Critically, however, despite the move from box-and-arrow to computational formats, neuropsychological evidence remains critical for assessing the adequacy of the models. Thus the most direct support for the predictive adequacy (and in a sense for its explanatory adequacy too) of the DRC model lies in the syndromes of phonological and surface dyslexia. For the Plaut et al. model too, neuropsychological evidence is its lifeline. Without the evidence from semantic dementia on the role of the semantic route in reading aloud, the model would be a historical curiosity only. However the viability of the Plaut et al. model has a cost for neuropsychological methodology. The model clearly shows that the idea that a dissociation necessitates a conceptual split in the functional architecture, even if the resource artefact explanations are not relevant, is premature. The Plaut et al. triangle model does not provide qualitatively different routes through the functional architecture for surface dyslexia and for reading without semantics, even though the DRC model and the Z–H–B models do. Much worse, the Plaut et al. model has great virtues but it abandons the idea that all subjects can premorbidly be considered as having identical cognitive systems, since it relies on plausible but *ad hoc* assumptions of

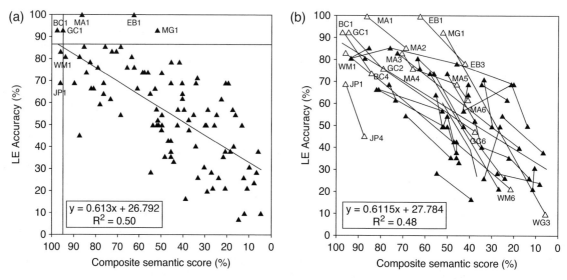

Fig. 4.19 The accuracy of the semantic dementia patients of Woollams et al. (2007) on reading of low-frequency exception words as a function of a composite measure of semantic knowledge. (a) 100 observations from 51 patients. The horizontal lines indicate two standard deviations below the control mean. Note that patients MA, EB and MG show no deficit in reading, despite impaired semantic knowledge. (b) 75 observations from 27 patients, with repeated observations on the same patient joined by lines. Note that patients MA, EB and MG show a similar decline in accuracy on low-frequency exception words to that of the other SD patients. Copyright © 2007 by the American Psychological Association. Reproduced with permission. Woollams et al, 2007, SD-squared: On the association between semantic dementia and surface dyslexia. *Psychological Review*, *114*(2), 316–339. The use of APA information does not imply endorsement by APA.

individual differences to account for the different patterns of reading aloud in surface dyslexia and reading without semantics. We now turn to this issue.

4.9 Assumptions Concerning Individual Differences

In the previous section we argued that the added complexity of incorporating a semantic route into models of reading aloud was productive. Can one say the same for using individual differences to explain away apparently conflicting patterns of data? This, by contrast, potentially opens a Pandora's box. In the original version of their model, Plaut et al. also considered a syndrome we have not discussed in detail—reading without semantics—in which patients can read aloud normally without understanding what they read. They stated, 'By our account ... the phonological pathway had developed a relatively high degree of competence without assistance from semantics' (Plaut et al., 1996, p. 99). To justify this they merely continued 'but this *post hoc* interpretation clearly requires some future, independent source of evidence'. Patterson et al. (2006) by contrast make a case, rather than a bland assumption: 'There is always variance around the regression line. ... If this variation is distributed normally, then a small number of cases will fall in the upper tail of the distribution, performing better than expected given their level of semantic impairment; in the rare case

'better than expected' may even be in the normal range' (Patterson, et al., 2006, p. 179). The findings of Woollams et al. (2007) enable one to examine the magnitude of the variance. In their data the spread in the patient results is somewhat greater than those in the simulation (see Figure 4.13). Moreover, three cases on first testing seemingly show the reading without semantics type of pattern (MA, EB, MG) (see Figure 4.19). However as their semantic abilities decline then the word reading performance of the three patients deteriorates in a parallel fashion to that of the group regression line. This supports the idea that there has indeed been some semantic contribution to their reading too. The idea that the reading without semantics pattern of performance occurs only in patients with a premorbidly greater reliance on the phonological route than the average subject is supported. More generally, the idea that individual differences cannot be ignored theoretically gains a lot of strength.

However, the conceptual move made by Plaut et al. has repercussions far beyond models of reading. It undermines assumption 4 discussed earlier. But this assumption is the foundation on which the methodology of cognitive neuropsychology depends. One cannot have a methodology based on individual cases if individual differences critically affect inferences to the functional architecture. And once the issue is raised over one syndrome, namely reading without semantics, then it can be raised elsewhere.

Take phonological alexia, the empirical bedrock on which the three routes of the DRC model are based. Van Orden et al. (2001) are brutal. They point out that developmental phonological alexia has frequently been described in subjects not suffering from neurological disease (see e.g. Temple & Marshall, 1983; Campbell & Butterworth, 1985; Howard & Best, 1996). They continue 'Lesions acquired after learning to read are not necessary to produce the symptoms. If not necessary, we may wonder whether acquired lesions are sufficient to produce these symptoms. [...] Nobody provides pre- and post-lesion data, so the available data are indeterminate' (van Orden et al., 2001, pp. 123–124). They go on to criticise the whole theoretical methodology of cognitive neuropsychology.[57]

Van Orden et al.'s arguments on phonological alexia are not convincing for all such patients. Thus, as we discuss in Section 5.10, Rapcsak et al. (2009) have shown that phonological alexia is a frequent sequelae of a lesion to the left parietal or left frontal cortex. However, the cases of phonological alexia held to be theoretically critical earlier in the chapter are those where the phonological output system is relatively intact. These are the cases of phonological alexia described by Caccappolo-van Vliet et al. (2004a, 2004b). They are patients with Alzheimer's disease, in whom the syndrome was becoming more severe, and not patients in whom an earlier deep dyslexia had recovered to phonological alexia. We have no evidence that van Orden et al.'s arguments apply to these patients but no evidence that they do not!

We will return to the issue of individual differences shortly. In fact, phonological alexia can occur with normal spontaneous speech following other lesions to a rather surprising site. Buiatti et al. (in preparation) found that phonological alexia frequently occurs in the acute state after *right* parietal lesions. This has major

implications for the Plaut et al. model. Buiatti et al. explain their findings by assuming that non-words, unlike words, are read aloud by decomposing them into smaller visual components, and that it is this decomposition process which is impaired in the right parietal patients.[58] Such a decomposition process is clearly straightforward for the DRC and Z–H–B models, but presents difficulties for the Plaut et al. model. Conceivably they could add a preparatory stage which selects the appropriate size of visual unit for entry to the phonological route,[59] but if so this would be a considerable modification which would necessitate reimplementation of at least their accounts of the normal reading data.

This means that phonological alexia cannot be explained away just in terms of oddities in the premorbid cognitive system of the patient. However one still has the more general issue of how to deal with individual differences. Patterson et al. (2006) take a counter-revolutionary stance, and argue that it has major implications for single case methodology. 'We nevertheless argue that selective emphasis on these exceptional cases is misguided because it fails to explain the majority of the evidence' (p. 179). Goldberg (1995) had earlier attacked the single case approach using two arguments related to those of Patterson and colleagues. First, he had argued that in general 'strong dissociations … must be approached with a degree of wariness, pending the demonstration of their high prevalence' (p. 195). They may be 'statistical aberrations' (Goldberg, 1995, p. 193), although the meaning of this term is obscure. Whatever they may be, Coltheart (2000) points out that there are many rare strong dissociations which are not 'statistical aberrations' within the performance of the individual patient; the results are clearly solid as they are repeatedly replicated within the patient's performance. If the results are 'statistical aberrations' compared with those of other individuals then they correspond to the cognitive system of the patient being premorbidly at the extreme of some distribution or qualitatively different from that of other subjects. So this argument reduces to the next. Goldberg's second argument is that 'the tacit assumption of the invariant (across individuals) nature of cognitive architecture […] is probably wrong' (Goldberg, 1995, p. 194).[60] Coltheart's response is 'if this assumption is wrong, then cognitive psychology (and cognitive neuropsychology) has no subject matter, since the aim of these disciplines is to discover the architectures for cognitive systems' (Coltheart, 2006a, p. 105).

---

[57] Van Orden et al.'s (2001) more general arguments are highly cogent. However, they are so sweeping, that all major cognitive neuropsychologists appear to have preferred to ignore them. It should, though, be noted that the problem of developmental disorders is not all pervasive. In other areas of cognition, it is highly implausible that one could attribute a pattern of performance found after the lesion just to cognitive characteristics that existed prior to the lesion. Otherwise it would have not been possible for the person to function in the way that they did. Consider amnesia as a simple example. A patient without an effective episodic memory is essentially helpless. Most studied neurological impairments are less subtle than the inability to read non-words! One can also treat the developmental disorder in the typical cognitive subtraction style of cognitive neuropsychology by making the analogue of assumption 5_N (see e.g. Temple & Marshall, 1983). However, this too is highly contentious (see e.g. Thomas & Karmiloff-Smith, 2002).

---

[58] To be discussed further in Chapter 8.

[59] See Làdavas et al. (1997a, 1997b) for related ideas to explain aspects of visual neglect.

[60] The assumption was far from 'tacit'. It was explicit (see Caramazza, 1986; Shallice, 1988a).

What presumably Coltheart means is that the current methodologies available in the two fields would fail, as it is clear one could have a well defined different architecture in each individual which current methods would not allow us to determine because they are idiosyncratic to the individual. Coltheart continues 'Fortunately for these disciplines, however, Goldberg provides no argument or evidence which shows that this assumption is wrong.' This argument is out of date. Since then Woollams et al. (2007) have shown that individual differences could well prove critical in explaining reading-without-semantics. Moreover, even before 2006, van Orden et al. had pointed out that we know from the study of developmental disorders that there are major quantitative and possibly qualitative individual differences in cognitive development so Coltheart's dismissive response will not do.

Returning to Patterson et al.'s negative perspective on the single case approach, bold as this is, one can interpret it in either a strong or a weak form. The strong form is that the policy of giving priority to the study of 'pure cases' manifesting striking selective disorders, in other words the methodology of choice during the history of cognitive neuropsychology, was a mistake. This would seem to involve the root and branch jettisoning of all the advances that cognitive neuropsychology has produced. There is though, fortunately, a weaker position, fairly compatible with the arguments of Patterson et al.. This is that there are a variety of methods available in neuropsychology and in particular the single case approach, the case-series approach, and the group study (where results are averaged across patients). All have problems when making inferences to models of the normal system, but so do all other methods available. In particular the individual difference problem is a severe problem for the single case approach. The case-series approach avoids that problem.[61] However, the case-series approach in turn suffers more from the problem of potential anatomical association of deficits even though this potential problem is dismissed rather cavalierly by Patterson et al. in their study. In addition, testing is almost inevitably more rigid and less comprehensive in a case series, so the core data will be less rich from the functional syndrome perspective, to be discussed shortly.

It is this second conclusion we will draw. We will take the less extreme position and assume, in line with

assumption 4, that there are no *qualitative* differences in the organisation of the cognitive architecture across individuals but that the underlying parameters may vary according to reasonably well-behaved unimodal distributions. This makes inferences based on the single case much more complex. Even if one ignores the problem that tasks can have qualitatively similar cognitive requirements but quantitatively different resource requirements, in that they differ merely in difficulty not in which subsystems they depend upon,[62] the Woollams et al. example of reading without semantics provides a clear type of difficulty. In this example, one cannot assume that in the average subject reading aloud does not depend upon semantics, because a patient like MA or EB, who is scoring at a clearly impaired level on semantic tasks, scores at 100% when reading low-frequency words. This is because the mapping between the task and the underlying architecture may itself be probabilistic in the sense that task performance depends upon a weighting of the contributions of different subsystems that varies across subjects. The critical distributions, as on the Plaut et al. triangle theory, may not be those of the observed scores but of a variable that is not directly observable, namely the relative weight the system gives to one process or system as opposed to another, in this example the phonological as opposed to the semantic route. If the phonological weighting is very high prior to the lesion then good performance on reading aloud is possible. But this distribution is not empirically observable—it is *theory dependent*. So one can never know in a theory-independent way whether an observed dissociation can be 'explained away' through entirely standard empirical measures of pre-lesion individual differences.

If we define a 'pure case' performance pattern as one that shows a completely selective loss of a single system, then the argument in FNMS was that the 'pure case' was the royal road to the uncovering of the organisation of the cognitive system, and that such patients are initially detected because they show classical dissociations across tasks. The arguments of Patterson et al. (2006) and Woollams et al. (2007) underline that a 'pure case', say a patient who exhibits reading without semantics, is only 'pure' in terms of a particular theoretical interpretation. However the argument presented in FNMS was that the classical or strong dissociation is only a preliminary filter to determining pure cases. There are many alternative ways in which they may be explained.[63] When alternative theories have been developed in the domain, then, the argument went, if different individual patients are theoretically critical

---

[61] In addition, as pointed out by Lambon Ralph (2004), one of the authors of the Patterson et al. (2006) study, computational models can predict changes in the nature of a deficit pattern with increasing severity. Unfortunately the only empirical claim we know of this type—that of Gonnerman et al. (1997) on category specificity (discussed in Chapter 6)—could not be replicated in a better controlled study of Garrard et al. (1998).

[62] See FNMS Chapter 10.

[63] See Figure 4.1 and FNMS Chapter 11.

for different theories, then the theorist needs to consider all patients treated as 'pure' by all competing theories. Van Orden et al. (2001) claim this was a pious hope that has singularly failed to be followed in practice. They do not provide evidence for this claim, and we consider it to be unfair; for instance Plaut et al. (1996) very directly confront the problems posed for their theory by patients showing reading without semantics and surface dyslexic patients like KT who have a very large difference between their ability to read regular and exception low frequency words.[64]

4.10 Towards a Revised Neuropsychological Methodology

Instead of the individual case approach, the methodology advocated, say, by Patterson et al. (2006) and Woollams et al. (2007) is the case series in which a series of patients drawn from category X are each treated in individual case fashion. Theoretical conclusions are then drawn from the overall findings. Thus a conclusion as to whether a patient (or patients) is or is not qualitatively different from the rest of the sample can be inferred by statistical methods rather than by inferential fiat.

However we immediately run into a problem of regress. How do we define category X? If one is an advocate of the DRC model, then surface dyslexia is a separate category from reading without semantics, if one of the Plaut et al. triangle model, then they should be combined. So what category X should be is theory dependent. One has the same problem as for pure cases. Thus one returns to the approach just advocated—that all patients with deficits in any related domain need to be considered—except the problem is far worse. Instead of considering all potential pure cases, all patients with deficits in the domain need to be considered both individually and as drawn from distributions. The case-series approach works very well for semantic dementia because there is a disease process which creates a large number of 'pure case' patients, that is patients held to have an impairment to the same single computational resource. This is a virtually unique situation in neuropsychology, so there are no grounds to assume that the methodology generalises.

One can provisionally summarise this discussion in two ways:

1 Computational theories are often sufficiently flexible and have many parameters, so they can often be patched to account for apparently conflicting results.[65]

2 Empirically single dissociations in individual patients, even if strong or classical ones, are an insufficient basis for making strong theoretical inferences, so—on the bases of dissociations alone—it is difficult to select theoretically key patients for investigation. Case series, in turn, are difficult to apply as it is unclear what the criteria should be for inclusion in the series.

From this provisional summary, one can propose two ways to confront the difficulties that have been found to occur in extrapolating from neuropsychological data to cognitive theory. The first presupposes that for a computational theory to be an advance it must explain the existing theoretically critical cases. However, its critical aspect is that the model also needs to give rise to what we will call *signature effects*, those where the model provides explanations of apparently counter-intuitive phenomena, as in the examples from Patterson et al. (2006), or makes predictions about such effects. We will give an example from single case approach in the next section.

On the second point, we may ask why do the semantic dementia patients prove such a rare but suitable vehicle for a case series? Why do they have qualitatively equivalent impairments? It is held by Woollams et al. to be because the disease process affects the same region of cortex. Atrophy and hypometabolism affect the anterior temporal lobes (Mummery et al., 2000; Nestor et al., 2006). We can therefore see it as an indirect application of assumption 3_N which we introduced earlier in the chapter.

Using assumption 3_N, one can, however, provide a strong supporting argument as to why functional syndromes based on dissociations exhibited in the individual case are theoretically critical. If they do correspond to a cleavage in the functional architecture, they will replicate in patients with lesions in the same brain area, assuming that this can be specified. Thus the case-series approach of Patterson et al. (2006) and Woollams et al. (2007) works because semantic dementia primarily affects a particular region of cortex, namely, the anterior temporal lobes as just discussed. It would further follow that reading without semantics would not pass as a functional syndrome, assuming that Woollams et al. are correct and that there is no macro-anatomical difference between the lesions of the patients with surface dyslexia and those exhibiting reading without semantics.

---

[64] For excellent examples in other domains predating van Orden et al. (2001) see Caramazza and Shelton (1998) or a number of the articles in Vallar and Shallice (1990).

[65] Our field is far from unique in this respect. For instance, consider the scathing analysis of Smolin (2006) of the state of play in string theory.

This anatomical argument reopens the possibility of strong neuropsychological evidence being provided by methodologies other than the case series. Thus if the data available on individual patients is not sufficiently robust to allow strong theoretical conclusions to be drawn assumption 3_N allows one to average over patients with similar lesions—the anatomically based group study. This methodology will be discussed further in Chapter 9.

Second, given converging evidence from other sources, one can turn the argument concerning individual case studies on its head. If other types of evidence, say from functional imaging, support the existence of an isolated computational system then the individual patient can be used to test different theories of the operation of the underlying process. The lesion site of the hypothetical pure case would, of course, need to be compatible with the localisation as determined by functional imaging, say. An elegant application of part of this strategy is provided by the work of Duchaine et al. (2006) on a normally employed man, Edward, who had a severe selective difficulty in identifying faces, prosopagnosia. A common account of prosopagnosia is that it arises from damage to a processing system specific to face recognition, but many competing accounts are available. For instance, the system damaged might be specific not to faces but to types of visual object in which one has become expert, of which faces would just be one example (e.g. Gauthier & Tarr, 1997). In six experiments Duchaine and his colleagues take four rival hypotheses of which the expertise hypothesis is one and show that Edward has no difficulty in visually processing stimuli, which while not being faces, should create difficulties if one or more of the other hypotheses were appropriate. For instance, he acquired the ability to recognise complex nonsense objects called *greebles* as rapidly as normal controls. The only problem, but a serious one, for the current argument is that Edward has a developmental disorder, not an acquired one, and had no localisable lesion![66]

4.11 The Putative Functional Syndrome as the Computational Target: Deep Dyslexia

Earlier in this chapter, using the criteria developed by Jacobs and Grainger, we argued that while predictive

adequacy is important, it is dangerous to place too much weight on it alone, given the softness of psychological evidence and the number of free parameters that a model like the DRC has. At least as much weight for computational models should be placed on simplicity and explanatory adequacy. This will be achieved if a number of key aspects of a functional syndrome derive from the core assumptions of a model. These would be the *signature effects* discussed in Section 4.8.

But what is a functional syndrome? The concept of the *syndrome* received an even worse press from cognitive neuropsychologists than did the group study. Cognitive neuropsychology ideologues who were opposed to group studies were also opposed to treating patients as examples of syndromes. The same type of argument was frequently presented that one can never know whether or not two patients are functionally equivalent, that they have the same functional impairment. Indeed historically, syndromes have fractionated into subtypes which are now considered functionally heterogeneous. A good example is conduction aphasia—one of the classic aphasia syndromes. This is roughly the inability to reproduce heard words which can be separately comprehended and produced. Conduction aphasia is now considered to fractionate into at least three types—repetition, reproduction and disconnection varieties.[67]

Thus functional syndromes—collections of symptoms that occur together repeatedly across patients—are a somewhat dangerous source of evidence. They may merely arise from associated deficits—the lesion affects multiple systems with some symptoms occurring because one functional system is damaged and other symptoms because of impairment to an anatomically close but functionally unrelated system. Moreover, if the combination of symptoms recurs continually across patients, the combination can still be an associated deficit; for instance, because of the involvement of one particular arterial territory within the vascular system.[68] However, when the same combination recurs without similar but critically different patterns being present in other patients, this increases the probability that it has a common functional cause, as well as a common anatomical one. It therefore encourages theorists to attempt to find an explanation for the pattern even though the

---

[66] There is as yet no equivalent study on acquired prosopagnosia (see Duchaine & Garrido, 2008). Striking double dissociations between face processing and object processing do exist in acquired cases such as between patient FB of Riddoch et al. (2008) and patient, CK of Moscovitch et al. (1997), but while FB's lesion fits reasonably well the imaging localisations, CK had sustained a head injury and the lesion was difficult to localise.

[67] See FNMS Chapter 7 and also Section 7.5.

[68] One example is the frequent co-occurrence of pure alexia and colour agnosia, the loss of the conceptual aspects of colour (Damasio & Damasio, 1983). Another is the Gerstmann's syndrome in which patients with left parietal lesions sometimes present with a particular cluster of deficits—right-left disorientation, acalculia (the difficulty in performing arithmetic calculations), pure agraphia and finger agnosia (where the patient has difficulty locating the relative position of fingers by touch)—see FNMS Section 2.6.

TABLE 4.1 Ten properties of the reading of deep dyslexic patients. (See Colheart, 1980b.)

1 Semantic errors (e.g. VIEW → 'scene', GONE → 'lost')
2 Visual errors (e.g. WHILE → 'white', BADGE → 'bandage')
3 Function-word substitutions (e.g. WAS → 'and', OFF → 'from')
4 Derivational errors (e.g. MARRIAGE → 'married', BUY → 'bought')
5 Nonlexical derivation of phonology from print is not possible (e.g. pronouncing non-words, judging whether two non-words rhyme)
6 Lexical derivation of phonology from print is impaired (e.g. judging whether two words rhyme)
7 Low imageability/concreteness words (e.g. JUSTICE) are much harder to read than high imageability/concreteness words (e.g. TABLE)
8 Reading of verbs is harder than of adjectives, which is harder than of nouns
9 Reading of function words is harder than of content words
10 Whether a word can be read at all depends on its context (e.g. FLY as a noun is easier than FLY as a verb)

testing of any model needs to be across all patients with relevant disorders, as in the case series method.

A functional syndrome may also arise from a common functional cause with this not necessarily being limited to damage to a single subsystem. Thus damage to different parts of a network of subsystems may give rise to similar symptoms for reasons which are functionally equivalent. For these reasons we use the terminology of a *putative functional syndrome* to refer to a set of symptoms which is a candidate for being derived from a common functional cause.

It is useful in this respect to consider the history of the first modern dyslexia syndrome, deep dyslexia. Deep dyslexia was a prime example of why cognitive neuropsychologists rejected syndromes. After the historically important initial description by Marshall and Newcombe of two patients with reading problems characterised as examples of the syndrome in 1966 and 1973 (see Sections 1.3 and 4.6), many more such patients were described. By 1993 Plaut and Shallice were able to refer to at least 35 cases in the published literature. As far as could be established from the experimental and clinical reports 10 properties held almost entirely for the reading of these patients (see Table 4.1). Yet there is a conceptual puzzle concerning deep dyslexia. Coltheart (1980a) puts the conceptual problem clearly 'The deep dyslexic not only makes semantic errors; he makes visual errors; he makes derivational errors, he lacks the ability to derive phonology from print, he has particular difficulties with low-imagery words and he also has difficulty with function words. There is no obvious relationship between these various symptoms' (Coltheart, 1980a, p. 326). He points out that it seems necessary to presume a variety of different loci of

damage within the left hemisphere. But, he continues 'If these symptoms arise at independent neurological loci, why is it that they do not occur independently in patients? Why, for example, do we not find patients who make semantic errors but no visual errors?' (Coltheart, 1980a, p. 327).

We will come shortly to Coltheart's answer to his own question. However, Coltheart et al. (1987) in a review drew the conclusion that standard box-and-arrow models of the disorder, such as that of Morton and Patterson (1980) (see Figure 4.20), could not give a principled account of why the required impairments on these models should co-occur. At about the same time a review by one of us was being still more dismissive, in explicitly supporting the associated deficits position. 'The attempt to provide a unitary functional account of deep dyslexia seems to be suffering the same fate as the attempt to characterize the disorder rigorously using a symptom-complex methodology. It is most plausible that the patients so labelled are functionally heterogeneous' (FNMS p. 116).

However, this deconstruction of the syndrome became less attractive in the light of a computational study carried out in the very beginning of modern connectionism. As discussed in Section 1.7, in 1983 Hinton and Sejnowski invented Boltzmann machines—the first type of connectionist system that both contained attractors and learned—and one of the networks they investigated was a very simple 3-layer feed-forward net, which mapped three-letter words (e.g. *bat*) into meanings (see Figure 1.18). What was critical was that the 'orthographic' and 'semantic' vector representations of the words were orthogonal. They found that a single lesion produced errors that showed a similarity to the correct word that reflected *both* the input (visual) and the output (semantic) dimensions of the net even though they were arbitrarily related.

Hinton and Shallice (1991) and then Plaut and Shallice (1993a) in much greater detail followed up this initial insight, by taking the triangle model, assuming that the phonological route was no longer operative, and then considering the semantic route. Plaut and Shallice investigated a variety of networks as implementations of the semantic route (see Figure 4.21). They used a 'toy' vocabulary consisting of 40 three- or four-letter concrete nouns.[69] Each noun had 28 orthographic features, seven

---

[69] Jacobs and Grainger (1994) claim toy models are not useful because they do not scale. However their argument is that technically simple (e.g. small) networks do not generalise to more complex (e.g. larger) networks. This is an argument about the networks not their environments. Nevertheless, models are always more simple then the real-world phenomena they attempt to capture; if they were not they would not be useful. Moreover, since the brain is orders of magnitude more complex

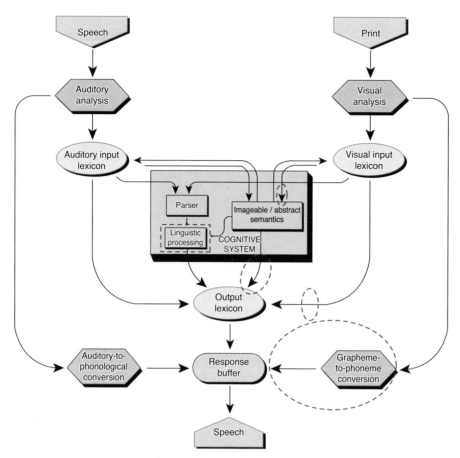

Fig. 4.20 A standard multiple route box-and-arrow diagram of the organisation of spoken and written language processing from the early 1980s, together with possible impairments to account for deep dyslexia (dotted ellipses). Based on Morton and Patterson (1980).

for each of the four letters. It also had 68 'concrete' semantic features including ones relating to size, shape, colour, hardness, taste, location where found, relation to the body, activities, its constituents and its function.[70] The networks were trained by the learning algorithm called back-propagation through time (see Section 1.7) over a series of seven time-slices for each word input.

When trained, the initial representation accessed in the semantic units—when the semantic system first becomes influenced by the input at time slice 3—is rather distant from the final representation. However, because of the clean-up recurrent aspects of the net, in a few cycles the semantic representation in the trained network becomes increasingly close to the correct

representation. In other words, as discussed in Section 1.7, the output of the net settles into a fixed attractor (see Figure 1.15). When the networks are lesioned they behave in a similar fashion to the Hinton and Sejnowski network. They quite frequently settle into an incorrect attractor, which can represent a unit that is visually similar—a *visual error*—or one semantically similar—a *semantic error*—or a *mixed error*—one both visually and semantically similar. This, however, should only occur when the lesion is placed before the level of the attractor. If, instead, one considers the 40–80i net (left centre), the set of connections Intermediate (I) → Semantic (S) is not followed by a set of clean-up units. Thus, after damage, one would not expect the representation to be 'cleaned-up' into another inappropriate item in the set. The output would instead tend to be a set of features that do not correspond to a word, and would thus be represented by the network (and presumably the patient) as an *omission* response. When the basic 40–60 net was compared with the 40–80i one, then the error rate was somewhat higher in the former than in the latter when the Orthography → Intermediate connections

----

than even the most complex neural network model, this argument, if accepted, would reject the entire field and not just toy models. Most critically, the argument ignores the Plaut and Shallice theoretical methodology of developing a theory of the models (see below).

[70] Semantic feature representations are frequently employed in psychological theorizing; see Smith and Medin, 1981.

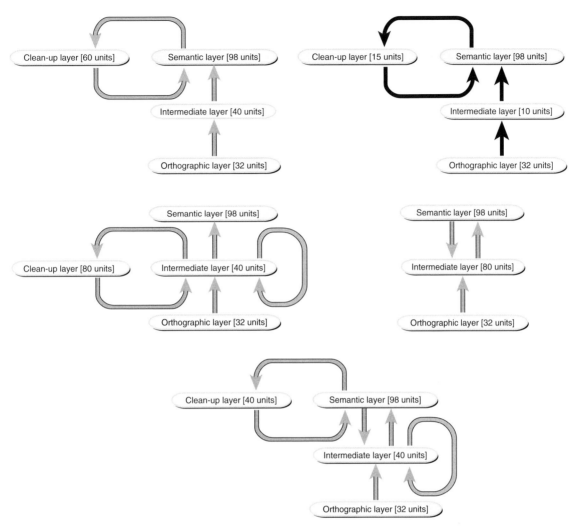

Fig. 4.21 Five network architectures used by Plaut and Shallice (1993a) in investigating the role of the semantic route in deep dyslexia.

were lesioned (7.2% vs 5.3%) but many times higher when the Intermediate → Semantic connections were lesions (3.5% vs 0.2%). The 40–80i net did not make substantive errors when connections following its clean-up layer were lesioned.

With the exception of situations when they do not make substantive errors, the networks made both visual errors and semantic errors wherever they were lesioned, just like deep dyslexic patients. This is rather counterintuitive; Figure 4.22 illustrates why a lesion near to the semantic system produces visual errors, if there are cleanup units at the semantic level. In addition, even stranger types of error that are exhibited by deep dyslexic patients also occur after single lesions to the network, such as the visual-then-semantic error (e.g. *sympathy* → *orchestra*, mediated by *symphony*) (Marshall & Newcombe, 1966; Coltheart, 1980b). Such errors are rare in the simulations, but they are in the patients too.

One final similarity between the behaviour of the patients and of the network was the effect of abstraction. Abstraction was crudely if simply simulated by providing an abstract word with a much less rich and extensive set of features—on average only 4.7 features were 'on'—compared with those for a concrete one—which averaged 18.2 features on. This is a somewhat one-dimensional view of abstraction. However Jones (1985) had shown that it was much harder to generate abstract than concrete predicates of words and argued that it represented an important quantitative difference between concrete and abstract representations, which was relevant for deep dyslexia.[71]

---

[71] The simulations involving abstraction used a more complex network than the earlier ones, in that it represented output as well as input processes.

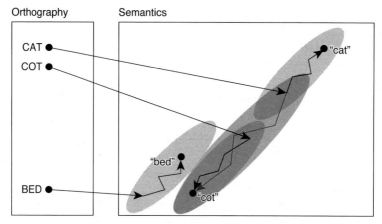

Fig. 4.22 Semantic lesions to the Hinton-Plaut-Shallice network may lead to visual errors. Attractor basins in semantic space are shown as ellipses with the trajectory of a point during settling shown by the zig-zagging lines in semantic space. The grey ellipses represents the attractor basin of 'cat', 'cot' and 'bed', while the red ellipse represents the modified attractor basin of 'cot' following a lesion to the semantic units. After such a lesion, the orthographic representation CAT maps to a point in semantic space within the modified basin of attraction of 'cot'. Adapted from: Deep dyslexia: a case study of connectionist neuropsychology. D.C. Plaut & T. Shallice, *Cognitive Neuropsychology*, 1993, *10*(5), 377–500, reprinted by permission of the publisher (Taylor & Francis Group, http://www.informaworld.com).

When the net illustrated in Figure 4.23 was trained on the abstract and concrete word stimulus set, it performed better on concrete than abstract words for lesions to the input pathway. The stronger attractors, which result from the richer input, protect the processing of concrete words somewhat. As can be seen from Figure 4.24, when the input connections (O → I and I → S) are lesioned the net produces a very strange effect. There are considerably more *visual* errors on abstract than on concrete words. In other words the *semantic* status of the word determines the likelihood of a visual error on the word.

Deep dyslexic patients show both these effects. They show large differences in their ability to read concrete versus abstract words: 73% vs 14% for KF (Shallice & Warrington, 1975); 67% vs 13% for PW and 70% vs 10% for DE (Patterson & Marcel, 1977). Moreover in deep dyslexic patients in whom it had been investigated, visual errors occurred more often on less concrete words (see e.g. Shallice & Warrington, 1980).[72]

Now there is one critical difference, which relates to the simplicity and explanatory potential aspects of a simulation, between these simulations and those concerning the phonological route discussed earlier in the chapter. Plaut and Shallice provide a theory of the nature of a system, which, they claimed, should give rise to the characteristics of deep dyslexia reading

if damaged. Their claim was that deep dyslexia reading has the following characteristics (see also Table 4.1).

1 Semantic, visual, mixed visual-and-semantic, visual-then-semantic, and *other* (unrelated) errors occur.

2 Concrete words are read better than abstract words.

3 Visual errors (a) tend to have responses that are more concrete than the stimuli, (b) occur more frequently on abstract than concrete words and (c) have stimuli that are more abstract than do semantic errors.

These characteristics, they propose, arise from damage to a system with the following properties:

1 Orthographic and semantic representations are distributed over separate groups of units, such that similar patterns represent similar words in each domain, but the similarity metrics of the two domains are not correlated.

2 Knowledge is encoded in connection weights that are learned by a procedure for performing gradient descent in some measure of performance on the task of mapping orthography to semantics.

3 Mapping orthography to semantics is accomplished through the operation of attractors (and the lesion does not seriously impair the connections which implement the attractors).

4 The semantic representations of concrete words are much 'richer' than those of abstract words (i.e. contain considerably more consistently accessed features).

These theoretical claims were not proved, but it was shown that the key characteristic 1 occurs with

---

[72] The complimentary effect of the responses of visual errors being more concrete than the stimuli has also been shown in three patients; see, e.g. Barry and Richardson, 1988.

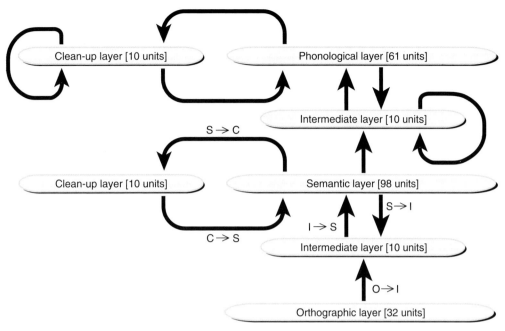

Fig. 4.23 The network architecture of the reading model giving rise to the error patterns shown in Figure 4.24. (See Plaut & Shallice, 1993a; Figure 19.)

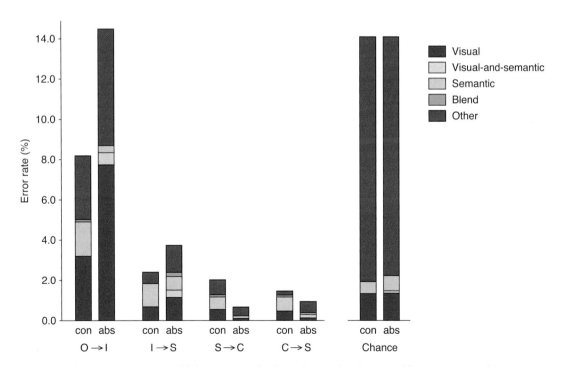

Fig. 4.24 Types of reading error for abstract (abs) and concrete (con) stimuli arising from lesions to different sites in one of the Plaut and Shallice networks (see Figure 4.23). The right-most columns show chance error-rates based on randomly selecting an output word for each input word. Adapted from: Deep dyslexia: A case study of connectionist neuropsychology. D.C. Plaut and T. Shallice, *Cognitive Neuropsychology*, 1993, *10*(5), 377–500, reprinted by permission of the publisher (Taylor & Francis Group, http://www.informaworld.com).

five different architectures that share these properties, with alternative output systems and with more than one learning algorithm (see Figure 4.21). Moreover, no counter-example has been produced. Thus accepting the Plaut–Shallice theoretical hypothesis, the relation between syndrome characteristics and properties of the model require far fewer specific assumptions and is more directly explanatory than the computational models discussed so far in the chapter.

That said, the position has been challenged in two ways. The first is a straight empirical challenge. The theoretical finding is that with lesions to this type of attractor network, it will produce visual errors as well as semantic ones. However, three patients who make semantic errors but not visual errors have been described, namely KE of Hillis et al. (1990), and RGB and HW of Caramazza and Hillis (1990). The account provided by Plaut and Shallice for the behaviour of these patients was to apply assumption 2 and argue that the patients adopted a procedure different from that typically used in reading aloud. They gave circumstantial evidence supporting their claims.[73]

The second challenge is that alternative accounts of deep dyslexia can be produced if one questions another of the basic assumptions, namely 5_N, that the damaged system is a proper subset of the undamaged system. A second popular theory of deep dyslexia put forward by Coltheart (1980a) and Saffran et al. (1980) is that it results from reading being carried out by a right hemisphere reading system, and as such, as Saffran et al. (1980) point out, not necessarily the normal reading system subtracted of some components.

The evidence for this position is mixed. Against it, at least one patient has been described who read in a deep dyslexia fashion and lost the ability following a left hemisphere stroke (Roeltgen, 1987). In favour of the hypothesis is that the right hemisphere of the two split-brain patients showed little sign of being able to carry out spelling-to-sound translation and yet the patients were able to match pictures of objects to printed words (Zaidel & Peters, 1981).[74] Moreover a child suffering from Rasmussen's encephalitis had to have her left hemisphere removed at the age of 15 to treat the resulting seizures. Her ability to read was studied by Patterson et al. (1989). Following the hemispherectomy her reading showed many similarities to that of deep dyslexic patients in that she appeared unable to carry out spelling-to-sound translation but could read aloud roughly 30% of presented words. She also showed a similar part-of-speech effect to deep dyslexic patients. On the other hand an imaging study of Price et al. (1998) of deep dyslexic patients did not support the hypothesis. When reading, their patients activated, normally or supranormally, the left posterior inferotemporal and the anterior temporal cortices, regions associated with semantic processing—as we will see in Chapter 6.

However, even if the right hemisphere is the material locus for the processing of the written word, as far as semantics is concerned, at least for some deep dyslexic patients, this explanation does not provide an information-processing account. It gives no explanation of the detailed error characteristics of such patients, such as how a word's imageability affects its propensity to give rise to a visual error. For those types of detail a computational model is required. Moreover the right hemisphere hypothesis is entirely compatible with the Hinton–Plaut–Shallice model. One just needs to assume that normal reading can utilise two similar sets of resources, but with the left hemisphere being the larger, particularly at the orthographic (or word-form) level.[75]

4.12 The Brain Bases of a Reading System: the Word-Form System

Can the localisation of a possible subsystem be used to fix its functional reality, as was suggested at the end of Section 4.10? Consider the visual word-form system. The DRC theory and the Plaut et al. triangle model differ subtly in the way they conceive of how the written word is processed prior to the accessing of phonological and semantic representations. On the DRC model (see Figure 3.4), there is a common set of letter units and these feed an orthographic input lexicon and a grapheme-phoneme rule system which

[73] The importance of considering atypical procedures will be discussed in the next section. In the case of KE it was argued that a limited set of stimuli drawn from a small number of categories were repeatedly used and so any potential visual error would be likely to fall outside the known set of categories; it would therefore be known not to be a potential stimulus. For RGB and HW, where the putative functional lesion lay between the semantic system and the phonological clean-up units (see Figure 4.23), the patients appeared to be attempting to characterise the meaning of the written word, which they appeared to understand, in their response; they were responding off-line. Tests of these claims were never carried out to our knowledge and indeed the patients may well have been no longer available.

[74] In the split-brain patient the corpus callosum has been sectioned at operation to attempt to reduce the effects of previously intractable epilepsy. In such patients information concerning words presented to the left visual field received by the right occipital cortex cannot cross to the left hemisphere.

[75] Further support for a model of accessing semantics of the Hinton–Plaut–Shallice type is provided by its ability to explain counter-intuitive phenomena relating to the speed of processing of words with multiple meanings by normal subjects. See Section 6.6.

are quite separate. In contrast on the Plaut et al. triangle model (see Figure 3.3) a single orthographic system is assumed to provide a point-of-entry to both the orthographic and the phonological routes.

The Plaut et al. triangle model is in this respect similar to one of the two more popular theories in its account of much the oldest of the acquired dyslexia syndromes. This is pure alexia, first described by the French neurologist Dejerine in 1892 and reported in hundreds of patients since (see, e.g. Kremin, 1982). Such patients may be able to identify written words reasonably well but very effortfully and laboriously, taking seconds to read a single word. Behaviourally their reading time is strongly and often roughly linearly affected by the length of the word, and in addition script presentation creates great difficulties (e.g. Staller et al., 1978; Warrington & Shallice, 1980).[76] In contrast, normal subjects read words with a naming latency of 500–600 msec, little affected by word length for relatively short words (Weekes, 1997).

In such patients these effects appear to arise from a compensatory strategy by which the patient attempts to get round their difficulty. The patients typically read letters better than words. Clinically, many pure alexia patients appear to attempt to read through naming the letters aloud or, more commonly, sotto voce; this is called letter-by-letter reading. There is strong evidence that some patients do use a so-called *reversed spelling* strategy (see e.g. Warrington & Langdon, 2002), at least in irregular languages such as English or French, explicitly using their knowledge of spelling to attain the identity of the word.[77] In other patients, however, a more purely visually based strategy may well be being used (Patterson & Kay, 1982; Hanley & Kay, 1996; Rosazza et al., 2007).

For nearly a century after Dejerine's description of the disorder the principal explanation was that the patient's reading difficulty arose from a disconnection of the systems responsible for reading from its source of input. Input from the right visual field would typically not be available because there was a lesion affecting the left occipital lobe and so the patient had a hemianopia; that is, loss of all input from that visual field. Input from the left visual field, in turn, was also thought to be unavailable, in this case due to a lesion of the fibres crossing the splenium—the most posterior part of the corpus callosum—from the right occipital cortex to reading centres in the posterior left hemisphere (see e.g. Hécaen & Albert, 1978).

An alternative perspective was put forward by Warrington and Shallice (1980).[78] They argued that the functional basis of the disorder was damage to a system responsible for the orthographic processing of letter strings including that of achieving the word's orthographic identity. This approach fits quite naturally into the triangle model and indeed is a related explanation to that given by Marshall and Newcombe (1973) for a related disorder, *visual dyslexia*, the forgotten third of the three syndromes they described in their famous paper. Much more solid evidence for a related position was produced by Cohen et al. (2003). They described four patients with lesions in the left occipital lobe. Two of these (patients F and A in Figure 4.25) showed the typical length effect in word reading characteristic of pure alexia (Figure 4.26). Two others with anatomically nearby lesions (D and M in Figure 4.25), showed in one case no word length effect and in the other case only a mild one (Figure 4.26). The lesions of patients F and A were slightly more lateral in the fusiform gyrus than those of patients D and M.

Critically the study also included a functional imaging experiment on normal subjects in which alphabetical stimuli—words or consonant strings—were contrasted with the presentation of chequer boards. A strongly left-lateralised network involving a variety of regions was obtained. However, within the occipito-temporal area the region activated overlapped with the lesions of patients F and A, and also of a globally alexic patient VOL (see Figure 4.25). By contrast the occipito-temporal area activated in normal subjects was more lateral than that of those patients who were not pure alexic, that is patients D and M.[79]

As will be discussed in the next chapter, Cohen et al. have found this left occipito-temporal region activated in a variety of functional imaging studies on normal subjects (see, e.g. McCandliss et al., 2003). They propose that it is organised as shown in Figure 4.27 (Dehaene et al., 2005). This may be seen as a brain-based

---

[76] See FNMS, Section 4.2.

[77] If reversed spelling is unavailable then the slow version of surface dyslexia discussed in Section 4.10 can occur.

[78] More recently it has been shown that at least part of the

problem in many pure alexics may precede orthographic processing, as many such patients have some visual problems apparently unrelated to orthography (see Behrmann et al., 1998). However in some patients there is strong evidence for the relative preservation of visual processing where this does not involve orthography (Chialant & Caramazza, 1998; Miozzo & Caramazza, 1998). In other patients an account which does not involve orthographic word processing is not plausible because of the relative preservation of visual span for letters by comparison with word reading, e.g. Warrington & Shallice (1980).

[79] The figure also shows the lesion site of a patient without hemianopia RAV2, who was alexic for information presented in the right visual field but showed no length effect for letter strings restricted to the right visual field; again the lesion does not lie in the area activated by a letter string in normal subjects.

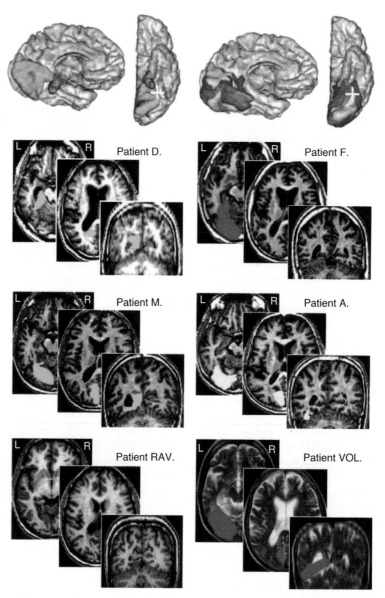

Fig. 4.25 Reconstructions of the lesions of six left-hemisphere patients described by Cohen et al (2003). Those in the right column were of patients with pure alexia; those in the left column had relatively unimpaired reading. Reprinted from L. Cohen, O. Martinaud, C. Lemer, S. Lehéricy, Y. Samson, M. Obadia, A. Slachevsky and S. Dehaene, Visual word recognition in the left and right hemispheres: Anatomical and functional correlates of peripheral alexias, *Cerebral Cortex*, 2003, *13*(12), 1313–1333, by permission of Oxford University Press.

extension of the classical McClelland–Rumelhart model of orthographic processing (see Figure 3.21).[80]

Behrmann, Plaut and Nelson (1998b) have also applied a model similar to the classic McClelland–Rumelhart one to account for the characteristics of pure alexia. Such a model predicts that partial damage

early in the system will in cascade fashion allow limited activation of higher structures to occur. Indeed if, in the spirit of Chapter 3, one takes the distributed analogue of the localist interactive activation model as far as the relation between orthography and semantics is concerned, namely the Hinton–Plaut–Shallice model, then the activation of broad semantic areas occurs when precise access to a particular semantic representation is not possible (Hinton & Shallice, 1991). Moreover, this is found in certain pure alexic patients who show partial semantic access for words they cannot read and

---

[80] See Rosazza et al. (2007) for supporting neuropsychological evidence for the different levels of processing involved in this model.

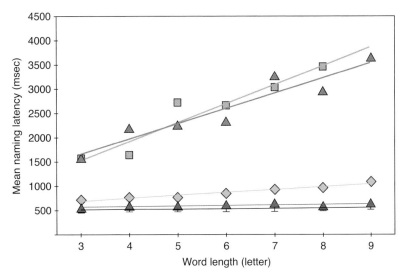

Fig. 4.26 Reading latency as a function of word length for control subjects (in black) and the patients of Cohen et al referred to in Figure 4.25. Colour coding for the patients is as in Figure 4.25. Reprinted from L. Cohen, O. Martinaud, C. Lemer, S. Lehéricy, Y. Samson, M. Obadia, A. Slachevsky and S. Dehaene, Visual word recognition in the left and right hemispheres: Anatomical and functional correlates of peripheral alexias, *Cerebral Cortex*, 2003, *13*(12), 1313–1333, by permission of Oxford University Press.

of which they do not know the precise meaning (see, e.g. patients reported by Shallice & Saffran, 1986; Coslett & Saffran, 1989; Coslett et al., 1993; McKeeff & Behrmann, 2004). For words they cannot read or identify such patients can make two-choice decisions about the category in which they lie well above chance. For instance, ML (Shallice & Saffran, 1986) was able to correctly categorise 94% of 50 towns and countries as being either in or not in Europe, and 93% of famous names as belonging either to authors or politicians. In certain of these patients Coslett et al. (1993) have shown the effects to occur only when the patient uses an appropriate strategy. Thus their pure alexic patient JWC took about 20 sec to read a five-letter word. When asked not to try to read a word but to guess whether it was or was not in a given category then he was 86% correct for foods and 85% for animals—by no means perfect but well above chance. If, however, he was asked to attempt to read the word aloud and only if he could not read it to say whether it is a food or not, then he performed completely at chance (52%) on the categorisation task. The induced strategy had a large effect on his performance.

The visual word form model can be viewed as realised computationally in the McClelland and Rumelhart interactive activation model, and more generally as the orthographic part of an expanded triangle model. However, critically it, and pure alexia which corresponds to the behavioural manifestation of its impairment, can be rooted materially in a particular part of the left fusiform gyrus, namely the Cohen et al. visual word from area.

4.13 **Methodological Conclusions**

Methodologically one can draw a number of conclusions. One, from pure alexia, concerns the linkage between function and anatomy. We begin however with another. As Coslett and Saffran have shown, the behavioural characteristics of pure alexia are critically dependent upon the strategy that the patient applies when trying to read words. Indeed the characteristic behavioural signs, for instance, that of a linear increase in word reading time with the number of letters in the word, simply reflects properties of the standard compensatory strategy rather than characteristics of the impaired system. Thus assumption 2, which separates the patient's strategy from the properties of the underlying functional architecture, is in practice critical.

However, as will be discussed in Chapter 9, we have no dictionary of procedures and no operational methods for determining which procedure is in operation. Thus the need to have recourse to notions like *procedure* as part of the explanatory framework of cognitive neuropsychology is a problem as far as the falsifiability of theories and their explanatory adequacy is concerned. Procedure-based explanations are almost inevitably intuitive and based on plausible *ad hoc* additions to processing theories rather than derived directly from them.[81] This is illustrated by the example of possible

---

[81] Some recent ideas in computational modelling are aimed to address this difficulty. The problem of procedure or strategy is particularly acute when evaluating models developed within a cognitive architecture (see Section 3.8), where it is generally

Putative area	Coded units	RF size and structure	Examples of preferred stimuli

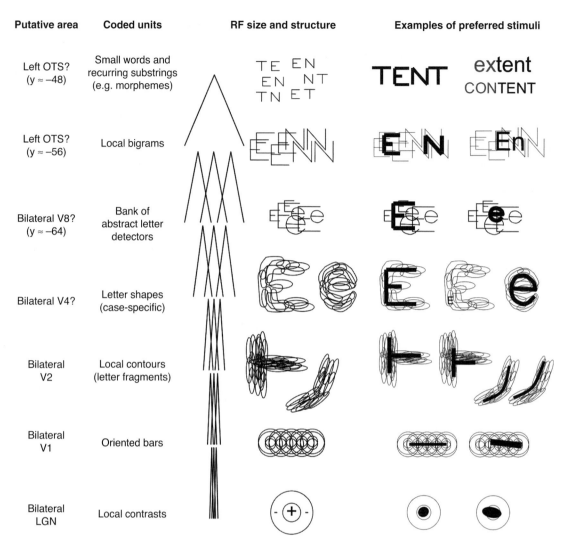

Fig. 4.27 The hierarchy of 'local combination detectors' proposed to support the word-form level of word recognition by Cohen, Dehaene and colleagues. Reprinted from *Trends in Cognitive Sciences*, 9(7), S. Dehaene, L. Cohen, M. Sigman and F. Vinckier, The neural code for written words: a proposal, 335–341, Copyright (2005), with permission from Elsevier.

strategies used by patients showing semantic errors without visual errors in reading.

At the same time, earlier in this chapter we have shown that the basic assumptions of cognitive neuropsychology, as initially laid out by Caramazza (1986), in

feasible to implement any number of strategies. Howes et al. (2009) suggest a principled solution—namely that the strategy applied is that which is in some sense optimal given the constraints of both the architecture and the task. The authors illustrate their argument with a re-analysis of psychological refractory period performance (also discussed in Section 3.8) which leads to a novel account of strategy selection within ordered dual-task situations.

practice need to be questioned in particular cases. Thus, the assumption that the system following the lesion is a reduced form of the normal system (assumption 5_N) has been extensively questioned in the case of the right hemisphere theory of deep dyslexia. In addition, in examples where there is a different pattern of performance with different modalities of input or output, one may need to consider the possibility that different hemispheres are involved in processing different types of stimuli or responses. Moreover assumption 4—that there is a qualitative identity across patients as far as their underlying functional architecture, and so the individual case study method can be applied—has been questioned both quantitatively as far as surface dyslexia and reading without semantics are concerned, and qualitatively as far as phonological alexia is concerned.[82]

It is clear that to operate the methodology of cognitive neuropsychology based on individual cases just assuming that the basic assumptions are all intact, while appropriate in the 1980s, would be ostrich-like today. Does this mean that one should abandon the cognitive neuropsychology method, and in particular the detailed analysis of the behaviour of patients with apparently theoretically interesting disorders? In our view this would be to throw the baby out with the bathwater. The inferential method based on the basic assumptions needs to be retained, but in any individual case the assumptions may be questionable. To compensate for this increased inferential fragility, we therefore need additional arrows in our methodological quill. One is provided by the possible development and application to neuropsychological data of computational models with higher levels of explanatory adequacy and their application to neuropsychological data such as relating them to functional syndromes with counterintuitive aspects, as was discussed for deep dyslexia. A second, as discussed for surface dyslexia, is the use of the case-series approach. A third, where we used the example of pure alexia again, aims to support the case-study approach by linking the functional systems that are postulated to account for behavioural data to their anatomical bases. Even when only a small numbers of cases are available, the functional reality of the particular subsystem—in this case the visual word-form system—is reinforced by showing that there is a consistent relation between the functional impairment and lesion location. Moreover, in this case the correlation is supported by parallel functional imaging studies in normal subjects. This is an application of assumption 3.[83] Finally, given that the gross organisation of the cognitive system is accepted in a particular domain, the individual pure case can be used to assess rival theories of the operation of the component.

This chapter has therefore introduced two methods of supporting functional considerations by anatomical ones when assessing the theoretical implications of neuropsychological data. The case-series approach can operate for computational as well as resource-based (box-and-arrow) theories. The second, the lesion-mapping approach, which has been introduced for pure alexia here, is critically linked to resource-based theories. We will see a further method—the group-study approach—in which there is averaging across patients with respect to behaviour and or lesion site in later chapters.[84] However, the natural next step is to consider anatomically-based methods for functional imaging of normal subjects. This is the topic of the next chapter.

---

[82] In principle this issue can be examined by using functional imaging. In practice it has not been.

[83] Price and Mechelli (2005) have presented functional imaging evidence which they hold argues against the assumption that a visual word-form functional subsystem has been isolated. We address these issues in more detail in Chapter 5.

[84] See in particular Chapters 9 and 10.

Inferences to the Functional Architecture from Functional Imaging

5.1 The Processing of Functional Imaging Findings

In the previous chapter we have seen that there are considerable problems in making solid inferences from neuropsychological findings to models of normal function. But why bother with this old-fashioned technique when modern technologies provide much more spatially precise findings and one can use them to study the normal brain directly?

There are two reasons. The first is that inferences from functional imaging evidence to models of normal cognitive function are, somewhat paradoxically, much more complex than those from neuropsychology. More critical is, however, the second reason. Functional imaging, just like human experimental psychology and cognitive neuropsychology, must make use of cognitive tasks, and cognitive tasks, as we have discussed extensively in Chapters 2 and 3, are very complex; and the behavioural aspects of functional imaging are those of normal human experimental psychology and so have relatively little power. There are no differential error types that lead to serendipity in neuropsychology. Indeed quite a number of highly experienced cognitive scientists have argued that functional imaging is in practice if not in theory of little or no use for assessing models of normal cognition (Bub, 2000; Harley, 2004; Page, 2006; Coltheart, 2006b).

A range of technologies exist that measure aspects of brain processes while the subject is carrying out a task. In this chapter, however, we will discuss just two—positron emission tomography (PET) and functional magnetic resonance imaging (fMRI)—the two that are the most reliable for ascertaining the anatomical location of the activation in adults. We will also use the term 'functional imaging' to refer to these two techniques. The most important widely used other methods are EEG and MEG; for further discussion of these techniques see Darvas et al. (2004). To relate the results of behavioural experiments which use these techniques to cognitive theorising would require chapters of considerably greater complexity than this and the last. Of the other technologies, optical imaging has had relatively weak spatial resolution; moreover its limited penetration depth means that so far it has been mainly used with babies, whose thin skulls allow it to be more effectively applied (Wolf et al., 2007). We can also anticipate the development of combinations of techniques such as TMS and fMRI (e.g. Bestmann et al., 2008) and also many new technologies. To give one example, it is now possible to use multiple-electrode grids implanted during operations for the control of epileptic seizures or to remove tumours. They can provide very interesting evidence of cellular activity in humans, particularly from the use of so-called *high-gamma* frequency ranges when combined with EEG analysis procedures (see Canolty et al., 2007). However rigorous analysis of their cognitive implications would be extremely complex.

There are two ways in which inferences from functional imaging to cognitive models are more complex than those from neuropsychology. The first, obviously, is how the measurements are carried out—the technology that has to be employed. The second, though, is the relation between the task and what is measured.

We will use the inferential framework developed in Chapter 4. To go from performance of a task to a measure such as provided by PET or fMRI of the neural processes involved can be viewed as requiring five steps.

1 Carrying out the task requires the use of a procedure (assumption 2 of Section 4.5).

2 Realising the procedure requires the operation of a particular set of cognitive systems and their connections.

3 The operation of each of the different systems entails that for each a specific region of the brain—its base region—becomes neurally more active.

4 The change in neural activity leads to an increase in blood flow into the region, which begins typically 2–4 sec after the neural activity has occurred (Kwong et al., 1992). This change in blood flow—the haemodynamic response—lasts for roughly 10–12 sec (Blamire et al., 1992) (see Figure 5.1).

5 The increase in blood flow is assessed by a change in a specific measure. For PET this is the quantity of a radioactive tracer in the blood. Commonly this is

^{15}O-labelled water but other agents can also be used (Jones et al., 1976). The most typically used ligand ^{15}O has a 2-min half-life, which allows a single scan lasting 30–60 sec to be taken once every 10 min or so. The exposure to ionizing radiation it produces is not trivial, so a very limited number of scans can be carried out on normal volunteers in an experiment without exceeding radiation doses. It provides a measure of regional cerebral blood flow (rCBF). For fMRI the most common measurement is of the quantity of oxygen in the blood. Increased blood flow in an area brings more oxyhaemoglobin (oxygenated haemoglobin) into the region in which the neural activity has taken place. This results in a decrease in deoxyhaemoglobin concentration in the blood, a signal that can be measured by MRI. The signal is called the Blood Oxygenation Level Dependent (BOLD) contrast mechanism.[1] fMRI does not involve radioactivity and creates no known dangers provided all metal is removed from the subject. The restrictions on the length of use of PET do not therefore have an analogue in fMRI.

In order for functional imaging to become an effective scientific method for the analysis of cognitive processes, two advances were necessary in addition to the development of the technology per se—one in experimental method and one in statistical analysis. The advance in experimental method was the use of experimental designs that decompose the overall cognitive process into subcomponents. In information-processing psychology, the chronometric method—the use of reaction times—had been employed to attempt to decompose the set of processes involved in a very simple task into its elements from the time of the Dutch psychologist Donders mentioned in Section 1.9. However the work of Donders was forgotten and it was the analyses of Saul Sternberg, discussed in Section 3.3, which led to the widespread use of reaction time decomposition in the 1960s. By the early 1980s the leading exponent of the method was Michael Posner (see Posner, 1978) and it was his cross-disciplinary collaboration with radiologist Marcus Raichle and his group in St. Louis that led to the introduction of the first widely used method for decomposing the complex overall rCBF signal averaged over a scan into components attributable to different computational processes. This was the subtraction method applied to the subcomponents of the reading process (Petersen et al., 1988; see Section 1.10). In fMRI the analogue to rCBF would be to use the BOLD signal averaged over a block of trials, at least in so-called *blocked* designs.

---

[1] The physics of how the BOLD signal is measured is not discussed in this book. See Huettel et al. (2009) sections 2–5. This provides a relatively elementary introduction to the topic.

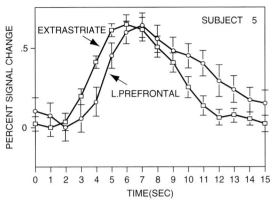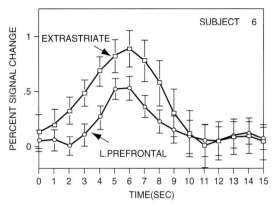

Fig. 5.1 The heamodynamic response function. The percentage signal change is shown for two cortical areas in two subjects. The subjects performed a simple word-stem completion task in which on each trial three letters are presented e.g. COU and the subject must produce a word e.g. COUPLE. The increase in signal strength begins approximately 2 sec after stimulus presentation, and continues for approximately 10–12 sec. Reproduced with permission from R.L. Buckner, P.A. Bandettini, K.M. O'Craven, R.L. Savoy, S.E. Petersen, M.E. Raichle and B.R. Rosen (1996) Detection of cortical activation during averaged single trials of a cognitive task using functional magnetic resonance imaging. *Proceedings of the National Academy Sciences of the United States of America*, 93(25), 14878–14883, 1996; figure 4, p. 14882. Copyright (1996) National Academy of Sciences, USA.

The complementary step to that of experimental design was in statistical analysis. Historically the experimental adequacy of many fields, such as agricultural research and experimental psychology, was revolutionised by the introduction of more powerful statistical methods derived from the analysis of variance. Functional imaging went through an analogous jump in its experimental adequacy. In the mid-1990s, formal procedures were introduced to enable proper statistical analysis of PET and fMRI imaging to be made, and so for findings to become properly replicable. A number of methods have been employed. However the first and much the widest used has been Statistical Parametric Mapping (SPM), developed by Karl Friston and his colleagues in the early 1990s (for an overview see Friston et al., 2007).[2]

The SPM procedure is complex (see Figure 5.2). It too goes through a number of stages. The first three pre-process the data before it is entered into a statistical analysis in the final two stages. A simple characterisation of the stages is as follows:

1 *Realignment.* The subject is lying in the scanner carrying out a simple task. He or she tries not to move. However, if physical movements do occur this results in shifts of the signal. In fMRI an initial preprocessing step for each subject is to realign each image to the standard prototypic structural image of the subject's brain. The imaged brain is treated as a rigid body capable of translation in three dimensions and of being rotated in three dimensions. Various procedures

exist for making an optimum estimate of any translation or rotation that has taken place due to the movement of the subject (see Ashburner & Friston, 2007).[3]

2 *Spatial Normalisation.* The brains of different subjects differ. Some investigators therefore co-register the data with the structural scans of the individual subjects. In addition, due to the noisiness of individual subject data, empirical generalisations relevant to theory frequently require comparisons involving multiple subjects. Some form of standardisation of the individual images is thus required before averaging across subjects. This stage of SPM therefore involves moving and warping the images derived from each subject to match some idealised or standardised brain. Up until 1999 this was the brain of one fairly elderly Frenchwoman mapped in detail by Talairach and Tournoux (1988). Now a standardised anatomical space currently derived from about 150 normal brains is probably the most used.

3 *Spatial Smoothing.* fMRI offers high spatial resolution. However, the spatial scale of haemodynamic responses is thought to be about 2–5 mm (Friston, 2007). In addition, the standardisation procedure, just discussed, cannot be perfect. Even after spatial normalisation, minor differences will remain as to

---

[2] In principled fashion SPM is implemented in regularly updated public access software. Different versions are labelled with the date they became freely available.

[3] See also Friston (2007) for dealing with other types of variance in fMRI time series that are not compensated by realignment. Given that the different slices are actually scanned at different times within say a 2-sec period, it is now also common to use interpolation algorithms to correct for the differences in the precise time at which individual slices are scanned. This can be done before or after movement correction.

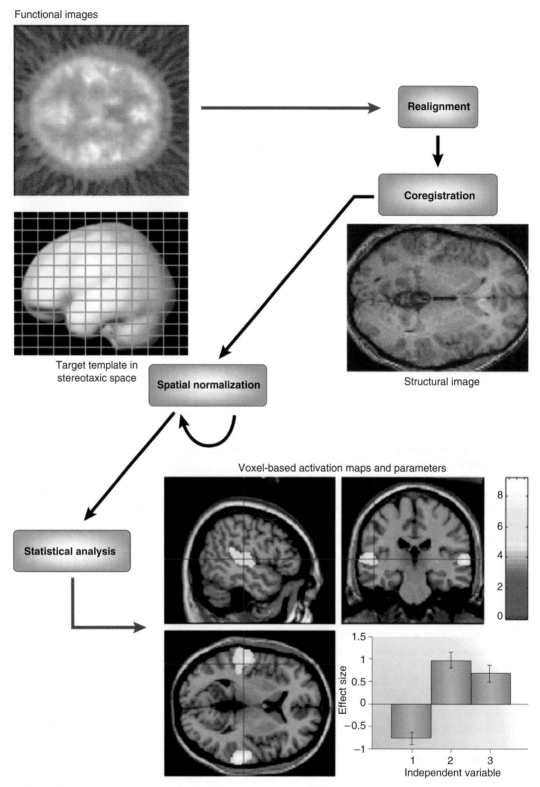

Fig. 5.2 Stages of image processing. Images are first realigned to the subject's structural scan. They are then normalised to a reference brain and spatially smoothed before application of statistical procedures such as the general linear model and statistical inference. Reprinted by permission from Macmillan Publishers Ltd: Nature Reviews Neuroscience (M. Brett, I.S. Johnsrude and A.M. Owen, The problem of functional localization in the human brain, *Nature Reviews Neuroscience*, 3, 243–249), copyright (2002).

the location of a given anatomical structure across brains. Smoothing—technically convolving the data with a Gaussian (normal) distribution—lessens the effect of any such minor differences. Moreover smoothing improves the signal-to-noise ratio, as the origins of the signals are frequently from structures several millimetres or more in extent, while noise can be assumed to have a higher spatial frequency.

4 *Application of a General Linear Statistical Model.* In this stage of the analysis a parametric statistical approach is used to assess the significance of the difference in activation between different conditions in comparison with within-condition error variance.

5 *Statistical Inference.* Stage 4 provides a t-value for each voxel in the 3D structure. However, such comparisons are being made across tens of thousands of voxels simultaneously. Therefore a higher threshold than that typical for statistical inference is required in order to conclude that there has been a significant change between conditions. There are various methods for determining significance (see Friston, 2007). One of the most widely used at present is to use the probability of a continuous cluster of a given size of voxels having a given activation difference (or greater) between conditions than would be expected under the null hypothesis. Thresholding procedures in use also differ. Currently the standard approach within SPM it to use two thresholds. The first is for whether any given voxel is activated differently in two conditions; a common criterion is the use of 0.001 uncorrected. The second is then applied; it is whether a cluster of such activated voxels is significantly larger than would be expected by chance, given the number of such activated voxels; a common criterion for this is .05 corrected for multiple comparisons.

SPM provides the investigator with a beautifully precise map of the regions that differ significantly between task conditions in activation, as we will colloquially call the rCBF or BOLD measures. How, though, does one relate the output of SPM to cognitive processes and in particular to the operation of isolable systems? Here one moves from the bright sunlight of precise and technically sound procedures to a murky world peopled by a majority of investigators who use only vague implicit assumptions together with a few brave iconoclasts proposing rather more rigorous perspectives. It would seem plausible that if a region is activated differently between two conditions, then, working back through the chain of inferences at the start of this section, differential use is being made of the different cognitive systems and connections across the two conditions. However the devil is in the detail. Indeed it is so much in the detail that some noted theorists have argued that functional imaging, despite the great sums spent on it,

has proved essentially useless as far as our understanding of cognition is concerned (Harley, 2004; Coltheart, 2006b). The majority of investigators find this view incomprehensible but the attempts to positively present a well-worked out inference procedure have been relatively few and little used in practice (e.g. Bub, 2000; Shallice, 2003; Henson, 2005; Poldrack, 2006). We will return to these arguments later in the chapter.

5.2 What is the BOLD measure?

The use of a procedure like SPM or any other of the packages available to analyse functional imaging data presupposes that the measured activation has a clear relation to cognitive processes. What, however, is the neurophysiological basis of the BOLD signal, say? Why should it have any relation to cognition at all?

In some situations BOLD seems to be closely related to the output activity of a region of cortex. Thus Rees et al. (2000) examined a situation similar to that we discussed in Chapter 2, namely how BOLD related to the coherence of visual movement. Subjects look at a set of moving dots. The situations vary according to how coherent is their motion—from 0% (i.e. random directions) to 100% when they all move in the same direction. In the movement sensitive area V5 there is a linear relation between the degree of coherence and the amplitude of the BOLD response. In research related to that discussed in Section 2.1 it was found that most V1 cells also show a linear relation between their response and the degree of motion coherence (Britten et al., 1993).

How widely such a simple relation holds between the neuronal output and the BOLD response is unclear. However, since the work of Rees et al., Nikos Logothetis and his colleagues have looked more closely at the neurophysiology of the BOLD response. Physiologically, the BOLD signal seems to be more closely related to what are called the *local field potentials* than the actual spiking of neurons (Logothetis & Wandell, 2004). The region of brain surrounding a set of neurons acts as a volume conductor—a generator of electrical potential. Given the electrical activity of the neurons the resistance of the extracellular medium leads to the creation of so-called *extracellular field potentials*. The extracellular field potentials in the low frequency range are called *local field potentials*. They are thought to reflect aspects of the electrical activity of the dendrites—the input regions of neurons.[4] For alert monkeys given a visual task, local field potentials were better predictors of the BOLD response than was spiking activity (Goense & Logothetis, 2008).

---

4 More specifically they reflect the weighted average of synchronised dendro-somatic components of the electrical activity (see Logothetis & Wandell, 2004).

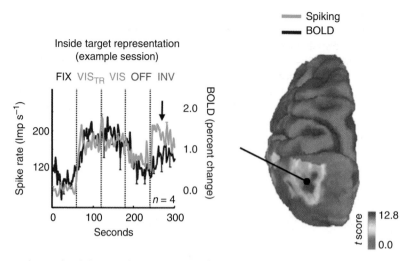

Fig. 5.3 Spiking response (in green) and change to the BOLD response (in purple) in the five conditions (see text) of the experiment of Maier et al. (2008). Reprinted by permission from Macmillan Publishers Ltd: Nature Neuroscience (A. Maier, M. Wilke, C. Aura, C. Zhu, F.Q. Ye and D.A. Leopold, Divergence of fMRI and neural signals in V1 during perceptual suppression in the awake monkey, *Nature Neuroscience*, 10, 1193–1200), copyright (2008).

This deviation of BOLD from actual neuronal spiking can be quite major. Thus Maier et al. (2008) studied in two monkeys *generalised flash suppression* where a brief target—a red disk—presented to a single eye is made to disappear phenomenally by the abrupt presentation to both eyes of a surrounding field of 200+ moving dots. They compared a number of conditions (see Figure 5.3). In two conditions VIS$_{TR}$ and VIS it was arranged that the target was seen by the monkey, for instance, by the target being presented to both eyes; that the target was seen was confirmed by experiments similar to those of Cowey and Stoerig (1995) to be discussed in Section 11.2. In other conditions the target was not seen, either because it was not presented (FIXation, OFF) or because it was subjectively invisible due to the surrounding field (INVisible). In this last condition the BOLD response to the target was indeed reduced to nearly the level of the OFF condition. However the spiking response remained at the same level as when the target was seen (VIS).

Why the dissociation between spiking activity and awareness should occur is a puzzle. However the experiment clearly shows that the BOLD response diverges from the spiking activity.[5] By contrast, for local field potentials the signal was reduced in the INV condition to below the two visible conditions, although the reduction was less than for the BOLD signal. A precise neurophysiological characterisation of the mechanism

underlying the BOLD signal and how it relates to local field potentials still, however, remains unknown.

This means that if we do not know what the BOLD signal corresponds to at the neurophysiological level, how it relates to cognitive operations cannot be certain at present. Thus as Rorden and Karnath (2004) discuss we have no definite grounds for assuming that an activated region is functionally necessary. They suggest that some regions may be being activated because they have strong connections to other regions required for the task. Indeed they float the plausible possibility that activations frequently seen in the right hemisphere in language tasks may occur merely because of their connections to corresponding regions of the left hemisphere but have no relevance for language processing. This is made more plausible given that BOLD corresponds better to the input to a subsystem than to its output (Kayser & Logothetis, 2010). In practice, Rorden and Karnath point out that a neurosurgeon would resect such right hemisphere regions without worrying about impairing language functions. One could see such activations as an evolutionary appendix-like legacy of the basically functionally bilaterally organised brains of our forbears.

How should one proceed? One approach is to follow Harley (2004) and Coltheart (2006b) by saying that this confirms the lack of utility of functional imaging findings for speaking to the validity of cognitive models. This, however, ignores a golden rule of cognitive neuroscience—that all empirical brain-based findings must currently rely on somewhat flaky inference procedures as far as cognitive conclusions are concerned. If we attempt to be too rigorous we make no progress at all.

---

[5] The deviation of BOLD from spiking rates seems to be less with temporal smoothing as typically used in a human fMRI experiment (Kayser & Logothetis, 2010).

A second alternative proposed by Henson (2005) is to treat imaging data as just 'another dependent variable'. He says 'I do not see any privileged status to the behavioural data; all types of data are in principle, observations about the system we are trying to understand, viz, the mind (with the implicit assumption of materialism). Put flippantly, accuracy and reaction times have been the 'meat and two veg' of experimental psychology; I am simply highlighting a larger range of dietary options' (p195).[6] There is though quite a difference between the two sorts of measure. Accuracy and reaction time have an integral link to cognitive models; for many cognitive models one can in principle estimate what they should be from the model, given that the model is sufficiently explicit. BOLD activation in say, part of the posterior parietal cortex is not in principle predictable from a standard type of cognitive model. It would be helpful to have other examples from science where a measure that was not understood was used effectively and rigorously to differentiate between theories. We think it preferable to provide a bridge law, even one that is probably inadequate in some situations as the work just discussed suggests; thus in cognitive neuropsychology the assumption 5_N is probably false for some patients but it has proved enormously useful heuristically. Moreover the assumptions can then be tested and if found to be inadequate replaced by something better. To start with the bridge law would require that the cognitive model be linked to neuroanatomy. Then, it requires a correspondence between processing in the model and the BOLD signal.

The anatomical correspondence is provided by assumption 3 of the previous chapter. For the second part of the bridge law we assume that the BOLD signal is a rough neurophysiological measure of a *cognitive* variable, namely the amount of *resource* required of a subsystem that a task is using, a concept introduced in assumption 5_{NR} of Section 5 in the last chapter.[7] This will be discussed further in the next section. Alternative bridge laws can, however, be proposed. Thus cognitive architectures such as ACT-R and 4-CAPS discussed in Section 3.8 explicitly attempt to relate processing within the model to functional imaging data. In fact, within 4-CAPS the notion of the net activation of the working memory elements of a cortical production system maps directly onto our notion of a resource. We discuss bridging laws in relation to ACT-R in Section 5.5.

An inference from the findings of a functional imaging experiment to a cognitive model requires, however,

more than a cognitive characterisation of the BOLD signal, it requires an experimental design. Starting in Section 5.6, we will consider a number of possible complex designs that address limitations of the first design widely used in functional imaging experiments—that of subtraction—itself discussed in Section 5.4. However to consider the adequacies and inadequacies of designs we need to introduce four more bridge assumptions similar to those used for neuropsychological findings in the last chapter.

5.3 The Inferential Framework

Two conceptual frameworks for relating functional imaging evidence to the organisation of the cognitive system have been proposed. These are the 'forward inference' or 'function-to-structure' approach of Henson (2005, 2006) and the 'reverse inference' or 'structure-to-function' approach of Poldrack (2006). The forward inference approach takes existing cognitive theories and attempts to use functional imaging evidence to differentiate between them. The reverse inference approach attempts to reason backwards from the presence or absence of 'activation' in a particular region across different experimental paradigms to its involvement in a particular cognitive function. We will return to these approaches later.

The approach to be adopted in this chapter is more in the spirit of the attempts to support reverse inference in Poldrack's sense, but at the same time being closer to Henson's forward inference approach in its presuppositions concerning function. Consider the set of assumptions used to justify neuropsychological methodology in Section 4.5. The first was essentially:

> 1. 'We assume that the mind is composed of weakly modular systems each of which computes a specific input-output function which we will call a basic I-O function.'

Poldrack's reverse inference approach implicitly makes some form of modularity assumption. Henson's forward inference approach appears not to do so. However, in the most detailed development of this approach Henson (2006) considers only theoretical contrasts which are essentially based on modular distinctions.[8] To our knowledge little conceptual analysis has been attempted of the relation between a connectionist model and functional imaging evidence.[9] However,

---

[6] 'Meat and two veg' is a reference to the delights of traditional British cuisine.

[7] Henson in fact uses the term 'function' in a rather similar sense to 'resource', though he leaves it undefined.

[8] One example considered by Henson (2005) is of the connectionist short-term memory model of Burgess and Hitch (1999) to be discussed in Chapter 7. However the functional imaging evidence Henson considers relates only to a functionally separable part of the model, namely the system which is the source of the internal timing signal.

[9] See, however, the discussion of the work of Fiez and Petersen in Section 10 of this chapter.

such models typically make no assumptions that relate to anatomical localisation and without some such assumption they can hardly relate to functional imaging findings which are inherently anatomically based.

A shortened version of the second assumption of Chapter 4 is:

> 2. *To account for task performance, one requires in addition to a model of the on-line processes, the specification of a procedure.*

This applies equally to functional imaging experiments. Subjects must internalise and obey task instructions.

The third assumption introduced in the previous chapter is a key one for functional imaging methodology:

> 3. *Specific computational operations depending upon an individual I-O system are anatomically relatively focally localised. In particular each of the I-O functional systems (F$_i$) is held to occupy a relatively restricted region of the brain (b$_i$), its base region. Within each hemisphere the base region can be viewed as a continuous sheet at a reasonably gross anatomical level.*

This is essentially an assumption much discussed in Chapters 2, 3 and 4. The final part of the assumption justifies the use of the continuous voxel method of determining whether areas of activation be considered significant, as discussed in Section 5.1.[10]

It should be noted that we are not assuming that each base region of the cortex subserves a single I-O function. Thus for any region b_i there can be a number of I-O functions whose base regions overlaps with it, as we discussed in Section 3.4.

Complementary to assumption 3_N for neuropsychology, which follows from assumptions 3 and 4, we have the following assumption:

> 3$_P$. *The base region of each I-O system is in an equivalent position in the brain of each subject with a normal cognitive system.*

This assumption is necessary if we are to use group data for making inferences to the normal cognitive system,[11] and nearly all functional imaging studies report group data. This assumption hides a whole host of potential problems. First, the existence of normalisation algorithms in say, SPM, testifies to the reality that brains are not quantitatively equivalent. However, while the gross macroanatomy of the brain is fairly

consistent across normal young adults in a culture, it can vary considerably on a more detailed level (Kennedy et al., 1998; Thompson et al., 1996). An example given by Devlin and Poldrack (2007) is that the number and size of transverse gyri in Heschl's gyrus in the superior temporal lobe, the seat of the primary auditory cortex, varies considerably across individuals (Rademacher et al., 2001).

However, what is more critical is the degree of individual variability in a typical cognitive experiment. Consider the study that essentially began the functional imaging of cognitive processes—that of Petersen et al. (1988). In one condition the subject is presented on each trial with a noun and has to produce a related verb. In an experiment of Crescentini et al. (2009), which used this paradigm, two critical frontal areas were found concerning the subtraction between this condition and a control condition of reading the noun aloud. These were the left inferior frontal gyrus and the supplementary motor area (SMA). If we now look at individual subjects, 10/14 activated a cluster of voxels in both areas significantly and 3 of the others activated significantly only a lateral prefrontal cluster (Crescentini personal communication). More critically, in both areas the distribution across subjects of activation levels in the verb production condition relative to the read condition baseline did not differ significantly from a normal distribution and there were similar means for the effect size and fairly small standard deviations (0.33 and 0.36 of the mean). Interestingly, there was no correlation across areas (Pearson $r = -0.02$) between the activation levels relative to the read condition baseline. This suggests that for the regions in the dominant hemisphere there was rough qualitative equivalence across subjects, which echoes the conclusion tentatively arrived at for neuropsychological data in Section 4.6. Overall, at least for within-hemisphere contrasts, this study provides some support for the assumption of qualitative similarity of the organisation of subsystems across subjects.[12]

However there is a complication. As the activation levels across the left and right ventrolateral areas were significantly correlated (Pearson $r = 0.62$) it would appear that the corresponding systems in the two hemispheres had related functions in this task. Yet only five subjects had significant activation somewhere in the right inferior lateral region (see Figure 5.4). More critically, the distribution of differences in activation between the two conditions in the right inferior frontal region differed significantly from normal. Indeed one

---

[10] An exception to this part of assumption 3 (assumption 3') would be complementary regions in the two hemispheres. Note that the continuity assumption does not work at a finer anatomical level, see Section 5.8.

[11] This assumption applies to anatomically based neuropsychological group studies too.

---

[12] For further evidence that supports cross-subject consistency see the discussion of the study of Boly et al. (2007) in Section 11.7.

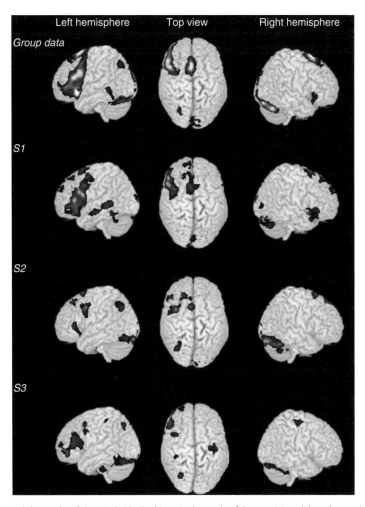

Fig. 5.4 The group results and the results of three individual subjects in the study of Crescentini et al. (2009) on verb generation. S1 activates both the let and right inferior frontal gyrii and also the supplementary motor area, S2 activates just the first and third of these regions and S3 only the first. (Crescentini, personal communication.)

subject had an effect size nearly 3 SDs greater than that of the group as a whole. This opens up the grizzly spectre of the lateralisation of function being prone to qualitative differences between subjects.

We now return to the delicate question deferred from the previous section, with respect to the cognitive levels of explanation, of what the BOLD signal measures. In the last chapter (Section 4.5), the concept *resource* was introduced. It derives from attempts to characterise what happens in dual-task studies as more or less emphasis is placed by the subject on one task or the other, for instance as the relative pay-off of the two tasks changes (see Norman & Bobrow, 1975; Navon & Gopher, 1979). In FNMS and Chapter 4 the concept was also used to relate to the effect not of reduced attention being paid to a task, but also to the reduced cognitive capacity of a subsystem resulting from neurological damage, for instance, as a dementing process occurs.

This type of neuropsychological assumption (5_{NR}) also has an analogue for functional imaging, which follows from proposals made by Just et al. (2001) and Shallice (2003):

> 5_{FR}. *The degree of activation measured by the BOLD signal in the relevant base area fulfilling a particular type of I-O mapping is monotonically related to the level of resource (r_n) required of a particular subsystem in order for it to fulfil its role in the carrying out of a particular task to a given accuracy level. (Resource is defined as in assumption 5_{NR} of Section 4.5 and the subsystem is assumed to have a basic I-O computational function.)*

Many authors make somewhat similar assumptions, although not so explicitly. Henson (2006) makes a related assumption in presupposing that the amount of a 'hypothetical function' varies with accuracy (positively), reaction time (negatively) and with activation levels.[13] It is not made specific in Henson's account that 'function' should be identified with the information-processing purpose of the relevant subsystem, in contrast to its anatomical localisation, but this is the natural interpretation. Moreover whether such functions are continuous as is the concept of resource is also unclear. Yet again it is difficult to see how otherwise it could have continuous variable consequences as required by the BOLD response. So, essentially Henson's (2005, 2006) conceptual framework seems to differ principally in terminology from the current one. We, too, will use 'function' to refer to the computational purpose of a subsystem in contrast to its material basis.[14] We are therefore left with a large but unknown number of resources $r_1 \ldots r_n$ with a set of base region localisations $b_1 \ldots b_n$, where the size of any b_i is unknown.[15]

Is 'resource' a plausible cognitive concept in a bridge law? As pointed out above, the concept of resource originally derived from the cognitive psychology of dual task performance. Consider, as an example, the effect of carrying out at the same time two tasks, which rely on different on-line cognitive systems. Just et al. (2001) gave subjects two such tasks. One was making true/false judgements about sentences relating to general knowledge. The other was the Shepard and Metzler (1971) mental rotation task (see Figure 5.5). The former task stressed predominantly left temporal structures and the latter predominantly right parietal ones.[16] Each task was run in blocks of 22.5 sec with either three sentences or four figures, respectively, presented at regular intervals during the period. In addition, subjects had a dual-task condition where both tasks had to be done together. All three conditions were compared with a rest baseline. The results are shown in Figure 5.6. Nine regions of interest in the cortex posterior to the motor strip were selected a priori on the basis of the literature. In all nine regions more voxels were more activated in the relevant single task condition than in the dual task condition.[17]

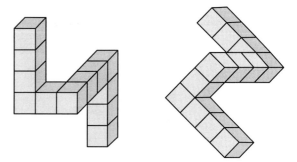

Fig. 5.5 Typical stimuli for the mental rotation task of Shepard and Metzler (1971). Subjects are required to state whether the stimulus on the right is a rotated version of that on the left.

We are dealing here with the number of voxels above threshold, rather than activation levels *per se*. It might also be argued that what might be happening is that subjects are just switching between the tasks so the reduced voxel volume just reflects less time on task. However, similar effects of increased attention to task leading to increased activation are very common. For instance, Friston (2007) reports an experiment in which subjects viewed monochromatic coloured stimuli that occasionally moved and changed colour at the same time. Subjects had either to attend to the colour change or to the movement. Figure 5.7 shows how the response in V5/MT depended on whether the subject was attending to the movement or not.

Moreover as one would expect from the neuropsychological discussions of resources in Section 4.5, greater task difficulty requires greater levels of resource available. Carpenter et al. (1999) used the same Shepard and Meltzer task as in the previous study but varied the angular difference between the two stimuli. As the tasks became more difficult the number of voxels activated in parietal cortex and also the percent increase in activation in maximally activated voxels both increased (see Figure 5.8). But, the reader may well argue, could not this just be because subjects took longer and so there was a longer signal to convolve with the haemodynamic response function? There is an internal test of this possibility. The fusiform region is also activated by presentation of the shape, probably because it is involved in the process of object recognition, but there is no task difficulty effect (see Figure 5.9) presumably because it is not centrally involved in computations which are critical for the task. Similarly, in Section 7.2

---

[13] See Henson (2006), figure 1.

[14] Price et al. (1997a) make an analogous assumption when they assume that 'there will be more neuronal activation in a functionally specialised region when a task demands the explicit involvement of the function than when it does not' (p. 265).

[15] It is assumed that the particular relation between BOLD and resource is specific to the individual region, as there may be anatomical differences, such as those concerning the vascular response, that differ between regions.

[16] Mental rotation tasks are discussed in Section 8.6.

[17] Unfortunately in its methodology the study effectively predates the use of SPM or an analogous statistical procedure. Moreover, statistical comparisons reported are between the single tasks combined compared to the dual tasks. For all nine

---

areas the effect was significant. However in general the regions were very much more widely activated in one single task condition than the other—by ratios of 8:1 to 29:1 in number of voxels—so the significant difference presumably generalises to the fairer comparison of one single task condition compared to the dual condition.

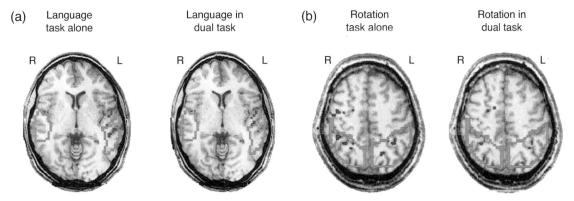

Fig. 5.6 A comparison of BOLD activation in single task and dual task conditions. (a) Language comprehension without and with a secondary task. (b) Mental rotation without and with a secondary task. In both cases, the number of voxels activated in the region of interest (outlined in green) is greater in the single task condition than in the dual task condition. Reprinted from *NeuroImage, 14*(2), M.A. Just, P.A. Carpenter, T.A. Keller, L. Emery, H. Zajac and K.R. Thulborn, Interdependence of nonoverlapping cortical systems in dual cognitive tasks, 417–426. Copyright (2001), with permission from Elsevier.

when we discuss priming we will see that repeated presentation of a stimulus in the same task conditions leads to a reduced BOLD response compared to the original operation; this fits with behavioural evidence such as speeding up of processing, in suggesting that the resource requirement is reduced on a second and subsequent operations. This can be explained computationally by a variety of possible mechanisms (see Section 7.2), such as the existence of short-term weights in a connectionist network which lead to more rapid accessing of the appropriate output representations.

One complication produced by this more concrete consideration of resources is that while a basic computational I-O function is held to have a single resource function relating its efficacy to activation levels, activation levels vary within the base region and even the size of the base region may vary. We will therefore add a subsidiary assumption:

> 5_{FS}. *Within each subregion of a base region fulfilling a particular type of I-O mapping there is an upwardly monotonic relation between its BOLD activation level and the single-valued resource requirements of the whole subsystem.*

In other words, the subsystem acts anatomically as a single entity, even if different parts are of differential importance to the whole; when different resource demands are made of the subsystem as a whole, there is no cross-over of activation values for one subregion compared to another across the relevant task conditions

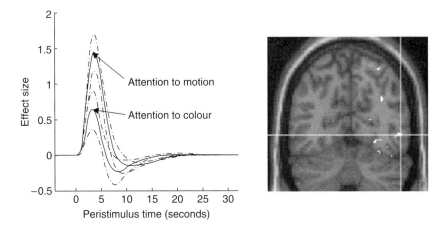

Fig. 5.7 BOLD response in V5/MT, modulated by task set. Stimuli were monochromatic images that occasionally moved and changed colour at the same time. Subjects attended either to motion or colour. Effect sizes were greater in the former condition than the latter. Reproduced with permission from Friston, K. (2007) Statistical parametric mapping; figure 2.6, p. 23. This chapter was published in Friston, K., Ashburner, J., Kiebel, S., Nicholls, T. & Penny, W. (Eds) *Statistical Parametric Mapping*. (pp. 10–31). Copyright Elsevier (2007).

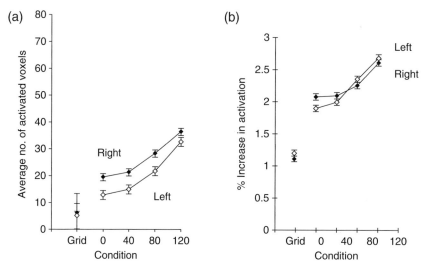

Fig. 5.8 The effect of task difficulty on the BOLD response in left and right parietal regions, as measured by varying the angular disparity in a mental rotation task. (a) The average number of voxels activated as a function of angular disparity. (b) The percentage change in signal as a function of angular disparity. The 'Grid' condition required subjects to visually scan a rectangular grid of small squares. Reproduced with permission from P.A. Carpenter, M.A. Just, T.A. Keller, W. Eddy and K. Thulborn (1999) Graded functional activation in the visuospatial system with the amount of task demand. *Journal of Cognitive Neuroscience*, 11(1), 9–24. Copyright © 1999, MIT Press Journals.

(see Figure 5.10).[18] Whether treating the BOLD signal as a measure of the cognitive resource employed by a particular subject in carrying out any particular task is appropriate remains an open issue. However the assumption provides an initial starting point to review the appropriateness of particular experimental designs. We therefore make the assumption here that the level of activation for a particular region corresponds monotonically to the amount of resource being employed. We know of no case in cognition where the assumption is clearly invalid, but we will discuss some potential problems later.

5.4 Early Advances in Macro-aspects of Experimental Design: Cognitive Subtraction

There are two different aspects of experimental design used in functional imaging experiments—a macro-aspect and a micro-aspect. The macro-aspect relates to the selection of the different conditions, in each of which there will be a different but related task, and in particular how the activations obtained in the different conditions are contrasted. The micro-aspect refers to how the trials, of which a condition is typically composed,

are organised, both with respect to the other trials in the same condition and to the trials in contrasting conditions. For instance, a major division is between blocked and event-related designs. In blocked designs, activation is summed across all of a given block of trials. In event-related designs, activation is summed across trials that are specified according to the nature of the stimulus, the response or the relation between them, without their being consecutive. Event-related designs generally have more empirical potential, allowing, for instance, the separation of the effects of a given trial from preceding ones; this can be done in various ways, such as the use of *jitter*, selecting the interval between consecutive trials from a statistical distribution.[19] Micro-aspects of experimental design are not considered in this book.

As far as the macro-aspects of experimental design are concerned, consider the study of Petersen et al. (1988) on functional imaging of word processing discussed in Section 1.10. The approach used in this study was the first major step that did not involve a technological advance in making functional imaging an effective science. It introduced a method—the subtraction method—by which an individual modular component in the functional architecture could be isolated by an imaging procedure. In the subtraction procedure we are concerned with what Price et al. (1997a) call the *cognitive component of interest*. The effects of this component are, however, necessarily conflated

---

[18] As we will see in Section 5.8, this assumption breaks down if one scales the subregion down to the size of a voxel. The assumption replaces a much more specific and less plausible assumption in an earlier treatment of this conceptual framework (Shallice, 2003).

[19] This allows the effects of the dependent variables to be deconvolved—see Huettel et al. (2009) for further discussion.

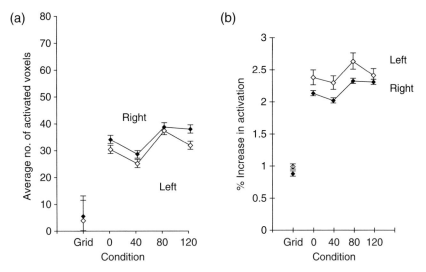

Fig. 5.9 In contrast to Figure 5.8, there is no significant effect of task difficulty on the BOLD response in left and right fusiform regions, as measured by varying the angular disparity in a mental rotation task. (a) The average number of voxels activated as a function of angular disparity. (b) The percentage change in signal as a function of angular disparity. The 'Grid' condition required subjects to visually scan a rectangular grid of small squares. Reproduced with permission from P.A. Carpenter, M.A. Just, T.A. Keller, W. Eddy and K. Thulborn (1999) Graded functional activation in the visuospatial system with the amount of task demand. *Journal of Cognitive Neuroscience*, *11*(1), 9–24. Copyright © 1999, MIT Press Journals.

with that of others in task performance. In subtraction an additional process assumed to depend on this subsystem is 'inserted' in one condition but not in another which in other respects is held to be the same. The statistical main effect of the cross-condition comparison is intended to localise this process.

In some situations the appropriateness of the subtraction procedure is clear. Thus Zeki et al. (1993) studied a visual illusion involving a rosette of wedge-shaped spokes emanating from a central grey circle. There are two conditions. In the experimental condition the spokes end at the grey circle while in the control condition they continue through (see Figure 5.11). In the experimental condition the subject has the impression

of 'enigmatic, circular motion', particularly in the outer of the three dark circles, but there is no such effect in the control condition.

One may consider the processes utilised in the control condition (C) to be:

$$P_1$$

and in the experimental condition (E):

$$P_2 + M$$

where M are the specific processes involved in the production of the perception of movement and P_1, P_2 (involving subsystems S_1 and S_2) are the processes that

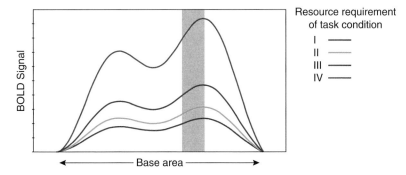

Fig. 5.10 Hypothetical activation levels within a base area such that assumption 5_{FS} is satisfied. It is assumed that for any subregion, indicated by the grey background, the activation levels across the task conditions with different resource requirements (I to IV), such as, say, for processing stimuli of different frequencies, are ordered in the same way.

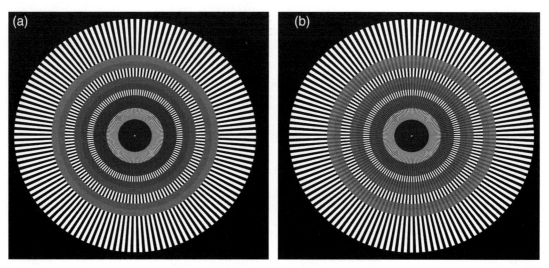

Fig. 5.11 Stimuli used by Zeki et al. (1993). Fixating on the centre of the left figure results in illusory rotory motion in the concentric circles. The illusory motion is not seen in the control figure (right). Reprinted with permission of Royal Society Publishing from S. Zeki, J.D.G. Watson, R.S.J. Frackowiak (1993) *Proceedings of the Royal Society of London B. Biological Sciences*, 252(1335), 215–222, Royal Society of London; figure 1, p. 216.

give rise to the other aspects of the perceptual experience. Since the two figures are so similar in other respects, P_1 and P_2 can be presumed to be virtually identical to each other.

In the experiment the activation produced in condition E can thus be presumed to be identical to that produced in condition C except for a significant difference in activation in a region which is inferred to be the seat of process M. This was identified with that of human MT/V5, the region discussed in Chapter 2. Subtraction logic is clear and straightforward in this experiment. The differences across conditions in the non-inserted processes involved in the task are apparently negligible and phenomenologically are qualitatively distinct from the effects of the insertion.[20]

In many applications of subtraction, however, the non-inserted processes are much less closely matched between the experimental and control conditions. Take the initial use of the methodology by Petersen et al. discussed in Section 1.10. One experimental condition was *Reading Nouns Out Loud*, intended to localise speech production processes, and a second control condition was *Viewing Nouns*. Possible decompositions of the two tasks are shown in Figure 5.12. Note that task decomposition requires a theoretical choice to be made. For simplicity we adopt a combination of the Coltheart et al. (2001) model of reading discussed in Chapter 4 and the Levelt et al. (1999) model of speech production discussed in Chapter 3. The processes other than those involved in

speech production (i.e. those downstream from the phonological output lexicon) are not identical across the two conditions. Not only is there an additional grapheme–phoneme rule system used (at least for regular words) in the former task, the resource values of each subcomponent probably differ systematically across tasks with $R_i > r_i$. Thus any interpretation which views all differences in activation as just the responsibility of the inserted speech production components becomes automatically suspect.

In fact the subtraction design has many other problems. It is easier to appreciate them from the perspective of resource assumptions.

1 Procedural differences (assumption 2) can occur in how tasks are carried out in the different conditions, so that different combinations of subsystems can be involved in the different conditions. Thus differences in task decomposition can lead to differences between the processes underlying the non-subtracted parts of the control (P_1) and experimental (P_2) tasks. Then, given the restricted base regions of cortex occupied by each of the different functional subsystem (assumption 3_F), it is likely[21] that there will be activation differences resulting from the operation of the S_1 and S_2 subsystems, when according to subtraction logic they should produce the same pattern of activation.

2 There can be changes in how a stage held to be common to both conditions is carried out across the two conditions. Consider, say, a perceptual stage of

---

[20] This example is taken from an excellent early critique of the logic of functional imaging methodology—that of Bub (2000).

[21] On assumption 3_F it is possible but unlikely for different possible subsystems to occupy overlapping base regions.

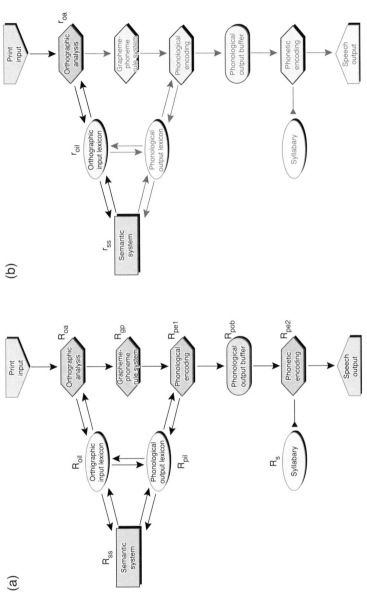

Fig. 5.12 Hypothetical decomposition using the Coltheart et al. (2001) model of reading aloud and the Levelt et al. (1999) model of speech production of the component processes involved in (a) Reading Nouns Out Loud and (b) Viewing Nouns in the study of Petersen et al. (1988). *R/r* correspond to the resource requirements of a given subcomponent for that task.

processing. Given the discussion in the preceding section about factors such as concentration and attention affecting resource levels in a system (assumption 5_{FR}) it follows that such resource differences would lead to BOLD activation differences between conditions. Thus activation differences can occur between P_1 and P_2 even when the same set of systems is involved. So in the experimental condition of the Petersen et al. study, the visual input lexicon system would be more active than in the control condition.[22] Technically even with procedural equivalence between conditions, the resource requirements of all non-critical components must be greater than or equal in the control condition than in the experimental condition. This is virtually never assessed.[23]

3 Bub (2000) raises another objection to subtraction methodology. He takes as an example a study of Price et al. (1997b), which compared a subject's ability to make a semantic decision on a word, with a putatively phonological decision, namely to decide whether a visually presented letter string had two syllables or not. Subtracting the semantic task from the phonological gave rise to significant activation bilaterally in the supramarginal gyrus, in the left precentral gyrus, the left cuneus and the right angular gyrus. What cognitive processes are involved? Price et al. suggest that 'in a syllable judgement task subjects are forced to attend to sublexical phonology in order to parse words into syllables. Possibly sublexical phonology is maintained in the phonological store whilst a decision is made' (Price, 1997b, p. 310). Bub instead suggests that the decision may be made orthographically using the pattern of consonants

and vowels in the letter string; in other words he criticises the interpretation of the processes held to involve this set of regions. However in the interpretation of behavioural experiments it is completely standard to produce this type of alternative account of the mechanism putatively giving rise to a particular empirical finding. In purely behavioural experiments it is dealt with by designing an experiment to distinguish between the two possibilities. This option is equally available for functional imaging experiments.

This third argument is not an in principle objection to subtraction methodology, even if it is practically important to appreciate that tasks are frequently opaque as to the subsystems they require. However, if either of the first two objections applies, then the subtraction inference is vitiated. For instance in the Petersen et al. example, the activation of component processes other than those involved in speech production ones, such as the visual input lexicon or the semantic system, could differ across conditions. One can therefore not assume that the localisation of speech production processes has been isolated by the subtraction.

Does this mean that the subtraction procedure is useless for cognitive theorising? If one can assume that the non-central components are virtually identical across the two conditions then it would be appropriate to draw theoretical inferences from it. But as we said earlier, the appropriateness of this condition is very rarely explicitly justified. However one could make this assumption on the plausible intuitive grounds that the other aspects of the process are unlikely to differ, as in the Zeki et al. example given earlier. Alternatively one may be engaged in testing theories that explicitly make the assumption. A third possibility arises if only one region is activated in the contrast, since the critical component of interest under theoretical investigation must presumably be carried out somewhere and that region is the obvious candidate. However this last possibility is a dangerous line of argument as it presupposes that the design is sufficiently sensitive to detect every process that theoretically differs between the conditions being compared.

We have discussed subtraction rather extensively as many other more complex designs are parasitic on it. From this stage on the argument presented in the chapter divides into two streams. In the next section we discuss alternative approaches to what in principle may be inferred from the results of functional imaging experiments in the light of the set of assumptions just made. Then we consider individual types of experimental design that have been used in functional imaging experiments.

---

[22] How the setting up of a given task leads to the particular resource demand placed on individual subsystems is currently an open question. We will assume merely that it is fixed given the procedure selected and the motivation level of the subject. Whether an actual resource difference is detectable in any given experiment will, of course, depend on a variety of procedural factors such as the number of subjects, the number of trials per condition and many other microdesign aspects. To add an extra complication, cascaded flow as in interactive activation models discussed in Chapter 3 (e.g. McClelland & Rumelhart, 1981), could lead also to a greater activation of semantic systems in the experimental than the control condition, when the visual input lexicon is more strongly activated.

[23] It could be argued that neuropsychological inference needs to be subject to a similar constraint. The difference is that performance of patients on theoretically sensitive tests in accuracy, at least, is normally relatively insensitive to minor differences in resource requirements of non-critical components across tests; in functional imaging these lead to activation differences given assumption 5_{FR}.

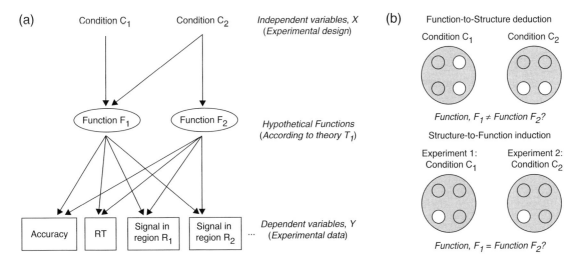

Fig. 5.13 Inference from findings to theory in experimental cognitive psychology and neuroimaging. (a) Dependent variables and their relation to the hypothetico-deductive method commonly used by experimental cognitive psychologists. (b) Function-to-structure deduction and structure-to-function induction. The circles represent schematic statistical parametric maps over four brain regions. The white circles represent regions reliably activated versus a common baseline condition, C_0. From R. Henson (2005) What can functional neuroimaging tell the experimental psychologist? *The Quarterly Journal of Experimental Psychology*, 58A(2), 193–233. Reprinted by permission of the publisher (Taylor & Francis Group, http://www.informaworld.com).

5.5 The Cross-over Interaction and Reverse Inference

Empirical findings have a range of functions in science. In basic science they broadly range from the casting of doubt on preconceived theoretical ideas, without necessarily strongly pointing to why, to the explicit testing and possible corroboration of a particular theory. An example of the first would be Galileo's 1610 extrapolation from his observations of three or four 'stars' close to Jupiter that they were its moons, so posing a major problem for Aristotelian cosmology. An example at the other extreme would be Eddington's travel to the island of Principe to observe the position of stars near the sun during the solar eclipse of May 1919 and so test an empirical prediction from general relativity and thereby provide evidence strongly supporting the theory (see Dyson et al., 1920).[24]

As we discussed in Section 5.3, Henson (2005) in a definitive account of inferences to theories of the cognitive system from functional imaging findings considers two different types of inference, which broadly relate to the two ends of the continuum just discussed. He uses the concept of *functions*, which are defined very generally as 'unobservable theoretical constructs' (p. 196) (see Figure 5.13a). For the present purposes they may be viewed as including the concept of resource used in this book. The first type of inference is what he calls *function-to-structure* inference. We have seen in the discussions of subtraction that a difference in activation between conditions in a single region could just be that one condition is merely more difficult than the other; it might for instance just use less familiar stimuli. Henson holds, however, that if two conditions C_1 and C_2 produce 'qualitatively different patterns of activity across the brain' (p. 197) then, in the terms of the current chapter, the cognitive processes underlying performance in conditions C_1 and C_2 differ in at least one cognitive resource. In this inference the actual localisations in the brain of the qualitative differences in BOLD that are found do not matter. For the second type of inference they do. This is the *structure-to-function* inference: 'if condition C_2 leads to a BOLD response in brain region R_1 relative to some baseline condition C_0 and region R_1 has been associated with function F_1 in a different context (e.g. in comparison of Condition C_1 versus C_0 in a previous experiment) then function F_1 is also implicated in condition C_2' (p. 198) (see Figure 5.13b).

---

[24] One of us argued in an earlier book—FNMS—that neuropsychology was important only for the first type of approach. This claim was strongly criticised by McCloskey and Caramazza (1991). Later studies both of theirs, e.g. Caramazza and Miceli (1990) on a disorder of spelling to be discussed in Section 7.6, and also ironically by one of us (Plaut & Shallice, 1993) on a model of deep dyslexia and reading-to-meaning—see Section 4.11), showed the argument to be incorrect.

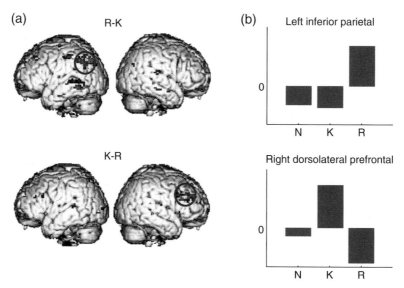

Fig. 5.14 Activations in left parietal and right dorsolateral prefrontal cortex in a study of recognition of a previously studied word list (Henson et al, 1999). (a) SPM images showing the difference between activation for responses where subjects recollected the stimulus (R) and ones where they just 'knew' correctly it had been present (K), and vice versa. (b) Bar charts showing the corresponding differences in magnitude of activation for the two responses, and additionally for stimuli correctly identified as new (N). From R. Henson (2005) What can functional neuroimaging tell the experimental psychologist? *The Quarterly Journal of Experimental Psychology*, 58A(2), 193–233. Reprinted by permission of the publisher (Taylor & Francis Group, http://www.informaworld.com).

Consider first the function-to-structure inference. Henson gives various examples. One is drawn from the study of Henson et al (1999) on *remember-know* judgements, where subjects were required to carry out a recognition memory task and in the same set of responses comment on whether they recollected the stimulus or merely 'knew' it had occurred. This is the paradigm we discussed conceptually in Chapter 2 and we will discuss further in Chapter 10. Figure 5.14 shows the activations in two regions—left parietal and right dorsolateral prefrontal—for responses where subjects recollected the stimulus, ones where they just 'knew' correctly it had been present and ones where they correctly said that this stimulus had not occurred. As we will see in Chapter 10 there are now both two process and single process models of the underlying memory trace, the two hypothetical processes being *recollection*, which is held to depend, on the subject re-experiencing in some way the event when the word was presented, and *familiarity*, where a specific phenomenal experience of the event is lacking. Henson (2005) argues that 'I think it would be difficult to explain these imaging data in terms of purely quantitative differences in memory strengths' (p. 202).[25]

From a resource perspective one might just say that two regions are activated and so there must be at least two resources involved. However we do not know the size of a base region. Moreover if a difficult task is compared with a very simple one the regions extracted from SPM, say, may be very large.[26] In addition, even though assumption 3 presupposes that base regions are continuous, since levels of activation can be conceived of as continuous functions which vary quantitatively in an uneven fashion within a region, it is possible that a region may illusorily fragment into apparently anatomically separate subregions, when operationalised using SPM or a similar analysis package.

However, the resource framework offers a simple solution parallel to the one adopted by Henson. If one compares the recollection condition (R) and the know condition (K) the activations obtained in the two areas form a cross-over interaction of activation which, given assumption 5_{FS}, (allows an inference of two separable resources to be drawn. Since BOLD is held to be a monotonically non-decreasing of function resource (for all subregions of a given region) then:

For part of region A (centred in left parietal):

resource (condition R) > resource (condition K).

Therefore for all of region A (which is of unknown extent) by assumption 5_{FS}:

---

[25] This is an unfortunate conclusion which does not follow from his argument. There is no need for the different regions to both hold memory traces. We will argue in Chapter 10 that one of them has a memory control function.

[26] This is probably because many different basic computational I-O functions are involved, but in any particular case the possibility of a very large single base region may be difficult to exclude.

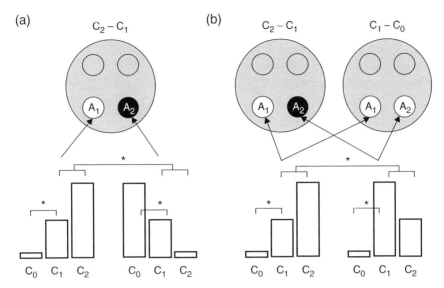

Fig. 5.15 Schematic SPMs and activity profiles. (a) A significant interaction between areas A_1 and A_2 and conditions C_1 and C_2. On Henson's (2005) account, the interaction alone is not sufficient to indicate a qualitative difference between the conditions, as an increase in the use of a single function under C_2 could result in activation in A_1 but deactivation in A_2. (b) A qualitative difference is supported, however, when in addition both areas are activated positively relative to a third condition C_0. From R. Henson (2005) What can functional neuroimaging tell the experimental psychologist? *The Quarterly Journal of Experimental Psychology*, 58A(2), 193–233. Reprinted by permission of the publisher (Taylor & Francis Group, http://www.informaworld.com).

resource (condition R) > resource (condition K).

Similarly for all of region B (centred in right prefrontal, and which is also of unknown extent):

resource (condition K) > resource (condition R).

Thus regions A and B have different resources and so different computational I-O functions.

In fact this example, one of four considered by Henson, may appear not to qualify properly using his more fine-tuned criteria. For Henson considers a cross-over interaction by itself to be insufficient. This is because a *function* for Henson differs in one important way from a *resource* as used here. A function is not restricted to having a monotonically non-decreasing relation with performance. Henson takes this position because a cross-over pattern may simply reflect that 'regions R_1 and R_2 have reciprocal connectivity in their implementation of function F_1. Then a pattern like in Figure 5.15a could still reflect a quantitative difference in the engagement of the same function F_1, even though that function 'activates' R_1 and 'deactivates' R_2.' He therefore proposes as required a pattern like Figure 5.15b with both regions having the same sign in the change from baseline.[27] This objection of Henson's to the

utility of the concept of resource implies that a function can involve two or more regions where activation has a different sign with respect to performance. We know of no example where such an account is required. Consider what is required by the neuropsychological analogue of the functional imaging example; it implies that a lesion which reduced resource would lead to improved performance on a task. While very occasionally there are claims of some such patient/task combinations (e.g. Kapur, 1996; Reverberi et al., 2005c), 99% of patients do worse rather than doing better if their task performance changes materially as a result of a lesion. We will therefore assume that within the individual subject, increased activation implies an increase in resource and leads to an increase in performance.[28] On this approach different resources would be considered to be involved in the critical situation considered by Henson if there were 'activated' and 'deactivated' regions.[29]

This approach shows that it can be justified to represent the pattern of performance across two different conditions as involving qualitatively different combinations of subsystems. On Henson's three conditions,

---

[27] This is the equivalent of what Dunn and Kirsner (1988) in a critique of inferences from double dissociations in neuropsychology call a 'reversed association'.

[28] This does not apply across subjects where an increase in activation can be associated with a decrease in performance, such as in the effect of ageing.

[29] An example would be lateral and medial regions in frontopolar cortex, held by Burgess et al. (2007) to control stimulus-independent and stimulus-dependent thought processes respectively.

approach C_0 and C_1 should be less than C_2 for area A_1 but C_0 and C_2 should be less than C_1 for area A_2 (see Figure 5.15b). In this case one can argue that other than subsystems involved in the baseline (C_0), the two experimental conditions (C_1 and C_2) involve different subsystems.

In neuropsychology a theory is not tested by a single experiment. Instead a complex set of tasks is used to provide a data base for inference to theory. The complementary approach in functional imaging seems to be present in Henson's function-to-structure mapping. This though can be treated as a special case of Poldrack's (2006) reverse inference, which we will consider instead.

Poldrack alludes to 'an epidemic of reasoning taking the following form:

1 In the present study, when task comparison A was presented brain area Z was active.

2 In other studies, when cognitive process X was putatively engaged, then brain area Z was active.

3 Thus, the activity of area Z in the present study demonstrates engagement of cognitive process X by task comparison A.

This is a 'reverse inference' in that it reasons backwards from the presence of brain activation to the engagement of a particular cognitive function' (p. 59).

This is a somewhat breath-taking set of assumptions, possibly made unduly blunt by the necessarily condensed nature of the vehicle—a Trends journal. As far as this book is concerned, the isolation and specification of the cognitive processes is why we are interested in functional imaging. Poldrack's second assumption somewhat bizarrely assumes we already have this information. More pragmatically, for very few cognitive tasks for which functional imaging has been used do we have more than the bare bones of a componential analysis of the systems underlying task performance.[30]

One can however recast Poldrack's position slightly and see it as the use of functional imaging for the complementary type of inference from Henson's 'function-to-structure' one. In other words it is a procedure for the testing of a given cognitive theory. As Poldrack points out the inference is not logically valid. To be logically valid statement (2), as Poldrack states, would need to be amended to include *if and only if*, but multiple functions are often attributed to individual brain regions—see Section 5.3. This would imply that all the other cognitive processes required to carry out task A do not involve brain area Z, which is in any case also a necessary assumption.

Poldrack therefore recasts the inference using Bayes' Theorem. Bayes' Theorem states that:

$$p(X|Z) = \frac{p(X).p(Z|X)}{p(Z)}$$

In this formula:

$p(X)$ = the probability of event X occurring, when one does not know anything about whether X occurred. This is known as the *a priori* probability (or more simply the *prior*). Typically $p(X)$ is not actually known but based on assumptions.

$p(Z)$ = the probability that evidence Z occurs. This is called the *base rate*.

$p(X|Z)$ = the conditional probability of X occurring given that Z has occurred. This is known as the *a posteriori* probability.

$p(Z|X)$ = the conditional probability of Z occurring given that X has occurred. This is assumed to be known.

Within statistics, in general, Bayesian approaches were long viewed as a conceptual framework providing a somewhat dubious alternative to more conventional hypothesis testing approaches (see, e.g. Jeffreys, 1961). They were held to be dubious because of the dependency of the outcome on the frequently unknown priors. This dependency may be overcome by expressing the change in probability of the event due to the presence of the evidence as the *Bayes factor*. This is the ratio of the posterior odds of the event to the prior odds of the event, where the odds of event E is given by the ratio $p(E) / (1 - p(E))$. The Bayes factor is independent of the prior probability of the event.

Over the last twenty years the approach has become enormously popular in a variety of fields. In ones related to computer science Bayesian approaches have, for instance, been used in models of perceptual categorisation, such as in so-called Helmholtz machines (Dayan et al., 1995), while in the cognitive psychological literature they have been used to described behaviour in a range of reasoning tasks (Oaksford & Chater, 2007). An application to the topic of inference from functional imaging experiments is therefore not surprising.

Poldrack uses an overall framework similar to that illustrated in Figure 5.13a.[31] He takes a somewhat more

---

[30] In addition we have the problem of what counts as a 'brain area'. This, however, is a general problem for all analyses of inferences from functional imaging findings for cognition and one Poldrack confronts appropriately.

[31] The only quasi-substantive difference is to replace Henson's vague term *function* with the more tangible *cognitive process*.

TABLE 5.1 Frequency of activation of a region of Broca's area as a function of fMRI study type. Data from the BrainMap database, as reported by Poldrack (2006). Reprinted from *Trends in Cognitive Sciences, 10*(2), R.A. Poldrack, Can cognitive processes be inferred from neuroimaging data?, 59–63. Copyright (2006), with permission from Elsevier.

	Language Study	Not Language Study
Activated	166	199
Not Activated	703	2154

complex form of Bayes' theorem and applies it to so-called *meta-analysis* in functional imaging:[32]

$$p(COG_X|ACT_Z) =$$

$$\frac{p(COG_x).p(ACT_z|COG_x)}{p(ACT_z|COG_x).p(COG_x) + p(ACT_z|\sim COG_x).p(\sim COG_x)}$$

where COG_X refers to the involvement of cognitive process X (or cognitive resource X to use the terminology of this chapter) and ACT_Z to activation in region Z.

Poldrack applies reverse inference to the issue of whether Broca's area is involved in language. He took a particular voxel (–37, 18, 18) in Brodmann Area 44 and created a cube of 20 mm cross-section centred on it. He then examined a database of functional imaging data (Fox et al., 2005) for whether experimental contrasts activated the region. The empirical results are shown in Table 5.1. What happens when we apply Bayes theorem? Poldrack assumes that we are ambivalent about whether some language tasks activate Broca's region, that is our prior probability is 0.5. He then derives an a posteriori probability that activation in Broca's region occurs because the task engages language functions of 0.69. This corresponds to a Bayes' factor of 2.26. On the basis of a convention analogous to the 0.05 significance level, a Bayes' factor of between 1 and 3 is held to imply a positive but relatively weak increase in confidence.[33]

This is a somewhat disappointing conclusion. If from over 350 positive contrasts in functional imaging experiments not to mention over 2800 negative contrasts the only conclusion one can draw is to obtain a slight increase in confidence for a relation that has been known in neuropsychology since the nineteenth century, then this is not a very impressive feat for functional imaging. This is even if one leaves on one side the question of what counts as a region, which can only be intuitively or pragmatically dealt with at present. However, a similar reverse inference procedure stripped of its Bayesian fig leaf can be used for cognitively more interesting analyses where the cognitive process is more constrained.[34] We will, for instance, discuss several meta-analyses of this sort, as in Section 9.4.[35]

Most critically, however, it is unclear how this type of inference can help to isolate what the component functions involved are. It requires a putative theoretical decomposition of the task to operate. The contrast with cognitive neuropsychology is clear. In cognitive neuropsychology a function putatively held to be impaired in a particular patient is characterised on the basis of the specific pattern of intact and impaired performance across a complex set of tasks. The inference procedure is far more complicated than the mere application of Bayes' theorem. Simple meta-analyses based on functional imaging reverse inference are unlikely to be sufficient. Fortunately there are theory-testing procedures other than meta-analyses which are much more solid and powerful. We will come to some of these shortly.

First though consider an alternative to the concept of resource or function that is used by John Anderson

---

[32] This is equivalent to the previous formula. The difference in the denominator on the right side of the equation arises from decomposing $p(ACT_z)$ into the sum of two weighted probabilities—the probability of ACT_z given COG_x and the probability of ACT_z given not COG_x.

[33] As noted above, this analysis is compromised by the possibility that non-linguistic processes might engage the region of interest. As we will see in later chapters, there is evidence that many non-linguistic processes do engage Broca's area. A second factor that affects the result is that by considering statistical significance as black or white Poldrack loses information about the level of significance of the individual studies contributing to the analysis. Worse still, if a study were to find an increase in activity in Broca's area below the 0.05 corrected level in a contrast involving language functions then this would count against the hypothesis, even if the result was only marginally non-significant.

[34] In fact, a simple chi-squared test may be performed on the data in Table 5.1 to test if there is an association between activation of the region in question and a linguistic component of the task. This association is highly significant: $\chi^2 = 71.59$, df = 1, p < 0.001.

[35] In one respect Poldrack's approach was much superior to the procedure used in most meta-analyses. These often just rely on activation maxima reported in published studies. Poldrack, by using a defined region-of-interest and a database, was able to determine definitely whether in any particular study part of the region was activated above threshold in the relevant contrast between conditions.

and colleagues. They relate processing within the ACT-R architecture discussed in Section 3.8 to the BOLD response. Recall that ACT-R consists of a central production system together with peripheral processing modules, including the manual module, the imaginal module, the goal module, and so on. Anderson (2005) associates these modules with regions of cortex based on informal converging evidence (of the sort appealed to by Poldrack's second assumption). Thus, the manual module is identified with a region of motor cortex centred on (–37, –25, 47), while the goal module is identified with a region of anterior cingulate cortex centred on (–5, 10, 38).[36]

This provides a first step to relating processing in ACT-R to imaging data. However, processing within an ACT-R module is all-or-none—for any model of a specific task in ACT-R at a given point in time a module will either be engaged or not engaged. How can this dichotomous variable be related to the continuous BOLD signal? Anderson and colleagues (2004b) assume that when a module is engaged it demands metabolic resources, leading to a rise in the BOLD signal, but that when the module is not engaged the metabolic resource demand drops to zero and the BOLD signal declines. Now, during each MRI scan, which lasts the order of a second, each module will be engaged for some fraction of the scan time (see Figure 5.16a). Anderson and colleagues therefore obtain a response function for each module/region of interest that is continuous over time by convolving the module's proportion of engagement during each scan interval with the haemodynamic response function (see Figure 5.16c). Thus the ACT-R approach does not attempt to model specific contrasts as might be obtained by the subtraction procedure or any of the more sophisticated designs considered in later sections of this chapter. Rather, it attempts to model the BOLD response over time and brain-space in each experimental condition (and there may be in principle be just one condition).

In our view Anderson's modules are too few and consequently the mapping of modules to cortex is too coarse. For example there are no modules that relate specifically to language processing, and no modules are mapped either to Broca's area or to the temporal cortices. But these criticisms reflect inadequacies of a specific version of ACT-R and its mapping to cortical regions; they might be addressed by a subsequent version of ACT-R. More critical would appear to be the dichotomous nature of the all-or-none involvement of modules. However, the transformation of this variable into the proportion of engagement per scan results in a continuous variable that is equivalent in many respects to our notion of resource. That is, it satisfies assumptions 1, 2, 3, 3_F and 5_{FS} of Section 5.3. The only real difference concerns the lack of specification of how ACT-R's bridging law might be extrapolated to neuropsychological inference.

5.6 Advances in Experimental Design: the Method of Specific Effects

Given the origin of the subtraction method in chronometric studies of mental processes (e.g. Posner, 1978) an obvious step forward is to use factorial methods, where the analogue of additive factors logic is used. The possible advantages of the approach were first articulated by Friston et al. (1996). They examined an object and colour naming situation in which four conditions were used:

A Saying Yes when a coloured shape is presented.

B Saying Yes when a coloured object is presented.

C Naming the coloured object when it is presented.

D Naming the colour of a shape when it is presented.

This can be viewed as a design involving two factors, namely a *Visual Process* (colour/object recognition) and a *Phonological Retrieval Process* (naming/saying Yes). Using standard statistical procedures of a two-way ANOVA, together with an early version of SPM, the authors contrasted a factorial design with a subtraction design involving (B–A) for processes concerned with object recognition and one involving (C–B) for processes related to naming. They show that the factorial design is more sensitive. The main effects in the factorial analysis are larger, at least for object recognition,[37] than the corresponding subtraction effects. This testifies to the greater statistical power of combining two comparisons instead of using one. They also find that most of the regions significantly activated in the analysis of main effects are also significantly activated in the interaction term (see Figure 5.17). They argue principally that the existence of an interaction indicates the inadequacy of the pure insertion involved in the subtraction design, and see it as a sign of the gross interactivity and non-linearity of brain processes.

Surprisingly, having criticised the use of subtraction and the assumption of pure insertion, the authors

---

[36] The localisation of the goal module to the anterior cingulate does not accord well with the discussion of the function of this part of the cortex in Chapter 9. See Anderson (2005) for a complete list of ACT-R modules and their localisations.

[37] This was before SPM was well developed and 0.05 (uncorrected) significance level were used.

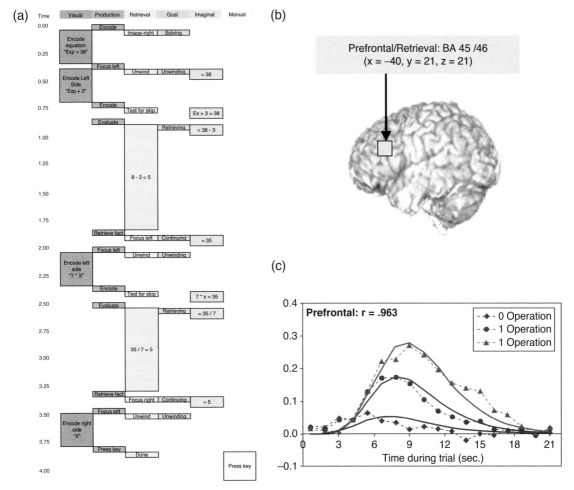

Fig. 5.16 (a) The time course in seconds of activity within ACT-R modules during the simulation of the solution of an algebra problem involving two operations (If $7x + 3 = 38$, what is x?). (b) The assumed location of ACT-R's retrieval module (light blue in the time course shown in panel a). (c) BOLD activity as predicted by the model (solid lines) and as observed (dashed lines) in the region associated with retrieval (BA 45/46) for algebraic problems involving zero, one and two operations. From Human symbol manipulation within an integrated cognitive architecture, J.R. Anderson (2005) *Cognitive Science*, 29(3), 313–341. Lawrence Erlbaum Associates. Reprinted by permission of the publisher (Taylor & Francis Group, http://www.informaworld.com).

seem to assume that interactions are less susceptible to multiple interpretations. They conclude that the interaction 'clearly implicates the inferotemporal regions in a phonological network during object naming, despite the absence of a main effect of phonological retrieval in this region' (p. 102). Considering resources involved shows that one should not draw this positive conclusion. Thus from a resource perspective carrying out the object naming task when compared with the Yes-saying Object task loads much more heavily on high-level visual perceptual resources, as well as phonological output lexical selection resources. The subject needs to attend to the visual shape more. The experiment is therefore not a useful task for trying to disentangle the two types of interpretation of

the interaction.[38] A more appropriate conclusion is that the control conditions are insufficiently close in non-critical respects to the experimental task, so that no theoretical inferences can safely be drawn from a factorial analysis alone.

From the perspective of the discussion of the subtraction design, the optimum result for straightforward inference is to have completely distinct regions for the two main effects and no significant interactions. Then for either of the main effects considered as subtraction

---

[38] Indeed a case has been made that the additive factors logic for dissociating components chronometrically is not generally useful when studying mental processes because interactions are the norm (Van Orden et al., 2001).

(a)

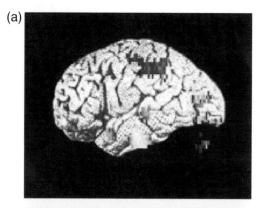

(b)

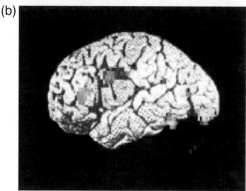

(c)

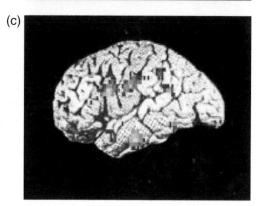

Fig. 5.17 Statistical parametric maps showing the main effects due to (a) object recognition and (b) phonological retrieval and (c) their interaction in the factorial analysis of the study of Friston et al. (1996). Many of the areas found to be activated in the main effects are also actived in the interaction. Reprinted from *NeuroImage*, 4(2), K.J. Friston, C.J. Price, P. Fletcher, C. Moore, R.S.J. Frackowiak and R.J. Dolan, The trouble with cognitive subtraction, 97–104, Copyright (1996), with permission from Elsevier.

designs, the argument that the activated region corresponds to the theoretically relevant process is supported. The activation of another region *by another contrast* indicates that the design is sufficiently sensitive to detect activation in the other region of cortex, so the restriction of activation to one specific region and not the other for each main effect is not due to a lack of

sensitivity. That the two effects involve different processing resources is supported.

A further problem for experiments with factorial designs raised by Aguirre and D'Esposito (1999) is that it rests on the assumption that the transformation from neural activity into the BOLD or rCBF signal should be linear. The example we gave earlier in the chapter of the work of Rees et al. on motion perception in fact fitted the linearity assumption well. Using chequerboard stimuli, Huettel and McCarthy (2000) later showed that if a second stimulus follows the first by 1 sec, then the BOLD response to it is reduced by 40%. This does not happen—at least with respect to short duration flashes of light—if stimuli are separated by 2.5 sec or more (Dale & Buckner, 1997) (see Figure 5.18). In fact these authors argued that the current evidence at that time was that the BOLD signal is generally linear with number of stimuli presented. However, D'Esposito and colleagues (1997) have produced examples where how one paces the trials affects the pattern of results with slower rates of presentation, although such effects could be due to strategic differences.

That the effects of more than one stimulus summate linearly when stimuli are presented separated by short intervals does not, though, imply that the relation between the BOLD response and a psychological variable is generally linear. Yet theoretical inferences from fMRI experiments quite frequently implicitly make a much stronger assumption than assumption 5_{FR}, which merely assumes the BOLD signal behaves monotonically with the level of each specific resource required for task execution. Instead, as Aguirre and D'Esposito point out, they assume that the relation between BOLD and a psychological variable is linear.

What this means is that one must differentiate three forms of interaction arising from factorial designs as far as their cognitive relevance is concerned (see Figure 5.19). Cross-over interactions we have already discussed in Section 5.5. Triangular interactions essentially depend on monotonicity, i.e. assumption 5_{FR}, not linearity. Trapezoidal interactions, however, depend critically on the delicate assumption of linearity.

Before attempting to review and simplify the conclusions about factorial design it is useful to introduce another type of multiple subtraction design—the parametric design—where a factor takes multiple values. The inferential conclusions about parametric design are very similar to those about factorial design. Henson (2007b) gives two interesting examples of a word-generation paradigm of the general type discussed in Section 5.3. Subjects generate one word by association from another in one condition. In the other, they just read the presented word. First he considers as a second factor—time on task. The results are shown in Figure 5.20. Here, in addition to one factor (generation minus read)

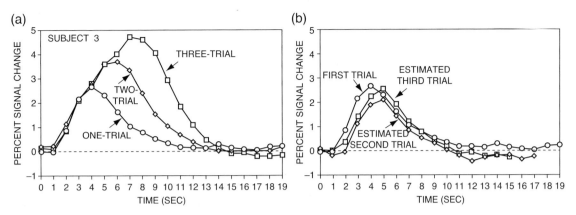

Fig. 5.18 The additive character of the heamodynamic response function measured in the visual cortex of a single subject when trials are spaced two seconds apart. (a) Raw data collected from runs consisting of one, two or three trials, where each trial involved presentation of a flickering checkerboard pattern. (b) The estimated contribution to the raw signal of each trial event. Reprinted with permission from A.M.Dale and R.L. Buckner (1997) Selective averaging of rapidly presented individual trials using fMRI, *Human Brain Mapping*, 5(5), 329–340. Copyright © 1997, John Wiley and Sons.

involving the left inferior frontal cortex, as in the experiment of Crescentini et al. discussed earlier, there is a second factor, which varies in a generally declining fashion across time.[39] Clearly such parametric effects potentially allow for stronger tests of theories than do simple main effects. At times the parametric effects can be non-monotonic as in inverted U-shaped effects of rate in generation tasks—Henson's (2007b) second example (see Figure 5.21).

Returning to factorial designs more generally, the presence of the interaction can provide empirical support for a theoretically framework. But this potentially involves making the assumption of linearity. It also depends upon the assumption—and it almost always is an assumption—that different values of a given factor do not make different resource demands on other factors.[40]

However, the strongest type of application of factorial or parametric designs is if they allow the application of what Bub (2000) calls the *method of specific effects*, where the activation of one region is affected by variable X but not variable Y and of another region by variable Y but not X.[41] A complex but powerful example comes from the study of Badre and D'Esposito (2007) on

the level of abstraction at which multiple potential responses compete in action selection. The study involved four different experiments (see Figure 5.22). In all, the subject had to make a four-choice response. In the simplest—the *Response* experiment—the subject must respond just according to the colour of the presented square. The four different colours were, however, mapped on to one, two or four different responses in different blocks of trials, so producing different degrees of response competition. In the *Feature* experiment, the subject was presented with an object in a coloured square and had to respond according to a feature of the object, say its texture, but again the degree of response conflict was increased by making which feature should be treated as positive depend upon the colour of the square. In the third experiment— the *Dimension* experiment—the coloured squares each contained two objects and subjects must decide whether they match along a given dimension with the relevant dimension again cued by the colour of the square. As before, response conflict was manipulated as indicated in the figure. Finally, in the *Context* experiment the task was the same as in the Dimension experiment but the frequency of the colour-to-dimension mapping was varied across the whole experiment from frequencies of 1.0 (C1) to 0.25 (C4). Subjects knew which mapping was relevant at the beginning of each block. For tasks with more abstract response competition, response competition at less abstract levels was maintained constant.

The design of the experiment varied control demands according to the dimension of abstractness-of-choice, and also quasi-parametrically according to the degree of competition. A change in degree of competition will presumably change the amount of a given resource that is required and indeed in all conditions reaction time

---

[39] That effects can vary so greatly with time in a study indicates the importance of counterbalancing and randomising conditions over time. Interestingly the effect of time-on-task is found elsewhere than the left inferior frontal cortex, the region shown being the left temporal cortex, probably relating to the gradually declining effect of perception of one's own voice.

[40] For an example of this theoretically driven inference logic see the study of Fletcher et al. (1998a) as discussed in Section 10.10.

[41] This is analogous to the critical variable variant on double dissociations in neuropsychological inference, discussed in FNMS Section 10.5.

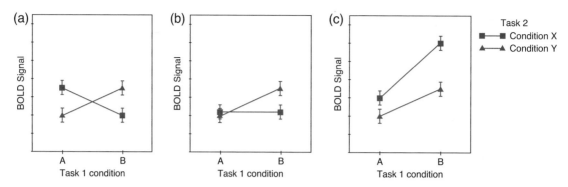

Fig. 5.19 A schematic illustration of three types of interaction that can occur with a standard factorial design: (a) cross-over interaction; (b) triangle interaction; and (c) trapezoidal interaction.

increases with increasing competition. Although the tasks vary in a variety of ways, each shows an increase in activation in at least one region with the greater degrees of competition (see Figure 5.23.)

The natural way to explain the pattern of results is to assume that each of the regions involves a different resource and that response competition (R) involves resource I, feature competition (F) resource II, dimension competition (D) resources II and III and context competition (C) resources III and IV. Then the appropriate parametric effects are explained. This conclusion, that there is a set of resources differing in degree of abstractness

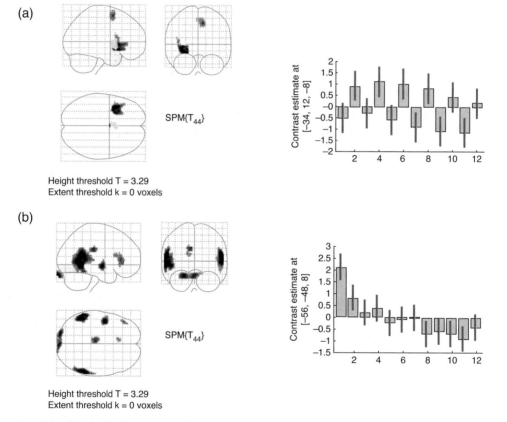

Fig. 5.20 Henson's (2007b) example of a parametric effect of a factor. In the experimental condition, subjects generated a semantically related word for each of a series of words presented visually. They read the visually presented words aloud as the control condition. (a) Shows the effect in left inferior frontal cortex of the categorical factor of (Generate – Read). (b) Shows the parametric effect of another factor—time on task—on the left superior temporal cortex. Reproduced with permission from Henson, R.N. (2007) Efficient experimental design for fMRI; plate 15, p. 312. This article was published in Friston, K., Ashburner, J., Kiebel, S., Nicholls, T. & Penny, W. (Eds) *Statistical Parametric Mapping*, pp. 193–210. Copyright Elsevier (2007).

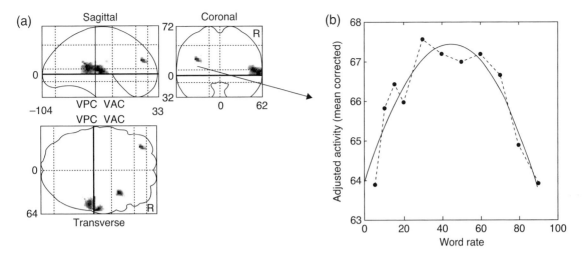

Fig. 5.21 Henson's (2007b) example of a non-monotonic effect with respect to a factor. The study is the same as for Figure 5.20. What is shown is the effect of a further factor—rate of presentation of the visual stimuli. The x-axis is words per minute. Note that when rates become high, issues related to those to be discussed in Section 9.2 may become relevant, as too may the inter-stimulus effects on BOLD discussed at the beginning of this section. When rates are low the process becomes much less effortful. Reproduced with permission from Henson, R.N. (2007). Efficient experimental design for fMRI; plate 17a, p. 312. This article was published in Friston, K., Ashburner, J., Kiebel, S., Nicholls, T. & Penny, W. (Eds) *Statistical Parametric Mapping*, pp. 193–210. Copyright Elsevier (2007).

and with base regions on a roughly anterior-posterior axis, fits with other studies on frontal cortex as we will see in Section 9.6.

It should, though, be noted that cross-over interactions of the sorts discussed with respect to Henson's analysis of forward inference have not been found. One needs therefore to consider whether the results can be explained using less than four quantitatively different resources involved in the execution of these tasks. In fact if one assumes different monotonic activation-resource functions for the different regions a single resource is sufficient (see Figure 5.24). The whole swathe from A to D would have to be a single base region; but as no operational definition of a base region exists this is conceivable. For region A, a qualitative difference from the other regions is in fact much more plausible given the data. For the other three regions, and in particular for the claimed qualitative distinction between regions B and C, the situation is much less clear. This is a somewhat analogous situation to that of *single* dissociations in neuropsychology where the assumption of different performance-resource functions for different tasks can explain the existence of a single dissociation by assuming only a single resource, unlike for a double dissociation.[42]

What is different about the current example is that there is no supporting argument as there can be for single dissociations (e.g. task difficulty) to buttress the idea that these different brain regions should have different

activation-resource functions. It is a hypothetical possibility. It does, however, make much less solid the inference that four resources are involved—one for each of the regions. The Method of Specific Effects is a rather slippery entity.

5.7 Advances in Experimental Design: Cognitive Conjunctions

The cognitive conjunction design, developed by Price and Friston (1997), is powerful and yet insufficiently used. It is the first design we have considered which does not derive fairly directly from designs used in human experimental psychology. It is specifically a theory-testing design in the sense that it is only useful if one makes the assumption that one particular subcomponent should exist and be the common component in a set of otherwise different tasks. We will give an example that will become theoretically relevant in Section 9.14. It relates to the attempt to assess whether there is a system involved in holding or realising intentions.

In Chapter 2 we discussed a study of P. Burgess et al. (2001) which attempted to isolate the brain systems involved in setting-up, holding and realising intentions. They used an elegant design. Subjects had to carry out two types of task. One type was an 'on-going task' in which they had to respond to roughly 30 stimuli. This task was performed under three conditions. In one condition it was the only task the subject had to perform. However, in two other conditions, subjects had to be ready to carry out a second task—a so-called

---

[42] See FNMS Chapter 10 for extensive discussion.

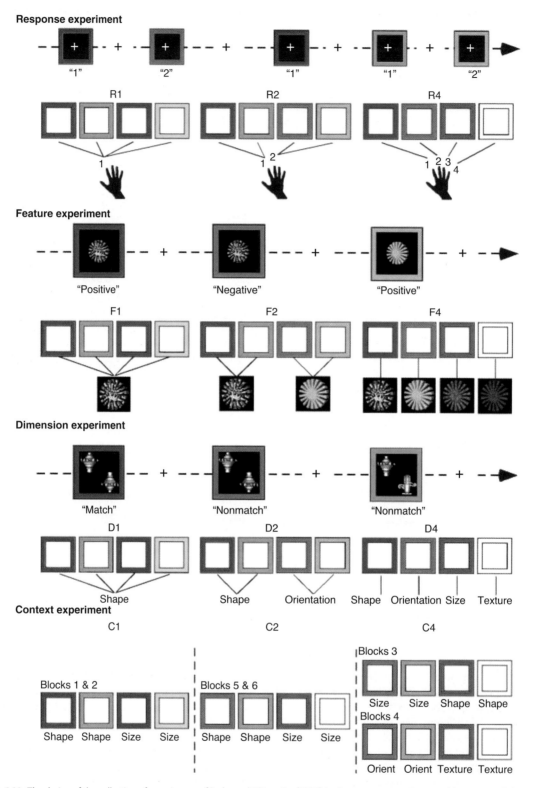

Fig. 5.22 The design of the collection of experiments of Badre and D'Esposito (2007). In the response experiment, subjects responded on the basis of the colour of the border of the square stimulus. Colours mapped to one, two or four responses, depending on the block. In the feature experiment, the colour of the stimulus border determined how the subject should respond to the feature contained within the square. The number of features that mapped to each response varied across blocks (one, two or four). In the dimension experiment, the stimulus boxes contained two figures, and subjects were required to indicate if the figures matched on one or more dimensions, as determined by the colour of the border of the square. The number of dimensions involved in the comparison varied across blocks (one, two or four). In the context experiment, the decision was based on a dimension (e.g., shape), cued by the colour of the border, with the cue-dimension mapping depending on the temporal context (i.e. the block), and with subjects having one, two or four contexts throughout the experiment. Response competition increases as illustrated by the change across conditions R1→R4, F1→F4, D1→D4 and C1→C4 respectively. Reproduced with permission from D. Badre and M. D'Esposito (2007) Functional magnetic resonance imaging evidence for a hierarchical organization of the prefrontal cortex. *Journal of Cognitive Neuroscience, 19*(12), 2082–2099. Copyright © 2007, MIT Press Journals.

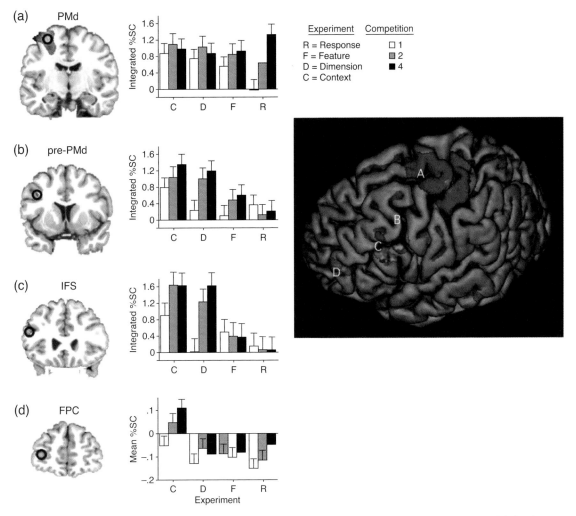

Fig. 5.23 Results of the study of Badre and D'Esposito (2007). (a) Greater response competition led to greater activation in left dorsal premotor cortex. (b) Greater feature competition led to greater activation in left anterior dorsal premotor cortex. (c) Greater dimension competition led to greater activation in left inferior frontal sulcus. (d) Greater context competition led to greater activation in left frontal polar cortex. Reproduced with permission from D. Badre and M. D'Esposito (2007) Functional magnetic resonance imaging evidence for a hierarchical organization of the prefrontal cortex. *Journal of Cognitiv Neuroscience, 19*(12), 2082–2099. Copyright © 2007, MIT Press Journals.

'intention' task. In one of these conditions—intention maintenance—subjects received instructions to carry out the intention task, but no stimulus that required it occurred during the scan. In another condition—intention realisation—stimuli that required an intention response occurred about once every six stimuli.

The elegance of the design was that Burgess et al. used the cognitive conjunction analysis procedure. The study employed four different pairs of 'on-going' and 'intention' tasks, each pair involving a different lower-level cognitive domain (see Figure 5.25). The results were based on conjunction analyses over the sets of tasks. Regions activated in less than the full set of four pairs of tasks in theory do not qualify. Using this method, holding any type of intention over time—even

when it is never realised—activated the right dorsolateral prefrontal region and the left and right frontal pole, when compared with just carrying out the on-going task by itself (Figure 2.3). The critical point is that the very great difference in on-line processing requirements between the different pairs of on-going and intention tasks means that the resource localised to these regions by the fMRI study is most likely to relate to the common element, namely setting up and holding intentions *per se* and not to any concrete manifestations of specific tasks.

What is very important methodologically is that unlike the previous designs considered, cognitive conjunctions do not require perfect matching across conditions of the resources involved in non-critical

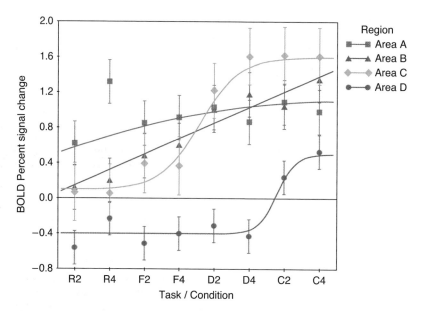

Fig. 5.24 Hypothetical resource-BOLD functions to show how some results of Badre and D'Esposito (2007) might be explained by differing monotonically increasing resource-BOLD plots for the different regions they implicate, for instance due to differences in blood supply. The x-axis represents the amount of a *single* hypothetical resource required to perform successfully in each of the eight conditions. The y-axis represents the hypothetical degree of activation that the use of a particular level of resource produces for a particular brain area For areas B and C, in particular, the possibility of a mere difference in this relation rather than a qualitative difference in function needs to be entertained. (Area D activation is arbitrarily magnified by 5, as the function of signal change (SE in Figure 5.23) used was different.)

components. Indeed there should be qualitative differences between them given non-critical components do not repeat in the (AB) pairs, which all contain the same critical experimental (A) versus control (B) contrast (see Figure 5.26).[43]

The concept of cognitive conjunction is straightforward. However its statistical implementation has varied considerably across applications. Consider two experimental tests (A_1, A_2) each with a matched baseline (B_1, B_2). In SPM 96 a cognitive conjunction was defined as there being a main effect of (A_1+A_2) versus (B_1+B_2) with the proviso that the interaction of A_1/A_2 versus B_1/B_2 was not significant (Price & Friston, 1997). So it is held that A_1 differs from B_1 and A_2 differs from B_2 in this region. This is termed the *interaction masking* procedure.

This procedure has the problem that both the A_1vsB_1 and A_2vsB_2 comparison may be highly significant but overall the pattern would not count as a conjunction if the interaction term is also significant. In addition, the procedure was considered dubious so a later statistical implementation (Friston et al., 1999) used the Minimum

Statistic compared to the Global Null procedure (MS/GN). This compares the individual *t*-values for A_1vsB_1 and A_2vsB_2 and takes the minimum of the *n* (in this case 2)

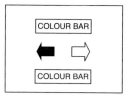

Arrows: Ongoing task: press in direction of black arrow. Intention: if colour bars are the same colour, press the third key.

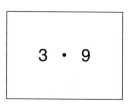

Numbers: Ongoing task: press the key that is in the direction of the larger number. Intention: if both numbers are even, press the third key.

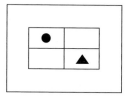

Shapes: Ongoing task: press the key that is in the direction of the shape which is not a circle. Intention: if both shapes appear in the lower quadrants, press third key.

Fig. 5.25 The four pairs of 'on going' and 'intention' tasks of Burgess et al. (2001). Reprinted from *Neuropsychologia*, 39(6), P.W. Burgess, A. Quayle and C.D. Frith, Brain regions involved in prospective memory as determined by positron emission tomography, 545–555, Copyright (2001), with permission from Elsevier.

---

[43] Bub (2000) points out that this design is somewhat analogous to the procedure in cognitive neuropsychology of showing that impairment occurs to roughly the same extent in somewhat different versions of a task as in the example of span for different types of material in the short-term memory syndrome (see Section 7.3).

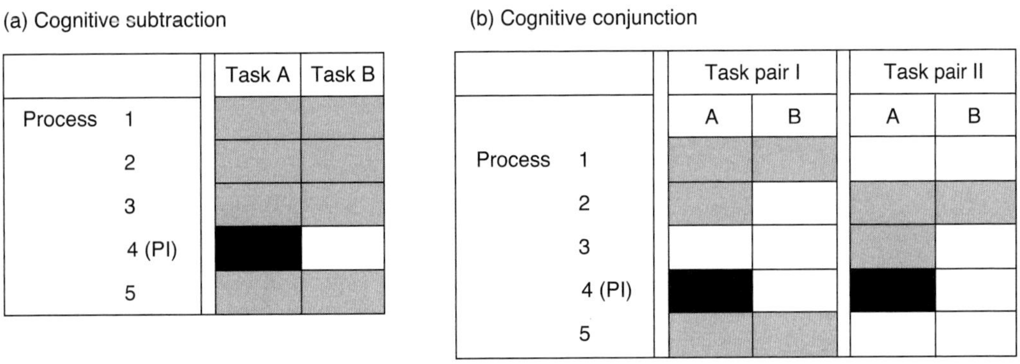

Fig. 5.26 Cognitive subtraction versus cognitive conjunction. Processes 1 to 5 are distinct but arbitrary task components. PI is the process of interest. Reprinted from *NeuroImage*, 5(4), C.J. Price and K.J. Friston, Cognitive conjunction: a new approach to brain activation experiments, 261–270, Copyright (1997), with permission from Elsevier.

t-values being greater than, or equal to, t_{min}, where t_{min} is derived from the distribution of the minimum of n t-statistics. This is a sort of reverse Bonferroni procedure. Nichols et al. (2005) argue that this procedure does not use the correct null hypothesis, namely that one or more of the individual comparisons A_1vsB_1; A_2vsB_2 is not different from zero. They therefore propose using a worst case procedure over the A_1vsB_1, A_2vsB_2 and so on comparisons to determine significance and hence set t_{min} at the standard 0.05 level (Miminum Statistic compared to the Conjunction Null: MS/CN).

They supported their procedure over the MS/GN one using the following pharmaceutical parable (Nichols et al., 2005, p. 655):

Three drug companies have each made a drug which they hope will reduce blood pressure. Each company has run a study comparing their own drug to placebo in people with high blood pressure. The three drugs are *A*, *B* and *C* and the three studies have yielded *t* values of 0.5, 1.1 and 1.3, respectively, when comparing drug to placebo. Thus, none of the individual compounds had a 'statistically significant' effect on blood pressure. This was painful for the manufacturers of drug *A* because the drug had been expensive to develop. The mood was despondent until a company statistician remembered having read a neuroimaging paper on 'conjunctions'. He suggested that instead of testing the drugs individually, they should test if *all* of the drugs had an effect. The MS/GN threshold for the minimum of 3 *t* values is 0.34, so the MS/GN test is highly significant. If the drug company interprets this test as a logical AND, they would think they had hard statistical evidence that their drug was effective, when this is clearly not the case.

But this parable is faulty. The three drugs are different. In the cognitive conjunction procedure the *same* critical component is tested with varying additional cognitive

components, so combining evidence over tests is legitimate. Moreover we agree with Friston et al. (2005) that the MS/CN procedure advocated by Nichols et al., while valid, is extremely conservative. As the number of tests increases so the probability that any one of those tests would not give a significant result, even if on average it would, will continue to increase. SPM in fact currently allows one to select which of the two cognitive conjunction procedures is applied.

Aguirre and D'Esposito (1999), in their review of the experimental designs used in fMRI, raise the following objections to the use of the conjunction design in some situations: 'Some cognitive processes, by their very nature, require the evocation of an antecedent process. For example, can working memory be meaningfully present if not preceded by the presentation of a stimulus to be remembered?' (p. 374). Thus the conjunction procedure could misleadingly add another process.[44]

This is an important objection. Consider a study of Monti et al. (2007), which used the logic of cognitive conjunctions without the formal conjunction analysis procedure. They were carrying out an investigation of deductive reasoning using logical connectives such as *and*, *or*, *not* and *if/then*. Inferences could be valid or invalid and subjects had either to confirm or reject them. They divided inferences into simple and complex types. A second factor was employed in cognitive conjunction style, namely varying the type of material— relating to faces, house, blocks or 'abstract' non-word entities. Thus, an example of the latter type of valid simple inference would be:

If there is either a sug or a rop then there is no tuk.
There is a sug.
Therefore there is no tuk.

---

[44] In fact working memory can utilise purely remembered stimuli. However this is a quibble as normally working memory operates on accurately perceived stimuli.

The critical step was to divide regions that were more activated in complex, than in simple, inferences into two types. One were those that were activated whatever the material. They called these content-independent regions. As we will discuss in Chapter 12, these involved a variety of left lateral prefrontal and inferior parietal regions; see Section 12.4 and especially Figure 12.8). The second, the content-dependent regions, were those held to form the material basis of the deductive processes used with the particular material. Following Aguirre and D'Esposito, carrying out a logical inference clearly requires verbal working memory. The left inferior parietal regions and left lateral frontal regions, other than Brodmann area 10, may well have been involved in holding material rather than deduction per se. Thus Aguirre and D'Esposito's criticism appears to be correct. However, the objection should relate more to the original theoretical isolation of the critical cognitive component—deduction in this case—rather than to the cognitive conjunction method. A more focussed study could attempt to differentiate between the theoretical possibilities.

A further possible problem can arise if the activation in one of the $A_i$vsB_i task contrasts does not correspond to the theoretically assumed underlying components, because of some complexity of the particular task. Then, since conjunction analysis by its essence will detect only activation contrasts that occur across *all* $A_i$vsB_i task pairs, there is a danger of a failure to detect a theoretically appropriate interpretation. It just needs one $A_i$vsB_i task component to be incorrectly assessed for this to happen. Moreover, because the contributions of individual $A_i$vsB_i task pairs are hidden in the overall statistic, this would be difficult to detect. In this way potential flaws in the componential analysis of the constituent tasks are more difficult to detect with cognitive conjunction analysis than for dissociation analysis in neuropsychology. The overall results of the procedure are further from the effects obtained on any particular task; this is because in dissociation analysis one compares performance on tasks directly and not in one overall set of statistics.

Overall, though, conjunction analysis provides a type of replication of processes which localise reliably and so points potentially to the existence of an isolable subsystem. The advantage of using it far outweighs the possible potential artefacts.

5.8 Behaviour-to-BOLD correlations

From the cognitive perspective a valuable method is to relate the degree of activation change in a subtraction across conditions to the behaviour of a subject or, more typically group of subjects. For instance, Kristjansson et al. (2007) investigated the neural basis of the pop-out

phenomenon, where a visual display with multiple elements contains one element that differs from all the others, which are identical. This makes perceptual aspects related to the oddball easier to detect; phenomenally they pop out. In one part of this study the authors considered trials where the colour of the target was repeated from the previous trial compared to when successive targets differed in colour and the investigators were interested in whether the odd stimulus popped-out more easily. In another part of the study the repeated aspect of the stimulus was its particular location.

Across the brain as a whole a small number of regions showed reduced activation following a repeat of the colour compared to a non-repeat, a typical effect of priming (see Figure 5.27a).[45] In addition, though, in two of these regions in the right hemisphere there was also a strong correlation across subjects between the reduced activation for the repeated colour or location of the oddball and the decrease in reaction time to detect it (see Figure 5.27b). That this pair of regions—the right frontal eye fields and the right intraparietal sulcus—show the behaviour-to-BOLD correlation—was used in the theoretical account of these phenomena, namely that these regions are part of the attention network discussed in Section 1.8. Such behaviour-to-BOLD correlations provide an additional type of information absent from most fMRI methodologies but present—in spades—in neuropsychology. They support the assumption of a causal role of these regions in behaviour, as one would expect if activation level does in fact correlate positively with the amount of a computational resource critical for task performance. Indeed that the positive behaviour-to-BOLD correlations were specific to the right hemisphere is consistent with the right hemisphere lateralisation of impairments of the neglect network—unilateral neglect—discussed in Section 1.8. The basic fMRI results themselves would not fit with the lateralisation of the function.

What can one say if there is no relation between BOLD level and behaviour, as indicated for the left hemisphere regions in Figure 5.27b? Consider the study of Tyler et al. (2010) on syntactic processing across the life-span. Subjects needed to detect the presence of a particular target word (e.g. *tooth*). This could be in random words, in a normal pairs of sentences or in syntactically correct but semantically anomalous sentences

---

[45] Priming is a frequently used functional imaging procedure with the aim of isolating a particular processing component; the repeated operation on the same stimulus is held to require less resource. However interpretations of reduced activation following a repeat of stimulus can be complex, as we will see in Chapter 7.

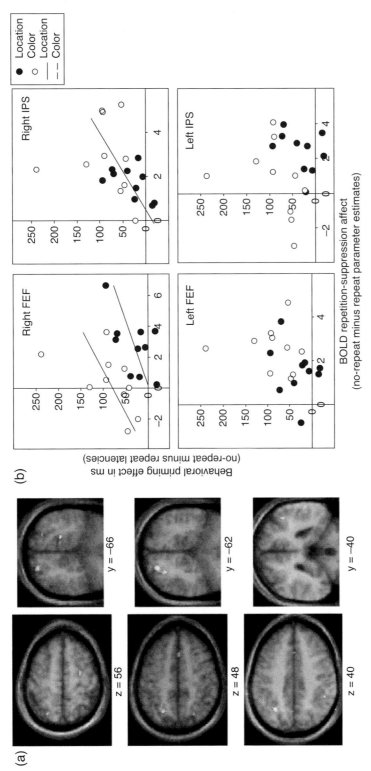

Fig. 5.27 Results of Kristjánsson et al. (2007). (a) Regions associated with priming of the colour of the stimulus on consecutive pop-out trials. (b) Scatter-plots showing behavioural effect size (vertical axis) plotted against the BOLD effect size for 10 participants for colour and location priming. Reprinted from A. Kristjánsson, P. Vuilleumier, S. Schwartz, E. Macaluso and J. Driver, Neural basis for priming of pop-out during visual search revealed with fMRI, *Cerebral Cortex, 2007, 17(7)*, 1612–1624, by permission of Oxford University Press.

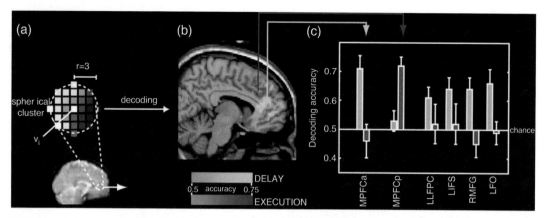

Fig. 5.28 The analysis procedure and results of Haynes et al. (2007). (a) For each voxel, a local neighbourhood was defined and the response pattern on a subset of trials was used to train a pattern classifier to recognise either addition or subtraction trials. (b) The green regions show medial frontal regions found to be associated with holding which operation (addition or subtraction) is to be performed for the duration of a delay period. The red regions show those regions which differentiated the two operation types during task execution. (c) Accuracy of the decoding (compared to chance) for several frontal regions for holding an intention (green) and executing an intention (red). Reprinted from *Current Biology, 17*(4), J-D. Haynes, K. Sakai, G. Rees, S. Gilbert, C. Frith and R.E. Passingham, Reading hidden intentions in the human brain, 323–328, Copyright (2007), with permission from Elsevier.

such as: *Stephen did not catch himself very much. Her tooth was driven because he had a weak nail and she couldn't heat anyone properly.* Both older and younger subjects were much faster with normal prose (267 msec) than with anomalous sentences (352 msec), but critically these latter stimuli were much faster than for random words (430 msec). Having correct syntax helped. In older subjects, for the normal prose compared to a non-verbal auditory control task, activation changes were restricted to the left temporal lobe. Yet for the anomalous sentences there was much more widespread bilateral temporal and frontal activation. In Chapter 8 we will see that the *left* inferior frontal gyrus (LIFG) plays a key role in syntactic processing. Why then should the right inferior frontal gyrus be activated? Behaviour-to-BOLD correlations begin to give an answer. For the LIFG the correlation between the BOLD response and RT is highly significant across subjects but for the RIFG it is not (Tyler, personal communication). This suggests that the relation between resource required and BOLD is different for the two regions. For the LIFG a big change in activation corresponds to a large change in the resource used, but for the RIFG this is not the case. As we discussed with respect to the Crescentini et al. study in Section 5.3, activation in a minor hemisphere for a task may be relatively non-functional.

An especially important type of behaviour-to-BOLD correlation design is the so-called multivariate pattern recognition procedure initially developed by Haxby et al. (2001) and applied powerfully to the nature of subjective visual experience by Haynes and Rees (2006). This technique is especially important as it bypasses all the problems inherent in any form of subtraction between conditions, which is a necessary component of all techniques discussed to this point. In multivariate pattern recognition one examines whether particular voxels are statistically significantly linked to particular responses.

Consider the example of the study of Haynes et al. (2007) on the type of intention a subject had generated. On each trial subjects are first given the free choice of deciding what task they will perform. Their choice is, however, limited to two: addition and subtraction. A variable time later two two-digit numbers are presented and the subject must perform the operation that they had previously chosen. Two seconds later, four numbers are presented, one of which corresponds to the sum of the original pair of numbers and another the differences between them. The subject must then indicate by a button press which number corresponds to the result of the operation they carried out.

It is now known which operation they had previously chosen a few seconds before. The critical analysis took each voxel and produced a spherical cluster of voxels centred on it with radius 3 voxels (see Figure 5.28). Seven of the eight runs of trials were then used to train a statistical pattern classifier to produce the best correspondence between a pattern of activity across the cluster with respect to generating an addition intention compared to generating a subtraction intention.[46] Then the pattern classifier was assessed on the eighth run. The process was repeated with each of the eight runs being used as the test run in turn and the average of the eight was taken. Doing this in turn for each voxel

---

[46] Technically this was a linear support vector pattern classifier (Cortes & Vapnik, 1995).

led to a spatial map of average decoding accuracy. For intention generation this is shown in green in the figure; for realisation of intentions it is shown in red. The highest decoding accuracy was 0.71 ($p < 0.001$) at the medial surface of the anterior prefrontal lobe, a region to be discussed in Section 9.14.

This statistical pattern classifier technique is a very interesting method. To rigorously draw inferences to cognition from findings using it would depend on assumptions about a more micro-level of modelling of brain function than the concept of *resource* allows. However, as far as base regions are concerned, this technique essentially confirms, using a very different paradigm and analysis procedure, the findings of the cognitive conjunction analysis of P. Burgess et al. (2001) discussed in the previous section. In Section 2.4 we gave the example of the findings of P. Burgess et al. as evidence that relatively localised systems could have abstract functions. The work of Haynes et al. uses a methodology not dependent on subtraction, but comes to a similar conclusion. Equipotenatiality is not a plausible candidate even for high-level functions.[47]

5.9 A Potential Weakness of fMRI Cognitive Paradigms

The new functional imaging beasts aimed at isolating cognitive subsystems and determining how they operate stand on two legs. One, the technical methodology for determining the location of where in the brain activation changes occur, is svelt yet strong, youthful and highly trained. The other, the cognitive paradigm, though rather elderly, can be well and skilfully exercised, but is often much more feeble than it appears. Unfortunately the utility for propelling functional imaging forward scientifically is dependent equally on both. Yet the creature is mentally extremely frisky, aiming to leap and jump with alacrity. More and more ambitious areas of cognition are being apparently made scientific by the development of novel paradigms and their being carried out in the scanner.

Take lying. Kozel et al. (2005) write 'Deception is ubiquitous in human societies' and claim it 'is essential for proper social interactions' (p. 605).[48] This universal process could seem amenable to detection by brain imaging. So a paradigm was developed of asking subjects to participate in a mock crime and then to deny it in the scanner. They were instructed to 'steal' either a watch or a ring, objects left in desk drawers, and then to place the 'stolen' object in a locker. In the scanner four types of question are asked of the subject—20 related to the ring, 20 related to the watch, 20 neutral such as 'Are you under age 50?' and 20 control such as 'Have you ever forged a signature?'. Subjects were instructed to answer the watch and ring questions as though they had not taken either and the other questions truthfully. Seven clusters of voxels showed an effect of the subtraction (Lie–True), where the item they had not stolen counted as the referent for the 'True' condition (see Figure 5.29a).[49]

Such complexity is characteristic of complex cognitive events taking more than a second or two. As we have seen subtraction designs have many problems. And the more complex the situation scanned, the less adequate will any control condition tend to be to allow 'Pure Insertion' to operate in an unbiased way, which in this case would be for the hypothetical cognitive components underlying lying to be satisfactorily realised. Yet, at least for the three largest cortical structures qualitatively the same cluster, although 30–50% smaller in size was also present for the (True–Neutral) comparison (see Figure 5.29b). Thus lying about an actual event involves essentially the same structures as telling the truth about the event. In no sense was a lie-network isolated. Yet the interpretation in the paper relates to the lying process such as 'These results imply that these regions are important for lying in humans. One possibility is that the anterior cingulate[50] monitors the reading and incorrect (deceptive) response to a question. The anterior cingulate modified the baseline behaviour of the prefrontal cortex for deception responses' (p. 611). From the study one has no stronger evidence for attributing this or any other property to the anterior cingulate than to any other of the clusters activated. Instead one sees sociologically a procedure often used in functional imaging papers of making an interpretation of activated regions based on hypotheses about the region's function derived from other studies without any constraining evidence from the study itself.[51] In fact the anterior cingulate is the structure most activated in functional imaging experiments (Paus et al., 1998). As we will see in Chapter 9, monitoring of response competition is only one of the hypotheses put forward for the computational operation carried

---

[47] Further support for these conclusions derived from the Burgess et al. study comes from neuropsychological findings; see specifically Burgess et al. (2000) and Roca et al. (2009), and more generally Chapter 9.

[48] Unfortunately no reference is given for this claim, only the statement that the lack of the ability is indicative of neuropathology (Spence et al., 2004), a very different matter.

---

[49] The selection of clusters used an alternative package to SPM, AFNI—Analysis of Functional NeuroImages (Cox, 1996).

[50] A key structure in the largest cluster.

[51] This is essentially an instance of the point made by Poldrack in his analysis discussed in Section 5.5.

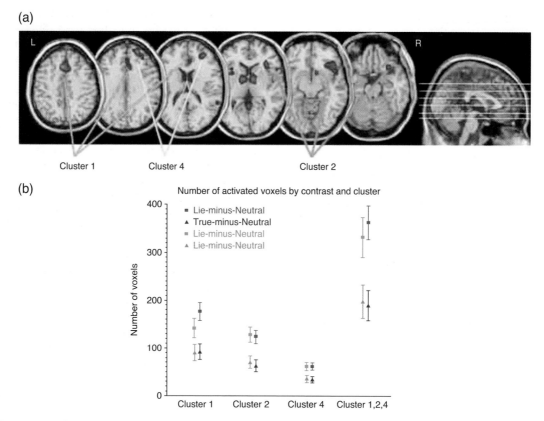

Fig. 5.29 Results from the fMRI study of Kozel et al. (2005) on lying. (a) Group analysis of lie minus truth showing anterior cingulate (cluster 1), right inferior orbitofrontal (cluster 2) and right superior frontal (cluster 4) activity. (b) The number of activated voxels by contrast and cluster. Error bars show one standard error above/below the mean. Reprinted from *Biological Psychiatry*, *58*(8), F.A. Kozel, K.A. Johnson, Q. Mu, E.L. Grenesko, S.J. Laken and M.S. George, Detecting deception using functional magnetic resonance imaging, 605–613, Copyright (2005), with permission from Elsevier.

out in the superior medial cortex—the area activated in cluster 1—and in particular the anterior cingulate.[52]

The reader may well argue that this example is based on cognitive subtraction, which was discussed earlier in the chapter as an inadequate methodology. But even if a superior design methodology, such as multivariate pattern recognition classification, had been used, would stronger cognitive conclusions be able to be drawn? The answer is almost certainly not. Again regions involved in Lie versus True comparisons are also likely to be involved in True versus Neutral. It is the cognitive paradigm that is most inadequate. Thus subjects may well feel guilt at obeying the instruction to carry out the mock theft, as in the famous Milgram (1974) experiments. The object reminds them of this. And the True condition may remind the subject of that, even though they took the other object. Or more prosaically the

Lying and True condition questions may lead to some confusion about what response should be given, and the confusion is greater with the 'stolen' object than the 'non-stolen' one.

But these suggestions are mere guesses. Any complex paradigm lasting a few seconds will almost inevitably allow many plausible guesses about the processes involved. Thus what is critical is to use paradigms that, ideally, have a natural history that is well understood and, most critically, are aimed to isolate subsystems that are computing what is plausibly a basic computational I-O process. 'Lying' seems an unlikely candidate, as do many other complex processes currently being investigated in the scanner under the rubric of new and fashionable disciplines. Without a putative task analysis, interpreting functional imaging results is little better than reading the tea leaves. When the basic set of mental component processes have been isolated and are understood, and only then, will it be really productive to use the scanner to investigate more complex situations. Otherwise we are attempting to do organic chemistry without knowing the basic set of elements.

---

[52] For incisive deconstruction of lying paradigms using the much superior detection of concealed information paradigm see Gamer et al. (2009).

5.10 **Combining Inferences from Neuropsychology and from Functional Imaging**

The basic argument of this chapter so far has been that we have new and very powerful techniques that give us beguiling evidence that one can isolate individual cognitive subsystems having specific functions and localise them in particular parts of the brain. However, despite the most impressive developments in imaging analysis and experimental design of the last twenty years, the inferences from statistical patterns of activation to the theories or models on the cognitive level and even for the existence of isolable subsystems (and so their localisation) is full of uncertainty, with many potential artefacts.

The tightness of the experimental design of functional imaging experiments is definitely improving. But relatively few experimenters use such a rigorous and sophisticated design as cognitive conjunction or multivariate pattern classification. And cognitive paradigms typically involve a number of cognitive subsystems and give rise to data that lack power. Worse, as we discussed in the last section, we now have a plethora of poorly understood experimental paradigms as the criteria for paper acceptance relate to the potential intuitive interest of the result and the technical satisfactoriness of the fMRI analysis and hardly at all to how well understood cognitively is the paradigm. And it is perfectly acceptable in the field to guess at the cognitive function of subsystems that might be producing unanticipated cortical activations. And looking at excellent examples of functional imaging research, Coltheart (2006b) has even argued that functional imaging has not as yet told us anything about the functional architecture of the mind saying, 'I'll claim that no functional neuroimaging research to date has yielded data that can be used to distinguish between competing psychological theories' (p. 323).[53] Moreover he takes the seven examples that Henson (2005) selected to show how evidence from functional imaging can be used to distinguish between competing cognitive level theories and produces strong counter-arguments against Henson's arguments in six cases.[54] The Harley–Coltheart position is generally

viewed in functional imaging circles as a modern equivalent of holding to a flat earth hypothesis. However no one to our knowledge has attempted to respond to Coltheart's deconstruction of Henson's examples or offered alternatives.

In our view, Coltheart's critique is subtly misdirected. He blames our stumbling progress on the left leg when it is the right that is weak. We are handicapped by behavioural data and cognitive paradigms, which while absolutely vital, are highly complex and lacking in power.[55] Functional imaging is doing the best that is technically possible with this flimsy base. However this state of affairs makes converging evidence absolutely necessary when one wants to draw theoretical conclusions about cognition from functional imaging research.

The simplest procedure is meta-analysis—combining in some way the results of all experiments which contain a subtraction based on what is normally a broadly defined contrast. We will consider examples in Chapter 9. However the standard critique of meta-analyses is that they are typically not theoretically sufficiently specific, and worse that they contain no internal quality control. More satisfactory is converging evidence using different fMRI methodologies as was obtained from the P. Burgess et al. (2001) and the Haynes et al. (2007) studies on the setting up and realising of intentions discussed in Section 5.8. Best of all, though is to obtain convergence with a completely different methodology—neuropsychology.

Neuropsychology, too, as we discussed in the last chapter has many potential artefacts. However, potential artefacts manifest themselves very differently in the two fields, as the methodologies are so different. Thus virtually the only things they have in common is the brain and the cognitive paradigm. And even the constraints over the organisation of tasks so that they can be run in the scanner are very different from those found for experiments outside the scanner with patients.

Thus we have one very simple way to check the overall inferences, given the basic assumption of the previous section—do the lesion sites in 'pure' syndromes correspond to the regions activated when the corresponding isolable subsystem is used in a functional imaging experiment? The idea of cross-checking localisation between neuropsychology and functional imaging is of course used as standard supporting evidence in papers

---

[53] See also Harley (2004).

[54] The examples relate to the remember-know debate (see Section 5.5 and Chapter 10), Otten and Rugg's (2001) study of subsequent memory effects during semantic or phonological study tasks, theories of the phenomenon of attentional blindness, bottom-up versus top-down approaches to repetition priming in face processing (see Section 7.2), verbal versus visuospatial slave systems in working memory (see Chapter 7) and 'simulation theory' versus 'theory theory' of representing other's intentions.

---

[55] Thus it is noteworthy that Coltheart in his paean of praise for purely behavioural evidence gives the example of whether the semantic system is needed for reading aloud. However the conclusion derived from behavioural evidence he claims to be clearly correct is not the one we arrived at in Chapter 4. Functional imaging evidence may cause us to change our view again, see later in this chapter.

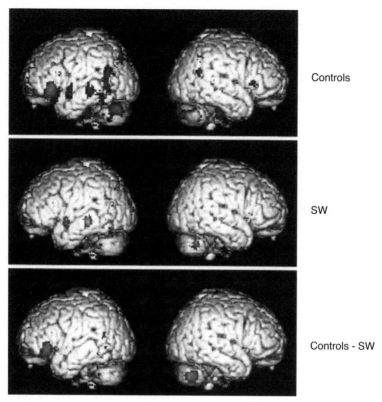

Controls

SW

Controls - SW

Fig. 5.30 Areas activated during the semantic decision task of Price et al. (1999). The normal system is illustrated in the top panel. The centre panel illustrates the areas where patient SW activates normally. The bottom panel illustrates the areas that SW fails to activate. Reproduced with permission from C.J. Price, C.J. Mummery, C.J. Moore, R.S.J. Frackowiak and K.J. Friston (1999). Delineating necessary and sufficient neural systems with functional imaging studies of neuropsychological patients. *Journal of Cognitive Neuroscience, 11*(4), 371–382; figure 2, p. 377. Copyright © 1999, MIT Press Journals.

on both topics. The argument being presented here is that it should be considered much more than supporting evidence. We will in later chapters treat the two as equally relevant—both requiring support for their functional inferences from the other.

The position being put forward considers cognitive neuropsychology and functional imaging as equal but qualitatively very different partners, which when combined are much more effective than when separate. And this can work well. We will consider the example of the reading system which was the focus of much of Chapter 4. First, though consider what happens when the methods do not converge.

In a series of papers, Price and her colleagues have discussed the problem that occurs when the outputs of the two methodologies do not match. Take, for instance, Price et al. (1999). They consider a region—the left frontal operculum—often associated with language production. But they are concerned with its functions relevant to semantics. As we will see in Chapters 7, 8 and 9, the region is often activated by semantic tasks, such as the initial task of Petersen et al. of producing verbs from nouns discussed earlier in Section 5.3, other

so-called deep encoding tasks (e.g. Kapur et al., 1994) and semantic selection tasks (e.g. Thompson-Schill et al., 1997) among others. Price et al. consider, in particular, a task in which subjects have to judge which of two concrete nouns (e.g. *chair, sofa*) is closer in meaning to a third (e.g. *table*). This study activated the left inferior frontal gyrus in normal subjects (see Figure 5.30). However they also showed that a patient, SW, who had a lesion entirely affecting this area on structural MRI, could carry out the task, if more slowly than normal subjects, but at a level within the range of normal control subjects. They also showed that when SW carries out the task the left inferior frontal region, hardly surprisingly, is silent. They say 'By combining functional imaging and neuropsychology we have demonstrated that the inferior frontal cortex is not necessary for the types of semantic decision SW is able to perform'. They continue 'Either (i) inferior frontal activation seen in normal subjects is incidental to the semantic component of task requirements or (ii) the semantic system can adapt to emulate the same cognitive functionality in the absence of viable frontal activity (for instance in SW the function of BA 47 may be executed by the

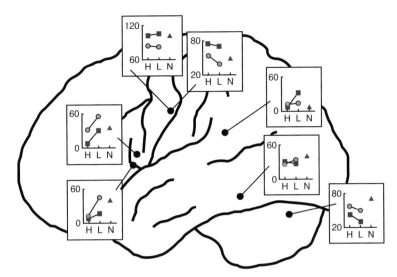

Fig. 5.31 The locations of the seven regions found by Fiez et al. (1999) that showed effects of frequency, spelling-to-sound consistency or lexicality in reading aloud. Graphs show mean regional activations across frequency (High, Low, Non-words) with inconsistent words indicated by green circles, consistent words by blue squares, and non-words by red triangles. Reprinted from *Neuron, 24*(1), J.A. Fiez, D.A. Balota, M.E. Raichle and S.E. Petersen, Effects of lexicality, frequency and spelling-to-sound consistency on the functional anatomy of reading, 205–218. Copyright (1999), with permission from Elsevier.

medial superior frontal cortex)' (p. 378). There is also even the additional possibility of individual differences either across the functional architecture of subjects[56] or—more likely—that the patient is carrying out the task using a different procedure and so different subsystems from normal subjects; after all the patient is slower.

In our view, if there is a mismatch between lesion evidence and functional imaging evidence, then little progress can be made in resolving it without a detailed componential task analysis. Even with it, one may well not be able to sort out which of the numerous possibilities are right. Mismatches between the cognitive products of different methods are thus not likely to prove fruitful.[57] However, the existence of such mismatches means that if much credence is to be given to either method we need to be confident that correspondences in theoretical interpretations between the two types frequently occur. We will therefore address the reading system discussed in Chapter 4 and consider in detail whether correspondences exist for the conclusions drawn there.

It is essential that any attempt to produce isomorphisms should operate between putative I-O computational subsystems and their localisations and not

between tasks. This means that a theoretical framework must be produced prior to any attempt to produce a mapping. The empirical alternative of producing a mapping between tasks is inadequate because task performance involves many subsystems. This can be illustrated by an attempt by Fiez and Petersen (1998) to link certain imaging studies, which activate inferior left prefrontal cortex, with phonological alexia, discussed in the previous chapter. They consider nine imaging studies which produce in all 147 maxima. They then intuitively group these maxima into clumps (see Figure 5.31) and consider as one putative region the left frontal operculum (BA 44 and 45 plus a part of the insula). This region is more strongly activated by reading pronounceable non-words than words, but also more by words exceptional in their spelling-to-sound patterns (e.g. *yacht*) than those regular (e.g. *mouse*). They appropriately consider a hypothetical function of the region from the perspective of then current models of reading. Indeed even more appropriately they do it twice for two different models, from the perspective of multiple route models such as that of Coltheart et al. (1993) and from the connectionist perspective of Plaut et al. (1996).[58] For instance, from a connectionist perspective the two sets of stimuli that activate the region more are those that would lead to a slower rise in activation of phonological output units than do regular words and so more activation overall when activation is integrated over time.

[56] This is made less plausible by the results of Crescentini et al. discussed in Section 5.3.

[57] This book generally does not discuss the use of functional imaging on neurological patients. For a guide to some of the potential complexities in interpretation of such findings see Wise (2003).

[58] These models are extensively discussed in Chapters 3 and 4. See especially Figures 3.3 and 3.4.

So far so good. They then argue, 'The syndrome of phonological alexia is particularly relevant for this discussion, because within the domain of reading it has been viewed as a relatively pure impairment in orthographic-to-phonological transformations' (p. 918), although they do add the rider 'though some reports have emphasised that phonological dyslexics have more general phonological deficits' (p. 918). Yet when they look to see whether all phonological alexia patients have damage to the left frontal operculum, about half the patients in their literature review do but for the other half the lesion site is elsewhere.

Now phonological alexia is a mixed syndrome; the same behavioural effect can occur for many reasons. Indeed if one considers a multiple route model of reading of the Coltheart et al. type (see Figure 3.4), then the non-lexical spelling-to-sound route has multiple stages. Thus many phonological dyslexics have greater difficulty when the output does not correspond to a word than when it does (e.g. *weem* vs *weet*) but for others the main problem is analysing complex graphemes (*shrich* is more difficult than *patimo*) (Derouesné & Beauvois, 1979).[59] Thus the possible correspondence has to be made broader on the imaging side.

Rapcsak et al. (2009) address the same topic—the anatomy of phonological alexia—more systematically and also with a more sophisticated neuropsychological approach. First, they consider their own sample of 31 patients selected for having a left hemisphere lesion. Nearly all the patients have had a stroke in which the lesion involved the region round the Sylvian fissure, which divides the temporal from the parietal and frontal lobes—standardly known as the perisylvian region. 21 of the patients manifested a pattern of phonological alexia, showing no difference between the reading of regular and irregular words but poorer performance with matched pronounceable non-words (see Figure 5.32). They then compared the relevant lesion sites within the perisylvian regions with regions activated by phonological processing as opposed to more general semantic or sentence processing in language in a functional imaging meta-analysis (Vigneau et al., 2006). The correspondence was impressive (see Figure 5.33). Moreover the authors argue 'different aspects of phonological processing may have been disrupted in our patients as a function of lesion location, suggesting that it might be possible to identify different subtypes of phonological dyslexia based on the exact nature of the underlying phonological deficit' (p. 587).[60] Thus Fiez and Petersen's

project of producing correspondences concerning the systems involved in phonological alexia, while not completely accomplished, seems promising.

Consider now the complementary syndrome surface dyslexia, where patients can read regular pseudowords but have problems with low frequency exception words. As we discussed in Section 4.7 this syndrome is most frequently found in conjunction with semantic dementia, which as we will discuss in the next chapter is associated with bilateral anterior temporal lobe atrophy, often worse in the left hemisphere. Thus we can assume this structure to be involved in the semantic reading route.

However, the syndrome also offers us the opportunity to check the anatomy of multiple route models for reading in another way. Wilson et al. (2009) imaged five surface dyslexic patients as they were reading low-frequency exception words, such as *yacht*, and compared them with controls. Surface dyslexic patients, as one would expect given the discussion in the last chapter, performed particularly poorly on low-frequency exception words with a mean success rate of only about 30%. Normal subjects were over 90% accurate in reading low-frequency exception words. Moreover many of the errors made by the patients were regularisations of the spelling of the exception words. Thus it is clear that these surface dyslexic patients were making use of a phonological route—possibly a non-lexical one if such exists—to read low-frequency exception words. On high-frequency words, though, the surface dyslexics were roughly 90% accurate.

Turning to the functional imaging findings, there is one region that showed an interaction of group by word type. This is the left intraparietal sulcus (see Figure 5.34), close to lesion site c of Figure 5.33. This region is activated in controls only for pronounceable non-words. In surface dyslexic patients it is activated in low-frequency words and pronounceable non-words, more than for high-frequency words. What then is the process being carried out in the left intraparietal sulcus? Wilson et al. argue that as it was not atrophied in the semantic dementia patients it involves compensatory operations for words that could not be identified semantically. They also note that it is particularly activated when regularisation errors occur. Also in their normal subjects the region is more activated in reading low-frequency regular words than low-frequency exception words, as previously found by Fiez et al. (1999). The region therefore seems to be involved in the operation of some form of phonological route. One possibility is that it is involved in the spatial decomposition of the letter string into sublexical units and somewhat less likely in the reintegration into a whole utterance. Such a spatial type of operation would fit the intraparietal sulcus location. It would be ironic if a functional imaging

---

[59] See FNMS Chapter 5 for discussion.

[60] To complicate matters somewhat neuropsychologically phonological alexia frequently occurs immediately after right parietal lesions (Buiatti et al., in preparation)—see Chapter 8.

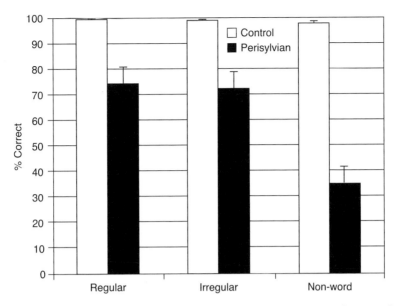

Fig. 5.32 The influence of stimulus type on reading performance in perisylvian patients and normal controls. Reprinted with permission from Rapcsak et al. (2009). This article was published in *Cortex*, *45*(5), S.Z. Rapcsak, P.M. Beeson, M.L. Henry, A. Leyden, E. Kim, K. Rising, S. Andersen and H. Cho. Phonological dyslexia and dysgraphia: cognitive mechanisms and neural substrates, 575–591. Copyright Elsevier SRL (2009).

study finally tipped the balance in favour of the 3-route reading theory of Coltheart et al. (2001) over the triangle model.

The location of semantic processing will be discussed in the next chapter and a correspondence between the two methodologies shown. This leaves the orthographic processing components of the traditional reading models.

As discussed in Section 4.12, Cohen, Dehaene and their colleagues have argued that there is a correspondence between a hypothetical visual word form system held to be damaged in pure alexia and a left fusiform region activated in normal reading. For instance, Dehaene et al. (2001) used a priming or adaptation type of functional imaging procedure referred to earlier in this chapter.

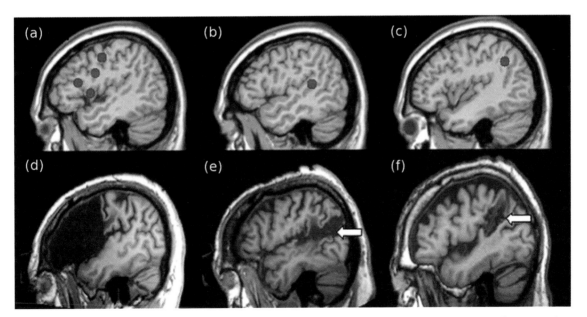

Fig. 5.33 The overlap between regions found to be associated with phonological processing in normals in a meta-analysis of Vigneau et al. (2006) (a, b, and c) and the lesion sites of patients with phonological dyslexia/dysgraphia (d, e and f). Reprinted with permission from Rapcsak et al. (2009). This article was published in *Cortex*, *45*(5), S.Z. Rapcsak, P.M. Beeson, M.L. Henry, A. Leyden, E. Kim, K. Rising, S. Andersen and H. Cho. Phonological dyslexia and dysgraphia: Cognitive mechanisms and neural substrates, 575–591. Copyright Elsevier SRL (2009).

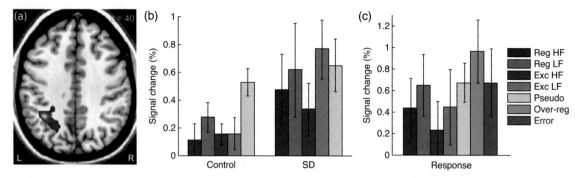

Fig. 5.34 Imaging results for controls and semantic dementia patients of Wilson et al. (2009) when reading regular (Reg) and exception (Exc) words of high (HF) or low (LF) frequency and pseudowords (i.e. pronounceable non-words) (Pseudo). (a) The left intraparietal sulcus (IPS) was the region to show an interaction of group by word type. (b) Signal change for high and low frequency regular and exception words and pseudowords for the two groups in the left IPS. (c) Signal change in semantic dementia patients for correct responses to the five conditions, over regularisation (Over-Reg) responses to exception words, and other miscellaneous errors (Errors). Reprinted from S.M. Wilson, S.M. Brambati, R.G. Henry, D.A. Handwerker, F. Agosta, B.L. Miller, D.P. Wilkins, J.M. Ogar and M.L. Gorno-Tempini, The neural basis of surface dyslexia in semantic dementia, *Brain*, 2009, *132*(1), 71–86, by permission of Oxford University Press.

Subjects were presented with word stimuli and had to make a semantic decision as to whether each referred to a living or man-made thing (see Figure 5.35). Just before the word was presented it was preceded by a priming word that was masked so that it was not seen. Subjects still responded more rapidly if the prime was the same word as the target, even if it was made physically different by being in a different case. At the same time if the prime was the same word, activation was reduced in the part of the left fusiform known as the visual word-form area. Oddly, there is little discussion in the paper as to why a reduction should occur in this condition, especially as prime and target are so close together in time and so their effects would overlap in the BOLD response. There seem two possibilities. One is to explain it by a habituation (or response suppression) phenomenon to be discussed in Section 7.2. The other is to use an interactive activation model; an initially different prime say HOUSE instead of RADIO would produce activation which will compete with the later ariving stimulus *radio* so that the activating process for *radio* itself would be slowed. Then the activation in the whole system when integrated over time in the HOUSE prime case would be greater than in the RADIO prime case.

Later papers by this group attempted to distinguish different levels of a visual word-form system. Thus, in a study of Vinckier et al. (2007), subjects had the simple task of detecting the occasional string comprised of four hash signs in a row. The study however was concerned with neural responses to stimuli to which subjects did not have to physically respond. The authors compared the activation induced by words with that produced by letter strings having different degrees of similarities to words and also to stimuli made up of symbol-like entities of somewhat similar shape to letters—so-called

'false font' (see Figure 5.36). Thus stimuli at the *bigram* level were composed of letter strings in which each pair of succeeding letters frequently occurred in words but the sets of four letters with which they were compared did not have this characteristic. Figure 5.37 shows the proportional activation relative to words of the 6 types of stimuli. The pattern of findings found for the left visual word-form area (Figure 5.37c) fit with a model put forward by Dehaene et al. (2005) (see Figure 4.27), which is essentially a brain-based extension of the classical McClelland and Rumelhart (1981) model of orthographic processing (see Figure 3.21). The location obtained for the visual word-form area, which involves all orthographic processing at above the level of the single letter, fits with the localisation of pure alexia discussed in Section 4.12.[61]

Objections have been raised to this correspondence from both sides. From the functional imaging side, Price and Devlin (2003) have argued that there is nothing specifically orthographic about the so-called 'visual word-form area' (VWFA), which they hold to be as relevant for processing other sorts of visual input as for objects. Thus when Price and Mechelli (2005) compared reading with the naming of line drawings, the visual word-form area is, if anything, more activated for object naming than for reading. However, while such studies show that the VWFA is also activated by visual stimuli other than words, it does not mean that the area is as specialised for object processing as for word processing. Object naming is a much more resource demanding—and a slower—task than reading single words aloud, and so one would expect greater activation with the former. Indeed, Ben-Shachar et al. (2007) have shown

---

[61] See also Binder et al. (2006), for related findings.

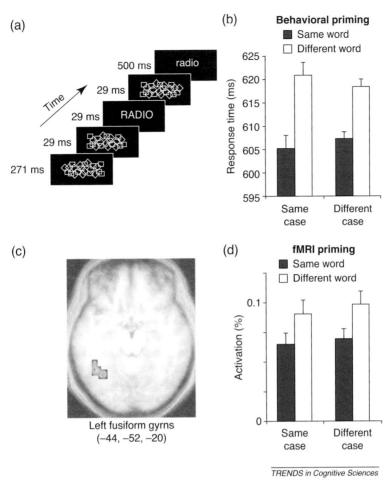

Fig. 5.35 Design and results of the Dehaene et al. (2001) study. (a) Subjects were required to make a semantic decision on the word (in this case *radio*) which may have been primed by a brief presentation of the same word in a different case 29 msec earlier. (b) The behavioural data show an effect of priming that is not dependent on the case of the prime/target. (c) The visual word-form area in left fusiform gyrus showed reduced activation on repeated word trials, characteristic of priming. (d) Activation of the left fusiform gyrus in the various conditions, showing effects equivalent to those in the behavioural data. Reprinted from *Trends in Cognitive Sciences*, 7(7), B.D. McCandliss, L. Cohen and S. Dehaene, The visual word form area: expertise for reading in the fusiform gyrus, 293–299, Copyright (2003), with permission from Elsevier.

the left but not the right VWFA region is significantly more sensitive to letter stimuli than to both visually closely matched line drawing and false font stimuli. Thus as Price and Devlin (2004) themselves point out, orthographic processing seems to be more lateralised to the left fusiform compared to object processing.

Complementarily, two objections have been made to using pure alexia to localise the visual word-form area. Behrmann et al. (1998a), in an exhaustive review, argued that pure alexic patients have problems in early visual processing. Thus five letter-by-letter readers studied by Behrmann et al. (1998b) were relatively much slower compared to controls at naming highly visually complex line drawings than low visually complex ones; they were more than 500 msec slower for the highly complex ones compared to a 150 msec difference for

controls. This claimed lack of exclusivity to the written word of the processing by pure alexics of visual stimuli echoes the concerns of Price and Devlin regarding the functional imaging evidence.

In addition attempts to localise pure alexia have not always honed in on a VWFA area. However, the most detailed study is that of Binder and Mohr (1992), who carried out an extensive anatomical analysis of three groups of patients: five global alexics, five letter-by-letter readers and seven patients with normal reading but lesions to the left posterior cerebral artery, close to those of the letter-by-letter reading group. They showed that two areas were critical for global alexia—a left fusiform region very close to the VWFA, as localised by Cohen et al. (2000) (see Figure 5.38), and a much higher region near the splenium. The critical letter-by-letter

Types of stimuli

	False font	Infrequent letters	Frequent letters	Frequent bigrams	Frequent quadrigrams	Words
Strings	0	0	0	0	0	high
Quadrigrams	0	low	low	low	high	high
Bigrams	0	low	low	high	high	high
Letters	0	low	high	high	high	high
Features	high	high	high	high	high	high
	ꓶꓩꓵꓯꓵꓲ	JZWYWK	QOADTQ	QUMBSS	AVONIL	MOUTON

Components of stimulus strings

Examples

Fig. 5.36 The experimental design and illustrative examples of stimuli used in the study of Vinckier et al. (2007). Six types of stimuli were used ranging from 'false-font' stimuli to real (French) words. Reprinted from *Neuron, 55*(1), F. Vinckier, S. Dehaene, A. Jobert, J.P. Dubus, M. Sigman and L. Cohen, Hierarchical coding of letter strings in the ventral stream: dissecting the inner organization of the visual word-form system, 143–156. Copyright (2007), with permission from Elsevier.

readers, however, just had the first type of damage. So the results fit well with later localisations of the VWFA.

Cohen et al. (2000) in a cleverly designed study provided further support for their position, which combined functional imaging and patients. Information about words which are presented to one visual field is initially analysed in the visual cortex of the appropriate hemisphere. However, from Dejerine (1892) on, in models of the reading system the final stages of orthographic processing—the word-form system in the current framework—are standardly assumed to take place in the left hemisphere. Cohen et al. therefore compared the reading aloud of words presented to the left hemifield with the equivalent procedure when they are presented to the right hemifield. A cognitive conjunction analysis was used. It was found that for a number of regions a purely unilateral activation was obtained. These included the left middle temporal gyrus and the left VWFA. However one could ask why, from a functional imaging perspective, should one treat the left VWFA as the seat of a putative word-form system? An elegant combination of methods answers that point. Cohen and collaborators reported investigations of two patients AC (Michel et al., 1996) and RAV2 (Cohen & Dehaene, 1996) who had lesions affecting the splenium of the corpus callosum. This would prevent information from the left visual field reaching the posterior left hemisphere. Indeed these two patients show activation of the same cortical regions as controls when the words are presented to the right or left visual fields. The one exception was the left fusiform region which both patients activated significantly in the right visual field condition, but for which there were highly significant differences for both between left and right visual field presentations.[62] We thus have converging lines of evidence for a critical process at the relatively early stage of reading taking place in the left fusiform region. Functional imaging has not yet definitively favoured a two-route over a three-route model or vice-versa but their common characteristics—and they are many—are supported by both methodologies.

5.11 Beyond Cross-subject Processing Systems

The evidence from the reading system shows that when the processing system is reasonably precisely characterised, functionally inferences from functional imaging and neuropsychological studies can be mutually reinforcing in a variety of ways. Moreover insofar as we have an agreed architecture, functional imaging allows the possibility to develop it in a variety of ways. We give one supporting example. Consider two further issues, to determine what strategies subjects are using and whether there are individual differences. As we discussed in the context of the Rapcsak et al. study, the intraparietal sulcus is not the only area where lesions give rise to problems with pronounceable non-words, the left inferior frontal cortex is also critical. And in

---

[62] RAV2 was 97% correct in the right visual field (RVF) and 2% in the left visual field (LVF). AC was better, roughly 95% in both, but took 714 msec on average for RVF presentation and 1800msec for LVF presentations. Earlier AC had presented with a deep dyslexia to LVF stimuli (Michel et al., 1996) so the stimuli used in the current experiment were concrete words.

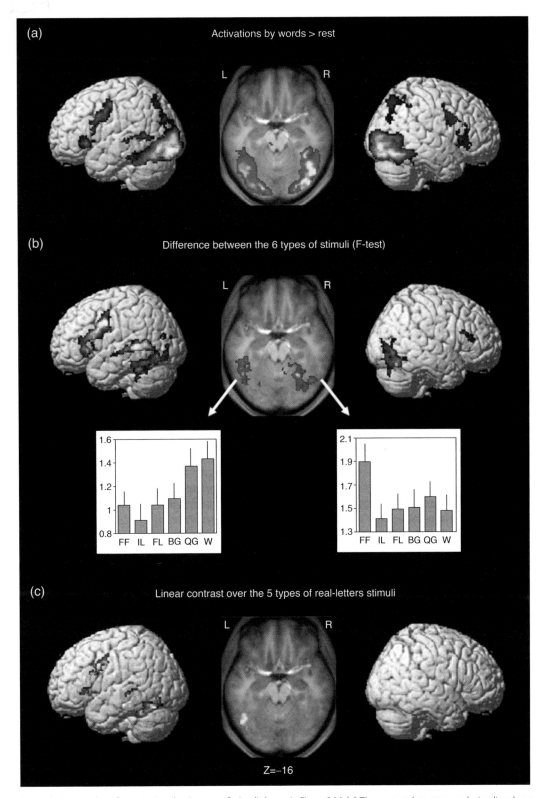

Fig. 5.37 Activation resulting from viewing the six types of stimuli shown in Figure 5.36. (a) The contrast between word stimuli and rest yielded approximately bilateral activation, primarily in ventral occipito-temporal cortex. (b) Regions showing a significant effect of stimulus type. Histograms show mean activation relative to rest for the six stimulus types in the left and right ventral regions. (c) Linear contrast over the different real-letter stimuli, showing regions whose activation increased with the similarity of the stimulus to real words. Regions showing this linear contrast include the visual word-form area, but not the homologous region in the right hemisphere. Reprinted from *Neuron*, 55(1), F. Vinckier, S. Dehaene, A. Jobert, J.P. Dubus, M. Sigman and L. Cohen, Hierarchical coding of letter strings in the ventral stream: dssecting the inner organization of the visual word-form system, 143–156. Copyright (2007), with permission from Elsevier.

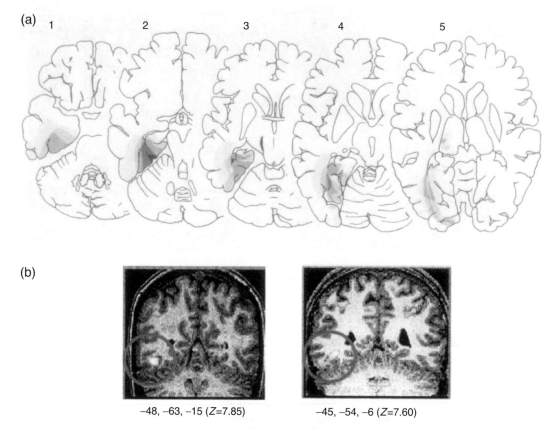

Fig. 5.38 (a) Lesion overlap in the global alexic patients of Binder and Mohr (1992). (b) Regions activated in two normal controls in the word reading study of Cohen et al. (2000). Fig. (a) reprinted from J.R. Binder and J.P. Mohr, The topography of callosal reading pathways, *Brain*, 1992, *115*(6), 1807–1826, by permission of Oxford University Press. Figure (b) reprinted from L. Cohen, S. Dehaene, L. Naccache, S. Lehéricy, G. Dehaene-Lambertz, M-A. Hénaff and F. Michael, The neural basis of surface dyslexia in semantic dementia, *Brain*, 2000, *123*(2), 291–307, by permission of Oxford University Press.

many studies this area has been found also to be more activated by reading non-words than real words (Fiez et al., 1999).

Heim et al. (2009) compared two tasks involving written words: one was lexical decision; the other was phonological decision, where the subject decided whether the phoneme with which the word started was technically a fricative (as in *sat* or *fat*) or a stop consonant (as in *pat* or *cat*). Then one of a number of procedures was used to assess whether brain regions were activated together in a task so as to operate more as a network. The method used was dynamic causal modelling (Friston et al., 2003).[63] In dynamic causal modelling, the activity in brain regions are treated as 'hidden' variables. The parameters relate to the degree of connectivity between regions, both generally and in particular

conditions. They are estimated by a Bayesian procedure (see Section 5.5), which bases its assumptions about prior probabilities on biophysical models of blood flow and broad estimates of a number of neural network characteristics such as the half-life of neuronal activity in a region.

Four different connectivity models are considered by Heim et al. (see Figure 5.39), involving three regions generally activated in these two tasks. These were an inferior temporal region, essentially the VWFA, and two regions in the inferior frontal gyrus, BA45 and 44, very speculatively held to be involved in an output phonological lexicon network and grapheme-phoneme conversion on the Coltheart et al. (2001) model.[64]

Two types of conclusion were drawn from the connectivity model findings. First, the same model does *not* fit all subjects. Qualitative individual differences exist.

---

[63] There are a variety of procedures that can be used to determine effective networks (assumption M5 in Section 3.5) operating in particular task conditions; see Harrison et al. (2007).

[64] In fact in a standard SPM contrast the phonological decision activated the inferior temporal region and BA44.

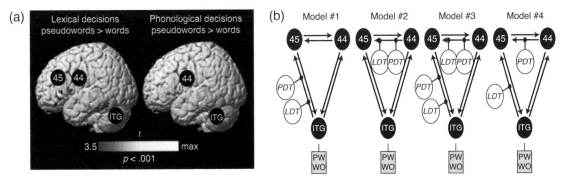

Fig. 5.39 (a) A conventional subtraction analysis of the difference between pseudowords (i.e. non-words) and words for a lexical decision task (LDT) and a phonological decision task (PDT). (b) Dynamic causal modelling of the interactions between the regions identified in (a). Heim et al. (2009) tested four models in which the connections between regions were held to be modulated by the different tasks. PW and WO indicate input of pseudowords and words into the left inferior temporal gyrus. Reprinted from S. Heim, S.B. Eickhoff, A.K. Ischebeck, A.D. Friederici, K.E. Stephan and K. Amunts, 2009, Effective connectivity of the left BA 44, BA 45, and inferior temporal cyrus during lexical and phonological decisions identified with DCM. *Human Brain Mapping, 30*(2), 392–402. Copyright © 2009, John Wiley and Sons.

In 12 out of 14 subjects model 1 is best; in two subjects, though models 2 and 3 were much superior to model 1. This type of result—showing a dominant but not completely similar pattern across subjects—supports the use of group and case-series approaches but presents problems for the single-case method. Second, the two tasks seem to modulate the fixed architecture in a similar way. Differences in results cannot be put down to purely procedural differences between tasks—they seem to reflect differences in the functional architecture.

Exploration of such issues we consider more for the future than for the more basic level of analysis with which this book is mainly concerned. However a critical theme of this chapter has been the need for an appropriate componential analysis of task performance; without it one cannot draw strong theoretical inferences from functional imaging findings. And as soon as we move away from studies of early perceptual processes to more complex areas of cognition any para-

digm will involve a variety of types of process. Thus the researcher cannot be a specialist in one area as the paradigms used and the activations produced will necessarily involve a variety of processes. Thus one requires a broad theoretical perspective. This book aims to provide a minimum set of types of process necessary for theorising on more complex cognition.

In the chapters that follow we will be concerned principally with inferences to cognition that can be drawn from the two cognitive neuroscience methods—neuropsychology and functional imaging. We have argued that drawing cognitive inferences from functional imaging, like the analogous process within neuropsychology, is subject to a host of potential artefacts. Our strongest theoretical conclusions will therefore depend on inferences where the two techniques support common theoretical claims about the organisation of the cognitive system. We have shown in this section that for an intensively investigated domain like reading the approach is a practical one. It works.

On the Semantic Elements in Thought

6.1 **The Structure of the Rest of the Book**

In the last three chapters we have laid out a theoretical and empirical methodology for the cognitive neuroscience of higher cognitive functions. The methodology may seem rather straightforward. However many disagree with aspects of it and some with virtually all. It would be an impossible task to review how well it can be applied with respect to all putative cognitive systems in our current state of knowledge. We have too many findings and too few principles with which to organise them. We will therefore take a number of critical areas and apply the methodology to them. In general our approach will be to take one area of a particular type and treat it in detail, rather than spread our attention equally across all such areas. This is to allow us to address the more abstract issues in sufficient depth.

The areas are, however, selected from a theoretical perspective. We aim to discuss how brain-based evidence can be integrated with cognitive theory, and so to show that the philosopher, Jerry Fodor, was wrong when he argued that the study of the brain has told us nothing of interest about the mind. Therefore the areas that we will principally consider are ones treated by symbolic cognitive science. The core of cognition is thinking and the areas we address are those most closely related to thought. We therefore tend to ignore, or better assume knowledge of, the more peripheral parts of the input and output processes.

We will tackle these issues on two levels. First, we will consider three types of computational element necessary for the operation of what we will call a *cognitive computational engine*, namely a physical entity capable of carrying out cognitive operations, such as those required by simple tasks such as making coffee, adding two numbers or understanding a straightforward sentence. This chapter and the next two will be concerned with such functions. Then we will argue that there are a number of systems whose role is to modulate the operation of these basic cognitive functions in nonroutine situations, of which the prototypic one is dealing with novelty. The last four chapters will deal with those systems.[1]

The concept of a cognitive computational engine derives from ideas of two of the most influential early theorists of symbolic AI, Allen Newell and Herb Simon. In the 1970s they abstracted what they saw as the essence of a system hypothesised to provide 'the necessary and sufficient means for general intelligent action' (Newell & Simon, 1976, p. 293). This they called a *physical symbol system*. Formally it 'consists of a set of entities, called symbols, which are physical patterns that occur as components of another type of entity called an expression (or symbol structure). Thus, a symbol structure is composed of a number of instances (or tokens) of symbols related in some physical way (such as one token being next to another). At any instant of time the system will contain a collection of these symbol structures. Besides these structures, the system also contains a collection of processes that operate on expressions to produce other expressions: processes of creation, modification, reproduction and destruction. A physical symbol system is a machine that produces through time an evolving collection of symbol structures. Such a system exists in a world of objects wider than just the symbol expressions themselves' (Newell & Simon, 1976, p. 292).

The physical symbol system as described by Newell and Simon is in the class of computational models defined by a Turing machine. However, Newell and Simon flesh these ideas out; they add two other central notions:

- *Designation*: an expression designates an object (outside the physical symbol system itself) if, given the expression, the system can affect the object or behave in ways dependent upon the object.

- *Interpretation*: the system can interpret an expression if the expression designates a process and if given the expression, the system can carry out the process.

In this and the following chapters we will assume that the working of human intelligence requires *a cognitive computational engine*, which derives from the idea of a physical symbol system but with some aspects of the earlier concept elaborated and other aspects restructured.

- *Elaboration:* a physical symbol system carries out processes that take some symbol structures as input and produce other symbol structures. For many cognitive operations it must rely on a finite working memory in which to store the intermediate products of the operations.[2] As a *cognitive computational engine* it must

---

[1] Historically the computational idea that the mind contains such high-level modulatory systems derives from Aaron Sloman, whose career took an unusual twist. He began academic life as a philosopher-of-mind and then became a computer scientist, even becoming identified with the use of a particular computer language, POP-11. In the 1970s he circulated a fascinating samizdat about the possible subsystems a high-level modulatory system might contain called 'Design for a Mind'. Unfortunately this was never published. For somewhat paler shadows of it, see Sloman (1978, 2000).

[2] If it were to have an infinite memory a physical symbol system would have exactly the same power as a Turing machine. With a finite memory, there are limits on the internal computations that a physical symbol system can perform. A Turing machine has an infinite tape which, at least in the von Neumann interpretation,

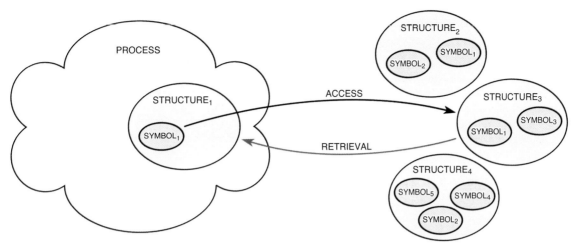

Fig. 6.1 Newell's conception of a symbol. Symbols form parts of structures and in virtue of this relation they allow processes to access or retrieve those structures.

also produce actions as outputs, where the actions are realised in the continuous four-dimensional space-time of the physical world. Thus a system with the computational requirements to carry out basic cognitive operations of a logical inference type must involve three types of entities: *symbols, working memory,* and *operations* which translate one symbol structure into another and into physical actions.

♦ *Restructuring:* a physical symbol system has the most basic and abstract properties required of a computational cognitive engine. However, it is a rather bloodless entity, remote from much of human cognition. It is suitable for abstracting the essence of solving problems that rely specifically on logical operations, such as cryptarithmetic or Sudoku. Yet it is less clear that it relates to the basic computational processes involved in selecting the next move when rock-climbing or in the appreciation of poetry, both highly demanding forms of thinking. A symbol by definition need have no relation to what it represents and strictly obeys Fodor and Pylyshyn's compositionality principle (see Section 3.7). However the representations used in human thought are semantically 'rich' (Doumas & Hummel, 2005). In *he buckled the belt* and *Orion's belt,* the same entity is referred to in the two expressions but the aspects that are present in thought do not strictly obey compositionality; they are not identical. In the concept of a cognitive computational engine we assume that the representations processed need to be conceived of as having properties redolent of wave-particle duality, complementarity, in having both symbolic and semantically rich properties.

We consider the three basic aspects of the cognitive computational engine in this and the following two chapters. They will be followed by chapters on Supervisory System processes, episodic memory, thinking and on consciousness, where additional highly specific properties are added on to the cognitive computational engine. We argue that these processing domains relate to the modulatory functions referred to earlier; they concern a variety of special types of processes which are held to modulate in a top-down fashion the operation of the basic computational cognitive engine.

6.2 The Term: Putting the Flesh on the Symbol

The limiting nature of the Newell–Simon approach is apparent when one considers the basic element or representation which is transformed by a process, the symbol. What is this *symbol* according to Newell? The key aspect for him is that it provides access to the outputs of operations carried out elsewhere (in time or space) in the system (see e.g. Figure 6.1). This is indeed a key aspect of the elements which the cognitive computational engine transforms by means of operations. However it has three types of limitation.

The first is that even to carry out this type of function the symbol needs to be somewhat more complex. Thus, in many programming languages, including COGENT, discussed in Section 3.6, we have a richer computational vocabulary, which is entirely compatible with the physical symbol system approach. In COGENT, the system has a variety of cognitive elements, representations capable of being held in working memory and, in particular, in taking different logical roles in cognitive operations. These include numbers, atoms (i.e. symbols with no internal structure),

is considered to be internal to the machine and so is not a physical symbol system.

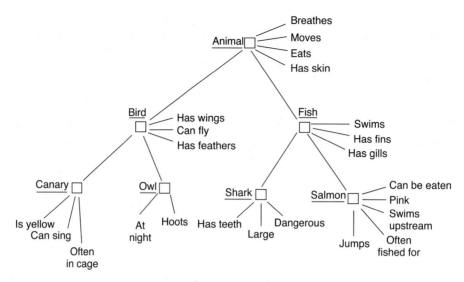

Fig. 6.2 A semantic network, in the style of Collins and Quillian (1969).

variables, compound terms and lists.[3] Moreover, as we will see, such an elaboration has brain-based consequences. Thus from the brain-based point of view numbers, say, have a different material basis from other types of cognitive atoms (see Section 3.4). In addition, the difference between numbers and other types of cognitive atom has a clear logical basis, and so numbers would form a natural subtype of symbol in a physical symbol system. Indeed, many of the cognitive atoms in the COGENT sense may themselves be divided into different types having as different a material basis as each does from number. Therefore each would thus carry with it a different type of conceptual implication.

Second, a somewhat related issue is whether the same cognitive atom may be known in more than one type of format (see Caramazza et al., 1990; Shallice, 1993). This could have conceptual consequences. What, for instance, is the relation between how we understand the word *ball* and what happens when we realise we are seeing *a ball*? Are the representations the same or are they separate but linked? In linguistics both views are represented; for instance, by Fodor et al. (1975) and Jackendoff (1987) on the one hand, and by Katz (1980) on the other. There is a similar split among psychologists with a unitary view having been upheld by Pylyshyn (1973) after Paivio (1971, 1986) had initially proposed a dual-code hypothesis.

The third question is how adequate is it to view the representation as a discrete entity, a conceptual atom. For certain theorists the relation between atoms may be carried by entities like the meaning postulates of Carnap (1947) and Fodor (1975), such as a *if X is a tiger then X is a mammal* or *if X is a bachelor then X is an unmarried man*. From this perspective, Newell (1990) says 'when processing "The cat is on the mat" ... the local computation at some point encounters "cat"; it must go from "cat" to a body of (encoded) knowledge associated with "cat" and bring back something that represents that a cat is being referred to, that the word "cat" is a noun (and perhaps other possibilities), and so on' (p. 74). Yet nowhere in Newell's major work *Unified Theories of Cognition* (1990) is there any real account of what information about *cat* other than 'noun-ness' is brought back.

Within linguistics and psychology there have been different approaches to how to characterise conceptual atoms, such as the semantic content of words. A few theorists, such as Fodor (2000), argue that there are no in principle objections to viewing the mind as a system in which the operations of all more central modules are characterisable by purely syntactic operations as in Newell's approach. Similarly, the links in a semantic network postulated by Collins and Quillian (1969) (see Figure 6.2) may be thought of as allowing the relation between words, say *tiger* and *mammal* or *unmarried man* and *bachelor* to be implemented by symbolic operations. Jackendoff (1987) refers to this type of approach as utilising a *deductive* strategy.

An alternative approach to the deductive strategy approach is to view the understanding of *tiger* as involving decomposition of the atom into elements of meaning. The earliest decompositional theory was that of Katz and Fodor (1963), which attempted to build the

---

[3] The set of primitives derives from the AI programming language PROLOG, mainly used in Europe and Japan, which is related in many ways to LISP, still primarily used in North America, which was itself stimulated by the early work of Newell and Simon.

meaning of a sentence by combining the semantic features of each unit in the sentence in accordance with the syntactic operations.[4] Later psychological theories of this type were those of Rips et al. (1973) and Smith and Medin (1981), and the approach has since then been widely used by connectionist modellers.[5]

Viewed more widely, if we consider language, then the inadequacy of treating words as conceptual atoms was exposed by Wittgenstein (1953) in *Philosophical Investigations*, which now provides the intellectual foundations for many post-modern philosophical approaches. At the very least it seems attractive to conceive of word meaning as something that, in addition to what one might call its symbolic aspects, needs to be represented in a high-dimensional space, which contains a distance metric.[6]

We address, in due course, each of these three possible ways in which the Newell-type symbol may be enriched. As we will move towards the position that in all three respects the symbol concept is unnecessarily restricted, we will use the less contentious if vaguer term *representation*—a term that, it will be argued, should be understood as having complementarily both symbolic and rich semantic properties. We begin however by considering the neural basis of representations.

6.3 The Selective Loss of Semantic Representations

Conceptual atoms or representations, as we are calling them, play two types of role with respect to operations. In the presence of the appropriate motivation they can help to elicit an operation. A red light leads to braking, a written word leads to reading. We will use the term 'trigger' for this role, and discuss it further in Chapter 9. The other role is that they can fill slots in how an operation is effected. When you pass a plate or add two

numbers, the mental equivalent of the operands are representations. Following the terminology of logic and computer science we will call them the *arguments* of the operation.

Considering the enormous range of motor and cognitive operations we can carry out there are many types of representations that can be used as arguments. However in many cases there are a number of levels of representations, two of which in particular are important. The first is the type of representation that categorises the perceptual input as an example of one of a set of known possibilities. The second allows access to links with the many different types of information known about the conceptual atom. Loosely, one is pre-semantic and the other is semantic.

An example of this difference in the domain of object recognition is Marr's (1982) distinction between the structural description and the semantic representation of the object. This is mirrored in Warrington's (1982) distinction between a perceptual categorisation stage of object recognition and a visual semantic one, which she holds to be manifest when damaged in apperceptive and associative agnosia, respectively.[7] In word representation, beginning with Morton's (1969) logogen model, virtually all models allow for different level representations at the orthographic and phonological levels on the one hand from the semantic level itself. In face recognition the same type of distinction exists in the classical Bruce and Young (1986) model (see Figure 6.3), which distinguishes a *face recognition unit*, which merely categorises a face as being a specific learned one, and a *person identity node*, which adds the knowledge about the person whose face it is. The separation of these systems is well supported by both neuropsychological and functional imaging evidence;[8] they lie in the lateral fusiform part of the temporal lobe and the anterior temporal lobe, respectively, predominantly in the right hemisphere (see Figure 6.4) (Haxby et al., 2000). Even in colour processing one can distinguish between pre-semantic systems in ventral area V4 or the nearby V8 where lesions give rise to the loss of the sensation of colour, achromatopsia, and systems in which the knowledge of an object's colour is realised (see Luzzatti & Davidoff, 1994).

In all these cases except one, the function carried out by the earlier system is to categorise the input as a particular one of a learned set or to fail to categorise it,

---

[4] Fodor (1975) himself later abandoned this approach in favour of atomic meanings for each word and meaning postulates allowing relations between words to be derived.

[5] For an excellent review see Harley (2008).

[6] Somewhat related to this perspective, there is increasing evidence from psycholinguistics that, even as apparently an autonomous process as parsing a sentence involves the parallel operation of different types of *constraint*—syntactic, semantic, discourse and frequency-based. In particular, when multiple syntactic interpretations of a sentence are possible, semantic factors are used on-line to select between them (e.g. Altmann et al., 1992; Trueswell & Tanenhaus, 1994; for review see Harley, 2008). Harley considers both parallel constraint-satisfaction models of sentential parsing and serial two-stage models. In the former semantics and syntax interact from the start of processing but in the latter only at the second stage. Harley's view is that currently the psycholinguistic evidence is compatible with both theoretical approaches.

---

[7] See FNMS chapter 8 but note that Farah (1990) gives the two clinical terms somewhat different processing referents. Although in the latter case the assumptions about underlying subsystems are equivalent to the current one.

[8] See Section 4.10 for discussion of aspects of prosopagnosia, the selective loss of the ability to recognise faces.

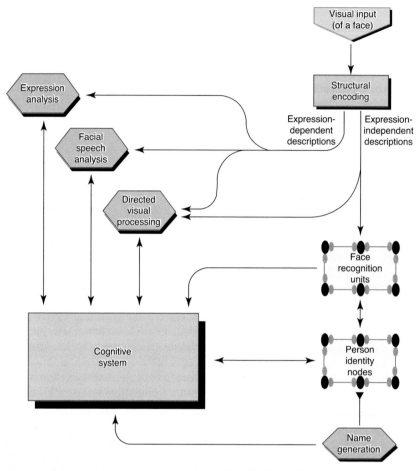

Fig. 6.3 The Bruce–Young model of face recognition. Structural encoding yields two forms of representation (expression-dependent and expression-independent), which are the inputs to the other processes within the model.

which implies that it is unknown.[9] The function of the second system related to semantics is more complex. In linguistics, semantics contrasts as a domain of language processing and competence with the domains of syntax, morphology, phonology and pragmatics. However, after the comparisons drawn between episodic and semantic memory by Tulving and Donaldson (1972), which were discussed in Section 2.2, the term has been used more widely in cognitive neuroscience to refer to the processes underlying other forms of knowledge too. 'Semantics' is thus a very slippery term with different but overlapping senses in different disciplines.

What is the neurobiological basis of semantics? The initial step was taken by Warrington (1975), who described three patients in the early stage of a dementing disease. The cognitive abilities of two of the patients, AB and EM, were in many respects well-preserved. Thus they had IQs of 122 and 117, respectively. Moreover, most critically, in

addition to their intact problem-solving and reasoning, tests showed that their pre-semantic levels of perceptual processing and also language operations involving syntax, orthography and phonology were all well-preserved.[10] So was episodic (autobiographical) memory.[11] However the knowledge that the patients had of everyday things was selectively grossly impaired. This was true whether the item was presented visually or verbally. Thus when pictures of two objects, such as a *needle* and a *trumpet*, or of two animals were presented and the patient was asked to point to one of them by name, e.g. *needle*, AB made 60% errors and EM 38%. Warrington also reported a dissociation within tests of knowledge. The patients were reasonably good at making a decision on the superordinate category in which a concept should

---

[9] This does not apply in the colour case where the representation is a position in a continuous multi-dimensional space.

[10] The same degree of detailed testing of atypical non-semantic representations discussed in Section 4.8 in the context of the Patterson et al. (2006) study was not carried out. Such effects of typicality would probably have been found but may be viewed as second-order ones.

[11] See FNMS Section 12.3 for further details.

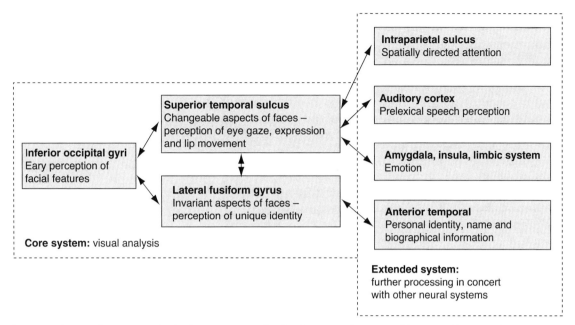

Fig. 6.4 Localisation of processes involved in face recognition isolated in the Bruce and Young model. Reprinted from *Trends in Cognitive Sciences*, *4*(6), J.V. Haxby, E.A. Hoffman and M.I. Gobbini, The distributed human system for face recognition, 223–233. Copyright (2000), with permission from Elsevier.

be placed, e.g. is a *cabbage* an *animal,* a *plant* or an *inanimate object*? In this test, EM made only 2% errors. If, however, they were asked about any specific attribute, e.g. is a *cabbage green, brown,* or *grey*, they were far worse; in this case EM made 28% errors.

Theoretically, Warrington drew upon the contrast between episodic and semantic memory, which had been articulated just before. She argued that her patients had a selective deficit of semantic memory. That there are such highly selective deficits of semantic memory is now standardly accepted (see e.g. Hodges et al., 1994). Indeed, in Chapter 4 we have already referred to the existence of the condition. One reason why the characterisation has been accepted is that it fits well with developments in the more clinical analysis of the syndrome. Thus, within the clinical literature, from a behavioural prespective, the term *primary progressive aphasia* was introduced by Mesulam (1982), building on a long neurological history going back to the early twentieth-century Czech neurologist, Arnold Pick, to describe a dementing illness which specifically affected language functions.[12] From an anatomical perspective, the term *fronto-temporal dementia* is now also used to describe the condition; fronto-temporal dementia often runs in families (Chow et al., 1999;

Spilantini et al., 1998) and differs markedly from standard manifestations of Alzheimer's disease in the way it presents (Bozeat et al., 2000). Most patients with fronto-temporal dementia are non-fluent, but there is a fluent subgroup who have been referred to as suffering from 'semantic dementia' (Snowden et al., 1989; Hodges et al., 1992; Gorno-Tempini et al., 2004). Patients with semantic dementia present as suffering from a selective loss of semantic memory (see Murre et al., 2001).

It can be argued that if the neuropathological characterisation of the dementing patient does not unequivocally determine that they have a dementia of the primary progressive aphasic type, let alone a semantic dementia, then the assignment of the patient to the clinical category is insufficiently rigorous. Indeed in a study of 18 clinically defined semantic dementia patients, Davies et al. (2005) found them to include patients who from a pathological perspective had motor neuron disease, Pick's disease and Alzheimer's disease. This heterogeneity could have major implications if the arguments about neuropsychological methodology in Chapter 4 are applied. If the criteria for assigning a patient to the semantic dementia category are not clear-cut than the methodology of the case series approach discussed in Chapter 4 is undermined.

Pragmatically the situation is more satisfactory. Thus Gorno-Tempini et al. (2004) studied 31 patients with fronto-temporal dementia. They were divided using standard clinical procedures into three groups—semantic dementia, non-fluent progressive aphasia,

---

[12] In fact patients with the classical neuropathological markers of Pick's disease are only a subset of those currently classified as exhibiting primary progressive aphasia (see Hodges & Miller, 2001a).

TABLE 6.1 Comparison of semantic dementia patients with two other sub-groups of fronto-temporal dementia patients (data from Gorno-Tempini et al., 2004; table 2, p. 339). All figures are percentage correct. 'Pyramids and Palm Trees' (Howard & Patterson, 1992) is a widely used inference test depending on knowledge of word or picture meanings. Thus the patient must say whether *pyramid* goes with *palm tree* or *pine tree*. 'Repetition' is a Western Aphasia Battery subtest.

	SD (n=10)	NFPA (n=11)	LPA (n=10)	Controls
Semantically Based				
Word Picture Matching	81[abc]	100	98	100
Naming	17[ab]	83	50[a]	?
'Pyramids & Palm Trees'	68[abc]	95	90	100
Phonological Production				
Speech Fluency	89[b]	54[a]	80[a]	100
'Repetition'	85	65[a]	72[a]	100
Syntactic Comprehension	91[c]	86	74[a]	100

[a] Indicates significantly less than controls.

[b] Indicates that the semantic dementia patients are significantly different from the non-fluent patients.

[c] Indicates that they are significantly different from the logopenic group. SD = Semantic Dementia. NFPA (Non-Fluent Progressive Aphasia), LPA (Logopenic Progressive Aphasia).

characterised by laboured articulation and agrammatism, and logopenic progressive aphasia, where the patient tends to produce slow syntactically simple sentences with frequent word-finding pauses. Behaviourally the distinction is clear (see Table 6.1). For all tests involving semantic processing, the semantic dementia group performed much worse than either of the other groups; by contrast tests involving fluent production or syntax but not semantics were better carried out by the semantic dementia patients than by one or other of the other two subgroups. Critically, there was also a difference in the areas of greatest atrophy (see Figure 6.5). The semantic dementia group had greater loss in the bilateral anterior temporal lobes confirming previous studies (e.g. Mummery et al., 2000; Chan et al., 2001). More specifically, Davies et al. (2005) have identified perirhinal cortex and posterior parahippocampal cortex as the most severely damaged regions of the anterior temporal cortex in semantic dementia. Thus the group is both anatomically and functionally specific.

That patients exist with selective deficits of semantic memory is therefore now well-accepted.[13] Thus semantic dementia seems to have the potential to localise semantic memory processes. One could then see whether the same localisation is obtained as for functional imaging of semantic processes in normal subjects, the methodology proposed in the last chapter. It would however be premature to move directly into this comparison. It is possible that the problems that semantic dementia patients have in semantic memory tasks do not result from damage to the representations in some semantic store. They may instead reflect problems in, say, access to it. One must first functionally characterise a disorder before it is useful to localise it for theoretical purposes. The detour is quite extended!

6.4 Contrasting Impairments of Semantics

In 1979 Warrington and Shallice compared the original three semantic dementia patients described earlier by Warrington (1975) with a different type of patient whose difficulty involved semantics. They argued that the original patients, who would now be described as suffering from semantic dementia, had a *degraded store* impairment. By contrast a further patient, AR, whose reading they described, was held to have a *semantic access* deficit. This contrast has been much more solidly established by studies of Warrington and McCarthy (1983, 1987), Cipolotti and Warrington (1995b), Warrington and Crutch (2004) and in particular Warrington and Cipolotti (1996). In these studies, however, it is held that the so-called 'access' problem actually arises in these patients from the storage system becoming refractory after the previous item has been retrieved.

Warrington and Shallice initially proposed four behavioural criteria for differentiating between degraded store and access deficits—they related to (i) effects of word frequency, (ii) the consistency of responding for a given item, (iii) the susceptibility to cueing from a semantically related word, and (iv) depth of processing, namely what type of information could be accessed if the word could not be properly identified. Warrington and McCarthy (1983) added a fifth criterion, how semantic identification is affected by presentation rate, and Cipolotti and Warrington (1995b) added two more, the effect of the semantic relatedness within a superordinate category, and whether the patient shows

---

[13] Indeed other dementing patients—particularly many with Alzheimer's disease—appear to have a related problem, except that it is compounded by additional difficulties in episodic memory (e.g. Martin & Fedio, 1983; Chertkow & Bub, 1990).

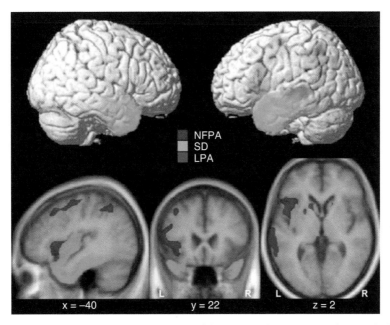

Fig. 6.5 Areas of significant atrophy in three groups of aphasic patients (when compared with 10 age- and sex-matched controls): non-fluent progressive aphasics (NFPA, *n* = 11), semantic dementia patients (SD, *n* = 10) and logopenic progressive aphasics (LPA, *n* = 10). Reprinted with permission from M.L. Gorno-Tempini, N.F. Dronkers, K.P. Rankin, J.M. Ogar, La Phengrasamy, H.J. Rosen, J.K. Johnson, M.W. Weiner and B.L. Miller (2004) From Cognition and anatomy in three variants of primary progressive aphasia. *Annals of Neurology, 55*(3), 335–346. Copyright © 2004, John Wiley and Sons.

a serial position effect with performance deteriorating through a block of trials (see Table 6.2). The access/refractory patients have also tended to have different aetiologies from the degraded store patients—the former type of deficit typically arises from the presence

of a cyst, a vascular difficulty or a tumour by comparison with a dementing illness such as semantic dementia for the latter type (see Warrington & Cipolotti, 1996; Campanella et al., 2009).

Rapp and Caramazza (1993), in a sweeping critique, rejected the distinction between semantic access and semantic degradation disorders as neither theoretically nor empirically well-founded. From a theoretical perspective they argued that the clinical empirical effects observed were not theoretically derived from the claimed basic cognitive impairments—damage to the stored representations versus access to them—using a 'fully-worked-out theory'. This they argued prevented the theories being properly evaluated using 'the putatively relevant evidence'. This became a potentially potent objection when combined with their second line of argument. They pointed out that the claimed criteria for distinguishing storage and access deficits had not at that time been applied consistently to any set of patients. Particular criteria had been applied to contrasts between individual patients, but that there were two contrasting patterns was, they argued, far from a clearly substantiated empirical phenomenon. This was an appropriate criticism of the earlier studies.

The critique of Rapp and Caramazza was made passé by the study of Warrington and Cipolotti (1996). They took four dementing patients with a similar pattern of difficulties. Their performance on a series of tests on their knowledge of words and everyday things was compared

TABLE 6.2	Characteristics held to distinguish semantic degradation and access/refractory disorders introduced by Warrington and Shallice (1979)[1], Warrington and McCarthy (1983, 1987)[2], Warrington and Cipolotti (1996)[3]. Susceptibility to cueing implies that a word is more likely to be processed correctly if preceded by a semantically related word; this criterion was not used in the later papers. Depth of processing refers to whether judgements about stimulus attributes are performed less well than judgements about superordinate categories.

	Semantic Degradation	Access/Refractory
Effect of Word Frequency[1]	Strong	Weak
Consistency[1]	High	Low
Susceptibility to Cueing[1]	None	Considerable
Depth of Processing[1]	Strong	Weak
Presentation Rate[2]	None	Considerable
Semantic Relatedness[3]	Weak	Strong

TABLE 6.3 Performance of four semantic dementia patients (S1-4) and two auditory semantic access patients (A1-2) (data from Warrington & Cipolotti, 1996).

	Rate of Presentation		Word Frequency		Semantic Relatedness		Serial Position Effect
	Fast	Slow	Low	High	Close	Distant	
S1	67	69	39	96**	69	65	NS
S2	63	66	42	87**	68	61	NS
S3	64	69	40	92**	59	74*	NS
S4	63	69	36	97**	67	69	NS
A1	49	73**	60	62	48	74**	p < 0.0001
A2	58	76*	70	64	60	75*	NS

NS: Not significant;

*$p < 0.01$;

**$p < 0.001$.

with that of two patients with a putative semantic access disorder. One had had a stroke, the second had had a tumour. The basic task used was picture-word matching. Four pictures are presented to the patients, all of them items in the same category, say four animals. A series of words is then presented, each occurring four times, but in a randomised order. The patient is required merely to point to the picture representing the word.

Three categories were used—objects, animals and foods. But for each category there were four different arrays, two levels of each of two factors being employed—frequency (high vs low) and the semantic relatedness of the set (close vs distant). Thus for the animals the high frequency closely semantically related set was *rabbit, donkey, cow* and *lamb* and the array with the completely complementary properties was *koala, shrimp, bison, walrus*. In addition the words were presented either at a fast rate with only one second between the patient's response and the next word or at a slow rate with the interval being 15 sec. The latter was *very* boring for the experimenter and subject alike. Each combination was presented three times to the patient.

The results were clear (see Table 6.3). The semantic dementia patients were *all* strongly affected by word frequency but not by semantic relatedness or speed of presentation. They did not show a serial position effect. For *both* of the putative access patients all the effects were just the opposite.[14] In addition, the semantic dementia patients were highly consistent in their performance across multiple presentations, as the earlier semantic dementia patients had been, while the access disorder patients were completely inconsistent across different presentations of the same stimulus.

The study, using five of the criteria shown in Table 6.2, establishes that there are indeed two very distinct patterns of impairments which affect the semantic system. Rapp and Caramazza's criticism of the empirical foundation of the storage/access distinction was severely undermined.[15] It could still be argued, that the 'semantic access' functional syndrome rests too heavily on selected individual cases. However, Campanella et al. (2010) using the case series methodology have shown that posterior superior temporal lobe tumours give rise to a pattern of difficulty in word-picture matching of an access type. Such patients are highly inconsistent in the words to which they respond correctly, and show no frequency effect but a strong semantic relatedness effect. Unlike most of the semantic access patients described as individual cases, though, they were not affected by rate-of-presentation.

Considering specifically semantic dementia patients, they are highly consistent across stimuli in terms of whether they can identify an item satisfactorily or not; this was first shown by Coughlan and Warrington (1981). In addition, whether an item has been retained in the store is highly dependent upon its frequency of occurrence. These two characteristics fit with what one would expect from a storage impairment. Critically, too, the selectivity of the semantic deficit which is characteristic of the early stages of semantic dementia provides us with a functional syndrome which, because of its relative purity, is a clear candidate for modelling.

---

[14] Except that patient A2 did not show a serial position effect.

[15] This still leaves unresolved the 'mixed' patients, such as KE (Hillis et al., 1990), who show high levels of consistency but no effects of word frequency. Notably both were stroke patients. If there is no additional localisation constraint, then it is our view that having a stroke *per se* is unlikely to lead to a specific functional syndrome, but see Jefferies and Lambon-Ralph (2006), to be discussed in Section 6.6, for a somewhat different view.

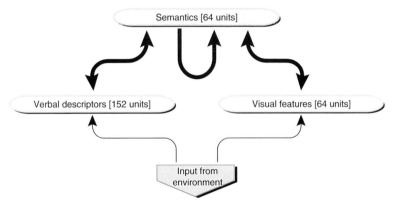

Fig. 6.6 The architecture of semantic cognition explored by Rogers et al (2004). The bank of verbal descriptor units consist of 40 name units, 64 perceptual units, 32 functional units and 16 encyclopedic units.

The access deficit tends to occur in more generally impaired patients; but the set of characteristics that patients of this type have in common is also a candidate for modelling.

6.5 Models of Disorders of Semantics

No model yet explains all aspects of the semantic dementia syndrome. However a promising beginning has been made. Rogers et al. (2004) trained a simple connectionist network (see Figure 6.6) in which semantic units were bi-directionally connected to verbal descriptor units and visual feature units. The model used a feature-based representation of semantics similar to that discussed in Section 4.10 (the model of Plaut and Shallice, 1993a), in which objects have a variety of different types of properties. Indeed the model is analogous to the Plaut and Shallice model with two input streams. One input stream is from verbal descriptors, the other from visual features. As far as the verbal descriptors are concerned, Rogers et al. divided the properties that concrete objects have into four types—perceptual characteristics (e.g. *has eyes, has wheels*), functional ones (e.g. *can fly, can roll*), encyclopaedic (*lives in Africa, found in the kitchen*) and name information.[16] In addition, the semantic units were connected to visual feature units; the representations of the set of objects across these units retained their actual visual similarity, as assessed by the number of visual features two objects have in common. Rogers et al. also followed Tyler and Moss

(2001), Garrard et al. (2001) and McRae and Cree (2002) in distinguishing between features that are shared with other items (like the number of legs an elephant has) and features that are distinctive to the item (like an elephant's trunk): 64 items—32 animals and 32 artefacts—were selected and ratings of the verbal and visual features obtained from normal subjects.

The network was trained by being presented repeatedly with the name, the visual pattern or the verbal attribution—the set of verbal perceptual, functional and encyclopaedic features—for each of 48 stimuli constructed with similar featural properties to those of the original 64 items. The model then settled for 7 time-steps, as in the Plaut and Shallice model, and the weights were then adjusted to improve performance by a small amount. After the model had learnt, lesions were made by removing connections, either inputs or outputs of the semantic system or ones internal to the semantic system. For a given proportion of connections lesioned, the responses of the model were classified as correct or as superordinate errors, semantic errors, cross-domain errors or omission errors. The results were compared with the average performance of 15 semantic dementia patients in whom naming performance had been studied as it deteriorated over time, a standard characteristic of a dementing illness (see Figure 6.7). The similarity seems remarkable. A number of other characteristics of semantic dementia were also simulated, such as ones which could be assumed to rely on accessing visual units, such as in the tasks of delayed copying and drawing.

How can we assess this simulation? First, the model is a toy model; it represents only a small part of the semantic system of a typical subject, but we have earlier argued that this is not a critical objection. Second, while the occurrence of semantic and, in particular, superordinate errors is a very well established part of the functional syndrome (Warrington, 1975; Hodges et al., 1995), Tyler et al. (2004b) have shown in a functional imaging study to be discussed in Section 6.8 that

---

[16] For a more detailed analysis of the different types of properties of objects see McRae and Cree (2002). The way Rogers et al. characterise functional features across both living things and artefacts in terms of an abstract property of the object (e.g. an *eagle* can *fly*) is neuropsychologically dubious (see Section 6.10). What tends to be neuropsychologically critical is whether the object has a function for a potential human agent. The *flying* of an *eagle* does not, although it does for the eagle!

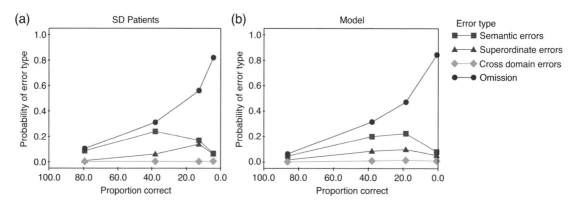

Fig. 6.7 Picture-naming errors averaged over longitudinal data from 15 semantic dementia patients (a) and the Rogers et al. model with lesions to between 10% and 35% of connections (b). Copyright © 2004 by the American Psychological Association. Adapted with permission. T.T. Rogers, M.A. Lambon Ralph, P. Garrard, S. Bozeat, J.L. McClelland, J.R. Hodges and K. Patterson (2004). Structure and deterioration of semantic memory: A neuropsychological and computational investigation, *Psychological Review*, *111*(1), 205–235. The use of APA information does not imply endorsement by APA.

in object perception, superordinate naming activates somewhat more posterior structures earlier in the ventral route, than item naming. They argue that complex conjunctive combinations of features are required for the latter process but not the former and that these conjunctive combinations are more anteriorly located. This pattern of localisations would generally fit with the assumptions of the Rogers et al. model, but the Tyler et al. study suggests that preservation of the superordinate might not be one of the characteristics of the syndrome that the model needs to explain. At the same time similar effects of superordinate knowledge occur in semantic dementia when words are presented (see Warrington, 1975), so an account of superordinate-preservation when subordinate characteristics are lost simply in terms of anatomical differentiation of the systems necessary for the two types of process is unlikely to provide a complete explanation.

The model was also given the task of sorting pictures or words into general categories—animal or man-made—and more specifically for an artefact whether it was a vehicle, household object or tool.[17] Unfortunately the model did relatively less well with words than with pictures (see Figure 6.8). Thus the model's simulation for pictures of the superordinate-preservation phenomenon is a valuable feature. However, given the lower adequacy of the model for words, and the failure to use

the same categories for model and patients, the fits are less impressive than they initially seem.

The authors go on to draw two strong conclusions from their modelling endeavour. First they argue that critical to the behaviour they observe is the attractor dynamics of the model which cause the representations of less typical items to migrate toward the centre of mass of similar items in their immediate neighbourhood in the multi-dimensional space of semantic representations. This effectively renders them more typical. 'Initially this collapse affects items with small well-separated clusters (such as the category of birds). As damage mounts these attractors will collapse into even more general states, which reflect the central tendency of a broader set of items' (pp. 229–230) This is just the type of effect obtained by Patterson et al. (2006) in a variety of cognitive domains, as discussed in Section 4.8 (see also Patterson, 2007). In other words, as in deep dyslexia with the model of Plaut–Shallice discussed in Chapter 4, we are seeing in this model of semantic dementia evidence for the theoretical assumption of the existence of attractor-based distributed networks. With the caveats mentioned above this seems a justifiable conclusion.

In addition, though, the authors claim that the results support another assumption of their model—that there is a unitary semantic system. No argument is presented as to why the effects obtained would not occur with a more complex internal structure to the semantic system especially as the effects arise by disconnecting it from other systems with which it has bi-directional links. Moreover no attempt is made to model patients who have so-called modality-specific and category-specific effects, to be discussed later. As critical a problem is that, while many aspects of the representation of each object in the stimulus set are carefully obtained from a property-generation study of normal subjects (Garrard et al.,

---

[17] Somewhat bizarrely the patients did not have the identical set of specific categories, tools being replaced by musical instruments. This is doubly unfortunate as in category specific disorders, to be discussed shortly, musical instruments behave differently from other man-made objects (see e.g. Warrington & Shallice, 1984).

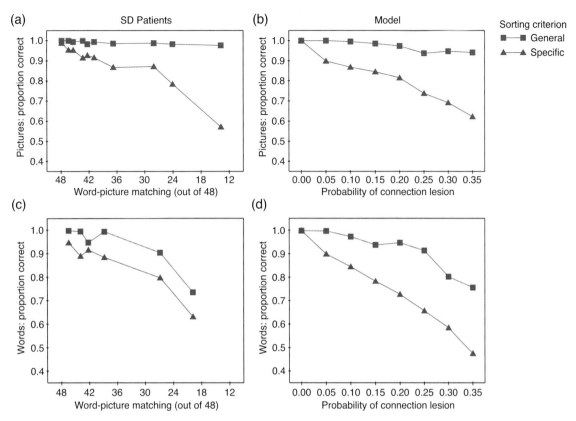

Fig. 6.8 Average sorting accuracy for picture and word stimuli for the semantic dementia patients of Rogers et al (2004) (a, c) and for their model (b, d). Copyright © 2004 by the American Psychological Association. Adapted with permission. T.T. Rogers, M.A. Lambon Ralph, P. Garrard, S. Bozeat, J.L. McClelland, J.R. Hodges and K. Patterson (2004). Structure and deterioration of semantic memory: A neuropsychological and computational investigation, *Psychological Review*, *111*(1), 205–235. The use of APA information does not imply endorsement by APA.

2001), the equally important quantitative aspects of the model—the number of units for each type—is apparently arbitrary. We have no way of judging to what extent the attractive fit comes from a highly specific set of numerical assumptions which are never justified. For instance, increasing the number of units in the semantic layer while keeping the other layers the same might well considerably change the quantitative predictions illustrated in Figure 6.7.[18] This is a serious methodological difficulty with the work and make this theoretical generalisations from the model to a single semantic memory system much less convincing than its support for the utility of attractor representations of concepts.

Despite the apparent success of the fit of the simulations, the assumptions made in the modelling jar with two very different aspects of the syndrome being modelled. First, semantic dementia is a condition in which the anterior temporal lobes atrophy severely. To simulate it as a so-called 'disconnection syndrome', as the authors do, appears to fly in the face of pathology. It is especially odd as much the same set of authors had themselves earlier modelled semantic dementia by ablating a certain proportion of semantic units by clamping them to zero (Lambon-Ralph et al., 2001).[19]

---

[18] To give a more specific example, the increase in omission errors in the model as proportion correct decreases is relatively easily engineered. An omission occurs when no name unit exceeds a threshold of 0.5, but the use of this particular threshold is not explained. Changing it will change the shape of the omission curve. Since the sum of the error types must be 1.0 when the proportion correct is zero, the increase in omissions necessarily pushes all the other error types down.

[19] A functional imaging study of semantic dementia patients has been titled 'disrupted temporal lobe connections to semantic dementia' (Mummery et al., 1999). However, the more detailed claim of the authors is that regions involved in naming, held to be the left posterior inferior temporal gyrus (BA37), are not activated. On this more specific conclusion the evidence does not speak to whether semantic dementia arises from a problem in a store or due to disconnections to or from it. Either position would predict the results.

TABLE 6.4 Effects of different forms of damage on the encoding of exceptions and generalisation performance on a variety of three layer feed-forward networks (see Figure 4.2). The 9-100-9 network had 9 input and output units which used localist coding and 100 hidden units. The 36-100-36 network had 36 input and output units and used distributed coding. The 36-600-36 network was similar but with 600 hidden units. The reading model network was that of Bullinaria (1994). (Data from Bullinaria & Chater, 1995.)

Form of damage	Network Type	Exceptions Lost (Mean)	Generalisations Lost (Mean)
Removal of connections	9-100-9	52.1	7.2
	36-100-36	82.0	2.9
	36-600-36	91.5	2.1
	Reading model	32.0	7.5
Removal of hidden units	9-100-9	31.3	7.2
	36-100-36	24.7	11.6
	36-600-36	31.0	11.2
	Reading model	26.9	5.5

Fortunately computational help could be at hand. A plausible assumption is that if one lesions a connectionist net by ablating a certain proportion of neurons in a layer, then this is roughly equivalent, qualitatively and quantitatively, to lesioning a (potentially different) proportion of the connections to and from the layer. Hinton and Shallice (1991) examined the effects of both disconnections and ablations in a feed-forward plus clean-up network, like the 40-60 net shown top left in Figure 4.21. For lesions to both the 40 intermediate units and the 60 clean-up units, the rate of production of different types of errors generally lay intermediate between the effects of disconnecting the set of hidden units from the systems before and after it. However, in potential conflict with this conclusion, Bullinaria and Chater (1995) using a single three-layer feed-forward network, as discussed in Section 4.3, found that removing connections led to a clear loss of exceptions as opposed to generalisations; a typicality effect analogous to that which Rogers et al. require, but this was less clear with removal of hidden units (see Table 6.4). Rogers et al. justify their lesion method by merely stating somewhat blandly 'To simulate cortical atrophy … we simply removed an increasing proportion of all the

weights in the model, a choice motivated by the fact that all weights are either intrinsic to the semantic layer or project into or out of this layer' (p. 217). As over 75% of the connections are with the input/output layers their justification of the choice of lesioning is inadequate.[20]

6.6 Degraded Stores and Atoms of Meaning

A second problem for the Rogers et al. model concerns a very different aspect of semantic dementia: the high levels of consistency that relevant patients show in whether or not they can identify a word or a picture (Coughlan & Warrington, 1981; Warrington & Cipolotti, 1996). For another domain of processing—that of the output phonological lexicon—Howard (1995) argued that consistency of responding across testing sessions was best explained in terms not of distributed representations, but in a localist framework in which the individual lexical entries were either normally present or lost. There are, however, strong empirical arguments to prefer a distributed representation account within the domain of semantics. First, the model of Rogers et al., which gives such generally good fits to data, is based on the idea that meaning is decomposable into elements or features. Second, the major error types are the superordinate error and the semantic error. Take the superordinate error, which is, as we have seen, a very robust aspect of the behaviour of semantic dementia patients. The patient given a picture of a *tiger* or, more critically given the earlier arguments, its name, knows it is an animal but little else about it. A distributed account explains this in terms of a subset only of the elements being preserved, enough to identify the category but not the item itself. On the contrasting view of meaning we discussed in Section 6.2—the atomic view of representation—to know that a tiger is an animal one must use a meaning postulate. But why is just that meaning postulate preserved in semantic dementia, rather than, for instance, that it has stripes? We know of no account.

Or why does a semantic error occur? What meaning postulate should produce an identity transformation but when impaired instead comes up with a semantic associate? If these patients really have lost aspects of their semantic representations, the semantic representation

---

[20] In fact, according to Lambon-Ralph (personal communication), Rogers et al. obtained very similar results from lesioning units in their amodal semantic store to those obtained by disconnecting. They reported the disconnection findings as they were less noisy!

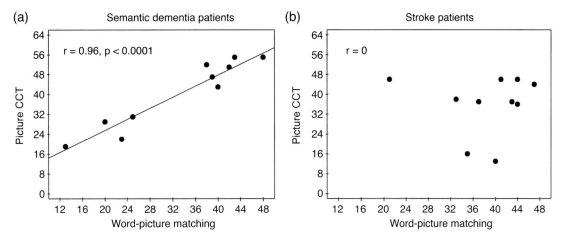

Fig. 6.9 Cross-task correlations between performance on a task of semantic association (the picture version of the Camel and Cactus Task, a test similar to the Pyramids and Palm Tree test (see text): Bozeat et al., 2000) and word-picture matching for samples of semantic dementia patients (a) and stroke patients (b). Reproduced from E. Jefferies and M.A. Lambon-Ralph, Semantic impairment in stroke aphasia versus semantic dementia: a case-series comparison, *Brain*, 2006, *129*(8), 2132–2147, by permission of Oxford University Press.

can hardly be atomic. Fodor claimed, in a discussion involving one of us, that what we learn of the brain has had no relevance for cognitive science. What we have learned from the brain seems to be that one of his core ideas is wrong!

If, however, we reject the localist, all-or-none account of semantic representations, this still leaves two problems. The first is why lesioning a distributed model should lead to a consistent pattern of performance for semantic dementia. Jefferies and Lambon-Ralph (2006) have shown, for instance, that this does not occur with an unselected group of stroke patients with semantic problems. Thus it is not an inherent consequence of having semantic problems when performance on one semantic task is compared with that of another. These authors took combinations of two tasks, which employed the same 64 concrete items, such as animal and household objects. For instance, one task could be word–picture matching and the other a relation of the Pyramids and Palm Trees Test.[21] The semantic dementia and the stroke patients behaved entirely differently (see Figure 6.9).[22] In this paper Jefferies and Lambon-Ralph (2006)

make a subtle shift of position from that taken by Rogers et al. two years before. They describe the Rogers et al. model, when referring to an amodal semantic store, as 'When *these units* or their connections are damaged, as they are in semantic dementia, then the core semantic representations become degraded'. We will shortly argue that when connections are damaged, access characteristics are observed. Consistency of performance across sessions, we suggest, depends upon the units in the storage system itself being damaged. However this remains to be demonstrated both empirically and computationally. Indeed, there is no source of potential variability in the Rogers et al. model; given an initial input the consequences are deterministic not stochastic so the model is incapable of confronting positively or negatively the issue of consistency. We will return to this point in the next section.

If we reject an entirely localist account of semantic representations, a second problem is that there seems to be a theoretical gap between distributed representations which semantic dementia suggests is the way that concepts are stored in the brain, on the one hand, and on the other, the conceptual atoms on which cognitive operations can be carried out so as to give entirely predictable results, i.e. Fodor and Pylyshyn's systematicity and compositionality (see Section 3.7). If a concept were to correspond just to a region in conceptual space with boundaries between the regions relating to neighbouring concepts, the system would not be very robust.

[21] In the Pyramids and Palm Trees Test of Howard and Patterson (1992), the subject must choose between a picture of a *palm tree* or a picture of a *pine tree* as to which goes best with a *pyramid*. Or the test can involve the equivalent word stimuli.

[22] Jefferies and Lambon-Ralph explain their findings with stroke patients in terms of loss of executive processes controlling semantic retrieval. However, no justification is given for considering the stroke patient group as consisting of a single functional syndrome. Indeed, their lesion sites were diverse. Instead they should serve merely as a control group to illustrate

the behavioural consistency of the semantic dementia group, and so echo the conclusions in this respect of Warrington and Cipolotti (1996).

Incidental changes—the state of arousal, the just preceding activity, time-of-day, degree of effort and many other variables—would tend to move the output of the process across a boundary. This would mean that an operation using an input at a particular point in semantic space would lead to different outcomes according to the state of hosts of these other variables. Compositionality and systematicity in Fodor and Pylyshyn's terms would be lost.

There is a possible way out of this problem, as discussed in Section 3.7, namely the assumption of attractors as the underpinnings of word meaning. Compositionality and systematicity relate to how the meanings of structures are built from substructures. If the lowest level representations are inherently variable, then it is unclear how the whole structure could respect such principles. The Rogers et al. network, however, has been trained to have a strong attractor structure. On an attractor framework, the output of any level of processing which has internally an attractor structure is from only a small subset of the total semantic space. The fixed points—the sinks of each basin of attraction corresponding to a particular learned item (see Figure 1.15)—are surrounded by an empty space of impossible outputs much like stars in the night sky; and the effects of the extra variables discussed above would be on the trajectory by which the sinks of the attractor basin are reached, not on the points of the semantic space that are eventually achieved. An attractor net, therefore, at least gives you a fixed, context independent, meaning for the lowest level representations. Compositionality and systematicity are not automatically excluded as possible ways in which the structure of the whole might be characterised.

And yet the argument in this last section is non-dialectical. The Wittgensteinian arguments of the beginning of this chapter have been forgotten. Compositionality applies to the meaning of words, but there are dimensions of word meaning which are not well captured by it. As we discussed earlier, a word like *belt* can have multiple analogical meanings. *Orion's belt* or the *beltway* around an American city are not materially graspable artefacts like a leather belt. Yet attractor nets of the types we have been considering can explain well analogical aspects of word meaning. Consider, as an example, the ability of such models to explain counter-intuitive phenomena relating to the speed of processing by normal subjects of such words having multiple related meanings. Rodd et al. (2002) have shown that whether words with multiple meanings are processed slower or faster than other words of similar frequency which have only a single core meaning depends on whether the multiple meanings are polysemously related, as in *belt*, or are unrelated homonyms, as in *bank*. Rodd et al. (2004) model this phenomenon in

terms of attractor nets with either a single broad attractor containing sub-attractors within it (Unambiguous Many Senses) or two unconnected attractors (Ambiguous Few Senses). In the latter case, settling into one of the attractors is slow, because of the competition between them; in the former case it is fast, because movement toward any one of the sub-attractors facilitates a generally correct trajectory in the semantic space (see Figure 6.10). Overall, returning to the Rogers et al. model, and considering both its positive aspects as well as its negative ones, it would be churlish not to accept that it represents an advance in our theoretical understanding of how the semantics of concrete items are implemented.

There is not a similarly convincing theoretical account for the complementary condition to semantic dementia, namely the semantic access disorder. Four different accounts have been put forward. The most detailed comes from an elegant model that gives flesh to the notion that representations become refractory, which has been developed by Gotts and Plaut (2002). In one major way this is a more complex model than those considered hereto; it involves neurophysiological assumptions about the operation of synapses within the context of an otherwise standard feed-forward connectionist model. Gotts and Plaut (2002) investigated a simple feed-forward model (see Figure 6.11) trained with the so-called back-propagation through time learning algorithm (see Sections 1.7 and 4.11).

The critical neurobiological assumption they made concerned so-called *synaptic depression*. When a presynaptic neuron in the cortex fires repeatedly, the rate of firing of the post-synaptic neuron decreases (Abbott et al., 1997). Recovery from synaptic depression typically takes 3–4 sec but complete recovery can take a minute or so (Finlayson & Cynader, 1995; Varela et al., 1999). It is known that the two neurotransmitters, acetylcholine and norepinephrin, have the effect of reducing neurotransmitter release at the synapse (e.g. Vidal & Changeux, 1993); this in turn should have the consequence of reducing the magnitude of the subsequent synaptic depression, since the supply of neurotransmitter will be less exhausted. The effect of the neuromodulators was simulated by Gotts and Plaut by changing the activation function of the units in their model; they changed the relation between the post-synaptic activity and the presynaptic input. To simulate an access deficit, they did this by reducing a neuromodulatory parameter, M, in the model (Figure 6.12); this led to greater synaptic depression and so the representations involved became refractory. With these assumptions they obtained a good account of both the semantic relatedness effect and the lack of a frequency effect (see e.g. Figure 6.13).

The Gotts and Plaut model has not gone unchallenged as an account of the semantic access patterns

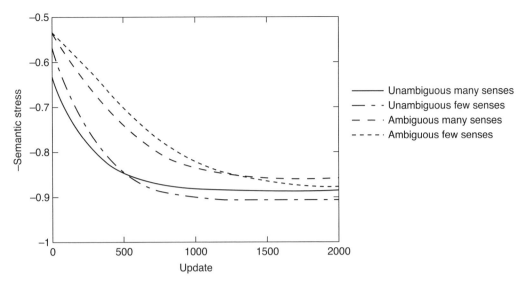

Fig. 6.10 Convergence of the model of Rodd et al (2004) during settling for different types of words. The vertical axis shows a measure of how close the activation in the semantic layer is to the local minimum within a basin of attraction while the horizontal axis shows the number of cycles since presentation. For words with a single core meaning (i.e. unambiguous) having many senses (e.g. *twist*—twist an ankle, twist the truth) tends to aid recognition, while ambiguity in words (e.g. *bark*—sound of a dog, surface covering of a tree) makes them harder. Different senses are encoded as random adjustment of a subset of features. Ambiguity is encoded as random set of semantic features for each meaning. Reproduced with permission from J.M. Rodd, M.G. Gaskell and W.D. Marslen-Wilson (2004) Modeling the effect of semantic ambiguity in word recognition. *Cognitive Science*, *28*(1), 89–104. John Wiley and Sons. © 2003 Cognitive Science Society, Inc.

of performance. Forde and Humphreys (2007) reject the idea that the pattern arises from representations becoming refractory. If this were the case they argue, one would expect that in multiple-choice word-to-picture matching a just preceding stimulus should be less likely to be selected as a response than a stimulus whose verbal label had not yet been presented. Instead they suggest an almost opposite explanation, namely that a preceding stimulus could have left an abnormally strong legacy—that *priming* processes to be discussed in the next chapter are exaggerated—and this in turn would produce a tendency to perseverate the preceding response. Ironically the idea that there is damage to the

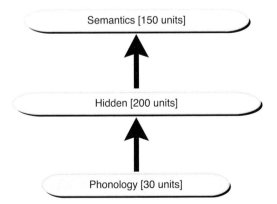

Fig. 6.11 The architecture of the three-layer feed-forward network used in the simulations of Gotts and Plaut (2002).

cholinergic input to the temporal lobe can be used to strengthen this account too. In Section 10.12, with respect to episodic memory, we apply the theory of Hasselmo and colleagues (e.g. Hasselmo et al., 1996) to the origin of what are called confabulations. Hasselmo et al.'s idea is that the cholinergic input to a system can act as a switch—when it is high, the system favours new input but when it is low, retrieval of previously processed information is favoured; in the present situation this would produce strong competing input at say a clean-up level from previously presented representations. In fact the errors of the semantic access patient, JM, of Forde and Humphreys favoured neither theory. In particular, when JM made an error he did not tend to point to the previously given stimulus, nor did he tend to point to a picture whose name was yet to be presented. He favoured the two possibilities at roughly the a priori chance. However, Campanella and Shallice (in press) produced an analogue of refractory semantic access disorder in normal subjects, and in this situation though, there is a significant tendency for error responses to be preceding stimuli and not still-to-be-presented ones. The issue is complex (see Gotts et al., 2002) and deserves more detailed empirical investigation.

To complicate matters further, the prototypic semantic access patients, e.g. VER of Warrington and McCarthy (1983), have had large left-hemisphere strokes with the territory of the middle cerebral artery gravely infarcted; this includes the likely site of the auditory word-form

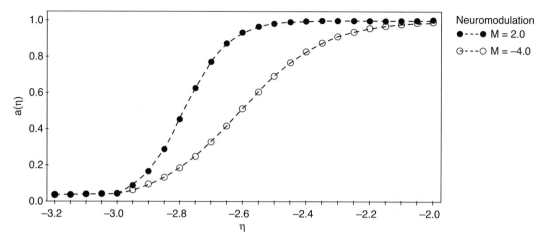

Fig. 6.12 Effects of neuromodulation on postsynaptic activity in the model of Gotts and Plaut (2002). η is the net input to a unit. Semantic access patients have low *M*, normal controls and semantic dementia patients higher *M*. Redrawn from S.J. Gotts and D.C. Plaut (2002) The impact of synaptic depression following brain damage: a connectionist account of 'access/refractory' and 'degraded-store' semantic impairments. *Cognitive, Affective, and Behavioral Neuroscience, 2*(3), 187–213.

area, near Wernicke's region in the superior left temporal lobe. Thus in a model of the word processing required in the word–picture matching task, such as that shown in Figure 6.11, one cannot plausibly assume that the input to the hidden units is normal; it is likely to be much weakened. Indeed one could explain the semantic relatedness effect by analogy with a model of Plaut and Shallice (1993b) which accounted for perseverations by adding so-called short-term weights to a model similar in structure to Figure 6.11 and then examining the effects of partial disconnections to the input stream.[23] As a final alternative, Jefferies et al. (2008) have argued that semantic access disorders may arise through damage to a specific control system concerned with selection between semantic alternatives, to be discussed in Section 9.13. Currently all these theoretical possibilities remain in contention.

Putting these alternative possibilities on one side for the moment and returning to the only well-developed model of semantic access disorders, that of Gotts and Plaut, it is clear that although quite different in detail this model is in principle compatible with the model of Rogers et al. which we have just discussed. Indeed the two groups of modellers may be viewed as producing simulations which could differ just in their implementation details but essentially are of the same basic model.[24]

Thus one could easily conceive of a model that combined the key characteristics of both. Indeed, Jefferies and Lambon-Ralph (2006) sketch an extended version of the Rogers et al. model (see Figure 6.14), which, as far as the functional architecture of semantics is concerned, is virtually identical to a model of Plaut (2002). Moreover, while there have been many competing accounts of the semantic access syndrome the idea of semantic dementia as leading to the loss of semantic representations themselves is widely accepted. Thus one can use the syndrome to begin to localise a semantic store.

6.7 Converging Localisations of the Semantic Store

We argued in the previous chapter that inferences from neuropsychological evidence to processing models and from functional imaging findings to processing accounts were both subject to many rather insecure assumptions. However the inferences were strengthened if they converged in isolating similar regions as the locus of key processing components. Take the semantic store, as held to be degraded in semantic dementia. Does the localisation of the pathology fit with that obtained by functional imaging studies of semantic memory in normal subjects?

---

[23] The model actually dealt with object-to-semantic processing, but it has a related structure to that in Figure 6.11. It is discussed in Section 7.2.

[24] By 'implementation details', we mean aspects of a model that are necessary for a complete, running, simulation, but which have no theoretical import and no significant effect on relevant aspects of the simulation's behaviour. An aspect of a model can be shown to be an implementation detail by providing

alternative implementations of that aspect and demonstrating that the alternative implementations produce the same behaviour, as discussed for the Plaut-Shallice model in Chapter 4 (Cooper et al., 1996). Unfortunately while it is common to treat aspects of a model as implementation details, there are few published simulations that adopt this methodology of actually varying them.

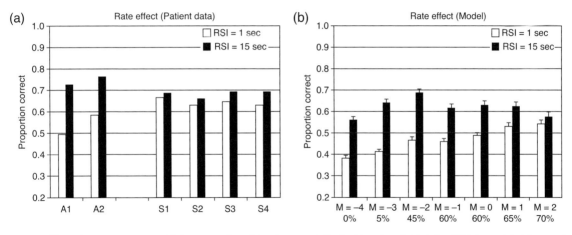

Fig. 6.13 Effects of presentation rate in (a) the patient data of Warrington and Cipolotti (1996; see Table 6.3) and (b) the model of Gotts and Plaut (2002) under different damage combinations. The values of the neuromodulation parameter (M) and the percentages of lesioned connections are listed for each damage combination. A rate effect occurs. When the RSI = 1 sec, performance is worse for patients A1 and A2 and the model when M < 2. Redrawn from S.J. Gotts and D.C. Plaut (2002) The impact of synaptic depression following brain damage: a connectionist account of 'access/refractory' and 'degraded-store' semantic impairments. *Cognitive, Affective, and Behavioral Neuroscience,* 2(3), 187–213.

Any pathological correlation carried out with a degenerative disease is made precarious because the disease is progressive in time. It is in practice virtually impossible to see all the subjects at the same point in the progression of the disease. However this problem was essentially solved by the application to structural imaging of the Price–Friston conjunction analysis (see Section 5.7). For a region of the brain to appear abnormal using conjunction analysis, all patients had to have an impairment in the region. Mummery et al. (2000) used Voxel-Based Morphometry (VBM), a technique developed by Wright et al. (1995) for detecting structural abnormalities in the brain. It is adapted from the statistical parametric mapping procedure standardly used for functional imaging (see Section 5.1). The great advantage of the voxel-based morphometry procedure is that it provides a rigorous quantitative means of amalgamating pathological findings across patients.

Six patients were scanned. All fitted the appropriate diagnosis for semantic dementia with selective loss of the meaning of words. Thus all were impaired in the Pyramids and Palm Trees Test discussed above. The abnormalities on the structural scans were remarkably similar (see Figure 6.15). Conjunction analysis showed four regions of the temporal lobe—mainly in the left hemisphere—to be damaged with maximal involvement at the temporal pole.[25] Later studies using a larger patient sample but somewhat less sophisticated methodology,

also saw the anterior temporal lobes as critical but, in addition, suggested the involvement of medial anterior temporal structures, and that the effects were bilateral (Gorno-Tempini et al., 2004).

We will treat the Mummery et al. localisations as the key lesion sites for semantic dementia. Surprisingly, though, the lesion sites do not overlap that well with those of another syndrome thought to involve problems in semantics. One of the classical aphasia syndromes initially described by Lichtheim (1885) is *transcortical sensory aphasia.* In transcortical sensory aphasia the patient is held to have fluent speech and normal reproduction of verbal material[26] but impaired comprehension of verbal material. The syndrome, which is not common, has not been as well-studied neuropsychologically as semantic dementia. In a definitive anatomical analysis based on CT scans and an extensive review of the literature Alexander et al. (1989) propose two areas to be critical—an inferolateral mid-temporal region (BA37) and a 'crescent of posterior association cortex, portions of Brodmann areas 39 and 19 at the temporal-parietal-occipital junction' (p. 89).[27] The inferior temporal lesions found in semantic dementia in the

---

[25] There were also more minor abnormalities in the ventromedial frontal cortex, the insula and the amygdala, all of which have reciprocal connections with the relevant regions of the temporal lobe.

[26] In more modern analysis of aphasia disorders a distinction should be made between *repetition* of a series of frequent short words and *reproduction* of single longer less frequent words, as the two dissociate (see Shallice & Warrington, 1977a). This distinction is not drawn when using the classical Wernicke–Lichtheim categories for categorising aphasia—see FNMS Chapters 3 and 7.

[27] This is a very similar localisation to that illustrated in the PET study of Price et al. (1997b). See Figure 6.17.

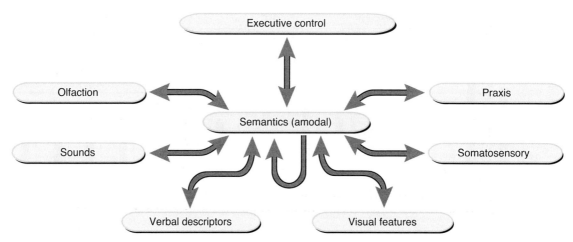

Fig. 6.14 The computational architecture of semantic cognition proposed by Jefferies and Lambon Ralph (2006). The architecture extends that in Figure 6.6 with units for additional modalities (sounds, olfaction, praxis, somatosensory) and executive control.

Mummery et al. study were in general anterior of BA37 and not all semantic dementia patients in their study had lesions involving the temporal–parietal–occipital junction. We will return to this puzzle following consideration of the functional imaging of semantic processing in normal subjects.[28]

One possibility is that some patients characterised as transcortical sensory aphasia have an access problem. As far as a semantic access disorder is concerned, we have until recently lacked a solid neurological predisposing condition to localise the syndrome. Patients VER, JCU and A1 suffered from a left middle cerebral artery lesion, while patient A2 had a left occipital and posterior temporal high-grade tumour. A series of six further high-grade tumour patients, who also showed the access pattern studied by Campanella et al. (2009), had a fairly similar lesion site to A1 (see Figure 6.16). As discussed in the previous section, this fits better with the disorder arising from damage to connections from phonological processing systems, which we will assume to be located near Wernicke's region in the left superior temporal cortex (see Scott & Johnsrude, 2003), and the semantic system, if that is assumed to be in the anterior left temporal lobe, than to a storage deficit. Thus much more tentatively we can say that the localisation of the access/refractory disorder is also compatible with an anterior inferior temporal lobe localisation of the semantic store.

There is now an extensive literature on functional imaging of normal subjects concerned with the localisation of semantic processes. Many of the tasks from which inferences about semantics have been drawn, activate semantic processing only weakly; an example would be the contrast between reading a word and a non-word, since word reading predominantly uses a non-semantic orthography-to-phonology route (see Chapter 4). In addition the tasks may recruit processes other than semantics in the critical comparison, e.g. in comparing language with non-language tasks. Only the studies with more powerful contrasts are of primary interest. One of the earliest such studies was that of Price et al. (1997b), which compared a subject's ability to make a semantic decision on written words with that of making a phonological decision. The semantic task was to decide whether the word, e.g. *PIG* corresponded to a living thing or not. The phonological task involved the decision of whether it has two syllables. A swathe of temporal cortex was found to be significantly more activated in the semantic than in the phonological task. The swathe ran from the left angular gyrus medial part of the anterior temporal lobe through to the temporal-parietal-occipital junction (see Figure 6.17). It is restricted to the left hemisphere. Price (2000) terms this swathe 'extrasylvian temporoparietal'.

A somewhat similar swathe was obtained about the same time by Vandenberghe et al. (1996) in a study where they contrasted a semantic judgement with a visual judgement for triads of words or pictures. In their task three words, e.g. *spanner, pliers, saw* or the corresponding pictures are presented on the screen. In the semantic condition subjects are given one word and must judge which of two other words is more related in meaning; in the visual condition they must judge which is equal in size on the screen. The findings in the

---

[28] It should be noted that one major class of explanation given for patients who fit this transcortical sensory aphasia symptom pattern is a disconnection between the phonological input lexicon and the semantic system; this is Lichtheim's (1885) explanation in more modern terms (e.g. see that of Geschwind et al., 1968, and Heilman et al., 1976).

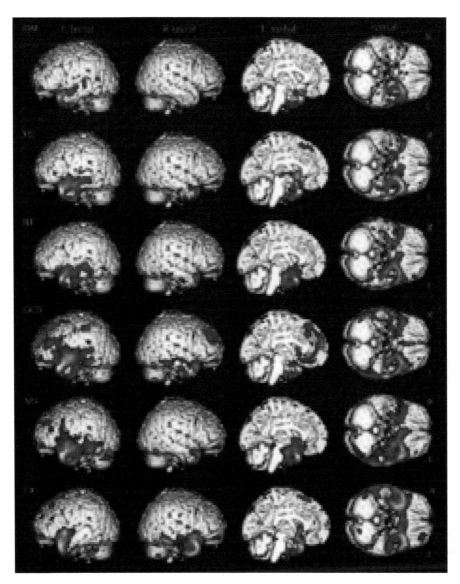

Fig. 6.15 Structural scans of six semantic dementia patients, showing the neural damage in each case. Note the atrophy of the anterior temporal cortices, generally bilateral, but also more on the left. Reprinted with permission from C.J. Mummery, K. Patterson, C.J. Price, J. Ashburner, R.S.J. Frackowiak, J.R. Hodges (2000) A voxel-based morphometry study of semantic dementia: relationship between temporal lobe atrophy and semantic memory. *Annals of Neurology, 47*(1), 36–45. Copyright © 2000, John Wiley and Sons.

semantic tasks were generally similar to those of the Price et al. study.[29]

When reviews were carried out of functional imaging experiments that contrast semantic with non-semantic processing where the contrasts are drawn broadly (e.g. by Binder & Price, 2001), many regions appear to be involved in semantic processing, although mainly in the left hemisphere: regions of the parietal cortex such as the angular gyrus (BA39), prefrontal

regions such as the superior frontal gyrus (BA8 and 9) and the inferior frontal gyrus, as well as the medial and inferior temporal gyri and the fusiform gyrus; in other words, large sections of the left hemisphere. However the contrasts made in nearly all the early studies such as Vandenberghe et al. (1996) are broad-brush; they are subject to the standard objections to subtraction designs discussed in Section 5.4 and potentially involve many computational processes.

It is conceivable that semantic processing has a mass action characteristic but the use of more focussed semantic tasks leads to the activation of more restricted areas. For instance, Tyler et al. (2004b) compared two

---

[29] The findings of Vandenberghe et al. were replicated by Mummery et al. (1999).

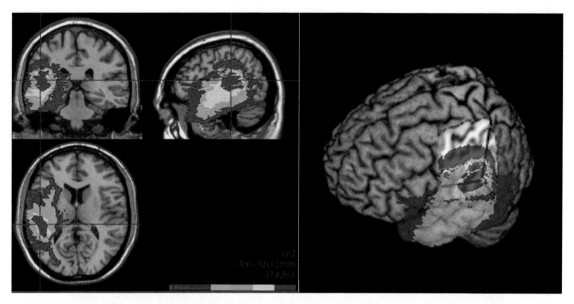

Fig. 6.16 Lesion overlap of the semantic access dysphasia patients of Campanella et al. (2009). The area common to patients with semantic access difficulties is in the left superior and middle temporal gyri. The left parietal cortex also tends to be undercut. (Red indicates maximum overlap). Reprinted with permission from F. Campanella, M. Mondani, M. Skrap and T. Shallice (2009) Semantic access dysphasia resulting from left temporal lobe tumours, *Brain, 132*(1), 87–102.

conditions both involving naming objects. In one condition the standard name was required, that of the so-called 'basic' level, e.g. *donkey* or *hammer*. In the other, subjects would just have to give the superordinate category *living* or *manmade*. The former is more resource-demanding at the semantic level. There was a significant activation difference between the two tasks only in the left inferior anterior temporal cortex—the left entorhinal and perirhinal cortices (see Figure 6.18). Animal studies have suggested that the perirhinal cortex integrates information received from different sensory systems and stores complex feature conjunctions (e.g. Desimone & Ungerleider, 1989; Bussey & Saksida, 2002). In addition, it corresponds reasonably well to the location of the semantic stores as derived from semantic dementia.

Overall the neuropsychological and functional imaging evidence reinforce each other well. Most of the evidence fits with the existence of an attractor-based storage system which holds known items, which in turn conjoin the many different features concrete objects have, and this appears to be located in the inferior left anterior temporal cortex. However, at least two anomalies exist within this characterisation that need to be resolved. First, as has been extensively discussed, the main computational model realises semantic dementia in terms of disconnections instead of loss of units *per se*. Second, both the neuropsychological and the functional imaging point in addition, to the involvement of a swathe of regions running more posteriorly in the left temporal cortex and particularly involving

the left temporo-parietal-occipital junction. We will return to these points later. On the whole, though, neuropsychological, imaging, computational and basic neuroscience accounts seem to be converging on a common picture.

6.8 Semantics and the Variety of its Possible Formats

The picture painted in the last section is beguilingly simple. Actually it is over-simple. Let us begin by considering whether a concrete object known verbally and know visually have the same representation. Rogers et al. are clear: 'Patients with semantic dementia are impaired on tasks regardless of the modality of testing … and typically do not show preservation of one (semantic) domain relative to another' (p. 230).[30] There has long been an alternative intellectual tradition in psychology that we think in one of two codes, verbal or visual (e.g. Paivio, 1971). But what might a visual form of representation mean? Take for instance, the developmental psychologist Jean Mandler (2004), who on the basis of experiments on babies argues that 'a mechanism of perceptual meaning analysis extracts and summarises a subset of incoming perceptual information from which it creates a store of meanings or simple concepts. These meanings

---

[30] Rogers et al. merely cite in support of this claim a paper by Lambon-Ralph et al. (2001), which contains no relevant findings and does not discuss alternative positions.

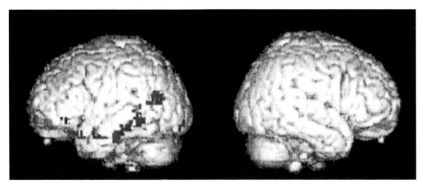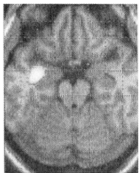

Fig. 6.17 The 'extrasylvian temporoparietal' region activated in semantic versus phonological contrast of Price et al. (1997b). The large superior blob is near to the temporo-parietal-occipital junction discussed by Alexander et al. and their more anterior 'crescent' is also clearly visible. Reprinted From C.J. Price (2000). The anatomy of language: Contributions from functional neuroimaging, *Journal of Anatomy, 197*(3), 335–359. Copyright © 2000, John Wiley and Sons.

are typically descriptions of what is happening in the scenes the infant observes, for instance, "self-motion" or "containment". Such meanings arise from attentive, conscious analysis of spatial information. [...] Thus, [such] image-schemas have three main functions: first, to create an explicit, declarative conceptual system that is accessible to conscious thought; second, to structure and give meaning to the images we are aware of when we think; and third, to provide the underlying meanings or concepts onto which language can be mapped' (p. 14).[31]

Mandler argues that such image-schemas provide a natural basis from which word-meaning can be built. Moreover in the models of semantic access outlined in Section 6.5, the features in the semantic store could be derived in some way from image-schemas. However other lines of work on normal subjects suggest that other word-meaning representations may have in part a different origin. Thus Gleitman et al. (2005) argue that the acquisition of vocabulary is set in motion by *word-to-world* pairing where the representations of the world could be Mandler's 'image-schemas'. Gleitman et al. however, continue, Armed with this stock of "easy" words, the learner achieves further lexical knowledge by an arm-over-arm process (which they call syntactic *bootstrapping*) in which successively more sophisticated representations of linguistic structures are built. Lexical learning thereby can proceed by adding *structure-to-world mapping* to the earlier available machinery, enabling efficient learning of more abstract items—the "hard" words' (p. 25). They illustrate this second process for perspective verbs like *chase* and *flee*

and for so-called mental-content verbs like *think* and *know* (for a related view see also Gentner, 2006).

This suggests that knowledge, even of words, is acquired by a variety of means and also that the semantic representations used in language might have some degree of autonomy. Related to this, some analysts of normal language processing (e.g. Vigliocco et al., 2004) explicitly make a separation between a conceptual level of representation, which would include image-schemas, and a feature-based lexical-semantic representation. Their main argument is that languages represent related meanings using different principles (see Talmy, 1975). For instance, English has a set of motion verbs, which express the manner of motion but not its direction (e.g. *crawl, creep, sneak*), but Romance languages such as Spanish have the complementary type of representation (e.g. *caer* (to fall down), *salir* (to exit). However judgements of similarity show similar patterns between the languages (Malt et al., 1999).[32]

Is there any brain-based evidence pointing to a possible difference in the neural bases of such two types of semantic representations? There has been a strong tradition in neuropsychology for a related separation between so-called *verbal semantics* or Vigliocco et al's *lexical-semantic* representations on the one hand and *visual semantics* which would correspond to Mandler's image schemas on the other (e.g. Warrington, 1975; Beauvois & Saillant, 1985). However until recently it was essentially derived from disparate individual cases, without the existence of a functional syndrome.

One such individual case was described in the study of Breedin et al. (1994), who investigated the knowledge of word meaning of a semantic dementia patient, DM. Prefiguring Vigliocco et al.'s later characterisation of a manner versus direction contrast in different languages

---

[31] It is not clear why Mandler limits her 'image-schemas', a term derived from cognitive linguists, such as Talmy (1983), to spatial information. Thus the 'image-schema' *ripe* applied to fruit, would principally be based on colour and texture information.

[32] For a related position see Barsalou et al. (2003).

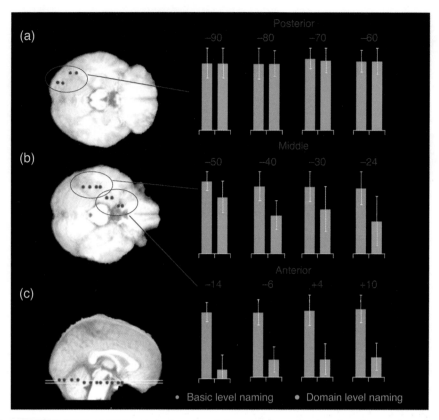

Fig. 6.18 Signal change during basic-level and domain-level naming relative to baseline at 12 points along the posterior to anterior extent of the left interior occipital and temporal cortices. The approximate location of each point is shown superimposed on axial (a and b) and sagittal (c) slices of a normalized brain. Figures above each plot indicate the position on the y (coronal) axis in MNI space. Both tasks yield similar signal strength in posterior regions (a), but basic level naming yields greater signal strength in more anterior regions (b and c). Reprinted with permission from L. K. Tyler, E. A. Stamatakis, P. Bright, K. Acres, S. Abdallah, J. M. Rodd, and H. E. Moss (2004) Processing objects at different levels of specificity, *Journal of Cognitive Neuroscience*, *16*(3), 351–362. Copyright © 2004, MIT Press Journals.

in the lexicalisation of actions, Breedin et al. constructed an odd-one-out test with different sets of verbs (see Table 6.5). The only set of these verbs on which DM had problems were those that differed in manner.

	DM	Controls (Mean)	Controls (Range)
Non-Relational Triples (e.g. *augment – diminish, lessen*)	25	26.6	(25–27)
Manner Triples (e.g. *gnaw – gobble, gulp*)	13	23.5	(20–26)
Relational triples (e.g. *convince, persuade, acquiesce*)	21	23.0	(19–26)

TABLE 6.5 Comparison of DM (Breedin et al., 1994) and five controls on three odd-one-out tests each consisting of 27 items. DM is well below the control range on manner triples but within it for the other two sets.

Breedin et al. adopt a position derived from Jackendoff (1987) and argue that DM has lost the perceptual aspects of conceptual representations.[33]

However sceptics could adopt the methodological arguments presented in Chapter 4 concerning the problems that potential individual differences can create for inferences based on individual cases. More convincing support for the distinction has, however, come from an unlikely source, namely the author who first demonstrated the overlapping activations for semantic judgements based on words and those based on objects, Rik Vanderberghe, with his collaborators (Vandenbulcke et al., 2006). These authors carried out two studies. One was a single case study of a patient JA2. JA2 had a lesion of the posterior right fusiform region (see Figure 6.19a where the lesion is shown in black). She showed a loss of knowledge of visual attributes of many different

---

[33] For semantic dementia cases with roughly the complementary pattern of deficits see McCarthy & Warrington (1988), although for one category only, and Lauro-Grotto et al. (1997).

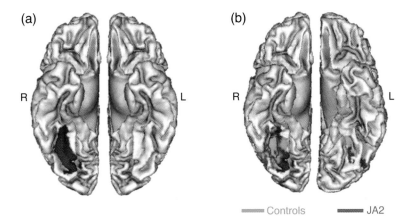

Fig. 6.19 (a) The lesion of patient JA2 (as viewed from below), who shows a selective loss of knowledge of visual attributes of many different semantic categories. The lesion site is shown in dark shading. (b) Picture-specific activation obtained in healthy controls (green) and for JA (red) superimposed on JA's brain. Reprinted by permission from Macmillan Publishers Ltd: *Nature Neuroscience* (M. Vandenbulcke, R. Peeters, K. Fannes and R. Vandenberghe (2006) Knowledge of visual attributes in the right hemisphere, *Nature Neuroscience, 9*(7), 964–970), copyright (2006).

semantic categories while being entirely normal in knowledge of other types of attributes (see Figure 6.20).[34]

To complement the case study, they carried out a functional imaging study with normal subjects. Subjects had to carry out two tasks. In one the task was based on the Pyramids and Palm Trees test, judging the odd one out of three stimuli when the critical dimension was semantic. In the other they had to make a size judgement of which of two stimuli to the left and right of a centre one matched it most closely in absolute size *on the screen*. The tasks were carried out with pictures and words in separate conditions. The area that showed an interaction between tasks (associative-semantic versus absolute size) and stimulus (picture, word) in normal subjects is also shown in Figure 6.19b. It can be seen that the functional imaging study on normal subjects led to the accessing of semantic information specifically for visual input in a virtually identical region of cortex to that involved in JA2's lesion. There is therefore converging evidence supporting the idea of a region of cortex in some sense carrying out semantic operations primarily on visual input. It is clear that this is very different from the amodal semantic area discussed in the previous section.

Sceptics could respond that what was being accessed in this task was the *visual features* system in the model shown in Figure 6.14. However, a task like Pyramids and Palm Trees, discussed in Sections 6.5 and 6.6, requires much more than merely knowledge of visual features. It requires, for instance, knowledge of which other sorts of objects are found in a related environment. And Mandler's

image schemas require knowledge of an object's likely behaviour. Another critical issue is whether these representations can be accessed independently of any amodal semantic area in the left anterior temporal cortex (see also Patterson et al., 2007). We return to this point later, following a discussion of dissociations within semantics which are more unexpected.[35]

6.9 Categorical Specificity: Selective Losses of Knowledge of Living Things

In the last section we presented initial evidence that there is more than a unitary semantics. However, essentially we just scratched the surface of an issue of great complexity. We did not specify visual semantics clearly. Thus Mandler's image-schemas are much more restricted in scope than the way neuropsychologists have characterised so-called *visual semantics*, which in some version could provide an almost completely parallel semantic system. The arguments for a more purely lexical semantics derived from the study of Gleitman et al. could easily be used to argue for some specialisation of abstract concept semantics. The content

---

[34] See Miceli et al. (2001) for a somewhat analogous case where the deficit was limited to colour.

[35] Plaut (2002) produced a very interesting model of the syndrome optic aphasia, where patients without an anomia know more about an object than they can verbalise if the object is presented visually. The model can be seen as a sort of halfway house between a Rogers et al. type of model and one which has separable visual and verbal semantics; in the Plaut (2002) model the distinction between a *visual semantics* and a *verbal semantics* is graded not all-or-none. Most of the evidence which supports a categorical distinction between the two systems is also explicable on Plaut's approach. The Vandenbulcke et al. evidence is perhaps the most difficult for his model.

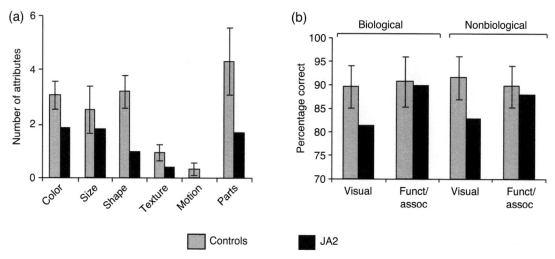

Fig. 6.20 Performance of JA2 and controls on a feature-generation task. JA2 generated fewer visual attributes than age- and education-matched controls, and this deficit affected all subtypes of visual attribute (a). She was impaired at generating visual features for both biological and nonbiological objects, but the impairment did not affect the generation of functional or associative features (b). Reprinted by permission from Macmillan Publishers Ltd: *Nature Neuroscience* (M. Vandenbulcke, R. Peeters, K. Fannes and R. Vandenberghe (2006) Knowledge of visual attributes in the right hemisphere, *Nature Neuroscience, 9*(7), 964–970), copyright (2006).

of representations in hypothetically separable systems which are in some sense 'semantic' needs to be addressed more directly.

We begin with the dramatic phenomenon of category specificity. Many patients have now been described who show a highly specific loss or preservation of particular parts of their semantic repertoire. They often present with a specific difficulty in identifying categories of items, such as animals or plants. Clinical reports of patients with a difficulty which would now be interpreted as examples of 'category specificity' were made by a number of neurologists beginning with Nielsen (1946). However these clinical descriptions were not supported by quantitative evidence and the dissociations they claimed seemed so implausible that little attention was paid to them. However by the late-1970s a new treatment became available for herpes simplex encephalitis, a very rare condition, which had previously been fatal in most patients who had the disease. The treatment—acyclovir—halted the disease but not before parts of the cortex had been affected in many of the patients. How much cortex was damaged depended upon the precise timing of the beginning of treatment. However the initial regions to be affected tended to be the anterior temporal lobes, particularly their medial surfaces. At that time Warrington and one of us established quantitatively in four such patients that they were very grossly impaired at naming or identifying living things, but identification of artefacts was relatively spared. To give the flavour of the impairment, JBR defined *briefcase* as a 'small case held by students' but when asked to define *parrot* could only say 'don't know'; SBY said that a *whistle* was a 'thing you blow to make a

piping sound' whereas a *kangaroo* was 'an animal that swims.' The effects were very large, e.g. 6% correct (living things) v 80% (artefacts) in identification for JBR; and remained so when the effects of word frequency and familiarity were partialled out. They occurred when the test was word-picture matching (see Figure 6.21) so the effects are not due to a problem in speech production. By 2003 at least 27 cases with this pattern had been described in the literature (see Capitani et al., 2003). In nearly all of the patients the impairment involved knowledge of animals, plants and foods, although testing of foods was often limited to fruit and vegetables. We will call this pattern as found, say, in a prototypic patient such as JBR (Warrington & Shallice, 1984; Bunn et al., 1997) the selective impairment of knowledge of living things. It should however be noted that this is specifically a label which does not necessarily relate to the origin of the disorder or even to some of its finer-grain characteristics.

Twenty years ago such findings were treated sceptically and attempts were made to explain them as due to combinations of some more basic and more obviously explicable effects such as the affected categories differing on item familiarity or in terms of the structural complexity of the visual stimuli (e.g. Funnell & Sheridan, 1992; Stewart et al., 1992) or, more interestingly, in terms of the relative 'density' of concepts in the category in semantic space (Gaffan & Heywood, 1993). In fact when the appropriate variables have been controlled, the category specific effects still remain (see e.g. Sartori et al., 1993; Farah et al., 1996; Forde et al., 1997; Bunn et al., 1998; Caramazza & Shelton, 1998; Kurbat & Farah, 1998; Borgo & Shallice, 2001).

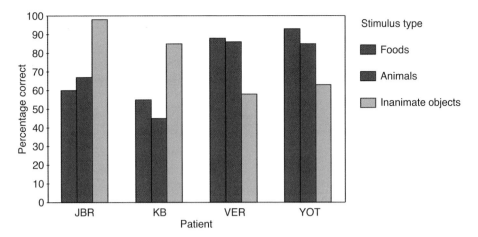

Fig. 6.21 Effects of semantic category on word-picture matching in two herpes simplex encephalitis (JBR and KB) and two vascular global aphasics with large lesions around the Sylvian fissure affecting at least both temporal and parietal cortices (VER and YOT). Data for JBR and KB from Warrington and Shallice (1984). Data from VER and YOT from Warrington and McCarthy (1983) and Warrington and McCarthy (1987), respectively. Chance = 20%.

However more recently lines of criticism have been developed somewhat resembling one that was discussed with respect to reading-without-semantics in Chapter 4. A number of attempts have been made to show that category specificity like reading without semantics is not a robust effect. Thus Laws (2005) argues that control groups have not been used to assess the degree of deviation from the norm in the performance of patients claimed to be category specific. In fact, studies in normal subjects using matched sets of stimuli, if anything, show better and faster naming of living than of non-living things (Laws & Neve, 1999), although slightly better performance for non-living things is found in questionnaire studies of knowledge of features (Capitani et al., 1993). Moreover the category effects in individual herpes patients other than JBR discussed above can be large (see Table 6.6). We will return to this issue later after discussing the neurological basis of the effect in patients.

In addition, a smaller set of patients have been described who show the complementary pattern of category specific effects. The first such patients were two global aphasic patients, VER and YOT, described by Warrington and McCarthy (1983, 1987). They showed a strong and robust superiority of living things in picture-word matching, in an identical test to that which showed a strong non-living superiority in the herpes encephalitis patients (see Figure 6.21). Later patients of this type have not been specifically anomic, e.g. JJ (Hillis & Caramazza, 1991), CW92 (Sacchett & Humphreys, 1992). In all, 18 patients of this type are listed by Capitani et al. (2003). One would need very large individual differences across the population to explain away the overall pattern.

But perhaps the effects still stem from premorbid individual differences? Maybe there are very large individual differences in this domain even though the classic methodology of cognitive neuropsychology implicitly assumed such differences did not exist. One pointer in this direction is that Barbarotto et al. (2002) have shown a strong interaction (in normals) between gender and category, such that men tend to be better at artefacts and women at some biological categories. However, a point in the opposite direction is that clinically prior knowledge does not seem to be that strong

TABLE 6.6	The contrast in naming living and non-living objects in seven herpes encephalitis patients		
Patient	**Source**	**Living Things**	**Non-living Things**
ER	Kolinsky et al., 2002	36%	83%
FI	Barbarotto, Capitani & Laiacona, 1996	13%	57%
Felicia	De Renzi & Lucchelli, 1994	40%	90%
JBR	Warrington & Shallice, 1984	6%	67%
LA	Silveri & Gainotti, 1988	30%	100%
Michaelengelo	Sartori & Job, 1988	33%	75%
RC	Moss & Tyler, 1998	9%	50%
SBY*	Warrington & Shallice, 1984	0%	75%

* Giving core concept as judged by referees, as SBY was anomic.

TABLE 6.7	Number of patients in the database of Capitani et al. (2003) who had a category-specific deficit affecting either one or more biological category, e.g. animals, fruit and vegetables or one or more artefact category.

	Herpes	Head Injury	Dementia	Stroke	Other/ Unclear
Living Things Deficit	27	8	11	7	8
Artefacts Deficit	1	0	5	11	0

a determinant of performance. Moreover controlling for gender-specific familiarity, as done by Albanese et al. (2000) and Samson and Pillon (2003), did not remove the category-specific effects.[36] From a more clinical perspective, individual differences do not seem a very plausible explanation. Michaelangelo, the patient of Sartori et al. (1993) who had lost the ability to identify animals, had been an active member of the World Wildlife Fund before his illness and a patient of Humphreys et al. who had a selective problem naming fruit and vegetables had been an expert on food (Humphreys & Forde, 2001).

More critically, if one examines meta-analyses of patients reported with a selective deficit of one or more living things categories (e.g. animals or fruit/vegetables) and compares them with those reported without selective impairments of artefacts, there is a clear difference in probabilities of particular aetiologies (see Table 6.7). In particular, herpes encephalitis, a very rare disease, is consistently associated with selective deficits of living things. This would not be expected if category specific effects arise just from premorbid individual differences in the organisation of the semantic system as Laws (2005) suggested may be possible. Herpes encephalitis thus plays the role for category specificity that semantic dementia does for generalised semantic memory loss. It provides the critical neurological base. In particular it is very hard to see how premorbid individual differences could give rise to the gross differences in aetiology for which syndrome they predispose the patient to develop

---

[36] Another front has recently been opened by Laws and Sartori (2005). They described two herpes patients who show a living things deficit on one test (e.g. feature verification) and a non-living things deficit on another (picture-naming). However no attempt was made to replicate the effects within the individual patient across sessions as is necessary for a reliable phenomenon. Moreover, inconsistency across tests in category-specificity appears to be the exception rather than the rule to judge from an early meta-analysis of Barbarotto et al. (1996).

after neurological disease. Thus one cannot discuss individual cases of category specificity with the herpes aetiology as merely patients in whom assumption 4 of Chapter 4 has essentially broken down, that is, as showing an idiosyncratic pattern of performance.

6.10 Knowledge of Living Things: its Localisation

Can the processes involved in storage of information and retrieval from storage concerning our knowledge of living things be localised? There are two ways to address this question—by consideration of the neuropsychological evidence and of course from the functional imaging literature. Consider first patients with a selective loss of knowledge of living things deriving from herpes simplex encephalitis. We will assume they have a degraded store deficit. The two of the original patients in whom it could be tested (JBR and SBY) were highly consistent in the items which they did and did not know across sessions.[37] If this functional interpretation is correct, this makes their lesion site directly relevant to the location of the store.

Gainotti (2000) was the first to produce a detailed and expert analysis of the localisation of the lesion sites. Essentially the same conclusions can be drawn from Capitani et al.'s slightly larger and neuropsychologically somewhat more definitive sample. Using the latter data, Table 6.8 divides patients into whether they have temporal involvement or parietal involvement or both. Statistically the living things deficit is more likely to involve the temporal lobes by comparison with the parietal when compared to the artefacts deficit. The artefacts deficit is also relatively speaking more likely to be specifically left rather than bilateral.[38] Thus the

---

[37] Barbarotto et al. (1996), reviewing patients with selective loss of knowledge of living things, apply an analysis procedure for identification or naming devised by Faglioni and Botti (1993) and argue that one herpes patient, Michaelangelo of Sartori and Job (1988), presented with an access disorder. In our view this is incorrect. Michaelangelo was tested six times for naming 20 objects and 20 living things. He showed some improvement over the retesting. However, if we take the three tests where a similar number of correct responses were given (tests 2, 3, 5) 17/20 stimuli showed the identical performance across the three trials—far above chance; tests 4 and 6 where performance was better also showed a similar 16/20 identical responses. Barborotto et al. report two other patients, LF and EA, who they hold to have a 'mixed pattern'. However, EA performed almost at floor on living things (e.g. 1% correct naming) so on living things a degraded store deficit cannot be ruled out.

[38] Gainotti (2000) argues that the degree of bilateral temporal involvement is underestimated as the evidence for a fair number of patients was only a CT scan.

TABLE 6.8 Stated localisation of lesion (considered with respect to the involvement of the temporal and parietal lobes only) for reported cases of specific living things deficit (divided by aetiology) and specific artifact deficit (see Capitani et al., 2003). There were two other Living Things Deficits patients (Other Aetiology) whose lesion locations were given—one left occipital and one left frontal and basal ganglia.

Living Things Deficit	Temporal			Tempero-Parietal			Parietal		
	Bil.	Left	Right	Bil.	Left	Right	Bil.	Left	Right
Herpes	14	9	2	-	-	-	-	-	-
Other Aetiology	9	11	-	3	1	-	-	2	-
Artifacts Deficit	1	6	1	1	2	-	0	6*	-

* All involve the left fronto-parietal lobes.

two syndromes differ with respect to localisation, as well as in aetiology.

There are 20 patients (using all aetiologies) where more detailed information was available to Gainotti. He notes that within the temporal lobes for the selective living things deficit damage is more centred on anterior (temporal pole, hippocampus, parahippocampal gyrus) and antero-lateral temporal cortex, with the posterior parts of the temporal cortex, particularly the posterior–lateral temporal cortex being relatively spared. On the superior–inferior dimension, it is the inferior temporal lobe that is damaged in all patients.

If one turns to functional imaging, the picture was very complex but is now becoming somewhat easier to interpret. Cappa et al. (1998), Martin et al. (1996) and Damasio et al. (1996) were the first groups to examine by the use of PET whether there was any anatomical specialisation related to the processing of animals. Thus Martin et al. compared naming of animals and tools, as representative living and non-living categories. In the subtraction, naming animals selectively involved the medial left occipital lobe and the inferior temporal regions. Cappa et al. and Damasio et al. obtained somewhat similar but not identical results. For instance the activation sites in the Damasio et al. study in the inferior temporal lobe were more anterior than those of Martin et al.

Damasio's study was particularly interesting as the critical activation site was compared with a lesion location analysis. Patients were compared who had selective damage in a task of naming animals by comparison with tasks of naming persons in books. Animals selectively activated the left infero-temporal cortex and the left temporal pole. Out of 97 patients with localised lesions 16 performed particularly poorly on naming animals. Their lesions were localised in a very similar area (see Figure 6.22) to the region activated in imaging of normal subjects.[39]

Later functional imaging studies on normal subjects, however, appeared not to confirm this degree of specialisation. Tyler and Moss (2001) summarised relevant studies as showing that 10 different regions are found in tasks with processing of natural kinds compared with processing of artefacts. However the range of tasks considered is too wide; the choice of baseline tasks in the studies reviewed often meant that the experimental and control tasks differed on many processes. Two studies illustrate the contrast. Chao et al. (1999) used a variety of tasks in the same set of subjects with fMRI. One was 'viewing' where the subject merely had to look carefully. A second was 'delayed match-to-sample', where a photograph is presented for 1 sec and then 0.5 sec later two photographs are presented and the subject must choose which of the two is identical to the initial one. The third task was silent naming. The fourth was silent reading to be followed by answering preset questions about the item, such as 'is it a forest animal?' Three regions showed unilateral or bilateral activations across all four tasks in at least some subjects.[40] These were the

representations. This would be equivalent to what Levelt (1989) calls the 'lemma' (see Section 3.5) rather than the semantic representations per se. Damasio et al. came to this conclusion because they measured the number of items subjects failed to name which they 'appropriately recognised, so that scores reflected true word-retrieval ability' (p. 499). However, if there is a correlation between the number of items in a category that patients have some idea of *but* cannot name *and* the number of items in a category they do not know at all, then one would have obtained the same results if a more direct test of item knowledge had been used. This is what herpes patients—and there are five in the study—are likely to show. No direct test of recognition for each category was in fact used. The functional imaging data clearly is compatible with both explanations. Thus the argument of Damasio et al. that we are not dealing here with a semantic deficit per se is very weak (for a related critique see Caramazza & Shelton, 1998).

[40] These were apparently not all the same subjects who showed the effects in different conditions!

---

[39] Damasio et al. argue that this region is critical not for semantic representations *per se* but for the mapping between semantic representations of animals and phonological lexical

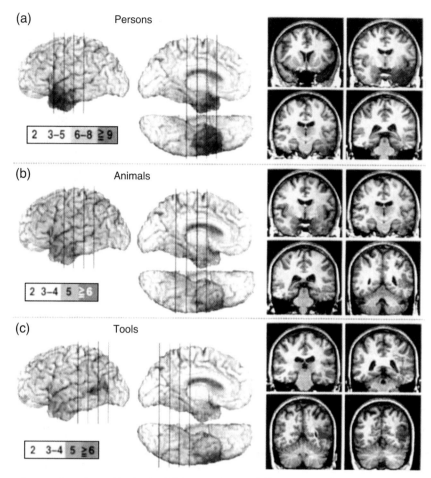

Fig. 6.22 Lesion overlap maps for patients with selective deficits in word retrieval, showing the overlap for patients with defective retrieval of words for persons (a), animals (b), and tools (c). This is derived from a group of 29 left-hemisphere patients with abnormal naming performance. Reprinted by permission from Macmillan Publishers Ltd: *Nature* (H. Damasio, T.J. Grabowski, D. Tranel, R.D. Hichwa and A.R. Damasio (1996) A neural basis for lexical retrieval. *Nature, 380*, 499–505). Copyright (1996).

inferior occipital gyrus, the lateral fusiform gyrus and the superior temporal sulcus, but more on the right than the left. Two of these regions—the second and third—are shown in the illustrative figure (see Figure 6.23).[41] This and a number of other studies, such as Martin et al. (1996) and Beauchamp et al. (2002, 2003), as well as that of Wheatley et al. (2005) discussed in the last chapter, have led Martin (2007) to propose that these regions are involved in conceptual processing, in this case of animate entities.

A more transparent procedure was adopted by Devlin et al. (2002). They argued that category-specific effects would be expected to be context dependent, in that responses in a particular brain region to a particular category will vary with both the task and the stimulus. They therefore took the results of seven previous PET experiments carried out by Price and her collaborators, in which each incorporated the distinction between living and non-living categories as one among a number of functions. They then carried out a multi-factorial analysis with category type as one factor. A second factor was stimulus type—words, pictures or both pictures and words. The final factor was the nature of the task, e.g. perceptual decision, semantic decision, syllable decision or word retrieval. This procedure made the findings especially important. It enabled data from more than 60 subjects to be used and gave the study far more statistical power at that time than any other on the topic. The main results are shown in Figure 6.24.

---

[41] This paper used an unusual statistical procedure which makes the reliability of the conclusions difficult to judge. Cross-subject Talairach co-ordinates are presented but no overall statistical analysis. We are told how many subjects passed a very low threshold ($p < 0.05$) for each task in each region but the criteria for including an activation in a region was not defined.

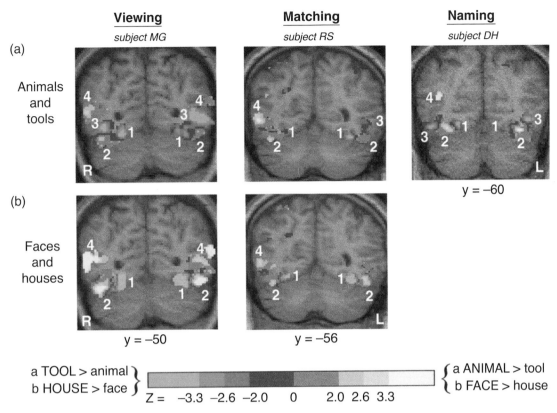

Fig. 6.23 Category-related activation related to (a) animals and tools and (b) faces and houses in three representative subjects of Chao et al. (1999). Critical regions are numbered as follows: 1, medial fusiform; 2, lateral fusiform gyrus; 3, middle inferior temporal gyrus; 4, superior temporal sulcus. Reprinted by permission from Macmillan Publishers Ltd: *Nature Neuroscience* (L.L. Chao, J.V. Haxby and A. Martin, 1999, Attribute-based neural substrates in temporal cortex for perceiving and knowing about objects. *Nature Neuroscience*, 2(10), 913–939.), copyright (1999).

They are not the areas found by Chao and Martin. Instead they are the left and right medial anterior temporal regions.[42] The effect is not independent of task. There was considerable variation in the activation of these regions across tasks as well as across stimuli. Indeed there was one type of task which did not activate these two regions, namely perceptual ones; this indicates the regions are specifically concerned with semantic processing. However, there was no suggestion that the regions were concerned solely with animals or with fruit and vegetables. Both types of stimuli seemed to activate these regions in certain tasks. Indeed the authors point out that similar medial anterior temporal regions had been activated in within-category dissociations involving

faces, their names or the names of common objects (Gorno-Tempini et al., 1998). So they argue that the regions are involved when an object has many features or attributes that need to be mapped onto a single conceptual representation (e.g. Meunier et al., 1993; Buckley et al., 1997). Living things have these multiple sensory dimensions.

By contrast, Devlin et al. found that naming tools specifically activates the left posterior middle temporal gyrus across all tasks except phonological and visual ones. This fits with many earlier studies (e.g. Damasio et al., 1996; Martin et al., 1996; Mummery et al., 1996; Cappa et al., 1998). Moreover three studies with different types of aetiology have all found a remarkably similar localisation for a specific deficit in the naming of tools or, in one case, manipulable artefacts, to the posterior superior left temporal lobe—in a varied aetiology study (Damasio et al., 1996) (see Figure 6.22), in dementing patients (Brambati et al., 2006) and in acute tumour patients (Campanella et al., 2010). So one has strong cross-method corroboration. In addition, at a lower threshold some imaging studies activate parts of the

[42] This localisation makes the use of a very large sample especially critical. These areas are subject to a so-called loss-of-signal artefact in fMRI (Jezzard & Clare, 1999) due to their proximity to part of the sinus system. This also means that the failure to find effects in these regions with smaller samples could well be a false negative effect.

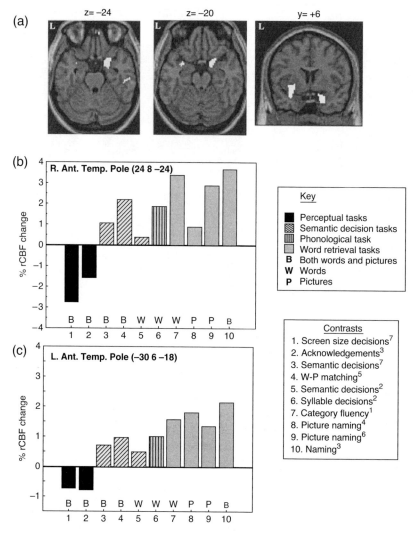

Fig. 6.24 Results of the metaanalysis of Devlin et al. (2002) of imaging studies of category specificity effects. (a) Areas more active during tasks involving living things than tasks involving artefacts. (b and c) effect size for the right and left anteriomedial temporal poles respectively. The only discrepant tasks are non-semantic perceptual ones. Contrasts are labelled with a letter to indicate whether the stimuli were words (W), pictures (P), or both (B). Reprinted from *Neuroimage, 15*(3), J.T. Devlin, C.J. Moore, C.J. Mummery, M.L. Gorno-Tempini, J.A. Phillips, U. Noppeney, R.S.J. Frackowiak, K.J. Friston and C.J. Price, Anatomic Constraints on Cognitive Theories of Category Specificity, 675–685, Copyright (2002), with permission from Elsevier.

left premotor cortex, again like many earlier studies (e.g. Martin et al., 1996; Grafton et al., 1997). Many studies have also found inferior parietal activation with pictures of tools (e.g. Chao & Martin, 2000; Okada et al., 2000). These are the structures that collectively form the object-manipulation system that was described in Section 3.4 and will be discussed further in Chapter 8. Indeed, digressing a little, listening to action verbs like *kick* led to activations specific to the individual effectors in a study of Tettamanti et al. (2005) (see Figure 6.25).[43]

Returning to tools, if one compares the tasks employed in the Chao et al. study and those employed in the Devlin et al. study, half the tasks in the former study are visual and do not require semantic processing.

---

[43] MEG experiments carried out at much the same time produce such effector-specific activations less than 200 msec after the end

of a critical disambiguating syllable, which argues against the idea that subjects are just imagining acting the word (Pulvermuller et al., 2005). However TMS experiments show interference effects only at about 500 msec not at 170 or 350 msec (Papeo et al., 2009), so the issue of whether subjects are consciously imagining the action in studies like that of Tettamanti et al. remains to be resolved. The patient data is the more convincing as far as on-line first-pass semantic processing is concerned.

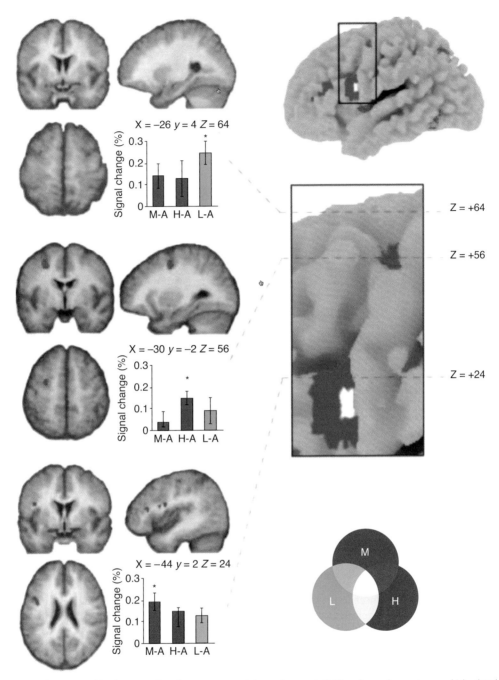

Fig. 6.25 Brain regions engaged by the processing of sentences containing action words. Subjects listened to sentences which related to actions performed with the mouth (M, blue), the leg (L, green) or the hand (H, red), such as those containing verbs like *lick* or *kick*. Somatotopic activation observed in Broca's area and the premotor cortex are shown in the enlarged section. Reproduced with permission from M. Tettamanti, G. Buccino, M.C. Saccuman, V. Gallese, M. Danna, P. Scifo, F. Fazio, G. Rizzolatti, S.F. Cappa and D. Perani; (2005) Listening to action-related sentences activates fronto-parietal motor circuits. *Journal of Cognitive Neuroscience, 17*(2), 237–281. Copyright © 2005, MIT Press Journals.

It is also not that clear what processes are involved in tasks where reading is followed by later questions. It is entirely conceivable that subjects generate an image, in which case perceptual processing will be required. For the present we will assume that the earlier locations that give rise to consistent activations in the Chao et al. study relate to processing at the perceptual categorisation or structural description levels. The more anterior regions activated in the Devlin et al. study are, however, consistently activated in semantic tasks and *not* in purely perceptual tasks. It seems more appropriate to see them as containing regions activated when processes dependent on semantic representations of living things are carried out.

The reader who has not become bogged down in anatomical detail will have jumped to one reassuring and one rather alarming conclusion. The reassuring conclusion is that the anatomical localisation of the regions activated by living things in normal subjects in the critical Devlin et al. meta-analysis corresponds at a reasonable level of approximation with Gainotti's localisation of the lesion in the corresponding category-specific effects in herpes simplex encephalitis patients. One has a solid brain-based correspondence for the neuropsychological dissociation. It becomes a solid empirical datum about which theorising is appropriate.

However at the same time there is an alarming aspect. The regions that are more activated for animals, as opposed to tools, in the Devlin et al. analysis are very similar to those associated with the seat of semantic dementia in Section 6.7. How does one then explain the sparing of knowledge of tools in the herpes syndrome when this type of knowledge is generally lost in semantic dementia? There seem to be a number of possible ways out of this dilemma. For the moment we will follow Martin and presuppose that the left middle temporal gyrus region, which shows specific activation for tools, is part of a system that has a conceptual role, as suggested by Martin (2007), and is not purely a structural description system involved in their perceptual encoding. If it were purely a structural description system, then non-visual knowledge of tools would be intact. This region might then be damaged in semantic dementia but not in the herpes syndrome. A second possibility is that semantic dementia, even if it does not lead to structural damage to such a region, leads to its functional deactivation, as it does for anatomically closely similar regions in Brodmann area 37 (see Mummery et al., 1999). Yet another possibility will be considered in the next theoretical section. For the present we will assume that this dilemma can be resolved and consider theories of the prototypic form of category specificity.

6.11 Theories of Category Specificity

A variety of explanations have been put forward for this double dissociation in the relative loss of knowledge and sparing of living things. However they fall into two main classes. One argues that there is a functional separation, and so localisational differences, between the different types of knowledge required by different semantic categories. The other argues that the internal structure of how different types of knowledge pertain to a semantic category differs for one type of category compared with the other. In this second class of theory it is presupposed that there is no necessary difference between where in the brain different types of knowledge is stored; they form neither psychologically nor anatomically isolable subsystems. We will consider three theories—two of the first type and one of the second. We begin, however, with the second type of theory.

On the second type of theory it is argued that semantic attributes have different patterns of connections with each other in different categories of knowledge and it is for this reason that categories are differentially sensitive to damage (Devlin et al., 1998; Tyler et al., 2000). In particular, Tyler and colleagues developed a position, initially put forward in a non-connectionist framework by De Renzi and Lucchelli (1994), that the form and function of artefacts are organised internally in a different fashion from those of living things. For artefacts it is held that distinctive functional information co-occurs with distinctive perceptual features. For example, a *bicycle's handlebars* are for *steering* and there are very few types of perceptual feature that have this function. Thus distinctive attributes of different types mutually support each other in a one (or few) to one (or few) way in a network. By contrast for living things functional information and perceptual information is shared in a many-to-many way by many members of the category; consider *seeing* going with *eyes*, for example. Thus members of different categories will have different patterns of correlated features; in artefacts distinctive attributes in perception go with distinctive attributes in function frequently in a way specific to the item; in living things they do not.

The attraction of these models is much increased by the way that at least one of them—that of Gonnerman et al. (1997)—shows cross-over effects of degree of damage of a category-specific form (see Figure 6.26). Thus Gonnerman et al. (1997) claimed that the effect their model predicts occurred empirically in a group of Alzheimer's patients they studied. However in a much more detailed empirical study, Garrard et al. (1998) found no relation between the overall degree of impairment and category-specific effects in Alzheimer's disease, which are at best rare in the syndrome, and certainly did not obtain a cross-over pattern.[44] In any case such models, while being compatible with anatomical differences in localisation of features, are much more strongly motivated if such differences do not exist. However, as we have seen in the previous section, they do.

---

[44] The Tyler et al. model predicts the opposite cross-over pattern with the main effect being a living-things deficit for most levels of impairment. This latter effect does occur for Alzheimer patients (Sartori et al., 2007).

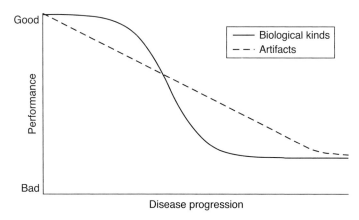

Fig. 6.26 Schematic illustration of the trajectories of increasing impairment for different types of word as the disease progresses for biological kinds and artefacts held to result theoretically from increasing random damage to semantic features in the model of the semantic system of Gonnerman et al. (1997). Reprinted from *Brain and Language, 57*(2), L.M. Gonnerman, E.S. Andersen, J.T. Devlin, D. Kempler and M.S. Seidenber, Double Dissociation of Semantic Categories in Alzheimer's Disease, 254–279. Copyright (1997), with permission from Elsevier.

Just as critically, this type of theory offers no intellectual leverage for explaining the difference in behavioural pattern between semantic dementia and the category specific form of herpes simplex encephalitis (see Table 6.7).

The more traditional theories of category specificity assume that the categorical difference reflects an underlying difference in localisation between relevant subsystems. The original position developed by Warrington, McCarthy and one of us (Warrington & McCarthy, 1983; Warrington & Shallice, 1984) was that the core attributes held to be the distinguishing key for how living things and artefacts are semantically differentiated were different. The core attributes of knowledge of living things, in general, were held to be their sensory features—shape, colour, texture, and in the case of animals the pattern of their walk, the sounds they make, in the case of foods their taste, and for plants smell (consider wild sage), or tactile sensations (for instance long grass). Thus the core attributes of the *crocus, daffodil* and *tulip* were seen as differing in their sensory characteristics.

By contrast, the core element of the meaning of artefacts was held to be their function—what they are used for. For instance, *chalk, crayon* and *pencil* on the one hand, can have a variety of colours, say; they differ critically with respect to the type of surface they are best suited to when used for drawing. In both cases there are differences in the more abstract information one knows about them—that pencils contain a type of graphite, that tulips are associated with Holland and so on—but these were viewed as additional non-core elements of meaning. It was held that these different core semantic elements are held in different subsystems which are located in different regions of cortex and which in turn have different patterns of connections to

other subsystems.[45] Caramazza and Shelton's (1998) theoretical position was different. They argued that there are a number of semantic domains which are evolutionarily critical for the human and so these categories—including knowledge of animals, knowledge of plants and knowledge of artefacts—have differentially localisable underlying systems in the brain. On this theory it is the concepts as a whole that are differently anatomically organised not their critical elements.

Is either of these positions compatible with the evidence? Take the earlier theory that different categories load differentially on different types of features and it is the feature-base which is differentially localised. Caramazza and Shelton (1998) made a blistering attack on this position which they claim to have 'refuted'. They have two main arguments. The first concerns the type of knowledge that patients have about items in these impaired categories. It seems obvious that on the sensory-functional theory one would expect that the selective impairment of knowledge of living things should be the most severe for sensory quality aspects of such knowledge rather than functional knowledge such as that *horses* are used to pull carts and that *cows* produce milk.

The natural place to derive more specific predictions would be from a simple connectionist model developed by Farah and McClelland (1991) in which there are separate sets of *sensory quality units* (called *visual units* by Farah and McClelland) and *functional units* (see Figure 6.27). Following the assumptions initially made when the sensory-functional theory was developed, living

---

[45] The theory used by Martin and collaborators to explain the pattern of functional imaging data, while based on the anatomical dorsal-ventral route theory, has many similarities to the sensory-functional position.

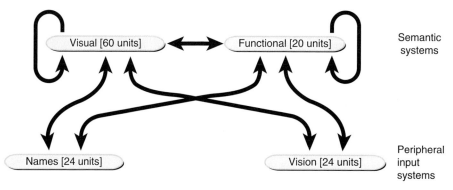

Fig. 6.27 The architecture of semantic cognition explored by Farah and McClelland (1991). The model was trained and tested on associating names to pictures for both living and nonliving things. As described in the text, the ratio of visual to functional units in the semantic representations of living things was on average 8:1. For non-living things the ratio was 1.8:1.

things within the model have relatively speaking more sensory quality features than functional ones when compared with artefacts. Farah and McClelland tested this by asking subjects to mark visual and functional descriptions in definitions of animals and living things. The ratio of visual to functional properties was far higher for living (8:1) than non-living things (1.4:1). Using these ratios in the setting up of the model has the consequence that, after it has learned, its knowledge of the sensory quality attributes of artefacts comes to be dependent on the more dominant functional units. For living things it is the other way round, the knowledge of the functional attributes is in part supported by the activity of the sensory quality units. This can be seen by the effect of damage to the two types of unit respectively (see Figure 6.28). Thus knowledge of the functional attributes *of living things* would be impaired following damage to the sensory quality units. The 'obvious assumptions' referred to earlier should not be taken at face value.

This argument was, though, rejected by Caramazza and Shelton, even though their criticism was of a part of it that is almost self-evidently true! They said the contrasting ratios are not justified empirically. They asked subjects to underline all sensory/perceptual descriptions and all functional *or associative* descriptions in definitions. Then they found the difference in ratios between artefacts and living things disappeared. Why did they make the change from *functional* to *functional or associative* descriptions? They argued that asking subjects to underline 'what it is for', for living and non-living things, which was in fact only a subset of what Farah and McClelland asked, 'will not provide a fair estimate of the nonsensory properties known for living things. This is because the use of an item—what it is for—is a highly specific property *typically found with artefacts but not natural kinds*' (italics added) so it 'will not provide a fair estimate of the nonsensory properties known for living things' (p. 18). What was the original theory?

'The evolutionary development of tool use has led to finer and finer functional differentiation for an increasing range of purposes. We would suggest that identification of an inanimate object crucially depends on determination of its functional significance, but that this is irrelevant for the identification of living things' (Warrington & Shallice, 1984, p. 849). This early statement is a little cavalier in its all-or-none characterisation. However, Caramazza and Shelton by decree simply state that Farah and McClelland's faithful operationalisation of this idea is 'unfair' to living things. They therefore test an alternative theory based on 'nonsensory properties,' a concept they dreamt up. After showing this to be empirically inadequate they claim to have refuted the original functional-sensory quality theory, a proper test of the theory having been excluded as 'unfair'! We will take Farah and McClelland's assumptions to be appropriate.

Knowledge of the two types of attributes has in fact been assessed in a number of patients, beginning with studies by Basso et al. (1988), Sartori and Job (1988) and Silveri and Gainotti (1988).[46] However the results are far from conclusive. In these early studies, the effects obtained were often large. Thus LA of Silveri and Gainotti named 58% of animals from functional description and only 6% from visual description. Moreover, Giulietta and Michaelangelo (Sartori et al., 1993) showed similar effects. Yet such early studies have been criticised on the grounds that the questions were not shown to be of equal difficulty (Caramazza & Shelton, 1998). Instead, Caramazza and Shelton put forward four other patients—FM2 and GR2 of Laiacona et al. (1993) and LF and EA3 of Laiacona et al. (1997)—who showed a contrasting pattern of effects; although much better at naming artefacts than living things, they showed similar

---

[46] Patient NV, however, of Basso et al. suffered from semantic dementia and not herpes simplex encephalitis.

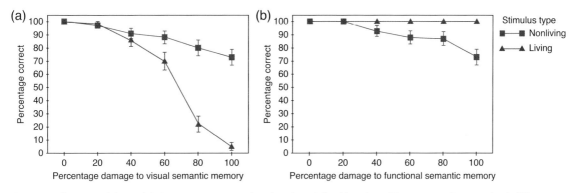

Fig. 6.28 Performance of the model of semantic cognition of Farah and McClelland (1991) on different types of input and with different levels of damage. Performance is measured in terms of the probability of correctly associating names with pictures. (a) Damage to visual semantic memory affects performance on living things more than non-living things. (b) Damage to functional semantic memory affects performance only on non-living things. Data from Farah and McClelland (1991), Table 3.

levels of performance when questioned about functional/associative or sensory aspects of stimuli. Capitani et al. (2003) list a further set of such patients. For the patients considered by Caramazza and Shelton, a test was used in which controls performed roughly equally well on the two types of question.[47] In fact, LF, one of the two herpes encephalitis patients considered by Caramazza and Shelton, did not even show the characteristic selective living things impairment properly; his mean performance for living things across two testing sessions was just in the normal range. For the second such patient, EA, the critical results are presented for living things and non-living things combined and he showed a floor effect. Thus the study does not discuss a single herpes encephalitis patient who showed the theoretically critical strong selective deficit for living things. Thus on the arguments of Chapter 4, it is technically irrelevant! In fact a few later patients provide some support for aspects of the Caramazza and Shelton position but even they produce complexities for their overall argument. Thus MU (Borgo & Shallice, 2003), a herpes patient showing a strong selective category specific effect, was indeed roughly equally bad for functional as compared with sensory quality judgements concerning living things, but was much better at functional than sensory quality judgements for the categories of edible substances (e.g. *mayonnaise, gorgonzola)* and

drinks (e.g. *beer, Coca-Cola*). Overall, Caramazza and Shelton empirically did an excellent job in undermining the positive earlier evidence for differential preservation of different types of knowledge in category specific patients. However the negative evidence they provide seems equally fragile.

The second line of criticism made by Caramazza and Shelton was much more solid. They pointed out that in some of the patients who had a selective loss of knowledge of living things the effects were even more specific and their impairment was limited to a single category. These were typically either of animals or of fruit and vegetables. A particularly clear case is patient EW, described by Caramazza and Shelton. EW scored at only 28–41% when naming animals in a variety of tests. By contrast she scored at least 80% when naming items from a variety of other categories including fruit (100%) and vegetables (100%). When items were matched for visual complexity and familiarity she scored 41% for animals and 94% for other items. She was also grossly impaired at deciding whether an apparent entity was real or not, but only for animals. In addition she made many errors on deciding whether a particular attribute was or was not a property of an animal. This was true whether the attributes were visual, associative or functional ones.

There have been three types of responses to descriptions of individual patients with more specific deficits than the more common but less specific loss of knowledge of living things. Warrington and McCarthy (1987) have argued that the sensory/functional domain is basically correct but needs further refinement. They argued that particular subdomains of sensory, functional and associative knowledge may make differential contributions to the way the semantic system is locally organised. Thus the core knowledge of plants may critically depend on colour. Humphreys and Forde (2001) have adopted a somewhat related position with a whole

---

[47] In fact, the performance of control subjects is by itself not a very adequate way to assess level of difficulty; the control patients would be expected to perform near ceiling, regardless of question type, as they do in the Caramazza and Shelton study. Moreover, most other patients considered by Caramazza and Shelton and by Capitani et al. were trauma, stroke or semantic dementia patients, not herpes encephalitis, which on the methodological arguments of Chapter 4 suggests that there may be a different functional basis for their syndrome, such as premorbid individual differences.

variety of featural subdomains assumed in their HIT (hierarchical interactive theory).

As we have seen, Caramazza and Shelton took a different line in arguing that certain types of knowledge are organised categorically in the brain. The three categories which they consider to be of sufficient evolutionary importance to be separately organised are knowledge of animals, of plants and of artefacts. This then explains why these categories are the ones that are found to be selectively impaired or spared.

There is, however, a third and simpler possibility. The more restricted category specific effects could as we discussed above just arise from individual differences in the degree to which knowledge of the different categories is represented in the mind premorbidly (Sartori et al., 2007). One simple way to refute this possibility is if the different types of specific deficits have different localisations. Neither the functional imaging nor the lesion location evidence shows any real indication of different specific localisations existing for knowledge of fruit and vegetables on the one hand and animals on the other. Gainotti (2000) notes that selective deficits of the 'plants' category was particularly clear in patients with *solely* left hemisphere strokes, but there were only four of these. This may merely mean that, generally, knowledge of plants is less over-learned or in the case of fruit/vegetables less differentiable and so is more susceptible to loss than is knowledge of animals. The anatomical similarity in the areas of the brain involved in the semantic processing of the relevant categories, if anything, supports the sensory-functional theory, rather than the evolutionary critical categories theory of Caramazza and Shelton. Moreover the most striking specific case, namely EW of Caramazza and Shelton, had a left fronto-parietal lesion, completely different from the standard lesion site for the category-specific herpes encephalitis syndrome. This suggests a quite different type of functional origin for the patient's problem rather than an animal-specific problem which is a component of the more commonly seen general living things deficit.

In functional imaging Marques et al. (2008) have tested knowledge of different types of attribute (surface form or type of motion) across different categories, and in particular compared the living versus non-living categories. They found strong effects of different types of attribute but no effects of category. Caramazza and Shelton's theory that knowledge is organised through evolutionarily critical categories has little solid support.

There is however yet another reason for doubting the theory of three evolutionarily critical categories. The range of category-specific impairment is not just limited to living things and artefacts. Other categories, which can also be selectively damaged or spared include,

for instance, parts-of-the-body (see e.g. Goodglass et al., 1966; Dennis, 1976; Shelton et al., 1998). Important, indirect support for the existence of body parts as an evolutionary separate domain comes from *autotopagnosia*—a condition that is well characterised as a deficit in the *visual* structural descriptions of the *human* body and its parts (Sirigu et al., 1991; Buxbaum & Coslett, 2001). Knowledge of parts-of-the-body could well be another evolutionary specialised system so this category-specific effect does not pose a problem for the Caramazza–Shelton position.

There are, though, other category-specific effects that do. Take, for instance, knowledge of geographical visuo-spatial information. Shallice and Saffran (1986) reported a pure alexia patient ML with a left posterior lesion who was incapable of reading aloud words unless given exposures of much more than 2 sec. Moreover, if asked to carry out a Peabody Picture–Word matching test, where one word must be matched to one of four pictures, then given 2 sec exposure of the word, he was virtually at chance (33/100). By contrast, when words were presented auditorily he was accurate. Yet when town names were presented visually and he had to locate the towns on a map he was as good visually as he was auditorily. He had a selective preservation of orthographic access to town-location knowledge.

One possible explanation of this pattern is that knowledge of town locations—a semantic task—is stored in the right hemisphere not the left. Converging evidence comes from the related task of naming countries.[48] In two patients, TM (Incisa della Rocchetta et al., 1998) and BF (Cipolotti, 2000), the patient had a selective sparing in production of country names, compared with other categories. Incisa della Rocchetta et al. (1998) speculated in a fashion consonant with the above argument that knowledge of country names was based on representations derived from visuo-spatial operations.

6.12 Herpes Simplex Encaphalitis and Semantic Dementia

There are converging lines of evidence for semantic representations being based on an attractor structure but with core attributes differing across word-type. From a neuropsychological perspective these lines of evidence stem from semantic dementia on the one hand and the category-specific impairments on the other, particularly those deriving from herpes simplex encephalitis. Yet the

---

[48] ML had many characteristics in common with the pure alexic patients of Coslett and Saffran discussed in Chapter 4. Indeed his preserved knowledge of town locations fits with their right hemisphere account of pure alexia.

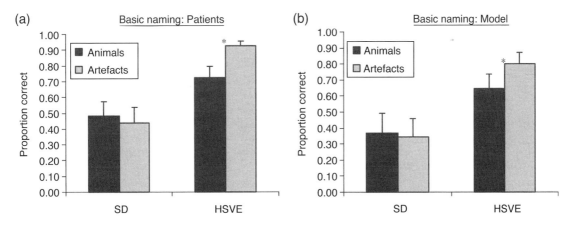

Fig. 6.29 Comprehension and basic naming performance for (a) patients and (b) the two variants of the model. Mean and standard errors of proportion correct for word-picture matching and basic-level naming of animals and artefacts are plotted for each patient group and for the semantic dementia (SD) and herpes encephalitis (HSVE) variants of the model. Reproduced from M.A. Lambon Ralph, C. Lowe and T.T. Rogers, Neural basis of category-specific semantic deficits for living things: evidence from semantic dementia, HSVE and a neural network model, *Brain*, 2007, *130*, 4, 1127–1137, by permission of Oxford University Press.

lines of evidence have so far been considered separately. What happens when they are combined? Then these lines of evidence if followed too far produce an apparent conflict. Semantic dementia and herpes simplex encephalitis both arise from lesions to the inferior anterior temporal cortices. Yet far from producing the same pattern of difficulties they produce contrasting patterns. A severe herpes encephalitis patient such as JBR or MV could be considerably better than a moderately severe semantic dementia patient on knowledge of artefacts but considerably worse on knowledge of living things (for examples see Noppeney et al., 2007).[49] How can one account for this putative double dissociation?

Half of the answer is given by a recent meta-analysis by Noppeney et al. (2007) using VBM, discussed in Section 6.7, of the lesions of four patients with herpes simplex encephalitis and six with semantic dementia. The herpes simplex patients were found to have decreased grey matter compared with both the semantic dementia patients and a control group in the medial parts of the anterior temporal cortices bilaterally just in the area that Devlin et al. (2002) have found to be particularly strongly activated by living things compared with artefacts in fMRI in normal subjects.[50]

This explains the relative deficit of the herpes patients on living things. It does not, however, explain their better performance on non-living things. Lambon-Ralph et al. (2007) make an ingenious suggestion. They take the model shown in Figure 6.14 and consider as a simplification just the part shown in Figure 6.6—that which is most critical for the relative preservation of artefact representations. Then they damage it in two ways. One is the way they simulated semantic dementia before—and we have already criticised—by lesioning connections to and from the semantic units. The other, to simulate herpes simplex encephalitis, is by adding an increasing amount of noise to these connections. They compare the effects obtained in the simulation with the performance of 8 semantic dementia patients and seven herpes patients on the naming of artefact and living thing stimuli. The correspondence (see Figure 6.29) is most impressive.

The devil, as in much cognitive experimentation, however, lies in the detail. The task was naming at the so-called basic *level*. *What* were the stimuli? Each domain was represented by six tight clusters of different examples (each belonging to basic categories such as *car* and *boat*), whereas the animals were organized in six tight clusters (corresponding to basic categories such as *bird*, *dog* and *fish*). The artefact clusters were appropriately more separated from each other than the animal clusters, which have many features in common; this led to the relative preservation of artefacts with noise. Also the model was trained with superordinate names (e.g. *animal*) and subordinate names for the individual examples (e.g. *collie*, a type of *dog*). However the test where model and patients were best compared—basic level naming— *car, fish* etc.) was very easy and the herpes simplex patients were essentially at ceiling for artefacts, so the nice quantitative fit is more apparent than real.

---

[49] Occasional semantic dementia patients have been described who did show the living things deficit typical of herpes simplex encephalitis. This, however, is a rare pattern for the aetiology (see Lambon-Ralph et al., 2003).

[50] By contrast the semantic dementia patients had lost more grey matter in the right lateral inferior temporal cortex.

Most critically there is no real justification as to why the two diseases should be realised in the model by the two forms of damage. At present this remains at most an interesting speculation for the difference between the syndromes.

A second possibility arises from the simple fact that herpes patients as a group are generally younger than semantic dementia patients. Thus it would be possible that the neural assemblies in their relatively preserved object manipulation system provide more adequate 'support' processes for the functioning of cortically distant groups of neurons as occurs on the Farah and McClelland model. Thus the assemblies in the damaged temporal cortices would receive greater support from an effectively functioning system controlling use of artefacts. However, whether this speculation holds up or not, the herpes syndrome appears to undercut the Rogers et al. position that accessing a representation in the semantic system in the inferior anterior temporal cortex is essential for retrieving semantic information about the concrete object. It appears that the spokes of the semantic wheel can be more autonomous than the hub model would assume.

Overall, then, category-specific effects fit well with a feature-based approach to semantics, as does semantic dementia. We cannot, therefore, like Fodor, assume that semantic representations can be treated purely as atoms of meaning, and so an approach to cognition treating its underlying operations as purely syntactic in type will be inadequate. Conversely, the attractor structure of concepts is also supported by the neuropsychological data. It would appear though too that the underlying network is not equipotential; concepts have a type of semantic core which can differ from one concept to another. The central core of the attractor for different types of concept could be based on features from a wide range of basic domains—shape, texture, colour, action, intention, spatial operation. Moreover concepts would be particularly sensitive to lesions which affect their core attributes, and so different types of concept would be susceptible to lesions in different regions of the brain.

6.13 On Abstract Concepts

So far we have been considering concepts that represent concrete objects. Can one simply extend the theoretical approach we have favoured to abstract concepts? Are there, for instance, just quantitative differences between the two types of representations? In the simulations of deep dyslexia of Plaut and Shallice (1993a), discussed in Section 4.11, impairments in the processing of abstract words were held to arise because such words were represented by a smaller number of features than

were concrete words. In a similar fashion, Barry and Gerhand (2003) have argued that concrete concepts have a higher degree of specificity than abstract ones. However other neuropsychological phenomena should make us wary of assuming that a merely quantitative extrapolation from the structure of concrete words can alone provide the conceptual base for the structure of abstract ones. For instance, as will see in Chapter 9, the ability to induce abstract rules or the ability to represent an abstract idea in another form is lost after prefrontal lesions, not temporal lobe ones. More directly, while there are many conditions such as deep dyslexia where concrete words are processed better than abstract ones by patients, some patients have been described who perform better at giving the core meaning of abstract words than of concrete ones. Thus the semantic dementia patients, AB of Warrington (1975) and DM of Breedin et al. (1994), produce contrasting success rates of 85% (abstract) versus 24% (concrete) and 59% (abstract) versus 46% (concrete), respectively, in giving their core meanings, and the herpes simplex encephalitis patient SBY of Warrington and Shallice (1984) similarly was successful with 94% (abstract) versus 50% (concrete).

Papagno et al. (2009) refer to nine other such cases described individually. However how general such a reverse concreteness effect is in patients is not known. The one relevant published group study was carried out by Yi et al. (2007) on 12 semantic dementia patients. On a test of matching one of four words to a description, the patients performed better on so-called cognitive verbs, mainly psychological or social interaction terms like *bore* or *refuse*, than so-called motion verbs like *push* or *ride*. The contrast was in some cases rather subtle. Moreover no equivalent effect was found with abstract versus concrete nouns. Somewhat ominously for a non-artefactual account, Lambon-Ralph (personal communication) in a series of 18 semantic dementia patients found none had the reverse concreteness effect. Indeed such effects just might (but no more than might!), following the general line of argument of Sartori et al. (2007), be attributable in these patients to an unusual differential representation of the two categories of words premorbidly. Thus AB was a high-level civil servant. However patient CAV of Warrington (1981), who was suffering from a left parieto-temporal glioma and who read abstract words much better than concrete ones, was a shopkeeper.

If we turn to functional imaging, abstract words have been contrasted with concrete in a number of studies using more than one task. The results are rather heterogeneous (see Papagno et al., 2009). However, if one restricts attention to conditions where there is not an obvious biasing between the tasks used with the different word-types, then on 8/11 studies there is left inferior

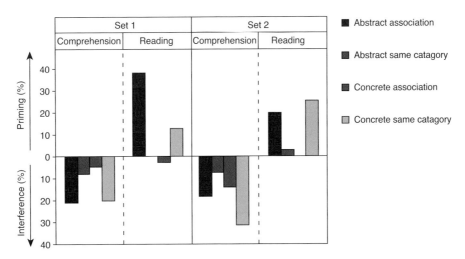

Fig. 6.30 Interference and priming effects shown in comprehension (matching spoken and written words) and reading for patient FBI of Crutch and Warrington (2007) as a function of word type. FBI was tested with two sets of words. Reproduced from *Brain and Language, 103*(1), S.J. Crutch and E.K. Warrington, Contrasting effects of semantic priming and interference in processing abstract and concrete words, 88–89. Copyright 2007, with permission from Elsevier.

frontal involvement, much the highest rate for any brain area.[51] Yet the left inferior prefrontal cortex is not the site that has been argued to be the hypothetical semantic hub for the representation of concrete concepts. Another system appears to be involved.

Not only are there anatomical suggestions of different underlying systems, there are also other neuropsychological signs that abstract words are represented qualitatively very differently from concrete ones. Such suggestive evidence comes from two studies by Crutch and Warrington (2005, 2007) working with two patients. One was an aphasic patient, AZ, assessed using a 5-choice spoken word-picture matching tests like those used in the study of semantic access/refractory disorders. The second was a deep dyslexic patient, FBI, assessed using analogous written word to spoken word matching tests. We will concentrate on the results of FBI, but those obtained with AZ were similar.

Crutch and Warrington contrasted two types of similarity effects with concrete and abstract words. The first type involved the tests used with semantic access/refractory disorders discussed in Section 6.4, namely where a group of stimuli are presented which are semantically related members of category, such as *yacht, dinghy, canoe, ferry, barge* for concrete words or *fury, anger, rage, annoyance, wrath* for abstract words. The contrasting situation was where the words are not all

from the same semantic category but have a semantic association; an example would be the *dagger, blood, ambulance, policeman, handcuffs* for concrete words or *democracy, republic, freedom, politics, election* for abstract ones. In addition to carrying out the written word to spoken word matching test, the patient has to read aloud the words in their sets. For a particular type of word one of the kinds of similarity effect has a major effect for both of the tasks. However the other kind of similarity had little effect. Essentially over the two experiments the critical similarity had a positive effect on reading but a negative effect on word matching. The striking result of the experiment was that for the concrete words the critical effect was similarity within a category but for the abstract words it was similarity amongst a group of associated words (see Figure 6.30).[52]

Crutch and Warrington argue that the difference in the critical dimension of similarity suggests that the representations of associated abstract words such as *politics* and *election* are more closely linked than ones in the same category, say *anger* and *rage,* while for

---

[51] This excludes, say, a D'Esposito et al. (1997) study, where quite different tasks are used for the two types of words, but includes as an extra Fletcher et al. (1996), where memory encoding was used for both.

[52] For the abstract words the result was clear in the sense that over two experiments, the four conditions that should have shown a significant positive effect on this characterisation all did so and none of the other four conditions did. For the concrete words the results were less clear; there was only a 3-1 difference. However, the concrete results need to be considered in the context of very similar findings in semantic access/retrieval disorder. Hamilton and Coslett (2008) in an apparently similar patient obtained no difference on these tests between abstract and concrete words.

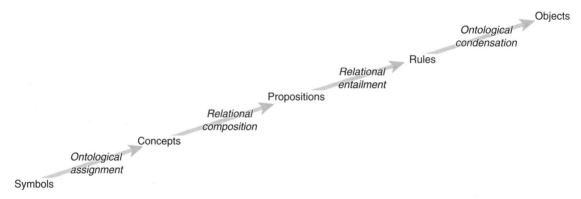

Fig. 6.31 Fox's 'knowledge ladder', showing the relation within AI between lower-level symbols and concepts and higher-level rules and 'objects'. An 'object' in this computer science sense may be thought of as a collection of rules.

concrete words two words in the same category are more closely linked than a pair of words that are associated. It is not clear what the authors mean by 'linked' in this context. We would draw a weaker conclusion namely that the underlying semantic representations of concrete words and of abstract words have a qualitatively different structure. A purely quantitative approach to the difference in meanings between the two types of word might explain the loss of within-category effects when moving to abstract words.[53] However it is unclear how such an explanation could deal with the association effect with abstract words.[54]

What could the difference be between the nature of the representations of concrete and abstract words? Consider, say, a *parrot* and a *sparrow*. The parrot is brightly coloured but the sparrow is drab. The parrot can be quite large for a bird but the sparrow is small. The parrot can squawk and the sparrow merely cheeps. These characteristics can presumably all be explained by biologists in terms of the different evolutionary niches that the two birds fill. However to the rest of us, that two of the possible eight combinations of characteristics correspond to actual birds is a matter of selecting arbitrarily two out of the eight possible triplets (*colour, size, call*). A feature-based representation such as those used in the Rogers et al. simulation could well underlie the contrast. But instead take *hope*. One might try to characterise it as a list of features: *hope* is *a human emotion, concerns a belief, is positive, relates to time*.

However the list of features, even if extended, fails to capture the real meaning of *hope*.

A more adequate characterisation of abstract concepts can be derived from AI approaches to knowledge. Fox (2005) summarises progress in knowledge representation (epistemics) over the last few decades in terms of a 'knowledge ladder' (see Figure 6.31). At the lowest level are atomic symbols that have no meaning in and of themselves. Meaning accrues through a series of abstraction operations:

(1) *ontological assignment* associates symbols that signify related things into categories by assigning them as exemplars of concepts;

(2) *relational composition* allows concepts to be composed into propositions or (to use Fox's term) descriptions through the use of relations between concepts;

(3) *relational entailment* allows the expression of generalisations over relations within propositions (e.g. that a relation is transitive); and ultimately,

(4) *ontological condensation* groups collections of rules into what computer scientists refer to as objects, or packages of encapsulated information that may be manipulated or queried through a well-defined interface.

Fox's ladder is capable of characterising some abstract concepts (e.g. that of a *task*), but for a concept such as *hope* it is necessary to go even further, from *epistemics* to what Fox refers to as *pathics*—mental states. Here, too, there has been significant progress driven by AI and formal semantics, leading to the widespread use of Belief–Desire–Intention (BDI) agents (e.g. Rao & Georgeff, 1995) and rigorous mathematical treatments of the underlying concepts in terms of modal logics (Blackburn et al., 2001). BDI agents are systems capable of generating behaviour based on three distinct types of propositional knowledge—*beliefs, desires* and *intentions*—while modal logics extend predicate calculus with

---

[53] The attractors would have a weaker bottom-up base; see Plaut and Shallice (1993a).

[54] Another type of difference is likely to involve the degree to which the concept is learned purely verbally—see the discussion of Gleitman et al. (2005), in Section 6.8. However, abstract concepts are not just learned verbally; consider geometrical concepts such as tangent or isosceles, the concept of a weak pawn or well-placed knight in chess or even the concept of a limit in mathematics.

modal operators (such as *necessity* and *possibility*) which are typically given a formal semantics in terms of possible worlds.[55] Returning to the concept of *hope*, its meaning might be characterised in modal terms as:

hope(p) if and only if *desire(p) & believe(possible(p)).*

The argument structure is essential to the characterisation, as are the logical form and operators *desire*, *believe* and *possible*. The list-like characterisation of the contrasting properties of *parrot* and *sparrow* would fail completely to do justice to the meaning of *hope*.

Clearly these contrasts between abstract and concrete words are not all-or-none, and indeed for some purposes, such as reading aloud, the feature-based account of abstract words may be conceptually adequate. However, the argument suggests that the implementation of the meaning of abstract words may require a very different type of computational basis and hence a different material basis in the brain from that for concrete words. We will return to the issue of BDI agents in Section 9.7 and the representation of pathic concepts in Section 11.1.

6.14 Conclusions

The overall conception of semantic representations that we have reached has four levels. We need a basic network of subsystems that each has different computational functions and different anatomical bases. The subsystems include ones concerned with the categorising of visual form, and of other visual qualities, similar ones for auditory and tactile sensory systems, and ones for object manipulation, and for spatial representations and transformations among others. Many semantic representations are based on neuronal assemblies that cross this network of subsystems. In this respect the overall structure corresponds qualitatively to that proposed by Allport (1985).[56]

In addition, though, we presume that the assemblies have an attractor structure spread across the individual subsystems, as for instance in the model discussed by Kropff and Treves (2008). Then the acquisition of individual attractors appears to be critically based on one or more of the subsystems discussed above—core subsystems for that concept—so its meaning representation

becomes an onion-like structure as far as the importance of different parts of the assembly is concerned with the inner layers of the onion being based in these core subsystems. Critical amongst these core subsystems is often one derived evolutionarily from the need to distinguish between visual representations of concrete objects. This subsystem has in turn to represent complex and apparently arbitrary conjunctions of attributes; this is the hub semantic system of Rogers et al. (2004) and Tyler and Moss (2001) that is damaged in semantic dementia. We assume it to be particularly relevant for the representation of concrete objects.

Finally, however, there is a fourth aspect where the inner structure of the representation of the concept is more critical for realising its meaning than mere number of arbitrarily coexisting features that it contains. Here the organising principle must be based on the internal logical structure of the concept. One example of these types of concepts are numbers, based on systems located in the intraparietal sulcus for estimating numerosity which were discussed in Section 3.4 and concepts known to be capable of being left intact in semantic dementia (Cappelletti et al., 2002). More generally we have argued that abstract concepts need to be viewed from the perspective of this organising principle. A consequence is that for such concepts the symbolic split we have made between concepts and operations becomes artificial. Before discussing operations per se, though, we need to consider the memory processes which thought requires and particularly those that are loosely known as working memory.

---

[55] Thus, propositions are interpreted with respect to a possible world. A proposition is *necessary* if and only if it is true in every possible world accessible from the current one, and *possible* if and only if it is true in at least one possible world accessible from the current one.

[56] See FNMS Chapter 12 for discussion. The swathe of activation in posterior left temporal and parietal cortices discussed in Section 6.5 could well correspond to the accessing of these aspects of the semantic representations.

CHAPTER 7

Short-term Retention, Buffers, Priming, and Working Memory

7.1 Introduction

Any cognitive task that does not just involve a series of responses each immediately triggered by the perceptual input requires one or more systems to store the products of intermediate operations. This is true of AI systems, both theoretical ones, such as the Turing machine, and real ones, such as production systems, and also of humans. For the last fifty years the topics of short-term memory and working memory have therefore been central both in cognitive psychology and later in cognitive neuroscience. However, the 'centrality' of the concepts has led to the application of the terms, particularly the latter, to what is in effect a range of overlapping referents.

As discussed in Section 1.4, when the domain began to be intensively investigated the initial perspective, drawing analogies from the computer systems of their times, was of an all-purpose *short-term store* or *primary memory* which held information while it was laid down in long-term memory (e.g. Waugh & Norman, 1965). Conceptions of short-term memory soon became more complex. On the initial perspective, using the computer science metaphor, the role of short-term memory was seen as passive. Thought, though, is active. So the conception of short-term memory was modified in two ways. Atkinson and Shiffrin (1968) hypothesized not two but three types of memory system: sensory buffer stores, a limited capacity short-term store and a long-term memory system. In this respect, Atkinson and Shiffrin's model was a typical so-called *modal model*, a term used by Murdock (1974) to describe the common basic ideas in many competing models of the late 1960s and early 1970s. However, the distinguishing contribution of Atkinson and Shiffrin was to separate out from these different stores so-called *control processes.* These are putative systems held to underpin active processes such as rehearsal, which occur in experiments on short-term memory, and to be functionally separable from their three types of memory store. Secondly, Baddeley and Hitch (1974) built on this by rejecting the idea of a single short-term store and replacing it by a central executive store and two slave systems—the articulatory loop and the visuo-spatial sketchpad. The slave systems in turn contain buffers; thus the articulatory loop contained a phonological buffer. The central executive store, in turn, had some of the functions attributed by Atkinson and Shiffrin to control processes.

At this point the field could have settled into Kuhnian normal science mode. Instead it began to fragment. To start with, Baddeley and Hitch made another apparently innocuous change. They renamed the field 'working memory' (i.e. an active concept) instead of 'short-term memory' (a passive one). At roughly the same time Craik and Lockhart (1972) continued the undermining of what was later seen as passive box-and-arrow models ('boxology') by partly erasing the distinction between processing and storage in their levels-of-processing theory which held quite appropriately that storage was a by-product of processing operations. The deeper within the system the processing of the input occurs, the more durable, it was held, is the storage. Again, however attention was directed away from the nature of short-term storage itself. To make matters more complex the obvious point was made that whatever is being stored in short-term memory depends upon learned representations, and so can be viewed as an activated part of long-term memory (Norman, 1968). Erroneously, the structural view of short-term memory as a separable system was held to be undermined (e.g. Crowder, 1993).

The conflation between storage and processing soon gathered pace. Daneman and Carpenter (1980) wanted to investigate how fluent reading depends upon working memory. They argued that traditional 1960s-type measures of short-term memory, such as digit span, were too passive.[1] Instead they argued that the function of working memory requires it to divide its capacity between processing and storage. They therefore developed a new measure—so-called *working memory span.* In the working memory span task a subject reads a string of sentences and, immediately after the last sentence, they must repeat back the last word of each.

Span is measured as the maximum number of sentences for which the subject is correct on two out of three trials. Unlike digit span, working memory span correlates highly with various measures of reading comprehension performance, such as tests of pronominal reference (Daneman & Carpenter, 1980; see also Caplan & Waters, 1999). However, that a measure can be reliable and correlate highly with another measure does not necessarily mean it has any simple relation to any single basic component of cognition.[2]

These trends within cognitive psychology soon received very powerful indirect support. As discussed in Section 1.2, Fuster and Alexander had described cells in prefrontal cortex of the monkey, which continue to respond in the interval between a food-well being baited with food and the time at which a response has to be made. In a most elegant development, Funahashi et al. (1989) trained monkeys to maintain fixation for from between one to six seconds and then to make an eye movement to a location that had been indicated before the delay. Cells in sulcus principalis of dorsolateral prefrontal cortex were active during the interval, as if they held a *mnemonic* receptive field corresponding to a particular part of the visual field of the monkey. Moreover lesions in sulcus principalis could lead to a so-called *mnemonic scotoma*: the monkey would be inaccurate in recalling the position where a stimulus was presented if it had been in that particular part of the visual field.[3] From these beautiful findings, Goldman-Rakic (1987) argued that the dorsolateral prefrontal cortex was the seat of 'working memory'.

These different lines of ideas coalesced into what may be called the 2000 'modal model'. In an excellently organised volume on working memory, Miyake and Shah (1999a) invited the main theorists in the field to write reviews of the field orientated around a number of key theoretical issues that had to be addressed. Miyake and Shah (1999b) were therefore wellplaced to write a definitive overview. However they also needed to be faithful to their contributors. They proposed the following 'all-encompassing definition of working memory' (p. 450):

> Working memory is those mechanisms or processes that are involved in the control, regulation, and active maintenance of task-relevant information in the service of complex cognition, including novel as well as familiar, skilled tasks. It consists

---

[1] Digit span is the number of random digits spoken to the subject at a one per second rate that can be echoed back without error.

[2] One obvious example is the concept of general intelligenc, *g*, which has had a torrid history as far as its referent is concerned, even though it correlates highly with other measures and is a very reliable construct psychometrically, but see Chapter 9.
[3] The term *scotoma* is used to describe the loss of vision in part of the visual field due to a lesion in, say, occipital cortex.

of a set of processes and mechanisms and is not a fixed 'place' or 'box' in the cognitive architecture. It is not a completely unitary system in the sense that it involves multiple representational codes and/or different subsystems. Its capacity limits reflect multiple factors and may even be an emergent property of the multiple processes and mechanisms involved. Working memory is closely linked to LTM [long-term memory], and its contents consist primarily of currently activated LTM representations, but can also extend to LTM representations that are closely linked to activated retrieval cues and, hence, can be quickly reactivated.

In other words, it is a very very complex beast indeed, half-defined apaphatically and characterised as involving a multiplicity of mechanisms. Given this complexity, it becomes unclear how useful a concept it is.

The philosophy of this chapter is almost the opposite to that of Miyake and Shah (1999b) in their overview and possibly may seem dispiritingly traditional to readers. We will be concerned with the way in which information is retained specifically over short intervals of time so as to allow other cognitive computational operations to take place. We will, even worse, use the old-fashioned language of 'boxes'. We will argue that three types of short-term memory process need to be distinguished:

1. The process of *priming*, whereby—to simplify for the present—the processing of a specific input by a cognitive subsystem results in that system (or the cognitive system as a whole) responding to the same or a related input more rapidly and/or more efficiently on a subsequent presentation. Thus, in repetition priming, subjects respond more quickly and accurately when required to respond to a stimulus (e.g. in an object recognition or categorisation task) on second and subsequent presentations (e.g. Tulving & Schacter, 1990; Dobbins et al., 2004). In semantic priming subjects respond more quickly to words that are semantically related to a prime than to other words (e.g. Marslen-Wilson & Tyler, 1997); for example, when their task is to recognise the words. Priming is also frequently examined in word-stem completion tasks,[4] where word-stems are more likely to be completed by primed items than by non-primed items (e.g. Horner & Henson, 2008).

2. Repositories of information, where information can be passively retained over short-intervals of time; such short-term repositories of information can conveniently be called *buffers*. These correspond to key components of Baddeley and Hitch's slave systems, such as the *phonological buffer*, which holds phonological information, and a system with a capacity for retaining visual patterns, which is a component of their visuo-spatial sketchpad, the *visual cache* to use Logie's (1995) term. A critical feature of such a system is that its memory characteristics are specific to the type of store. Thus it was shown by Mitchell (1972) that information retained in an auditory–verbal short-term store, later to be called an *input phonological buffer*, is structured on the basis of its time of occurrence or at least in terms of the order in which items arrive; however, by contrast a visual short-term store is primarily spatially *not* temporally organised.[5]

3. Systems where short-term retention of information has the role of activating and selecting what we will call thought or action schemas, following the model of Don Norman and one of us (1980, 1986). In other words, short-term retention is of the relevant part of the control structure for action or thought. This function is analogous to that of the working memory in a production system (see Section 1.7); on each cycle of operation of the system, the conditions of each production are checked against such a working memory and, if they are satisfied by its contents, the production fires and an external or internal action ensues.[6] In Chapters 8 and 9 the position will be developed that these working memory and production memory functions are anatomically combined in a common system—that of selection of action and thought schemas.

Now Miyake and Shah's (1999b) definition of working memory combines all three of these characteristics. The position being put forward here is that all, or virtually all, of the cognitive subsystems in the cerebral cortex have working memory characteristics in some Miyake and Shah sense. However, both the subsystems themselves and the processing domains they are concerned with differ according to which of the characteristics 1, 2 or 3 or some combination of the three apply.

Why do we take this view? First, apparently similar processing domains do not contain isomorphic sets of subsystems with respect to these properties. Take the comparison between faces on the one hand and words

---

[4] In stem completion tasks a subject is presented with a set of words such as *scorch* to remember. Later s/he is cued with the first three letters of the word e.g. *sco.*

[5] In fact as Kintsch et al. (1999) discuss, while some of the models of working memory in Miyake and Shah's book are neutral about the existence of such buffers, most actually do support their existence. Whether such buffers are physically separate from processing systems will be discussed later.

[6] This is a simplification. In many production systems conflict resolution occurs between selection of a production and action ensuing (see Section 1.7 and McDermott & Forgy, 1978).

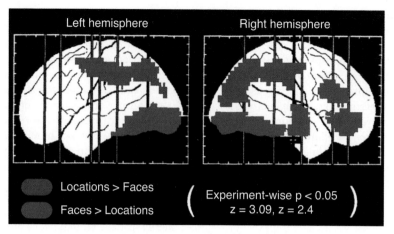

Fig. 7.1 Areas showing differential activation in the face and location working memory tasks of Courtney et al. (1996). Different regions of prefrontal cortex are implicated in the two tasks, but non-frontal regions are also differentially implicated. Reprinted from S.M. Courtney, L.G. Ungerleider, K. Keil and J.V. Haxby, Object and spatial visual working memory activate separate neural systems in human cortex. *Cerebral Cortex*, 1996, *6*(1), 39–49, by permission of Oxford University Press.

or spatial locations on the other. There are now many studies looking at working memory for faces and comparing them with working memory for words or spatial locations (for a review and meta-analysis see Wager & Smith, 2003). Consider the technically elegant and tightly controlled early PET study of Courtney et al. (1996; for related studies see also Courtney et al., 2007). In the encoding phase, subjects saw three faces selected from a set of 24 each presented at one of 24 possible locations (using an irregular 4×6 array) at a rate of 1.5 sec per stimulus; 0.5 sec later a face is presented at a particular location. In one condition the subject must say whether that face had been presented in the set of three. In the other condition the task was to make the equivalent judgement just about location. The results of the direct comparison between the two tasks are shown in Figure 7.1. The principal findings are summarised as demonstrating 'that both face and location working memory tasks activate frontal cortex, but that the regions activated by each task are distinct' (Courtney et al., 1996, p. 44). Much less attention is given to the massive differences between the two tasks in the posterior part of the cortex. The theoretical summary given is that 'one of the three components in the Baddeley and Hitch (1974) working memory model, the visuo-spatial sketchpad, can be further subdivided into two functionally and anatomically distinct systems for visual object working memory and visual spatial working memory' (p. 47–48).

Yet there is a very different account of the data, namely that unknown faces, unlike locations, lack a buffer and subjects therefore need to use with some difficulty their long-term episodic store in this so-called working memory study. Thus performance on faces is much worse and much slower than on locations. Moreover, when compared to a very non-demanding sensorimotor control

task with virtually no working memory requirement, the spatial location working memory task, unlike the faces one, did not give rise to frontal activation, just parieto-occipital. This could also be because the spatial location task is essentially buffer-based. It does not need supervisory processes. Short-term memory for faces by contrast does. Faces therefore differ from spatial locations absolutely in their type 2 characteristics.

Why is the second account more plausible? In a very early study, Warrington and Taylor (1973) tested a small group of subjects on immediate and delayed recognition of faces and surnames. In one task, participants were presented with a series of up to four faces or five surnames and then required to identify the stimuli in an array consisting of twice as many foils as targets. In a second task, participants were presented with three stimuli and required to recognise them in an array of targets and foils either immediately or after a 30-sec delay. Faces and words (i.e. surnames) behaved differently, as shown in Figure 7.2, with immediate recognition being poorer for faces, but with no appreciable affect of delay on face recognition. Warrington and Taylor's study also contrasted memory for faces and names in amnesics and age-matched controls. The amnesics differed from the controls on face memory but not on memory for surnames, further illustrating differences between the processing domains.[7] Thus words and faces differ in their type-2 buffer characteristics. In Section 7.4 we will discuss the extensive evidence that

---

[7] In other work it has been found that memory for serial order of faces shows similar primacy effects to that of serial order of words (Smyth et al., 2005), but in the case of faces the recency effect is limited to a single item.

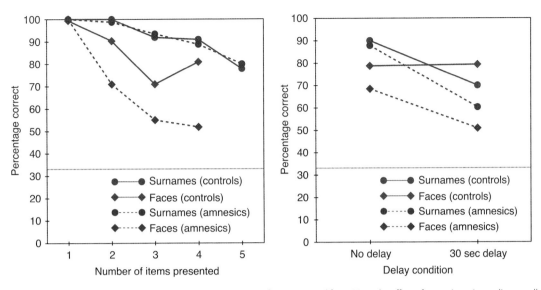

Fig. 7.2 Performance of controls and amnesics on recognition tests of surnames and faces. Note the effect of amnesia on immediate recall of faces but not of surnames. Data from Warrington and Taylor (1973).

spatial locations, like verbal material, has type 2 buffer characteristics, as one would expect on the Baddeley-Hitch model.

For what types of material would buffers be useful? Patients with impaired short-term memory for words have difficulty comprehending complex sentences (e.g. Caplan & Waters, 1999; Cecchetto & Papagano, in press). One therefore needs a phonological buffer to allow certain types of language operations to take place (see Section 7.3). By contrast there is no major computational reason why primitive humans should need to hold sets of novel faces for short intervals of time. Thus if we do need to store a group of previously novel faces it is unlikely that they will only be relevant for a few seconds at most, or that the sequential order of those faces will be important. Take meeting a novel football team. One needs to be able to continue to identify them for nearly two hours. It is pointless to store for only 10–20 sec that it was the balding would-be Cristiano Ronaldo who has just fluently accelerated past you; he may not reappear in your patch for another 15 min, upon which he will then repeat the aggravating manoeuvre as easily as before unless your mind contains a longer-term trace.

Buffers then on this view do not exist for all types of representations. Their existence depends on the particular computational operations that the representations are typically called upon to serve. Thus to compare directly how short-term retention of information occurs for faces and for words without taking into account how they may differ with respect to underlying buffers could easily lead one astray.

Most of this chapter will be concerned with buffers. Type 3 working memory processes will be considered in Chapter 9. However priming processes are the simplest type of short-term memory process. We will begin by considering them.

7.2 Short-term Retention by Priming

The simplest way in which information is retained by the cognitive system is by means of priming. As discussed with respect to functional imaging in Section 5.3, priming occurs in stimulus–response paradigms (e.g. lexical decision) in which presentation of one stimulus (the prime) results in a more rapid response to a subsequent related stimulus, but it also occurs in response-generation paradigms (e.g. stem-completion). Critically, priming need not be associated with any awareness of the underlying processes—indeed it is standardly assumed that awareness of the underlying processes implies that something more than priming is occurring. Moreover the process does not just operate in the short-term. Thus in certain situations priming has been shown to last for more than a year (Cave, 1997).

Historically, a major distinction has been drawn between so-called perceptual and conceptual priming (see e.g. Schacter & Buckner, 1998). The former is strongest when the cue and the target are perceptually identical as in perceptual recognition tasks but is independent of the degree of semantic processing required in the generation of the response. By contrast, the latter is insensitive to variations in presentation (such as font, in the case of visually presented verbal stimuli) but is greatest when extensive semantic processing of the cue and target is required. Patient studies provide some support for the perceptual/conceptual distinction. Thus, even quite severe Alzheimer's patients typically

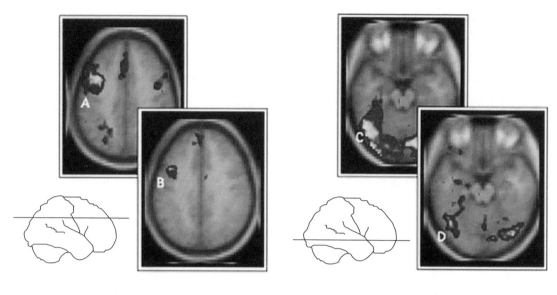

Conceptual priming   Perceptual priming

Fig. 7.3 Conceptual and perceptual priming. In each pair of images, one (upper left) shows the difference in BOLD response between novel items and a low level reference task, revealing all areas activated by the task. The other (bottom right) shows the direct comparison between the novel and repeated items, revealing those areas in which activation levels are reduced as a consequence of priming. Left prefrontal areas that activate for novel items (A) show reductions in activation for repeated items (B), perhaps as a reflection of conceptual priming. In contrast, an area in extrastriate visual cortex that is activated by presentation of novel visual words (C) shows reduced activation with repeated visual words (D), perhaps as a reflection of perceptual priming. The schematic of the brain on the left shows the approximate level from which the section is taken. Reprinted from Neuron, 20(2), D.L. Schacter and R.L. Buckner, *Priming and the brain.* 185–195, Copyright 1998, with permission from Elsevier.

show normal perceptual priming together with impaired conceptual priming (Gabrieli et al., 1994). The opposite dissociation has been reported in several patient studies. Gabrieli et al. (1995), for example, report patient MS, a large portion of whose right occipital lobe was removed in order to treat epilepsy. In a visual word recognition task, MS showed normal levels of recognition accuracy, but in contrast to controls and patients with focal lesions not involving the right occipital cortex, he failed to show any priming effect. In addition, MS showed normal levels of priming in both an auditory word recognition task and a word-stem completion task with auditory presentation of the primes and visual presentation of the word-stems. This latter task was held, not very convincingly, to tap conceptual priming. On the basis of the performance of MS and the Alzheimer patients of their earlier study, Gabrieli and colleagues conclude that perceptual and conceptual priming may dissociate. Their experiment also followed studies of normal subjects (e.g. Morton, 1979; Clarke & Morton, 1983) in showing that perceptual priming is specific to the modality of input.[8]

Support for the perceptual/conceptual distinction has also been garnered from a number of imaging studies (e.g. Squire et al., 1992; Blaxton et al., 1996; Gabrieli et al., 1996; Buckner et al., 2000). For example, in a PET study in which subjects were initially required to count the number of T-junctions in a set of words (the primes), Schacter et al. (1996) found a reliable bilateral decrease in activation of the extrastriate visual cortex during a subsequent word-stem completion task for primed completions as compared to non-primed completions.[9] This, the authors argued, reflected perceptual priming. In contrast, in a related task in which conceptual priming was held to apply, Buckner et al. (2000) found repetition related decreases in left inferior frontal and left inferior temporal activity. The results of the studies of Schacter, Buckner and colleagues are summarised in Figure 7.3.

The above patient and imaging studies appear to argue for separable priming processes, with the locus of (visual) perceptual priming being occipital and that of conceptual priming being left inferior frontal/inferior temporal. However, other studies suggest that the perceptual/conceptual contrast may be an overly crude

---

[8] See Carlesimo et al. (1994) for an acquired dyslexic patient showing a similar dissociation between visual and auditory perceptual priming.

[9] As discussed in Section 5.3, priming is associated with a *decrease* in the relevant rCBF or BOLD signal.

distinction. Postle and Corkin (1999), for example, compared priming for low and high familiarity words in two tasks: a word stem completion task and a perceptual identification task. In both tasks study methods appropriate for perceptual priming were used. A simple distinction between perceptual and conceptual priming would suggest that in both tasks priming should be equally sensitive to familiarity. This was found not to be the case. Priming in the perceptual identification task was not dependent on familiarity, while priming in the word stem completion task was. This result may be explained by assuming that perceptual identification relies on early, prelexical processing (and hence is sensitive to prelexical features of the input but not lexical features of the input), while word stem completion relies on lexical processing (and hence is sensitive to lexical properties of the input, such as familiarity).

Functional imaging studies have further shown that priming need not be limited to extrastriate visual cortex or inferior frontal/temporal regions. Thus, using videos of actions as stimuli, Grafton and Hamilton (2007) found repetition-related decreases in activation in parietal areas—regions commonly held to be involved in action (see Section 8.5). Also when using pictures of faces or real and nonsense objects as stimuli, Henson et al. (2000a) and Vuilleumier et al. (2002) found such effects in mid-fusiform regions—regions commonly held to be involved in face and object recognition (see Section 6.3). Taken together, these findings suggest that priming is not well-characterised by the simple perceptual/conceptual dichotomy. Rather, they argue strongly for a more general view of priming—the component processes view (Tenpenny & Shoben, 1992). This is that priming is a property of processing in a particular cognitive component where a current input to that component shares features with a recently processed input to it. This is held to be a general characteristic of cognitive subsystems.

The component process view of priming is of course also consistent with the modality-specific deficits in perceptual priming observed by Carlesimo et al. (1994) and Gabrieli et al. (1995)—visual and auditory perceptual processing are different component processes and therefore may be independently impaired. The neuropsychological perspective, however, offers a second line of support for the component process view. From the neuropsychological perspective, priming can manifest itself negatively in the phenomenon of perseveration. This can be found with respect to damage to many types of systems, including action generation (e.g. Humphreys & Forde, 1998), different stages of language production (e.g. Cohen & Dehaene, 1998), and executive functioning (see FNMS Section 14.5). Cohen and Dehaene (1998) demonstrate that, across several patients who show perseverations at different levels of language production (phonological, lexical, and numeric when reading numbers composed of digit sequences), the probability of making a perseverative error to a particular stimulus declines exponentially as function of time since that stimulus. The same exponential function has been found to hold between the size of the priming effect and the number of items between the prime and the target in repetition priming (McKone, 1995). From this, Cohen and Dehaene conclude that perseverative errors derive from the failure of the correct response to suppress a primed response. Minimally, this implies that priming can occur at various stages within language production. If the explanation holds for perseverative errors more generally (e.g. in action generation, executive functioning, etc.) then it further suggests that priming may also occur in processes responsible for these other functions.[10]

There have been four main proposals of how priming might operate computationally. Originally the dominant view was of the automatic retention of activation which declined over time or the spreading of activation to nearby representations (e.g. Schvaneveldt & Meyer, 1973), and this is the mechanism advocated by Cohen and Dehaene (1998). However, it can also be viewed within the context of a connectionist model as resulting from the existence of *short-term weights*. These are a type of weight of a connection in a network which is strengthened by Hebbian learning. The learning rate parameter has a high value and the weight's strength decays exponentially at a fast rate. Short-term weights thus encode the network's recent processing history. In a network with attractor dynamics, they ensure that, should the network be exposed to the same input twice in relatively quick succession, it will settle into the relevant basin of attraction more quickly on the second presentation.

The short-term weights account can explain a variety of diverse aspects of perseveration syndromes. Take optic aphasia, which has been associated with left occipital lesions extending to the splenium (Caramazza & Mahon, 2006). Optic aphasic patients have a specific difficulty in naming pictures, despite being able to demonstrate recognition of the depicted stimuli (Beauvois, 1982). In this task they produce a variety of errors, including semantic errors, perseverative errors (responding with the name of a previously presented picture or a semantically related word) and unrelated errors (producing an incorrect response that is neither a semantic associate nor a previous picture). Visual errors (responding with the name of a visually similar

---

[10] This relates to the Forde and Humphreys account of semantic access disorders considered in Section 6.6.

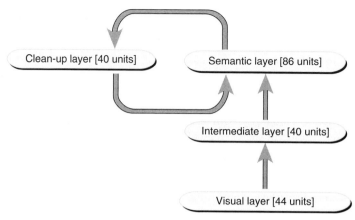

Fig. 7.4 The architecture of the optic aphasia network of Plaut & Shallice (1993b).

object) are rare. Plaut and Shallice (1993b) simulated this error pattern using short-term weights within a recurrent connectionist network (see Figure 7.4). Clean-up units, associated with the semantic units of the network, ensured that the semantic system exhibited an attractor structure. Following training[11] the network was able to generate the appropriate semantic representation for each input. When a proportion of connections in the network were lesioned, however, the network produced errors similar to those of patients, with a particularly high proportion of perseverative errors.

A third potential computational mechanism underlying priming has been proposed by Kinder and Shanks (2003; see also Berry et al., 2006, 2008). Neuropsychological studies have shown that priming dissociates from episodic memory processes. Thus, amnesic patients may show preserved priming in the face of gross impairments in episodic recall (Warrington & Weiskrantz, 1970, 1978).[12] Shanks and colleagues challenge the view that these dissociations imply that separable systems are responsible for priming and recognition memory. Thus, Kinder and Shanks (2003) take as an example a simple recurrent network model that learns sequences of stimuli using standard back-propagation of error (see Sections 1.7 and 4.11). Following training, for each point in a letter sequence the network predicts the next letter.[13] The accuracy of this prediction

is used to provide a measure of both priming and recognition accuracy. It is then demonstrated that a reduction in the network's learning rate results in an impairment of recognition but not priming, while an impairment at input (in the form of degraded input representations) results in a reduction in priming but not recognition.[14]

Priming in this approach is not directly related to any simple computational mechanism. It results from the way the network's prediction accuracy is transformed into a measure of priming (which itself is indirect), and the way that this is sensitive to the integrity of the input but not the network's learning rate.

The model demonstrates that dissociations in output measures do not necessarily imply separability in the processes that generate those measures.[15] However, there are strong reasons to question whether it offers a general account of priming. First, the measure of priming produced by the model is the change in identification rate given prior exposure, and not the change in response time. The model can therefore not be directly related to priming experiments in which RTs are the main dependent variable, such as those involving perceptual identification (e.g. Gabrieli et al., 1995, experiment 1) and lexical decision (e.g. Marslen-Wilson &

---

[11] The network was trained to generate semantic patterns for 40 different objects, where the objects corresponded to different vectors at the input layer. Back-propagation through time was used to train the network to settle into an attractor state for each input. Following the processing of each input pattern, the short-term weights were adjusted as described in the text. All patterns were presented 9000 times during training.

[12] See FNMS Section 15.3.

[13] That is, given the string-initiation marker as input, it generates as output the first letter of a string on which the network

was trained. Given this first letter, and the string's context as encoded by feedback connections in the layer of hidden units, the network then generates the second letter of the trained string, and so on.

[14] Berry et al. (2006) demonstrate that this single system approach can also account for various attentional manipulations on priming and recognition, while Berry et al. (2008) extend the approach to fluency—that is, that in recognition tests hit and false alarm responses are faster than miss and correct rejection responses.

[15] For a somewhat analogous lack of transparency concerning connectionist nets, see the discussion of abstract errors in deep dyslexia, in Section 4.10.

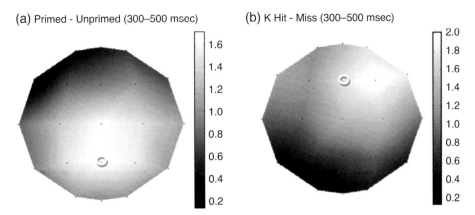

Fig. 7.5 (a) Mean ERP priming signal (operationalised as the difference between primed and unprimed conditions, collapsed over correct "know" responses and misses). (b) Mean ERP recognition signal (operationalised as the difference between correct "know" responses and misses, collapsed over primed and unprimed conditions). Reproduced with permission from A. Woollams, J.R. Taylor, F. Karayanidis and R.N. Henson (2008), Event-related potentials associated with masked priming of test cues reveal multiple potential contributions to recognition memory. *Journal of Cognitive Neuroscience*, 20(6), 1114–1129. Copyright © 2008, MIT Press Journals.

Tyler, 1997). Second, the modelling work considers only recognition memory (and then only recognition of sequences); yet as argued above priming is widespread and appears to occur in many cognitive subsystems, not just those that underlie recognition memory. Third, in an ERP study using priming of masked stimuli and a remember/know paradigm.[16] Using these paradigms Woollams et al. (2008) found a number of distinct neural signals associated with the repetition of a stimulus. Most critically, within the 300–500-msec window following target presentation, a significant difference was found between the ERP signal associated with priming and the signal associated with recognition. Priming was operationalised as the difference between the primed and unprimed conditions (see Figure 7.5a). Recognition was operationalised as the difference between correct 'know' responses and misses (see Figure 7.5b). The topography of the latter was more frontally localised than the former. In fact, using the paradigm Woollams et al. isolate four distinct neural signals which, they speculate, might contribute to recognition memory. This appears to directly contradict the suggestion of Kinder and Shanks that recognition memory is the product of a single memory signal (i.e. prediction accuracy).

A final mechanistically plausible account of priming is that it involves the creation and strengthening of direct stimulus–response (SR) links. Logan (1990) noted parallels between repetition priming and developing automaticity, and suggested that repetition priming effects may be *stimulus-driven*. They may be due in part to the creation of stimulus-specific SR links which bypass more central cognitive processes. This would facilitate speeded responding to previously encountered stimuli. Building on this idea, Dobbins et al. (2004) investigated reduced activation arising from repetition priming in an fMRI study of categorisation in which subjects were required to categorise visually presented stimuli on the basis of whether they were 'bigger than a shoe-box'. After a number of trials in which some items appeared multiple times (allowing the authors to assess priming effects), the categorisation rule was reversed (to 'smaller than a shoe-box'). Behaviourally, priming was found in the initial condition and this was reflected in reduced neural responses (i.e. repetition suppression) in both prefrontal and fusiform cortices. Following rule reversal, behavioural priming was still present, but reduced, for items presented before the reversal. This behavioural reduction was no longer accompanied by reduced activation within the fusiform cortex, while the effect remained in prefrontal cortex. The authors argue that these findings support a mechanism of priming as involving the learning of direct stimulus–response mappings. This supports the position that the fusiform activation when reversal does not take place allows prefrontal cortex to be effectively bypassed rather than providing 'tuning' of object recognition processes to task-relevant features in the input.

However, the absence of reduced activation in the fusiform cortex across conditions in the study of Dobbins and colleagues is surprising. Many previous studies in which the design aimed to minimise learning of stimulus–response mappings have found reduced activation effects in fusiform cortex (e.g. Schacter et al., 1996; Henson et al., 2000a, 2003; Schott et al., 2005). Moreover, in a partial replication of the Dobbins et al. study, Horner and Henson (2008) examined rule reversals which switched stimulus–response mappings. They found reduced activation in both prefrontal cortex *and*

---

[16] Remember/know paradigms are a form of memory procedure discussed in Sections 2.3 and 5.5; see also Chapter 10.

fusiform cortex. A computational analysis of the task suggests two potential processes where re-processing of a stimulus might be faster the second time around: in perceptual identification, at a presemantic level, and in classification by size. The former process can be related to the priming effect in fusiform cortex, the putative locus of the face recognition units of the Bruce–Young model considered in Section 6.3. So, given the other priming results discussed above and, notwithstanding the null result of Dobbins et al., priming here may plausibly be effected through tuning of connections (as might result from, for example, strengthening of short-term weights). The reduction in prefrontal cortex activity, on the other hand, may reflect 'caching' of the classification result, such that the classification process itself (and its associated prefrontal activity) can be bypassed when a stimulus is presented again.

We will not consider priming further. We will assume that all subsystems—with the probable exceptions of peripheral ones such as early visual areas (see Schacter & Buckner, 1998)—when presented with the same input and in the same task situation, produce the same output more rapidly. No doubt the parameters vary from subsystem to subsystem. It will, however, be argued in the next sections that the operation of buffers requires *more* than mere priming.

7.3 The Phonological Input Buffer

Now let us return to verbal material and the next level of temporary memory processing—the buffer. Normal subjects can repeat back without error a few letters, words or digits, up to a certain number, their *span*, traditionally for English digits, seven. As a mechanism, priming alone is insufficient to account for this ability. Furthermore, as discussed briefly in Section 1.9, there is a well-described functional syndrome of selective impairment of auditory–verbal storage. Immediately after presentation, such patients cannot recall short strings of familiar verbal units, such as words or sentences at the normal level; their span is much reduced. The problem affects recognition as well as recall (Warrington & Shallice, 1969), and the deficit is more severe when the items being recalled are inherently meaningless such as letter or digit strings but is manifest for any sort of verbal material (see Shallice & Valler, 1990). Moreover gist can be retained when the surface phonological form is lost (Saffran & Marin, 1975).

In initially unrelated research on memory in normal subjects, Baddeley (1966a, 1966b) had shown that immediate recall of five-word sequences was greatly affected by the phonological similarity of the different words, but not by their semantic similarity—the *phonological similarity effect*. In contrast delayed recall of a ten-word sequence showed the opposite pattern. Thus the idea of a phonologically-based short-term store and a semantically based longer-term store was born. The impairment of auditory–verbal short-term memory patients fits exactly with what would be expected of the loss of a phonologically-based short-term store. Thus, such patients may be characterised as having:[17]

1 A selective deficit of span in contrast to normal or relatively normal performance on other verbal skills.

2 A comparable performance level for all strings of unconnected verbal items, e.g. digits, letters, words, when presented auditorily.

3 Intact word perception.

4 Their span deficit not arising from a speech production deficit.

A functional impairment of the phonologically-based short-term store would not be expected to compromise word perception or speech production (points 3 and 4), but it would be expected to lead to reduced span for all types of unconnected auditorily-presented verbal stimuli (points 1 and 2).

Initially in developing their theory of working memory, Baddeley and Hitch (1974) had viewed the phonologically-based store as a special output store—the *phonemic response buffer* (Baddeley & Hitch, 1974, p. 77) or the *articulatory buffer* (see Baddeley et al., 1975). However, Levy (1971) had shown that short-term retention of visually-presented information is much reduced if controlled rehearsal is prevented by constantly repeating the same word—*articulatory suppression*—while the stimuli were being presented. This was not the case for auditorily-presented material which was relatively unaffected by suppression. Salame and Baddeley (1982) thus revised the Baddeley–Hitch working memory model to make the phonological buffer an input store.[18] The resulting model of auditory–verbal short-term memory, known as the phonological loop model, is shown in Figure 7.6.[19]

---

[17] See FNMS Chapter 3, Vallar and Shallice (1990) and Vallar and Papagno (2002) for more detailed descriptions of the functional syndrome, and in the third case a meta-analysis of 25 patients.

[18] The empirical evidence that Salame and Baddeley (1982) used to support this change in the model primarily relied on the deleterious effect of speech which did not have to be attended—*the unattended speech effect*. Their explanation of this particular paradigm is much disputed. However the findings of Levy (1971) still stand.

[19] The Baddeley–Hitch model is supported by a number of additional empirical effects not described here, such as the *word-length effect*, and the interactions of these effects with articulatory suppression. However, these effects are normally argued to relate to the rehearsal process, rather than the phonologically-based store.

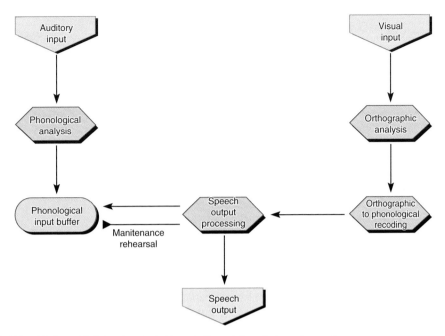

Fig. 7.6 The Baddeley–Hitch model of the phonological input buffer and the articulatory loop system.

The conception of the Baddeley–Hitch phonological buffer as an input store is also supported by the functional deficits of short-term memory patients. These patients show similar deficits in recognition situations to recall (Shallice & Warrington, 1970; Vallar et al., 1997). Moreover as specified above in the fourth characteristic of the functional syndrome, a number of them had normal or virtually normal spontaneous speech (see e.g. IL, Saffran & Marin, 1975; JB, Shallice & Butterworth, 1977; PV, Vallar & Baddeley, 1984; and LA, Vallar et al., 1997).[20]

Now the existence of a putative functional syndrome is only the starting point for a theoretical interpretation. This interpretation of the behavioural difficulties of these patients in terms of impairments to a phonological buffer was challenged by Allport (1984). Allport took a position related to that of the levels-of-processing perspective of Craik and Lockhart (1972), arguing that the problems faced by the patients in short-term memory tasks derived from a more basic perceptual problem. He was not saying that such patients do not perceive the words and so do not remember them. His objection is more complex. He is saying that a reduced span is a side-effect of a reduction in the capacity of phonological processing; that there is no modular division between phonological processing and short-term phonological memory. Indeed certain of the short-term memory patients such as JB do have mild phonological processing problems. However others such as PV (Vallar & Baddeley, 1984) have shown quite normal performance on tests similar to that used by Allport, for instance scoring 100% in a test in which she had to carry out a same/different judgement on pairs of non-word syllables; when they differed it was by only either one or two phonetic features. EDE (Berndt & Mitchum, 1990), TB (Baddeley et al., 1987) and LA (Vallar et al., 1997) are similar.

Even for those patients of this type with mild phonological processing difficulties there are two problems with Allport's position. Martin and Breedin (1992) worked with one of the patients, EA. EA had a much reduced span and previously Friedrich et al. (1984) had followed Allport's perspective in attributing the problem to a difficulty in developing abstract, speech-based phonological codes in perception. Martin and Breedin took three other patients with phonological processing problems that were qualitatively and quantitatively similar to that of EA—AA, MP and MW—and compared their auditory–verbal short-term memory capacities with those of EA. It can be seen from Table 7.1 that despite phonological processing difficulties comparable to EA (and JB) they were much superior to EA on auditory-verbal short-term memory tasks. Moreover they showed a superiority of span for acoustically dissimilar to acoustically similar letters, and the superiority of auditory over visual input in short-term recall, both of which are typical of normal short-term memory (see Baddeley, 1986). EA like other STM patients (e.g. Shallice & Vallar, 1990) showed neither effect. Patients with mild phonological processing problems do *not* necessarily present with grave short-term memory problems. The results

---

[20] In the case of JB spontaneous speech was analysed quantitatively. In the other patients there is only a clinical rating.

| **TABLE 7.1** | The percentage of lists (of size 2 to 5) recalled correctly for rhyming and nonrhyming letter sequences for four patients and a group of five matched controls. All patients have similar phonological processing difficulties, but for AA, MP and MW (and unlike EA) these difficulties do not impair recall. |

	Auditory			**Visual**		
	Non-rhyming	**Rhyming**	**Difference**	**Non-rhyming**	**Rhyming**	**Difference**
EA	38	20	18	50	58	−8
AA	68	58	10	70	53	17
MP	95	68	27	60	50	10
MW	75	50	25	80	48	32
Controls	86	50	36	79	58	21

Reproduced from: Dissociations between speech perception and phonological short-term memory deficits, R.C. Martin & S.D. Breedin, *Cognitive Neuropsychology*, 9(6), 509–534, 1992, Psychology Press. Reprinted by permission of the publisher (Taylor & Francis Group, http://www.informaworld.com).

fit much better with the patients being cases of impairment of the phonological input buffer. Allport's explanation for the functional syndrome is therefore not plausible.[21]

On the Baddeley–Hitch theory the phonological loop subsystem of the working memory has subcomponents other than the phonological buffer which allow processes such as rehearsal to occur (see Figure 7.6). Often in phonological (input) buffer patients rehearsal also appears to be impaired (Vallar & Papagno, 2002), but this is not necessarily the case. Thus, patient LA (Vallar et al., 1997) showed two effects, which supported the idea that he could rehearse. First, for a two (!) digit serial recall test on which he was 97% correct, his performance fell to 80% correct if he could not rehearse by being forced to repeat an irrelevant syllable ('blah'). A second effect related to rehearsal concerned the making of phonological judgements, such as stress assignment on words. Burani et al. (1991) had shown that the ability of normal subjects to make such judgements is also impaired by articulatory suppression. LA was well within the control range for two such tasks—stress assignment and judging whether two written words start with the same sound (e.g. *candela* (candle, starting with /k/) and *ciliegie* (cherries, starting with /ch/)). In contrast there was a second patient, TO, who also had a reduced span. He showed no effect of articulatory suppression on his serial recall of four digit lists. However he was grossly impaired on the two phonological judgement tasks for words (see Table 7.2). Thus one has a quite different pattern between a typical phonological input buffer patient (LA) and a patient who is held to be unable to rehearse (TO). A similar patient, MC, with a rehearsal deficit, has been reported by Papagno et al. (2007).

The neuropsychological evidence therefore supports the existence of a separable input store in which information is encoded in phonological form. What, though, is the purpose of this store? Patients with severe phonological input buffer deficits can have near normal comprehension (see e.g. PV of Vallar & Baddeley, 1984), so the integrity of the phonological input buffer is not essential for basic comprehension, at least for less complex sentences. Phonological buffer deficits also do not necessarily interfere with morphological processing (Kavé et al., 2007). However, phonological input buffer patients do typically show comprehension deficits when tested with complex sentences.[22] Thus, PV, who had a digit span of three, performed poorly when required to judge the truth or meaningfulness of sentences such as the following:

1 *The world divides the equator into two hemispheres, the northern and the southern.*

2 *One cannot reasonably claim that sailors are often lived on by ships of various kinds.*

Critically, PV had no difficulties with long sentences whose constituents were semantically easily distinguishable. One possibility is that the phonological input buffer serves as a general back-up store for holding phonological information which is difficult to comprehend semantically on the first-pass, such as in noisy environments or when sentences contain lists of semantically similar material and where order and completeness are critical (see FNMS Section 3.7).

Baddeley (2003b) questions whether the back-up role of the phonological buffer in comprehension is of sufficient functional significance to provide the advantage needed to support the buffer's evolution, and argues

---

[21] A complex individual difference-type of argument might be developed to account for the overall pattern, but until that is motivated as it was for reading-without-semantics in Section 4.9 it remains completely *ad hoc*.

[22] The same holds for patients with functional impairments elsewhere in the phonological loop. Thus, MC, of Papagno et al. (2007), who has a selective rehearsal deficit, is also impaired at comprehension of complex sentences.

TABLE 7.2 Accuracy scores for LA, TO and matched controls (showing mean with range in brackets) on the stress assignment and initial sound tasks of Vallar et al. (1997). Both patients had reduced span, but only TO was also impaired on the phonological tasks.

	Stress assignment	Initial sound
LA	0.87	0.97
Controls	0.90 (0.87–0.94)	0.87 (0.81–0.94)
TO	0.74	0.87
Controls	0.95 (0.90–1.00)	0.94 (0.90–1.00)

Reprinted from *Neuropsychologica*, Vallar, de Bettac, and Silveri, The Phonological short- term store-rehearsal style: Patterns of improvement and correlates, 1997 with permission from Elsevier.

that an alternative function of the phonological input buffer is in language learning. Thus PV was found to be impaired at learning Russian vocabulary, but not at learning arbitrary paired associates where the individual words were known (Baddeley et al., 1988), and in normal subjects other factors that impair phonological buffer tasks (e.g. articulatory suppression) also impair foreign language learning (Papagno et al., 1991). However, this view does not explain why the phonological buffer's span is typically substantially greater than what would seem to be required for vocabulary learning (i.e. two items). Thus, in sentence repetition the surface structure of 15 to 20 words can be retained in span, depending on the clause structure of the sentence (Jarvella, 1971). With simple clause structure this can amount to two sentences (Glanzer et al., 1981). Moreover in STM patients, e.g. IL (Saffran & Marin, 1975), JB (Butterworth et al., 1990), PV (Vallar & Baddeley, 1984) and EA (Martin et al., 1994), this ability to retain the surface form is lost in a comparable way to the digit span deficits. This all suggests that a short-term phonological buffer must have considerable capacity. We speculate, therefore, that while the phonological buffer may initially have evolved to support language learning, its capacity has subsequently increased to support comprehension of complex sentences, possibly in conjunction with the increasing complexity of language.

Can the phonological input buffer be localised? Vallar and Papagno (2002) reviewed the localisation of the lesions of patients in the literature with selective auditory–verbal short-term memory deficits as characterised by points 1 to 4 earlier in this section (see Table 7.3). All but one has left-hemisphere lesions.[23] Furthermore, in all cases the lesions affected the parietal lobe and in all but two the temporal lobe. Where more detail was

available the localisations overlap in the posterior inferior parietal and posterior superior temporal regions (see Figure 7.7). When Baldo and Dronkers (2006) directly contrasted ten left inferior parietal patients with eight left inferior frontal ones they found that the parietal patients had a grossly reduced span when they pointed to digits (approx. 2) by comparison with more than 5 for the frontals and nearly 7 for the controls.

Functional imaging gives a highly compatible position. A series of studies (e.g. Grasby et al., 1993; Paulesu et al., 1993; Smith et al., 1996; Jonides et al., 1998; Postle et al., 1999; Henson et al., 2000b) also found that the left supramarginal gyrus (BA 40) is activated when the resources of a phonological buffer system are required. Consider the original PET study of Paulesu and colleagues. Subjects were scanned under two experimental conditions. In the first condition, they were presented visually with six random phonologically distinct consonants at a rate of one per second and instructed to memorise the letters. Two seconds after the last letter was presented, a probe was presented and subjects were required to indicate whether the probe had or had not been in the list of presented letters. In the second condition, subjects were required to judge whether consonants, again presented at a rate of one per second, did or did not rhyme. Both conditions were contrasted with control conditions in which the stimuli were shapes (Korean characters). The first task was held to engage both subvocal rehearsal and the phonological buffer, while the second was held to engage subvocal rehearsal but not the phonological buffer. A clear difference in the regions activated was found across tasks, with Broca's area (left BA 44) differentially activated when subvocal rehearsal was required and left supramarginal gyrus (BA 40) activated when the phonological loop was required.

Moreover the correspondence is not merely of two independent approaches. Paulesu et al. (1999) scanned the patient JB when carrying out the control task of the earlier Paulesu et al. study. The regions activated fitted well with those that would be expected from the probable localisation of the other components of the phonological loop. In addition, patients who have been described with complementary problems involving other component subsystems of the phonological loop tend to have lesions which fit with the Paulesu et al. (1993) position on their localisation. Thus TO of Vallar et al. (1997) discussed above, who is held to have a rehearsal deficit, has lesions in left inferior frontal areas including Broca's area and the left anterior insula. MC of Papagno et al. (2007), another rehearsal impairment patient, also has a lesion affecting the left anterior insula.[24]

---

[23] The exception, patient EDE, had a so-called *crossed aphasia* after her stroke. This is a disorder of language that arises from a right hemisphere lesion.

[24] Dronkers (1996) argues on the basis of a meta-analysis that left anterior insula is specifically associated with early articulatory

TABLE 7.3 Lesion localisation for short-term memory patients. X (or a brain region) indicates the lesion site.

Patient	Aetiology	Source	Lesion site			
			Frontal	Temporal	Parietal	Occipital
KF	Head injury	Post mortem		×	Inferior	×
JB	Meningioma	Surgery		Sup. / Mid.	Inferior	
WH	CVA?	Brain scan		×	Inferior	
LS	Head injury	Angiography			×	×
IL	CVA?	Brain scan?			Posterior	
MC	CVA	CT scan		Post. / Sup.		
PV	CVA	CT scan	×	×	×	
EA	CVA	CT scan		Posterior	×	
RAN	CVA	CT scan			×	
ER	CVA	CT scan		×, insula	×, insula	
RR	CVA	CT scan		×	×	
SC	CVA	CT scan		×	×	
LA	Head injury	MR scan		Sup. / Mid.	Inferior	
JO	CVA?	Brain scan	×	×		
TB	CVA?	CT scan		×		
EDE	CVA	CT scan		×	×	
RoL	CVA	CT scan		×	×	
HB	CVA	Not stated		×	×	
MMG	CVA	Not stated	×		Posterior	
Anon$_1$	CVA	MR scan		Superior		

Data from: Vallar & Papagno, 2002; Howard & Nickels, 2005; Takayama et al., 2004.

rTMS[25] has also been applied in an attempt to localise the processes related to the phonological input buffer. The results available at present are less clear cut. Romero et al. (2006) applied rTMS over BA 40, BA 44 and a control location while participants performed the phonological judgement tasks of Burani et al. (1991; see Table 7.2), a digit span task and a pattern span task. The phonological judgement tasks were intended to invoke the rehearsal process but not the phonological input buffer. The digit span task was intended to invoke both rehearsal and the phonological input buffer. The pattern span task was intended as a control, tapping response processes and visuo-spatial short-term memory processes. rTMS over both BA 40 and BA 44 led to significant performance decrements in both the phonological judgement tasks and the digit span task in comparison with the pattern span task. This is consistent with a localisation of *either* BA 40 *or* BA 44 for the phonological input buffer, but it also suggests involvement of *both* areas in rehearsal, contrary to the frontal localisation of rehearsal suggested by neuropsychological studies such as those of TO (Vallar et al., 1997) and MC (Papagno et al., 2007). However, from a computational perspective, as rehearsal is an operation on the content of the store it must also involve the store itself.

Thus, the patient and imaging work appears to give a consistent picture—one that both supports the theoretical construct of the phonological input buffer and localises it to left BA 40 and posterior superior temporal

planning, a process plausibly related to subvocal rehearsal. See Blank et al. (2002) for consistent functional imaging evidence on the localisation of speech production processes.

[25] rTMS—Repetitive Transcranial Magnetic Stimulation—involves administering a relatively rapid sequence of TMS pulses to a region of cortex, generally for the duration of a complete trial. In this way a cortical region can be effectively lesioned in a healthy subject for an extended period of time.

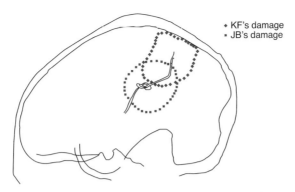

♦ KF's damage
▪ JB's damage

Fig. 7.7 Schematic composite diagram of two short-term memory patients based on neurosurgical investigation, showing: (a) the angular artery of KF, (b) the macroscopically-damaged area of KF, and c) the meningioma of JB. Reproduced from *Neuropsychologia, 9*(4), E.K. Warrington, V. Logue and R.T.C. Pratt, The anatomical localisation of selective impairment of auditory verbal short-term memory. 377–387, Copyright 1971, with permission from Elsevier.

cortex. This picture is challenged, in two different ways, by an imaging study of Ravizza and colleagues (2004) and a theoretical review by Buchsbaum and D'Esposito (2008).

Ravizza et al. (2004) show that dorsal and ventral portions of the inferior parietal cortex are differentially sensitive to task conditions used in a memory task that contrasted verbal and non-verbal memory under conditions of high and low load. The task was based on the *n-back task*, in which subjects are presented with a series of stimuli and must detect when the current stimulus matches the stimulus presented *n* items earlier in the series. In the low-load condition, subjects were required to detect a specified stimulus in a series of stimuli. This is sometimes referred to as n-back with *n* = 0, but is equivalent to item recognition. In the high load condition, *n* was set to 3 (so subjects had to detect when the current stimulus matched the stimulus presented 3 items earlier in the series). Visually presented stimuli were either English letters (verbal) or Korean letters (presumably nonverbal for the English-speaking subjects). The more superior part of inferior parietal cortex was found to be sensitive to load bilaterally but not to the type of letters.[26] In contrast, the more ventral inferior parietal cortex was found to be insensitive to load in the verbal condition. At the same time, Broca's area did show the expected effect of modality (greater activity for verbal than non-verbal stimuli) and load (greater activity for high-load than low-load). Ravizza et al. argue that if BA 40 (or part thereof) was the neural correlate of the phonological short-term store then it should be sensitive to both load and condition. Since neither dorsal nor ventral regions of inferior parietal cortex show the required sensitivity, the study appears to argue

against either a phonological short-term store or its localisation to BA 40.

The problem with this study is its use of the n-back task. This complex task is potentially open to subject-specific and load-specific variations in strategy. It is far from clear that the resource loadings it imposes on the phonological input buffer are that much greater in 'high-load' than 'load-low' conditions. Thus, as we discussed above for the Glanzer et al. (1981) study, three items is not a large load in the phonological input buffer. However, in the 3-back condition subjects must use retrieval strategies potentially involving counting or complex updating. Indeed, Kane et al. (2007) have shown that n-back performance correlates poorly with measures of memory span. Ravizza et al's data are therefore not relevant to the issue of localisation of the phonological short-term store.

We turn now to the theoretical challenge of Buchsbaum and D'Esposito (2008), who argue first, following Becker et al. (1999), that the localisation evidence is not as consistent as has been suggested here, and second, that the theoretical construct of a phonological input buffer is flawed. The alternative proposed by Buchsbaum and D'Esposito is that phonological short-term memory is the product of the interaction between the neural processes that underlie speech perception and those involved in production. The left temporo-parietal region treated above as the locus of the phonological input buffer is, on this view, conceived of as an *auditory-motor interface*; it is held to be responsible for binding 'acoustic representations of speech articulatory counterparts stored in the frontal cortex' (Buchsbaum & D'Esposito, 2008, p. 774).

Certainly, some imaging studies have been interpreted to suggest that more superior and posterior parietal areas are involved in phonological short-term storage. However, these studies have generally used n-back tasks rather than span. For example, Awh et al. (1996) localise

---

[26] The left dorsolateral prefrontal cortex showed a similar effect.

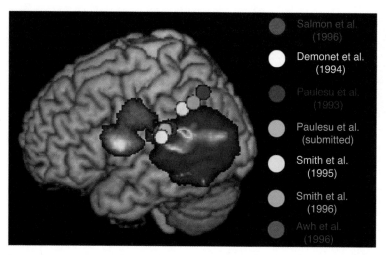

Fig. 7.8 Region activated in STM patient JB in the phonological control task not loaded on STM of Paulesu et al. (1993) (in red), together with (i) the region generally inactive in the patient due to the lesion (in blue), and (ii) the maxima of activation in regions held to involve phonological short-term memory in seven studies on normal subjects Note the similarity of the locations obtained in the Paulesu et al. and Demonet et al. studies with that of the overlap of the two lesions indicated in Figure 7.7. (With thanks to Eraldo Paulesu for permission to publish the figure.)

the phonological short-term store to left superior posterior parietal regions. Yet the memory and control tasks used in Awh et al.'s experiments were relatively complex and not very demanding of the resources of the phonological input buffer (e.g. a contrast of the 2-back task with a search task that was argued to require a lower memory load). Without a proper task analyses of all experimental conditions, it is unclear whether the neural components isolated in this study truly correspond to any notion of a phonological short-term store. Moreover these posterior superior parietal regions are outside the area of damage in at least one auditory–verbal STS patient—JB (Paulesu et al., 1999; see Figure 7.8). We thus dispute the claims of Buchsbaum and D'Esposito concerning localisation.

Buchsbaum and D'Esposito's attack on the phonological input buffer as a construct is largely based on their presupposition that any such buffer should not be localised within regions near to those commonly associated with language. The rationale for this derives from the relatively minor linguistic deficits typically associated with short-term memory patients (see Vallar & Shallice, 1990). However somewhat illogically, Buchsbaum and D'Esposito continue by suggesting that the short-term memory deficits of such patients can effectively be disregarded as statistical outliers! The rationale is a completely *ad hoc* argument without supporting evidence such as that provided for reading-without-semantics in Section 4.9. Indeed the study of Baldo and Dronkers (2006) conclusively shows that reduced span is typical of left inferior parietal patients. Moreover, as acknowledged by Buchsbaum and D'Esposito, replacing the phonological input buffer store with an auditory-motor interface which binds representations to ones in a phonological output buffer fails to address evidence for

separate input and output buffers, as discussed in Section 7.5. Such a view, too, would need to explain what phonological trace is used in our very considerable capacity—at times of 20 words or so—for veridical reproduction of surface structure—the phonological form—in immediate sentence recall (Jarvella, 1971; Glanzer et al., 1981), and why short-term memory patients, such as IL or JB, lose this ability to reproduce surface structure but can perform much better at immediate recall of gist (Saffran & Marin, 1975; Butterworth et al., 1990). That a phonological buffer, which can have such a large capacity if accessed via appropriate semantic and syntactic retrieval cues, is on the input side of the speech system is much more plausible than its being on the output side; in that case it would be expected to be of the order of a phonological phrase in capacity. Moreover, as discussed earlier, short-term memory patients do have problems in acting on sentences heavily loaded with information—it is just that their difficulty is not specifically syntactic. The case made by Buchsbaum and D'Esposito is inadequate.

Given that the concerns of Ravizza and colleagues and of Buchsbaum and D'Esposito are unfounded, one therefore has convergent cognitive neuroscience evidence for one buffer—the phonological input buffer. Two further questions follow. First, which other buffers are there? And second, can cognitive neuroscience evidence elucidate the functioning of buffers at Marr's algorithmic level?

7.4 The Visuo-spatial Sketchpad

Strong evidence exists for a number of other buffers. Consider Baddeley and Hitch's *visuo-spatial sketchpad*, the

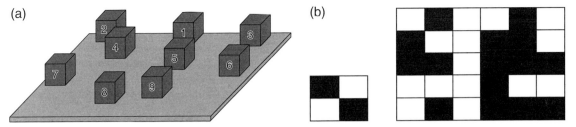

Fig. 7.9 (a) The Corsi span test apparatus. The numbers on the blocks are visible to the examiner only and facilitate recording of subject performance. (b) Example stimuli from the Visual Patterns Test of Della Sala et al. (1999). Panel b reprinted from *Neuropsychologia, 37*(10), S. Della Sala, C. Gray, A. Baddeley, N. Allamano and L. Wilson, Pattern span: a tool for unwelding visuo-spatial memory. 1189–1199, Copyright 1999, with permission from Elsevier.

visuo-spatial analogue of the phonological loop. Initial evidence for this component of the working memory model came from studies of dual-task interference. Subjects were able to combine a verbal memory task with a secondary spatial tracking task with relatively little impact of the tracking task on verbal memory performance. In contrast, performance on a visuo-spatial memory task (remembering the positions of numbers in a matrix) was significantly affected by the secondary spatial tracking task. The converse was found when the secondary task was verbal rather than spatial (Baddeley et al., 1975).

Patients with selective deficits of visuo-spatial short-term memory have also been described (e.g. De Renzi & Nichelli, 1975; Hanley, Young & Pearson, 1991; Carlesimo et al., 2001b; for review see Della Sala & Logie, 2002), further supporting the existence of a functionally separable visuo-spatial memory. Classically, such patients have severe deficits on the Corsi span test—a visuo-spatial analogue of digit span in which subjects must touch a sequence of pegs in a display containing nine of them (see Figure 7.9a) after the examiner has tapped out the sequence. However, performance on the Corsi span task has been shown to dissociate from that on a purely visual short-term memory task without a spatial component. Some measure of visual short-term memory, beyond Corsi span, is therefore required. One option is provided by the *visual patterns test*, as described by Della Sala et al. (1999). This test requires subjects to reproduce a pseudo-random chequer-board pattern within a matrix ranging in size from 2×2 squares to 5×6 squares (see Figure 7.9b). Visual pattern span is the number of filled cells in the most complex pattern perfectly recalled by the subject. In contrast to Corsi span, visual pattern span does not require the retention of sequential order information.

The correlation between Corsi span and visual pattern span in a group of control subjects was found to be relatively low (0.27 and 0.35 for two versions of the visual patterns test). More critically, a group study of 69 patients revealed two patients who scored above the median on visual pattern span but below the 5th

percentile on Corsi span, and one patient who showed the reverse dissociation (see also Grossi et al., 1993).

Della Sala and colleagues have also provided experimental evidence for the dissociation between visual pattern span and Corsi span using dual-task interference. Subjects (healthy university students) first completed each of the span tasks with 10 sec between presentation and recall. They then completed the span tasks a second time, but with the 10-sec retention interval filled with a visual or spatial task (viewing abstract paintings or copying a spatial sequence). Performance on the visual patterns test was affected more by the visual task than the spatial task, while the opposite pattern was observed for performance on the Corsi task (see Figure 7.10).

The distinction between visual and spatial short-term memories is reflected within the general framework of the Baddeley–Hitch working memory model by what Logie (1995) refers to as the *visual cache* and the *inner scribe*. Logie's inner scribe serves both as a spatial short-term store and as a process that is able to refresh the visual cache (with the refresh function paralleling the rehearsal function within the phonological loop). Klauer and Zhao (2004), however, present experimental evidence both for separate visual and spatial short-term stores and for separate rehearsal functions.

As we will see, the theoretical analysis of visuo-spatial short-term memory is less advanced than that of auditory–verbal short-term memory. Possibly as a result, the anatomy is rather poorly characterised neuropsychologically. Group studies that have compared unilaterally lesioned patients on visuo-spatial tasks with short-term memory requirements (DeRenzi & Nichelli, 1975; DeRenzi et al., 1977; Feigenbaum et al., 1996) have generally found right lesioned patients to be more impaired than left lesioned patients, but not significantly so. Della Sala et al. (1999) replicated this non-significant disadvantage for right hemisphere patients in both the Corsi span and visual pattern span tasks (see also Della Sala & Logie, 2002). However, individual case studies support a right hemisphere localisation, at least for elements of spatial short-term memory. For example, Carlesimo et al. (2001b) report MV, who sustained right fronto-parietal

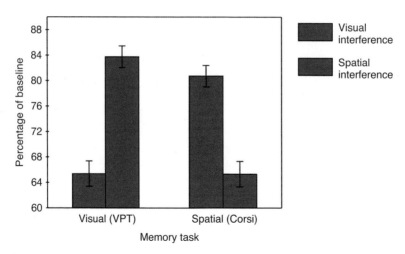

Fig. 7.10 The effect of secondary task interference during the retention interval on performance in the Visual Patterns Test and the Corsi Test. In all conditions performance is expressed as a percentage of baseline performance obtained from a condition with no secondary task. Subjects were healthy university students. Reprinted from *Neuropsychologia, 37*(10), S. Della Sala, C. Gray, A. Baddeley, N. Allamano and L. Wilson, Pattern span: tool for unwelding visuo-spatial memory. 1189–1199, Copyright 1999, with permission from Elsevier.

damage following a stroke. MV's digit span was within the normal range, as was his long-term visuo-spatial memory as assessed by immediate and delayed reproduction of a very complex geometrically-organised shape—the Rey figure A. He performed poorly, however, on the Corsi task, scoring below the 5th percentile. MV was not tested on the visual pattern span task, but Carlesimo and colleagues argue on the basis of other visual short-term memory tests that he has a selective spatial, but not visual, short-term memory deficit. In particular, MV scored better than age-matched controls in a test in which he was first presented with an ordered sequence of 3 to 7 shapes and then required to arrange the full set in the order given.

A separate research tradition has investigated how the visual complexity of objects interacts with the capacity limitations of visual short-term memory, and in particular whether visual short-term memory is feature-based (and hence limited by the number of features to be stored) or object-based (and hence limited by the number of objects to be stored). Behavioural studies support object-based encoding, with visual short-term memory being able to store equally many single feature objects as two-feature objects (e.g. Luck & Vogel, 1997). This is further supported by fMRI studies which have varied the number of single-feature objects. Thus, Todd and Marois (2004) found a correlation between the number of objects to be stored and activation in the intraparietal and intraoccipital sulci. They later showed a correlation between individual visual short-term store capacity and posterior parietal activation (Todd & Marois, 2005).[27] Building on this and using multi-feature objects

that varied in colour and shape, Xu (2007; see also Xu & Chun, 2006) found activation in the inferior intraparietal sulcus to be dependent on the number of objects stored in visual short-term memory, but activation in the superior intraparietal sulcus was dependent on number of stored features (see Figure 7.11). This suggests that visual short-term memory cannot be understood in terms of a single buffer, perhaps with a rehearsal process, containing a set or sequence of object descriptions. Rather, visual short-term memory appears to be subserved by a network of processing regions operating at both featural and object levels. The latter will require mechanisms to bind features of a single object into a unitary representation.[28]

Input buffers, as their name suggests, are held to operate on representations relatively close to perceptual input and to maintain those representations for subsequent processing. They may be contrasted with output buffers. When cognitive systems produce potential outputs at a more rapid rate than the effector systems can follow, it is necessary to hold the products of the central system online or the central systems will have to repeat the same operations. Systems that function as output buffers are therefore required in the control of skilled action—consider the processes involved in piano playing or fencing—or in speech, or in complex amalgams of the two—writing and typing

---

[27] These studies varied the feature, *colour*, with the task requiring short-term association a set of colours with up to 8 spatial locations,

all presented simultaneously. The task thus varies somewhat from the neuropsychological studies, which involve the feature *shape*.

[28] One might equally view storage and reproduction of a sequence of single-feature objects as requiring binding—in this case binding of object elements occurring at the same time, possibly linked by visuo-spatial attention to the item (see Treisman & Gelade, 1980, and Sections 1.8 and 9.3).

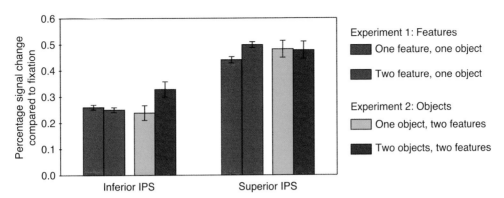

Fig. 7.11 Comparison of BOLD signal change from two experiments of Xu (2007). First, subjects were required to store feature information for one object with one feature compared to one object with two features. There was no difference in activation of inferior intraparietal sulcus (IPS) but significantly greater activation was observed in superior IPS for the two feature case. Second, subjects were required to store information concerning one object with two features contrasted with two objects with one feature each. Activation in superior IPS was independent of the number of objects, while activation in inferior IPS was greater when the features related to separate objects. Data from Xu (2007).

(see e.g. (i) Sternberg et al., 1988; (ii) Sperling, 1967; Morton, 1970; (iii) Ellis, 1979, 1982; Wing & Baddeley, 1980; Rumelhart & Norman, 1982).

From a functional imaging perspective it is difficult to study the operation of output buffers. Quite apart from the problem of movement artefacts, which are more severe for action than for speech, any successful output buffer operations will lead to a sequence of further output processes. To determine which activated region corresponds to which output process, including the operation of an output buffer, would require a complex paradigm. With neuropsychological methods the task is easier. The buffer can be overloaded by using particular types of stimuli such as long items or complex forms such as, in the case of speech, clichés, which operate as single representations at the appropriate level (McCarthy & Warrington, 1984). These neuropsychological methods have been supplemented by extensive computational modelling of the operation of output buffers. We will therefore address output buffers and two types of output buffer in particular—the phonological output buffer and the graphemic output buffer—in some detail. After discussing output buffers more generally, we will address the question of their operation, before returning to consider the operation of the phonological input buffer. We will then consider the possibility of semantic and episodic buffers, concluding with discussion of the involvement of structures located in prefrontal cortex in working memory processes.

7.5 The Phonological Output Buffer

The first major successful theoretical prediction in the history of neuropsychology was probably the German neurologist Ludwig Lichtheim's (1885) proposal of the existence of a third aphasic syndrome in addition to what are now known as Broca's and Wernicke's aphasia, which were briefly discussed in Section 1.3. Lichtheim

separated a centre for 'auditory word-representations' from one for 'motor word-representations' (see Figure 1.1) and argued that the syndromes described in the preceding two decades by Werniche and Broca could correspond to damage to each of these. Then he argued there must be a direct connection between them, as children learn to produce a word with the right sound, and so made the prediction that there should be a syndrome which corresponds to damage to this connection. This he held was conduction aphasia, which he in turn described.

The principal deficit of conduction aphasic patients was predicted to be a selective difficulty in repetition of a heard word or utterance. However, conduction aphasic patients, in addition to having this selective deficit, were also generally fluent and produced *literal paraphasias*—a phonological approximation to the intended utterance in which the individual phonemes are appropriately articulated (e.g. in the French patient of Dubois et al., 1964, 'dans mon chandarsin', where 'chandarsin' was argued to be a telescoping of 'champ' and 'jardin'). This latter characteristic did not fit the simple Lichtheim-style theoretical account. Shallice and Warrington (1977a) argued that the clinical syndrome of conduction aphasia should be divided into two forms. One would be a difficulty of repeating a number of high-frequency items (span) but with the ability to produce individual long low frequency items preserved. The second form would have the complementary characteristics. Span should be intact but individual long low frequency forms should present difficulty to the patient. It was argued that the two forms represented damage to an input and an output phonological buffer, respectively.[29] The short-term memory

---

[29] In 1984 McCarthy and Warrington proposed a third disconnection type which corresponded more directly to Lichtheim's conception of 99 years before.

TABLE 7.4 Percentage of items repeated, read and written correctly for IGR and LT.

IGR: Non-words

Length	Repetition	Reading	Writing
4-5 letters	90%	88%	80%
6-7 letters	78%	82%	74%
8+ letters	67%	85%	62%

LT: Words

Length	Repetition	Reading	Writing
2 syllables	75%	84%	65%
3 syllables	59%	76%	50%
4 syllables	45%	66%	52%

LT: Non-Words

Length	Repetition	Reading	Writing
2 syllables	40%	64%	42%
3 syllables	27%	38%	24%
4 syllables	8%	19%	8%

Data from: Caramazza et al., 1986; Shallice et al., 2000.

syndrome discussed extensively in early sections would correspond to the first syndrome. In the second, it was proposed, the literal paraphasias would occur, which are clinically accepted to be part of conduction aphasia. Shortly thereafter, Damasio and Damasio (1980) indeed described patients who had the conduction aphasia pattern of spontaneous speech and repetition—both full of literal paraphasias—but also had normal spans.

The first descriptions of a patient with an impaired output phonological buffer, which was experimentally well characterised, was given by Caramazza et al. (1986), in their Italian patient IGR. In fact, IGR was a very mild case. His errors were initially entirely limited to the production of pronounceable non-words, like *cantevi*. The elegant methodological innovation of the paper was to show that the errors in the production of non-words were very similar, whichever of three tasks were used—repeating non-words, reading non-words aloud and writing non-words to dictation. This was shown to be the case both when one examined the effect of quantitative variables—say number of syllables—and when one looked qualitatively at the type of errors. Errors consisted of single substitutions, insertions, deletions and transpositions of phonemes. Tables 7.4, 7.5 and 7.6 show results of two patients, IGR and a more severe patient—LT of Shallice et al. (2000)—who shows qualitatively the same problems but also exhibits them with words.

A number of patients of this sort have now been described. In some, the effects are restricted to non-words as in IGR (e.g. MV: Bub et al., 1987; RR: Bisiacchi et al., 1989), while in others there is an effect on words as well, as in LT (e.g. GC: Romani, 1992; RN: Wilshire & McCarthy, 1996).[30]

As mentioned above, the methodological novelty of the study of Caramazza and colleagues was to show this qualitative and quantitative similarity in the performance of IGR across the three tasks.[31] Caramazza et al. reasoned that the locus of the deficit would be a stage in common in the flow of information through the systems responsible for performance of each of the three tasks. Thus it cannot be on the input side of the system because the tasks differ in their input characteristics. Moreover it cannot be too late in the speech output processes as writing is also affected.[32]

In addition, the patients have the following characteristics in common:

1 There are no marked semantic class effects.

2 There is a marked effect on the errors of length of the word/non-word unit in all basic tasks (see Table 7.4).

3 Errors are predominantly phonemic—substitutions, insertions, deletions and transpositions (see Table 7.6).[33]

4 Errors are predominantly single errors of one of these types, but are at times double errors or ones that involve more complex sets of the basic operations (see Table 7.5).

5 Such errors tend to bear a phonological relation to the correct phoneme.

6 The ratio of errors on consonant and vowel is roughly the same for a patient across tasks.[34]

The effect of length and the nature of the errors point to a system that holds phoneme-based information

---

[30] Vallar et al. (1997) also interpret their patient TO as having a phonological output buffer impairment, and this would fit with the general position taken here. Unfortunately the tasks carried out on patients of the IGR type have not been carried out on TO, or the tasks used with him on them.

[31] The method can be seen as the equivalent in neuropsychology to the cognitive conjunction design of functional imaging (see Section 5.7).

[32] The slight superiority of reading can be explained by the patient using a strategy of processing one syllable at a time.

[33] In writing these error types are naturally realised as letters.

[34] See Shallice et al., 2000, for further details of the characteristics. GC and RN were not tested in as much detail as the other patients in these respects. It should also be noted that MV was unable to write.

TABLE 7.5 The percentage of single, double and complex errors made in the repetition, reading and writing of nonwords and words by two graphic buffer disorder patients: IGR from Caramazza et al., 1986, and LT from Shallice et al., 2000.

	Repetition		Reading		Writing	
	IGR	LT	IGR	LT	IGR	LT
Nonwords						
Single	61	44	83	59	77	35
Double	18	27	17	26	18	28
Complex	21	32	–	25	5	37
% Correct	76	30	85	45	71	28
Words						
Single	–	50	*	64	76	53
Double	–	25	*	24	24	23
Complex	–	25	*	12	–	24
% Correct	100	61	98	77	97	56

*= too few observations to be useful.

Data from: Shallice et al., 2000.

for output as the potential site of the impairment. This was the claim made by Caramazza et al. (1986). It is supported by the way that errors tend to increase with syllables within a word or non-word, which fits with an interpretation in terms of an abnormally weakening trace. Moreover the existence of transposition errors also fits this account; they are frequent in auditory memory span when capacity is exceeded (see e.g. Ryan, 1969). The pattern of findings thus fits with the impairment of a speech output buffer, which is implicated in spoken (and written) production regardless of input modality (see Figure 7.12).[35]

Four questions may be posed about this interpretation. Why should the buffer be considered to be an output buffer? Why should some of the patients not show the effects with words but only with non-words? How does such a buffer relate to the speech production system as a whole? And how would such a buffer work?

Consider first the status of the buffer as an output buffer. Traditionally in cognitive psychology and neuropsychology it was standard to argue that the phonological input system and the phonological output system were separate with the two systems having different

buffers (see, for instance, Monsell, 1984).[36] Yet, this position has been increasingly questioned (e.g. Allport, 1984; Page et al., 2007). However, LT and GC—if tested by the use of probe recognition methods or digit sequence repetition—had normal or near normal spans. Could the impairment of these patients, though, be attributed to damage to systems that follow a single input-output store in the speech system? If so, one would not be able to explain easily the virtually identical pattern of performance that exists for writing and repetition, which involve quite different output systems. Just as critically, it would not explain why phonological input buffer patients do not show the same problem in repeating single words. The double dissociation between the two types of patient is much more easily explained in terms of two distinct stores.

When IGR was first described, the fact that his deficit appeared for non-words but not for words led Caramazza and his colleagues to suggest that the use of the phonological buffer was only required if word order was critical. The production of single words and even short sentences would, it was argued, be carried out without the buffer. Bub et al. (1987) came to a different theoretical conclusion: 'incompletely specified traces for a meaningless sequence trigger a higher-level interpretative mechanism, which evaluates the response options. Since the potential candidates at this level of representation are morphemes that provide the best possible fit to the description in the response buffer, the output selected will be a word that is a close phonological approximation to the target' (p. 95). So words will be retrieved even when non-words of similar structure will not be. Moreover if any phonemic representations in an output system are supported by an attractor structure, as discussed in Chapters 4 and 6, then the main potential candidates will instead be those representations that correspond to an attractor basin, i.e. morphemes. On this view if the patient's deficit were more severe it would affect words too. It is possible to plot the performance of patients whose deficit did not affect words and ones where it did on the same curve—supporting the idea that the two types of deficit just differ in the amount of relevant resource that is lost (see Figure 4.5).

A more complex issue is how a buffer such as this relates to the general speech production system as a whole. Mechanisms that hold phonological information, at least with the capacity of a clause, have been postulated from research with a more linguistic orientation focusing on speech errors in normal subjects (e.g. Fromkin, 1973). From the perspective of say a model such as that of Levelt (1989), as discussed in Section 3.5,

---

[35] Caplan and Waters (1992) point out that the errors that reproduction conduction aphasics make in spontaneous speech may be more complex as they may involve lexical insertion into sentential structures.

[36] This issue is extensively reviewed in FNMS Chapter 7.

TABLE 7.6 The percentage of different types of single errors made in the repetition, reading and writing of nonwords and words by two graphic buffer disorder patients: IGR from Caramazza et al., 1986, and LT from Shallice et al., 2000.

	Repetition		Reading		Writing	
	IGR	LT	IGR	LT	IGR	LT
Nonwords						
Substitution	81	75	81	79	68	68
Insertion/Add.	11	8	13	7	13	17
Deletion	3	7	6	10	17	11
Transposition	5	9	–	4	2	4
Total	63	110	70		114	94
Words						
Substitution	–	71		88		75
Insertion/Add.	–	12		4		16
Deletion	–	10		5	–	10
Transposition		6		1	–	8
Total	*	108	*	81		122

Only conditions where 10 or more errors were made are included.

*= too few observations to be useful.

Data from: Shallice et al., 2000.

the phonological output buffer sits at the interface between the formulator and the articulator (see Figures 3.15 and 7.12). Thus, following a long tradition (e.g. Levy, 1971; Baddeley & Hitch, 1974; Baddeley et al., 1975; see also Section 7.3), Levelt proposes an 'articulatory buffer', which holds a phonetic plan for the forthcoming word or phrase, as supplied by his formulator component. This positioning of the articulatory buffer, which is made explicit by Postma (2000), is consistent with the location of the phonological output buffer within recent diagrammatic presentations of the phonological loop model, which indicate that 'spoken output' is generated from the contents of the phonological output buffer.

This leaves the final question yet to be considered; namely how a buffer of this type might work. This question is more easily tackled after discussion of another putative output buffer—the graphemic output buffer—and its involvement in the act of writing.

7.6 The Graphemic Output Buffer

The study of the graphemic output buffer might seem a rather recherché topic. However writing and typing are highly important skills. They represent along with driving (or cycling), cooking and cleaning the most widely used overlearned complex motor skills in advanced industrial

societies and the acquisition of complex skills is one of the hallmarks of modern humans (see Chapter 8). Moreover writing is much easier to study than many motor skills as the relevant units of representations—which can be damaged at many levels[37]—are manifest in the output. It is also easier to study than speech output.

It was standardly accepted by the end of the 1970s that the writing process, from the orthographical lexicon down, had a quite distinct material basis from the phonological system, even if the two are interconnected (see e.g. Morton & Patterson, 1980; Ellis, 1982; Figure 7.13). This has been rediscovered more recently, but on the basis of elegant new evidence. Patients have been described who regularly make qualitatively different semantic errors to the same stimulus according to whether they are speaking or writing (see Hillis et al., 1999). That the errors are semantic suggests that the impairment is 'high' in the system, that they are different suggests that the downstream systems are different.[38]

If fluent writing has a separate material basis from fluent speech, then the system that is involved will also need to hold temporary representations at a number of

---

[37] See FNMS Chapter 6.

[38] It is conceivable that the two types of error derive from processing in different hemispheres.

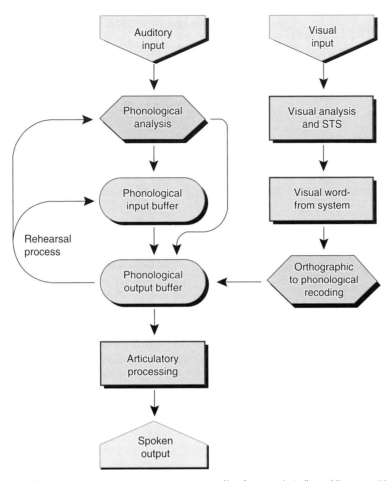

Fig. 7.12 The architecture of the phonological short-term memory systems. (See, for example, Vallar and Papagno, 1995.)

different levels. In two classic papers Ellis (1979, 1982) analysed the nature of the writing slips of normal subjects and showed that the types of errors they make differ according to the properties of the letters that are involved in an error. Thus some errors depend upon the similarity of the physical form of the letters—the graphemic motor patterns—such as certain types of substitution, e.g. *within* → *mi*...[39] Other errors depend upon the selection of the particular form of the letter—the so-called allograph or overall structure of the produced letter; *T* and *t*, for instance, differ but so do different forms of the same case of letter—in writing one of us, for instance, uses two different forms of *f*, one which loops below the line and the other which does not. A third error type, a haplography, involves a string of letters that is omitted between two identical letters as in *depending* → *dending*. This error only occurs when the identical letters are the same allograph; *Depending* → *Ding* based on omission between the *D* and the *d* does not occur. Finally there are letter transpositions, often

'supported' by carrier letters, as in *J. Neurol. Neurosurg.* → *J. Seuro*..., where the *ur* acts as a carrier or *Pye Cambridge* → *Pyce*..., without a carrier. Here the allographic form of the letter is not the level at which the error occurs; instead the maintenance of letters appears to be at an abstract graphemic level of representation in a graphemic buffer.

The first well-described patient characterised as having an impairment of the graphemic buffer was patient LB (Caramazza et al., 1987; Caramazza & Miceli, 1990). Since then, around 20 patients have been described, who have shown a number of similar characteristics (for reviews see Sage & Ellis, 2004, and Cipolotti et al., 2004). The deficits exhibited by the patients have many similarities in their different domain to those of the phonological output buffer patients just discussed:

1 There are no major effects of semantic class or regularity of the sound-to-spelling mapping.[40]

---

[39] The specific errors given here are from Ellis's original study.

[40] Patient MC2 of Annoni et al. (1998) did show an effect of the second of these variables.

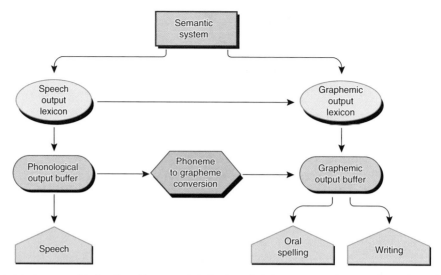

Fig. 7.13 A typical dual-route model of spelling with separate lexical and non-lexical routes converging upon the graphemic buffer. (See, for example, Sage and Ellis, 2004.)

2 There is a marked effect of word length in spelling either when assessed by writing or by spelling aloud (see Figures 7.19 and 7.22).

3 Errors are qualitatively the same with words and non-words with errors on words being quantitatively somewhat fewer.

4 Incorrect responses predominantly involve single errors (substitutions, insertions, deletions and transpositions; see Figure 7.20) but are at times double errors or more complex ones. For instance 49.2% of LB's errors were single (Caramazza et al., 1987) and 44.3% of AS's (Jónsdóttir et al., 1996).

5 Patients make characteristic types of errors when there are words with doubled letters, so called geminates. These include moving the geminate to the neighbouring letters as in *freeze → frezze; summit → sumiit* (from AS).

All of these characteristics are closely complementary to those produced by the phonological output buffer patients discussed in the previous section, except for the last one.[41] One very neat result was also found in one of the patients by Miceli et al. (1995). Their patient, AZO, had been a professional stenographer before her stroke. Stenographic production is faster than handwriting because many highly frequent letter groups are omitted or abbreviated. Moreover the symbols themselves can be

produced faster. AZO showed very similar characteristics across the two quite different sorts of script, supporting Ellis's arguments that the code which is being used in the graphemic output buffer is at quite a high level of the output system.

How might the characteristics of the two types of syndrome be explained? Two different types of account have been given. The first approach was that of Caramazza and Miceli (1990). Their graphemic buffer patient, LB, was Italian. They found that the patient wrote words with a particular syllabic structure, much better than other ones of the same length. The good syllables were ones with a so-called simple consonant–vowel structure (e.g. CVCVCV like *tavolo*); LB was 73% correct in writing six-letter words as opposed to 56% correct with otherwise comparable words with a more complex structure. It is standardly accepted by phonologists that the phonological representations of words involve a number of levels, known as tiers (see e.g. Clements & Keyser, 1983). Caramazza and Miceli adapted this approach to the orthographic structure of words as indicated by Figure 7.14. They had a symbolic model of the orthographic organisation of the words. A typical error would occur when a specific letter was lost, but the nature of the error is on this view still constrained by the whole structure (see Figure 7.15).

In two English patients, no effect of syllabic structure was found (Kay & Hanley, 1994; Jónsdóttir et al., 1996). Moreover, Jónsdóttir et al. argued that the difference between the two types of patient might lie in the relation between phonology and orthography, which is much closer in Italian (where the sound-to-spelling relationship is regular), than in English (where it is not). Specifically, they suggest that differences between the

---

[41] The equivalent of characteristic 3 is in fact only found with a subset of the phonological output buffer patients, but, as argued in Section 7.5, the failure to find it in all has been attributed to a quantitative difference in the degree of impairment, namely a resource problem.

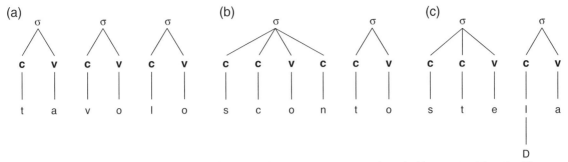

Fig. 7.14 Tiered graphemic templates for three types of Italian words. C = consonant, V = vowel, D = doubling. Reprinted from *Cognition*, 37(5), A. Caramazza and G. Miceli, The structure of graphemic representations, 243–297, Copyright 1990, with permission from Elsevier.

spelling performances of the patients may arise from a difference in the degree to which phonological information in the two languages constrains spelling, rather than from any syllabic structure intrinsic to the graphemic buffer. This interpretation receives further support from an analysis of the writing of YK, a dysgraphic patient reported by Kim et al. (2007) who wrote Korean and English. YK produces consonant/vowel transposition errors in English but not Korean. Kim and colleagues suggest that the preservation of CV structure in Korean, which involves spatially well-formed configurations of symbols, is supported by spatial processing which was preserved following the patient's left-hemisphere lesion.[42]

Indirect support for the argument that there may be critical differences between languages in the way the cognitive system deals with orthography comes from a striking functional imaging study on reading of Paulesu et al. (2000). Neurologically healthy native English and Italian speakers were scanned while reading words and non-words. Behaviourally, the Italian speakers were much faster for both words and non-words than the age- and IQ-matched English speakers. Paulesu and colleagues argued that this reflected the more regular phonology-to-orthography mapping of Italian. These behavioural differences were also reflected in the imaging results. Italian speakers showed greater activation of left superior temporal regions when reading both words and non-words, while English speakers showed greater activation of left posterior inferior temporal gyrus and left anterior inferior frontal gyrus when reading nonwords (see Figure 7.16). Paulesu and colleagues suggest that the superior temporal regions highly active in the Italian subjects reflect phonological processes required if reading uses a syllable-by-syllable procedure. The inferior temporal regions highly active in the English subjects probably reflect greater resources

devoted to processing of the whole visual word-form (see Chapter 4). The critical region is slightly lateral to the visual word-form area discussed in Chapters 4 and 5.

Returning to writing, this supports the idea that phonological mediation is more critical in Italian subjects in orthographic processing, as suggested by Jonsdottir et al. The theory of Caramazza and Miceli is in any case concerned only with the representations held in the graphemic buffer. It does not give any account of how the representations, especially when damaged, are realised in behaviour. Additional processing assumptions are required for this, but those assumptions are poorly developed in their approach compared with the assumptions about the representations themselves.

An alternative approach derives from a class of localist connectionist models, called *Competitive Queuing* (CQ) models, invented by Houghton (1990). They are themselves a development of the architecture introduced by Rumelhart and Norman (1982) in their model of typing, which in turn relates to ideas produced by MacKay (1970) to explain speech errors. Houghton's approach is a potential solution to Lashley's famous problem of how the appropriate serial order of movements in rapid behaviour is produced. He was concerned with behaviour too rapid for simple chaining of elementary responses to work, as in playing the piano. Houghton's solution was to separate out two types of input to the basic nodes or item representations from which a selection has to be made. These nodes correspond to letters in the case of writing. One type of input is obvious; it concerns the presence or absence of the items that compose a known larger unit accessed earlier in the writing process—a word-form or lemma, say. So in writing *house* this input would tend to elicit *e, h, o, s, u*. The second input is more subtle; it provides a *rough* timing signal for when the appropriate letter is to be produced.

In Rumelhart and Norman's model, the timing signal was merely carried out by a measure of the distance from the beginning of the word. However in most patients errors most often appear in the middle of sequences— the serial position curve of errors is concave upwards.

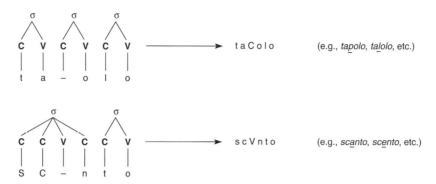

Fig. 7.15 Graphemic output errors resulting from adherence to a tiered graphemic template as shown in Figure 7.14 for the Italian words tavolo and sconto. Reprinted from *Cognition, 37*(5), A. Caramazza and G. Miceli, The structure of graphemic representations, 243–297, Copyright 1990, with permission from Elsevier.

Houghton replaced this timing signal dominated by the beginnings of words by two signals—one dependent upon the distance of where one is from the beginning of the word, the other dependent upon the distance of where one is from the end (see Figure 7.17). The timing signal relating to the beginning of the word is the represented by the I (for 'initiate') node, and the one dependent upon the distance from the end of the word the E (for 'end') node.

In the original Houghton (1990) procedure each new sequence that is learned involves separate pairs of units. In the learning phase these two timing inputs—I and E—are varied for each letter position of the word. The appropriate output at any particular position is associated by Hebbian learning (see Section 1.6) with that combination of I and E inputs. At the retrieval phase, the sequence of timing states, each of which represents a given position, is reproduced. At each position the output letter node that is most highly active controls behaviour, provided that its level of activation exceeds a preset threshold. This is done on the CQ approach by the activation in the item nodes in a particular domain being copied into an internally competitive output system such that at most one output node

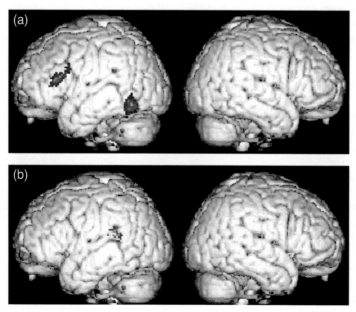

Fig. 7.16 Anatomical differences between regions active in English and Italian reading systems. (a) Those regions where English subjects produce greater activation when reading nonwords. These include the left inferior posterior temporal areas and the anterior portion of the inferior frontal gyrus. (b) The left planum temporale regions, more active generally in reading in Italian subjects. Reprinted by permission from Macmillan Publishers Ltd: Nature Neuroscience (E. Paulesu, E. McCrory, F. Fazio, L. Menoncello, N. Brunswick, S.F. Cappa, M. Cotelli, G. Cossu, F. Corte, M. Lorusso, S. Presenti, A. Gallagher, D. Perani, C. Price, C.D. Frith and U. Frith, A cultural effect on brain function, 2000, *Nature Neuroscience*, 3(1), 91–96), copyright (2000).

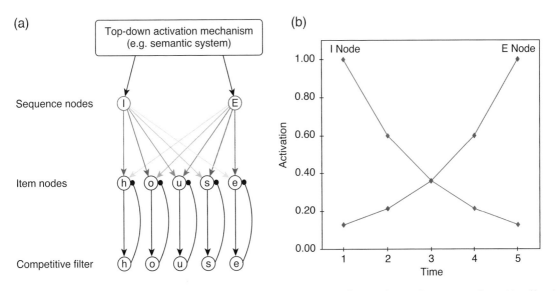

Fig. 7.17 The Competitive Queuing mechanism of Houghton (1990). (a) The structure of the mechanism, showing inputs from Initiate (I) and End (E) nodes to the letter nodes. (b) The activation of I and E nodes over the course of one learning or recollection trial for a five letter word.

is selected at a given point in the output process. The corresponding item node for the selected output must then be inhibited so as to become temporarily refractory. This is to prevent the system perseverating on that output.

To be more specific, consider the application of the CQ approach to spelling. Then if one rejects the Caramazza and Miceli claim concerning the existence of orthographic syllable structure, at least as a major aspect of the writing of English, then the key output units would be letter nodes, without an orthographic syllabic structure supporting them. The full model is shown in Figure 7.18.[43]

As just discussed once a letter has been produced it is necessary to inhibit the node previously activated. If not, there will be a tendency for perseveration to occur in selection. This is because the timing signals are only roughly calibrated and so the combination will be nearly as relevant for the next position as it is for the current one. In addition the item nodes retain a trace of their activation state when the previous letter is produced. This inhibitory effect makes it very difficult for the system to learn a sequence of two identical letters as the node is inhibited after the first of the two. The approach makes the striking prediction that a special mechanism is needed for pairs of identical letters. Indeed such a mechanism clearly exists given the strong evidence for a geminate marker such as *sneeze* →

snezze and *pepper* → *pepper* in AS (Jónsdóttir et al., 1996; see also Caramazza & Miceli, 1990; Houghton et al., 1994; Tainturier & Caramazza, 1996).

The assumption of an end node increasing in activation as one moves towards the end of the word might seem an implausible assumption. It is implausible in the original form of the model, where one-trial learning is assumed. However given that the length of the word is also something to be learned, then it should be noted that prefrontal units have been described which behave in a somewhat analogous fashion to I and E units. Thus in 'working memory' delay tasks of the type discussed in Section 1.2 where a signal is presented to cue a response that an animal must make some seconds later, the response of units in the critical relevant region of prefrontal cortex can show various patterns of behaviour (Fuster, 1973; Fuster et al., 1982). Some show a peak firing rate at the beginning of the delay period and then a graded decline in firing. This is what would be required of an I node. Others show the complementary pattern as required for an E node (see Averbeck et al., 2002). Now these units are in dorsolateral prefrontal cortex, not where timing signals for writing are most plausibly located. However they indicate that the neural circuitry does have the potential to support such timing signals.

Other theorists have replaced the I and E node signals with an alternative type of rough characterisation of the temporal or ordinal position of an item in a sequence, such as a vector which changes gradually over time (e.g. Burgess & Hitch, 1992; Glasspool, Shallice & Cipolotti, 2006). At retrieval the same sequence of vectors is reproduced. The essential aspect of the CQ models are of learning to specify which of the set of more elementary units

---

[43] The separate item and letter layers in Figure 7.18 (when contrasted with Figure 7.17) allow words with repeated letters to be produced, such as *pasta*, while the geminate mechanism allows words with double letters, such as *spaghetti*.

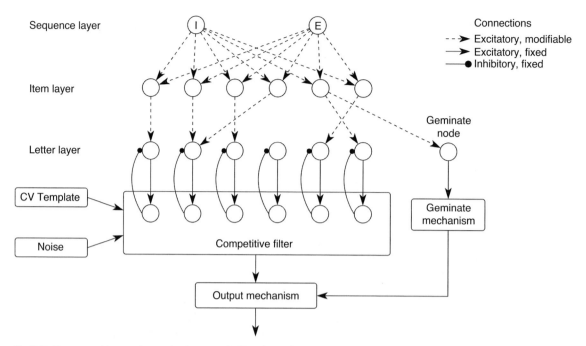

Fig. 7.18 The competitive queuing mechanism as applied by Glasspool and Houghton (2005) to a model of spelling. The model augments the basic mechanism with separate item and letter layers, and includes a geminate node for spelling words with double letters. Reprinted from *Brain and Language*, *94*(3), D.W. Glasspool and G. Houghton, Serial order and consonant-vowel structure in a graphemic output buffer model. 304–330, Copyright 2005, with permission from Elsevier.

out of which the whole large unit is composed—letters or phonemes in the case of words—should be selected at a given time by using an association with the appropriate value of a rough timing signal. The sequence of states of the timing signal acts as the cue for retrieval to elicit each of the elementary units at its appropriate time.

As far as spelling is concerned, if noise is added to the model then it reproduces the characteristics of the graphemic buffer disorder (see Houghton et al., 1994; Shallice et al., 1995). It shows a strong effect of word length on performance (see Figure 7.19). It shows the same error types (see Figure 7.20). It also shows similar effects to the empirical data with respect to the geminate marker moving to adjacent letters.[44]

The original model was localist, with a one-to-one mapping between nodes in the various layers and words or letters. Moreover it required that each new unit learned had a separate set of I and E nodes. This seems neurally implausible. However, a distributed network version of the same basic theory has been developed by Glasspool et al. (2006) and Machtynger (2006) (see Figure 7.21). The distributed version is much more complex than the localist one. However it makes much clearer the basic two-route conception of item and

position information being carried separately. Moreover it captures the basic phenomena of the graphemic buffer syndrome, although somewhat less well than the simpler localist model.[45] Thus because of its complexity and the necessarily greater computational requirements this produces, the Glasspool et al. (2006) model does not incorporate a geminate marker subsystem and so cannot spell words with immediately repeating letters. However, Machtynger (2006) does include such a mechanism in his distributed model.

The distributed model has one major empirical advantage. The graphemic buffer syndrome is mimicked in the model by impairing the operation of the competitive filter so that the letter produced is not necessarily the most active letter node at that instant. There are though many other sites within the model where a failure in its operation can be introduced. One such site selected by Glasspool and colleagues was the connections from the semantic representations to the word identity units—hidden layer 1 in Figure 7.21. This lesion site led to a pattern of behaviour with some similarities to the previous one. For instance, qualitatively the same error types occurred although deletions were much more frequent. However there were major differences. Errors increased linearly towards the end of the

---

[44] The way that the geminate marker in the model works is that if at any time it becomes above threshold then the letter being activated at that time is doubled in the output string.

[45] However unlike the localist model it tends to preserve consonant/vowel status in substitutions.

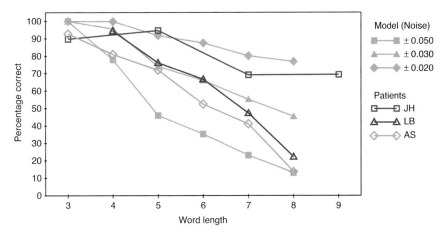

Fig. 7.19 A comparison of performance of the CQ model with different levels of noise (grey) and three patients (shown in colour). With noise of ± 0.030 the model performs at a similar level to patients LB and AS. From: Can neuropsychological evidence inform connectionist modelling? Analyses of spelling, T. Shallice, D.W. Glasspool and G. Houghton, *Language and Cognitive Processes*, 10(3/4), 195–225, 1995, Psychology Press, reprinted by permission of the publisher (Taylor & Francis Group, http://www.informaworld.com).

word. Moreover, Machtynger (2006) demonstrated that if the semantic representations of abstract and concrete words are realised by using different numbers of features, as carried out by Plaut and Shallice (1993a) in the simulation of deep dyslexia discussed in Section 4.10, then there was a strong effect of this variable; the system was considerably more likely to spell a concrete word correctly than an abstract one. This effect was not found when the operation of the competitive filter was impaired, or in the original model of Glasspool and colleagues.[46]

Now these effects in the model resolve an empirical problem that had been posed by patients showing the graphemic output buffer error pattern. The patients described as *Graphemic Buffer Disorder* essentially fall into two types, GOB type A and GOB type B (Cipolotti et al., 2004), a classification prefigured by Ward and Romani (1998), who pointed out the difference in the serial position curves between their patient BA and also patient HR of Katz (1991) on the one hand (Figure 7.22a) and those of patients like LB and AS on the other (Figure 7.22b).[47]

Across patients this difference in serial position curves is strongly linked to three other effects (Table 7.7). One is whether the patients show a large difference between the way they spell words and non-words, with the prototypic patient like HR or BA being unable to spell non-words, or whether non-words are spelled like words except a little bit worse, like LB and AS. The second effect was whether—like HR, or not—like LB—the patients showed an effect of semantic or syntactic variables in their spelling. Thirdly, Ward and Romani showed that their patient BA makes a high rate—approximately equal to the rate of substitutions—of a new error type—so-called *fragments*—where the response is at least two letters shorter than the word (e.g. *sulphur* → *sulp*; *moth* → *bu*). These have been found in other patients of this type (e.g. in patient DA of Cipolotti et al., 2004), but do not tend to be found in the more classical graphemic buffer patients.

When patients performed very poorly with non-words or showed effects of semantic variables this has typically been dismissed as an irrelevant associated deficit. However if one considers the second 'lesion site' of the Glasspool et al. simulation discussed above, namely that between the semantic units and the word identity units, then we obtain the pattern described by Katz (1991) and by Ward and Romani (1998). Consider the novel error type described by Ward and Romani—fragments. For lesions at the competitive filter level they made up 2% of all errors. For lesions at the semantic system-to-word identity level they make up 40–70% of all errors depending upon the degree of damage. Thus the model predicts the existence of a second functional syndrome, which has indeed been found.[48]

---

[46] Machtynger (2006) also found that use of the Plaut and Shallice type semantic representations produced a more robust fit of the model to the basic data. Thus, the good fits of the Glasspool et al. model are highly dependent on the particular set of parameters used. This is not so for the Machtynger model. Thus, what might appear to be implementation details affect the model's neuropsychological predications.

[47] For discussion of these points see Cipolotti et al. (2004).

---

[48] Ward and Romani consider weak activation of the letter-node units in a CQ model as a possible explanation of their variant of the Graphemic Output Buffer syndrome (i.e. GOB type B). They reject this possibility on the grounds that they expected that the model would predict greater difficulty with words where the same letter occurs twice but does not have a

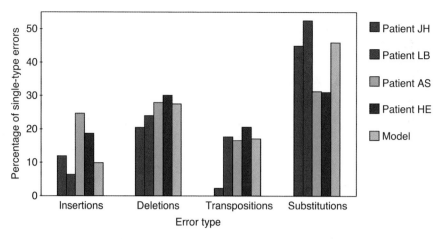

Fig. 7.20 The proportion of error types produced by four patients (JH, LB, AS and HE) compared with the CQ spelling model (averaged over 10,000 trials with noise at ± 0.030, which approximates the degree of impairment of LB, AS and HE, but not JH). From: Can neuropsychological evidence inform connectionist modelling? Analyses of spelling, T. Shallice, D.W. Glasspool and G. Houghton, *Language and Cognitive Processes*, 10(3/4), 195–225, 1995, Psychology Press, reprinted by permission of the publisher (Taylor & Francis Group, http://www.informaworld.com).

A final point in favour of the model concerns an apparently very different type of agraphia syndrome—deep dysgraphia. This is the complementary syndrome to deep dyslexia, discussed in Section 4.11, but with a similar combination of characteristics.[49] It was first described by Bub and Kertesz (1982). In complementary fashion to deep dyslexics, patients make semantic errors in writing, such as writing *clock* in place of *time*. They write concrete nouns much better than verbs, function words or orthographically possible non-words. In the standard way of thinking about the agraphias, deep dysgraphia occurs following impairments at a high level of the system. Since in the prototypic cases (e.g. Baxter & Warrington, 1985) the patient has intact comprehension, the impairment cannot be in the semantic system itself, so it would need to be to the connections from the semantic system to the lexical level of the orthographic system. Moreover an analogous model to that of Plaut and Shallice for deep dyslexia would lead to the deep dysgraphia pattern if an impairment occurred between the semantic level and output systems. However this would just repeat in a different model where the second type of impairment was made in the Glasspool et al. and Machtynger models.

Therefore the prediction follows that deep dysgraphic patients ought also to be GOB type B patients; that is they should make graphemic buffer errors. In all deep dysgraphic patients where the researchers have provided sufficient information for this to be checked the patients behave as predicted (see e.g. Friederici et al., 1981; Baxter & Warrington, 1985).[50] It would appear that whether experimenters reported their patients as being 'deep dysgraphic' or having a form of 'graphemic output buffer' depended on whether they concentrated on what the patient could write or instead how they went wrong.

Thus if we see the localist CQ model and the Glasspool et al. (2006) model as providing compatible implementations at different grains of the mapping from semantics onto letter outputs, then the collection of models works well. It predicts not only the broad pattern of performance in graphemic output buffer disorder, but also a new form of disorder with a related error pattern, which includes a new error type—fragments; the family of models moreover predict that this new form of disorder will be equivalent to an apparently quite different form of agraphia—deep dysgraphia—which it seems to be.

7.7 The Phonological Input and Output Buffers Again

Having discussed the graphemic output buffer in some detail the question naturally arises as to whether the same type of model is appropriate for the two more basic short-term memory domains considered earlier in

---

double-letter geminate (e.g. *paper*) when compared with control words (e.g. *table*). They assumed that *paper* would produce more errors because of the inhibition given to the repeated letter node (e.g. *p*) after the first occurrence of the letter; this they thought would make it more difficult to activate the letter a second time. They found no such effect in BA. However while such an effect seems a priori plausible, there was no such effect in the simulation either (Glasspool et al., 2006).

[49] See FNMS Section 6.6 for more details.

---

[50] The one patient whose performance does not clearly fit is patient FM of Tainturier and Caramazza (1996). Unfortunately full serial position curves are not given for this patient.

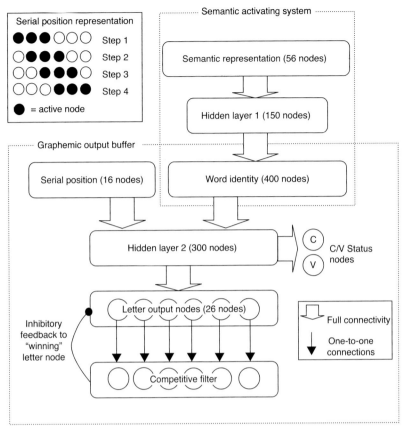

Fig. 7.21 Glasspool et al's (2006) distributed version of the competitive queuing model of spelling. (Compare Figure 7.18.) From: Towards a unified process model for graphemic buffer disorder and deep dysgraphia, D.W. Glasspool, T. Shallice and L. Cipolotti, *Cognitive Neuropsychology*, *23*(3), 479–512, 2006, Psychology Press, reprinted by permission of the publisher (Taylor & Francis Group, http://www. informaworld.com.)

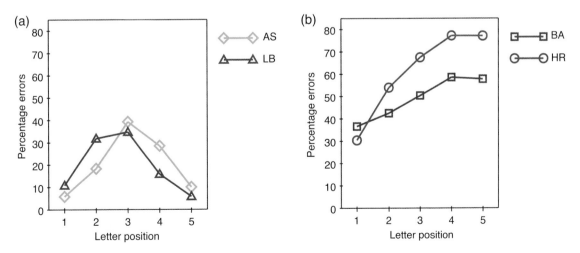

Fig. 7.22 The distribution of spelling errors as a function of position in word for two distinct types of graphemic buffer patients. (a) Data from AS (Jónsdóttir et al, 1996) and LB (Caramazza et al, 1987). (Graphemic buffer type A.) (b) Data from BA (Ward & Romani, 1998) and HR (Katz, 1991) (Graphemic buffer type B.) Position is normalised for length of word, so, for example, the middle letter of a word, regardless of length, corresponds to position C. (For details of the normalisation procedure see Caramazza et al., 1987. For an improved method see Machtynger & Shallice, 2009.)

TABLE 7.7 Characteristics of two distinct types of graphemic buffer disorder (GOB).

GOB type A	GOB type B
Errors most common at centre of word	Errors most common at end of word
Spells non-words almost as well as words	Unable to spell non-words
No effects of syntactic or semantic variables on spelling	Strong effects of semantic and syntactic variables on spelling
Fragment errors are rare	Fragment errors are frequent
Proto-typical patients: LB, AS	Proto-typical patients: HR, BA, DA

the chapter. The domain of the input phonological buffer is an excellent one for modelling because over the last forty years a wide variety of phenomena have been described concerning the detailed aspects of how normal subjects perform in span tasks (e.g. Baddeley, 1986; Page & Norris, 1998). A variety of models have been developed to account for these phenomena.

If one considers how the *order* of the items is reproduced when a subject repeats a list of items, then models have used one or other of three main principles. The first approach is to use traditional associative principles, by chaining of each item to the next, as in the TODAM model of Lewandowsky and Murdock (1989). The second is to base the order of items on the relative strengths of item information, with earlier items having greater strength, as in the Primacy Model of Page and Norris (1998). It has however been argued on the basis of error patterns made by normal subjects in immediately recalling a list of items that neither of these approaches is satisfactory (see (i) Henson et al., 1996; (ii) Henson, 1999; for review see Henson, 1998). The chaining approach has problems with explaining how particular types of sequence are remembered. The theoretically critical finding is the so-called sawtooth effect where sequences of acoustically similar and different items are interleaved (as in, e.g. RBLTHE … where B, T and E rhyme) compared with sequences which are all acoustically different (as in, e.g. RKLMHQ …). Subjects are worse when repeating the acoustically similar items than for the corresponding items in control sequences of all acoustically different items, but they are not worse on the interleaved acoustically different items contrary to what one would expect on a chaining approach (Baddeley, 1968; Henson et al., 1996; see Figure 7.23).[51] The primacy model in turn has problems

when grouping is introduced as in XBR .. HTL; transposition errors occur between items in the same position in different groups (Henson, 1998).

The third approach is to represent and retain the position of each item in the sequence, as for graphemic buffer models. A variety of different models which represent either the temporal position or ordinal position of each item—either absolutely or relatively—have been proposed (e.g. Lee & Estes, 1981; Neath, 1993; Brown et al., 2000; Botvinick & Plaut, 2006a; Botvinick & Watanabe, 2007). The models have many similarities (see Henson et al., 2003, and Burgess & Hitch, 2005, for discussion). We will concentrate on two because they are most directly compatible with the output buffer models considered above and because functional imaging experiments have been devised to localise their components. They are the first model of this genre, that of Burgess and Hitch (1992, 1999), and the Start-End model of Henson (1998).

On the Burgess and Hitch model, phonological storage occurs through the changes in short-term weights from phonemic representations to and from lexical representations. Articulatory rehearsal corresponds to the recycling of information around the loop from input to output phonemic representations (see Figure 7.24). Two classical phenomena within short-term memory theory are simply explained. One is the phonological-similarity effect (see Section 7.3). The other is the word-length effect, that span is negatively correlated with word length (Baddeley et al., 1975). The former is held to arise from confusions in the input- and output-phoneme layers of the model, and the latter through decay of short-term weights while the recycling process occurs.

These representations alone would, however, not be able to organise the order of the phoneme sequence. For this reason an additional set of units is required which provide a timing signal; this operates in an analogous fashion to the timing inputs of the CQ models just discussed. The model captures a host of detailed phenomena of normal phonological short-term memory well (see Burgess & Hitch, 1992, 1999).[52]

---

[51] Page et al. (2007) argue that the sawtooth effect derives from the output system and so would be irrelevant for understanding the operation of the phonological input buffer.

---

[52] Despite the model's strengths, two criticisms can be made of the Burgess and Hitch model. First, the model does not have separate input and output buffers. It is therefore only able to account for phenomena that relate specifically to the input phonological buffer. More critically, where the model does not explain an effect, it is possible to argue that the locus of the effect is, for example, in the phonological output buffer and therefore not relevant to the model. Second, the model in its standard form is unable to deal adequately with the Hebb paradigm. This involves repeating the same list to be recalled every few trials within the context of many different lists. Recall performance on the repeated list improves. Burgess and Hitch (2005) attempt

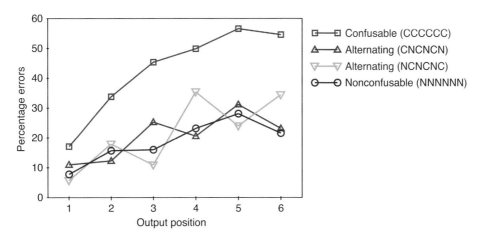

Fig. 7.23 The saw-tooth effect. Errors in immediate serial recall for six item lists consisting of confusable (C) and nonconfusable (N) items. The error rate is generally high when all items are confusable. When confusable and nonconfusable items alternate, errors are more frequent on confusable items than nonconfusable items, but the nonconfusable items are no worse than in pure nonconfusable lists. Data from Henson et al. (1996).

Henson's Start-End Model (SEM; Henson, 1998) shares some of the core assumptions of the Burgess and Hitch model, particularly the fundamental assumption of a separation in short-term memory between item information and order information. The main distinguishing features of SEM are: (1) the use of two context signals—a start signal and an end signal—analogous to the signals provided by the I and E nodes of CQ models (see Figures 7.17 and 7.18); and (2) its statement as a mathematical, rather than an algorithmic, theory. The model is able to capture a similar range of effects as that of Burgess and Hitch, though the use of start/end coding of position allows the model to capture potentially puzzling empirical effects concerning substitution errors between sequences of varying length, which Henson (1999) found respected the position of an item relative to both the start and the end of a sequence.

Both the Burgess and Hitch (1992, 1999) and Henson (1998) models assume some kind of timing or context units, and an attempt has been made to provide functional imaging evidence concerning these units. Henson et al. (2000b) argue that a key region for the timing signal is in left premotor cortex. Unfortunately the constraints of fMRI at the time meant that visual presentation had to be used. Yet two of the critical phenomena relating to order are critically dependent on the modality of input. One, the so-called grouping effect, is where input is presented in groups as in 249.573.627 rather than in a completely regular series, as used in normal span. Grouping facilitates recall but changes the pattern of errors greatly, both qualitatively as well

as quantitatively. However the extra inter-stimulus time necessary to create the organisation of a group is of the order of 100 msec (Frankish, 1974). Such a difference is not well registered in visual short-term memory (see Mitchell, 1972), which is much more attuned to spatially than temporally structured changes. Second, the pattern of recall changes greatly if an extra irrelevant item is always added to the list, e.g. 46982710. This is a phenomenon that occurs with auditory but not with visual input. It was originally explained by assuming an extra peripheral acoustic store, which held an additional auditory item (Crowder & Morton, 1969). However this explanation has problems.[53] Instead a better explanation is that it interferes with an auditory timing marker (Henson, 1998; but see Frankish, 2008). If, then as these phenomena suggest, the key aspect of the timing signal is derived from the auditory input then it will not be detected by using visual displays. Thus in our view we do not as yet have any neuroscience evidence on where in the brain the main internal timing signal for span originates.

We would argue that the information-processing concept of *buffer* can be thought of as having two properties when mapped into a connectionist framework. It corresponds to the combination of a mechanism specifically geared to the short-term retention of a type of information together with a mechanism for efficiently retrieving the information once stored. Using this

---

to address this by arguing that the effect is due to long-term learning, and is thus not relevant to the basic model.

[53] Henson (1998) lists several effects that the assumption of a so-called Precategorical Acoustic Store (PAS) cannot explain, including modality effects (Penney, 1989), effects of lip-read stimuli (Campbell & Dodd, 1980) and effects of dynamic or changing stimuli (Glenberg, 1990).

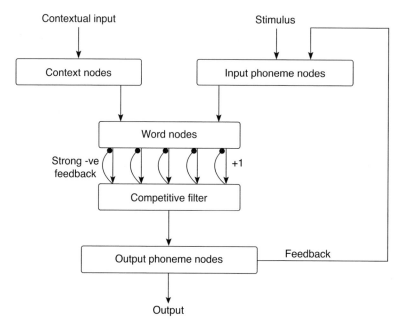

Fig. 7.24 The Burgess and Hitch (1992) model of Baddeley and Hitch's phonological loop. Reprinted from *Journal of Memory and Language*, *31*(4), N. Burgess and G. Hitch, Toward a network model of the articulatory loop. 429–460, Copyright 1992, with permission from Elsevier.

cross-framework correspondence, if one considers why there should be a phonological input buffer system, then one major lacuna of all the models is that they treat span as a purely memory phenomenon. They do not consider the buffer's function as a possible back-up store for holding the first-pass representation of an utterance in language perception/comprehension, and its role in their short-term retention as in the Jarvella effect as discussed in Section 7.3.[54] This function must be realised computationally using the phonological characteristics of the input signal. This is yet to be done.

Where a real integration between speech processing and the phonological input buffer has been made is in the domain of the phonological output buffer. Hartley and Houghton's (1996) model of word production follows an earlier model of Dell's (1988) in having separate sources of activation representing, on the one hand, phonemic content, and on the other, its place in the syllabic structure. The two sources separately activate phoneme-level units through a *content* pathway and a *structural* pathway (see Figure 7.25a). In this respect the basic idea is clearly similar to the distributed CQ model discussed in the previous section. Writing,

however, is in evolutionary terms a very recent acquisition of the human species, while speech is clearly part of our genetic make up. So the Houghton and Hartley model, which is localist, uses a much more complex structure for providing sequence information than does the CQ spelling model just discussed.

The structural pathway has two levels. The higher level represents the *syllable group*. The organisation of the structure of the utterance into a sequence of syllables is carried out by a CQ mechanism similar to that described for spelling. Within each syllable however the structural activation of phonemes is carried out using a more complex structure (see Figure 7.25b). As a syllable is being uttered, the representation in the structural pathway changes. The representation of each individual phoneme's position is based on the phonological characterisation of the English syllable as described by Fudge (1969), namely that the syllable has three components: (1) an *onset* composed of two consonant slots, (2) a *rhyme* composed of a *peak*—the vowel—and the *coda*—also two consonant slots and (3) a *termination*. The phonemes that can go in the six slots are determined acoustically according to their *sonority* (see e.g. Selkirk, 1984), which relates to the energy of the sound they represent. Thus the liquids *w*, *l*, *r*, *m*, *n*, *η* have intermediate sonority and go next to the vowels which have high sonority.[55] How the system identifies

---

[54] This is a characteristic problem of the over-specialisation of research in cognitive neuroscience. An exception is the model of Page et al. (2007), who consider the relation between short-term memory errors and speech errors. However they assume that the primary function of the principal short-term phonological store is in speech production and do not consider the neuropsychological evidence or the sentence memory experiments discussed in Section 7.3.

[55] There are only five slots in the 'wheel' of Figure 7.25b because terminations, which relate specifically to inflectional endings, are not implemented.

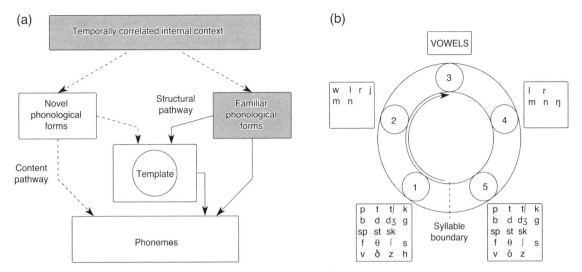

Fig. 7.25 (a) The general architecture of the Hartley and Houghton (1996) model of short-term retention of phonological information in speech production. Components shown in grey have not been implemented. (b) The cyclical within-syllable template at the core of the model. Reprinted from *Journal of Memory and Language*, 35(1), T. Hartley and G. Houghton, A linguistically constrained model of short-term memory for nonwords. 1–31, Copyright 1996, with permission from Elsevier.

which slot of the five a given phoneme should go in is not tackled by the model. The model assumes that the syllabic structure is given, and then, applying that, learns the order of phonemes in a given word. As in the previous localist CQ model the model learns each word separately. Training of each word is by single-trial Hebbian learning.

A model like this transcends the barren ideological dispute between supposedly innate structural positions and supposedly *tabula rasa* connectionist ones. How does it do in practice when confronted with the behaviour of phonological output buffer patients? Table 7.8 shows its performance on repeating non-words when compared with three of the phonological output buffer patients discussed in Section 7.5. The balance between single and double phoneme errors is fairly good. The ratio of substitutions is also appropriate. Deletions are, however, somewhat too frequent and exchanges (i.e. transpositions) too few. The main problem is probably that the within-syllable ordering induced by the symbolic structural pathway is too strong. Thus, if one compares the model with the CQ models of writing discussed in the preceding section, the Hartley–Houghton model has a much stronger constraint on the ordering of constituents than do the models in the writing domain. As a consequence it produces fewer exchange errors than the writing models. This, however, explains in a very simple way why phonological output buffer patients in general produce a very high rate of substitution errors— more than 60% in all patients performing in the 20–90% correct range for repetition, reading and writing (see Table 7.6). For comparable absolute error rates in graphemic buffer patients the rate of substitutions is much lower (30–55%; see Figure 7.20). Instead one has more

errors in writing where the ordinal position of the phoneme is not fixed—deletion, insertions and in particular exchanges.[56]

Now, as discussed earlier, we have little in the way of lesion location or functional information on the output buffer. One cannot therefore see whether any of the hypothetical components introduced in these models can be located in a specific brain region. However the neuropsychological evidence fits the model well.

7.8 The Episodic and Semantic Buffers

In 2000 Baddeley augmented the Baddeley–Hitch working memory model with one further buffer, the *episodic buffer*. This is neither an input nor an output buffer but is intended instead to support the temporary binding of information from the phonological and visuo-spatial buffers and long-term knowledge into integrated, unitary, episodes (see Figure 7.26). What is the evidence for this buffer and what are its properties?

Above it was noted that existing computational models of (auditory-visual) short-term memory fail to address the store's function in supporting other aspects of cognition such as understanding complex sentences. In particular, there is no account of why span for semantically related words or for words structured within a sentence should be so much greater than span for unrelated items. This in fact reflects a more general difficulty with the original Baddeley–Hitch model, as there was no means within that model for long-term knowledge (e.g. of semantic relatedness or syntactic

---

[56] For further discussion see Shallice et al. (2000).

TABLE 7.8 The rates of single and multiple phoneme errors produced by the simulation of Hartley and Houghton (1996) and three graphemic buffer disorder patients discussed in Section 7.5.

	Expected on Simulation	LT	IGR	RR
Single Phoneme Errors				
Substitution	55	47	62	75
Deletion	21	4	2	13
Insertion	1	4	8	0
Transposition	0.3	6	4	6
Multiple Phoneme Errors				
Double substitution	6	16	18	0
Substitution & Deletion	8	4	1	6
Substitution & Insertion	9	4	2	0
Other double transpositions/insertions	0	13	1	0

All figures are percentages.

From: The selective impairment of the phonological output buffer.
T. Shallice, R.I. Rumiati and A. Zadini, *Cognitive Neuropsychology*, 2000, *17*(6), 517–546, Psychology Press. Reprinted by permission of the publisher (Taylor & Francis Group, http://www.informaworld.com).

form) to influence short-term recall. One role, therefore, of the episodic buffer is to enable long-term knowledge to influence or support reconstruction of material from other buffers. Thus, in sentence repetition (and presumably comprehension of complex sentences), the episodic buffer is held to allow integration of phonological, syntactic, semantic and pragmatic knowledge into coherent episodes.[57] More generally, the episodic buffer is held to support both binding of information from multiple (sensory) sources into integrated representations, and chunking, allowing immediate memory capacity to be expanded by recoding multiple items into a single chunk (Miller, 1956).

Baddeley cites neuropsychological evidence in support of his episodic buffer. Two densely amnesic patients, KJ and DB, were found to show near normal immediate prose recall despite their severe amnesia. On immediate recollection of the ideas in a section of prose, these patients were able to recall 12 and 9.5 'idea units', respectively—within the normal range but far more

than might be attributable to any verbal short-term store (Baddeley & Wilson, 2002). These patients were further shown to have high intelligence and preserved executive functioning. Amnesic patients without preserved executive functioning were shown to be impaired on immediate prose recall. The argument, then, is that preserved executive functioning allows patients to build and temporarily maintain within the episodic buffer representations of events that integrate multiple sources of knowledge (including, for example, long-term story grammar or script knowledge: Schank & Abelson, 1977).

If the episodic buffer is to be a useful theoretical construct, and not a rag-bag for memory phenomena that do not fit neatly into either the phonological loop or the visuo-spatial sketchpad, it is necessary to clarify its properties, limitations, interactions with other components of the model and internal functioning. Baddeley (2003a; see also Repovs & Baddeley, 2006) is clear on the hypothesised properties. The episodic buffer is assumed to have limited capacity, to employ a multi-modal representational code, and to be accessible to conscious awareness. In this sense, the episodic buffer has the properties of a global workspace, as postulated in several contemporary theories of consciousness (see Section 11.11). However, many questions remain to be addressed. For example, while the episodic buffer's capacity is assumed to be limited, what that capacity may be, or even how it should be measured, remains to be determined.

Given these uncertainties, no attempts have as yet been made to model the episodic buffer.[58] However, tentative neuroscientific evidence has been adduced for some of its putative functions. Two fMRI studies have contrasted BOLD activity in tasks that involve the binding together of verbal and spatial information with analogous tasks that do not require binding. Prabhakaran et al. (2000) presented subjects with a display consisting of four letters and four spatial locations identified on screen by a pair of brackets. In the bound

---

[57] This suggests that the role of the phonological short-term store in language comprehension may be more than a simple back-up store. The role may be to hold items in an immediate verbal memory until they have been integrated into the episodic buffer, with the episodic buffer serving as the back-up store for comprehension. Either way, an auditory–verbal short-term store impairment will impair complex sentence comprehension.

[58] Several models of feature binding have, however, been proposed. The proposed mechanism of temporal binding (von der Malsburg, 1981) is often invoked for binding together features of an object within perceptual experience (e.g. Engel & Singer, 2001) or of subsystems carrying out one temporally specified part of a more complex process (Gross et al., 2004). Baddeley (2000) endorses this approach as a potential mechanism to operate within the episodic buffer, However it remains generally contentious, largely due to intrinsic computational difficulties in maintaining and discriminating synchronous neural firing (e.g. Shadlen & Movshon, 1999; O'Reilly et al., 2003; LaRock, 2007). O'Reilly et al. (2003) present several alternative mechanisms that are more compatible with existing connectionist models of cortical function.

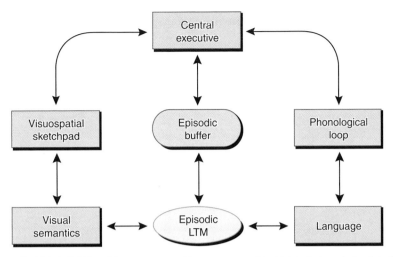

Fig. 7.26 The structure of Baddeley's (2000) multi-component working memory model, which includes an 'episodic buffer' which allows binding of information from multiple sources into integrated episodes.

condition, letters appeared at the locations (i.e. within the brackets), while in the separate condition letters were presented near a fixation point. Participants were required to memorise both the letters and locations, and after a delay subjects were then presented with a letter at a location. In the bound condition they were required to indicate whether the letter had appeared at that location. In the separate condition the task was to indicate if both the letter and location had been presented. Unsurprisingly accuracy was greater in the bound condition, but this condition also yielded greater right prefrontal activation. Zhang et al. (2004) also found greater right prefrontal activation in a task involving the use of integrated representations of auditorily presented digits and visuo-spatially presented locations. Repovs and Baddeley (2006) interpret these findings as supporting a right frontal localisation for the binding function of the episodic buffer. However, the results could equally be explained in terms of greater involvement of right prefrontal cortex in tasks requiring sustained attention and monitoring (see Section 9.10).

It is clear from the limitations of the original Baddeley–Hitch model that some augmentation or extension of the model is required if the working memory framework is to remain viable. Randi Martin and colleagues (e.g. Martin et al., 1994; Martin & He, 2004; Martin, 2005), working from the perspective of language comprehension and its deficits, have developed an alternative approach to some of the difficulties that motivated the episodic buffer. This approach is based on the concept of a *semantic buffer*.

Martin et al. (1994) described two patients EA and AB, with auditory–verbal short-term span of only 2 to 3 items. Martin et al.'s initial argument for a semantically-oriented buffer relied on the fact that EA was found

to have a slightly higher span than AB when tested with concrete words, while AB was found to have the higher span when tested with letters (see Table 7.9). The argument was that EA's performance on concrete words was supported by semantic influences. When tested with letters, such influences would be absent. Consistent with this interpretation, EA performed significantly better with words while AB's span was similar when tested with words and non-words. Furthermore, while EA scored higher than AB on a category span test, held to tap semantic short-term memory, AB scored higher than EA on a rhyme span test, held to tap phonological short-term memory.[59] AB was subsequently shown to be impaired in the comprehension and production of sentences that required retention of multiple word meanings (Martin & Romani, 1994; Martin & Freedman, 2001). A similar patient, ML, is described by Martin and He (2004). Two further short-term memory patients, HB and MMG, who both show improved span with high imagability words, have been reported by Howard and Nickels (2005). Furthermore, work with unimpaired subjects has demonstrated a correlation between measures of comprehension and *conceptual span*, a span measure intended to reflect an individual's semantic buffer's capacity (Haarmann et al., 2003).[60]

---

[59] In the rhyme span test, subjects were presented with a list of up to seven words, followed after a short delay by a probe. They were required to answer 'yes' if any word in the list rhymed with the probe and 'no' otherwise. The category span test followed the same procedures, with the probe being a category name and subjects being required to answer 'yes' if any word in the list was from the category specified by the probe and 'no' otherwise.

[60] Conceptual span measures how many semantically similar items a subject is able to recall, given a category probe. In this

TABLE 7.9 Performance of EA, AB and matched-controls on a range of span tasks. Concrete words: percentage of correct 2 to 6 item lists, with auditory presentation and picture pointing responses; letters: percentage of correct 2 to 5 item lists, with auditory presentation; 3 letter words and 3 letter non-words: mean percentage of correct 2 item and 3 item lists recalled, with lists comprising uncommon 3 letter words and non-words formed by rearranging the letters of those words, auditory presentation; rhyme span and category span: estimated length of lists for 75% correct performance based on linear interpolation.

	Concrete Words	Letters	3 letter words	3 letter non-words	Rhyme span	Category span
EA	39.4%	27.5%	42%	15%	2.65	2.82
AB	37.5%	39.0%	50%	45%	4.62	2.19
Controls	–	76.5%	68%	49%	7.02	5.38

Data from: Marin et al., 1994.

One could account for Martin's apparent dissociations in at least four ways that are broadly compatible with the Baddeley–Hitch framework. First, one may postulate a purely semantic buffer, analogous to the phonological input buffer. Such a buffer would, presumably, be capacity limited, represent items in a semantic code, and possibly require some support for rehearsal or refreshing. This is Martin's preferred position (see Figure 7.27), and is captured computationally in the model of Haarmann and Usher (2001). Second, one may account for the effects within Baddeley's revised multi-component model by postulating that semantic effects arise from binding of phonological and semantic information within the episodic buffer, and that it is this binding that is impaired in Martin's semantic buffer patients. Third, one may postulate that representations within the phonological input buffer may be supported by semantic influences (see Butterworth et al., 1990). Fourth, and most interestingly, the effects may be interpretable in terms of impairments to unification processes of language production to be discussed in Section 8.8. These last two positions, and their implications, remain to be explored.

If the arguments of Martin and colleagues are correct and the semantic buffer is an isolable component of the cognitive system, then the function of the semantic buffer is to support language comprehension and production. It should therefore be possible to situate the semantic buffer in a model of language comprehension and production such as that of Levelt (see Figures 3.15 and 7.12). Within that model, the semantic buffer would seem to provide the necessary functionality to support retention of the preverbal message during the operation of the formulator component. Levelt's model does not, however, deal with comprehension, which the semantic buffer is also held to support. An extension to

the model is therefore required to fully integrate it with the findings of Martin and colleagues.

There is, therefore, substantial evidence of shorter-term storage beyond the peripheral buffers associated with input and output processes. However, the concepts of both the episodic and the semantic buffer remain incompletely specified, with the evidence in support of each being somewhat tentative and not entirely satisfactory. This may be attributed to the putative location of these buffers within the cognitive system. Being less peripheral, they are more difficult to study. They also cannot be studied without a clear position on the structure, function and properties of the peripheral buffers to which they relate.

7.9 Deconstructing Working Memory and Prefrontal Cortex

Many readers may have found the chapter so far rather strange. The prefrontal cortex has hardly been mentioned. Yet, does not everybody in the field know that the basic structure responsible for working memory is the prefrontal cortex? As briefly mentioned in Section 7.1, this became the dominant view in neuroscience in about 1990 following the dramatic experiments on monkey prefrontal cortex conducted in the lab of Patricia Goldman-Rakic (see for example, Goldman-Rakic, 1987; Funahashi, Bruce & Goldman-Rakic, 1993), which in turn were greatly influenced by the studies of Joachim Fuster, discussed in Section 1.2. In those studies, cells in dorsolateral prefrontal cortex were shown to fire during a delay interval while monkeys retained the location of a food source.

In a series of studies, Goldman-Rakic and colleagues used not only single-cell recording but also complementary studies of lesions to the main sulcus in the prefrontal cortex—the sulcus principalis which is in area 9/46 of the monkey brain.[61] As discussed in Section 7.1, lesions

---

sense it measures resistance to semantic interference, rather than the number of semantically unrelated concepts that a subject is able to simultaneously encode.

---

[61] For frontal cortex we will use the revised Brodmann-type nomenclature devised by Petrides and Pandya (1994).

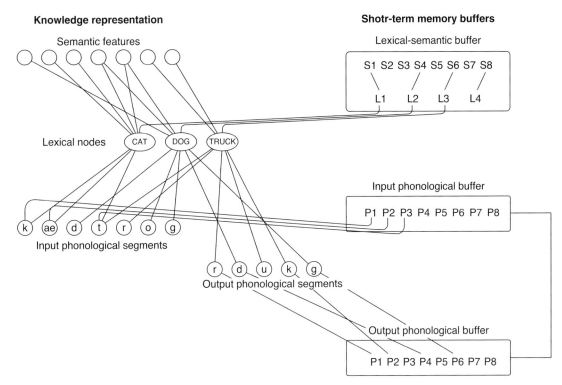

Fig. 7.27 The model of language processing and short-term memory of Martin et al. (1999), illustrating the role of the proposed semantic buffer in language processing and its relation to input and output phonological buffers. From: Short-term retention of lexical-semantic representations: Implications for speech production, R.C. Martin and M.L. Freedman, *Memory*, 9(4/5/6), 2001, 261–280, Psychology Press, reprinted by permission of the publisher (Taylor & Francis Group, http://www.informaworld.com).

in this area led to the monkey developing what the authors called a 'memory scotoma' in 'memory fields' analogous to those found in visual perception in area 17 (Funahashi et al., 1993). For instance, Figure 7.28 shows the findings of an oculomotor working memory task studied by Funahashi et al. (1993). The monkey fixates and a spot of light is presented at one of eight positions in the peripheral visual field. After a delay of 1.5, 3 or 6 sec the monkey must move its eyes to the target. If the light had been presented to one part of space the monkey was very inaccurate at making the eye movement, even though the monkey had no problem in control tasks with no memory component. Goldman-Rakic (1987) argued that the dorsolateral prefrontal cortex held a representation of the animal's recent spatial environment as a working memory.

Does working memory necessarily have a major prefrontal involvement? The functional imaging evidence itself seems clear. Spatial working memory tasks tend to lead to greater activation in dorsolateral prefrontal cortex (e.g. Zarahn et al., 1999).[62] Yet this line of research

appears to be in conflict with the positions on spatial working memory taken earlier in this chapter. A resolution was potentially available very early in the neurophysiological literature, where Michael Petrides (1994) had indirectly challenged the Goldman-Rakic position. He argued that the mid-dorsolateral prefrontal cortex, which includes the principal sulcus—the area investigated in the Funahashi et al. studies—was involved in the manipulation and monitoring of working memory representations, and not in the holding of working memory representations *per se*.[63]

There are, in fact, several reasons to question the role of prefrontal cortex in working memory, at least as it relates to digit span, where *manipulation* processes are less heavily involved. First, the basic Goldman-Rakic task involves only a single item being retained. Span involves multiple items. The Goldman-Rakic results can be explained in terms of the monkey maintaining attention

---

[62] Some authors (e.g. Courtney et al., 1998) have argued that the critical area is area 8, just anterior of the frontal eye fields, and not 9 or 46.

[63] It appears the debate between Petrides and Goldman-Rakic was complicated by their referring to subtly different lesion sites as the studies of Goldman-Rakic and colleagues were concerned with what is now known as area 9/46 and those of Petrides the slightly more anterior, mid-dorsolateral region of 46 proper (Petrides, personal communication).

to a position in space; related effects are found in dogs in an analogous task in the sense that the dog orientates its body physically in the appropriate direction (Konorski & Lawicka, 1964). Second, in humans, span can be relatively unaffected after prefrontal lesions Thus D'Esposito and Postle (1999) carried out a meta-analysis of all studies in which patients with frontal lobe lesions had been compared with a normal control group on the standardised digit span task from the WAIS battery. Digit span clearly counts as a working memory maintenance task. Eight such studies were found involving 115 patients. In none of the studies was a significant deficit found in the frontal patients. By contrast, one study—that of Ghent et al. (1962)—included a group of patients with posterior cortical lesions. They *were* impaired, particularly three patients with left hemisphere lesions. Third, what is affected by prefrontal lesions is any manipulation which requires operations upon the contents of the short-term store (e.g. WAIS backward span, where the subject must repeat back the digits in the reverse order).

The *coup de grâce* was provided by functional imaging. When retention is contrasted with operating on the contents of short-term memory, it is the operations that activate prefrontal cortex more, while retention tends to activate parietal cortex more—essentially the Petrides position—that was supported by later functional imaging studies. Thus, in the verbal domain D'Esposito et al. (1999) contrasted 'maintenance' in short-term memory of letters with their 'manipulation'. Subjects were presented with five randomly ordered letters simultaneously. The letters were followed immediately by a cue 'forward' or 'alphabetise' and after an 8-sec delay by a probe consisting of a letter and an integer representing a position in the list. Subjects had to respond by pressing a button for 'match' or one for 'mismatch'. The 'alphabetise' cue indicated that the probe would refer to the alphabetic order of the set of letters and that manipulation of the set was required. In the 'forward' condition the probe referred to the same order as at presentation. The results were clear (see Figure 7.29). In all subjects the manipulation condition led to greater activation of dorsolateral prefrontal cortex throughout the delay period than the maintenance condition.

An elegant confirmation that the same contrast is found in spatial working memory was obtained shortly thereafter by Rowe et al. (2000). The experimental paradigm they used was rather original (see Figure 7.30). Three dots are presented. After an interval, which varied across trials, a line appears. The subject's task is to move a cursor to the position of the dot that, if presented at the same time, would lie on the line. The authors contrasted 'maintenance regions' continuously

active during the delay period with 'selection regions' active only while the cursor was being positioned (see Figure 7.31). Maintenance regions were mainly parietal.[64] The regions active at selection were predominantly in the lateral prefrontal cortex. Thus the position of Petrides that the involvement of prefrontal cortex in working memory tasks concerns manipulation of its contents rather than retention per se seems to have won the day.

High-level cognitive operations often clearly do require that a considerable amount of material be temporally stored. However, the relation between storage and manipulation is complex. Those complexities are highlighted by computational or process accounts of working memory tasks that involve high-level cognitive operations. There are a number of lines of investigation, but as yet no definitive position. We give two contrasting examples. Consider first the *12-AX task*, a task extensively modelled by O'Reilly and colleagues (e.g. O'Reilly & Frank, 2006; Hazy et al., 2006, 2007), which is derived from a task much used in studies of the anterior cingulate by Carter and colleagues (e.g. Carter et al., 1998), to be discussed in Chapter 9. In 12-AX task subjects view a sequence of the letters and digits including the items 1, 2, A, X, B and Y. They must respond by pressing a 'yes' key if the stimulus is the target and pressing the 'no' key otherwise. When the digit '1' appears the target is 'X', provided it is immediately preceded by an 'A'. When the digit '2' appears the target is 'Y', provided it is immediately preceded by a 'B'.

To produce good performance on the 12-AX task, subjects must maintain both the current rule and the previous stimulus in working memory. These items must be maintained there as long as required, but it must also be possible to selectively and rapidly update parts of working memory. Thus, the record of what is the last stimulus must be updated with each new stimulus (unless the new stimulus is a digit). On the basis of these requirements, O'Reilly, Frank and colleagues (e.g. Hazy et al., 2007) argue that working memory consists of a set of independently updatable registers, which they refer to as *stripes*.[65] Each stripe is held to be part of a cortico-subcortical loop, which either maintains the stripe's contents or allows updating of those contents,

---

[64] Maintenance was also associated with bilateral activation of area 8.

[65] Within the simulations reported by O'Reilly, Frank and colleagues, each stripe stores one letter or digit, so the model may appear to be a neurally-motivated descendent of slot theories of working memory of the late 1960s (e.g. Neisser, 1967). However, they suggest that cortico-subcortical loops may support as many as a few thousand stripes, so in no way is the capacity determined by the number of slots.

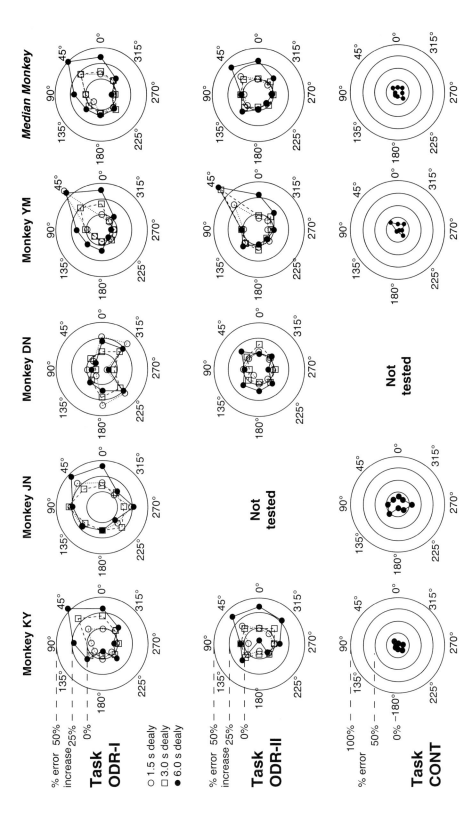

Fig. 7.28 Summary results from four monkeys with unilateral frontal lesions on two oculomotor delayed response tasks (ODR-I and ODR-II) and a control task (CONT). Monkeys were required to maintain fixation on a central target while a cue was presented for 0.5 sec in the peripheral visual field. The fixation target remained visible for a short delay period, after which the monkey was required to make a saccade to the position of the cue. In the control task the cue remained on for the full duration of the trail. The plots show the increase (post-lesion minus pre-lesion) in error rates for different radial locations of the cue. From: S. Funahashi, C.J. Bruce and P.S. Goldman-Rakic, 1993, Dorsolateral prefrontal lesions and oculomotor delayed-response performance: Evidence for mnemonic "scotomas", *The Journal of Neuroscience*, 13(4), 1479–1497. Figure 2, p 1482.

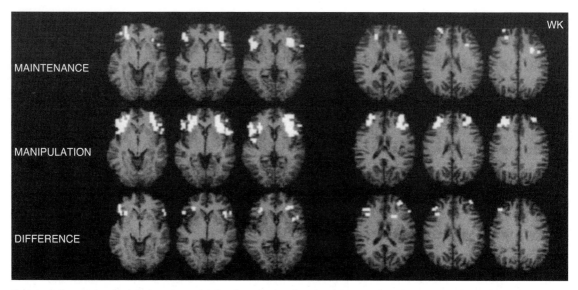

Fig. 7.29 Delay-correlated activity from three axial slices from the dorsolateral and the ventrolateral PFC in one subject of D'Esposito et al. (1999). The top row represents delay-period activity in maintenance trials compared to baseline; the middle row represents delay-period activity in manipulation trials compared to baseline; and the bottom row represents the difference, where delay-period activity was greater in the manipulation than the maintenance trials. Reprinted from *Brain and Cognition*, *41*(1), M. D'Esposito, B.R. Postle, D. Ballard and J. Lease, Maintenance versus manipulation of information held in working memory: An event-related fMRI study. 66–86, Copyright 1999, with permission from Elsevier.

with the decision to maintain or update being dependent on the current stimulus and learned through a procedure based on reinforcement learning (see Figure 7.32). The viability of the theory has been demonstrated through a complex connectionist implementation (for details see e.g. O'Reilly & Frank, 2006), but the critical elements of the approach for the current discussion are the memory requirements, namely maintenance and rapid updating of task-relevant representations through a process referred to as *active gating*. The model essentially deals with maintenance of information, which we have argued is not the principal function of lateral prefrontal cortex. It does not attempt to account for manipulation of information within working memory as might be involved in, for example, Backward Span. Moreover so far there does not appear to be much comparison of the behaviour of the model with empirical data from humans.[66]

The storage requirements of symbolic cognitive architectures, such as those as described in Section 3.8, are very different. These architectures are capable of performing a range of tasks which make intensive use

of working memory. They do so without emphasising functions such as maintenance and updating. How do they achieve this? Consider ACT-R. It contains a number of different buffers, but nothing that is directly equivalent to the input or output buffers discussed earlier in this chapter. Recall that ACT-R has a modular structure in which a central production system controls the interactions between a set of informationally encapsulated sub-systems (see Figure 3.25). Each subsystem has an associated buffer, and the central production system coordinates behaviour by writing to or reading from these buffers. Thus the central production system might write to the buffer associated with the manual module, causing the manual module to produce a response (e.g. a key press). Alternatively it might write to the visual-location buffer, thus orienting attention to a specified visual location, or read from the visual-object buffer, and thereby extract the features of the object at the currently attended location.

All ACT-R buffers are able to store just one 'chunk', where a chunk is a template with filled slots (Neisser, 1967) that represents an atomic proposition (e.g. that 'the capital of France is Paris', or that the currently attended item is the word *pheasant*). Buffers can store only a single chunk, but there are no hard limits on the number of slots within a chunk. Given this, how might the 12-AX task be performed by ACT-R? One can envisage several possible alternative approaches, each corresponding to a different set of ACT-R production rules. Plausible alternatives are likely to draw on ACT-R's auditory (or

---

[66] The account of working memory provided by O'Reilly and colleagues may also be criticised theoretically. For example, it provides an approach to representing atomic elements but no way to represent relations between those elements. Many more complex working memory tasks appear to require the representation of structured information. Such tasks are currently beyond the scope of the model.

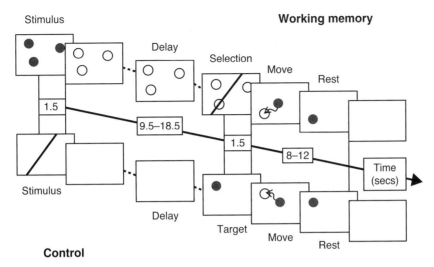

Fig. 7.30 The structure of working memory and control trials in the task of Rowe et al. (2000). In working memory trials three red dots were initially presented for 1.5 secs. The screen then went blank for a period of between 9.5 and 18.5 sec, during which subjects were required to remember the locations of the three dots. (The outlines of the dots as shown in the figure were not visible during this period). A line was then presented for 1.5 sec that would have passed through one of three dots. A red cursor then appeared and subjects were required to use a joystick to move the cursor to the position of the dot that the line would have passed through. In control trials the sequence of presentation of the stimuli was reversed, so the line appeared first. This could be ignored. After the delay one red dot was presented and subjects were then required, as in working memory trials, to move the cursor to the position of this dot. Reprinted from J.B. Rowe, I. Toni, O. Josephs, R.S.J. Frackowiak and R.E. Passingham, 2000, The prefrontal cortex: Response selection or maintenance within working memory? *Science, 288*(5471), 1656–1670.

visual) input module, its manual (or vocal) output module, its central production system, and two further ACT-R modules, the *retrieval* and the *imaginal* modules:

1. The retrieval module implements in ACT-R a form of memory which includes both semantic memory and episodic memory components.[67] Like other ACT-R modules, it is informationally-encapsulated and accessed through a buffer that is able to store a single chunk. If the central production system writes a chunk to that buffer, the retrieval module stores the chunk by copying it to an unlimited-capacity, long-term, declarative store. If the central production system writes a partial chunk (i.e. a template with some unfilled slots) to the buffer, the retrieval module will attempt to complete or elaborate that chunk with the most appropriate information from the long-term declarative store. Once the chunk in the retrieval buffer has been filled-in (i.e. once retrieval from long-term memory has taken place), the central production system may read the complete chunk and act accordingly. All chunks in the declarative store have an associated activation value which decays with time but is boosted if and when the chunk is retrieved. The activation level determines whether the chunk can be retrieved and, if so, how long that retrieval takes.

2. The imaginal module allows temporary storage of the results of cognitive processing that are not represented in the external world. Like the other modules, it includes a single-item buffer where the item can have a complex structure—a chunk—but unlike the retrieval module there are no processes attached to this buffer. Thus, central cognition can place a chunk in the buffer and then retrieve it at some later point.

As shown in Figure 3.25, Anderson et al. (2008b) speculatively place the retrieval module in ventrolateral prefrontal cortex and the imaginal module in posterior parietal cortex.[68]

Given this organisation, a plausible approach to the 12-AX task in ACT-R might involve maintaining the current response rule (i.e. whether the current target is 'X' preceded by 'A' or Y' preceded by 'B') in the retrieval buffer and the last stimulus in the imaginal buffer (see Figure 7.33). The two different response rules would be considered declarative knowledge. One would then require a set of productions to retrieve the appropriate response rule from declarative memory into the

---

[67] Technically this is called a *declarative memory*, to be discussed in Chapter 10.

[68] In accordance with the earlier part of the chapter, it would be reasonable to assume that (i) the imaginal module fractionates into left-lateralised phonological and right-lateralised spatial components, (ii) chunks in each are encoded in terms of phonological or spatial templates, respectively, and (iii) decay operates on the contents of each module's buffer.

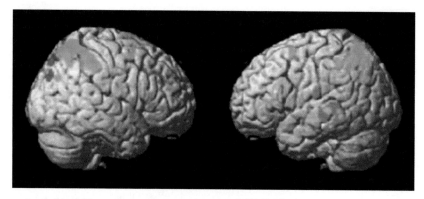

Fig. 7.31 Regions associated with working memory maintenance (green) and selection (red) in the study of Rowe et al. (2000). See text and Figure 7.30 for details. Reprinted from J.B. Rowe, I. Toni, O. Josephs, R.S.J. Frackowiak and R.E. Passingham, 2000, The prefrontal cortex: Response selection or maintenance within working memory? *Science, 288*(5471), 1656–1670.

retrieval buffer whenever a digit was presented. A second set of productions would be required to assess whether the current stimulus (temporarily held in either the auditory or visual input buffer) and the previous stimulus (recorded in the imaginal buffer) fit the requirements of the response rule (held in the retrieval buffer). If they do, then the motor output is triggered. Finally, a third set of productions would be required to copy, at the end of each trial, the current stimulus from the relevant input buffer to the imaginal buffer. This account would predict, amongst other things, that performance on the 12-AX task should be associated with ventrolateral prefrontal and posterior parietal activity.[69]

Such an approach using ACT-R can be criticised on several grounds. Most notably the implementation of tasks in ACT-R is under-constrained, so one can frequently develop many variant models of the performance of a given task within the architecture, each with different characteristics. There is at present no principled way of selecting between them theoretically. (see Howes et al., 2009). It is, however, the storage requirements that are most relevant to the current discussion. For the 12-AX task, there are two types of requirement: (1) temporary storage of information, which occurs in the buffers associated with modules, and which is used by productions that require multiple sources of information; and (2) storage in declarative memory of chunks, which need to be periodically refreshed if they are to remain accessible over the longer-term. Similar storage requirements hold for other complex working memory tasks, such as backward span, the n-back task, and even for sentence comprehension (Lewis et al., 2006).[70] Thus, a second criticism which follows is that ACT-R provides no immediate explanation of why prefrontal lesions, as we will see in Chapters 9 and 12, do not affect all tasks with complex working memory requirements uniformly.

The ACT-R model of the 12-AX task uses preprogrammed production rules and a network of informationally-encapsulated functionally-specialised modules. In contrast the model of O'Reilly, Frank and colleagues of the same task employs reinforcement learning and cortico-subcortical loops to achieve similar behaviour. These differences obscure the fundamental similarities between the memorial functions shared by the models. In both cases, maintenance and selective updating are key functions. The role of prefrontal cortex in supporting these functions, and more generally in performing operations on the contents of working memory, will be discussed further in Chapters 9 and 11.

7.10 Conclusions

The short-term retention of information or processing state is an essential aspect of much cognitive behaviour.

---

[69] Because of the modular nature of ACT-R and the way that productions match against the contents of buffers from multiple modules, the firing of a production serves a binding function equivalent to that used by Baddeley (2000) to motivate his concept of an episodic buffer. Thus, when an ACT-R production fires it temporarily binds the buffer elements matched by its conditions and generates, for example, a new buffer element derived from the bound elements.

[70] The ACT-R model of sentence comprehension of Lewis and colleagues (2006) is particularly interesting in this respect. This model is extremely impressive, both in its coverage of linguistic phenomena and in its use of ACT-R's retrieval module. It uses the module's retrieval latency and activation decay properties to explain a wide variety of linguistic puzzles concerning the relative processing difficulty of different constructions. It does not, however, make explicit use of serial order information in comprehension. It therefore has no need for the processes that support memory span, including those related to the imaginal buffer. A puzzle for the account is therefore why comprehension of complex sentences should be impaired in short-term memory patients.

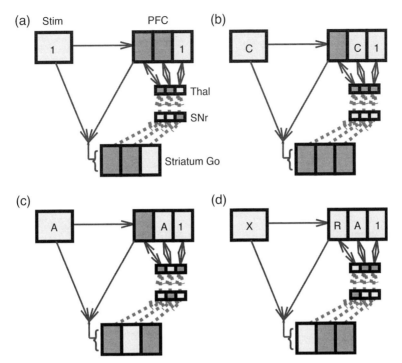

Fig. 7.32 Operation of the PBWM model of O'Reilly and Frank (2006) on the 12-AX task. When a stimulus is presented, it is retained within a stripe within PFC, provided the corresponding stripe in the striatum fires. Thus the striatum controls which information is retained within working memory and hence which information can contribute to responses. Reproduced with permission from R.C. O'Reilly and M.J. Frank, 2006, Making working memory work: A computational model of learning in the prefrontal cortex and basal ganglia, *Neural Computation*, *18*(2), 283–328. Copyright © 2006, MIT Press Journals.

Without it, one's responses would be entirely deter-mined by the current stimulus and long-term knowl-edge. There would then be no possibility for behaviour to be facilitated by the reprocessing of a stimulus, to be conditional on a sequence of inputs, or to be pre-pro-grammed when rapid output is required. These condi-tions represent situations where priming, input buffers and output buffers, respectively, allow a richness in behaviour that would not otherwise be possible. In all three cases, patient studies have provided detailed insights into the properties and functioning of the under-lying systems, while computational studies have allowed complex theories to be specified and evaluated in consid-erable detail. In the cases of priming and input buffers, neuroimaging evidence has supplied further supporting evidence concerning both localisation and functioning within specific tasks. The area of short-term retention therefore provides powerful support for the use of con-verging evidence within the cognitive neurosciences.

We have discussed a group of computational models in which the concept of a buffer is deepened consider-ably. For the rest of this book the concept of a buffer can be thought of as having two properties. The first is a mechanism for the short-term retention of information; for instances by continuing activation of representations or by the setting up of short-term as well as long-term

associative weights. The second is some mechanism for reactivating a set of such short-term traces. This requires the use of a dimension distinct from that of the content of the items to cue the retrieval process. This can, for instance, be time, as in the case of phonological buffers, or space, for the visuo-spatial short-term stores. However, for some types of material it is likely that no such dimension exists; in this case there is no buffer holding multiple items, as discussed in Section 7.1.

In addition to isolating a set of peripheral (i.e. input and output) buffers, it has also been emphasised that those buffers are sensitive to structural characteristics of their contents. Thus, phonological coding in the phono-logical input buffer makes the contents of that buffer susceptible to interference from phonologically related forms, while the phonological and graphemic output buffers appear, on the basis of patient error data, to be tailored towards the regularities in their respective domains (e.g. the syllabic structure of the patient's native language or the consonant-vowel structure present in the spelling errors of Italian graphemic buffer disorder patients). That buffers should be sensitive to these regu-larities is, no doubt, a trade-off between the susceptibil-ity to error that arises from interference or confusions within the buffers and the processing advantage that results from biases towards the regularities. Furthermore,

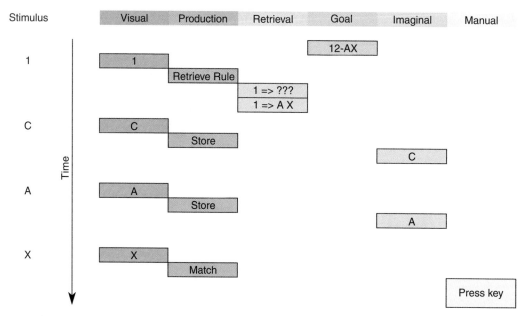

Fig. 7.33 The flow of information between modules for typical stimuli in a simplified ACT-R implementation of O'Reilly et al.'s 12-AX task. The current rule (1=>AX) is maintained in the retrieval buffer while the previous stimulus is stored in the imaginal buffer. An alternative implementation could use the goal buffer to maintain the current rule. Modules are shown in colour-coded columns, following the convention of Figure 5.16a. Time, shown on the vertical axis, is not to scale.

computational accounts have shown how such regularities may be encoded, whether it be explicitly through Hartley and Houghton's syllabic wheel (Figure 7.25b), or implicitly in trained connection weights as occurs with consonant-vowel structure in Glasspool et al's graphemic output buffer model (Figure 7.21).

There are two further situations, beyond those of input and output, were the holding of information over the short-term is critical, namely when it is necessary to combine or bind information from multiple sources, and when it is necessary to maintain task, goal or control signals over time in order to guide or maintain coherent, purposive behaviour. The properties of buffering in these situations are more difficult to study, given the relative distance of such buffering from input and output processes. Substantial theoretical (e.g. Baddeley's multi-store

model) and computational (e.g. Anderson's ACT-R) progress has nevertheless been made in these areas. Bringing this theoretical and computational progress together with neuroimaging and patient work remains a significant challenge. The second of the above forms of short-term retention comprises the maintenance and updating of multimodal or amodal representations for the control of other cognitive processes. This was referred to in the introduction as type-3 short-term memory. It will be discussed in further detail in Chapters 9 and 12. For now though our discussion of buffers has made it possible to turn attention to cognitive operations—the processing of information and the generation of behaviour that is sensitive to stimuli that are no longer present in the perceptual environment.

On Operations

8.1 Introduction

The work of transforming the combination of a task and a percept into an action is effected by operations, i.e. transformations between representations and from representations to behaviour. How operations might be explained, however, is an area in which cognitive science has been at its most theological over the last two decades. Prior to 1986 it was largely assumed that cognitive operations could be adequately characterised in terms of rewrite rules (see Section 1.5). This was most explicit with respect to syntactic operations in Chomskyan linguistic theory (e.g. Chomsky, 1965). Part of the appeal of rewrite rules is their ability to specify relations between symbolic structures in precise and computationally tractable terms. However, while it is obvious that the motors of human cognition have complex innate underpinnings, it is even more obvious that the human is *par excellence* an organism dependent upon learning. It is clear that an understanding of operations will almost certainly require some mixture of the two (i.e. of innate underpinnings shaped by learning), and that that mixture will probably be complex and may well differ for different areas. Therefore it is appropriate to investigate how far systems based on neurally-derived learning principles can be adapted to carry out cognitive operations that might have been expressed 25 years ago in terms of rewrite rules.

The first attempts to do this were by Dave Rumelhart and Jay McClelland (1986) in the area of past tense learning—learning that the past tense of *jump* is *jumped* and *kick* is *kicked* but that the past tense of *go* is *went*, and so on. Their approach became treated as a '*Trahison des Clercs*'. Rumelhart and McClelland demonstrated that a simple connectionist network using the back-propagation learning algorithm (see Section 1.7) could not only acquire the mapping between base and past tense forms, but in doing so it could explain why children progress through a phase of over-regularisation (where 'ed' is incorrectly added to the base form of irregular verbs, such as 'go', to give 'goed' or even 'wented') and how the past tense mapping can, once it has been acquired, be generalised to novel verb stems. The demonstration undercut the traditional structuralist approach. The result over the last 25 years has been an intellectual battle reminiscent of the First World War Battles of Ypres, fought to claim or reclaim or rereclaim particular phenomena for one type of explanation or the other.[1]

This chapter will argue, through examining a range of operations, that both types of explanation have a role. To provide some context for this argument, however, it is necessary to first consider two constraints on operations, namely:

(1) innate biases that constrain subsequent organisation within and between subsystems; and

(2) processes of learning or automatisation that result in qualitative differences in the mechanisms supporting an operation after automatisation as compared with before automatisation.

There are many examples of operations where, following a developmental process that may well occur in essentially the same fashion in all normal members of a culture, particular specialised subsystems come to carry out the operations. Visuo-motor skills, such as reaching for an object and bringing it to the mouth, or linguistic skills, such as producing correct adjective–noun agreement when generating a noun phrase, would be good examples. For these operations, which we refer to as *subsystem internal operations*, we assume that specialised subsystems come to carry out the operations. In addition we assume that to understand how the system works in the adult one can consider the adult state directly without being particularly concerned with the developmental process.

Many skills we carry out no doubt have certain innate properties underlying them. However in skills such as reading, writing, driving and playing card games, there is a level of control that is transparently the result of a learning process. We will refer to these as *transparently*

learned operations. The distinction between subsystem internal operations and transparently learned operations is not that there is no learning of subsystem internal operations. Rather, we assume that the learning of subsystem internal operations is primarily the result of species-wide developmental processes, and not the result of a particular form of explicit instruction. Most critically, the two perspectives are complementary.

A second argument of this chapter is that the transformations of representations involved in operations are highly complex and normally involve multiple sources of information. As such, they cannot be fully understood without consideration of the systems within which they occur. We will take as examples operations within the domains of skilled action and language, domains with intriguing similarities but also major differences. In both cases we will consider operations in the context of wider cognitive systems. In so doing, we aim to demonstrate yet again that, pace Fodor, brain-based techniques provide an important source of evidence in the development of cognitive theory.

But is it appropriate to consider language and action to be two different areas cognition? It is actually common for patients with left-hemisphere lesions to have impairments in both areas. However, there are also many reports of patients with impairments to action but not language and vice versa. Thus, in a group study of 699 consecutive left-hemisphere patients, Papagno et al. (1993) found 149 patients with language impairments who were not impaired in action, and 10 with the reverse dissociation. Disorders of language and action therefore doubly dissociate. Thus we treat the two domains separately, beginning with action.

8.2 From Motor Skills to Learned Action Sequences: Theoretical Alternatives

Humans have a number of types of operation that other higher primates do not have or have only to orders-of-magnitude less. A key one is the capacity for acquiring a large set of motor skills involving use of objects, which not only differ from each other but are each internally complex. Take as an example an object standard in Western cultures—the table knife. We know how to cut with it, and moreover how to apply appropriate pressure for the type of food so that the force is just sufficient and that the food does not disintegrate. We know how to spread a paste using it, how to push objects with it—both larger pieces and more mass-like entities such as peas. We know how to open a jar with one, how to extract a substance with high viscosity like jam. And this ignores situations where we use it in a place of a more appropriate object like a screwdriver

---

[1] Pinker (1999), one of the participants, uses a different martial metaphor—that of David and Goliath. Unfortunately he does not say which side is which!

when one is not available. And the table knife is just one of a very large number of artefacts that we use with appropriate actions frequently in daily life. Just consider how many different words for artefacts we have and in many cases the different types of action we have for each. By contrast only one ape habitually uses tools—the chimpanzee (McGrew, 1993). In McGrew's early analyses the maximum number of habitual types of tool-specific actions used by chimpanzees in one population was eleven (but see Whiten et al; 1999).[2]

The cognitive neuroscience literature on action is not as clearly structured from a theoretical perspective, as say that on reading or semantic memory. Empirical research has not generally been organised as an attempt to test rival theoretical positions. Or to be more precise there have been a variety of theories in the area but individual empirical studies tend to be related to one or other of these theoretical frameworks rather than attempting to select between rivals. In part this is because actions by humans involving use of artefacts may be understood from the perspective of at least three different domains:

1 The control of the physical movements that the intended action requires. This relates to actions as the product of the body, which is a biomechanically complex object, operating in a cluttered continuous three-dimensional space with varying sets of objects; in many skills—sports and work processes in particular—the objects on which the movements are operating are also in motion.

2 The selection of the appropriate operations in the context of the alternative learned operations that can be produced, where we are considering a finite set of learned alternatives rather than control of effectors which move in continuous space. This selection operates on multiple levels. Consider the alternative uses of the table knife discussed above.

3 How voluntary is the selection of one or other of the operations selected for the second perspective, i.e. the intentional-automatic contrast. This will mainly be considered in Chapters 9 and 12.

To provide structure to the discussion we consider the domains first from a broad theoretical perspective and then relate the theoretical framework to neuropsychological and functional imaging evidence.

Our understanding of action viewed from the first perspective has advanced rapidly in the past fifteen years. Wolpert and Ghahramani (2000) in an important review characterise these advances as involving a number of principles (see also Bays & Wolpert, 2007). The first is the use of *internal models*. Thus, Wolpert and Ghahramani differentiate three forms of sensori-motor loop (see Figure 8.1). Given the current state of the motor system,[3] a state of the current environment and a task, i.e. a state of the environment to be achieved, the computational problem is to estimate the motor command(s) to be generated in order to achieve the task; this is the so-called *inverse model*. The second stage is to determine what the forthcoming states (of both the motor system and the environment) will be after the action is made, given the previous state, the motor command and the environment; this is the *forward dynamic model*. Finally, given the current state, the motor command and the environmental context it is possible to estimate the sensory feedback to be expected from an action; this is the so-called *forward sensory model*.

To illustrate, consider pouring tea into a mug held in the other hand. The system needs to predict where the mug will be at the time the tea should be coming into contact with it; this requires a forward dynamic model. But the system also needs to know how to get the mug and teapot in the right position, producing sufficient tilt on the teapot to control the flow of tea. This requires an inverse model. Finally, the motor system needs to predict sensory feedback so that it may be compared with the sensory feedback that is actually received in order to evaluate the success of the action. This requires a forward sensory model.

But, how can the current state of the motor system and environment be estimated? Sensory signals about the location of objects in the environment and proprioceptive feedback from previous acts take time to arrive at the brain. Moreover they can be contaminated by noise. One solution to this problem of estimating the current state is the so-called Kalman filter model shown in Figure 8.2. The model uses the difference between predicted and actual sensory feedback to amend the current state predicted from a forward dynamic model. The amended current state provides an estimate for the actual current state. The model works well for empirical studies on estimation of hand position, posture and head orientation. Thus, van Beers et al. (1999) found good concordance between estimates of hand position generated by a Kalman filter-type model and those of subjects who were seated at a table and required to move one hand that was underneath the table (and

---

[2] They employed: sticks to fish, ant-dip, honey-dip, flail and throw, missile-throw, self-tickle and start-play; leaves to sponge, groom and as napkins; stems to comb (Goodall, 1986).

[3] The motor system contains about 600 muscles. If these are just considered to be either contracted or relaxed, this gives 2^{600} possible muscle configurations. The state of the system is therefore assumed to be a so-called *reduced description* with far fewer than 600 dimensions, which captures essential aspects of the very complex higher-dimensional space.

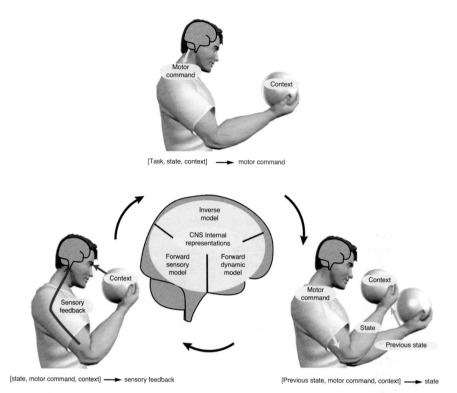

Fig. 8.1 The three types of internal model suggested by Wolpert and Ghahramani (2000). he inverse model allows the system to determine an appropriate motor command given both a task and the current state of the motor system. The two types of forward model then allow the system to predict the subsequent state of the world and the motor system and the expected sensory feedback that would follow. These are required when performing actions on objects, sequences of actions at speed, and when detecting error. Reprinted by permission from Macmillan Publishers Ltd: *Nature Neuroscience* (D.M. Wolpert and Z. Ghahramani, 2000, Computational principles of movement neuroscience. *Nature Neuroscience*, 3(11), 1212–1217), copyright (2000).

hence out of view) to landmarks on the table (for further discussion see Wolpert & Ghahramani, 2000).

A second principle of the lower-level control of intended skilled movements is that of optimisation. For instance why, when one makes a reaching movement, does the hand take a particular trajectory? Several models of motor control have been developed where the key assumption is that control operates so as to minimise some cost function (e.g. Flash & Hogan, 1985; Uno et al., 1989; Harris & Wolpert, 1998). In general the optimal cost function will depend on the task. Thus, in the model of Harris and Wolpert (1998) it is assumed that for reaching movements the cost function is the error in the final position of the arm. Harris and Wolpert further argue that the amount of noise in the motor system depends upon the magnitude of the motor command to the muscles. This, combined with their cost function and the principle of optimisation, results in a model that accounts very well for trajectories of both arm movements and associated eye movements.[4]

Forward and inverse models require some representation of the context, or state of the world, in order to generate motor commands and predict subsequent internal states and expected sensory feedback (as in Figures 8.1 and 8.2). Accurate maintenance of context leads to a third principle, namely the use of Bayesian estimation. Wolpert and Ghahramani (2000) show that the Bayesian formalism may be used to estimate the likelihood of subsequent contexts given the current context and the difference between predicted and observed sensory feedback. Thus, if the difference between predicted and observed sensory feedback is great (e.g. when picking up a box that is lighter than anticipated), Bayesian estimation allows one to deduce which of several possible contexts is most plausible (e.g. that the box is empty rather than full).

---

[4] Optimisation has also been argued to be critical in the integration of multiple sources of sensory information so as to

minimise noise in estimates of, for example, spatial position. Thus, behavioural studies suggest that proprioceptive and visual estimates of hand position are combined in a weighted average that minimises spatial error, given that both estimates may be independently affected by noise (van Beers et al., 1999; Bays & Wolpert, 2007).

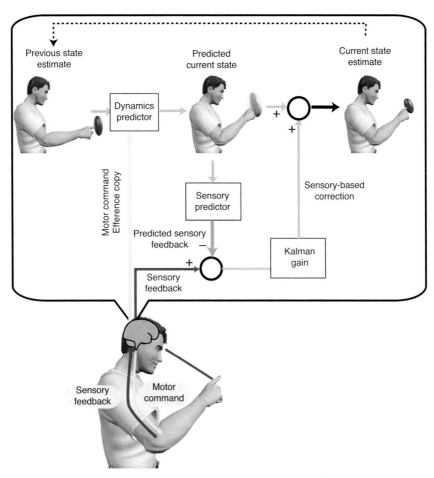

Fig. 8.2 The Kalman filter model for iteratively estimating the current state (for example of an effector) based on a prediction from its previous state and sensory feedback. Reprinted by permission from Macmillan Publishers Ltd: *Nature Neuroscience* (D.M. Wolpert and Z. Ghahramani, 2000, Computational principles of movement neuroscience. *Nature Neuroscience*, 3(11), 1212–1217), copyright (2000).

The computation concerned with motor skills is then heavily dependent upon the physics of the environment, the forces produced by our set of 600 muscles, and sensory and motor physiology. It clearly requires special purpose systems, which perform highly complex and specific computations. Harris and Wolpert assume that optimisation is actually achieved by a learning process that depends upon experience of repeated movements. However complementarity is required; such a learning process will require special purpose hardware with considerable innate specification. For example, Kawato (1999; see also Wolpert & Kawato, 1998) has argued that the cerebellum contains multiple forward and inverse models that compete when learning new motor skills (with the model that minimises the difference between predicted and actual feedback winning the competition), and this position has been supported by fMRI studies of the cerebellum (Imamizu et al., 2003). The cerebellum also appears to be a key organ as far as optimisation based on spatial

position is concerned. Kitazawa et al. (1998) have shown that Purkinje cells in the cerebellum produce complex spike discharges at the end of short-lasting movements that encode relative errors in those movements. Such signals are critical for the optimisation process when spatial error is the key element in the error function.

The parietal cortex too, however, may be associated with operations on an internal model. It is useful to return to the issue of its neural connectivity discussed in Section 3.4. The existence of dorsal and ventral streams in the cortical processing of visual information is now well established. Recent work, however, suggests that the dorsal stream itself can, at least in the monkey, be subdivided into two (or possibly more) sub-streams—a dorsal–dorsal pathway and a ventral–dorsal pathway (Rizzolatti & Matelli, 2003). The former projects from V6 to dorsal premotor cortex via the superior parietal lobule, while the latter projects from V5/MT to more ventral regions of premotor cortex via the inferior parietal lobule.[5] Pisella et al. (2006) and Rushworth et al. (2006), using images constructed with diffusion tensor tractography, provide evidence for a similar decomposition of pathways through the human parietal lobe. Given this connectivity, Pisella and colleagues argue that the route through superior parietal cortex is primarily concerned with immediate visuomotor control, while that through inferior parietal cortex is primarily concerned with more complex planning and programming of action.

As far as internal models are concerned, what is the evidence that the parietal lobes are also implicated in such functions? While the learning of internal models has been associated with the cerebellum (as discussed above), several studies suggest that the parietal lobes are also implicated in functions associated with internal models such as prediction. For example, in a study conducted by Sirigu and colleagues (1996), four apraxic patients with unilateral parietal lesions were asked to imagine certain movements and estimate how long they would take. While precise lesion sites varied across patients (ranging from left inferior parietal to right superior parietal), all were systematically impaired in their estimates of movement time in comparison to the actual time taken by them for the movement. The impairment in motor imagery was attributed to a failure to generate or monitor a forward model.

Buxbaum et al. (2005) have also suggested a link between motor imagery and internal models. Specifically, they investigated the relation between motor imagery and ideomotor apraxia, a disorder of action discussed in detail below. They argued that the former requires intact functioning of internal models. The latter would be the product of deficient internal models. More specifically this would produce an impairment in the ability to *pantomime* the use of an object.[6] In a group study involving eight left parietal apraxic patients, five left parietal aphasic patients and three healthy age-matched controls, Buxbaum and colleagues found, as hypothesised, a strong correlation ($r = 0.75$) between accuracy on a motor imagery task and the imitation of object-related actions.

---

[5] As can be seen from Figure 3.8, which is mainly concerned with the dorsal–dorsal pathways, this is still a very considerable simplification.

[6] In a pantomiming task, the subject must produce a characteristic action, e.g. hammering, without the object, which may or may not be present, being used. Some authors refer to pantomimes as *transitive gestures*, where 'transitive' indicates that the gesture is normally performed on or with an object. Transitive gestures are then distinguished from *intransitive gestures*, such as performing a military salute or waving, which are not performed on an object.

The extent to which internal models are implemented within parietal cortex remains unclear. The lesions of Buxbaum et al.'s (2005) apraxic patients were generally large, affecting up to 15 Brodmann areas in a single patient. A more specific localisation is suggested by patient PJ, described by Wolpert et al. (1998), who had a large cyst in her left superior parietal lobe. PJ was able to report the location of her right arm only if it was recently in motion or in view. When the arm was stationary and out of view, the impression of where it was would gradually fade such that, after a few tens of seconds, PJ was unable to report its position in space or, for example, whether a constant force was being applied to the arm. Equally, PJ produced large errors when asked to make slow pointing movements. Wolpert and colleagues interpreted PJ's deficit in terms of a failure of storage of the state estimate of the arm, as would be required by a control system operating with internal models.

The involvement of superior parietal processes in the control of reaching movements is consistent with this view. Take optic ataxic patients, who have a selective deficit in reaching to objects presented in the peripheral visual field, particularly in the one opposite to the lesion. The deficit is usually associated with superior parietal lesions (Battaglia-Mayer & Caminiti, 2002; but see Karnath & Perenin, 2005), and functional imaging also suggests the existence of a 'reach region' in posterior superior parietal cortex (Connolly et al., 2003). Optic ataxia could well arise from the loss of a superior parietal system encoding the future direction and velocity of effectors (Archambault et al., 2009)—the inverse model.

Optic ataxia has, however, also been associated with a deficit in online adjustments to movements. Thus, Pisella et al. (2000) demonstrated that an optic ataxic patient, IG, was impaired relative to healthy controls when required to reach to a target whose location was perturbed after the reach was initiated. IG produced two distinct movements—one towards the original target position and a second to the final target position, while the controls produced a single smooth movement that was adjusted on-line. However, IG, an ischemic stroke patient, had bilateral lesions affecting upper and lateral occipital regions, superior parietal regions and also encroaching on inferior parietal cortex, so it is far from clear how tightly linked the online adjustment problem is to the basic misreaching.

IG's deficit may, though, be understood in terms of internal models. In a reaching study reported by Desmurget et al. (1999), single TMS was applied over the left intraparietal sulcus while healthy participants pointed with their right hand towards either a stationary or a moving target. Participants' hands were occluded. When TMS was applied, movements towards moving targets were disrupted, but movements towards stationary targets were accurate. Desmurget and colleagues suggest that failure with moving targets was the result of disruption of feedback loops that support prediction, and hence allow correction, of an ongoing movement. Prediction is of course the function of forward dynamic and sensory models. A similar explanation might be applied to IG's deficit.[7] Overall, these studies suggest the possibility that more superior and posterior regions of the parietal lobe may be associated with the use of internal models. As we will see in Section 8.4, more complex actions would be associated with the intraparietal sulcus or inferior parietal regions.

8.3 Higher-Level Control of Action

In the terminology of the introduction to this chapter, the level of control of motor skills associated with internal models is the product of subsystem internal operations; it is supported by particular specialised systems and is acquired by most members of a culture following standard developmental processes. This type of operation contrasts with other aspects of the control of action over time. At any moment in time there are a range of actions which one might perform. Thus, as discussed above, if one is holding a knife then one may use it to slice, spread, lever and so on. Mechanisms are therefore required to select, at a particular instant in time, an appropriate operation in the context of an overall task and the alternative learned operations that can be produced. This selection is the focus of the *contention scheduling* theory (Norman & Shallice, 1986; Cooper & Shallice, 2000), which assumes that actions are structured hierarchically through schemas—control units for partially ordered sequences of actions or other lower-level schemas, which, when performed in the appropriate order, achieve some goal. At the lowest level action schemas control motor skills such as grasping and twisting (e.g. to open a jar), but at higher levels schemas, such as those used in preparing tea by filling and boiling a kettle, and so on, play a causal role in structuring more complex behaviour.

The term *action schema* derives from Bartlett (1932), who argued, referring to playing tennis, that 'How I make the stroke depends upon the relating of certain new experiences, most of them visual, to other immediately preceding experiences and to my posture or to balance of postures ....When I make the stroke, I do not … produce something absolutely new, and I never merely repeat something old' (p. 201–202). One can see the behaviour as depending on optimally satisfying many simultaneous constraints. Bartlett, and later Schmidt (1975), viewed the underlying process as a *schema*. We will use the term to avoid the too restrictive term *program*.[8]

We have demonstrated the feasibility of contention scheduling as a mechanism for the sequential selection of actions over extended periods through a computational implementation (Cooper & Shallice, 2000; Cooper et al., 2005). The model includes nodes that correspond to action schemas of varying levels of complexity, including nodes corresponding to single acts and nodes corresponding to complex schemas such as required for preparing a mug of instant coffee. Schemas compete for the control of behaviour through a mechanisms based on interactive activation (see Section 3.3). Thus, schemas are represented by nodes within a network, where each node has a continuous activation value. Schema nodes receive excitatory input from a variety of sources, including environmental triggering of object-appropriate schemas, 'parental' excitation from super-ordinate schemas in the hierarchy, and intentional excitation from systems related to the willed control of action—to be discussed in Chapter 9. In addition, a self-excitation process is necessary to ensure that, with suitable initial impetus, a schema's node will become highly active. Inhibition between competing schemas (such as schemas with overlapping resource requirements or schemas involved in alternative ways of achieving the same goal) operates to ensure that only one schema from a set of competitors may be highly active at any point in time. Figure 8.3 shows the full set of influences.

Evidence for the different sources of excitation within the contention scheduling theory comes from a variety of areas. For example, that environmental triggering of individual actions is possible is suggested by a series of experiments reported by Tucker, Ellis and colleagues (e.g. Tucker & Ellis, 1998; Symes, Ellis & Tucker, 2007). Thus, Ellis and Tucker (2000) had normal subjects produce either a power-grip or precision-grip response to a range of objects, where the response type was determined by a tone presented 700 msec after visual presentation of the stimulus (e.g. low pitch indicating power grip). Power-grip responses were produced reliably faster than precision-grip responses, when a power grip was appropriate for the visually presented object (e.g. a tennis racquet compared to a pen), and vice versa. That this triggering also operates at the level

---

[7] See also the imaging study of Culham et al. (2003).

[8] The term *schema* has a very complex history in psychology. It was used by German neurologists of the late-nineteenth century, such as Wernicke, but came to prominence with the ideas of Head and Holmes (1911) on the *body schema*—an organised model of ourselves, which was then taken up by Bartlett (1932) in speculations on the organisation of the memory of complex events and who extrapolated it to the control of action.

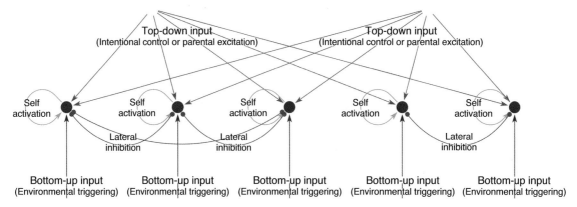

Fig. 8.3 Sources of excitation and inhibition operating on schema nodes within the contention scheduling model of Cooper and Shallice (2000). Four sources may operate on any node: top-down input from the supervisory system (red), bottom-up input from the representation of the environment (brown), self activation (green), and lateral inhibition from competing schema nodes (blue).

of temporally extended action sequences (i.e. schemas) is suggested both by certain neuropsychological disorders and by action lapses in normal subjects. One relevant disorder is utilisation behaviour (Lhermitte, 1983), where a patient tends to spontaneously use objects, such as a jug of water and glass in ways appropriate to the object, with no apparent motivation to do so and even when explicitly instructed not to.[9] A second is anarchic hand syndrome (Della Sala et al., 1991), where one of a patient's hands, typically the left, may perform complex purposeful actions in conflict with the patient's stated intentions. The interactive-activation framework is particularly attractive for the selection of actions because it allows the integration of these various influences (plus self activation and lateral inhibition) into a single activation value. Action selection then reduces to the question of whether the activation of a schema node exceeds a threshold. If it does, this allows the excitation of component schema nodes or, at the lowest level, triggers the performance of the corresponding act. At this level it is assumed that the model feeds into mechanisms such as those discussed in Section 8.2.

Self-activation and lateral inhibition solve one computational problem—that of selecting one schema from a set of competing alternatives. However there is a second problem, namely how to select schemas over time in order to achieve coherent behaviour. Within contention scheduling, this is solved by a combination of mechanisms. First, when their corresponding action or schema has been performed, inhibition of nodes prevents an action being repeatedly selected. This inhibition is analogous to that within the competitive queuing models of the graphemic and phonological output buffers discussed in Sections 7.6 and 7.7. Second, the control

a schema exercises over its component schemas depends upon goal pre-conditions and post-conditions. So, excitation of a component schema by a source schema that has been selected (i.e. parental excitation) requires more than just the existence of a component schema which satisfies a subgoal of the source schema. The subgoal's pre-conditions must be satisfied too, while the subgoal's post-conditions (the required result of the action) must not be (see Figure 8.4). Thus, when buttering a slice of toast, one subgoal might be to obtain a suitable knife. A pre-condition for this is to have a free hand. A post-condition is that the knife be held. If there is no free hand, or if a suitable knife is already held, then schema nodes for picking up a knife will not receive excitation from the super-ordinate schema.

A third computational problem concerns the selection of objects on which the action will take place and the effectors with which to act. Within the model this is achieved through additional interactive-activation networks in which nodes correspond to effectors and to representations of the objects required for the task or present in the immediate environment. Bi-directional links between the effector network, object representation networks and the schema network support positive feedback loops between schemas, effectors, and appropriate object representations. The complete model is shown in Figure 8.5a.

The interactive-activation network model of contention scheduling is able to account for the performance of temporally extended action sequences such as those involved in meal preparation and other activities of daily living. Figure 8.6 shows the activation profiles of schema nodes throughout the task of preparing a cup of coffee when provided with a cup of hot water and individual packets of the various ingredients; this task is aimed to simulate the ability of patients to use a hospital breakfast tray, which has been investigated

---

[9] See Chapter 9.

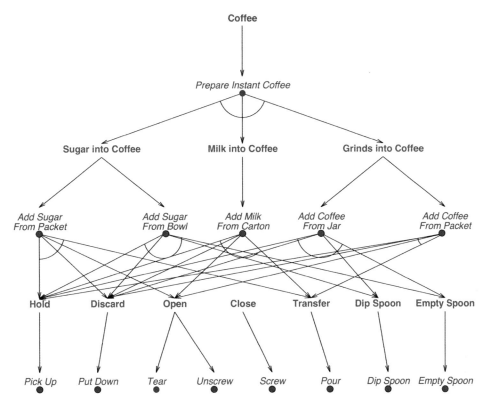

Fig. 8.4 A schema hierarchy for the routine task of preparing instant coffee within the contention scheduling model of Cooper and Shallice (2000). Goals are shown in red. Nodes in blue correspond to schemas. From: Contention Scheduling and the control of routine activities. R.P. Cooper and T. Shallice, *Cognitive Neuropsychology, 17*(4), 297–338, 2000, reprinted by permission of the publisher (Taylor & Francis Ltd, http://www.tandf.co.uk/journals).

empirically by Schwartz et al. (1991). The node corresponding to *prepare instant coffee* remains active throughout the duration of the task. Within this period, nodes corresponding to three subschemas (*add coffee from pack*, *add sugar from bowl* and *add milk from carton*) are activated at different stages of the task, while within each of these subschemas additional lower-level schemas (corresponding to basic level actions such as *pick-up* and *put-down*) are activated in sequence. The representations of the various objects used throughout the task show similar fluctuations in activation, such that, for example, the cup remains active as a target throughout the task, while the milk carton is active as a source only during execution of the *add milk from carton* subschema.

As described below, the contention scheduling model is able to account for a variety of neurological disturbances

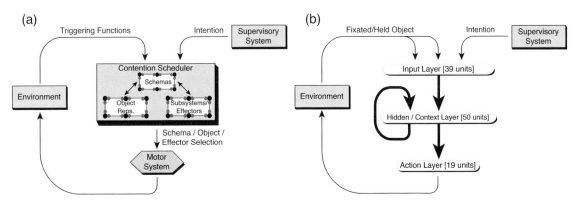

Fig. 8.5 (a) The interactive activation model of contention scheduling of Cooper and Shallice (2000). (b) The simple recurrent network model of routine action selection of Botvinick and Plaut (2004).

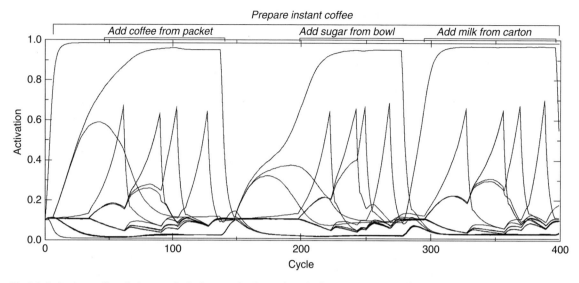

Fig. 8.6 Activation profiles of schema and subschema nodes during the task of preparing instant coffee in the contention scheduling model of Cooper and Shallice (2000). From: Contention Scheduling and the control of routine activities. R.P. Cooper and T. Shallice, *Cognitive Neuropsychology, 17*(4), 297–338, 2000. Reprinted by permission of the publisher (Taylor & Francis Ltd, http://www.tandf.co.uk/journals).

to action selection. However, Botvinick and Plaut (2004) have developed an alternative computational account of the selection of actions through time. They demonstrate that a simple recurrent network can be trained with a standard connectionist learning procedure (back-propagation through time; see Section 1.7) so as to produce the same kind of extended sequences of acts performed by the interactive activation network model. The Botvinick and Plaut model (see Figure 8.5b) has a layer of input nodes, which represent the current state of the environment (in terms of features of the object that the model is currently fixated on and the features of the object, if any, that is currently held). It has an output layer in which nodes represent actions, such as *fixate-on-sugar-packet* or *pour-held-object-into-fixated-object*. In addition there is an internal context layer with recurrent connections. Once trained, the model successfully reproduced action sequences of up to 37 steps (as required by Botvinick and Plaut's version of the coffee-preparation task).

What are the critical differences between the two models? It may appear that one is localist and one is distributed. However, in Chapter 3 we argued that this was a simple matter of modelling convenience. Simple recurrent networks may be trained to exhibit attractor dynamics such that, given an input, the network settles to one of several stable states. These states, and the competitive dynamic that operates between them, are functionally analogous to nodes within an interactive activation network. The basic architectures therefore merely represent alternative approaches—less and more sophisticated respectively—to how to implement

the competition element of the contention scheduling mechanism.[10]

A far more significant difference between the models results from the eliminativist stance that Botvinick and Plaut take towards schemas, hierarchical organisation and goals. Within the Cooper and Shallice model these are explicit constructs that play causal roles in regulating the flow of activation within the action selection system and between that system and the motor system. Within the Botvinick and Plaut model, they are epiphenomenal regularities that can be observed in the output of the action-control system. We return to the importance of this difference in Section 8.4 in the discussion of certain forms of apraxia and in Chapter 9 on the modulation of contention scheduling by a supervisory system.[11]

---

[10] Botvinick and Plaut, however, do not use recurrent network attractor dynamics to capture the response selection element of sequential behaviour. Rather, they use the dynamics of their model to capture the sequential aspects of action selection over time. Thus, when two actions are equally plausible given both the immediate preceding actions and the input from the environment (i.e. the representation of fixated and held objects), the Botvinick and Plaut model generates weak outputs for both actions (Cooper & Shallice, 2006a), rather than attempting to resolve the response competition through a settling process.

[11] A third difference between the models concerns the use of a separate interactive activation network for the representation of objects within the Cooper and Shallice (2000) model. This allows competition not only between actions, but also between the representations of objects on which to act.

The sequential selection of action within well-learned tasks is a transparently learned operation. The simple recurrent network model of Botvinick and Plaut (2004) suggests that standard connectionist learning techniques can capture aspects of the learning process underlying it. Indeed, when tested with low levels of noise affecting hidden unit representations, the Botvinick and Plaut model was able to reproduce faultlessly each of the sequences provided in its training set. However, the model's learning process is in many ways implausible. For example, the model is trained to imitate complete sequences that happen to consist of smaller, purposeful subsequences (such as adding sugar to a cup), yet there is no explicit representation of the subsequences or their purpose. Moreover, learning operates under the assumption that subsequences are not acquired prior to or separately from the acquisition of sequences that contain them, in contrast to development theories of skill acquisition (e.g. Fischer, 1980; Greenfield, 1991). Consequently, the model has difficulty in transferring subsequence knowledge to new situations, even after 20,000 iterations of the training procedure. It is also prone to catastrophic interference, where the acquisition of a new task over-writes existing task knowledge.[12]

The deficiencies of Botvinick and Plaut's learning regime stem from their eliminativist approach to schema and goal representations, but Ruh, Cooper and Mareschal (submitted) have demonstrated that the deficiencies are not intrinsic to the connectionist approach. Thus, in a modified version of the Botvinick and Plaut model explicit goal representations are assumed as a third type of input to the simple recurrent network (and predicted goals representations that may be fed back into the system are assumed as a second type of output). Ruh et al. have shown that hierarchically structured, goal-directed, sequence learning can be accomplished by such a network through connectionist learning techniques, namely back-propagation combined with reinforcement learning,[13] in such a way that the resultant network can be instructed at multiple levels (i.e. at the level of individual actions, at the level of subtasks such as adding sugar to a beverage, or the level of entire tasks such as preparing a specific beverage). The connectionist view of action selection is therefore complementary to the symbolic view, in which action schemas and their goals are treated as discrete symbols. Given this theoretical background, we turn now to consideration of empirical neuropsychological evidence.

8.4 **On Apraxia**

Apraxia is a disorder that is distinct from paralysis and plegia, in which the patient is unable to make appropriate actions to objects. It was first convincingly described by the German neurologist Liepmann (1900), who later made the most frequently used major subdivision into types of apraxia, in particular between *ideomotor apraxia* and *ideational apraxia* (Liepmann, 1908).[14] While the existence of apraxia is now uncontested, all attempts to provide more specific clinical categorisation have been challenged and remain highly controversial. However, to simplify, in ideomotor apraxia single gestures can be impaired and the disorder can be seen in the reproduction of meaningless as well as meaningful acts. By contrast, ideational apraxia involves the performance of meaningful actions and is perhaps most clearly manifest in the carrying out of meaningful sequences of behaviours.

The difficulties in the study of apraxia have derived in part from a long-standing dispute related to classification/description. The terms *ideomotor* and *ideational* apraxia have continued to be used in different ways by different authors. Thus some authors (e.g. Heilman & Rothi, 2003) treat pantomiming of gestures, either to command or in response to viewing a tool or object, and also the use of single objects, as tests of ideomotor apraxia. The deficit is most pronounced when pantomiming, but still apparent in single object use. To these authors, ideational apraxia is a disorder of the sequential organisation of action that is most apparent in the use of multiple objects. Moreover, Heilman and Rothi (2003) distinguish between ideational apraxia and conceptual apraxia, with the latter characterised by content errors in both the pantomiming and use of objects (e.g. use of a screw-driver as a hammer).[15] Others however (e.g. De Renzi & Lucchelli, 1988) see ideational apraxia as a more general disorder of object use, demonstrable by errors in the use of both single and multiple objects, and with sequential disorganisation being neither a necessary nor sufficient component of the disorder.

The terminological confusion is compounded by the range of behaviours on which apraxic patients may show deficits. Thus dissociations have been reported in

---

[12] See Cooper and Shallice (2006a, 2006b) for more details, and Botvinick and Plaut (2006b) for a response.
[13] See also Botvinick et al. (2009).

[14] Leipmann's original term for ideomotor apraxia was *ideo-kinetic* apraxia. He further distinguished these forms of apraxia from *limb-kinetic* apraxia (Liepmann, 1920) in which the patient is slow or clumsy in making fine finger movements. Some investigators consider this to be a mild form of hemiparesis (see Buxbaum, 2001).
[15] To complicate matters even further, Luria (1966) uses the term *frontal apraxia* to refer to those patients with frontal lesions who produce sequential errors of type seen in Heilman and Rothi's ideational apraxia.

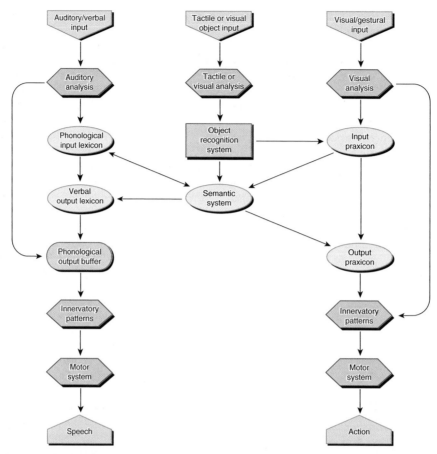

Fig. 8.7 Heilman and Rothi's (2003) proposed model of the action system. (See Heilman & Rothi, 2003, Figure 11.4.)

a number of different forms. One is the imitation of meaningless contrasted with meaningful gestures (e.g. imitation of an arbitrary hand gesture versus imitation of a military salute) (Goldenberg & Hagmann, 1997). A second would be performing a transitive gesture (e.g. pantomiming the use of a key) to command contrasted with imitation of the same gesture (Ochipa et al., 1994). Third, pantomiming object use can be contrasted with actual use of objects (e.g. pantomiming brushing ones teeth versus actually using a toothbrush) (De Renzi & Lucchelli, 1988). Finally, use of single objects is contrasted with use of multiple objects that are typically employed together (Poeck & Lehmkuhl, 1980). In some cases, these dissociations may merely reflect an effect of task difficulty, but in others the existence of double dissociations suggests the existence of functionally separable subsystems.

A second difficulty has been that theorists in general have talked past each other using very different types of conceptual framework. One approach, adopted by Rothi et al. (1991), has been to update Liepmann's ideas by using the analogy of multiple route models of reading (see Chapter 4) to construct a model of praxis processing.

The model, as updated by Heilman and Rothi (2003), is shown in Figure 8.7. As in the case of reading, support for the utility of this type of model comes from the study of patients with striking dissociations.

The first dissociation separated two forms of ideomotor apraxia according to whether recognition of gesture was impaired or intact. Heilman, Rothi and Valenstein (1982) carried out a group study of patients who performed poorly on a gesture-to-command task, which they held to be diagnostic of ideomotor apraxic.[16] They examined the ability of these patients to recognise gestures. Apraxic patients with more anterior lesions or with nonfluent aphasia were less impaired at this task than patients with posterior lesions or with fluent aphasia.[17] This dissociation between intact gesture

---

[16] The commands included both intransitive gestures, such as forming the sign for hitchhiking, and transitive gestures, such as opening a door with a key.

[17] Non-fluent aphasia was held to be diagnostic of relatively anterior lesions, while fluent aphasia was held to be diagnostic of relatively posterior lesions. At the time even CT scans were not generally available for all patients in neuropsychological

recognition and impaired gesture to command does not seem likely to arise merely from differences in task difficulty. Thus Bell (1994), in a study of 23 patients with left hemisphere lesions, found no correlation between the recognition and the imitation of pantomimes (i.e. transitive gestures). So Rothi et al. (1991) followed models of reading, such as that shown in Figure 4.3, by separating an *input praxicon* from an *output praxicon*, where the term 'input praxicon' refers to a system for recognition of actions and that of 'output praxicon' for schema-like action-control entities; on the model, these praxicon representations function as the equivalent of lexical items in the action domain.[18] However the existence of such dissociations, without clear evidence that the impairment is to the praxicon itself, is insufficient to establish the existence of separable input and output systems; they may merely reflect disconnections to and from a single system.[19]

In addition, however, Rothi et al. wanted to explain how patients can exist who in a counter-intuitive fashion can imitate a gesture that they cannot comprehend or discriminate. Rothi, Mack and Heilman (1986) had described two patients of this type with occipito-temporal lesions, who are presumed to have damage to the central object recognition route in their model.[20] Building on arguments developed by Roy and Square (1985) they added to the developing model *object recognition* and *action semantics* systems, with the latter being concerned with 'conceptual knowledge related to tools, objects and actions' (Rothi et al., 1991, p454). It has a family resemblance to the visual semantics of Chapter 6. Patients who could not comprehend gestures that they could imitate were held to have damage affecting access to action semantics from gestural input, but with neither the input nor output praxicons being damaged.

The presence of a route from the object recognition system to the praxicon systems was supported by the existence of three patients described by Heilman (1973) who were unable to pantomime an action to command, despite intact language comprehension. However, when presented with the object they could pantomime its use flawlessly. Thus multiple routes to the output praxicon are required.

A further dissociation was first described by Ochipa, Rothi and Heilman (1989). Their patient misused tools, for instance, brushing his teeth with a spoon, but could name the tools normally. They suggested this could result from an impairment of their action semantics system.[21] Related patients to the one studied by Ochipa et al. have since been described by Motomura and Yamadori (1994) and Heilman et al. (1997).[22] Further evidence for a distinction between a conceptual system (i.e. action semantics) and a production system (i.e. the output praxicon) is reviewed by Mahon and Caramazza (2005).

This type of model, however, gives little insight into how the mapping from action knowledge to the realisation of motor movements actually occurs. An updating of Liepmann's model by Buxbaum (2001) is promising in this respect. On Buxbaum's model (see Figure 8.8) gesture representations can be of two types, namely actions characteristically used with objects and *non-transitive gestures*, such as making the hitch-hiking sign. These representations are held to consist of two components, a stored portion, which is invariant over instances of the gesture, and a dynamic portion, which codes a specific instance of a gesture or act. Thus, the left component of Buxbaum's model—labelled 'dynamic portion of gesture representation'—contains a 'dynamic representation of the body forming the basis for the calculation of numerous frames of reference centred on the body parts involved in a given action' (p. 451). On the model, this type of representation is employed in the production of body-centred forms of spatiomotor coding, which in turn is used in the processing of all gestures, regardless of whether they are meaningful and regardless of whether a tool is held. These forms of representation are, however, held to be most critical when the procedures are not supported by other forms of information (e.g. for meaningless gestures).

We will identify Buxbaum's 'dynamic body schema' system with the processing domain of inverse and forward models described in Section 8.2. Poizner and his colleagues have carried out a number of studies that are suggestive of deficits at this level (see Poizner et al., 1997). They show that the low-level aspects of movements

---

group studies, so, as was then standard, Heilman and colleagues used behavioural correlates to grossly localise the lesion.

[18] The word 'praxicon' is a neologism created in the domain of action by analogy with the word 'lexicon'.

[19] The conceptual issue is discussed with respect to phonology in FNMS Chapter 7.

[20] The single-case study findings on apraxia are less rich and developed than those on, say, reading and semantics discussed in Chapters 4 and 6. It is therefore necessary to forego some of the methodological refinements developed in Chapter 4 and merely assume that individual differences, say, are not a factor in inferences from the dissociations described.

[21] This would be different from the output praxicon as the latter could be activated directly via gesture classification from the input praxicon.

[22] To be convincing, critical patients held to have semantic impairments, for instance the patient described by Ochipa et al. (1989), would need to be of the semantic degradation type (see Chapter 6). Otherwise an 'access' interpretation would be possible without the need to assume separate systems.

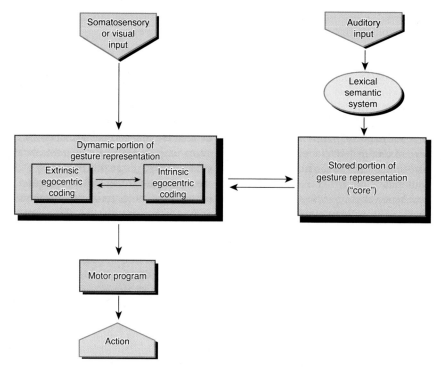

Fig. 8.8 Buxbaum's (2001) updating of Liepmann's model of the organisation of action systems. (See Buxbaum (2001) figure 2.)

by apraxics are disordered. For instance, Poizner and Soechting (1992) analysed the hand and arm movements involved in winding up a car window with the left hand (see Figure 8.9). The control participant showed smooth circular movements repeated about a well-defined centre point. The apraxic, who had a large left perisylvian lesion affecting frontal, temporal and parietal lobes, produced repeated circular movements but with continually changing amplitudes and spatial orientation. That a periodic behaviour is realised at roughly the correct rate but in a different fashion from one cycle to the next suggests (but does not prove) that the source of the deficit lies in the dynamic system, to use Buxbaum's terminology.[23] Further support for a link between ideomotor apraxia and deficits in the generation or use of internal models is provided by studies such as those of Sirigu et al. (1996) and Buxbaum et al. (2005), discussed in Section 8.2, which link deficits in motor imagery with ideomotor apraxia.

In her model, Buxbaum (2001) follows Rothi et al. (1991) in having, in addition to the dynamic system, a system of stored gestures. However, her theoretical position is more minimalist. The representation and storage of features, which do not vary and are involved

in differentiating one type of learned action from another, becomes the responsibility of a single system that she labels the 'stored portion of gesture representation ('core')'.[24] Damage to this system is identified with what Buxbaum calls *representational ideomotor apraxia*, in which patients have a problem in gesture identification as well as gesture production. These patients are held to have lesions to Brodmann areas 39 and 40 of the left parietal lobe.

There are two potential problems for Buxbaum's account. First, she needs to explain the findings of studies held to support the model of Rothi and her colleagues in terms of possible disconnections of this system from input or output. A second potential problem concerns dissociations between the production of meaningless and meaningful gestures—a contrast that we hold relates to the contrast between ideomotor and ideational apraxia. Thus, Goldenberg and Hagmann (1997) described two patients where the dissociation was clear. One, LK, had suffered from two left parieto-occipital haemorrhages, with the lesion from one involving the angular gyrus. The other, EN, had a lesion restricted to the inferior portion of the left angular gyrus. Both were grossly impaired in imitation of meaningless gestures but were normal on producing meaningful

---

[23] Alternatives would be a higher-level specification of the rhythm that was correct but a loss of other aspects of the core representation (see below) *or* a refractory deficit at the level of the core representation.

[24] In her paper she also appears to call it the 'central praxis system', although the referent for this term is not entirely clear.

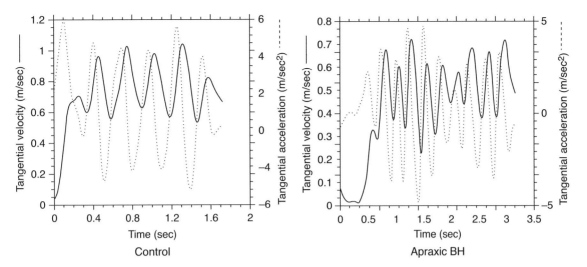

Fig. 8.9 Tangential velocity and acceleration of the hand of a control subject and the apraxic patient BH when performing a *winding* gesture. The control produced smooth regular movements while the movements of BH were erratic. Reprinted with permission from H. Poizner and J.F. Soechting, 1992, New strategies for studying higher level motor disorders. In D.I. Margolin (ed.) *Cognitive Neuropsychology in Clinical Practice.* By permission of Oxford University Press.

gestures (both from imitation and to verbal command—see Table 8.1 and Figure 8.10). Rather similar patients have been described by Heilman et al. (1986) and Buxbaum, Giovanetti and Libon (2000).[25]

We will therefore assume that the systems involved in the reproduction of meaningful gestures have some degree of functional specialisation when contrasted with the systems involved in the reproduction of meaningless gestures. However there are many ways in which this type of functional specialisation might be realised. In particular, while there is no agreed task analysis for the imitation of meaningless gestures, such an analysis seems likely to involve segmentation processes and the ability to characterise and retain multiple segments in an active short-term memory system. Neither of these processes would be involved in imitating meaningful gestures, where the subcomponents would be known and chunked into a single schema. So it is not clear in what way Buxbaum's model would need to be extended to deal with this dissociation.

To dismiss as theoretically opaque the occurrence of specific problems in the imitation of meaningless gestures does not mean one should take a similar approach

for the complementary type of impairment—imitation of meaningful gestures. In other ways, too, the approach of Buxbaum and her colleagues is one of conceptual minimalism. Thus, Buxbaum, in collaboration with Myrna Schwartz and Mike Montgomery (Buxbaum et al., 1998), essentially marginalises the concept of 'ideational apraxia', which we are associating with impairments in producing meaningful actions. Is ideational apraxia therefore a useful concept? It is productive to work backwards with respect to this question.

First, consider whether there is any lesion location specifically involved in the systems underlying actions with meaningful objects. De Renzi and Lucchelli (1988) provided evidence it was a left-parietal syndrome. However, Buxbaum et al. (1998) argued that there are 'several reasons to question the assumption that the left hemisphere is specialised for complex actions with objects' (p. 618) In particular they showed that a group of patients with right hemisphere lesions were at least as impaired on a new test they developed—the Multiple Level Action Test (MLAT)—as a group of left-hemisphere patients. In a further study it was shown that closed head-injury patients—generally with more anterior lesions—were similarly impaired on the MLAT (Schwartz et al., 1988). However, even the simplest version of the MLAT test involves three unrelated primary tasks—making a slice of toast with butter and jam, wrapping a present and packing a lunch box. In addition, the many objects that need to be used are placed on a U-shaped table in front of the patient.

We are therefore dealing with a much more complex situation than would occur if only a single-source schema were required, which would be the case on a

[25] Goldenberg and Hagmann's (1997) localisation of this deficit to the left angular gyrus is somewhat inconsistent with more recent work by Goldenberg and Karnath (2006), in which a deficit in the imitation of *hand* postures is localised to left angular gyrus but a deficit in the imitation of *finger* positions is attributed to lesions of the left frontal gyrus. Critically, Goldenberg and Karnath were concerned with imitation of novel gestures, and several other studies suggest a role for left frontal gyrus in the generation of novel finger positions.

| TABLE 8.1 | Scores (in all except symbolic gestures out of 20) for patients LK and EN on the apraxia tests of Goldenberg and Hagmann (1997). Control data is shown in the right-most column. Reprinted from *Neuropsychologia, 35*, Goldenberg, G. and Hagmann, S. The meaning of meaningless gestures, a study of vision imitative apraxia. Table 1, Copyright (1997), with permission from Elsevier. |

Test	LK	EN	Controls (range)
Imitation:			
of hand positions with own hands	11	3	18-20
of hand positions on a manikin	10	5	14-20
of finger configurations	19	11	15-20
of pantomimes of object use	17	18	
Gestures on verbal command:			
pantomimes of object use	18	17	14-20
symbolic gestures	12	12	10-12
Use of objects	20	20	19-20

trial of a more typical ideational apraxia task, involving, say, the presentation of a candle and matchbox. The importance of this difference is shown by a study of Hartmann et al. (2005), in which left- and right-hemisphere patients both failed on a complex naturalistic task (preparing coffee). By contrast, dissociations between the patient groups were seen on simpler tasks; the left-hemisphere patients had problems in retrieval of functional knowledge, such as knowing which of four objects should be paired with a potato peeler, while for the right-hemisphere patients their difficulties were in keeping track of multi-step actions, as

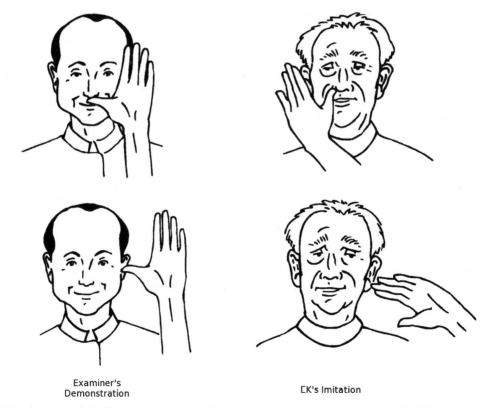

Examiner's
Demonstration

EK's Imitation

Fig. 8.10 Sample errors made by EK when imitating gestures. The examiner's demonstration is shown on the left. EK's imitation of the gesture is shown on the right. Reprinted from *Neuropsychologia, 35*, G. Goldenberg and S. Hagmann, The meaning of meaningless gestures: a study of visuoimitative apraxia, pp. 333–341, Copyright (1997), with permission from Elsevier.

required when solving a novel mechanical problem—opening a 'treasure box'—using an ordered sequence of actions.

The functional distinction between ideomotor apraxia and ideational apraxia is also supported by the study of De Renzi et al. (1968). 160 patients with left-hemisphere lesions took part, together with 45 patients with right-hemisphere ones. In the *ideational apraxia* test the patient was asked by word and gesture to take an object in their hands and show how to use it. The objects or pairs of objects ranged from a hammer (simplest) to a candle and matchbox (most complicated). Even the most severe aphasic had no difficulty understanding what was required. All the controls and right-hemisphere patients performed perfectly (14/14 items) on the test. However, 45 of the patients in the left-hemisphere lesion group (i.e. 28%) made one or more errors. These 45 could hardly be all those who had lost the core gesture knowledge on Buxbaum's theory. This is because 11 of those failing the test were in the normal range on the ideomotor apraxia test. Yet the ideomotor apraxia test of De Renzi and colleagues in fact requires meaningful gestures such as to 'make the sign of the horns to designate a cuckold', for which Buxbaum's core system would be needed. This suggests that Buxbaum's core system would be relatively intact for these 11 patients. Moreover some dissociations were gross—such as patients obtaining 5/14, 2/14 and 4/14 on the ideational apraxia test compared with 20/20, 19/20 and 18/20 with the ideomotor apraxia test and the correlation between performance on the two tests accounted for only 16% of the variance.

It is conceivable that in some of these ideational apraxic patients an associative agnosia in Warrington and Taylor's (1978) sense—an inability to know what the object is—could have been responsible.[26] However this is a very rare condition; thus Hécaen and Angelergues (1963) found only 4 such patients in a series of 415 patients with lesions. So it could not account for so many patients having a problem on such a simple test.[27]

The number of patients who scored very poorly on this test, while being normal or near normal on a movement imitation test held to assess ideomotor apraxia, was even more dramatic in a second study, that of De Renzi et al. (1982). In a very large left-hemisphere series involving 150 patients, 11 patients were found to have large discrepancies between the two tests, with the ideomotor one being performed better. Overall there

appears to be a specific problem concerning learned actions with meaningful objects that occurs following left-hemisphere lesions and that cannot be easily reduced to the operation of Buxbaum's 'dynamic body schema' system.

We will therefore restrict use of the term 'ideomotor apraxia' to an impairment in the generation or use of internal models of the Wolpert and Ghahramani type. How then might ideational apraxia be explained? Early ideas on ideational apraxia can be seen as corresponding to impairments to particular components of the contention scheduling system. For instance, De Renzi and Lucchelli (1988) found that there was a strong correlation between the ability of a patient to use single objects and the ability to use multiple objects. They held that ideational apraxia derived from a deficit in accessing part of the semantic repertoire of object features, an 'amnesia of usage' which affected knowledge of the specific way the object is used.[28] In a rather complementary fashion, Lehmkuhl and Poeck (1981) emphasised knowledge of the sequencing of subcomponent acts. They described five aphasic patients who failed on tasks such as making a cup of coffee and also had difficulties on a task which required them to place a series of pictures of the component actions in order.

In fact ideational apraxic patients can perform well when they are required to realise their conscious knowledge of sequencing actions as contrasted with implementing the processes themselves. Thus Rumiati et al. (2001) described two patients, DR and FG, who performed well below the normal range on the ideational apraxia test of De Renzi et al. (1968) discussed earlier which involves the use of objects.[29] Both patients performed completely normally at matching objects with pictures of actions (e.g. given the objects *fish*, *ham*, *sandwich* and *crash helmet*, which goes with the action of *fishing*? DR 40/40; FG 39/40) or at matching objects and verbal descriptions of functions (e.g. given four objects, a *hammer*, *screwdriver*, *spanner* and *pliers*, which is used to put nails into walls? DR 32/33; FG 33/33). Moreover both could sequence a set of photographs of component sub-actions of simple multiple object tasks such as lighting a candle (see Figure 8.11) much better than they could realise it in practice (DR: sequencing photographs 90%, production of actions 33%; FG: sequencing photographs 75%, production of actions 13%). By contrast a patient with a prefrontal lesion, WH2, showed the opposite pattern (sequencing photographs 58%; production of

---

[26] See FNMS Chapter 8 for discussion.

[27] Many individual patients have been described with ideational apraxia who do not have any problems in object perception. See, for example, Ochipa et al. (1989) and Rumiati et al. (2001).

[28] A similar position had been advocated by Morlaas (1928) much earlier.

[29] One patient, DR, also performed poorly on the De Renzi et al. ideomotor apraxia test; the other, FG, performed in the normal range.

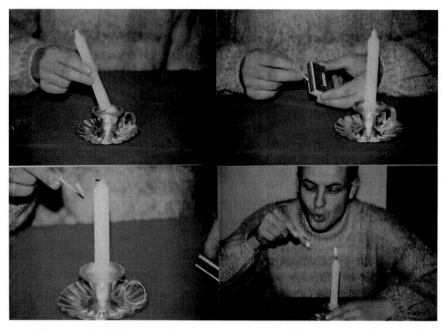

Fig. 8.11 Stimuli used in Rumiati et al's (2001) picture ordering task. From a random ordering, subjects are required to place the pictures in this sequence, which reflects the conventional order of steps in the use of the objects. (Figure supplied courtesy of Raffaella Rumiati.)

actions 85%).[30] The two types of task appear to involve separable subsystems.

The contention scheduling model depicted in Figure 8.5a looks very different from the model of Rothi et al., but there are considerable similarities. The input praxicon could correspond to object trigger representations and the output praxicon to schemas in the contention scheduling model. This latter model may also be seen as having different aspects which relate to the De Renzi and Lucchelli and to the Lehmkuhl and Poeck positions on ideational apraxia. Thus 'amnesia of usage' for objects could correspond to loss of the object trigger network. Sequencing of subactions depends on the appropriate interplay of activation and inhibition in the interactive activation network controlling schema selection and between this and the interactive activation networks corresponding to object representations. Indeed if one looks at the errors made by the two patients in carrying out multiple object tasks (see Table 8.2) 38% of DR's and 35% of FG's involve sequencing of subcomponent actions. These types of error occur when generalised noise is added to the networks of the contention scheduling model (Cooper et al., 2005), but they also occur when the flow of activation between the object representation and schema networks is partially lesioned. Thus, Cooper (2007b) implemented schema networks for five of Rumiati et al.'s (2001)

simple multiple object tasks. When activation flow from object representations to schemas was reduced by damage approximately 40% of the model's errors involved incorrect sequencing of subcomponent actions. Similar results held when activation flow in the reverse direction was impaired.

In addition, however, two types of errors occur in these patients, which can be termed 'conceptual', following the usage of Ochipa et al. (1989). In one type—the *misuse* class—the patient carried out an action appropriate for a related object, e.g. *hammering with a saw* ($misuse_1$) or for a different type of use of the activated object, e.g. *cutting an orange with a knife as though it was butter* ($misuse_2$). In the other—the *mislocation* class—the patient performed the correct action but either in the wrong place, e.g. *pouring from a bottle onto the table* instead of into a glass ($mislocation_1$) or on the wrong part of the correct object, e.g. *striking the match inside the matchbox* instead of against the side of the matchbox ($mislocation_2$). DR and FG showed different profiles under this categorisation of errors. Specifically DR produced a high proportion of misuse errors (and in particular $misuse_2$ errors), while FG was more prone to producing mislocation errors (and in particular $mislocation_2$ errors).

On the model, the ratio of misuse to mislocation errors depends on the relative strengths of the schema-to-object and object-to-schema links. $Mislocation_2$ errors are disproportionately common when the former are lesioned. The reason is that when activation flow from schemas to object representations is impaired or

---

[30] Zanini et al. (2002) have shown that this is a typical prefrontal pattern.

TABLE 8.2 Means (and standard deviations) of the number of errors of each type produced by two ideational apraxic patients on a battery of multiple objects tasks, together with best fits to each patient of the contention scheduling model (see Cooper, 2007b). The patient data are based on four attempts by each patient at the battery of 10 tasks as reported by Rumiati et al. (2001). The model data are based on eight attempts at 5 of those tasks.

Error Type	Patient DR	Model: $S_E = 0.00$ $O_E = 0.40$ $N = 0.075$	Patient FG	Model: $S_E = 0.10$ $O_E = 0.10$ $N = 0.075$
Sequence errors	4.75 (1.26)	4.91	10.50 (4.65)	9.97
Misuse$_1$	–	–	0.72 (1.50)	0.08
Misuse$_2$	5.00 (2.00)	3.63	1.25 (1.50)	1.95
Mislocation$_1$	1.75 (0.50)	0.40	2.50 (1.73)	3.75
Mislocation$_2$	–	1.16	5.75 (0.96)	5.40
Tool omission	0.75 (0.96)	0.48	1.50 (0.58)	1.09
Pantomime	–	–	0.75 (0.96)	0.17
Perplexity	0.25 (0.50)	0.29	5.75 (1.71)	2.29
Toying	–	–	2.50 (1.00)	0.34
Total errors	12.50 (3.70)	10.87	31.25 (11.30)	25.04
RMS fit to data		0.756		1.492

DR had a large unilateral ischemic lesion affecting the left frontal, temporal, and parietal cortices. FG had a unilateral cortical-subcortical haemorrhage of the left superior parietal lobule.

noisy, the limited activation so provided is generally sufficient to activate all aspects of the object which it is correct to use (e.g. the matchbox), but in the presence of noise it is not sufficient to specify reliably the correct part of that object (e.g. the rough side of the matchbox when it is appropriate to strike the match); this produces mislocation$_2$ errors. By contrast, misuse$_2$ errors are disproportionately common when the object-to-schema links are lesioned. When activation flow from object representations to schemas is weakened, object representations are unable to provide sufficient excitation to disambiguate in a reliable fashion between different potential schemas for a given goal (e.g. different schemas for cutting); this leads to misuse$_2$ errors. The model is therefore able to simulate not only the general pattern of impairment seen in ideational apraxia, but also the finer detail of the performance of patients DR and FG (see Table 8.2). Thus impairment to different parts of the model can explain different classes of the conceptual errors occurring in ideational apraxia.

The use of such a model as a vehicle for explaining ideational apraxia can be challenged in two contrasting ways. First it can be said to underestimate the complexity of the empirical domain. Second it can be held to be unnecessarily complicated in what it does explain. On the first point, Goldenberg and Hagmann (1998) explored how well patients can select and use novel tools (see Figure 8.12). For instance, patients were asked what was the best tool to attach to a cylinder in order to lift it out of its socket: 22 patients with right-hemisphere lesions and 42 with left-hemisphere ones were tested. The right-hemisphere patients were completely normal at tool selection but the left were impaired (Controls 12/12; RH 11.6/12; LH 9.5/12). Within the left-hemisphere group it was the left-parietal patients who were principally impaired, with only 19% making normal tool selections. These scores were similar to ones obtained from pantomiming familiar actions involving an object such as rubbing out with an eraser or pouring liquid from a bottle, where only 23% of the left parietal group behaved normally. This implies that the schemas for action selection must be triggered not only by objects with a known function but also by other objects which afford the function well. However, the action required is in some sense quite abstract, even though it is not dependent upon specific knowledge of the objects. The patient has to realise, for instance, that the most leftwards of the three 'tools' in the middle panel of Figure 8.12 is unsatisfactory because of the torque that the cylinder would create. In other words the simple domain of having object triggers for eliciting schemas has to extend into the much more abstract domain of practical naïve physics. Such an extension to the contention scheduling model seems in principle possible but has not been essayed thus far.

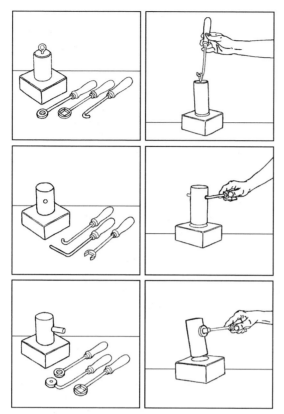

Fig. 8.12 Three examples from the novel tools test of Goldenberg and Hagmann (1998). Subjects are required to select and use an appropriate tool to remove the cylinder from its base. In each case the right panel shows correct performance. Reprinted from *Neuropsychologia*, 36(7), G. Goldenberg and S. Hagmann, Tool use and mechanical problem solving in apraxia, pp 581–589, Copyright (1998), with permission from Elsevier.

Ironically, a second objection is that the model is unnecessarily complicated in its explanation of skilled action. Botvinick and Plaut (2004) demonstrated that their simple recurrent network model, when lesioned through the addition of noise to hidden unit activations, can also reproduce a range of action selection errors including sequence errors similar to those made by DR and FG. Their model learns, as well as producing actions in the steady state, and also uses fewer concepts to provide an account of sequential action selection. Moreover, as described above it accounts for sequential action without explicit recourse to concepts such as goals, schemas or hierarchical structuring. It therefore might appear to provide a more parsimonious account of the ideational apraxic deficit.

In fact, while the Botvinick and Plaut model is able to provide an adequate account of sequential errors in ideational apraxia, it provides a poor account of conceptual errors. In the simulation of disorganised action reported in Botvinick and Plaut (2004), the great majority of errors were omissions (77%) or sequence errors

(15%). The remaining 8% of errors included a variety of different types. In a reimplementation of the Botvinick and Plaut model, Cooper and Shallice (2006a) found fewer than 2% of errors involved Ochipa et al.'s conceptual errors—object substitutions (i.e. misuse or mislocation errors).[31] Cooper and Shallice went on to argue that the relative scarcity of substantive non-sequence errors in the behaviour of the Botvinick and Plaut model arises in part because the model lacks separable object representations which can impact on action selection. In addition concepts such as that of *goal* and *schema* play an essential role in the explanation of misuse errors. It therefore seems that the contention scheduling model is not overly complicated.

8.5 Localisation of Action Related Subsystems

We have argued that operations performed by the action system may be understood at two levels—that of internal models and that of the sequential selection of motor skills within a routine task. The argument is supported by theoretical concerns and by evidence from neurological breakdown. We turn now to consideration of where the processes or subsystems responsible for the different elements of action control might be localised.

As we have seen, at a very coarse level, patient studies of ideomotor apraxia generally associate the syndrome with lesions of left parietal cortex (BA 5, 7, 39, 40). Thus, LK and EN, the ideomotor apraxic patients of Goldenberg and Hagmann (1997), both had lesions affecting the left angular gyrus (BA 39), while BG, a primary progressive apraxic patient reported by Buxbaum et al. (2000), had substantial atrophy of the superior parietal cortex (BA 5, 7). These areas are also the areas reported to be affected in group studies of deficits in skilled movement (Haaland et al., 2000) and meaningless imitation (Buxbaum et al., 2005). Patient studies of ideational apraxia similarly implicate left parietal cortex. In the group study of De Renzi and Lucchelli (1988) the deficit was related primarily (though not exclusively) to lesions affecting the tempo-parietal junction (BA 39/40).

This coarse localisation is supported by numerous functional neuroimaging studies. The first such studies

---

[31] Errors in the Botvinick and Plaut model tend to reflect the capturing of behaviour by some other learned potential trajectory in 'action space' so that behaviour moves into that other, inappropriate, trajectory. However, Botvinick and Plaut (2004) were attempting to simulate Schwartz et al.'s (1998) more general action disorganisation syndrome, rather than ideational apraxia per se. They therefore did not use the error classification of Rumiati et al. (2001), and so a precise figure for conceptual errors is not available from their simulations.

relating to the levels of processing impaired in ideomotor and ideational apraxia were carried out by Decety et al. (1994) and Jenkins et al. (1994). In an extensive meta-analysis, Grèzes and Decety (2001) considered the findings of these and 28 other imaging studies of the action system, including eight of action execution, six of *action simulation* (i.e. mental rehearsal of a motor act without overt movement), eight of action observation, and eight of action verbalisation. The primary result was significant overlap between the areas involved in action execution, simulation and observation. Large areas of cortex, including the supplementary motor area, the dorsal premotor cortex, the supramarginal gyrus, and the inferior and superior parietal lobules, were implicated in all three types of task. This is compatible with the patient studies just discussed. It also fits with the *mirror neuron* concept of Rizzolatti et al. (1996a), which has been very influential recently (e.g. Rizzolatti & Sinigaglia, 2010). This is derived from the observation in the monkey, that viewing an action activates neurons which are also involved in certain levels of action production. The original reports of mirror neurons were concerned with area F5 of the monkey premotor cortex, the human homologue of which is standardly agreed to be Broca's area (BA 44, 45). More recently, however, Fogassi et al. (2005) have reported neurons with mirror properties in monkey parietal cortex.[32]

Returning to the Grèzes–Decety meta-analysis, however, it is unfortunately critical that it does not allow fine-grained localisation of the specific action-related sub-processes contributing in each case, since multiple component processes are involved in each task and what those component processes are is not well specified. In an attempt to localise such processes more precisely, Hamilton and Grafton (2006, 2007, 2008) conducted a series of action observation studies using a priming paradigm. The paradigm depends upon *repetition suppression*—a form of adaptation or habituation whereby reduced activation occurs when an operation is repeated (see Section 7.2). A first study contrasted situations where an observed reaching/grasping trajectory was fixed but where the object being grasped varied, and vice versa. Reduced activation occurred in the left anterior intraparietal sulcus when the object (and grip) was the same, but the trajectory varied, and in the right superior precentral gyrus when the trajectory was the same but the object (and grip) varied (see Figure

8.13a). Minimally, this study implies that different cortical areas are relevant for different aspects of action understanding. The superior parietal location when the trajectory is the same fits with the localisation of the production of forward models discussed in Section 8.2. A second study (Figure 8.13b) generalised the result by varying the grip instead of the trajectory, while in a third study (Figure 8.13c) the means (e.g. pushing or pulling) was varied while keeping the outcome of the action fixed (e.g. closing the sliding lid of a box), and vice versa. Since all three studies did not require subjects to actually produce actions it is possible that the results do not generalise to action production. However, together the studies suggest that different cortical areas are recruited for the interpretation, and possibly for the production, of different aspects of the organisation of an action (i.e. trajectory, grip, goal, etc.).

Several imaging studies have sought to isolate processes related specifically to more complex aspects of the organisation of actions. Thus, Choi et al. (2001) contrasted neural activity during pantomiming of tool use gestures, such as using a razor or toothbrush (when presented with the tool name) with repetitive oppositional movements of the thumb and fingers (when presented with an unrelated function word). They found significantly greater activity not only in the left superior parietal cortex but also in the angular gyrus (as well as greater left premotor, left SMA and bilateral cerebellum activation) during the pantomime condition. A similar study by Moll et al. (2000), contrasting pantomiming of tool use with production of complex meaningless movements, associated pantomiming with increased activation of the left intraparietal sulcus and dorsolateral frontal cortex. The apparent conflict between the findings of these studies may be the product of scanning requirements and differences in methods. For example, in the Choi et al. study, all pantomimes and finger movements were made with the hand between the waist and chest, even if the pantomime would normally have been performed near the face, as in using a razor. Pantomimes were therefore performed in a non-standard spatial location and orientation.

Nevertheless, it has been demonstrated by Hermsdörfer et al. (2007) that pantomiming and actual tool-use evoke similar neural activity. They separated processes related to stimulus presentation, preparation and execution in a study where each phase lasts several seconds. Short video-clips of objects were shown to subjects during the stimulus presentation phase. By comparison to rest, this led to extensive bilateral occipital activation (presumably due to the visual presentation), bilateral superior parietal activation (with greater significance on the left, in accordance with Choi et al., 2001), left inferior parietal activation, bilateral activation of the inferior/middle frontal gyrus and left dorsal

---

[32] In fact differentiating whether a single system controls both input and output from a pair of systems with a relatively automatic flow of information between them is extremely hard. We are not convinced that the evidence currently available is conclusive. See FNMS Chapter 7 for discussion of the conceptual problem in the realm of language and also Lingnau et al. (2009) for a novel approach to the issue.

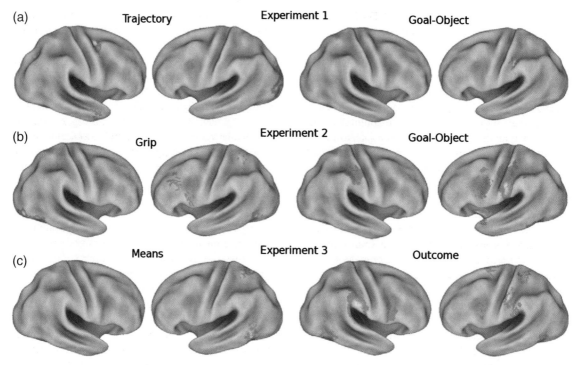

Fig. 8.13 Areas showing repetition suppression in the three action-observation studies of Hamilton and Grafton. (a) Regions associated with fixed hand trajectories (left) and fixed target/goal objects (right). (b) Regions associated with fixed grip types (left) and fixed target/goal objects (right). (c) Regions associated with fixed means (pushing or pulling) (left) and fixed outcomes (box open/closed) (right). See text for additional details. Reprinted from *Human Movement Science, 26*, S.T. Grafton and A.F. de C. Hamilton, Evidence for a distributed hierarchy of action representation in the brain, pp 590–616, Copyright (2007), with permission from Elsevier.

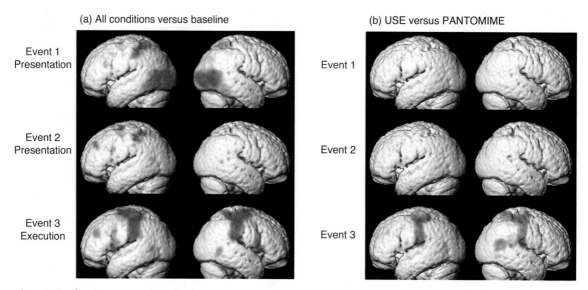

Fig. 8.14 Significant contrasts in the study of tool use versus pantomime of Hermsdörfer et al. (2007). (a) Activation contrasts for tool presentation, action preparation and action execution compared to a baseline resting condition. Red regions indicate significant differences (*p* < 0.05, corrected). (b) Activation contrasts for the three phases for actual tool-use minus pantomimed tool use. The reverse contrast did not reveal any significant activation differences. Reprinted from *NeuroImage, 36*, J. Hermsdörfer, G. Terlinden, M. Mühlau, G. Goldenberg and A.M. Wohlschläger, Neural representations of pantomimed and actual tool use: Evidence from an event-related fMRI study, pp T109–T118, Copyright (2007), with permission from Elsevier.

premotor activation (see Figure 8.14a). During a preparation interval, significant activation was observed in the region of the left intraparietal sulcus, bilaterally in the dorsal premotor cortex, and in left frontal regions. Finally, during execution significantly greater activation was seen in the premotor and motor cortices, superior parietal cortex, middle frontal gyrus, middle temporal gyrus, the basal ganglia and cerebellum (all bilaterally). The principal difference between pantomime and actual tool use occurred in the final condition, with greater bilateral activation of motor, superior parietal and temporal regions during actual tool use (see Figure 8.14b). Similar regions have been found in other studies of tool use (e.g. Johnson-Frey et al., 2005), strongly supporting the hypothesis of a left hemisphere network involving superior parietal, inferior parietal and premotor cortices for the control of skilled action.[33]

The problem with interpreting these studies is that many functional processes and many brain regions are involved. One has no principled way of determining the specific mappings between function and brain area.[34] Rumiati and colleagues (2004) report a PET study aimed specifically at fractionating components of the skilled action network. Four conditions were contrasted in a 2×2 design: pantomiming an observed action (i.e. imitating it: IA); pantomiming on visual presentation the typical use of an object or tool (IO); naming an observed action (NA); and naming an object or tool (NO). Rumiati et al. argued that IA involves recognition of the pantomime and generation of the corresponding action, while IO involves recognition of an object, triggering of the corresponding action by that object, and generation of the action. In an analogous fashion they argued that NA and NO are similar with naming replacing pantomiming. The contrast (IO + NO) – (IA + NA) therefore reflects the activity due to object recognition less pantomime recognition, while the contrast (IA + IO) – (NA + NO) reflects the activity due to pantomime minus naming. Most critically, the interaction term, (IO – IA) – (NO – NA), reflects the neural activity related specifically to the triggering of an object-related action by an object, i.e. the link from object representations to schemas posited within the contention scheduling theory.

Only one region was found to be significantly activated by condition IO (pantomime to object), but not by either condition when a pantomime was presented, namely a dorsal region of the left inferior parietal lobule (see Figure 8.15). Furthermore, this region was suppressed relative to rest in condition NO (object naming). This region therefore appears to be the locus of triggering of skilled actions by objects. A second parietal region, slightly ventral to the first, was found to be activated during conditions requiring a pantomime response but suppressed relative to baseline when a naming response to an object was required. This region therefore appears to be associated with the generation of object-related actions, regardless of the stimulus, i.e. with the generation of action schemas.[35, 36]

A further strand of support for involvement of the left inferior parietal cortex as the location of action schema units in the contention scheduling sense, or more likely their triggering, is provided by a set of monkey studies of action observation. Using single cell recording in the monkey, Fogassi et al. (2005; see also Fogassi & Luppino, 2005) found that many inferior parietal neurons coded acts differently depending on the context (i.e. the super-ordinate schema) in which the act was performed. Thus, cells showed different firing patterns when grasping was performed in the context of bringing food to the mouth than when it was performed in the context of moving food to a container near the mouth. Similar results held for the observation of motor acts (i.e. many cells in monkey inferior parietal cortex also had mirror neuron properties).

Other evidence, however, points to the neural basis of action schemas themselves as involving premotor cortex. This position fits with the standard characterisation of the region in the monkey literature (see, for example, Passingham, 1997, for a review). Thus, cells in

---

[33] The left inferior frontal gyrus was also activated in some of these studies. Goldenberg and Karnath (2006) have argued that apraxic patients who have specific difficulties in the imitation of finger positions frequently have damage to this region, while Alexander et al. (2005) found that patients with lesions in this region made more errors than frontal patient controls in acquisition of a 5-alternative finger-selection choice reaction-time task. The putative skilled action network may therefore also involve left inferior frontal gyrus, at least as far as skill acquisition is concerned, but see Chapter 9.

[34] This type of difficulty is an increasingly severe problem as the cognitive domains become more complex, as we will see in subsequent chapters.

---

[35] Three prefrontal regions were also highlighted by the interaction. A ventrolateral prefrontal region was more involved with the less natural task for each stimulus, while activity in the anterior cingulate and an area of left dorsolateral prefrontal cortex paralleled task difficulty. The roles of these areas are discussed in the Chapter 9.

[36] Peigneux et al. (2004) report a second PET study aimed at fractionating the components of skilled action. They specifically sought to isolate the components of Rothi et al.'s (1991) model of apraxia discussed in Section 8.4 (see Figure 8.7), again using a factorial design. Unfortunately, however, interpretation of the results is compromised because the authors do not report error rates across conditions and it is unclear how visual processing of familiar and novel gestures may be equated for difficulty.

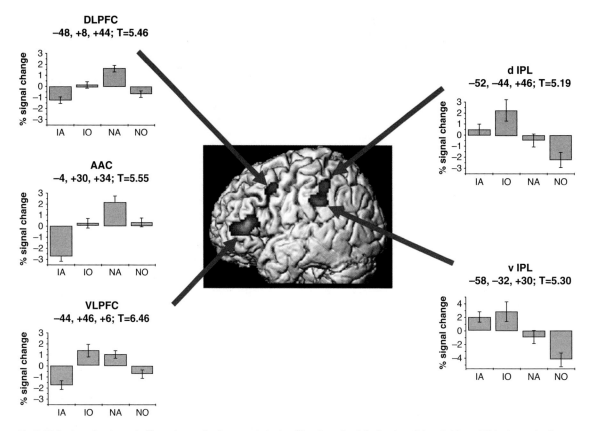

Fig. 8.15 Regions showing a significant interaction between imitation (I) and naming (N) of actions (A) and objects (O) in the study of Rumiati et al. (2004). Reprinted from *NeuroImage*, *21*, R.I. Rumiati, P.H. Weiss, T. Shallice, G. Ottoboni, J. Noth, K. Zilles and G.R. Fin, Neural basis of pantomiming the use of visually presented objects, pp 1224–1231, Copyright (2004), with permission from Elsevier.

this region are active while the monkey prepares a response in conditional motor learning i.e. giving response A to stimulus X and response B to stimulus Y (Wise & Mauritz, 1985). Moreover the region has been found to be active in a large number of imaging studies of action, including several of those referred to above (for reviews see Kellenbach et al., 2003; Johnson-Frey, 2003a). For instance, in the Rumiati et al. (2004) study, bilateral ventral premotor cortex activation was observed in both conditions involving the production of a pantomime (in contrast to those involving production of a name). The relative roles of the parietal and premotor cortices in the neurobiological basis of triggering and activating schemas remain to be resolved. From a connectionist perspective with sets of hidden units lying between input and output, the parietal sets of units would be relatively speaking more loaded on triggering functions than premotor ones, with the opposite tendency for schema activation functions. However these effects would be far from all-or-none. We return to this issue in Chapter 9. Contention scheduling itself (i.e. the activation and selection of subschemas through top-down biasing) may be implemented by subcortical loops

linking premotor cortex and the basal ganglia (Alexander et al., 1986).[37]

8.6 The Right Hemisphere, Spatial Analysis and Spatial Operations

Consider another type of operation that is critical for successful action. Take the example of repairing a chair. You are working on one leg of the chair, but for physical convenience you put the chair in a new position— perhaps rotating it or turning it upside down. Which is the leg you are working on? Operations like these are the bedrock of many practical human skills. Moreover an abstraction from them creates geometry.

_____

[37] Gurney et al. (2001a, 2001b) argue that the basal ganglia implement an action selection mechanism with some similarity to contention scheduling. One possibility is that competition between schemas—a key element of contention scheduling—is resolved within the basal ganglia, but evidence for this is currently weak. An alternative possibility is that action selection in the basal ganglia may operate at the level of behaviours such as feeding or grooming, rather than at the level of motor actions.

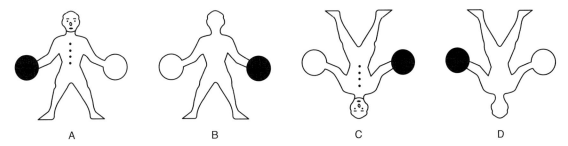

Fig. 8.16 Stimuli from the "manikin" task, adapted by Ratcliff (1979) from Benson and Gedye (1963). On each trial subjects are required to say which of the manikin's hands (left or right) holds the black disk. Reprinted from *Neuropsychologia*, 17, G. Ratcliff, Spatial thought, mental rotation and the right cerebral hemisphere, pp 49–54, Copyright (1979), with permission from Elsevier.

We will approach them by considering impairments of action following right parietal lesions. In studies of imitation, for example, Goldenberg and Strauss (2002) report that lesions of the left parietal region affect the ability to imitate both hand and finger positions, while lesions of the right parietal cortex affect only the ability to imitate finger positions. Furthermore, a high proportion of imaging studies of action have found right lateralised activity in one condition or another. Thus, Decety et al. (1997) found extensive right activation, including right inferior parietal activation, when subjects observed meaningless gestures with the intention of either imitating or memorising them. How might these findings be explained? Goldenberg and Strauss (2002) argue that greater perceptual discrimination is required in the processing of finger positions than hand positions. This in turn requires greater spatial processing, which they suggest is reflected in right parietal activity. Similar comments apply in interpreting the Decety et al. study: analysis of meaningless gestures would appear to require spatial processing beyond that required by meaningful gestures, resulting in increased right cortical activity in the meaningless condition.

Can one give a deeper characterisation? Consider, for example, the task of mental rotation. Spatial operations involved here dissociate from those operations involved in motor imagery which might be thought to have a spatial component. Tomasino et al. (2003) described nine unilateral patients with visual processing deficits as assessed by the VOSP battery (Warrington & James, 1991; see Figure 4.18 for one subtest). The four right-hemisphere patients all scored below the 5th percentile of control scores on the *manikin task*, which fitted the results of a pioneer group study by Ratcliff (1979). In this task, patients are shown line drawings of a figure holding a black disk in one hand (see Figure 8.16). The figure can be either upright or inverted and facing either towards or away from the patient. The patient's task is to decide which of the figure's hands is holding the black disk. By contrast, all five left-hemisphere

patients scored in the normal range. In complementary fashion, the right-hemisphere patients all scored in the normal range on a task that required them to decide whether rotated drawings of a hand corresponded to the left or the right hand (Luria, 1966). The left-hemisphere patients were all impaired on this task. This is a task where it appears you match the hand with one of your own hands; in the manikin task you operate entirely on the representation of an external object.

The right-lateralisation of *purely external* spatial operations is supported by imaging and TMS studies. Using PET, Harris et al. (2000) scanned subjects who were performing a forced-choice two-dimensional mental rotation task in which 10%, 40%, 70% or 100% of letter-like stimuli were presented either in canonical or mirror-reversed form at an angle ranging from 0° to 320°. The subject had to judge whether the stimulus was canonical or mirror-reversed. The only region whose activity was found to correlate with the percentage of stimuli requiring rotation was the right intraparietal sulcus (IPS). A follow-up study (Harris & Miniussi, 2003) compared the effects of rTMS over left IPS, right IPS, and a sham midline condition. Response times were significantly slowed only in the right IPS condition and then only when the TMS pulses were applied approximately 400 msec after stimulus presentation.

Case studies allow us to specify 'external' spatial transformation processes in more detail. Several individual patients with specific impairments in mental rotation have been studied. Thus, Bricolo et al. (2000) describe PAO, a patient with an extensive lesion of the right perisylvian area following a cerebrovascular accident. PAO performed within the normal range on tests of attention, language, action and memory, including visuo-spatial short-term memory as assessed by the Corsi Block Span test. However he was grossly impaired on some visuo-spatial tasks, particularly those involving the mental rotation of figures. For example, his performance on the manikin task was at chance when the figure was not both upright and facing towards him, as was his

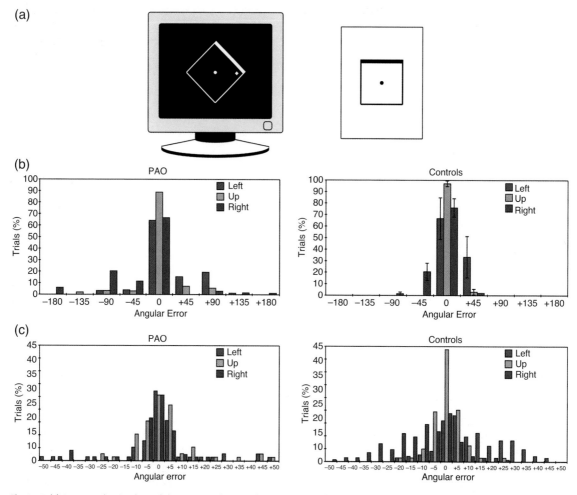

Fig. 8.17 (a) An example stimulus and the response sheet used by Bricolo et al. (2000) in their study of patient PAO. (b) Responses of PAO and controls grouped into gross 45° bins. (c) The central part of that response distribution grouped into fine 5° bins. Adapted from Selective space transformation deficit in a patient with spatial agnosia, E. Bricolo, T. Shallice, K. Priftis and F. Meneghello, *NeuroCase, 6(4), 307–319,* 2000, Oxford University Press. Rreprinted by permission of the publisher (Taylor & Francis Group, http://www.informaworld.com).

performance on a three-dimensional version of mental rotation shown in Figure 5.5 (Shepard & Metzler, 1971).[38]

Bricolo et al. showed PAO a series of images depicting a square with the top marked by a thick line and a point marked within the square. The square was presented on a PC monitor at one of three angular rotations (vertical, 45° left or 45° right), and the patient's task was to mark the position of the point on a template provided by the experimenter (see Figure 8.17a). PAO's angular errors, and those of controls, are plotted in Figures 8.17b and

---

[38] For patients with similar deficits in mental rotation, see patient ELD of Hanley et al. (1991), patient MG of Morton and Morris (1995) and patient VQ of Toraldo and Shallice (2004). Note though that ELD was impaired on the Corsi Block Span test, while MG's lesion was mainly left parietal, extending to medial regions.

8.17c. While controls occasionally erred by up to 45°, many of PAO's errors were much greater. Thus 29% of his responses were more than 50° wrong, compared to 6% for normal controls. However, if he was in the right ballpark, he was as good as controls (see Figure 8.17c). Following a distinction originally made by Kosslyn et al. (1992), Bricolo et al. (2000) argue that spatial information is encoded in both metrical and categorical forms. Metrical coding concerns quantitative effects of distance to nearby distinctive points in a continuous metric space. By contrast, categorical coding relates to the qualitative organisation of local space using (completely nonverbal) concepts such as left/right, above/below, close-to/distant and between. PAO's impairment is held to the latter but not the former. Whether this reflects a problem of categorical *operations* or of categorical *spatial representation* is at present unclear. A group

study of Buiatti et al. (in press) supports the localisation of categorical spatial operations to the right parietal lobe, consonant with PAO's lesion.[39]

We return now to the findings of Goldenberg and Strauss (2002). The imitation of finger positions was specifically affected by right hemisphere lesions. To imitate finger positions you need to know the categorical coding of fingers in relation to each other. A right-hemisphere localisation of categorical coding can explain this finding too. How it is carried out computationally is as yet unclear. However, a spatial version of the competitive queuing model (see Section 7.6) may suffice. Either way, it is likely to require a different type of process from the hierarchical organisation of skilled action that the left inferior parietal lobe provides.

8.7 **Morphological Operations**

It has been argued that the control of action involves a number of different types of operation—creation of inverse and forward models for motor control, triggering of schemas by the representation of objects, binding of object representations to the argument roles of schemas, and also spatial operations. These operations have different computational requirements and this leads to distinct neural localisations for the different types of operation. This is to be expected if such operations are implemented neurally by special-purpose subsystems. It is the realm of language, however, to which we now turn, which is *par excellence* the domain of special-purpose operations.

As we discussed when considering Levelt's theory of language production in Section 3.5, language involves many types of computational process. We will consider two in detail—morphological operations and syntactic ones.[40] We begin with the morphological ones concerning how the specific form of a word is selected.

Morphology concerns how words are created out of their component elements; consider, for instance, the English word *unfriendliness*, which is composed of a stem (*friend*) and one morphosyntactic affix (*-ly*), a negative

affix (*un-*) and a derivational affix (*-ness*), or the English word *jumped*, which is composed of a stem or base verb (*jump*) and one inflectional affix (*-ed*). We consider this specific type of operation because it is a relatively simple domain by comparison, say, with syntax, but also because the domain has been the focus of a very intense debate over the last twenty-five years, and the smoke is only now beginning to clear. The conflict has not as yet been won or lost, but two clearly differentiable positions have emerged.

As we discussed at the beginning of this chapter, prior to the mid 1980s, morphological operations had generally been assumed to be rule-based (e.g. Chomsky, 1959b; Pinker, 1984). That is, morphologically complex words such as *jumped* were constructed from, or decomposed into, their parts by the applications of rules. There were well-known exceptions to the rules. For instance, in the case of English past tense formation, where the rule is add 'ed' to the base form of the verb to generate the past tense, it applies only to regular verbs and not to verbs such as *sing*, *have* or *eat*. The existence of such exceptions implies, on the rule-based account, some separate mechanism or table of exceptions that is invoked when processing those exceptions.

In the 1980s, Rumelhart and McClelland (1986) produced a model that aimed to show that rules did not have to be explicitly realised in a mechanism to give rise to rule-following behaviour. Their model (see Figure 8.18), a multi-layer feed-forward connectionist network, became probably the most discussed and most controversial model of any cognitive process.

The model was given the present tense of verbs (e.g. *start* or *come*) as input and had to produce the past tense (e.g. *started* or *came*) as output. The model had three parts—a network that encoded the phonological form of the verb into a standard type of representation, which could form an input for a learning component of the model and for which no two verbs had the same representation; it is called a Wickelfeature representation in Figure 8.18.[41] The second part of the network is

---

[39] Kosslyn et al. had claimed that categorical spatial operations were left-hemisphere processes.

[40] Another computational process which has been extensively discussed in the literature is the translation of semantically represented information into a phonological form. The standard model of this process, other than that developed by Levelt and colleagues (1999), is that of Dell and colleagues (Dell, 1986; Dell et al., 1997a; Foygel & Dell, 2000). They put forward an interactive activation model which is analogous but in a different domain to the interactive activation model of McClelland and Rumelhart (1981). We do not consider it in detail because of the conceptual similarity to that reading model. For empirical and conceptual criticisms see Ruml and Caramazza (2000).

[41] All words need to have distinct representations at input and output. As input and output units are binary one could do this by having five units for the first letter, five for the second and so on, but this would not capture important generalisations such as that the regular past adds a /d/, /t/ or /^d/ depending on the last phoneme of the stem. This is because this approach does not represent the ends of words in a similar fashion, and so the system would have to learn to add that regular past tense ending in the right place separately for words of different length. It would also mean restricting stems to no more than five phonemes. McClelland and Rumelhart had the idea of employing a method invented by the American psychologist Wayne Wickelgren (1969) who noted that words could be unequivocally represented by the triples they contain. Thus for letters,

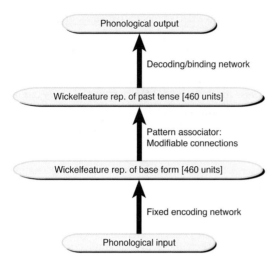

Fig. 8.18 The Rumelhart and McClelland (1986) model of the formation of the past tense.

a simple pattern associator of the type discussed in Section 1.7.[42] The third part is a mechanism for decoding the network's internal feature representations back into a phonological form. Only the second part learns. The critical aspect of the network is that regular forms of the past tense e.g. *started* are produced by exactly the same procedure as irregular ones, e.g. *came*.

The net learned to produce the appropriate past tense for a corpus of 420 verbs, 336 regular and 84 irregular. After 200 training trials about 99% of the features of the regular past tenses are correctly produced and over 95% of the irregular ones. Moreover the net showed many interesting features. Novel stems were regularised, as they are by native speakers. Moreover the way

the net responded to so-called 'irregulars' early in learning had many characteristics in common with children learning the past tense. Early in training the net would over-regularise as in producing *camed* for the past tense of *come*; preschool children do the same (Ervin, 1964).

The network also showed other interesting behaviour when given related irregular verbs. Thus, Bybee and Slobin (1982) divided the irregular verbs into several classes. One class was verbs that do not change in the past tense, e.g. *heat*, *cut*, *hit*. Another was verbs that undergo an internal vowel change, e.g. *give → gave*; *break → broke*. Bybee and Slobin showed that when preschool children are given the present tense form and asked to produce the past they tend to leave the verbs with a t/d ending unchanged but to add the regular suffix to the others. A related sensitivity to the final phoneme of the present tense was shown by the model (see Table 8.3).

Rumelhart and McClelland were not tentative about this achievement. They considered they had shown that rule-following was simply the behavioural manifestation of the superposition of related associations, that 'rules' were mere surface descriptions of behaviour *and* that there was no separability between formation of the regular and the irregular past tense. These claims led to one of the most detailed and systematic critiques in the history of cognitive science, that of Pinker and Prince (1988).[43] The critique highlighted twelve inadequacies, partly empirical and partly conceptual, of the Rumelhart and McClelland model, ranging from the model's explanation of over-regularisation errors in young children's speech production (e.g. producing *broked* as the past tense of *broke*) to representational problems, which meant that the model could not represent certain words.

Proponents of the connectionist approach produced a whole slew of models in response to Pinker and Prince's arguments (e.g. MacWhinney & Leinbach, 1991; Plunkett & Marchmann, 1993; Hare et al., 1995; Joanisse & Seidenberg, 1999), with each model attempting to address a different set of criticisms. That none of these models retain most of the basic implementation details of the original Rumelhart and McClelland model (i.e. representational assumptions, such as the use of Wickelfeatures, specific architecture or training regime) is testament to the fact that the arguments of Pinker and Prince were essentially correct as far as the rather primitive original form of the model is concerned. More critically, while the later models have successfully

---

rather than phonemes, the word can be used as the collection {-wo, wor, ord, rd-} where the four units form an unordered list. The authors then coded the 460 Wickelphones (i.e. Wickelgren triples for phonemes) in a manner roughly compatible with English phonology as binary strings across the 33 input and output Wickelfeatures of the net. In fact this method was an initial step allowing modelling to get a start on an ingenious idea, and quite different input representations can be used which leave the essence of the model unaffected (see e.g. MacWhinney & Leinbach, 1991; Plunkett & Marchman, 1993). Oddly Pinker (1999) in his popular book on the topic makes a great song-and-dance about the inadequacy of the Wickelfeature representations. They are not central to the issue. See for example the discussion of the Joanisse and Seidenberg model later in this section.

[42] The pattern associator maps directly from an input Wickelfeature representation of the base form of the verb to an output Wickelfeature representation of the past tense form. An intermediate layer is not necessary. Formally, this is because the mapping problem is linearly separable. Informally, it is a result of the consistency of the mapping and the fact that the Wickelfeature representation consists of more units (460) than there are items (with only 420 verbs).

[43] Pinker has gone over much the same ground in his popular book *Words and Rules* (1999). The earlier article is what should be read if only for the brilliance of the way the argument is developed.

TABLE 8.3 Sensitivity of past-tense formation in preschool children and the Rumelhart and McClelland model to verb endings. Preschool children data are from Bybee and Slobin (1982). The model data are from McClelland and Rumelhart (1986). What is critical is the ordering of conditions, and in particular the crossover interaction, as within the model there is no implementation of the mapping from response strength to number of responses.

	Stimulus not ending in t/d (e.g., give, break)		Stimulus ending in t/d (e.g., cut, hit)	
	Regular response (gived, breaked)	No-change response (give, break)	Regular response (cutted, hitted)	No-change response (cut, hit)
Preschool children (Number of responses)	203	34	42	157
Model (Mean response strength, trials 21-30)	0.52	0.11	0.32	0.41

addressed the representational inadequacies of the original network, it remains problematic whether, by using a connectionist approach, one can account for the developmental U-shaped learning profile of how the English past tense is acquired. The system needs to first produce correct irregulars, like *broke* and *hit*, then to over-extend the regular rule, producing overregular forms like *broked* and *hitted*, before finally correctly treating irregulars as exceptions to the rule. In general, connectionist models achieve this only through implausible manipulations of the training regime.[44]

Two main positions have emerged from the debate. McClelland and his supporters (e.g. Joanisse & Seidenberg, 1999, 2005; McClelland & Patterson, 2002) remain committed to the view that a single mechanism is involved in mapping word stems into inflected forms (whether the inflection signals tense, aspect or agreement). This mechanism they hold to be modelled well by a connectionist network that maps speech input to speech output—possibly modulated by other systems such as semantics—and it learns those mappings through a gradient descent algorithm. The current instantiation of this theory, which includes recurrent connections to clean up internal representations and learns by means of back-propagation through time, is shown in Figure 8.19.

The alternative '*Words and Rules*' approach, as supported by Pinker and colleagues (e.g. Pinker & Ullman, 2002), is that irregular forms are stored as appropriately marked lexemes within a mental lexicon, but that regular inflected forms are derived from, or decomposed into, their stems using an appropriate rule (such as the

'+ed' rule for past tense verbs). Regular stem forms are held also to be stored within a mental lexicon. While this approach might appear less parsimonious than that of McClelland and colleagues, it is in fact more compatible with grammatical theory at levels beyond single words. Thus, on this approach the processes involved in forming the past tense of a regular verb (e.g. *jumped* from *jump*) are no different in form from the processes involved in forming the infinitive (*to jump*). Furthermore, there is no prohibition on high-frequency regular (or even infinitive) forms being encoded in the lexicon, providing redundant representations for such forms.[45]

One type of evidence that has been considered critical in the debate is that provided by cognitive neuroscience. Pinker (1999) has argued that such evidence presents great difficulties for the McClelland and Rumelhart approach. For instance, double dissociations have been described between the ability to produce regular and irregular forms.

Marslen-Wilson and Tyler (1997) investigated a priming paradigm with a single-case approach. They studied two patients with specific difficulties in grammatical production—agrammatism—JG2 and DE, and a third patient, TS, who was also agrammatic but with more widespread damage. On each trial they presented the subject with two 'words', a prime followed 250 msec later by a target, and subjects were required to decide, as quickly as possible, if the target was a word. There were eight different kinds of trials, pairing regulars, irregulars, semantically related and phonologically related items, each in control and test versions (see Figure 8.20). The experiment was neatly designed. The test words were always in the uninflected present tense and the

---

[44] In the original Rumelhart and McClelland model, this was achieved by initially training the model on 10 high-frequency verbs, 8 of which were irregular, then adding 410 further verbs to the training set, the vast majority of which were regular. The downturn in the model's performance on irregulars occurred when the training set changed.

[45] A major criticism of the Words and Rules theory is that as yet no computational implementation has been developed, though Pinker accepts that the lexicon, with stem forms and irregulars, may well be based on a connectionist-style pattern associator (e.g. Pinker & Ullman, 2002).

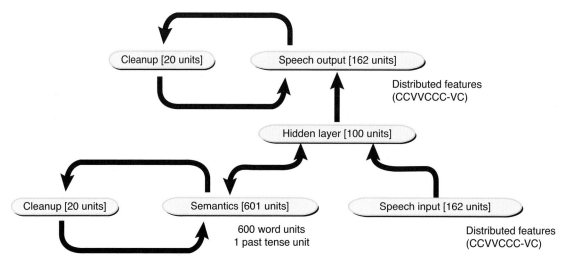

Fig. 8.19 The single mechanism model of Joanisse and Seidenberg (1999) for mapping base verb forms to past tense forms. (See Joanisse and Seidenberg, 1999, figure 1.)

non-word targets were all phonologically legal with a similar range of phonological relations between primes and word targets and between primes and non-word targets. It was the primes, to which no response was required, that differed according to condition. Thus, a regular test trial could take the form *jumped → jump*. This could be contrasted with a regular control trial (e.g. *locked → jump*). Control subjects showed significant priming for both regular and irregular verbs, with no interaction. JG2 and DE, on the other hand, showed normal levels of priming for irregular verbs, but significant levels of interference for regular verbs; they were slower if the prime and target had the same root than if they did not. In contrast, TS produced the opposite pattern, with normal levels of priming for regular verbs but no significant priming for irregulars. Moreover a significant triple interaction was found between patient, regularity and priming for both the comparison of DE and TS and for the comparison of JG2 and TS.[46]

These effects were replicated by Tyler et al. (2002a) in a group study involving five non-fluent aphasic patients (including JG2 and DE). The patients, who all had damage affecting left inferior frontal gyrus (BA44), showed significant priming (both individually and collectively) for irregulars but not for regulars. Marslen-Wilson and Tyler interpret their results as support for separable mechanisms in the processing of regular and irregular verbs, consistent with the Pinker and Ullman position but not the position of McClelland, Seidenberg and colleagues.

In accordance with Marslen-Wilson and Tyler's interpretation, difficulties with lexical decisions involving inflection in neurological patients are not confined to situations where production is required. Thus ML, a pure alexic patient of Shallice and Saffran (1986), who in a lexical decision task performed well for uninflected words (e.g. *window* versus *fancil*), accepting correctly 84% of uninflected stems and incorrectly only 38% of uninflected pseudostems. However he was completely at chance at detecting incorrectly affixed words, accepting as correct almost the same proportion of properly and improperly inflected stems (e.g. *windows* versus *windowing*; 79% versus 70%). This suggests, as do the findings of Marslen-Wilson and Tyler, that a process of 'affix-stripping' is occurring. However both of these studies involve the perception of inflected words not their production.

If one turns to production, a group study which appears to provide major difficulties for the McClelland and Rumelhart position was carried out by Ullman et al. (1997). Subjects were presented visually (or, if they had reading difficulties, auditorily) with sentence pairs such as 'Every day I *dig* a hole. Just like every day, yesterday I ___ a hole'. They had to say the missing word.

---

[46] More detailed inspection of the results produce some unexplained effects. The significant interaction with TS, came about mainly because of the great slowing of JG2 (174 msec) and to a lesser extent DE (94 msec) when presented with a regular past tense prime by comparison with a control prime. One possibility is that with only 250 msec between prime and target JG2 and DE who are both deep dyslexics were confused by the presentation of the same item with and without an affix so close together. A more recent study by the same group (Longworth et al., 2005) which examined priming between semantically related verbs in stem and past tense form (e.g. prime: *blamed*, target: *accuse*), and hence avoided rapid presentation of similar items, failed to find interference in the regular case. The three-way interaction was, however, preserved.

Condition	Test prime	Control prime	Target
Regular past	jumped	locked	jump
Irreguar past	found	shows	find
Semantic	swan	hay	goose
Phonological	gravy	sherry	grave

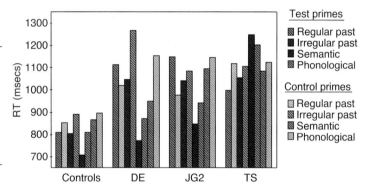

Fig. 8.20 Stimuli and results of the experiment of Marslen-Wilson and Tyler (1997). In the experimental conditions, primes were related to the target in one of four ways. In control subjects, regular and irregular past tense forms primed lexical decision of the base form, as did semantically and phonologically related primes. DE and JG2 showed a *reverse* effect for regular past tense forms but normal priming with irregulars (and semantic and phonological primes). In contrast, TS showed normal priming for regular and irregular past tense forms, and for phonological primes, but a reverse effect for semantic primes. Data from Marslen-Wilson and Tyler (1997).

A number of different patient groups were studied. The results of the most critical groups are shown Table 8.4. The Alzheimer and posterior-lesioned aphasic patients were worse at irregular than regular verbs, and tended to produce over-regularisation errors. This may reflect a deficit in retrieving irregular forms from the lexicon.[47] This supports the idea that such patients use a rule to produce at least some of the regular past tense forms. However Parkinsonian and anterior aphasic patients showed the opposite pattern of performance, with more errors on regulars than on irregulars. Anterior aphasic patients tended not to inflect regulars at all, leaving them unmarked for tense.

It is not disputed that some non-fluent aphasics show more errors when generating regulars than irregulars, or less priming when processing (i.e. an advantage for irregulars). However, as pointed out by Joanisse and Seidenberg (1999), the regular past tense forms used by Ullman et al. appeared more phonologically difficult than the irregulars, so any deficit observed with regulars may be due to a phonological processing deficit. Moreover, a connectionist model of the Rumelhart-McClelland type would predict the Alzheimer pattern in a straightforward way—mild to moderate damage to either hidden units or connections is likely to affect the processing of irregulars more than regulars. In order to demonstrate that the double dissociation was not fatal to the connectionist approach, Joanisse and Seidenberg (1999) developed a recurrent connectionist network

with dedicated semantic units and clean-up connections in both the semantic and phonological output units (see Figure 8.19). Once trained, damage to semantic units (implemented in a complex fashion) led to a selective impairment in the production of irregulars, while damage to phonological clean-up units led to insignificantly worse performance on the production of regulars than irregulars (see Figure 8.21).[48]

Joanisse and Seidenberg's account of the advantage for irregulars remains contentious. Tyler et al. (2002b) investigated the phonological deficits of four of the non-fluent aphasics from their earlier study (including patient DE). They found substantial variability in the severity of the phonological deficits of the patients as measured in a phonological segmentation task where a particular phoneme had to be isolated from the rest of the word. However, there was little variability in their patients' deficits on regulars, as measured by RT differences on a same/different auditory judgement task with pairs of regular and irregular verbs. Equally, the advantage for irregulars persisted when the phonological complexity of regulars and irregulars was controlled. However, a similar study involving a further 10 non-fluent aphasics by Bird et al. (2003) failed to replicate this. Here, all patients were found to show an irregular advantage on initial testing, but that advantage disappeared when the phonological complexity of the stimuli was controlled. A recent metaanalysis of production tests (Faroqi-Shah, 2007) also failed to find evidence of an irregular advantage.

---

[47] Tyler et al. (2002a) report similar results for a group study of four herpes simplex encephalitis patients. All patients in this study had (bilateral) damage to the inferior temporal gyrus (BA20). A single case, patient AW, who showed a similar deficit on the production of inflected forms (both nominal and verbal) is reported by Miozzo (2003). AW's lesions affected frontal white matter, medial and superior temporal areas and the basal ganglia.

---

[48] Lesioning was done by combining severing of a proportion of connections between the semantic layer and the clean-up units and adding noise to the activation of units in the semantic layer. This implementation procedure is not justified.

TABLE 8.4 Performance of four patient groups on irregular and regular verbs in a generation task.

	Alzheimer's disease (n = 5)	Posterior aphasia (n = 6)	Parkinson's disease (n = 5)	Anterior aphasia (n = 6)
Irregulars:				
Correct	60%	70%	88%	55%
Over-regularisation	27%	7%	0%	0%
Regulars:				
Correct	89%	83%	80%	20%

Data from Ullman et al. (1997).

A much more detailed study of Tyler et al. (2005a) suggests why the discrepancy may occur. They used the four types of test illustrated in Figure 8.20 on a group of 22 patients with predominantly left-hemisphere damage. The lesions sites of the patients who showed the smallest effect of 'regularity' priming using Voxel-Based Morphometry (see Section 6.7) are shown in Figure 8.22a. They involve the left inferior frontal cortex. It is noteworthy that the effect of size of phonological priming is not significant (see mauve line, Figure 8.22b, top). By contrast if one selects patients who show phonological priming then it is the left insula that is critical and these patients do not show a 'regularity' priming effect (see Figure 8.22b, bottom).[49] This suggests that phonological processing involves a separate system from morphological processing. It is conceivable the difference in lesion site is due to the contrast between perception and production. More plausible, though, the attribution of the regularity effect to phonological processing derives from the anatomical contiguity of the left inferior frontal gyrus and the insula. Patients who show a correlation between phonological priming and the regularity effect would have large lesions encompassing both areas. Overall the Joanisse and Seidenberg account does not seem to be supported.

A further complication is introduced by a claim of Seidenberg and Joanisse (2003) that their model does, on occasion, produce a reliable advantage for irregulars. The advantage though depends on chance settings of the initial weights and the specific connections lesioned. Thus, Seidenberg and Joanisse raise the possibility that patients who show the advantage for irregulars do so due to idiosyncrasies of the neural implementation of their verb processing system. As discussed in Chapter 4 such an explanation cannot be automatically excluded for individual case findings. It is, though, more difficult to use it as an explanation of multiple case/mini-group

findings such as Tyler et al. (2002b).[50] In addition though it tends to make the connectionist model essentially unfalsifiable, with all patterns of data predicted.

The individual case and mini-group analyses of Marslen-Wilson, Tyler and colleagues, and of Shallice and Saffran therefore suggest that certain neurological patients have difficulty with regularly inflected forms. Given the criticisms that have been made of the reliance on individual cases in this area (see, e.g., Plunkett & Bandelow, 2006), this makes the study of Tyler et al. (2005a) on a larger set of patients of particular importance. However, it would be premature to claim that this study is definitive.

It appears that additional sources of evidence are required to differentiate between the accounts, and naturally functional imaging has also been used to tackle the issue. However the results do not reflect well on the approach, with studies being argued to support both the single mechanism (e.g. Desai et al., 2006; Joanisse & Seidenberg, 2005; Sach et al., 2004) and the dual mechanism accounts (e.g. Beretta et al., 2003; Jaeger et al., 1996; Laine et al., 1999; Tyler et al., 2005a, 2005b). For example, in a generation task in which phonological complexity was controlled, Desai et al. (2006) using fMRI found greater activation in several areas (including bilateral posterior IFG (BA44), the precentral gyrus, anterior insula, IPS and the basal ganglia) during production of irregulars than of regulars, but no areas were more active in the opposite contrast. Desai and colleagues interpret their results as supporting the single process theory, suggesting that the additional activation in the case of irregulars was due to greater attentional demands—unsurprisingly RTs were slower and error rates were higher in the irregular condition than in the phonologically matched regular condition, suggesting that the irregular condition was in some way the more difficult of the two. Problematic, though,

---

[49] See Shafto et al. (2007) for a similar effect on the normal elderly.

[50] However, the patients whose performance was reported by Tyler et al. were not an unselected series.

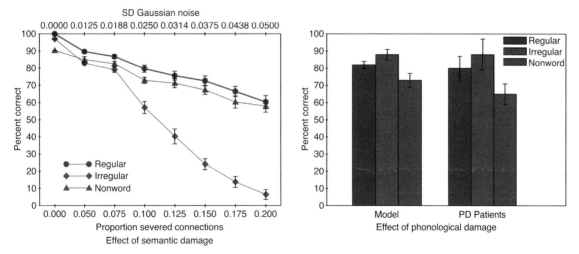

Fig. 8.21 Effects on the production of regular, irregular and non-word past tense forms of semantic (left) and phonological (right) damage to the model of Joanisse and Seidenberg (1999). Simulation data are in all cases averages over 10 different lesions. For semantic damage, severity was manipulated by increasing simultaneously both the proportion of severed connections between semantic and clean-up units and by adding noise to the activation of units in the semantic layer. Phonological damage was simulated by severing 30% of connections to/from the phonological layer. The right panel also shows data from Parkinson's Disease patients, from Ullman et al. (1997). Adapted with permission from M.F. Joanisse and M.S. Seidenberg (1999), Impairments in verb morphology after brain injury: a connectionist model, *Proceedings of the National Academy of Sciences of the United States of America*, 96(13), 7592–7597. Copyright (1999) National Academy of Sciences, USA.

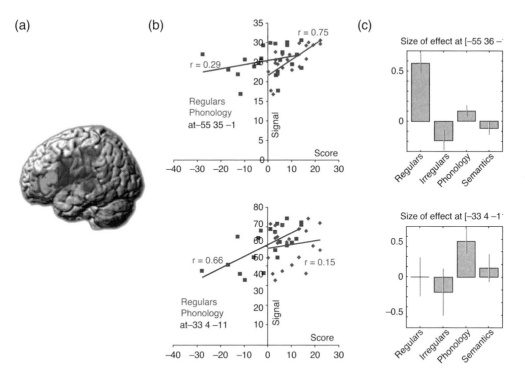

Fig. 8.22 (a) Cortical areas that correlate with priming for regularly inflected verbs at three thresholds (green: *p* < 0.001; blue: *p* < 0.01; red: *p* < 0.05). (b) Scatter plots showing correlations at two voxels between signal intensity and behavioural scores in phonological (phonology; mauve) and inflectional (regular; blue) priming conditions of the lexical decision task of Marslen-Wilson and Tyler (1997). The upper plot is based on (−55, 36, −1), within left inferior frontal gyrus (BA47). The lower plot is based on (−33, 4, −11), within the left insula. (c) Effect sizes for the four conditions at the two voxels shown in (b). Data are from 22 mainly left-hemisphere patients of Tyler et al. (2005a). Reprinted from L.K. Tyler, W.D. Marslen-Wilson and E.A. Stamatakis (2005), Differentiating lexical form, meaning, and structure in the neural language system, *Proceedings of the National Academy of Sciences of the United States of America*, 102(23), 8375–8380. Copyright (2005) National Academy of Sciences, USA.

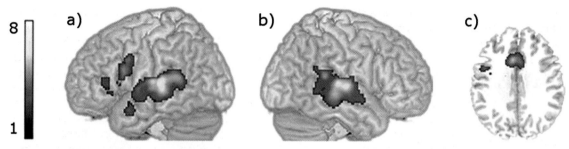

Fig. 8.23 Areas found in the Tyler et al. (2005b) same-different auditory judgement study to be more active when processing regulars than irregulars. The areas include (a) left superior temporal gyrus and left ingerior frontal gyrus, (b) right superior temporal gyrus, and (c) anterior cingulate cortex (predominately on the left). Reprinted with permission from W.D. Marslen-Wilson & L.K. Tyler, Morphology, language and the brain: the decompositional substrate for language comprehension. *Philosophical Transactions of the Royal Society B: Biological Sciences*, 362, 823–836 (figure 6, page 832), 2007, The Royal Society.

is that while Desai et al. (2006) report numerous comparisons between their conditions, they do not report what is potentially the most informative interaction term (*generate-regular–read-regular*)–(*generate-irregular–read-irregular*) and its reverse. These terms should reflect any differences in the generation of irregular and regular past tenses. So this study is not convincing.

In contrast, Tyler et al. (2005b) used event-related fMRI with the same-different auditory judgement task used in a study of Tyler et al. (2002b) reported above. They found several areas to be more active during processing of regulars than irregulars, including a fronto-temporal network, linking anterior cingulate, bilateral superior temporal gyrus and a left inferior frontal cortex area different from that of Desai et al. (see Figure 8.23). The authors argue that these areas support morphonological segmentation and grammatical analysis—additional processing that is required when processing inflected forms.

Given the apparently contradictory nature of the Desai et al. (2006) and Tyler et al. (2005b) studies, it is useful to consider one further study, that of Joanisse and Seidenberg (2005). This, like the Desai et al. study, was a generation study, but here generation was covert, in an effort to minimise the problem of movement artefacts to which fMRI is highly susceptible. Both regular and irregular stems yielded similar bilateral activation in the posterior temporal lobes, but (and in stark contrast to Desai et al.) greater activation was observed during the generation of regular past tense forms. This additional activation was in the inferior frontal gyrus (bilaterally), a region activated (in the left hemisphere) in the study of Tyler et al. (2005b), and indeed it would appear to corroborate their theoretical claims. Instead, Joanisse and Seidenberg provide an alternative interpretation. They argue that it reflects the additional phonological complexity of the regular past tense forms, and suggest that the inferior frontal gyrus and inferior temporal lobe support phonological and semantic processing respectively. The localisation of the hypothetical

phonological complexity effect is however in conflict with the VBM findings of Tyler et al. (2005b) discussed above.

The imaging findings are at worst contradictory and at best open to multiple interpretations, although on balance they are less tortuously explained by the dual process account. Further support for this position is provided by two recent ERP studies. Newman et al. (2007) recorded ERPs while subjects read English sentences containing various anomalies, including violations of one or other of regular past tense inflection (e.g. 'Yesterday I *frown* at Billy'), irregular past tense inflection (e.g. 'Yesterday I *grind* up coffee'), phrase structure (e.g. 'Yesterday I drank Lisa's *by* brandy the fire') and lexical semantics (e.g. 'Yesterday Daniel sipped his *sarcasm* for hours'). In comparison to matched control sentences containing no anomalies, violations both of regular past tense and of phrase structure elicited a Left-lateralised Anterior Negative (LAN) component.[51] Violations of irregular past tense and lexical semantics did not. Lück et al. (2006) report very similar results from an ERP study of German regular and irregular noun inflection. Both studies support the idea that regular inflectional morphology is a syntactic rather than a lexical process.

How can one assess the debate? In our view, the weight of neuroscience evidence currently points to the existence of some sort of separability for the different types of operation for the production of the regular (rule-based) as opposed to the irregular forms of a word, as the most detailed study, that of Tyler et al. (2005b) would suggest. However the evidence is not conclusive. Here there is a situation which justifies Fodor's scepticism.

---

[51] Left-lateralised Anterior Negative components occur between 150 and 500 msec after the stimulus, and are distinct from the N400. They have been reported in a number of studies involving violations of syntactic structure (e.g. Hagoort et al., 2003b; Barber & Carreiras, 2005).

Applying the methodological arguments of Chapter 5, no functional conclusion can be drawn from the localisation evidence, and in many ways, the situation is no better now than it was more than a century ago when Broca and Wernicke identified the left inferior frontal gyrus and left superior temporal gyrus as key language areas. But the debate has at least been focussed by the neuroscience studies coupled with computational studies such as that of Joanisse and Seidenberg (1999).

If one accepts the arguments of Pinker, Ullman, Tyler, Marslen-Wilson and others, then Rumelhart and McClelland were probably right about the irregulars being generated or analysed through a connectionist-style pattern-associator, and their approach has illuminated many aspects of this system. Pinker and Ullman (2002) explicitly accept this, but the definitive localisation of the process remains illusive. However Pinker and Prince were probably right about the separability of the rule system and the irregular system. This is supported by those imaging studies that use the most sensitive tests (Tyler et al., 2005a, 2005b), as well as the ERP studies of grammaticality violations. These implicate inferior frontal gyrus (particularly on the left) as the seat of the rule system. But how does the rule system actually work? Cognitive neuroscience has so far told us little. And how are the two systems integrated? We do not know.

There was a further aspect of Pinker and Prince's (1988) critique that we have not as yet discussed. Many of their criticisms were based on adult use of the regular past tense. In particular they argued that the use of the regular past tense for novel verbs depends upon the linguistic environment and that this occurs perfectly easily and naturally for the speaker. Thus so-called 'thinly disguised adjectives and nouns' take the regular form. Pinker and Prince gave a whole set of different types of example. For instance, if a proper name can be used as a verb, as in 'Clinton tried to out-Kennedy Kennedy', then it is regularised—'Clinton out-Kennedied Kennedy'. This is true even if the proper name is derived from an irregular verb. Pinker (1999) gives the example of the Attica Prison riots in 1971. They could be said to have 'out Sing Singed Sing Sing' and not 'out Sing Sang Sing Sing'.[52] Moreover, take German where the irregular forms, for adult speakers of the language, form an even higher proportion of the frequent verbs than they do in English. Indeed only 45% of the commonest German verbs are regular. Similar phenomena concerning the effect of the linguistic environment on regularisation occur to those found in English (see e.g. Marcus et al.,

1995), and an even more complex situation exists in the plural of German nouns (see Clahsen, 1999).

However the most critical problem for such models in our opinion is that, if Pinker and Prince are correct and that regularities occurring in morphology are appropriately characterised in terms of concepts such as 'noun or adjective thinly disguised as a verb', then there is no handle within a typical pattern-associator model with which to relate such generalisations. Concepts such as 'noun', 'adjective' and the like have no correspondence within the world of quasi-neural units and sub-symbolic learning algorithms. Note, however, that there has been no demonstration that some more complex mechanism of a broadly connectionist type might not be better in this respect.[53] Even here, though, we are in danger of sinking into an empirical quagmire. Are the Pinker and Prince generalisations valid? Ramscar (2002) argues that they are not, and that semantic and phonological similarity are critical to the use of the regular or irregular form. Pinker and Ullman (2003) are dismissive of Ramscar's empirical results, but if Ramscar is correct, sub-symbolic learning algorithms may be able to learn the necessary relationships through cueing from semantic and phonological similarity. It remains to be demonstrated whether this is in fact the case.

What Rumelhart and McClelland were trying to do—to produce known generalisations about cognition, in this case language behaviour, as a manifestation of a more detailed neurally-inspired model—is highly appropriate. It seems, though, that the basic assumptions of the lower-level system need to be more complex than simple associations between patterns. More generally, from the perspective of the separate systems approach it appears that inflectional morphology, as a combinatorial system, is best understood as being in the same processing domain as other grammatical

---

[52] Attica and Sing Sing are both New York prisons in which inmates have rioted.

[53] Also note that no equivalent argument to the one about 'noun or adjective thinly disguised as a verb' has been made about the situation often considered analogous to the past tense, namely the reading of words with irregular spelling-to-word correspondences (see Chapter 4). In this area a connectionist model (Plaut et al., 1996), and a hybrid one, that of Zorzi et al. (1998), remain two of the strongest candidates. The closest analogue of this type of model in the inflectional domain is that of Westermann and colleagues (e.g. Westermann & Goebel, 1995; Westermann et al., 1999). These models, like the Zorzi et al. model, use a combination of direct input-output connections, which learn to encode regulars, and connections via hidden units, which learn to encode irregulars. With such a model it would be fairly straightforward to prime or inhibit the 'irregular route'. The real issue is not, however, whether connectionist principles can learn the regular mapping—they clearly can. It is whether inflectional morphology should be treated within the same processing domain as phrase-level syntactic structure.

(i.e. syntactic) processes. Indeed, linguistic generalisations provide some of the strongest evidence that they are produced through separable operations, and not much of the apparently more solidly scientific cognitive neuroscience evidence. The fMRI evidence in particular is far from compelling.

To summarise, as in the case of action, morphological operations may be understood as the result of sub-symbolic and symbolic processes working in tandem, with the language system being differentiated into what linguists call a lexicon and a grammar. Given this, the issues concerning the past tense can be subsumed under the much more global issue of the relation between syntactic processing on the one hand and lexical processing on the other. It is to this issue which we now turn.

8.8 Syntactic Operations: Comprehension

In all of cognition, the paradigmatic example of unconscious rule-following behaviour is the use of syntax. Traditionally in cognitive science, under the influence of theories of generative grammar, syntactic operations have been viewed as taking place fairly autonomously from the compiling of lexical semantic representations. It was assumed that, during comprehension, the outputs of the two types of process were integrated fairly late in the processing stream (e.g. Frazier & Rayner, 1982; Frazier, 1987). However more recently, theorists influenced by computational techniques of incremental interpretation of an utterance (e.g. Altmann & Steedman, 1988), constraint satisfaction and especially connectionism have tended to conflate the two types of operation. Thus McClelland et al. (1989) implemented syntactic and semantic constraints in the same network, arguing that the two types of process are 'inextricably interwoven in the connections' (p. 313). (For related perspectives see also: Bates and MacWhinney (1989); MacDonald et al. (1994); Seidenberg and MacDonald (1999).)

Does the cognitive neuroscience evidence point to separable processes for syntactic and semantic operations during comprehension? The original clinical picture of the Broca's aphasic patient was that they had severe problems in producing speech, particularly its syntactic aspects (including function words and inflections: Goodglass and Kaplan, 1972; see Section 1.3). However, comprehension was held to be normal. More recently, the category of 'Broca's aphasic patient' has been argued to be a functionally heterogeneous one, there being considerable variability in the degree of syntactic disorder (i.e. of agrammatism in production) (Berndt et al., 1996). Complementarily, in a classic paper Caramazza and Zurif (1976) showed the generalisation about comprehension to be unfounded. If one

uses so-called *reversible sentences* e.g. 'the girl kissed the boy', where the sentence would be equally easily interpretable if the noun phrases are switched, then (agrammatic) Broca's aphasic patients can have great difficulty in selecting a matching picture.[54] They have particular difficulties with reversible passives, e.g. 'the girl is kissed by the boy' (e.g. Schwartz et al., 1980b). However they can perform almost normally on non-reversible sentences such as 'the boy kicked the ball' (e.g. Berndt et al., 1997), and their performance on comprehending individual lexical items, in particular nouns, can be virtually perfect. Thus, these patients are able to use semantic cues (semantic plausibility) but not syntactic cues (in this case, word order) to control the assignment of thematic roles[55] to the subject and object of a sentence.

By contrast, in patients with semantic impairments, syntactic operations can be spared.[56] The most detailed analysis is that carried out by Breedin and Saffran (1999) on a semantic dementia patient DM, who was discussed in Chapter 6. In that chapter it was shown that DM had a much reduced knowledge of the semantics of concrete words. However in their later study Breedin and Saffran showed by a variety of means that the syntactic processing of the patient was intact. Thus Table 8.5 gives his performance on subtests of the Philadelphia Comprehension Battery. His poor performance on tests dependent upon word meaning is very clear. By March 1995 he was scoring well below the aphasic group. Consider, though, the *reverse role distractors* test, where word order is critical. A sentence such as 'The policeman shoots the robber' is presented with two pictures, one of the policeman shooting the robber and the other with the roles reversed. DM's performance was above the normal mean. What is critical in this set of pictures is that the two concrete nouns are semantically very different from each other.

Experimental tests confirmed this pattern. Even when DM could no longer distinguish between the meaning of pairs of words (e.g. *lion, tiger*) he performed perfectly (240/240) at pointing to the correct animal in a picture given the instruction 'The lion carried the tiger. Show me the tiger.' However on ten trials where the instruction did not match the picture, as the picture showed the animals in the incorrect roles, he always pointed incorrectly. Thus he was using the syntax of sentence to identify the target rather than the word meanings.

---

[54] To complicate matters, the same pattern of performance was also shown by a group of five non-agrammatic conduction aphasics (Caramazza & Zurif, 1976).

[55] Thematic roles, such as *agent* or *patient*, are relations between the subject, object or indirect object of a sentence and its main verb.

[56] See FNMS Section 12.3 for early evidence of this contrast.

TABLE 8.5 Percentage of correct responses of DM on subtests of the Philadelphia Comprehension Battery at several points in time. The rightmost columns show performance of aphasics and controls. There are 60 items in each of the subtests shown.

	DM			Aphasics (n = 56)	Controls (n = 23)
	March 1992	**July 1993**	**March 1995**		
Tests of semantics:					
Within category lexical comprehension	88%	88%	75%	92% (14%)	99% (2%)
Synonymy judgement	80%	63%	56%	76% (18%)	96% (5%)
Tests of syntax:					
Grammaticality judgement	92%	95%	95%	83% (12%)	97% (3%)
Reverse role distractors	98%	98%	97%	73% (15%)	96% (5%)

Data from Breedin and Saffran (1999).

Breedin and Saffran also used a word-monitoring paradigm developed by Marslen-Wilson and Tyler (1980) in which subjects are required to detect a probe word in a following sentence that is syntactically scrambled, semantically anomalous or normal (see Table 8.6). Normal subjects were on average 22 msec faster in detecting the target on the syntactically correct but semantically anomalous sentences (condition b) than on the scrambled sentences (condition c). DM showed a 22-msec speed-up when first tested and 15-msec speed-up when tested a second time 7 months later. However when semantic information is added normal subjects speed up further—on average by another 64 msec (range 19–139 msec). DM, however, only improved by a further 11 msec on first testing session and 8msec on the second—on both occasions well outside the normal range. Thus he shows the normal improvement given the addition of syntactic constraints but obtains no further help from semantic ones, even though semantic ones are the more useful for the normal subject. Furthermore a detailed qualitative analysis of the quantitative aspects of DM's speech (proportion of closed-class words, complexity of auxiliary constructions, etc) showed it to be essentially normal.

A variety of other studies have shown evidence that semantic dementia patients are much less impaired syntactically than semantically (e.g. Hodges et al., 1994; Kertesz et al., 1998; Garrard et al., 2004). Thus, as far as concrete nouns are concerned, there is a classical double dissociation between lexical semantic and syntactic operations involved in the assignment of thematic roles. This suggests that certain of the underlying processes are separable (see Section 4.2).

Can we localise the separable syntactic process? Certain neuropsychological group studies have suggested a specific locus for syntactic operations in comprehension. In particular, Dronkers and her colleagues (2004) conducted an extensive analysis of 64 left-hemisphere stroke patients on 11 subtests of the receptive version of the Curtiss–Yamada Comprehensive Language Evaluation (CYCLE-R: Curtiss & Yamada, 1988) using voxel-based lesion-symptom mapping (VLSM: Bates et al., 2003).[57] In the CYCLE-R test, subjects are auditorily presented with a sentence and required to select a matching picture from an array of three or four line drawings. Subtests assess comprehension of different syntactic constructions, such as simple declarative sentences, subject relative clauses, agentless passives, and so on. When composite scores were analysed, five areas were found to be associated with impaired comprehension: middle temporal gyrus, anterior superior temporal gyrus, superior temporal sulcus/BA39, BA46 and BA47. The results are shown in Figure 8.24. Analysis of individual subtests appears to show some degree of specialisation. Thus patients with middle temporal gyrus (MTG) lesions performed worse on comprehension of possessives and simple declarative sentences than patients without MTG lesions. By contrast, BA46 was only implicated in the comprehension of more complex constructions such as double-embeddings and object or subject relatives. Lesions to Broca's areas (BA 44/45) and Wernicke's area (BA22) were not found to contribute to the patients' deficits.

A difficulty with interpreting these findings, however, is that patient performance on the subtests of the CYCLE-R does not doubly-dissociate. Rather, the subtests may be ordered in terms of difficulty, with patients who fail, for example, object relatives generally also

---

[57] VLSM, like VBM, involves computerised voxel-by-voxel reconstruction of patient lesions onto a standardised template and then correlating lesion site with patient performance on each dependent measure in a manner analogous to standard imaging techniques. The difference is that VLSM makes an all-or-none choice for each voxel.

TABLE 8.6 Stimuli from the word monitoring task of Breedin and Saffran (1999). Subjects were required to detect a probe word in each of the three conditions. In the examples given, the probe is *crown*.

Condition	Stimuli
Normal	People came from all over the world to see the coronation. The bishop placed the *crown* on the king's head.
Anomalous	World took from all over the life to use the mobster. The shelf kept the *crown* on the apartment's church.
Scrambled	Over took to the mobster world the life from all use. Shelf on the church *crown* the apartment's the kept.

failing double-embeddings, but not vice versa. Indeed, more generally, group studies of comprehension deficits tend to show a similar rank ordering of difficulty of different syntactic structures, regardless of aphasic classification (Caplan & Hildebrandt, 1988).[58]

A somewhat contrasting pattern of results has been obtained by Caplan et al. (1996). The comprehension performance of a group of 60 stroke patients (46 left hemisphere and 14 right hemisphere) and 21 neurologically healthy control subjects was examined on a set of sentence types which involved a range of syntactic operations (including many that overlap with the CYCLE-R subtests). Patients had to act out the sentences using toy animals or dolls. Patients with left-hemisphere damage performed more poorly than patients with right-hemisphere damage, who in turn performed more poorly than control subjects. Within the left-hemisphere group, patients with more anterior lesions, in particular of Broca's area, did not differ in their pattern of performance from those with more posterior lesions. Size of lesion was not an important variable.[59] The authors suggest two possibilities. First, that a critical area lies close to the line separating the posterior from anterior lesions. This would fit reasonably well with the position of Dronkers and her colleagues. Alternatively they suggest that syntactic operations in sentence comprehension may invoke a network in the perisylvian region. Indeed localisation studies such as those of Dronkers et al. ignore the possibility that certain disorders might arise because of disconnection between parts of the network (Catani et al., 2003).

Early functional imaging studies were more consistent. A set of four studies which manipulated the syntactic complexity of a presented sentence was reviewed by Hagoort et al. (1999). They showed a similar pattern of localisations. Thus in one—a study by Stromswold et al. (1996)—subjects were required to judge the grammatical acceptability of sentences which, though of equal length, differed in structural complexity (e.g. 'The juice that the child spilled stained the rug' is syntactically more complex than 'The child spilled the juice that stained the rug'). Half of the sentences contained a semantic anomaly that had to be detected. The critical contrasts in all four studies involved the left inferior frontal region (see Figure 8.25).

These studies are often interpreted as supporting the idea that syntactic processing in comprehension involves Broca's region. However there are two reasons for raising doubts about this conclusion. First, there is no model of the on-line processing in the tasks. Plausibly though such a model would involve post-syntactic operations related to verbal working memory. Thus in the example just given, subjects may repeat the embedded sentence in order to comprehend it. Therefore there is an additional process which potentially involves the left inferior to middle frontal cortex that could be involved in the more difficult condition. Indeed the activation sites of at least two of the studies surveyed by Hagoort and colleagues, those of Caplan et al. (1998) and Stowe et al. (1994), are close to those implicated in memory encoding experiments to be discussed in Chapter 10. Second, there is no explanation of the discrepancy with the lesion results of Caplan and colleagues discussed above. It would appear that we are again in a situation where conclusions from neuroimaging and neuropsychology do not agree, and, following the principles laid down in Chapter 5, no conclusions about the cognitive architecture can therefore be based on the localisation evidence.

An alternative hypothesis is that left IFG is specifically involved in the representation of verbs. Selective difficulties in retrieving verbs rather than nouns have long been known (e.g. Miceli et al., 1984; McCarthy & Warrington, 1985; Zingeser & Berndt, 1990). Moreover, using rTMS, Shapiro et al. (2001) found that verb production was affected more than noun production when it was applied over left frontal cortex. Following on

---

[58] Dronkers and colleagues also do not report any lesion-site subtractions between patients impaired on one sentence type and patients not impaired on that sentence type (following the method of Rorden and Karnath, 2004; see also Rorden et al. 2007). Such subtractions have the potential to provide further evidence for the isolation of specific subprocesses.

[59] An earlier study—that of Vanier and Caplan (1990)—found a similar effect for production.

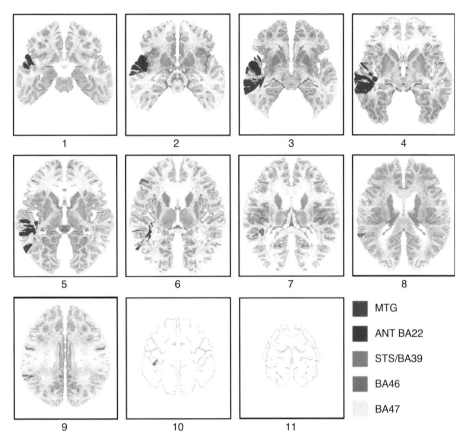

Fig. 8.24 Results of the VLSM analysis of Dronkers et al. (2004) of 64 left-hemisphere stroke patients. All patients completed the CYCLE-R battery. Damage to any of the five marked areas was found to impair performance. MTG = Middle Temporal Gyrus; STS = Superior Temporal Sulcus. Reprinted from *Cognition*, 92(1–2), N.F. Dronkers, D.P. Wilkins, R.D. Van Valin, B.B. Redfern and J.J. Jaeger, Lesion analysis of the brain areas involved in language comprehension, pp. 145–177, Copyright (2004), with permission from Elsevier.

from this, Shapiro and Caramazza (2003) reported an ischaemic stroke patient, RC, with extensive left posterior frontal lesions affecting Broca's area and nearby regions. RC was impaired on a sentence completion task when required to generate an inflected form of a verb (e.g. *judges*, as in 'These people judge, this person …') but not the phonologically identical inflected form

of the same noun (e.g. *judges*, as in 'This is a judge, these people are …'). Subsequently, Shapiro et al. (2006) reported an fMRI study of noun and verb production in normal subjects. Verb production led to increased activity in left prefrontal cortex and the left superior parietal lobule. The latter activity is interpreted as reflecting action-related aspects of verbs, while the

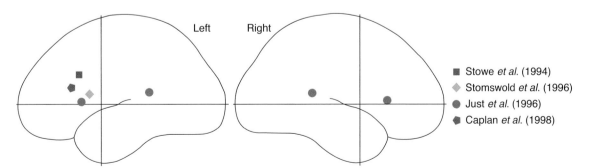

Fig. 8.25 Regions found to be differentially involved in processing complex syntactic constructions, as found in a metaanalysis of studies of syntactic complexity by Hagoort et al. (1999). Adapted with permission from P. Hagoort, C.M. Brown and L. Osterhout, 1999, The neurocognition of syntactic processing. In C.M. Brown and P. Hagoort (Eds), *Neurocognition of Language*. By permission of Oxford University Press.

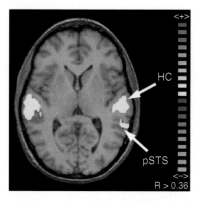 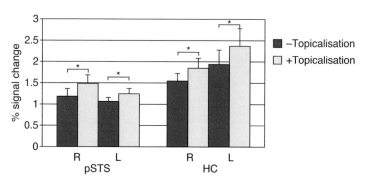

Fig. 8.26 Topicalisation effects in posterior Superior Temporal Sulcus (pSTS) and Heschl's Complex (HC). The statistical parametric map (left) shows the relative contribution found by Ben-Shachar et al. (2004) of the +topicalisation conditions (in yellow) versus the –topicalisation conditions (in blue) in posterior temporal regions of interest. Mean percentage signal change in bilateral posterior STS and Heschl's complex is shown on the right. Error bars denote one standard error of the mean. Reprinted from *NeuroImage*, *21*(4), M. Ben-Shachar, D. Palti and Y. Grodzinsky, Neural correlates of syntactic movement: converging evidence from two fMRI experiments, 1320–1336. Copyright (2004), with permission from Elsevier.

former, and the previous two studies, are argued to reflect the representation of verbs in left IFG. In contrast, and in line with the arguments presented in the previous section, Tyler et al. (2004a) argue on the basis of an fMRI study of semantic relatedness of written stimuli that nouns and verbs do not differ in the (inferior temporal) localisation of their neural representation, but that activity differences in left IFG reflect greater morphological processing of inflected verbs.

More recent imaging work has suggested that areas beyond Broca's region (or left IFG more generally) may be involved in syntactic operations related to comprehension. For example, Ben-Shachar et al. (2004) scanned subjects when performing an auditory comprehension task using five types of stimulus sentence (baseline, dative-shifted, so-called topicalised direct object, so-called topicalised indirect object, and baseline with an adjunct, all in Hebrew).[60] When compared with baseline and dative-shifted constructions (e.g. 'John gave the red book to the professor from Oxford' and 'John gave the professor from Oxford the red book'), topicalised constructions (e.g. 'The red book John gave to the professor from Oxford') resulted in greater activity in left IFG, but also in left ventral precentral sulcus and bilaterally in posterior STS (see Figure 8.26). Given that topicalised constructions are considered to be syntactically more complex than baseline equivalents due to the non-standard position of the object of the main verb, a plausible interpretation is that greater involvement of these areas is required in the processing of

complex or 'marked' syntactic constructions than of simpler syntactic constructions.[61]

Superior and medial temporal regions have also been found to be preferentially activated during the processing of local syntactic ambiguities. Rodd et al. (2004) (see also Tyler & Marslen-Wilson, 2008) studied MRI activation during processing of sentences containing a local syntactic ambiguity, such as 'Flying kites …'. This is syntactically ambiguous in that it can be a verb phrase (as in 'Flying kites is fun') or a noun phrase (as in 'Flying kites are dangerous'). Moreover one continuation or the other may be preferred in different contexts. The two versions can be compared if disambiguating continuations, such as 'are' or 'is', are provided. Processing of the non-preferred continuation, which was argued to require syntactic reanalysis of an initial fragment, led to increased activation of left IFG, left MTG and, to a lesser extent, right STG. Semantically ambiguous sentences led to increased activation of a subset of these areas restricted to the left IFG (see Figure 8.27; see also Rodd et al., 2005).

Both the imaging results and the patient studies support the hypothesis that language processing involves a set of mostly left lateralised regions including all three of the lateral temporal gyri, but they do not argue strongly for any specific localisation of syntactic operations. However we have not attempted to characterise syntactic operations from the perspective of theoretical linguistics. It is plausible that such a characterisation

---

[60] A dative-shifted sentence is one involving a dative verb, such as give or sell, where the indirect object precedes the direct object. A topicalised sentence is one where the object of the main verb occurs as the first constituent of the sentence.

[61] Ben-Shachar et al. interpret their results in terms of the Chomskyan linguistic theory of movement and trace co-indexation (see below). We find the interpretation in terms of general syntactic construction difficulty more parsimonious and more consistent with the aphasic comprehension data discussed above.

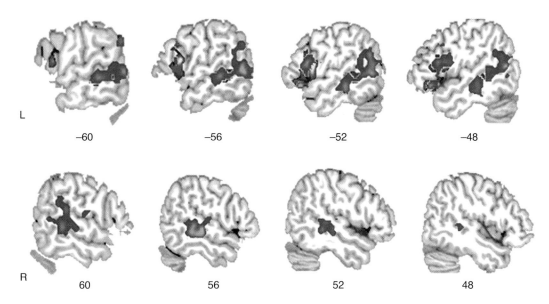

Fig. 8.27 Saggital slices showing the effects of processing syntactic (blue) and semantic (red) ambiguity in left and right hemispheres. Reprinted with permission from L.K. Tyler & W.D. Marslen-Wilson, Fronto-temporal brain systems supporting spoken language comprehension. *Philosophical Transactions of the Royal Society B: Biological Sciences, 363,* 1–18 (figure 6, page 1046), 2008, The Royal Society.

could reveal distinct syntactic operations which might be differentially involved in different linguistic constructions, and differentially localised.

One speculation, which is based on an essentially linguistic framework and that has received great attention from a cognitive neuroscience perspective, is the 'trace-deletion hypothesis' of Grodzinsky (1984, 2000), who argues that Broca's aphasia as a syndrome is a *natural kind*.[62] He claims that Broca's aphasics have a problem in a specific syntactic operation; this is the operation required to associate a noun phrase that is realised in a non-standard position with its thematic role.[63] Thus, consider the sentences:

(1) Who did Lorraine describe to Annette?

(2) Who did Sally describe Maria to?

Within Government and Binding theory (Chomsky, 1981), the version of Chomskyan linguistic theory

current when Grodzinsky initially developed his account of the Broca's aphasic deficit, a noun phrase that is not realised in its standard (canonical) position in a syntactic structure would form a *trace* (indicated by *t* in sentences 1′ and 2′ below), namely a phonologically silent entity which would occupy the canonical position of the sentential subject. The trace is co-indexed with *who*, as indicated by the shared subscripts. In terms influenced by an earlier conceptual approach in linguistics this involves a transformation; such sentences are held to involve *syntactic movement*. So one can represent this aspect of the syntax of sentence (1) and (2) as:

(1′) Who$_i$ did Lorraine describe t_i to Annette?

(2′) Who$_i$ did Sally describe Maria to t_i?

Syntactic movement occurs in a variety of constructions. For instance, a so-called 'verbal' passive such as:

(3) The boy was pushed by the girl.

requires two traces, as in:

(3′) [The boy]$_i$ was [$_{ve}$ t_j pushed t_i] by [the girl]$_j$.

Semantic interpretation of a sentence with syntactic movement requires assignment of traces to the thematic roles of the main verb. This assignment, Grodzinsky argues, is impaired in Broca's aphasics because traces are not properly maintained. The Broca's aphasic must therefore fall back on default interpretation strategies (e.g. of assigning a sentence initial noun phrase to the thematic role of *agent*). Grodzinsky (2000) thus gives a set of constructions where Broca's aphasics are said to be unimpaired, and a set where they are said to be at chance (see Table 8.7). He summarises:

---

[62] In other words, in the terminology of Chapter 4 it is a functional syndrome.

[63] Grodzinsky's position is closely tied to Chomskyan linguistic theory. As that linguistic theory has evolved—through Government and Binding (Chomsky, 1981) to Minimalism (Chomsky, 1995)—the statement of Grodzinsky's position has changed. Thus, in earlier statements of Grodzinsky's theory (Grodzinsky, 1984, 2000), the Broca's aphasic deficit was held to be one of 'trace deletion', while in its most recent incarnation (Grodzinsky & Friederici, 2006), Broca's aphasics are held to have a selective impairment of the MOVE$_{XP}$ operation. The essence of Grodzinsky's position, however, has remained constant. For consistency we use the terminology of Government and Binding theory.

TABLE 8.7 Corresponding constructions held by Grodzinsky (2000) to cause differential difficulties for Broca's aphasic patients.

Constructions with performance above chance		Constructions with performance at chance
Active:	⇔	Passive:
The girl pushed the boy		*The boy was pushed by the girl*
Subject relative clause:	⇔	Object relative clause:
The girl who pushed the boy was tall		*The boy who the girl pushed was tall*
Show me the girl who pushed the boy		*Show me the boy who the girl pushed*
It-cleft (raised subject):	⇔	It-cleft (raised object):
It was the girl who pushed the boy		*It is the boy who the girl pushed*
Active (with *in* prepositional phrase):	⇔	Passive:
The boy was interested in the girl		*The woman was unmasked by the man*
Active (with *by* prepositional phrase):		
The woman was uninspired by the man		

'It thus appears that most aspects of syntax, whether pertaining to basic relations or to the more intricate dependencies, are intact in the comprehension of Broca's aphasics, with one salient exception: syntactic movement—grammatical transformations' (p. 5) That is, what Broca's aphasics cannot do is construct thematic roles when a lexical item has a role in the syntactic structure different from its canonical position in a sentence, as indicated, by the co-indexation shown in (1'), (2') and (3').

Grodzinsky's main evidence has concerned the passive. Grodzinsky et al. (1999) surveyed 42 different patients derived from 17 different studies of the active/passive. The results are presented in Figure 8.28. The surveyed studies involved two-choice tests of comprehension. Chance performance was therefore 50%. Grodzinsky points out that the actives have a mode of 100% while the passives have a mean and median of 55%, supporting his trace deletion hypothesis.

A variety of objections can be raised to Grodzinsky's theory. For example, as briefly mentioned earlier, Broca's aphasic patients do not produce a single prototypic pattern of performance (Berndt et al., 1996; Caramazza et al., 2001; Luzzatti et al., 2001). Indeed Cappa et al. (2000) argue that there is no convincing evidence that Broca's aphasia is a clear-cut functional syndrome—a cognitive natural kind. One cannot appeal to neurology to define Broca's aphasia. It has been well known since the work of Mohr et al. (1978) that Broca's aphasia, at least in chronic patients, requires a lesion which is much larger than Broca's area. There is also no account of how severity, such as that reported in the Dronkers et al. (2004) study discussed earlier, might impact upon performance. This is because the theory draws a binary distinction between completely impaired and unimpaired performance on the co-indexation of traces. It is clear that the Grodzinsky theory—at least in its straightforward version—is incorrect.

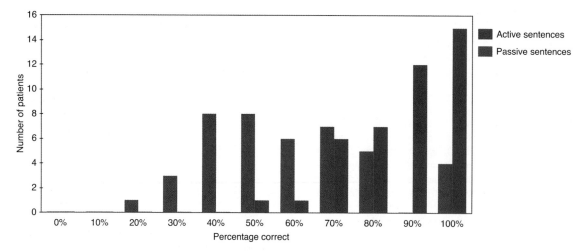

Fig. 8.28 Frequency histogram showing the number of patients (out of 42) at each performance level in a survey of two-choice comprehension tests of active and passive sentences by Grodzinsky et al. (1999). Data from Grodzinsky et al. (1999).

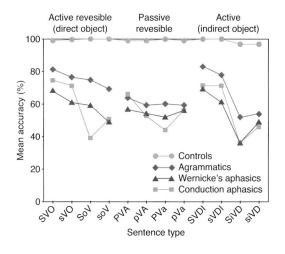

Sample stimuli		
Type	*Example*	*Literal translation*
Active reversible sentences		
SVO	Mario cerca Flora	Mario seeks Flora
sVO	Lui cerca Flora	He seeks Flora
SoV	Mario la cerca	Mario her seeks
soV	Lui la cerca	He her seeks
Passive reversible sentences		
PVA	Flora è cercata a Mario	Flora is sought by Mario
pVA	Lei è cercata a Mario	She is sought by Mario
PVa	Flora è cercata da lui	Flora is sought by him
pVa	Lei è cercata da lui	She is sought by him
Active sentences with indirect object		
SVDI	Mario dà un regalo a Flora	Mario gives a present to Flora
sVDI	Lui dà un regalo a Flora	He gives a present to Flora
SiVD	Mario le dà un regalo	Mario her gives a present
siVD	Lui le dà un regalo	He her gives a present

Fig. 8.29 Mean comprehension accuracy of controls and three patient groups on 12 sentence types. Comprehension was tested with a sentence to picture matching task. Chance performance in all cases was 25%. Adapted from C. Luzzatti, A. Toraldo, M.T. Guast, G. Ghirardi, L. Lorenzi and C. Guarnaschelli, 2001, Comprehension of reversible active and passive sentences in agrammatism. *Aphasiology*, 15(5), 419–441.

It is also clear that, at least on passive reversible sentences, the difficulties that Broca's aphasic patients have are quite unrelated to the most obvious manifestations of their syntactic competence in speech production. Thus Luzzatti et al. (2001) found the same pattern of performance on reversible passives in a group of ten Wernicke's aphasics and six conduction aphasics (see Figure 8.29), echoing the earlier findings of Caramazza and Zurif (1976). This is just what one might expect given the dissociations between syntactic operations in comprehension and speech production first noted by Miceli et al. (1983).[64]

Moreover the linguist, Kay (2000), while accepting Grodzinsky's empirical claims at face value, argues that they do not necessarily entail a hypothesis relating to syntactic movement, traces or 'trace deletion'. He takes the traditional route of the *logical subject* in linguistics and argues that the interpretation strategy of the typical Broca's aphasia is 'logical subject first'. Note that, by analogy with the case of letter-by-letter reading in pure alexia discussed in Section 4.12, the behavioural manifestation may not transparently reflect the underlying computational impairment. Indeed a 'logical subject first' strategy might arise for a whole set of reasons different from syntactic disabilities, such as impairments of working memory capacities or even a failure to interpret certain lexical items.

A second great problem with Grodzinsky's approach is that he has no task analysis. Following the syntactic analysis, thematic roles must be correctly assigned but that information must be retained while the process of

matching with the high-level visual semantic representations in the picture is carried out. Grodzinsky has nothing to say about these necessary additional processes and so he has not checked that they can be normally implemented in Broca's aphasia patients. Essentially like a good follower of Chomsky he has only a competence theory. The patients unfortunately however manifest performance.

Despite these conclusions, Grodzinsky's attempt to relate the comprehension deficits of Broca's aphasics to linguistic theory is appropriate. One difficulty is that while Chomskyan linguistic theory remains dominant, as mentioned in Section 1.7 it is not the only option within theoretical linguistics. A range of alternative frameworks has been proposed (e.g. Lexical Functional Grammar: Bresnan, 2001; Categorial Grammar: Steedman, 1996; Head-driven Phrase Structure Grammar: Pollard & Sag, 1994; Tree-Adjoining Grammar: Joshi & Schabes, 1997). The common feature of these (and recent versions of Chomskyan theory) is the use of highly structured lexical entries, i.e. representations of words in which syntactic category information is supplemented with information concerning number, agreement and, in the case of 'phrasal heads' such as nouns or verbs, the types of syntactic element required to complete the phrase.[65] With such highly structured

---

[64] See FNMS Section 7.6.

[65] Thus, a verb such as *chase*, which may head a verb phrase, requires a single noun phrase that is either unmarked or of accusative case to form that verb phrase. In contrast, a verb such as *promises* requires both a noun phrase (such as *Tracy*) and an additional infinitive verb phrase (such as *to wash the dishes*) to form a complete verb phrase (to give *promises Tracy to wash the dishes*). See the structures in Figure 8.30 for a further illustration.

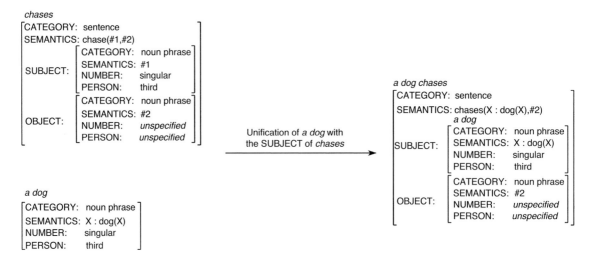

Fig. 8.30 An illustration of unification, adapted from the linguistic framework of Head-driven Phrase Structure Grammar (Pollard & Sag, 1994). When the structure corresponding to *a dog* is unified with the SUBJECT of the structure corresponding to *chases*, the values for the SEMANTICS attributes are bound. If the phrase is completed by an object noun phrase, such as *a rabbit*, then this will be unified with the OBJECT attribute and hence the semantic content of *a rabbit* will be unified with the variable #2. Note that the structure corresponding to a plural noun phrase or one that is not in the third person would not unify with the SUBJECT of *chases*, capturing the ungrammaticality of a construction such as *The dogs chases…*

lexical entries, syntactic rules such as 'S → NP VP' may be eliminated in favour of a handful of very general rules of grammar (see the discussion of X-bar theory in Section 1.7) or more general structure-building operations.

The lexicalist approach is reflected in Grodzinsky's recent work (Grodzinsky & Friederici, 2006). This follows the more recent minimalist theory of Chomsky (e.g. Bošković & Lasnik, 2007) in which the 'building blocks of syntactic knowledge' are reduced to five syntactic operations—LEX, MERGE, MOVE$_{XP}$, MOVE$_{VP}$ and BIND. Grodzinsky's stated goal is to localise each of these operations at the neurological level. He holds that only one of these, MOVE$_{XP}$, is impaired in Broca's aphasic patients. An alternative approach linking lexicalist syntactic theory with brain-based studies of comprehension is provided by Hagoort (2005). This is conceptually very different, as it is not limited to competence alone. It builds on a variety of approaches in different domains, including Joshi's Tree-Adjoining Grammar (Joshi & Schabes, 1997), Jackendoff's proposal of a single general grammar rule, UNIFY-PIECES (Jackendoff, 2002), and Vosse and Kempen's computational account of human sentence processing (Vosse & Kempen, 2000).

Unification is a well-established information-theoretic operation in which compatible or mutually consistent information is merged (see Figure 8.30). The operation is central to a number of formal theories of syntax (see Pollard & Sag, 1987, 1994). It is also straightforward to develop and implement sentence processing algorithms using unification (for examples in COGENT

see Cooper, 2002, chapter 7). For such algorithms to have psychological plausibility, however, they must account for a range of psycholinguistic findings. The results that have received most attention relate to the resolution of syntactic ambiguity. Vosse and Kempen (2000) present a computational model that embodies an algorithm aimed primarily at accounting for this data. The model is of particular interest as it has also been used to account for the comprehension deficits of aphasics. The algorithm makes substantial use of a 'unification space'—a kind of short-term working store in which representations of alternative constituent structures compete through a process of lateral inhibition (similar to the mechanism underlying competition within the contention scheduling model discussed in Section 8.3 and the competitive queuing models of Sections 7.6 and 7.7; see also Chapter 3). Thus, in processing a sentence such as *The woman sees the man with the telescope*, lexical frames associated with the nouns and verb are activated and the different ways in which the three noun phrases can be mapped to the thematic roles of the verb compete. This competition is influenced by several factors. One is word order, with an interpretation in which the agent precedes the verb being preferred. Another is the need to form a coherent structure in which function words such as *with* are incorporated (see Figure 8.31). If such a structure can be formed, it will be hierarchical, with the noun phrases being so-called *sub-constituents* of the verbal lexical frame.

The functioning of the Vosse and Kempen model is governed by a number of parameters that specify

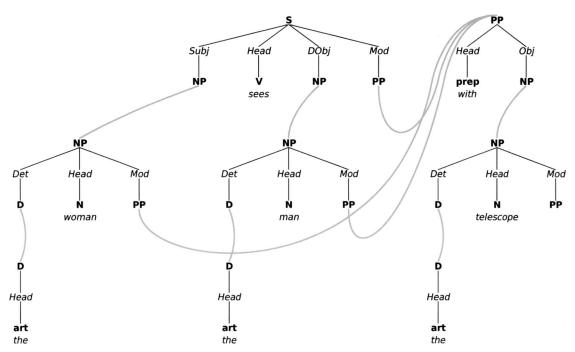

Fig. 8.31 The structures (in black) and a subset of the unification links (in blue) employed by the Vosse and Kempen model when parsing *The woman sees the man with the telescope*. Unification links associated with the same sub-constituent (here, the three links associated with the prepositional phrase *with the telescope*) compete with each other, such that when the model settles only one is highly active.

how the relative strengths of alternative constituent structures interact. For example, one parameter determines the rate at which activation of lexical nodes decays. Another determines the resilience of unification links, which is held to increase with the distance between its constituents; this favours local dependencies over long-distance dependencies. A sentence is said to be successfully processed when the activations of all unification links settle into a stable state. In this case only one link from each set in competition will have high activation, with the highly active link in each set specifying the preferred interpretation of the sentence. Vosse and Kempen determined optimal values of the parameters such that the model could -successfully process a range of standard constructions (including those commonly assessed in agrammatic comprehension studies). They were then able to account for the impaired performance of aphasic patients by varying key parameters (including lexical decay and sensitivity of unification links to inhibition). They used the performance of 144 aphasic patients studied by Caplan et al. (1985). The fit of the impaired performance of the model to patient data is shown in Table 8.8.

Vosse and Kempen's account of comprehension deficits is not grounded in any particular theory of the deficit. Their fit to the data is obtained by an essentially unguided search through the model's five-dimensional parameter space.[66] The quality of the fit is patchy—good for most constructions but poorer for some. Moreover a gross simplification is made in assuming that aphasics can be characterised in terms of a single parameter varying from normal to grossly agrammatic.

The lack of theory underlying the modelling of the impairment of patients limits the extent to which the model can be held to capture the comprehension deficits of agrammatic patients.[67] Nevertheless, Hagoort et al. (2003b) have argued that competition in the model's unification space between alternative syntactic structural representations is consistent with ERP findings concerning the effects of syntactic ambiguity in comprehension. Thus, ERP studies have shown that syntactic violations during sentence processing normally result in a positive shift in the ERP signal approximately 600 msec after presentation of the syntactically invalid word; this is known as the P600/SPS—syntactic positive shift (see Figure 8.32). Agrammatic aphasic patients do not show this effect (Hagoort et al., 2003a).

---

[66] The model has a total of thirteen parameters. Only five of these are varied in the patient simulations. No theoretical reason is given for holding the remaining eight constant.

[67] Haarmann et al. (1997) provide an alternative computational account of the comprehension deficits of agrammatic patients in terms of a resource deficit. Empirically, their account is of comparable adequacy to that of Vosse and Kempen.

TABLE 8.8 Comparison of the performance of agrammatic aphasic patients and the Vosse and Kempen (2000) model on eight sentence types. Patient data is from Caplan et al. (1985), corrected for chance, as reported in Vosse and Kempen (2000).

Construction	Patient data	Simulation data
Active: *The elephant hit the monkey*	73%	78%
It-cleft (raised subject): *It was the elephant that hit the monkey*	71%	69%
Passive: *The elephant was hit by the monkey*	36%	47%
Dative: *The elephant gave the monkey to the rabbit*	52%	67%
It-cleft (raised object): *It was the elephant that the monkey hit*	20%	20%
Subject relative clause: *The elephant hit the monkey that hugged the rabbit*	36%	58%
Dative passive: *The elephant was given to the monkey by the rabbit*	31%	30%
Object relative clause: *The elephant that the monkey hit hugged the rabbit*	17%	19%

Hagoort (2003) suggest that the P600/SPS is related to the time it takes to establish sufficiently strong unification links, with the amplitude of the signal being modulated by the amount of competition.

Since the Vosse and Kempen model can incorporate both syntactic and semantic constraints within its unification space, it is also able to account for immediate effects of semantic violations. These give rise to a strong N400 signal which is independent of the P600/SPS, suggesting that syntactic and semantic constraints are independent but continuously integrated.

Building on this work, Hagoort (2005) argues for three functional subprocesses underlying language processing: lexical memory, unification of linguistic information, and control (see Figure 8.33). Lexical memory is held to provide syntactic frames for the constituents that make up a phrase or sentence. If this is the case, one could assume that the deficits of certain patients would correspond to loss of the syntactic constraint system, which would return us to a purely syntactic interpretation of one form of agrammatism. However, Hagoort localises this component to the posterior superior temporal cortex (i.e. Wernicke's area), but the evidence for this localisation is somewhat weak, although it fits with the findings of Luzzatti et al. (2001) discussed earlier in this section. Unification is held to bind frames into parts of other frames; fMRI studies suggest this process occurs within left IFG (Hagoort et al., 2004). This localisation is also consistent with many of the imaging studies cited above and, through the aphasic simulations of Vosse and Kempen (2000), the classic localisation of

Broca's aphasia.[68] Their model applies in production as well as comprehension. As far as production is concerned, control is held to be involved mainly in discourse and the planning of communicative intentions, analogous to subprocesses of the *conceptualiser* level of Levelt's model discussed in Section 3.5. Related issues will be addressed in Chapter 9.

The general picture that arises from our consideration of syntactic operations is far from conclusive. The brain-based evidence implicates regions in the left inferior frontal gyrus, and bilaterally in the superior and middle temporal gyrii (i.e. similar areas to those involved in morphological operations), but the functional roles of these regions remain heavily disputed. Most critically, there is a lack of convergence between imaging and patient studies. There is even no clear picture of the functional deficit underlying the comprehension difficulties of agrammatic patients. Theoretical and computational linguistics would appear to be well-placed to inform this debate, but Grodzinsky's trace-deletion hypothesis is unable to account adequately for the variability found in comprehension deficits. The approach of Vosse, Kempen and Hagoort is in this respect more promising, but a great deal remains to be done to

---

[68] This account fits with a classic account of agrammatism—that of Linebarger et al. (1983)—namely that the problem for agrammatic listeners is not in actually constructing syntactic representations, but in providing them with a semantic interpretation.

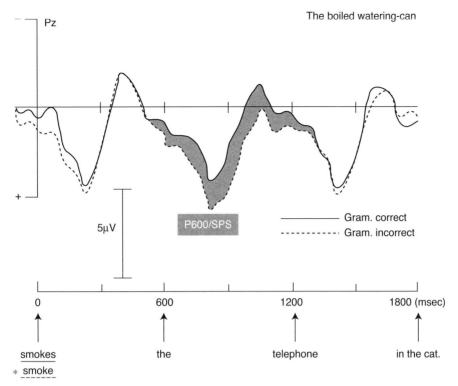

Fig. 8.32 The P600/SPS (syntactic positive shift), as revealed by violated number agreement in a nonsense sentence. Comparison of ERP Pz electrode responses to *The boiled watering-can smoke/smokes the telephone in the cat* reveals a positive peak approximately 600 msec after the agreement violation. Reprinted from *NeuroImage*, 20(S1), P. Hagoort, How the brain solves the binding problem for language: a neurocomputational model of syntactic processing, pp S18–S29, Copyright (2003), with permission from Elsevier.

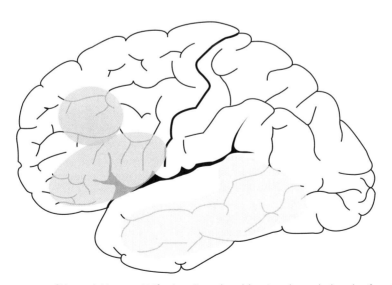

Fig. 8.33 The three components of Hagoort's Memory–Unification–Control model projected onto the lateral surface of the left hemisphere: Memory (yellow) in left temporal cortex, Unification (blue) in left inferior frontal gyrus, and Control (grey) in dorsolateral prefrontal cortex and (not shown) anterior cingulate cortex. Reprinted from *Trends in Cognitive Sciences*, 9(9), P. Hagoort, On Broca, brain, and binding: a new framework, pp 416–423, Copyright (2005), with permission from Elsevier.

properly anchor this work in theoretical linguistics, functional imaging, and patient studies.

8.9 **Conclusions**

We have considered a range of cognitive operations, focussing in four domains: action, spatial processing, morphology and language comprehension. In the first case, the computational task facing the cognitive system is to generate a sequence of motor commands subject to constraints imposed by the motor system, the environment, and typically the context of an intended task. In the second case, it is to map between different representations of physical space. In the third case, the computational task is to map between presumed lexical representations of word forms and their (inflected) phonological realisations. In the final case, it is to generate an interpretation of the linguistic input subject to morphophonological, syntactic and semantic constraints. In at least three of these case cases, the relevant operations are well characterised in terms of constraint satisfaction, the possible exception being spatial operations.

Many other types of cognitive operation exist in other cognitive domains. Indeed, as discussed in Sections 3.5 and 8.7, other cognitive operations are involved in language production, where a representation of a preverbal message (Levelt et al., 1999) is transformed into speech or writing. Such operations cannot be considered in isolation from those involved in comprehension, but the relation between the two is not transparent (see e.g. Hickok & Poeppel, 2004; Howard & Nickels, 2005).

Hierarchical structures appear to play critical roles in two cases. In the case of action they reflect the goal/subgoal structure of purposeful behaviour, while in the case of language comprehension, hierarchical structure reflects the constituent structure of the sentence or sentence fragment. Beyond these similarities, however, there are substantial differences between the computational tasks in the domains. Further differences emerge when other operations such as those related to mental rotation are considered, where hierarchical structuring and constraint satisfaction are less clearly relevant since we are dealing with transformations in 2D or 3D space, which are both qualitatively and quantitatively organised. These computational differences are reflected in evidence of distinct, special purpose, subsystems, each with its own localisation.

There are in fact strong relations between action and language that we have not explored in this chapter. Myrna Schwartz (1995), for example, noted that in both cases analogous structures exist. Thus the arguments or thematic roles of verbs within language correspond to the objects to which actions are applied (see also Schwartz et al., 1991). Thus, both language and action can be conceived of in similar terms. In particular they both have structure, with the *head* of the sentence, the main verb, having an analogous argument structure to action. Both, though, also require constraint satisfaction. Both therefore present the neural machinery with similar computational challenges. Moreover, it has been speculated that the evolutionary and neural basis of language is founded on action (Rizzolatti et al., 1996a), and more specifically imitation. While imaging studies described in this chapter provide some support for this position, with similar areas implicated in language and action processes, dissociations between deficits of action and language suggest that the relation between the two is considerably more complex.

Returning to the issue with which we opened this chapter—that of the characterisation of operations as rewrite-rules versus associative mappings—we see that for action and language neither approach is adequate by itself but that an account of cognitive operations needs to have characteristics of both. This is so whether the operations are subsystem internal (and hence the result of normal, species-wide, developmental processes) or transparently learned (and the result of explicit instruction). With the possible exception of categorical spatial operations, which remain much less well explored, each domain has its specific structural characteristics, potentially captured through rewrite-rules. In addition, other aspects of the domains are captured in the computational process of constraint satisfaction, operationalised as a continuous competitive process between discrete states. Current models implement those states as either symbols with activation values that compete through lateral inhibition, or as learned, mutually exclusive, attractor states. This is consistent with the view of representation and buffers emerging from Chapters 6 and 7.

At the neural level, evidence suggests a strong degree of functional specialisation for cognitive operations, with networks of regions implicated in each case. The specific regions involved, however, reflect the particular computational requirements of one part of a multifaceted overall process.

On Supervisory Processes

9.1 **Introduction**

In Chapter 8 we considered how fairly simple operations involving interactions with objects are carried out by the system called 'Contention Scheduling'. The evolutionary success of humans as a species depends critically on their ability to acquire a large variety of skills for using objects, a qualitatively different level of abilities than that available to our closest ape relatives (see McGrew, 1993). Just as critical, though, especially for the evolutionarily recent explosion in numbers of the human species since the Upper Palaeolithic, has been our ability to confront novel situations creatively (Amati & Shallice, 2007).

There has long been a school of thought within neuropsychology that the prefrontal cortex (PFC) is critical for our ability to act appropriately in non-routine situations. Thus Bianchi (1922) characterised the monkey with a large frontal lesion as having lost the ability to coordinate the different elements of a complex activity. Goldstein working at a roughly comparable period with soldiers with wounds affecting the frontal cortex described them as 'having a difficulty in grasping the whole of a complicated state of affairs, well able to work along old routine lines. But they cannot learn to master new types of task; in new situations … at a loss' (quoted in Rylander, 1939, p. 20). This line of thought concerning prefrontal function was developed clinically most deeply by the Russian neuropsychologist Luria (1966) who in World War II was confronted with large numbers of soldiers with wounds producing prefrontal lesions. He held that the prefrontal cortex was involved in programming all complex non-routine aspects of behaviour, including the preliminary synthesis of a situation, the construction of an appropriate plan, and the monitoring of its application.[1] More succinctly, Luria characterised the functions of the frontal lobes, by which he meant the prefrontal cortex, as the programming, regulation and verification of behaviour.

Luria's perspective on prefrontal function was put into an information-processing conceptual framework by Norman and Shallice (1980, 1986) and Shallice and Burgess (1996), who argued that the contention-scheduling system, discussed in Chapter 8, is modulated by a supervisory system (see Figure 8.5) that comes into play in three broad types of situation. The first is where the situation has important novel elements and routine schemas cannot be relied upon; this would include decision-making. A second is where the difference in pay-off between a successful and an unsuccessful action in the situation would be considerable, as in coping with dangers, dealing with precious fragile objects or the like. The third is where the situation elicits a strong tendency to carry out an inappropriate action, as in overcoming temptation.

How in fact, can non-routine situations be confronted by a cognitive system? In symbolic AI, architectures based on classical planning systems attempted to take the optimal path by considering all plausible contingencies. They were found to be slow and brittle; they could easily be upset by minor unforeseen differences from what they expected (see Russell & Norvig, 1995, for review). In the 1980s this made very appealing decentralised reactive-planning systems, such as those of Brooks (1985, 1991), which used many procedures each specific to a particular type of situation (see Figure 9.1). However, more recently a number of defects of reactive-planners have become clear (see Glasspool, 2005). Being highly reactive to the immediate situation they cannot follow long-term plans or have multiple long-term goals (Gat, 1998). Moreover, as they have no abstract characterisation of their behaviour they are difficult to program for new or complex operations.

In response, researchers began to work with three-layer architectures (e.g. Gat, 1991; Elsaesser & Slack, 1994). In a three-layer architecture, such as that of Gat (1998), the lowest layer consists of a Brooks-style reactive controller (see Figure 9.2). The highest level is a 'deliberative' system which is capable of reasoning and goal-directed behaviour. The middle layer assembles sequences of single behaviours that enable it to attain a higher-level goal using different lower-level behaviours each specific to a context. Glasspool (2005) argued that the middle-layer of the Gat-type architecture is in fact analogous to contention scheduling on the current approach and the highest level corresponds to the supervisory system. So the current planning frameworks used in symbolic AI have a set of systems on different levels which resemble those in the model.

Returning to the human cognitive system, the basic ideas of the Norman–Shallice model are found in a variety of other theories. In attention research, Shiffrin and Schneider (1977) provided evidence for a distinction between controlled and automatic processing. Logan (1988) later showed that race models assuming a competition between two processes could fit reaction time findings in tasks such as arithmetic ones, where an answer can be arrived at either by applying a rule or from memory. Moreover, as we will see in Chapter 12, two-process accounts of reasoning have been developed

---

[1] When normal subjects are presented with a novel problem, the first stage consists of a provisional investigation to obtain the broad structure of the situation, to generate lines of attack on the problem and to set goals. This was amply demonstrated in one of the greatest studies of problem-solving ever undertaken, that of De Groot (1966) on selection of chess moves by chess masters. Patients with lesions to the frontal lobes are held by Luria (1966) to have a 'profound defect' (p. 283) in this first 'preliminary investigation phase of problem-solving'.

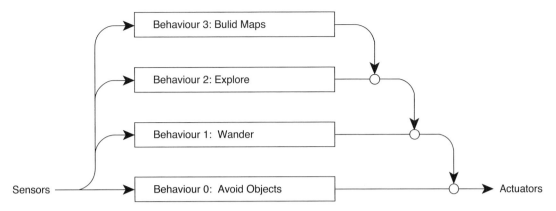

Fig. 9.1 The reactive planning *subsumption architecture* of Brooks (1985). High-level behaviours, such as building a spatial map, rely on low-level behaviours (e.g. exploring) which in turn rely on lower-level behaviours (wandering, and ultimately object avoidance), but can also inhibit them.

that assume it operates either by connectionist associative operations or by rule-based ones (Sloman, 1996).

Turning to the brain basis of one aspect of the Norman–Shallice theory, the position that the prefrontal cortex modulates lower-level systems, which can operate partially autonomously, is now standardly accepted (see e.g. Miller & Cohen, 2001). Thus the more abstract the representation that has to be acquired, the more distant from input and output processes, then the more lateral prefrontal neurons are heavily involved. There is, however, a complication. Consider the experimental paradigm of Wallis et al. (2001). On each trial, a monkey is presented with a picture and a cue. The cue tells the monkey whether the rule is that the picture should be the same as on the previous trial or different. However, the monkey has two cues for a given rule, match or non-match; for instance, a rule might be signified by either a drop of juice or a low tone. This is so that the investigator can differentiate between a neuron responding to a given physical cue and its responding to a rule being applied (see Figure 9.3). On any given day the monkey only has four pictures, but these change from day to day. The small number of pictures on any given day allows one to see whether neurons are consistently responding to one picture. On average, 41% of prefrontal neurons respond to rules, 24% to individual cues and 13% to pictures. By contrast, for inferotemporal neurons 12% respond to rules, 21% to individual cues and 45% to pictures (Wallis, 2008). However, it is not only prefrontal neurons that respond to rules, premotor ones do as well, and if anything even more of them (48%). Wallis points out that an extensive training period is required in order to reach steady-state performance in monkey experiments. The characteristics of steady-state performance do not specifically reflect what is involved in the acquisition of a rule in confronting novelty, which on the supervisory system approach would be the critical function for PFC. After training,

rules would also be represented as schemas in contention scheduling and this could be the reason for the premotor activation. Moreover, as far as prefrontal functions are concerned, Asaad et al. (1998) investigated in the monkey the acquisition of associations between objects and particular eye movements, which had to be made after a certain delay. They found that prefrontal neurons fired much more for a newly acquired association than

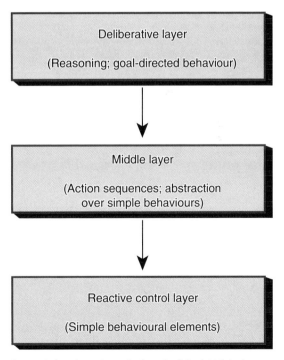

Fig. 9.2 A three-layer planner in the style of Gat (1998). In the absence of super ordinate control, the reactive layer allows the robot to perform simple behaviours conditional on its environment. The middle layer may bias the reactive layer towards sequential behaviours. The deliberative layer may bias the middle layer towards specific goal-directed behaviours.

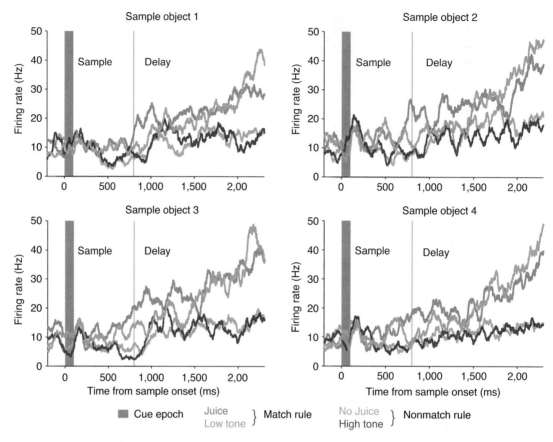

Fig. 9.3 Firing rate of a neuron in monkey PFC exhibiting rule-selectivity. The neuron was more active on match trials (blue, green) than on non-match trials (red, orange), regardless of the cue/sample object. Reprinted by permission from Macmillan Publishers Ltd: J.D. Wallis, K.C. Anderson & E.K. Miller (2001) Single neurons in prefrontal cortex encode abstract rules, *Nature, 411*, 953–956. Copyright (2001).

one that had been overlearned in previous sessions. Prefrontal neurons were sensitive to novelty.

9.2 The Modulation of Contention Scheduling

As far as humans are concerned, a variety of sources of evidence support the idea that prefrontal cortex (PFC) has a role in modulating the operation of lower-level systems which implement routine behaviour—contention scheduling. These may be divided into two types according to whether they involve simple tasks or more complex ones. As far as simple tasks are concerned, the most dramatic examples come from the effects of lesions to the PFC. The most basic is the *grasp reflex*, a standard clinical neurological sign of a prefrontal lesion. The examiner strokes with a finger the palm of the patient's hand and repeats this four times. If the patient grasps the finger, the examiner says, 'Why are you grasping? I have not asked you to do it'. In a study of De Renzi and Barbieri (1992) seven trials were given with three such negative remarks being made if grasping occurs. On each trial a score of 2 is given for a strong

grasp and 1 if the examiner's finger is touched by the patient. Patients were considered to exhibit the grasp reflex if they scored higher than 6.[2] In a very large series of over 400 patients, those with posterior cortical lesions never exhibited the grasp reflex, but 26% of those with a lateral frontal lesion did, as did 66% of those with a medial frontal lesion.

An analogous result was obtained in the ocular-motor domain. Paus et al. (1991) presented subjects with meaningless figures in central vision. On 11 of the 40 trials in which the figures were presented, stimuli also occurred in the periphery. The subjects had to look at the central figures and ignore the peripheral ones. Control subjects had no difficulty doing this. Patients with lateral prefrontal lesions were somewhat worse. However patients with unilateral medial frontal lesions made saccades to the peripheral stimuli, which should be ignored, on about 80% of trials when the stimulus was on the opposite side to their lesion.

---

[2] Nearly all such patients had a score of at least 10.

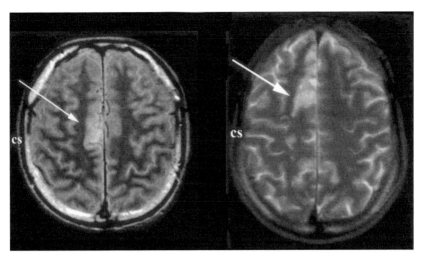

Fig. 9.4 MRI scans of the two patients of Gaymard et al. (1998), showing anterior cingulate lesions. Both patients were impaired on the anti-saccade task. (cs = Central Sulcus; left/right are reversed in the scans.) With kind permission from Springer Science+Business Media: *Experimental Brain Research*, Effects of anterior cingulate cortex lesions on ocular saccades in humans, 120(2), 1998, 173–183, B. Gaymard, S. Rivaud, J. F. Cassarini, T. Dubard, G. Rancurel, Y. Agid and C. Pierrot-Deseilligny, figures 1 and 3a.

A later study of Milea et al. (2003) attempted to localise the effect further within the medial prefrontal cortex in what is called the *anti-saccade task*. The subject must move his or her eyes away from a stimulus presented randomly to left or right 25° peripherally from the fovea, instead of making the natural movement toward it. The subjects were six patients being operated on for low-grade tumours located in the medial prefrontal cortex. Three made large numbers of errors post-operatively but the other three did not. The excisions made for the critical three involved a structure, to be a discussed later in the chapter, on the medial wall of the frontal lobes, the anterior cingulate. Two patients having a similar deficit and with analogous lesions had been reported by Gaymard et al. (1998) (see Figure 9.4). Thus in these studies, patients with lateral frontal lesions are impaired compared with controls, but patients with medial prefrontal lesions are far worse, possibly particularly due to damage to the anterior cingulate. Moreover, as one would predict, the anterior cingulate is also activated in functional imaging studies of the anti-saccade task (Doricchi et al., 1997; Paus et al., 1993).

Why the medial part of the prefrontal cortex should be particularly sensitive to such failures to inhibit a natural tendency fits with its role in the so-called *energisation* of non-routine processes to be discussed later in the chapter. However could it not be argued that this is a specific problem in inhibiting highly automatised responses and which would not generalise to other sorts of routine behaviour?

This would be an erroneous conclusion. A more complex direct sign of prefrontal damage, where the response that occurs when it should be inhibited varies with the concrete situation, takes place in so-called *uti-lisation behaviour*. Eslinger (2002) characterised these actions as being:

1 Unintended, disinhibited.

2 Solely triggered and compelled by objects in the environment.

3 Taken without regard to the patient's needs or social context.

4 Manifesting the limited capacity of the patient to over-ride the actions triggered by objects, particularly in early recovery phases.

This type of behaviour was first described by the French neurologist Lhermitte (1983). The standard procedure used by Lhermitte was to place, without giving any instruction, a glass and a jug of water on his desk in front of the patient who is seated on the other side. A normal subject would just look puzzled. Many prefrontal patients, however, poured the water into the glass and drank it, while Lhermitte never observed this with patients with posterior lesions. Lhermitte's procedure was open to a potent objection. How are patients to understand what the doctor wants them to do? The inference that, if doctors want patients to produce some behaviour they would ask them to do it, requires that the patient interpret the doctor's thought processes, which in turn would involve what is known as a 'theory-of-mind' function (see Section 11.1). An alternative possibility, similar to Lhermitte's own account, is that the behaviour results from the revealing of the operation of contention scheduling alone, when the supervisory system is not functioning.

A failure to understand the doctor's intentions cannot explain utilisation behaviour as it appears in another form. It can also occur when there is no explicit or implicit need to use objects and indeed when there is an explicit requirement to do something else. This is so-called 'incidental utilisation behaviour' (e.g. Shallice et al., 1989; Brazzelli & Spinnler, 1998; Boccardi et al., 2002). Thus patient LE of Shallice et al., not only showed incidental utilisation behaviour during testing sessions, but manifested it while at home, opening and closing cupboards, making tea for non-existent visitors, continually adjusting the central heating system, and so on. It is generally agreed that frontal lesions are necessary to produce utilisation behaviour (see Eslinger, 2002), with the strong suggestion that medial regions are more critical. Given that a failure to understand task requirements can hardly be the critical factor, at least for incidental utilisation behaviour, the syndrome fits just what would be expected of the behaviour of a contention-scheduling system operating without modulation from a supervisory system.

Reason (1979) called analogous errors produced by normal subject in action lapses 'capture errors'. The classic example given by William James (1890), is of going upstairs to change and finding oneself in bed. In diary studies in which normal subjects record their own lapses and rate them on certain scales, Reason (1984) showed that such errors occur when subjects rate both the captured and capturing behaviours as highly familiar and rate their own mental state as 'distractable'. This corresponds to situations where, for each action considered alone, contention scheduling can control behaviour and the supervisory system is otherwise occupied, an analogue in normal subjects to utilisation behaviour in prefrontal patients.

Can one obtain more solid evidence of the modulation of contention scheduling by higher cognitive systems than this cluster of clinical syndromes and diary studies? If one turns to more complex tasks, a study that provides tighter on-line control of behaviour is that of Jahanshahi et al. (1998), which employed TMS in the task of *random generation of digits*. In the random-generation task, subjects must produce a number between 1 and 9 at a given rate. In the study it was one every 1200 msec. In addition, the subject must make the sequence as random as possible, that is, the sequence must not satisfy any rule for too long or too frequently. Baddeley (1986), who had earlier invented the task, argued that as there are no external stimuli involved, any rule that is operating in the production of any one response would be controlled by a schema. The task requires that any such schema must be inhibited before the next response is produced and an alternative one activated. On the model these two steps would both involve the supervisory system. The most over-learned schemas in this situation are counting up or down by one. Jahanshahi et al. (1998) showed that a single TMS

pulse to the left dorsolateral prefrontal cortex, when compared with a sham TMS control, led to a rough doubling in the rate of such responses.

In a follow-up study using fMRI Jahanshahi et al. (2000) varied the speed of generation. The degree of randomness in the string of responses decreased dramatically as the required rate increased from 1 per 3 sec to 1 per 0.5 sec. The function was mirrored in the activation shown in one area of cortex, which was again the left dorsolateral prefrontal cortex (Figure 9.5). Thus, with the complication to be discussed later in the chapter that the theoretically critical effect occurred in a different part of the prefrontal cortex—the left dorsolateral region—the set of findings can be seen as a tighter analogue of utilisation behaviour and fit well with what one would expect on the model.

When the contention-scheduling system is not being modulated by a higher-level supervisory system, then responding is dominated by the familiarity and frequency of application of rules or task-contingencies. Can one also provide evidence for a direct link between prefrontal cortex and the successful confronting of novel situations? One of the earliest functional imaging studies to explore the issue was that of Jenkins et al. (1994). Subjects had to learn by trial-and-error sequences of eight key presses, using a pad with four keys. In one condition they learnt the sequence before having PET scans, with an extra 10 trials being given after perfect performance was achieved. Alternatively, they learned the sequence during the scan with a 'bonus' of a totally new sequence to learn if they were successful. These conditions were both compared with rest.

When the sequence was well learned before the scan, the most anterior regions activated were the lateral premotor cortex and the supplementary motor area. No prefrontal region was activated. In contrast, when the sequence was in the process of being learned, there was strong activation in many areas of prefrontal cortex bilaterally (areas 9, 10, 46, 47). A typical pattern of results is shown in Figure 9.6. The prefrontal cortex was only involved when the sequence was novel. A similar effect in the verbal domain was found at much the same time by Raichle et al. (1994). Again, successfully coping with a new situation—giving a verb to go with a particular noun—produced activation in prefrontal cortex. Practice on the task with the same stimuli led to loss of the prefrontal activation. These are both fairly low level tasks. However we will see in Section 12.5 that much the same happens with problem-solving.

9.3 The Three Attentional Systems of Posner and Petersen (1990)

Is the stress given in the previous section to the contrast between routine and non-routine situations unnecessary?

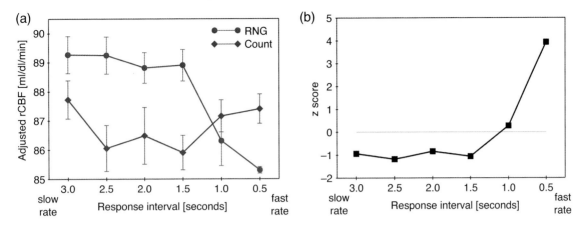

Fig. 9.5 Data from Jahanshahi et al's (2000) study of random number generation. (a) The rCBF response in left DLPFC (−34, 40, 24) during random number generation (red line) and the control task (counting, blue line) at six different response rates. (b) The degree of randomness at different response rates, as measured by the tendency to produce counting responses (e.g. 3, 4 or 3, 2). Random generation corresponds to z = 0 (shown in grey). Reproduced from *NeuroImage, 12*(6), M. Jahanshahi, G. Dirnberger, R. Fuller & C.D. Frith, The role of dorsolateral prefrontal cortex in random number generation: a study with Positron Emission Tomography, pp713–725. Copyright (2000), with permission from Elsevier.

Maybe the essence of prefrontal functions can be distilled more simply. There are at least two and a half such possibilities. In the 1990s overwhelmingly the most popular response in the neuroscience community as to the function of prefrontal cortex would have been to stress its role in working memory. However we have already argued in Section 7.9 that this emphasis is misplaced, at least as far as storage of multiple items is concerned.

A second apparent alterative for an over-arching idea for understanding prefrontal functions is to take the elementary basis for the 'working' aspect of working memory as attention. Thus in Chapter 1 we briefly referred to the proposals of Corbetta and Shulman (2002) that when attention is caught by a sudden external stimulus (*exogeneous attention*) a different network is involved from when it is directed top-down, say due to task instructions (*endogenous attention*). The theoretical position of Corbetta and Shulman, shown in Figure 9.7, is based on a number of meta-analyses of different paradigms, which all involve regions of prefrontal cortex. These paradigms include moving the focus of attention

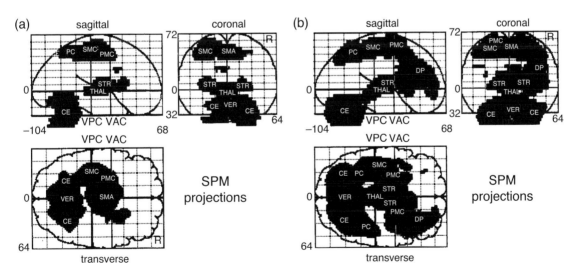

Fig. 9.6 Effects of motor sequence learning from Jenkins et al. (1994). (a) The contrast between performing a known/old sequence and rest. (b) The contrast between performing a new sequence and rest. Dorsolateral prefrontal activation (DP) is found in the latter contrast but not the former. Reproduced with permission from I.H. Jenkins, D.J. Brooks, P.D. Nixon, R.S.J. Frackowiak, and R. E. Passingham, 1994, Motor sequence learning: a study with positron emission tomography. *The Journal of Neuroscience, 14*(6), 3775–3790; figure 3a, p. 3778 and figure 4a, p. 3781.

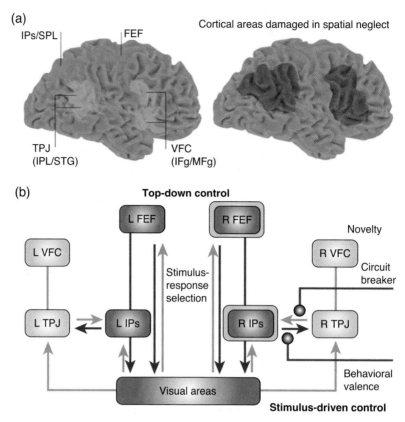

Fig. 9.7 (a) Dorsal (blue) and ventral (orange) frontoparietal networks held by Corbetta and Shulman (2002) to be involved in attention and their relation to lesions found in unilateral spatial neglect patients. (b) Corbetta and Shulman's neuroanatomical model of top-down and stimulus-driven control of attention. Reprinted by permission from Macmillan Publishers Ltd: M. Corbetta & G.L. Shulman (2002) Control of goal-directed and stimulus-driven attention in the brain. *Nature Reviews Neuroscience, 3,* 201–215. Copyright (2002).

to a previously unattended spot (Arrington et al., 2000; Corbetta et al., 2002)[3] and orienting towards rarely occurring targets—so-called vigilance (Corbetta & Shulman, 2002).

However the first of these situations can be viewed as a form of responding to novelty, if on a much more local scale than is typically implied, or more critically on the supervisory system theory, in coping with a non-routine situation where a strong incorrect bias has to be overcome. The second type of paradigm, and indeed also the basic theoretical position on endogenous and exogenous systems involved in the spatial directing of attention, emphasises that attention cannot be viewed as the province of a single system but instead comprises multiple complementary systems.

Phenomenologically, attention varies on a number of dimensions (see Evans, 1970). It may be voluntarily or spontaneously drawn to an object, the endogenous/exogenous distinction just discussed. Attention may be

oriented towards action, thought or perception. It may be shared between activities or concentrated on one task, and for perception it may be narrowly focused on one part of space or diffusely oriented towards a wide area. To what extent do these different aspects of attention involve the same or different neural mechanisms? There have been a variety of proposals for the existence of multiple attentional systems. By far the best known model—that of Posner and Peterson (1990)—asserts that there are three interacting neural systems of attention. One—*the orienting system*—has the role of allowing the overall system to orient spatially to critical stimuli.[4] A second system was initially characterised in terms of response selection, for instance when focussed attention is required in selection-for-action, as when responses must be made to very rapidly occurring signals as in a so-called *serial reaction time* paradigm in which the next of a long series of stimuli is presented almost immediately after the previous response occurs,

---

[3] Technically this involves reorienting to a so-called invalid target in the paradigm of Posner (1980).

[4] This system is in part divisible into the endogenous and exogenous systems of Corbetta and Shulman.

or when there is difficulty in response selection, as in the Stroop task.[5] Later the system became characterised as involving *executive attention* (Posner & Di Girolamo, 1998; Fernandez-Duque & Posner, 2001). The third system—the *alertness system*—ensures the alert state necessary for carrying out tasks efficiently when vigilance is needed because environmental stimulation is low, as classically exemplified in the work of a sentry or a radar operator.

Initially these three aspects of attention processing were characterised as the products of systems held to be centered on specific locations. The first was held to be in the parietal lobes, and if damaged produced unilateral neglect as discussed in Section 1.8. The second involved a structure on the medial surface of the prefrontal cortex discussed in the previous section, the anterior cingulate, much activated in functional imaging studies. The third was thought to be located in the right dorsolateral prefrontal cortex. However later (e.g. Fan et al., 2002, 2005) the systems became characterised as 'networks' with somewhat broader cortical localisations defined more by specific neurotransmitter pathways; the orienting system became parieto-frontal, the executive system both medial frontal and lateral prefrontal, and the alerting system right fronto-parietal (Fernandez-Duque & Posner, 2001; Fan et al., 2002).

Most recently, the localisations of the three networks have been held to be derivable empirically from a single neuroimaging study, that of Fan et al. (2005), who used a single task—the attention network test (ANT) (see Figure 9.8). This test was held to provide a means of exploring the efficiency of the orienting, executive and alertness networks. Within a single reaction time task, it allows three sets of variables to be distinguished; these sets have been found to be relatively independent in behavioural studies (Fan et al., 2002). The variables linked to the *orienting* network activated parietal sites, as would have been expected, but also the frontal eye fields, which is compatible with the findings of Corbetta and Shulman. The variables related to the *executive control* network continued to activate the anterior cingulate but also several other brain areas, particularly in prefrontal cortex. Those held to map to the *alerting* network showed strong thalamic involvement and 'activation of anterior and posterior cortical sites.' However there was no longer a clear role in alertness for the right, as opposed to the left, hemisphere or for the right prefrontal cortex in particular. As the paper does

not discuss in detail the discrepancies from the earlier localisations, particularly with respect to alertness, we will consider primarily the more classical Posner-Petersen approach to localisations of the claimed three attentional systems.

That spatial orienting involves the inferior parietal lobe, particularly on the right, is widely accepted both from functional imaging of normal subjects and from the anatomy of the unilateral spatial neglect syndrome discussed in Section 1.8 (see e.g. Corbetta & Shulman, 2002; Mort et al., 2003; Driver, Vuilleumier & Husain, 2004; but see also Karnath, Ferber & Himmelbach, 2001).[6]

There is much less uniformity of agreement about the other two attentional systems or networks proposed by Posner and his colleagues. This disagreement, as we will see, relates to both functional and anatomical aspects. Thus various alternative functional hypotheses to that of mediating executive attention have been put forward about the attentional role of the medial prefrontal system, and in particular the anterior cingulate. It has been argued that the anterior cingulate is involved in monitoring response conflict (e.g. Botvinick et al., 1999), in the facilitation of supervisory operations (Posner & Di Girolamo, 1998), or in the cortical arousal of the sympathetic nervous system (Critchley et al., 2002). Moreover, as will be shown later in this chapter, impairments of the medial and lateral prefrontal cortex have quite different characteristics. So if the medial and lateral parts of the prefrontal lobes are part of a common 'executive network' they probably contain subsystems with different properties in different sections of the network.

As far as the alertness system is concerned, Rueckert and Grafman (1996) showed that patients with predominantly right frontal lesions are indeed significantly slower than controls on a simple RT task with varying inter-trial intervals of 2 up to 18 sec and also miss significantly more targets (3% vs 0.5%). In a continuous performance task, the patients with right frontal lesions also miss more targets than do normal subjects in the second 5 min of the 10-min task. This can be seen as fitting the original characterisation of an alertness system of Posner and Petersen. However patients with predominantly left frontal lesions perform in an intermediate fashion, not significantly different from either the right frontal group or the controls. Moreover, as discussed earlier, the new characterisation of the alertness network by Fan et al., does not give the right frontal cortex any special role, which may be a consequence of functional imaging being less likely to detect lateralisation (see Section 5.2). In addition, we will see

---

[5] In the Stroop task subjects have to name the colour in which a word is printed. In its so-called incongruent or incompatible condition, the word is a colour name but it is printed in a different colour ink. Subjects are considerably slower and less accurate than if they are naming a colour patch.

---

[6] Neglect can also involve parieto-frontal disconnection see Doricchi and Tomaiuolo (2003).

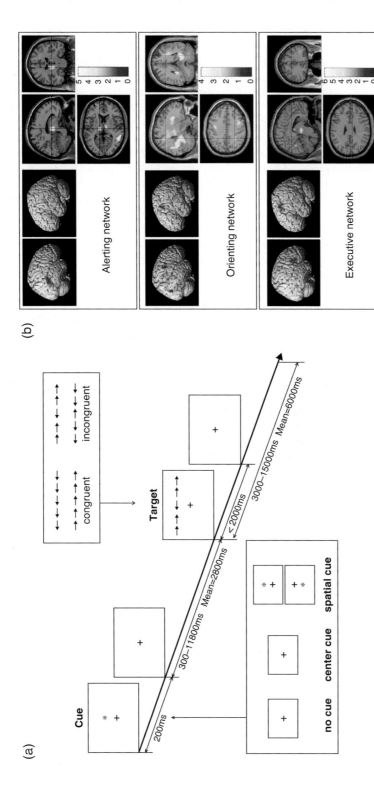

Fig. 9.8 (a) The experimental design of Fan et al. (2005). There are three conditions, differentiated by the cue (or its absence) which is presented for 200 msec. After a variable delay, a target arrow is presented. This is flanked by arrows which may be congruent or incongruent. Subjects then have 2000 msec to respond by pressing the left or right response buttons. A central fixation cross remains on screen for the entire trial. (b) fMRI results for the three attentional networks based on contrasts of centre cue versus no cue for the alerting network, spatial cue versus centre cue for the orienting network, and incongruent flanker versus congruent flanker for the executive (conflict) network. Reprinted from *NeuroImage*, *26*(2), J. Fan, B.D. McCandliss, J. Fossella, J.I. Flombaum and M.I Posner, The activation of attentional networks, 471–479. Copyright (2005), with permission from Elsevier.

in Section 9.10 that the empirical situation from neuropsychology is also considerably more complicated.

There is little doubt then that attentional and supervisory functions overlap. However the problems, particularly those concerning localisation, that have developed within the three attentional network model means that it is no longer a sufficiently solid conceptual basis for it to replace the supervisory system approach.[7] More critically, attentional processes, just like those involved in working memory, are only a subset of the higher-level processes necessary for confronting non-routine situations. We therefore move to a very different type of alternative theoretical framework.

9.4 The Lateral Prefrontal Cortex as the Seat of '*g*'

At the beginning of the last section, we referred to two and a half alternatives to the emphasis on confronting non-routine situations, stressed in Section 2 of this chapter. The 'half' referred to a rather different approach of the same level of complexity as that for confronting non-routine situations but which can in turn be treated as a potential capacity required by an organism coping with such situations.[8] This is the theoretical position of Duncan (2001, 2010), which operates on a number of different levels—cellular neurophysiology, a system-level characterisation, psychometrics and by analogy to AI. The highest level aspect of Duncan's position derives from his use of a traditional concept from psychometrics, the study of mental testing, namely '*g*' (Duncan et al., 1995). From the time of Spearman (1904) one major current of thought in psychometrics, probably the most major current, has been that confronting any intellectually demanding tasks involves a common core set of processes, whatever the processing domain they involve—language, visuo-spatial, mathematical, musical or whatever. Moreover when one examines

individual differences in the performance of such tasks then a part of the variance in the spread of scores across the population is attributable to the efficiency of these core processes—so-called Spearman's '*g*'.[9]

The main evidence that Duncan et al. (2000) provide for the localisation of '*g*' comes from a functional imaging experiment which compared performance on three types of task that theoretically load heavily on '*g*' but which have no apparent structural (i.e. lower-level) processes in common. All three were odd-one-out tests. However, one concerned designs with shapes, the second concerned relations between letters in a string, and the third concerned spatial relations. Each of the three was then compared with a structurally similar task that loaded much less on '*g*'. In all cases the lateral prefrontal cortex was significantly activated in the subtraction (see Figure 9.9).

The neural bases of '*g*' processing are held to be in so-called *multiple demand regions*. Duncan and Owen (2000) performed a meta-analysis of the functional imaging studies then published where task analyses of two conditions led to subtractions involving only a single variable related to one of the following factors: task novelty, response competition, working memory load, working memory delay and perceptual difficulty. They then compared activations for all pairs of conditions that differed on only one of the dimensions. An example would be that a condition with response competition was contrasted to an otherwise identical one without it. They found that as far as anterior structures were concerned, the maxima all lay in the anterior cingulate cortex and in two swathes down the lateral prefrontal cortices (see Figure 9.10). More specifically, these second sets of maxima clustered around the middle and posterior part of the inferior frontal sulcii (IFS) and more ventrally along the frontal operculum. Critically, however, even though the five different types of contrast seem very different to each other they did not localise differentially within these regions. The areas of activation all overlapped.[10]

The claim that these multiple demand regions are the seat of '*g*' is a contentious interpretation of the functional imaging evidence, given the chequered

---

[7] The two approaches can in any case be linked. Thus Posner and Di Girolamo (1998) argued that the executive attentional system could be characterised as the system required to potentiate the operation of a supervisory system. We will return to a similar conceptualisation later.

[8] Other major roles that have been ascribed to the lateral prefrontal cortex such as producing rule-following behaviour (Bunge & Wallis, 2008) or in the implementation of strategies (Genovesi & Wise, 2008) are more directly linked to the more global function of the confronting of non-routine situations as we will see in Section 9.12. Similarly the position of Koechlin and colleagues that it is involved in episodic control, when 'the signals for guiding action selection … are attributable to a past event, instigating a temporal 'episode' in which a new set of rules apply' (Koechlin & Summerfield, 2007, p. 230) has a more complex family resemblance to that of confronting novelty.

---

[9] For most of its long life the '*g*' theory of Spearman has been in confrontation with the theory of multiple intelligences (Thomson, 1935; Gardner, 1993). There has also been a long history of attempts to produce a neuroscientific analysis of '*g*' of which Duncan's is the latest.

[10] Duncan (2010) extends the number of multiple demand regions. There are currently held to be five such regions: the posterior inferior frontal sulcus, the anterior insula and adjacent frontal operculum, the pre-supplementary motor area (pre-SMA) and the anterior cingulate, 'in and around' the intraparietal sulcus and part of anterior lateral prefrontal cortex.

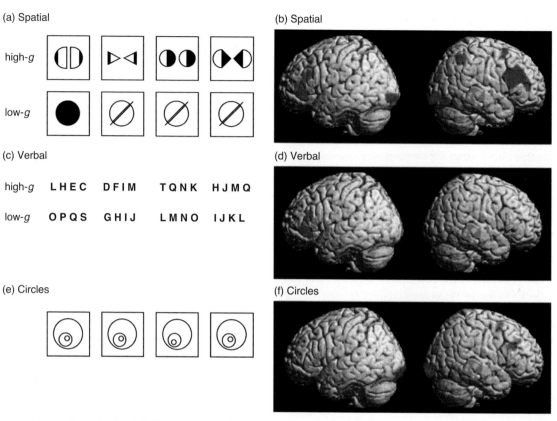

Fig. 9.9 Multiple demand regions linked by Duncan et al. (2000) to 'g'. (a) Sample high 'g' and low 'g' spatial tasks, and (b) their contrast as revealed by fMRI. (c) Sample high 'g' and low 'g' verbal tasks and (d) their contrast as revealed by fMRI. (e) A difficult task involving spatial relationships between circles (not shown is an easy variant), and (f) the contrast in BOLD activity between hard and easy circle tasks. From J. Duncan et al, 2000, A neural basis for general intelligence. *Science*, *289*(5478), 457–460. Reprinted with permission from AAAS.

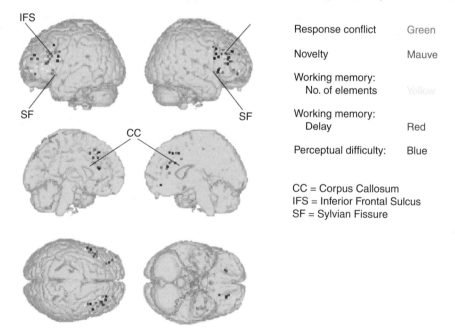

Fig. 9.10 Frontal activations from 'pure' experiments involving one each of five types of single constructs, as reported in the metaanalysis of Duncan and Owen (2000). Reprinted from *Trends in Neurosciences*, *23*(10), J. Duncan and A.M. Owen, Common regions of the human frontal lobe recruited by diverse cognitive demands, pp. 475–483. Copyright (2000), with permission from Elsevier.

history of the 'g' concept (Evans & Waites, 1981). However it describes well the evidence that Duncan reviews. Within the Spearman tradition 'g' is held to be the unitary core of confronting intellectually demanding tasks. Yet the multiple demand regions can be differentially activated across different tasks. For instance, as we will see, damage to medial prefrontal structures and lateral ones lead to very different types of disorder. They are not functionally equivalent. Thus the core concept Duncan uses appears to fractionate into more specific functions. 'g' is not an adequate conceptual tool for sculpting the mind, even if, possibly as the product of a set of multiple demand regions, it is pragmatically useful in psychometrics. However, the flexibility and innovative thinking required by a task which loads heavily on 'g' are indeed key functions of lateral prefrontal cortex. One can extract the essence of Duncan's position without necessarily accepting the concept of 'g'.

A further strand of support for Duncan's overall thesis, as it applies to the lateral prefrontal region, derives from the properties of cells in this area. He points out that a reasonable generalisation is that whatever arbitrary task the monkey has been trained to carry out, a substantial proportion of the neurons will show selective responses to some aspect of the events involved in task execution. This includes studies using rule switching (Asaad et al., 2000), spatial delayed responses (Funahashi & Inove, 2000), sound-colour matching (Fuster et al., 2000) and visual same-different comparisons (Wallis et al., 2000). For instance in a two-choice task where the monkeys needed to associate specific objects with eye movements, 80% of lateral prefrontal cells responded to object identity, direction of the saccade, or both. Typically cells responding to different triggers are spread across a wide section of lateral prefrontal cortex and are intermingled. Such cells according to Duncan are reprogrammable. They can respond to different aspects of the situation in two tasks which the monkey can perform (Miller & Cohen, 2001).

Duncan (2010) follows Luria in seeing the function of the multiple demand units as the programming of non-routine behaviours. He draws an analogy between the functional role of this region and that of the working memory of an AI production system model such as Soar (Newell, 1990), discussed in Section 1.7. The elements of Soar's working memory represent states of the environment and its goals at various levels as well as cognitive elements that have been added by production rules which have been executed just before.[11]

As we need to consider the separate function of each multiple demand systems, the 'g' approach is not specific enough. Three aspects of Duncan's conceptual framework will, though, be adopted in this chapter. The first is the great potential flexibility with respect to the properties of task events that the lateral prefrontal cortex provides. The second is that at least part of its general purpose function relates to the programming of novel behaviour. The third is the potential for a conceptual link with symbolic artificial intelligence and particularly production systems as considered in Chapter 1, which the analogy with Soar working memory provides.

9.5 The Interface Between the Supervisory System and Contention Scheduling: Task Sets and Source Schemas

To base the principal characterisation of prefrontal functions on a more specific process such as working memory or attention, or on a more general higher-level one such as 'g,' in all cases leads to a problem. We will continue therefore to use the supervisory system framework in which a particular system is held to have the function of coping with any sort of non-routine contingency by modulating lower-level processes in the 'routine' system, contention scheduling.

If we conceive of the two systems as mediating routine processing (by contention scheduling) and non-routine processing in (the supervisory system by modulation of contention scheduling), respectively, there is a key issue that must be faced. This is what form should, or even can, a system for non-routine processing take? Dan Dennett (1998), the philosopher-of-mind, characterised the first version of the supervisory system theory as 'an ominously wise overseeing homunculus who handles the hard cases in the workshop of consciousness' (p. 288). Can one do better than postulating an empty box?

Before confronting this question we will begin with a more tangible, if still tricky problem. The supervisory system is held to produce output which activates (or inhibits) higher level schemas in contention scheduling. This must involve both a set of schemas in contention scheduling and their presence as cognitive elements in the output of the supervisory system. Where might they be situated in the brain? This is a complex issue as the two are deeply inside the overall system, neither close to input nor output. Worse, activation is assumed to cascade from one to the other. So they will often be activated together. Indeed, we saw just this happening with respect to rule-following responses of prefrontal and premotor neurons in the monkey experiment of Wallis et al. discussed in Section 9.1.

---

[11] Soar's working memory to which Duncan alludes is far from isomorphic with the ACT-R working memory discussed in Section 7.9.

Consider a concrete example. Take the workers at an old fish market, like those in Grimsby or Trieste. The fish arrives at the quay and it is sorted by colour and shape into, in Trieste, say, bass, bream, turbot, swordfish and a variety of others with no well-known English name such as *scorfano* ('scorpion fish'). The sorting task for the workers on the quay was, we can assume, generally automatic. We can give an analogous if less colourful task to a typical experimental subject, by asking them to sort, say, a set of cards by the shape or colour of a design on them, although even if they receive what passes for extensive practice in most cognitive experiments, it will presumably be carried out in a less automatic fashion then sorting of fish in the situation referred to above.

Behaviour in this sorting situation is controlled by what is now often called a 'task-set' devised by combining two classical German terms *Aufgabe* (*Task*) and *Einstellung* (*Set*), which were standard theoretical concepts for the German Wurzberg School of psychologists of a hundred years ago (see e.g. Ach, 1905; also Humphrey, 1951, for a most subtle and clear account in English). 'Task-set' corresponds to the term used earlier in this book of 'action or thought schema'.[12]

In the contention scheduling model the highest level of routine control is a schema we will call a source-schema. It will be active throughout the period a routine task is being carried out, as for the *Prepare Instant Coffee* node in Figure 8.4. However this depends on the task being completely routinised. If it is not, then the operation of the task will require the continuing activation of a cognitive element within the supervisory system which is not autonomously triggered by the perceptual and motivational systems. We will elide the issue of which of these alternative types of unit we are discussing until later in the chapter, and instead use the theoretically neutral term of *task-demand units*. Where roughly in the brain are they located?

One method to attempt to determine this has been by investigating which areas of the brain are activated when a task has been signalled but before it has started. Holding an instruction to create an intention to act is also likely to involve higher-level processes. However these processes could well be less specific to the individual task being carried out than the task-set units themselves. With this theoretical perspective, Sakai and Passingham (2003) gave an instruction on each trial as to which of four working memory tasks to carry out, two being verbal and two spatial. One pair of tasks involved reproducing the order of the stimuli. The other pair required it to be reversed. The subjects then saw a set of four stimuli each containing a letter and a red square. Six seconds after the last stimulus they received a memory probe to which they had to respond. The memory probe showed two of the stimuli—e.g. the positions of two of the squares—and an arrow. Subjects had to respond according to whether the arrow matched the temporal order in which the stimuli had been presented. Subjects had been trained for 20 min before testing began, so the tasks were somewhat automated. Frontopolar regions showed a similar pattern of activation across tasks (see Figure 9.11), so they became candidates for supra-task-set processes, as we will discuss in Section 9.14. In dorsolateral prefrontal cortex there was a difference across tasks but it related to difficulty not type of task. However, the inferior frontal gyrus (Broca's area) was activated much more in the verbal tasks and the posterior superior frontal sulcus (Brodmann area 8) much more in the non-verbal ones.

A problem with drawing inferences from this type of paradigm is that if preparation involves cascading activation, it would be liable to lead to partial activation of the lower-level systems to be used even before the stimuli have been presented. Indeed more posterior regions such as the superior temporal gyrus and the superior parietal lobe showed the same patterns as Broca's area and Brodmann area 8, respectively. However, as the latter two areas are the most anterior regions with a function apparently specific to the individual task, we will treat them as providing putative localisations for the task-demand units.

Another dimension has been added by Koechlin and Jubault (2006), who contrasted activation of schemas at different levels of a hierarchy analogous to that of contention scheduling. The single-schema task was to produce a sequence of five patterns of key presses following the occurrence of a green coloured square and to stop it when a red square occurred. Compared with a single repetitive key-pressing task, this led to activation—during task execution and particularly at initiation and

---

[12] Schema, discussed in Chapter 8, instead was how Osgood (1953), in one of the finest twentieth-century textbooks of psychology, rendered in English the so-called total aufgabe (total task) of Selz (1913), who followed the Wurzberg school. The leading theoretician of the Wurzberg School, Ach, had held that in carrying out a single task like Give Co-ordinate: Parson → ? (Chaplain) the task-set of giving a coordinate combines with the association of Parson → Chaplain to produce the response. Selz rejected the idea of two separate tendencies—a so-called 'determining' (task) combining with a 'reproductive' (association) one. Instead he argued that the Total Task of Task + Stimulus elicited a single Wissen (knowing) previously stored in memory. Today one might consider it a Production, with the Total Task as the contents of working memory and any other goal specification that satisfies its conditions. However whether the task and stimulus should be conflated remains contentious. In Soar the goal and stimulus would be part of working memory while in ACT-R the goal would be stored separately in the goal buffer. Ironically, moreover, some aspects of prefrontal function may fit well with an approach more analogous to Ach than to Selz (see Ruge & Braver, 2008).

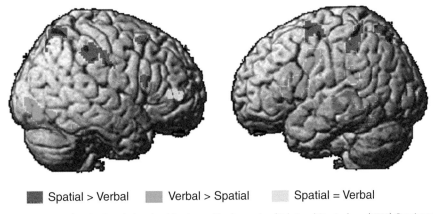

Spatial > Verbal   Verbal > Spatial   Spatial = Verbal

Fig. 9.11 Areas showing sustained activation during the delay interval in the study of Sakai and Passingham (2003). Reprinted by permission from Macmillan Publishers Ltd: K. Sakai and R.E Passingham (2003) Prefrontal interactions reflect future task operations. *Nature Neuroscience,* 6(1), 75–81. Copyright (2003).

termination—in Broca's area and its right-hemisphere homologue (see Figure 9.12).[13]

In addition, though, subjects had to produce a more complex set of responses. These were organised as a 2-level hierarchy with the higher level of the hierarchy cued by one of the letters A, B or C. The initiation and termination of the super-ordinate task activated regions slightly more anterior to the part of Broca's area activated in the simple task. This was in Brodmann area 45. Koechlin and Jubault interpret this set of results as indicating a physical axis of an increase in level in the control hierarchy as one moves forward in the inferior frontal cortex.

Other interpretations are, however, possible. Thus the super-ordinate task involved alphabetic material and the single task did not. More critically, the super-ordinate task appears to have been less well learned; the error rate was nearly double that in the single task (4.4% vs 2.5%). Koechlin and Jubault claim that the two tasks were 'appropriately over-learned' due to 56 presentations of each 'chunk' of trials on a preceding day. The evidence was that reaction times were no faster on the last series of trials than on the first series on the experimental day. However as will be discussed in Section 9.11 in a demanding 500-trial five-choice serial reaction time task, in which the next stimulus appears 200 msec after the preceding response, Alexander et al. (2005) found no change in reaction time across 5 blocks of 100 trials each. Yet the error rate of a left lateral group of frontal patients, particularly those with ventral lesions was significantly higher in the first 100 trials only.

Automatisation had not occurred in this group, even though reaction time had asymptoted. Koechlin and Jubault's argument that the task was 'appropriately overlearned', if this means automatic, appears flawed. The posterior–anterior dimension could then relate to degree of automatisation and not level in a control hierarchy as claimed. The BA 45 activations would thus be of task demand units in the supervisory system and the slightly more posterior Broca's area ones would be of source schemas.

These two studies both localise task-demand units and schema representations in the same gross area of the brain of the ventral premotor cortex and the neighbouring posterior prefrontal cortex. However the inferences from both sets of results can be criticised. Can one obtain converging evidence? A very popular paradigm over the last fifteen years for studying cognitive control processes has been that of task-switching. The task-switching paradigm is an information-processing abstraction of clinical neuropsychology tests such as Wisconsin Card-Sorting (Milner, 1963)[14] and the Extra-Dimensional/Intra-Dimensional Shift Test of the CANTAB battery (Owen et al., 1990), where on certain trials the dimension of the stimulus to which a subject attends must change. These tasks are known to be sensitive to lateral frontal lesions (Milner, 1963; Owen et al., 1990), and indeed Hampshire and Owen (2006) have shown in a functional imaging study that the mid-ventrolateral is the critical region for an attentional shift.

The clinical tasks, however, also tend to involve abstraction and working memory processes in addition to task-switching per se. In the mid-1990s researchers

---

[13] Virtually the same area as the other area identified by Sakai and Passingham, although here characterised as superior premotor rather than Brodmann area 8, was also activated, although here specifically at the initiation and termination of sequences.

[14] The Wisconsin Card-Sorting task is a test of a patient's ability to change task-set. It is described in Section 1.3 and in more detail in Section 12.6. Typically a lateral prefrontal lesion produces a tendency to perseverate the previously active task-set.

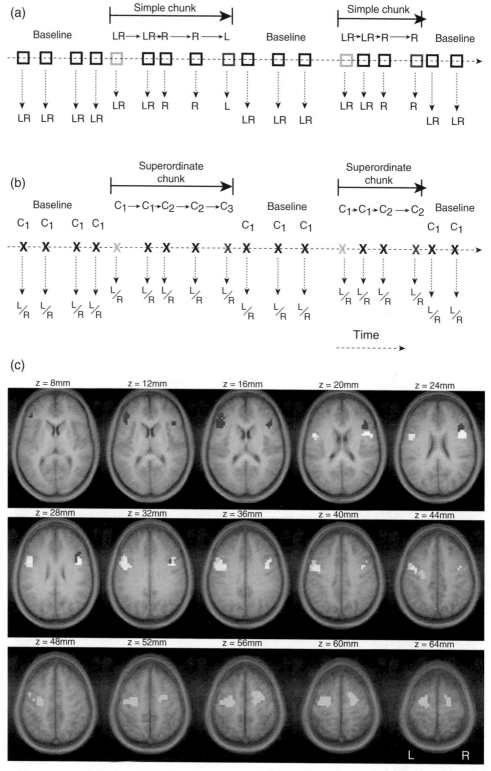

Fig. 9.12 Design and results of Koechlin and Jubault (2006). Figures (a) and (b) show a series of trials in the simple (a) and superordinate (b) conditions. The vertical arrows represent the responses that subjects made on each trial. The Cs in (b) refer to simple tasks. Figure (c) shows the lateral frontal activations involved in transitions between single motor responses (green) in beginning or ending a simple chunk (white, yellow) and in transitions between them (orange, yellow) and in beginning or ending superordinate chunks (red). Reprinted from *Neuron*, 50(6), E. Koechlin and T. Jubault, Broca's area and the hierarchical organization of human behavior, pp. 963–974, Copyright (2006), with permission from Elsevier.

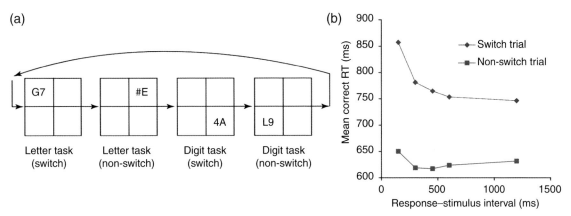

Fig. 9.13 (a) Stimuli illustrating successive trials of the Rogers and Monsell (1995) task switching study. Each stimulus had two characters – prototypically a letter and a digit. When the stimulus appears in the upper half of the screen, subjects must respond to the letter. When it appears in the lower half, they must respond to the digit. Trials cycle through four types, producing alternating switch and non-switch trials. (b) Mean RT on switch and non-switch trials, for five different inter-trial intervals. Increasing the inter-trial intervals beyond 600 msec had little effect on the switch cost. Reprinted from *Trends in Cognitive Sciences, 7*(3), S. Monsell, Task switching, pp. 134–140. Copyright (2003) with permission from Elsevier.

produced experimental paradigms which can be called more 'process-pure', since they honed in much more onto task-switching per se (e.g. Allport, Styles & Hsieh, 1994; Meiran, 1996). The most used of these paradigms is that of Rogers and Monsell (1995), where the subject has a visual display as shown in Figure 9.13. The stimuli—always a digit and a letter—are presented in each of the four cells in turn on successive trials moving in a clockwise direction. Whenever the stimuli are in the top two squares, the subject must respond to the letter; for instance; by indicating whether it is a consonant or vowel. For the next two stimuli in the lower two squares the digit is the critical stimulus and say, an odd/even decision is made, with the alternating pattern—of two trials per task at a time—continuing through the block of trials. Trials where the task switches take longer than the equivalent ones where it repeats; but this difference becomes less if the interval between the end of one trial and the beginning of the next increases (see Figure 9.14).

Early work on task-switching was dominated by two rival accounts of the so-called 'switch-cost' of having to switch between tasks. Rogers and Monsell (1995) argued for a top-down process of *task-set reconfiguration*, which they held to be required whenever a source schema or task set was changed. Allport et al. (1994) by contrast argued that the slowing occurred as a result of the need to inhibit the previously active schema.

In fact on a relatively simple model put forward by Gilbert and Shallice (2002) (see Figure 9.14) the two theoretical variables can be seen to be only indirectly related to behavioural data. Task set reconfiguration—if it exists—would be manifest in the processes preceding the top-down control input, and so its relation to behaviour would be mediated by a cascade of other processes.

Inhibition of previous task-sets could also require top-down control input, but how strong it would need to be could also depend on the bottom-up activation from input and output units. We will use the model to situate the later discussion.[15]

After the initial papers of the mid-1990s, the task-switching group of paradigms grew rapidly in popularity. Once again, it became apparent that, just as Tulving and Madigan had foreseen in 1970 in their idea of the *functional autonomy of methods* (see Section 1.4), there were hidden complexities in this apparently simple type of paradigm (see Monsell, 2003, for review). One study, which isolates several important factors, is that of Braver et al. (2003). It investigated task-switching between two semantic tasks—making *manmade or natural* judgements about the meanings of concrete nouns and *large or small* ones. In so-called 'mixed' blocks a cue to which task was active was presented 2 sec before a word with a so-called *jitter* interval of from 0.5 to 5.5 sec

---

[15] Allport and Wylie (2000) investigated how switching between tasks was influenced by the particular stimuli that had occurred on a previous run of the other task. Subjects alternated between short runs of two tasks. One is the Stroop task, described in Section 9.3; subjects had to name the colours in which a word was printed. For the other they had to read aloud the words which were the names of colours. Some of the colours which the subject had to name had also occurred in the reading task. Allport and Wylie found that on trials which switched from reading to colour naming, subjects were slower to give the colour name if it had occurred recently in the other task than if the colour name had not occurred in the previous block of trials. This provides further evidence of the automatic triggering of schemas by associated perceptual triggers of schemas which then have to be inhibited (see Chapter 8).

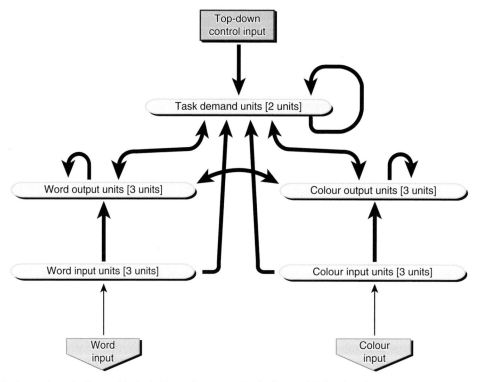

Fig. 9.14 The interactive activation model of switching in the Stroop task of Gilbert and Shallice (2002).

before the next task cue.[16] These mixed-task blocks, where both tasks were active over the block, were compared with single-task blocks, where only one task was active. Within the mixed-task blocks, *switch trials* were compared with *repeat* ones. Fast responses for a given task situation were also compared with slow ones.

The analysis carried out by Braver et al. enabled them to isolate regions in frontal cortex which produced greater sustained activity across a mixed-task block compared with single-task block trials but little transient effect within a trial (see Figure 9.15a; yellow regions). These regions will be discussed in Section 9.14. In complementary fashion, they could also isolate regions that overall saw no sustained increased in activation on mixed-trial blocks compared with single-trial ones but showed sizeable transient changes in activation within a block (see Figure 9.15a; red regions). The latter included a group of inferior left lateral frontal regions, of which the most posterior was close to that of Koechlin and Jubault's super-ordinate regions. The patterns of activation over the course of a trial in this area are shown in Figure 9.15b. It can be seen that in the preparatory period between the cue and the target, activation is higher when the subjects are fast on a trial

compared with when they are slow, while the opposite effect occurs after stimulus presentation has occurred. There is however no effect of trial type.[17] Braver et al., argue that this fits with what would be expected of a model such as that shown in Figure 9.14. The transiently activated regions just discussed—the inferior left lateral prefrontal ones—would correspond to the location of task-demand units discussed earlier.[18]

A broad-brush approach has also been used. A meta-analysis was carried out by Derrfuss et al. (2005) on functional imaging of what they call 'switching studies', specifically on 16 task comparisons where in one switching condition subjects must 'update their task representations based on cue information'. Derfuss et al. took the peak coordinates of the comparison between the switching condition and a non-switching one and treated them not as simple points but as the peak of 3D Gaussian probability distributions. A map is then created that gives for each voxel the probability that one or more of the maxima that entered the meta-analysis was

---

[16] The use of jitter allows one to disentangle the contribution to activation of events in the current trial from those of the preceding trial; see Section 5.4.

[17] The only area where there was any sign of task-set reconfiguration with switch trials producing more activation than repeat ones was, counter-intuitively, the left superior parietal cortex, far from a plausible seat for top-down control input.

[18] Further support for this simple type of model can be obtained from striking effects where the stimulus occurs prior to the task-cue, a paradigm investigated by Ruge and Braver (2008).

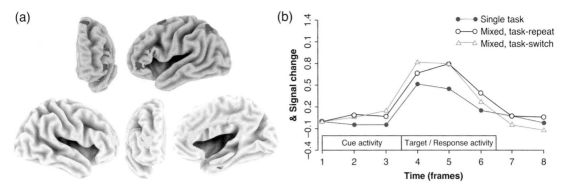

Fig. 9.15 (a) Regions obtained by Braver et al. (2003) in their study of task switching. Regions shown in yellow showed sustained activity across blocks rather than transient activity within a block. Regions shown in red showed the reverse contrast, i.e. more transient activity. (b) The activation of the left lateral prefrontal cortex over the course of the different types of trial. Reprinted from *Neuron*, 39(4), T.S. Braver, J.R. Reynolds and D.I. Donaldson, Neural mechanisms of transient and sustained cognitive control during task switching, pp. 713–726, Copyright (2003), with permission from Elsevier.

located at the voxel. This gives rise to a so-called activation likelihood estimate (ALE) map. This map is then compared to ALE maps derived from randomly distributed activation maxima. The null hypothesis of the random distribution could be rejected for a small region of the so-called inferior frontal junction (IFJ) lying on the inferior posterior lateral frontal cortex just anterior of the premotor cortex (see Figure 9.16). Brass et al. (2005) argue that this region is a key area for 'cognitive control'; however they do not elaborate theoretically what this involves, merely saying rather poetically that it is 'our ability to orchestrate our thoughts and actions in accordance with internal goals' (p. 315).[19]

Apart from the vagueness of the conclusion, there is a range of problems with it as far as it relates to any hypothetical processes involved in task-switching. An initial relatively minor problem is that the left and right IFJ are not the only regions that are above threshold in the meta-analysis. So are the anterior cingulate/superior medial region and a fairly inferior right prefrontal area anterior of the IFJ. More problematic for our present purposes is that the meta-analysis does not just include task-switching studies, it also includes imaging studies based on Wisconsin Card-Sorting, which as we saw also involve other complex processes, and in addition ones based on reversing stimulus-response contingencies which do not involve changing task-set at all. Even worse, of the 7 actual task-switching studies included, only 2 activated the IFJ and in one of these there were 13 different maxima!

If functional imaging does not provide a decisive answer to this question of where high-level schemas and the corresponding elements within the supervisory system are localised, can neuropsychology help? The answer is as yet no. Four studies with more than 10 frontal subjects have been run on task-switching (Rogers et al., 1998; Mecklinger et al., 1999; Aron et al., 2004; Shallice et al., 2008a). All studies found left lateral frontal patients to have problems in task-switching and one (Aron et al.) found them for right frontal patients too. However the left frontal regions held to be critical in both cases where more detailed anatomical claims are made is the middle frontal gyrus rather than the inferior frontal gyrus (Aron et al., 2004; Shallice et al., 2008a). Moreover as we will see later, the latter study, at least, pinpointed the relevant function which was impaired as involving task-learning *per se* and so was not directly relevant to localisation of task-demand units.

Whatever the inferior frontal junction region is held to do, the Derfuss et al. meta-analysis does not provide strong evidence that it corresponds to the location of task-demand units as specified so far. Indeed if Sakai and Passingham, and even Koechlin and Jubault, are right and different types of task-demand units are located in different brain regions, then there would be no common denominator for their localisation and the meta-analytic logic of Derrfuss et al. would not be an appropriate way to obtain information about them. We will therefore provisionally accept, as the most plausible interpretation of somewhat ambiguous data, that the *task-demand units* located in Broca's area or the premotor region as obtained, say, in Koechlin and Jubault's subordinate tasks are functionally *schema* units in contention scheduling. By contrast, when as in Koechlin and Jubault's super-ordinate tasks or Braver et al.'s transiently activated units, task-demand units are located in the posterior part of the lateral prefrontal cortex; they

---

[19] Derrfuss et al. (2005) support this conclusion by showing that the left IFS is also the main region above threshold in a meta-analysis of the Stroop colour-word task, which also makes heavy demands on cognitive control.

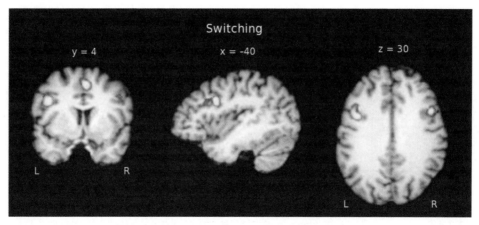

Fig. 9.16 Results of the metaanalysis of task switching studies by Derrfuss et al. (2005). The main finding was involvement of the inferior frontal junction. Reprinted from J. Derrfuss, M. Brass, J. Neumann and D.Y. von Cramon, 2005, Involvement of the inferior frontal junction in cognitive control: Meta-analyses of switching and stroop studies. *Human Brain Mapping*, 25, 22–34. Copyright © 2005, John Wiley and Sons.

would correspond to the location of cognitive elements in the lower levels of the supervisory system, which could be called *task-set* representations.[20] It should be emphasised that these anatomical to functional correspondences are as yet not solidly based.

9.6 On the Internal Organisation of the Supervisory System: a Hierarchical Approach

There have been enough preliminary discussions in this chapter. We must confront the central question. Consider a system that attempts to cope in practice with non-routine situations and has available to it a vast repertoire of knowledge, and of well-learned actions and cognitive operations and procedures. In addition it can control language production processes. What form should it take? There have been essentially two approaches as to how one might conceive of hypothetical subsystems engaged in supervisory operations.

Much the most fashionable approach is to use the framework of cognitive control related to that of task-switching and to replace the hierarchical relation between the supervisory system and contention scheduling by multiple layers of control levels. This echoes the hierarchy of TOTE (Test Operate Test Exit) units suggested for action control by Miller et al. (1960) fifty years ago. A key addition is that anatomically the hierarchy is an extension of that proposed by Fuster (1989)

(see Figure 9.17) into prefrontal cortex. The control systems are held to be realised on some posterior to anterior axis within the lateral prefrontal cortex (see Figure 9.18). Experiments to assess this type of conceptual possibility typically attempt to differentiate between tasks according to the position of their critical component in an apparent hierarchy of control.

An excellent example of the empirical evidence used to support such a conception comes from the study of Badre and D'Esposito (2007), which was discussed with respect to its methodology in Section 5.6. Subjects had a set of four choice reaction-time tasks (see Figure 5.22). The tasks, however, differed on how abstract was the critical choice involved. The critical highest-level choice required in a given task was thought of as involving one particular level of control. However the tasks were roughly downwards compatible in the control hierarchy in that the relevant dimension of a lower level of the hierarchy of processing in one task occurred as a critical level in another task. At the same time, the degree of conflict for the subject at each level was manipulated. For instance, in the easiest 'Response' experiment, the four colours could be mapped onto 1, 2 or 4 responses in different blocks of 8 trials.

Behaviourally the higher the level of control the longer the reaction time and the higher the error rate, although error rates were generally low. Also the more the degree of competition, the slower the reaction times were in general. As far as the fMRI findings are concerned, the authors concentrated on the four regions shown in Figure 5.23. The reported activations are in left frontal cortex.[21] It can be seen that the four

---

[20] Alternatively such representations could correspond to higher-level source schemas within contention scheduling. However higher-level schemas in contention scheduling also need to be controlled by units with temporary memory capacities, which we assume are not available in premotor cortex for durations of a few seconds or more.

[21] Frontal activations were also observed in left SMA (response competition conditions only), and right mid-dorsolateral PFC (context competition conditions only).

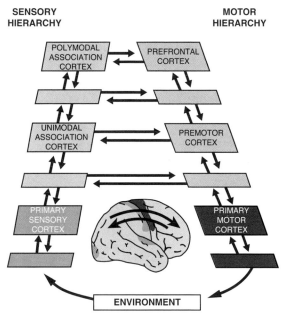

SENSORY HIERARCHY

MOTOR HIERARCHY

POLYMODAL ASSOCIATION CORTEX

PREFRONTAL CORTEX

UNIMODAL ASSOCIATION CORTEX

PREMOTOR CORTEX

PRIMARY SENSORY CORTEX

PRIMARY MOTOR CORTEX

ENVIRONMENT

Fig. 9.17 Fuster's account of the functional organisation of the cortex, in which prefrontal cortex sits at the top of a hierarchy of mappings between lower-level sensory and motor areas. Reprinted from *Neuron*, *30*(2), J. Fuster, The prefrontal cortex – an update: Time is of the essence, pp. 319–333, Copyright (2001), with permission from Elsevier.

regions differ in the lowest level of control which shows an effect of competition. Moreover what they call the pre-PMD (dorsal pre-premotor cortex; region B on Figure 5.23) is virtually equivalent to the inferior frontal junction of Brass et al. (2005) discussed earlier in the chapter (Section 9.5). The results overall fit with the idea of four different levels of control each stressed by a different type of competition. In addition there are similar effects for competition at the higher levels of control too at this inferior frontal junction region and to a lesser extent in the somewhat lower and more anterior inferior frontal sulcus (region C in Figure 5.23) but not for the dorsal premotor region (region A on Figure 5.23).

This seems to fit with a model of cascading inputs between different levels as might be expected if each level were just a new set of hidden units roughly analogous to models suggested by O'Reilly et al. (2002). However, this could be too superficial a view. First, statistical support for the existence of Badre and D'Esposito's parametric effects of competition is greatly assisted by the presence of no competition conditions at all levels. Whether their two above zero competition conditions give rise to statistically different activation levels, particularly in the case of feature and dimension competition, is unclear; so the results need to be rephrased in terms of presence or absence of competition at different levels.

Second, and more critically, two regions clearly differ qualitatively from the others; we are not dealing just with a simple quantitative relation between levels. The dorsal

premotor region (region A) is not in a cascading relation with more anterior regions. For instance, the dimension effect for region B is large but there is no suggestion of the effect at region A. It appears to be a *qualitatively different* processing domain, and this fits with its being in a region concerned with what we referred to earlier as contention scheduling.

In addition, the analysis carried out on the most anterior region (region D) differs in one respect from the others. For three of the regions (regions A, B and C in Figure 5.23) what is shown is the percentage change within a trial. For the fourth, the most anterior region (region D in Figure 5.23), it can be seen that the value is much smaller. This is because the percentage of signal change was averaged over the whole block. Therefore the effects obtained in region D are not directly comparable to the effects in the other three regions. Moreover a considerably more anterior site was obtained than in a logically equivalent condition of an earlier study of Koechlin et al. (2003). Figure 9.15 discussed in the previous section with respect to the findings of Braver et al. (2003) also indicated that the frontopolar cortex seems to be involved in potentiating multiple task schemas across a block. We will discuss the region further in Section 9.15.

This leaves two regions, which given the arguments in Section 5.6 cannot be adequately separated functionally in a principled fashion given these findings. The first is the inferior frontal junction (pre-PMD), discussed extensively with respect to activation of source schemas in Section 9.5. Such a characterization for the region fits

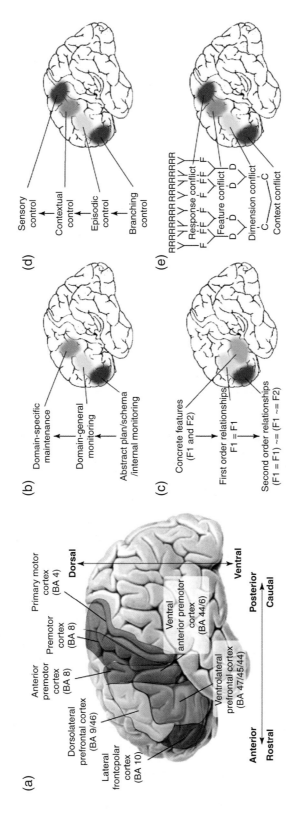

Fig. 9.18 The major anatomical sub-divisions of the frontal lobe, emphasising an anterior–posterior organisation (a) and a summary of theoretical positions on a possible anterior–posterior gradient (b, c, d and e). (b) The working memory perspective (e.g. Smith & Jonides, 1999). (c) The relational complexity view of Christoff et al. (2003). (d) The cascade model of Koechlin and Summerfield (2007). (e) The representational hierarchy view of Badre and D'Esposito (2007). Reprinted from *Trends in Cognitive Sciences, 12*(5), D. Badre, Cognitive control, hierarchy, and the rostro-caudal organization of the frontal lobes, pp. 193–200. Copyright (2008) with permission from Elsevier.

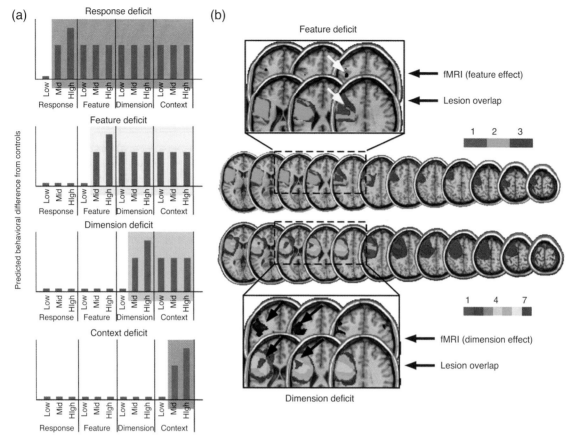

Fig. 9.19 Badre et al's (2009) analysis of the relation between patient lesion site and performance on their task involving four levels of control. (a) Four regressors, corresponding to idealised deficits at each of their four levels of control, were constructed for the analysis. (b) Lesion overlap analysis found the peak for dimension deficit patients to be anterior to the peak for feature deficit patients, mirroring the earlier imaging results. Reprinted by permission from Macmillan Publishers Ltd: D. Badre, J. Hoffman, J.W. Cooney and M. D'Esposito (2009). Hierarchical cognitive control deficits following damage to the human frontal lobe. *Nature Neuroscience*, *12*(4), 515–522. Copyright (2009).

well with the processing required when the colour of the square signals that feature is relevant. The second region is a somewhat more inferior and anterior part of the inferior frontal sulcus, which we have argued corresponds to the lowest level of representations in the supervisory system. A qualitative difference between these regions could well relate to a difference on the anterior–posterior dimension in the degree of control, depending on how well the task schemas have been acquired as discussed in Section 9.5. However even

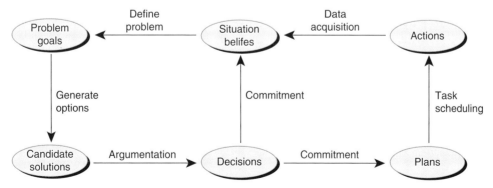

Fig. 9.20 Fox's domino architecture, showing how the six computational domains map between the various databases. In a COGENT implementation the arrows would each involve a process.

simple task-switching studies have many levels of complexity (see Monsell, 2003) so that, given the inference problems discussed in Section 5.6, such a conclusion must be highly speculative without a more detailed functional analysis of the tasks involved.

That the idea of a hierarchy of control in the spirit of Miller, Galanter and Pribram has considerable force is demonstrated by a study of Badre et al. (2009) using essentially the same combination of tasks, but now adapted for patient use. They compared the performance of 12 patients with focal frontal lesions with controls. In 62% of the 4-condition-by-12 patient combinations, the patient's performance was impaired, in that they scored more than 2SDs worse than the controls. However if a lower-level task gave rise to an impairment, then there was a 91% chance of the patient being impaired on a higher-level task, a significantly higher value.[22] Moreover when patients were allocated to subgroups by a best fit to a regressor procedure (see Figure 9.19), then the lesion sites were strikingly similar to the corresponding functional imaging sites found in Badre and D'Esposito (2007). Again, however, the evidence is most solid for the two middle levels. It would appear from Figure 9.19 that 10/12 patients were of these feature-impairment or dimension-impairment types.

Despite the powerful support coming from the studies such as those of Badre, D'Espositio and their colleagues just discussed, we need a complementary approach to that of a processing hierarchy. Consider the posterior regions of the cortex. For them the idea of hierarchy provides a useful conceptual framework, for instance for the inferior temporal cortex. However, for posterior cortex as a whole the idea of a single hierarchy would be far too simplistic. At least as important is the existence of processing systems with qualitatively different properties which mutually interact but do not merely involve computational domains that differ only in level. It is to this way of conceiving of the relation between supervisory subsystems to which we now turn.

9.7 On the Internal Organisation of the Supervisory System: the Domino Analogy

In Section 9.6 we left a much larger issue untouched. In *The Modularity of Mind* (1983) Jerry Fodor took the position that unlike the input systems, what he called the *central systems* involved in thought could not be modular. Fodor takes the example of theory production in science. This argument, grossly simplified, begins with the claim that there can be no limits

to what sort of information might be relevant in producing a plausible novel approach in scientific reasoning. Scientific inference is, he argues, conceptually unbounded. Take *On The Origin of Species* (Darwin, 1859). All sorts of apparently unrelated facts are considered in the argument from effects of domestication to what is now known as the Cambrian fossil explosion to animal morphology and to the distribution of species on oceanic islands.

However, Fodor takes scientific argument as merely a paradigm case. He extends the claim even to the processing involved in understanding a sentence. And he would certainly apply it to the systems used in confronting non-routine situations. The inferential system involved cannot have an informationally encapsulated input. Thus it cannot be modular.

This argument has been extensively criticised (see e.g. Cain, 2002). Most critically it takes too restricted a view of what a modular system might be. Consider Fodor's concept of a central system underlying thought. We hold in contrast to Fodor that its internal architecture could be broadly modular, but that there would need to be four core properties of a modular system if it were to provide the architecture to carry out central cognitive processes in the Fodorian sense:

1 Each subsystem would carry out a specific type of abstract computation (properties M2 and M7 from Chapter 3).

2 Each of these types of computation would be markedly different from that carried out by any other subsystem. By a *markedly different* computation we mean that one cannot take the neural implementation of one of the computations and, with relatively little modification, produce a neural implementation of one of the other computations (see Section 3.5, footnote 35).

3 Each of these types of computation is one that is frequently carried out by the intelligent agent which possesses the central system (see Section 3.5).

4 Certain individual central subsystems have potential access to the full range of outputs of the input systems, of semantic and episodic memory systems, and to the 'dictionary' of the intelligent agent's range of cognitive and higher-level motor skills. By *potential access* we mean that the relevant cognitive elements are not *in principle* unavailable to the subsystem as they would be if the input to it were informationally encapsulated (see the discussion in Section 2.5).

Why do we see these as core properties? Consider an evolutionary or learning process. For dedicated hardware in a brain to be devoted to a specific type of computation it must be one that is heavily used. If relatively little extra modification were required to implement a second frequently used computation, then a brain could

---

[22] It is not clear whether this effect must almost inevitably arise because of the logical relation between the tasks.

efficiently combine the two into a core computational component, possibly with an additional computationally light ancillary system or systems. As we will see in the next chapter, such a manoeuvre may well be true of the systems used for navigating around an environment and those involved in episodic memory (see also Section 2.2). Finally the position accepts the Fodorian argument that certain central subsystems need not be informationally encapsulated but does not accept that this implies there is only one central system.

Is it plausible that confronting non-routine situations might involve a set of such frequently used types of computations carried out in different subsystems? It is! Working from an Artificial Intelligence perspective, Fox and Das (2000) have produced a general account of how an artificial cognitive system can confront non-routine situations. The account is informed very directly by its application in concrete situations, namely medical decision-making and the organisation of longer-term treatment and care.

Fox and Das provide an account of what cognitive capacities are required by what they call a *third-order agent*. If a system operates by evaluating some function and responding on the basis of its evaluation then it is a *zero-order agent*; thus a thermostat is a zero-order agent. A *first-order agent* adds to this by containing an explicit model of the environment and its intended actions. A *second-order agent* contains more than one such model and so can be more adaptive than a first-order one by being able to compare alternative interpretations of the world and consider alternative plans of action. Finally, *third-order agents* 'are second-order agents that maintain a higher-order (meta) model of their beliefs and desires, including the justifications for their beliefs and intentions and the expected consequences of their intended actions' (Das et al., 1997, p. 412). Such capacities are not available to a simple production system operating in the fashion of contention scheduling—additional systems are required (see Newell, 1990).[23]

The recent line of work referred to above, that of Fox and Das (2000), contains both a general account of how to implement so-called third-order agents—ones that have a higher order model of their beliefs and can

justify their actions—as well as the specific applications of such a model to a variety of medical decision-making situations. Their model is called the *domino model* from its shape (see Figure 9.20). It consists of a collection of databases (nodes) and computational operations or functions (arrows). It operates in the following fashion. First it maintains a database of beliefs about a particular environment; in the medical context this includes patient data. Certain beliefs (e.g. unexplained weight loss) cause the system to raise goals (e.g. to explain the abnormal weight loss). Such goals lead to problem-solving to find candidate solutions (e.g. weight loss may be caused by cancer or peptic ulcer) and arguments are constructed for and against the candidates, by instantiating general argument schemas on the situation model (patient data) and general domain knowledge (medical knowledge). As additional data are required a point may arise where an assessment of the arguments for and against the various candidates permits the system to commit to a most probable hypothesis (e.g. cancer). This is accepted as a new belief, which, while it is held, guides further problem solving and action. Since the new belief concerns an undesirable—indeed life-threatening—condition another goal is raised, to decide on the best therapy for the patient (Fox & Das, 2000, pp. xxv–xxvii).

This triggers a further cycle of reasoning which again involves the left-hand part of Figure 9.20. 'As before candidate decision options are proposed (surgery, chemotherapy, etc.) and arguments are generated for and against the alternatives. In due course a commitment may be made to a single therapy (e.g. chemotherapy)' (Das et al., 1997, p. 415). Now the process extends to the right half of the figure. Clinical therapies, such as chemotherapy, are complex procedures executed over time. Such therapies can usually be modelled as hierarchical plans that decompose into atomic actions (e.g. administer a drug) and subplans (e.g. take baseline measurements, administer several cycles of therapy, and then follow up the patient for a period). The framework acknowledges this by providing ways of representing plans and specifying the control processes required during plan execution. In particular, the atomic actions of a plan must be scheduled.

So far the argument fits with many frameworks based on common-sense for the segregation of the subprocesses of planning in real-world situations (e.g. Ben-Yishay & Diller, 1983). What is critical about the domino model is that each stage is held to correspond to a different computational domain, each of which is sufficiently distinct to require a different 'logic' and a different underlying set of axioms. The stages are:

1 *(Defining problem stage)* The first computational domain is that required to specify the goal that the agent will

---

[23] Dennett (1996) proposes a somewhat similar hierarchy of 'minds', ranging from Darwinian minds, which have only hardwired behaviours and 'learn' on an evolutionary timescale, through Skinnerian and Popperian minds, to Gregorian minds, which are able to reflect on and learn from the behaviour of others. The computational nature of the order of agents conception is more suitable for the current discussion. And of course a hierarchical structuring of agents could well relate to the theories of the hierarchical organisation of prefrontal processing discussed in Section 9.6.

aim to achieve. This involves abstracting from the current situation those aspects that the agent will aim to improve.

2 *(Generate options)* The second computational domain is that required to produce possible procedures (candidate solutions) for attaining the goal.

3 *(Argumentation)* The third computational domain is that involved in producing arguments to select between the possible procedures in order to make a decision to act.[24]

4 *(Commitment)* The fourth computational domain is that necessary for the agent to commit to one possible procedure on the basis of the arguments from the third computational domain and articulate the selected procedure into a series of individual steps which are potentially implementable.

5 *(Task scheduling)* The fifth computational domain is that necessary in realising the steps as actions at the appropriate time.

6 *(Data acquisition)* The sixth computational domain is that used in checking that these actions are indeed assisting in realising the goal or goals. If not, the cycle begins again. A new goal is set up either to patch the existing procedure or to abort it and replace it by another.

What does it mean that different logics are required for the different domains? For instance, the selection between different candidate options to produce a decision uses a so-called *logic of argument*. This is a variant of intuitionistic logic (van Dalen, 1986). There is a set of inference rules which are used to construct arguments. In this logic the arguments do not prove their consequences but merely indicate support or doubt (Fox et al., 1993; see also Fox, 2009). They can be combined to produce a partial-ordering relation among the candidates being entertained by the system, so specifying what are the best ones, what are the next best, and so on. If, instead one considers the stage of going from plans to actions, this involves first assessing a set of preconditions, namely whether the basic conditions hold for the putative action to be carried out. The second stage then requires the realising of subtasks which involves scheduling constraints concerning the ordering of subtasks and specifying situations under which the actions will be aborted. Contrast these two stages of decision-making of deciding on a plan and implementing it. The first works in a domain of prioritising among alternatives, while the second operates in terms of time

and resources. The computational functions operating in the two domains have very different properties and dimensions. Yet each is very frequently used.

Applying our modular approach to Fodorian central systems discussed above, it becomes plausible that a neurally-based cognitive system faced with similar computational challenges to that of the Fox and Das package will implement its set of solutions as a set of neurally separable systems. The situation is seen to be abstractly similar to the way that syntactic operations and visuo-spatial processing—one producing a discrete single-dimensional output, the other operating in continuous two-or-three dimensional spaces—are implemented by different hardware in the brain.

The argument just made from considering Fox and Das's model can be viewed as operating on two different levels. First, it may be seen as corroboration from engineering an AI system that there are potential computational benefits in a modular structure for prefrontal cortex given it has the overall function of confronting non-routine situations. Second, the model suggests some specific computational functions that these subsystems may need to carry out. In the rest of this chapter we aim to show that the conclusions of the more abstract level of argument hold. Then we treat the Fox and Das proposals for the organisation of the domino model at the second, more concrete, level much more tentatively, as a set of hypotheses that need to be considered in the light of empirical cognitive neuroscience evidence. The conclusion will be that they are fine as far as they go, but that further processes need to be added. In the next few sections, together with sections in Chapters 10 and 12, we will therefore consider the following as potential computational primitives—active monitoring (required by data acquisition), commitment, option-generation, decision-production and argumentation, task scheduling and problem-definition. We take them in this order as the interpretation of the empirical evidence is increasingly uncertain as one moves along the list. In Chapters 10 and 12 we add computational functions not considered in Fox and Das's skeleton third-order agent.

There is, though, a problem. Much of the evidence for a heterarchical approach comes from an empirical method little discussed to this point, namely the neuropsychological group study. As a preliminary step for the more detailed discussion we introduce this method in the next section.

9.8 The Neuropsychological Group Study

In earlier chapters we have used individual case dissociations as evidence for separable systems. This

---

[24] This concept of 'argument' corresponds to the traditional sense and not to the concept of a function's argument, used in COGENT and in Chapter 8.

methodology works less well for prefrontal systems.[25] We need therefore to introduce a methodology for isolating subsystems based on localisation-based neuropsychological group studies.[26] The inferential methodology to be adopted is analogous to one considered in the context of single case studies (see Chapter 4). It is to take a set of tasks which in different combinations require the use of different subsets of a set of processing resources. In such a group study procedure a set of tasks are used with as far as possible a common set of input and output processes. If performance of different tasks in the set is compromised due to lesions in different sites then this provides analogous evidence to that of double dissociations in single case studies.[27]

There are various problems in applying this methodology. The first is that lesions in different locations may have different properties other than their location. They may, for instance, tend to occur in patients of different ages or aetiologies or they may differ in size. The second is that even when there are double dissociations, attempts to localise the key computational components of a given test can be indirectly confounded by associated deficits—due to lesions 'counted as' of area X actually also involving area Y. Third the sensitivity of a measure to lesions in a particular area will depend on the number of patients with damage there.

These are not just a problem if localisation uses presence or absence (however defined) in specific areas. Correlations between behavioural measures and the amount of damage in particular areas (Aron et al., 2004), which do not depend on parcellation of areas a priori, are also subject to the same problems, and the third for instance is a more severe difficulty. This is so even if use is made of sophisticated packages such as Voxel Behaviour Mapping (VBM) (see Section 6.7) or Lesion-Behaviour Mapping (LBM) (see Section 8.8)—which differ in whether the lesion is realised manually on slices or not. However the most important reason for not relying solely on such methods is that they do

not allow the results of multiple experiments to be easily compared as the critical group becomes different in each. They should be a second string methodology to be used when critical components have been isolated.

A particular application of the neuropsychological group methodology approach to the frontal cortex articulated by Stuss et al. (1995) was to tackle the underlying organisation of the anterior attentional systems using a conceptual framework that was a hybrid of the supervisory system approach and that developed by Posner and Petersen a few years before. It was hypothesised that a set of basic processes required in attentional tasks would be localised to different regions of prefrontal cortex. A series of empirical studies, known as ROBBIA, were set up to examine the performance of patients with lesions in different parts of prefrontal cortex on a set of simple tasks with common structural resource requirements. In this set of studies patients with prefrontal lesions were divided into four groups—left lateral, right lateral, superior medial and inferior medial—according to the general location of the lesions (see Figure 9.21).[28]

9.9 On Energising

We begin with processes somewhat orthogonal to those considered in the chapter so far, and consider first *energisation*. When the type of subgrouping procedure just described was used with frontal patients a striking feature was that three of the groups showed no slowing on many of the reaction time tasks. Take carrying out a 5-choice serial reaction time task in which the subject must press one of five keys each lying directly below one of five lights. The really demanding part of the serial reaction time task, though, is that there is only a 200- msec interval between the response to one light being made and the next light coming on. Surprisingly, frontal lobe patients do not slow up over 500 consecutive trials, and three of the subgroups are just as fast as controls (Alexander et al., 2005). One subgroup, however, the Superior Medial group was 30% slower than the others (see Figure 9.22a). This type of effect is a highly consistent finding over a variety of studies (Stuss et al.,

---

[25] Why this is the case is discussed in FNMS Section 14.4.

[26] Twenty years ago strong arguments were produced against making inferences to theories of normal function from neuropsychological group studies where group membership was defined by behavioural characteristics (e.g. Caramazza, 1986). Group studies with membership defined by localisation of lesion are much more robust inferentially (see FNMS Chapter 9).

[27] Formally, cross-over double dissociations are critical (see FNMS Chapter 9) but this will tend to be the case if the dissociations obtained are 'classical', as they are in the studies to be described shortly. There is nothing to prevent functional imaging studies using the same methodology (see the discussion of Henson's criteria in Chapter 5). The use of a wide set of fairly closely matched studies, characteristic of cognitive neuropsychology, is not however standard in functional imaging.

---

[28] Pragmatically the number of groups is limited by the need to have at least roughly 10 patients per group, given the inevitably large differences in factors like age and education in a typical group of patients. This division was originally developed by Stuss et al. (1998) using a statistical procedure—the CART—which in cluster analysis style makes the most consistent division between subgroups to give the clearest differential effect of a variable, which happened to be verbal fluency. However the medial-lateral contrast is such an important functional divide in prefrontal functions that it has continued to be used in other tasks.

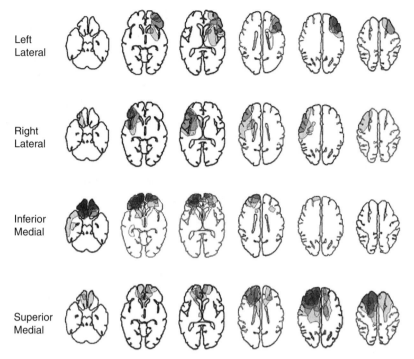

Fig. 9.21 Lesion locations (left-right reversed) of the patient groups considered in the ROBBIA series of studies. Reprinted with permission from T. Shallice, D.T. Stuss, T.W. Picton, M.P. Alexander and S. Gillingham (2008), Multiple effects of prefrontal lesions on task-switching. *Frontiers in Human Neuroscience*, 1(2), 1–12. Copyright (2008), the authors.

2002, 2005; Alexander et al., 2007; Picton et al., 2007; Shallice et al., 2008a, 2008b). Moreover, as we will see later in the chapter, many factors which lengthen reaction time exacerbate the Superior Medial deficit.

What might this energisation process involve? For routine tasks, say when walking along a very easy and safe path, where contention scheduling can operate in unmodulated fashion, the activation of the appropriate systems can be assumed to occur bottom-up. If, however, contention scheduling operating without top-down control would not produce an appropriate response or would, say, operate too slowly or with insufficient accuracy, other processes will be needed. These processes correspond to those considered in the ergonomics literature

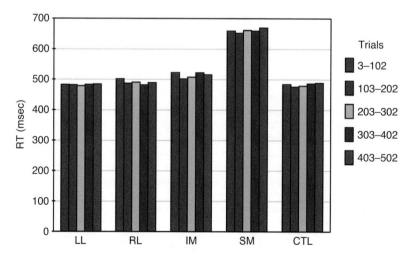

Fig. 9.22 Mean reaction times for controls and four patient groups in the 5-choice serial reaction time task of Alexander et al. (2005), binned into 100 trial bands. None of the groups show any slowing over the task, but the Superior Medial patients are slower than all other groups throughout the entire experiment. Data from Alexander et al. (2005).

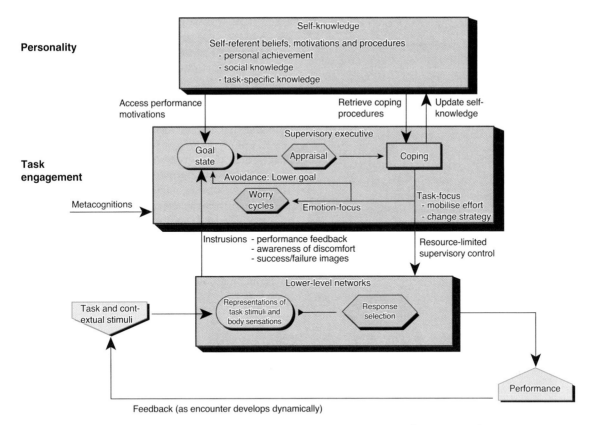

Fig. 9.23 The model of the interaction of task engagement and personality of Mathews et al. (2010). The concept of *Energisation* corresponds to the *mobilise effort* part of *Task Engagement*.

as responsible for *cognitive effort* (Hockey, 1993) or, more specifically within the supervisory system approach, the *mobilise effort* part of the Task Engagement processes of Matthews et al. (2010) (see Figure 9.23). When a task is carried out not only do the individual schemas and their arguments have to be selected, but the isolable systems that are required must also be activated and general parameters like speed-accuracy trade-offs set. Moreover this configuration must be sustained if the stimulus situation does not continually trigger action. Energisation carries out these more global functions.

Without supervisory control, contention scheduling has the potential to be captured by any random aspect of the stimulus situation. Where the cognitive demands of the task are simple or extremely well learned, then lateral prefrontal cortex is not critical for adequate task execution. However, preventing inappropriate capturing of behaviour by irrelevant aspects of the stimulus situation is still required, and impairment of the energisation system will lead to such captures taking place. This is why behaviours like the grasp reflex or utilisation behaviour discussed in Section 9.2 occur with medial prefrontal lesions more than lateral prefrontal ones.

The Superior Medial region is, though, a large area of prefrontal cortex. It includes the anterior cingulate.

This position is closely related to the position of other theorists on the anterior cingulate, particularly those who view it as part of an arousal network; these include Paus et al. (1997), Sturm and Willmes (2001) and Mottaghy et al. (2006). Certain versions of the Posner-Petersen attentional theory are also related. Thus Posner and Di Girolamo (1998) view the function of the anterior cingulate as providing general facilitation when supervisory system processing is required.

That the anterior cingulate has a mediating effect on other structures rather than being directly involved in top-down control of task performance has been elegantly shown by MacDonald et al. (2000). They had subjects prepare for a Stroop stimulus. Prior to each trial they were instructed on whether they should read the stimulus word or name the ink-colour. Subjects were scanned after the trial instruction and before the appearance of the stimulus. Left dorsolateral regions, but not the anterior cingulate, showed elevated activation during this interval if the trial required naming of the ink colour (the more difficult condition); it can be presumed that left dorsolateral regions were involved in preparing for the ink-naming task by the activation of appropriate task-set representations. The anterior cingulate was, however, more activated in the critical

Stroop condition *after* the stimulus arrived. As was later shown by Kerns et al. (2004) its role was to activate the dorsolateral region. Subjects who showed greater activation of the anterior cingulate on trial *n* showed increased activation of the dorsolateral prefrontal cortex on trial *n+1* (see Figure 9.24). Instead of direct top-down activation the role of the anterior cingulate fits better with a slower energising function.

The anterior cingulate is not at all the only structure within the superior medial regions. Moreover, it is not the only structure that has been associated with some form of energizing function. In general, though, it is rather difficult to differentiate by neuropsychological means between the functions of structures on the medial frontal surface because lesions arising from vascular accidents, in particular, often affect much of the medial surface. Moreover, TMS, for instance, cannot be used to study the anterior cingulate. It is too deep on the medial surface. TMS can however be used to investigate another structure on the medial surface, called the pre-SMA (supplementary motor area) (see Figure 9.25a). Thus, it has been known, since the work of Sternberg et al. (1978) that if the subject must produce a rapid sequence of motor responses, the reaction time to make the first response, but not later ones, is lengthened with increasing complexity of the sequence. It is assumed that the subject must compile the action schema prior to the first response. If the sequence is longer than the capacity of the relevant short-term memory buffer being used, then subjects tend to chunk the sequence into subsequences and a similar slowing occurs prior to each chunk being produced (see Figure 9.25b). Kennerley et al. (2004) examined how TMS over the pre-SMA affected the ability of subjects to produce such a long sequence of motor responses. They found, in a somewhat analogous fashion to the slowing of reaction time in the studies discussed above, that reaction time is indeed slowed. However, the slowing occurred

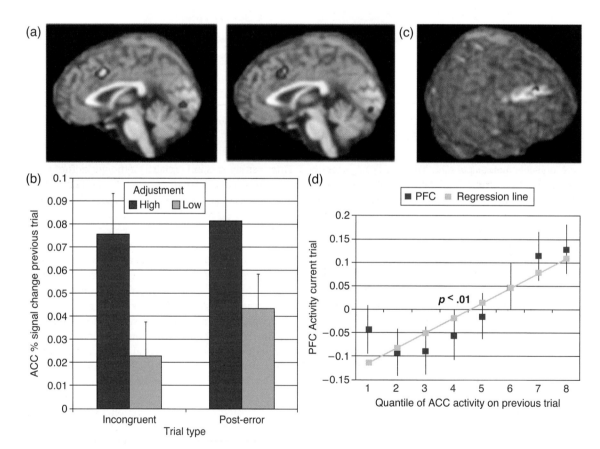

Fig. 9.24 The involvement of the anterior cingulate in the Stroop task. (a) Anterior cingulate activation was observed on (left) incongruent and (right) error Stroop trials (compared with congruent and no error trials). (b) Signal change in the anterior cingulate cortex on high adjustment trials (faster RT for incongruent trials and slower RT for post-error trials) is greater than on low adjustment trials. (c) The area of right middle frontal gyrus found to be more active during high adjustment (post-conflict and post-error) trials than equivalent low adjustment trials. (d) Anterior cingulate activity on trial *n−1* predicts lateral prefrontal activity on trial *n*. From J.G. Kerns, J.D. Cohen, A.W. MacDonald III, R.Y. Cho, V.A. Atenger and C.S. Carter, 2004, Anterior cingulate conflict monitoring and adjustments in control. *Science*, 303(1023), 1023–1036. Reprinted with permission from AAAS.

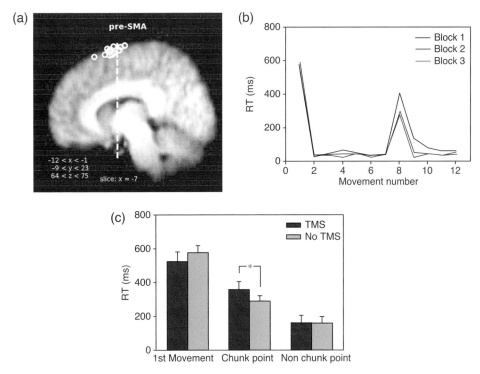

Fig. 9.25 (a) Composite image showing the pre-SMA locations at which TMS was administered in the study of Kennerley et al. (2004). (b) A plot of RT against movement number for one subject, suggesting that the subject chunked a sequence of 12 movements into a subsequence of 7 movements followed by another subsequence of 5. (c) RT at different points in the sequence when TMS was (and was not) applied over the pre-SMA. Adapted with permission from S.W. Kennerley, J. Sakai and M.F.S. Rushworth (2004). Organization of action sequences and the role of the pre-SMA. *Journal of Neurophysiology*, 91(2), 978–933. Figure 3a, p981, Figure 4, p983, and Figure 6, p985.

only at chunk points, points at which they broke down a long sequence into subsequences. Responses within chunks were unaffected by TMS (see Figure 9.25c). Thus energisation might well be implemented at different points on the medial surface with respect to different positions in the hierarchy of control within lateral prefrontal cortex.[29] As far as the pre-SMA is concerned this would be at the level of motor chunks within contention scheduling, while for the anterior cingulate it would be at the level of selection of task-set representations, as in the Kerns et al. study of the Stroop task.

9.10 On Active Monitoring and Checking

Returning to the processing systems localised in the lateral frontal cortices, it has been known since the 1990s that tasks involving estimation of time present problems to frontal patients. Why should this be the case? Rao et al. (2001), for instance, compared two tasks using the

same set of tones in a well-balanced design. The stimuli were two pairs of 50- msec tones. In the first task the subject must make duration comparisons of the interval between the first two tones and that between the second two. In the second task a pitch judgement is made about whether the second tone in the second pair is higher or lower than the other three. Using fMRI, Rao et al. examined when in a 10- sec interval, different regions of the brain were more activated in one task or the other.

Compared with an undemanding control task requiring listening and responding to tones, many regions are more activated in time perception tasks, but most of these are also activated in the pitch judgement task. A right mid-dorsolateral frontal region is however selectively involved in time but not pitch perception. Earlier, Mangels et al. (1998) had proposed that an analogous effect is due to monitoring. Instead Rao et al. argued that the right prefrontal cortex is carrying out a working memory function. Indeed as we do not have a componential analysis of the task, any account must be speculative.

Two ROBBIA studies both supported a monitoring impairment account of a specifically right lateral frontal impairment in time-related tasks, which, however, like the Mangels et al. studies involved somewhat longer intervals. Thus Picton et al. (2006) studied the

---

[29] Such a possibility has been suggested by Kouneiher et al. (2009).

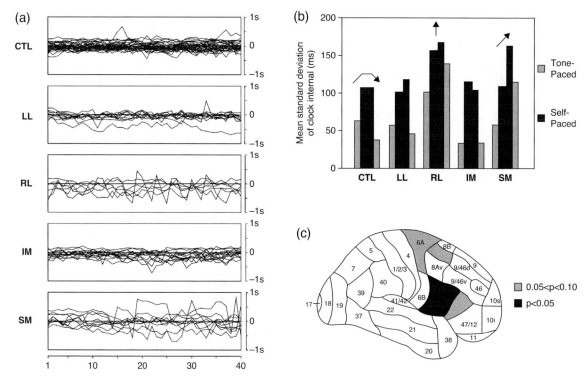

Fig. 9.26 (a) Tone–response intervals for all patients in the final tone-paced block of the study of Picton et al. (2006). There was more variability in the responses of Right Lateral (RL) and Superior Medial (SM) patients than of the other groups. (b) Mean variability of subject timing signals across the four blocks for each group of subjects. Right Lateral patients showed greater variability than other groups across all four blocks, while Superior Medial patients showed an increase in variability as the experiment progressed. (c) Localisation of lesions significantly associated with timing variability in the tone-paced condition. Reprinted from *Neuropsychologia*, 44(7), T.W. Picton, D.T. Stuss, T. Shallice M.P. Alexander and S. Gillingham, Keeping time: Effects of focal frontal lesions, pp. 1195–1209, Copyright (2006), with permission from Elsevier.

ability of patients to produce 50 taps at a 1.5- sec rate. This is done both in paced fashion by synchronising the taps with a series of tones and also by continuing a brief sequence of bleeps in an unpaced situation. A more natural rate would be a faster one, closer to 1 per sec, so the subject would have to carefully monitor their actual rate, with a failure leading to too rapid responding. Patients with Right Lateral prefrontal lesions tend to be too quick; they underestimate the intervals in the tone-paced blocks, echoing the results of earlier TMS studies of perception of intervals from 2 to several seconds (Koch et al., 2003; Jones et al., 2004). However in addition to the underestimation, Right Lateral frontal patients are also more variable than controls in the tapping intervals they produce. This occurs in both tone-paced and in self-paced tapping, which strengthens the plausibility of a difficulty in active monitoring as a possible account of their problem (see Figure 9.26).[30]

A second ROBBIA study (Shallice et al., 2008b) concerned vigilance. It involved the simple task of counting the number of bleeps occurring at a slow but variable rate, on average 1 per 3 sec. There were trains of 8–22 such bleeps. Right Lateral patients were not impaired. This does not accord with the 'vigilance' account of the functions of the right dorsolateral prefrontal regions that follows from the Posner–Petersen three-attention system model discussed earlier. However in a second task they had to count rapid sequences of bleeps occurring at a rate of roughly 3 per sec. Then the Right Lateral patients were significantly less accurate than controls, but without showing consistent underestimation.[31] The Right Lateral failure generally occurred for string lengths greater than 10, when subjects need to adjust their counting rate to cope with the extra length of each word; this fits with impaired active monitoring.

---

[30] By contrast with the Right Lateral patients, who do not consistently over or under estimate, Superior Medial patients were also more variable in their tapping rate, but not initially. They

only became so in the last two blocks, supporting the energising interpretation of superior medial impairments.

[31] The Superior Medial patients did, however, show consistent underestimation, again fitting an energisation account.

The argument that the right lateral prefrontal cortex is involved in the control of active monitoring or checking is compatible with the findings we have just described, but the findings do not tightly constrain this type of explanation; tapping rhythms and counting beeps could be derailed for a variety of reasons. This makes another of the ROBBIA studies especially important. This concerned the so-called *variable foreperiod* paradigm, where subjects prepare over an interval of a few seconds for a stimulus. This interval varies unpredictably, say obeying a rectangular distribution, from trial to trial. In this type of situation, it has been known for nearly 100 years that subjects respond faster with the longer intervals than the shorter (Woodrow, 1914). This effect is thought to be due to subjects deliberately changing their level of preparation as the varying interval gets longer, because the conditional probability of a signal occurring increases during a trial (Karlin, 1959; Drazin, 1961). At the same time, though, there are trial-to-trial sequential effects; subjects are faster if the previous foreperiod is short.

More recently, it has been argued by Los et al. (2001) that the speeding up over longer foreperiods can be explained, by analogy with certain conditioning phenomena, as a direct consequence of more basic sequential effects. They argue that the expectation for shorter foreperiods suffers extinction if followed by a longer foreperiod, but the expectation for longer foreperiods is not affected by an immediately following shorter foreperiod. However, Vallesi and Shallice (2007) showed that the reductions in reaction time with increasing foreperiod develop in children at a later age than

sequential effects, indicating that the foreperiod effects have a different cause. Indirectly this finding supports the more classical account that subjects actively monitor on each trial that no stimulus has yet occurred and, if it has not, increase their level of preparation. Such an active monitoring process would not be required if the warning interval is fixed over a block of trials.

Stuss et al. (2005) showed that performance of these two apparently very similar paradigms—variable or fixed within a block of trials—is impaired by quite different lesion sites. If the interval is fixed over a block of trials, then there is an optimum interval of about a second with performance slowing if it is longer (in a different block). Patients with Superior Medial lesions are of course the slowest group. In addition they slow significantly more than the other groups if the warning interval is 3 sec rather than 1 sec. This fits with an impairment of energisation (see Figure 9.27a).

If, however, one makes a slight change in the procedure and makes the interval variable within a block instead of between blocks, a quite different group is impaired. In another condition of the experiment subjects had a rectangular distribution of intervals from 3 to 7 sec within the same block. In this variable foreperiod paradigm there is again one patient group that do not show the normal pattern, which as discussed above is a speeding up of reaction time by 30–40 msec for longer preparatory foreperiods compared with shorter ones. In this case, though, the Superior Medial group show the same improvement as do normal subjects. It is the Right Lateral group that do not improve (see Figure 9.27b). Moreover this effect is found not only with choice

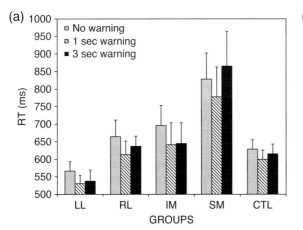
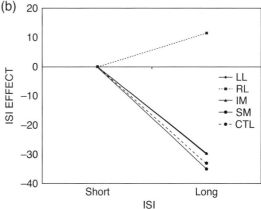

Fig. 9.27 (a) Mean reaction times for all groups in the Stuss et al. (2005) study of choice reaction time with *fixed* foreperiods. The Superior Medial (SM) group are slower overall, but they also differ from the other groups by showing significant slowing with 3-sec warning compared to 1-sec warning. (b) The change in reaction time in *variable* foreperiods for each group on long warning signal to stimulus trials (> 5 sec) compared to short warning signal to stimulus trials (< 5 sec). Right Lateral (RL) patients were slower on long trials than short. All other groups, including the Superior Medial group, showed the opposite pattern. Reprinted from *Neuropsychologia, 43*(3), D.T. Stuss, M.P. Alexander, T. Shallice, T.W. Picton, M.A. Binns, R. Macdonald, A. Borowiec and D.I. Katz, Multiple frontal systems controlling response speed, pp. 396–417, Copyright (2005), with permission from Elsevier.

reaction time as well as simple reaction time, but has been replicated using other patient populations (Vallesi et al., 2007a), by using TMS in normal subjects (Vallesi et al., 2007b) and indirectly by fMRI (Vallesi et al., 2009).

Why might this effect occur? On each trial where there is a longer foreperiod, two processes are necessary. First, the subject must realise that no signal has yet occurred. Second, they must increase their degree of preparation as the conditional probability of the stimulus occurring in the *next* interval of time has increased. Since the Right Lateral group prepare appropriately when there is a fixed interval throughout a block, it is presumably the first of these processes that does not function. Indeed, appreciating that nothing has yet happened, when it could have done, requires active monitoring—one of the two main processes held by Petrides (1994) to involve the mid-dorsolateral prefrontal cortex.[32] This paradigm suggests that it is predominantly a right lateral frontal process in humans.

Computationally what might active monitoring involve? 'Monitoring' is used by many theorists in many different contexts. According to Petrides, it involves '(a) an expectation of what must or will occur, and (b) verification of what has occurred against the expectation' (p. 74). On our approach, too, we assume its most basic role is in error detection. The critical process here is that of detecting a discrepancy between two states of affairs, most frequently states of the world, and also involving the efficacy of the strategy that you are adopting. As we will see shortly, these states of affairs need to be rather abstractly defined. When a discrepancy is detected, a new goal is set up which is either to 'patch' the 'bug' or to abandon the goal.

When carrying out a complex task the environment often forces us to realise that an error has been made. One just cannot go on. However, we also frequently detect errors that are less evident in everyday life situations. For instance, Rizzo et al. (1995) examined how people correct their many errors when learning a programming language. They propose a 4-stage process of coping with error. The first is to realise that there is a mismatch between one's goal and current reality. The second stage is to explicitly detect that the mismatch is arising from one's own behaviour. The third is to identify what error was made. The final stage is to recover from the error. Checking is involved in the first two of these stages.

Detection of mismatches, the first stage, can be complex. First, what is the mismatch between? An error, or

better an inappropriate behaviour, can be because some characteristic of the eventual goal is undermined, or of a subgoal, or of a subsubgoal and so on. This undermining can be because a necessary aspect of the final goal is being lost through the current action (see Figure 1.9 for an example) or because a resource necessary for a later part of the procedure is being used up. It can be because progress is too slow, or too difficult, or too expensive. It may be because it would require assistance from others. A mismatch may be based on an abstract property of the action, such as the length of time an operation is taking. It can require a comparison with the intuitive value a result should have. It can even involve inferences (Rizzo et al., 1995; Burgess and Shallice, 1996c). It is essentially that of checking for a mismatch between two rather abstractly defined states of affairs. The first is the situation created by current behaviour or one likely to be created by it or by the behaviour required in the carrying out of the plan. The other is that entailed by the eventual goal or any of the hierarchically organised set of subgoals necessary to achieve it. And this mismatch can involve a variety of criteria. In other words it requires many matching operations to be carried out *in parallel*. Moreover, if a mismatch occurs for any one of them, it should lead to an interruption in the ongoing behaviour. There are different degrees of active monitoring and checking. Thus at a lower level it involves an increased sensitivity to the task relevant aspects of the environment. At a higher level it involves explicitly making sure that inadvertent errors have not occurred, as frequently occurs as the final stage in complex problem-solving (see e.g. De Groot, 1965). We will for the present assume that a single control system is involved in both types of process, and will use the term of Petrides *active monitoring* to cover both. Critically if the process detects a mismatch, ongoing behaviour is interrupted for an attempt to produce a patch or to abandon the subgoal.

We have shown that the right lateral effects in the variable foreperiod paradigm are neatly explained by assuming the impairment is one of active monitoring. Here the patch would be to increase preparation. However if any cortical area is involved in active monitoring then one can go further and make predictions about the types of situation in which the region should be involved, namely:

1 In situations of uncertainty.

2 After a provisional solution has been achieved.

3 When a plausible alternative has to be rejected.

Failures should lead to:

4 A failure in criterion setting.

5 Capture errors, namely action lapses in which an alternative series of actions is carried out instead of the intended one (see Reason, 1984).

---

[32] The other he sometimes called manipulation and at other times planning. They are somewhat related to the task-setting and strategy implementation functions, to be discussed later in the chapter.

Moreover:

6 The process should be more specific than cognitive effort.

The last of these has already been shown in the comparison between the variable and fixed foreperiod effects, as the systems underlying fixed foreperiod effects correspond to those responsible for cognitive effort. Examples supporting the other five predictions will be discussed in Chapters 10 and 12 on episodic memory and on thinking.

One example from the domain of language is of particular interest with respect to prediction 1. This is because language processing primarily involves left-hemisphere systems, so that a right lateralised process in language comprehension cannot just be explained in terms of a generalised hemispheric bias. Sharp et al. (2004) compared two types of language task on individual words presented with two sorts of speech input. One language task involved semantic processes, namely a decision about which of two words is closest in meaning to another (e.g. *beach*: *island*, *mountain*). The other

task involved a decision about equivalence in the number of syllables the word possesses (e.g. *hammer*: *tool*, *trailer*). The two sorts of speech input were whether the words were presented in clear speech or distorted speech, namely so-called *vocoded* speech, which sounds like a hoarse whisper but can be understood after a brief period of training.

A variety of left-hemisphere regions and no right-hemisphere ones were activated in the semantic-syntactic contrasts between the two pairs of basic tasks. For both basic tasks, however, the distorted speech led to significantly greater activation in regions of the right lateral prefrontal cortex (see Figure 9.28). Moreover activity in the right lateral prefrontal cortex was significantly negatively correlated with performance; the worse the subject did on the basic tasks the greater the right prefrontal activation. The more uncertain the subject was, the greater the activation. This is not what one would expect if dealing with vocoded speech was in some way piggy-backing on systems dealing with intonation, which are held to be right lateralised (Ross and Monnot, 2008). Instead, the effect follows directly

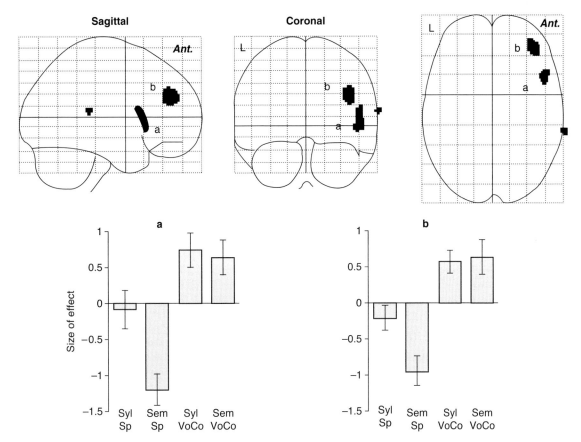

Fig. 9.28 The effect of vocoded speech versus nonvocoded speech in the study of Sharp et al. (2004) with semantic and syllabic judgements. Peak voxel differences were found in two regions: (a) right ventrolateral PFC (−50, 18, 0) and (b) right dorsolateral PFC (40, 42, 30). Reprinted from D.J. Sharp, S.K. Scott and R.J.S. Wise, Monitoring and the controlled processing of meaning: Distinct prefrontal systems, *Cerebral Cortex*, 2004, *14*(1), pp. 1–10, by permission of Oxford University Press.

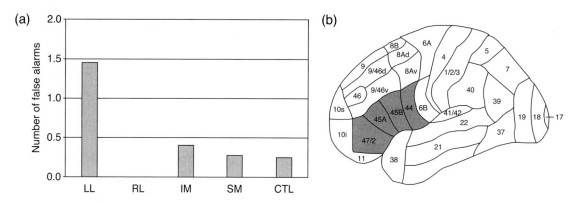

Fig. 9.29 (a) False alarm rates for the four patient groups and controls over the first 100 trials on the 5-choice serial reaction time task of Alexander et al. (2005). The Left Lateral group made three times as many false alarms as any other group. (b) Regions associated with the impairment shown in (a).

from prediction 1 on the localisation of active monitoring systems.

9.11 **On Task-setting**

One characteristic of the right frontal impairments found in the ROBBIA set of tasks is that they occurred throughout the experiment. By contrast with superior medial deficits, which tended to get worse later in a study, right lateral deficits remained constant. In contrast to both of these patterns of deficit, two effects found in left prefrontal patients reflected greater problems in the patients earlier in the task rather than later.

Figures 9.29 and 9.30 give the errors made by Left Lateral patients in two different tasks, showing performance at particular stages in learning the task. The first is the 5-choice serial reaction time task of Alexander et al. (2005), discussed in Sections 9.5 and 9.9, where Left Lateral prefrontal patients are as fast as controls. The second is the task-switching study of Shallice et al. (2008a), also discussed in Section 9.5. In both paradigms, the Left Lateral patients, unlike the Superior Medial patients, react as fast as normal controls throughout the experiment. However in both studies the Left Lateral patients make significantly more errors than controls on the first block of trials.[33] Their error rate rapidly declined to normal levels in later blocks.[34]

The Left Lateral group acquires the appropriate habitual task-set more slowly than, say, the Right Lateral prefrontal group.[35]

What does task-setting involve? In the task-switching study of Shallice et al. (2008a) the paradigm used was a variant of one initially developed by Meiran (1996) (see Figure 9.30). Using a production system framework, as discussed in Section 1.7, and COGENT, as discussed in Section 3.6, a set of IF/THEN rules and arrangement of processes at least as complex as those in Figure 9.31 are required to carry out the task. In the figure, the IF-side elements correspond to both (i) the output of the perceptual system and (ii) the equivalent of the contents of a production system working memory, while the THEN-side elements correspond to operations. The contents of brackets refer to arguments, i.e. variables that are set when a rule is applied. (See Section 3.6 for further details.)

On the supervisory system framework each of the production rules will need to be realised as a schema when automated. The impairment shown by the Left Lateral group could be in specifying the necessary set of productions. This would correspond to the programming function that Duncan attributes to his multiple demand units. Or it could be in initially explicitly holding

---

[33] And significantly more than the other frontal patient group in the Alexander et al., study.

[34] In the Shallice et al., study another group made a significantly higher number of errors than controls. This was the Inferior Medial group but this group did not show any decline in number of errors across later blocks. This effect was interpreted in terms of an impairment of another system—related to attentiveness or caring. The computational function of this system would be that of maintaining the subject on task. In a sense it is a complimentary function to that of the Active Monitoring system which has the function of interrupting

tasks if that is necessary. The Care system is responsible for maintaining the subject on the task they ought to be carrying out. It is the cognitive correlate of the motivational functions of the orbital prefrontal cortex (see Shallice et al., 2008c).

[35] Aron et al. (2004) came to a similar theoretical conclusion from the other large study of task-switching in frontal patients. Their inference was made from the larger reaction time switch costs found in their study. These costs were not reproduced in the Shallice et al., study which used a different task-switching paradigm. However, as a Superior Medial group was not distinguished from the lateral frontal ones in the Aron et al., study, it is possible that their Left Lateral switch cost effects are due to contamination from medial lesions.

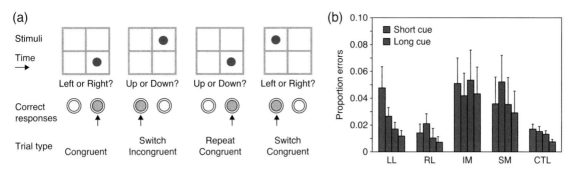

Fig. 9.30 (a) Correct responses and trial types for a sequence of trials of the cued switching task of Shallice et al. (2008a). (Compare Figure 9.13) On Upper/Lower trials subjects were required to respond with a left button press if the stimulus occurred in the upper half of the display and a right button press if it occurred in the lower half of the display. On Left/Right trials subjects were required to respond with a left button press if the stimulus occurred on the left side of the display and a right button press if it occurred on the right side of the display. A cue ('Upper of Lower?' or 'Left or Right?') was presented on screen prior to each trial to indicate which task was to be completed on that trial. Subjects completed one short cue block, where the cue was presented 200 msec before the stimulus, followed by two long cue blocks, where the cue was presented 1500 msec before the stimulus, followed by a final short cue block. (b) Errors of patient groups and controls over the four blocks. Results of each group are plotted from left to right in the order that the blocks occurred in the experiment. Reprinted from T. Shallice, D.T. Stuss, T.W. Picton, M.P. Alexander and S. Gillingham (2008), Multiple effects of prefrontal lesions on task-switching. *Frontiers in Human Neuroscience*, 1(2), 1–12. Copyright (2008), the authors.

the set of productions in a working memory (e.g. possibly using verbal mediation) or implementing them if that is required because the schemas (or productions) were not adequately automised. Or it could have been in the automisation process itself possibly in conjunction with the cerebellum. The two experiments discussed here are not sufficiently subtle to be able to distinguish which of the three putative processes are left lateralised.

1. IF: Cue is in *Perceptual Subsystem*: *Input*
   THEN: send process_text to *Perceptual Subsystem*: *Process*

2. IF: text(upper) or text(lower) is in *Perceptual Subsystem*: *Output*
   THEN: add attend(vertical) to Working Memory

3. IF: text(left) or text(right) is in *Perceptual Subsystem*: *Output*
   THEN: add attend(horizontal) to *Working Memory*

4. IF: attend(vertical) is in *Working Memory* and
           stimulus(AnyColumn, high) is in *Perceptual Subsystem*: *Output* and
           not blocked(_) is in *Control Buffer*
   THEN: send press(button(left)) to *Motor Subsystem*

5. IF: attend(vertical) is in *Working Memory* and
           stimulus(AnyColumn, high) is in *Perceptual Subsystem*: *Output* and
           not blocked(_) is in *Control Buffer*
   THEN: send press(button(right)) to *Motor Subsystem*

6. IF: attend(horizontal) is in *Working Memory* and
           stimulus(AnyColumn, high) is in *Perceptual Subsystem*: *Output* and
           not blocked(_) is in *Control Buffer*
   THEN: send press(button(left)) to *Motor Subsystem*

7. IF: attend(horizontal) is in *Working Memory* and
           stimulus(AnyColumn, high) is in *Perceptual Subsystem*: *Output* and
           not blocked(_) is in *Control Buffer*
   THEN: send press(button(right)) to *Motor Subsystem*

8. IF: instruction(long_cue_condition) is in *Working Memory*
   THEN: send blocked(short_time_period) to *Control Buffer*

9. IF: instruction(short_cue_condition) is in *Working Memory*
   THEN: send blocked(longer_time_period) to *Control Buffer*

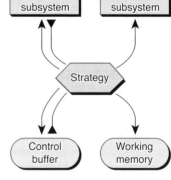

Fig. 9.31 A minimal set of COGENT rules for the *Strategy* process required by the task switching study of Shallice et al. (2008a). Some process similar to rules 8 and 9 is required to overcome the effects on rules 4–7 of task-set inertia (i.e., the continuing activation of schemas from the previous trial). The most difficult condition, which is the Short Cue one, must rely heavily on rule 9 to overcome these priming effects.

One issue is whether the left lateralisation arises just from the material being processed, such as in verbal mediation. One sign that this idea is not sufficient comes from the study of Buiatti et al., discussed in Section 8.6, which compared the performance of pre-frontal, premotor and parietal patients on the Bricolo et al. rotation task illustrated in Figure 8.17. Two groups of patients preformed significantly worse than the others—the right parietal and the left prefrontal—but their pattern of performance differed markedly. The errors of the right parietal patients were metrically appropriate with respect to a landmark such as a corner, but were qualitatively wrong, often involving rotation in the wrong direction; they are typically categorical errors. The prefrontal group that had problems, by contrast rotated in the right direction but rather wildly; they made metric errors. There was no evidence that they utilised the appropriate strategy of determining the relation of the point to an appropriate landmark, such as the top-right corner and using that to mediate where the dot should be after rotation. They did not set up the appropriate mental program. But this was the left prefrontal group not the right, again supporting the hypothesis that left lateral processes are involved in task setting.

9.12 On Strategies

The three tasks discussed in the last section are all simple. The processes involved seem too simple and too basic to correspond fully to the stage of generating options in a Fox–Das-type of framework. What is an 'option' that is generated in the Fox and Das model? It is a course of action which will potentially satisfy the problem goals specified by the *defining problem* stage. More specifically in the medical decision-making example it corresponds to a possible course of action to satisfy the already specified problem goals, which could consist, say, in a course of treatment.[36] In everyday language this would be the production of a possible *strategy*.

It would be surprising if this were the process malfunctioning in the two ROBBIA tasks with impaired task-setting as there appears to be relatively little need to develop a conscious strategy of how to approach the tasks, although maybe this is required in the Bricolo et al. rotation task. However, strategy production is a necessary early stage in task setting. Moreover there are important frontal systems involved.

A strategy differs from a source scheme in contention scheduling in at least two ways. First, it will often *not* correspond to a well-learned existing unit of action control (source-schema + object arguments) but may

involve a combination of them together with *if-then* contingencies. Second, it may operate over a longer time span than a routine act typically takes. In addition, as we will discuss in Chapter 11, while the operation of a source schema need not be conscious, a strategy is typically conscious when it is initially articulated so that it can be voluntarily effected or amended.

Either the attainment or the application of such strategies, or both, is impaired in patients with frontal lobe lesions.[37] This was first shown by Owen et al. (1990). They used a complex spatial working memory task, which was in fact a fairly straightforward computer game—part of the so-called CANTAB Battery. In it, subjects had to look for 'treasure' in randomly placed boxes on the monitor in a series of searches. On different trials there were 2, 3, 4, 6 and finally 8 boxes on the screen, the organisation of boxes being fixed for a trial. At any time during a trial the subject can select any box to open. A trial is, however, composed of a set of searches, the number in the set being the number of boxes on display. In any one search only one box has the 'treasure', so the subject has to look through the boxes until they find it. Then a new search begins with the treasure now only available in another box where it has not previously been. The trial ends when treasure had been found once in each of the boxes on the screen.

A good subject tends to adopt the strategy of searching over boxes in a fixed spatial pattern for each cycle for that trial, and then modifying the search pattern appropriately when treasure is found in a box by missing out that box on future searches in the trial. Use of the strategy lessens the memory load. Frontal patients use this strategy significantly less often. The seemingly rather insensitive measure of strategy adoption used was of how consistent subjects were on the first box opened on those trials involving 6 or 8 boxes. Frontal patients score significantly worse on the measure. As critically, the measure correlates strongly in patients with the number of errors made on those trials suggesting that an inadequate strategy is a major cause of the poor performance of frontal patients on the task.

A second study that gave related results was that of Burgess and Shallice (1996c) on the so-called Hayling B test. Subjects are presented with a sentence frame—a sentence missing its final word—which is, however, strongly constrained by the frame, such as *The ship sank very close to the ….* The test was designed with the idea of trying to isolate the problem of inhibiting a prepotent response. This is standardly assumed to be the core difficulty frontal patients have on the classical

---

[36] It also corresponds in an earlier cycle of processing in the domino to a possible diagnosis. We will return to this point later.

[37] At a neurophysiological level Genovesio et al. (2005) following Wise et al. (1996) have shown that cells in prefrontal cortex are active when monkeys use a particular strategy.

Wisconsin Card-Sorting task. However, it was found that when normal subjects are given a number of sentence frame problems of this type, they discover that it is hard to remove the prepotent response (e.g. *coast*) from their mind once it has occurred to them. They therefore often come up with the strategy of thinking of a word before the sentence frame is presented. Typically either they look round the room and select an object or think of a word related to the one they have just given. When the next sentence frame is presented, they check rapidly that the word they thought of is unrelated to any word in the sentence frame or its natural conclusion. If it is unrelated they give it as the response. Prefrontal patients report the use of this strategy much less frequently than do the normal subjects or patients with posterior lesions. Moreover their response fits with one of the two commonly used strategies less often than the responses of non-frontal subjects (bilateral frontal patients: 13%; unilateral frontal: 28%; posterior: 38%; controls: 38%), with unilateral frontal patients showing significantly fewer such responses than posterior or control groups.

The use of the search strategy in the Owen et al. study means that subjects must have abstracted that they will have a memory problem if they search randomly. Similarly in the Hayling task they need to realise that after they have heard the sentence frame they will have difficulty producing an appropriate response given the task requirements. So a critical prior stage in the production of an appropriate strategy is abstracting over what typically occurs in the situation, given the subject's typical behaviour and thought.

In these studies we are seeing the failure of a primitive strategy to be used. It is most plausible given the work reviewed in the previous section that the failure lies in the acquisition of a new strategy, rather than in its implementation. However the acquisition process is much more difficult to study, since it is liable to occur only once in a standard experiment and in such a situation one cannot effectively average over multiple critical trials. Moreover, novel strategy acquisition appears to be preceded by a process of abstracting over the types of difficulty that occur with attempts to use already known procedures to tackle the problem situation. Abstraction again is clinically known to be grossly impaired in patients with prefrontal lesions. For instance, they cannot give the meaning of a proverb (Benton, 1968), saying for instance that the meaning of *too many cooks spoil the broth* is that *if there are too many people in the kitchen, they get in each other's way*.[38]

In Chapter 12 we will provide some evidence that a critical step in developing an appropriate strategy—abstraction, which is necessary to determine the critical aspects of earlier inadequate solution attempts—is also a left prefrontal process. Thus the differential capacities of the left and right lateral prefrontal cortex appear to extend into the types of tasks that Fox and Das were considering.

9.13 On Selection

In 1997, a most elegant experiment was carried out by Sharon Thompson-Schill and her colleagues. Subjects were required to select which of two alternative words went more appropriately with another word. In addition the dimension on which appropriateness was judged changed from one condition to another. The critical comparison involved a *high-selection* condition in which both alternatives were associated to the target, but it was the nature of the association that was critical e.g. *COLOUR: tooth: tongue, bone*. By contrast the difficulty of a *low-selection* condition was generated by having four alternatives but with only one of them associated to the target e.g. *SIMILAR: flea: tick, well, shoe, school*. This high-selection condition led to greater activation in the left inferior frontal gyrus, which was held to be required by the process of selecting between competing alternatives in semantic memory (see Figure 9.32). Moreover such effects were not limited to comparisons between presented alternatives. Similar effects were also found in generation and classification tasks. Thompson-Schill and colleagues therefore argued that the left inferior frontal gyrus was involved in selection between competing alternatives. This is one of Fox and Das's computational domains, although Fox and Das considered it with respect to much more complex selection processes.

At about the same time as the study of Thompson-Schill et al., Robinson et al. (1998) were studying in patient ANG a striking neuropsychological condition, dynamic aphasia, first analysed by Luria (1966).[39] The core feature of dynamic aphasia is a severe reduction in the amount of spontaneous speech, which is disproportionate to any impairment of the core elements of the language mechanisms concerning the processing of syntax, semantics, morphology and phonology; in 'purer' cases these processes can be completely intact. Moreover, in the main form of the syndrome[40] the patient's performance is intact if the task does not involve language. In two patients (ANG: Robinson, Blair & Cipolotti, 1998; CH: Robinson et al., 2005) it was

---

[38] Roca et al. (2009) in a neuropsychological group study found that the impairment is particularly severe in frontopolar lesions.

[39] Dynamic aphasia corresponds reasonably closely to transcortical motor aphasia in the Wernicke–Lichtheim scheme for characterising the aphasias.

[40] See Robinson et al. (2006) for other variants.

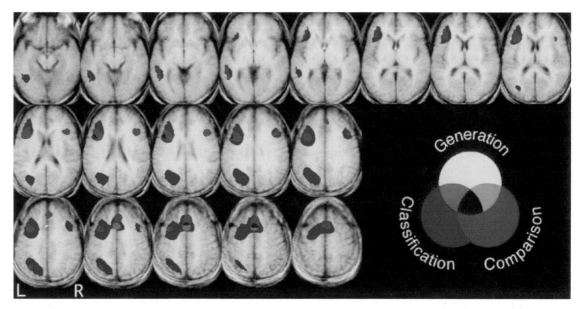

Fig. 9.32 Results of the study of Thompson-Schill et al. (1997). Colours show regions where the BOLD response was significantly greater in the high selection condition compared to the low selection condition for the generation, classification and comparison tasks. Reprinted with permission from S.L. Thompson-Schill, M. D'Esposito, G.A. Aguirre and M.J. Farah, 1997, Role of left inferior prefrontal cortex in retrieval of semantic knowledge: a reevaluation, *Proceedings of the National Academy of Sciences of the United States of America*, 94(26), 14792–14797. Copyright (1997) National Academy of Sciences, USA.

shown that the patient could produce sentences normally if there was no competition at some stage in the language production system. So, when they were presented with a single picture to describe, both patients scored at 100%, but when the task was to generate any sentence containing a given word, CH scored only 55% and ANG a mere 13%. A similar effect occurs at the single word level. Stimuli invented by Bloom and Fischler (1980) were also used with CH. They had produced norms for the number of alternative words that control subjects use to complete a sentence frame (i.e. a sentence minus its last word). Thus a sentence like *Water and sunshine help plants* … has few plausible completions in contrast to a sentence like *There was nothing wrong with the* … which has many. CH scored well in the former type, (92%) but very poorly in the latter (53%). And indeed on the classic neuropsychological word fluency test (Milner, 1963) where subjects have to generate as many words beginning with a given letter as possible in a minute both patients scored below the level of the worst 1% of controls.

Robinson et al. (1998) argued in a related fashion to Thompson-Schill and colleagues that the problem lay in selection between competing verbal responses.[41]

Moreover, a later group study (Robinson et al., 2010) showed that patients with left inferior frontal gyrus lesions were selectively impaired when compared with patients with other frontal lesions on high-competition tasks such as those discussed in the previous paragraph. This result echoed an earlier finding by Thompson-Schill et al. (1998) who found that four patients with left inferior frontal lesions were selectively impaired in generating verbs from nouns when the nouns induced multiple verb competitions (e.g. *cat*) compared to verbs with low selective demands (e.g. *scissors*).

Hardly surprisingly alternative formulations have been proposed to the global 'selection' account given by Thompson-Schill et al. (1997) and Robinson et al. (1998). Thus Martin and Cheng (2006), on the basis of a patient ML3 who had a lesion involving the inferior frontal gyrus, supported a proposal of Badre and Wagner (2002) that the left inferior frontal gyrus could be involved in 'controlled semantic retrieval'. Here the proposal is that a task like that of Thompson-Schill et al. (1997) requires top-down specification of the appropriate schema. Martin and Cheng compared three conditions in a verb retrieval task in which subjects were required to produce an associated verb when presented with a noun.[42] They found that ML3, like the controls, was no faster in a high-selection condition where items were strongly associated (e.g. *door-open; door-close*) than in a corresponding

---

[41] In a later paper (Robinson et al., 2005, the competition was placed at the level of conceptual preparation stage in the Levelt model of language production discussed in Chapter 3. (See also Warren et al., 2003.)

[42] The task is discussed in Section 5.3.

low-selection condition (e.g. *apple-eat*). It was only high-selection low-association conditions where they were slow (e.g. *rug-roll*; *rug-lay*).

Now ML3 is reported as having a slow speech rate (Martin & He, 2004), but it is unclear whether he had the clinical symptoms of a dynamic aphasic patient. Moreover, intuitively, virtually any of the parameters controlling the operation of an interactive activation system would, if moved towards a more impaired level, produce greater effects under low-association high-selection conditions than for the high-association conditions. Thus in the absence of a simulation the result does not seem to be very critical theoretically.

Further support for a similar idea appears to come from an imaging study of Badre et al. (2005). They used a related paradigm to that of Thompson-Schill et al. In a *judgement specificity* condition, they examined how selection was affected when the appropriate response had to be based on more than just an association by having it be determined by a dimension of relevance (e.g. same colour: *coal: tar? leek?*) rather than by just being semantically related. However, unlike Thompson-Schill and her colleagues, they also considered the effect of *associative strength* between the stimulus and the correct alternative (e.g. *candle: flame* vs *candle: halo*). One of their findings was that having to select the correct response on the basis of a particular dimension of similarity led to activation in what they termed mid-ventrolateral prefrontal cortex. They interpreted this in line with Thompson-Schill and colleagues as relating to a response selection process. Having to select a weak associative strength response as opposed to a strong one led to greater activation in this region but also in a more anterior ventrolateral region (see Figure 9.33). Badre et al. explain this finding in supervisory system style in terms of a need for greater top-down activation when making decisions that rely on weak associations. One could interpret this as greater activation being required of task-set representations (see Section 9.5). However, the inference that there is separable function related to associative strength and not selection in the more anterior region is dubious. We are not here dealing with clearly anatomically distinct regions or with cross-over interactions (see Section 5.5). There is even a non-significant trend of the selection variable too for that region. Moreover, across all variables considered, the more anterior region produces a smaller percentage change in blood flow than did the mid-ventrolateral region, and so is more likely to be less sensitive to any particular variable, such as the selection one. Finally, Crescentini et al. (2009) found only marginal support for an extra effect of association strength as far as the inferior frontal cortex is concerned. Thus at present it does not appear to be possible to be more specific about the process carried out in the left inferior frontal gyrus,

other than that it is involved in selection between alternatives in non-routine tasks and that task-specific representations, other than low-level schemas, such as task-set units may well be localised there.

The findings of Thompson-Schill et al., and Robertson et al., and their successors support the existence of a subsystem or subsystems specialised for selection between competing alternatives. *Commitment*—the decision to select between competing alternatives—is a key process in the Fox and Das model. The process initially studied by Thompson-Schill et al. appears, however, to involve a much less sophisticated selection device than that envisaged by Fox and Das in their model. No relation to arguments appears to be required. For instance, might it not be realisable by an interactive activation model? In fact, even in the sort of situations considered by Robertson et al. this would be a considerable over-simplification. Thus, if selection were to be operative at the conceptual preparation stage of the Levelt model of speech production a much more complex process than interactive activation alone would probably be required. One possibility is to view the selection between competitors as one aspect of the more global unification process of Vosse and Kempen (2000), which requires the choice of one potential structure over other potential structures. (See Section 8.8.)

However, even assuming that selection depends on a simple interactive activation model, impaired selection abilities—with relatively intact performance if production requires little need to select between competing alternatives—could come about for a variety of reasons. The simplest could be to reduce the activation of each

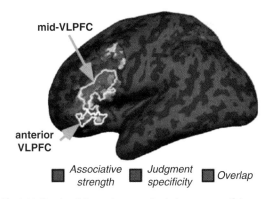

Fig. 9.33 Results of the study comparing judgement specificity and associative strength of Badre et al. (2005). Selection of a weak associative strength response activates anterior VLPFC. Judgement specificity leads to a region being activated similar to that of the selection regions of Thompson-Schill et al. (1997), shown in Figure 9.32. Reprinted from *Neuron*, 47(6), D. Badre, R.A. Poldrack, E.J. Paré-Blagoev, R.Z. Insler and A.D. Wagner, Dissociable controlled retrieval and generalized selection mechanisms in ventrolateral prefrontal cortex, pp. 907–918, Copyright (2005), with permission from Elsevier.

alternative. It could also arise from reduced inhibition between alternatives leading to any later systems being jammed by multiple outputs. Interactive activation networks typically have a positive feedback process producing self-activation by active units; a reduction in this parameter would also weaken the selection between competitions. One can even envisage the possibility that the existence of competition can induce increased top-down potentiation of this parameter or of a parameter controlling inhibition or both. Indeed a related account to this is given by Botvinick et al. (1999) for the function of the anterior cingulate.

Thus even assuming that selection is implemented by a simple interactive activation model there are clearly many subprocesses that could be involved. However, from an overall perspective the work of Thompson-Schill et al., Robertson et al., and their successors make the existence of a subsystem or—more likely—subsystems specialised for selection between competing alternatives, as proposed by the Fox and Das approach, more plausible.

9.14 Anterior Prefrontal Cortex, Intentions and Cognitive Modes

The Thompson-Schill study, like many of those discussed in this chapter, involved the more posterior parts of the prefrontal cortex. Let us move instead to the most anterior parts. There have been many single-cell recording studies of the dorsolateral and ventrolateral regions of prefrontal cortex. However, according to Ramnani and Owen (2004) there were none at that time of the frontal polar regions. It is technically much harder to carry out such a study in the monkey. However with the arrival of functional imaging, activations have increasingly been recorded from the frontopolar region in humans. Thus to take reasoning tasks as an example, a meta-analysis carried out by Christoff and Gabrieli (2000) found frontopolar activation to be present as frequently as dorsolateral. Yet activations of this area were also found in a variety of other tasks. These included so-called *self-ordered pointing* (Petrides & Milner, 1982), a self-organising working memory task,[43] tasks requiring information to be generated about the self, and also more familiar tasks such as episodic memory retrieval and certain more standard working memory tasks.

Many of these tasks, such as self-ordered pointing, are relatively complex and so with a very few exceptions

componential analyses of the tasks do not exist. In the absence of such componential analyses, neuropsychological findings, particularly strong dissociations, provide an easier basis for initial analysis. One noteworthy early study was that of Eslinger and Damasio (1985) who described patient EVR. EVR had previously been an accountant but after the removal of a large bilateral orbito-frontal meningioma he became incapable of organising himself effectively in everyday life. Thus he went bankrupt, and drifted through various jobs, was divorced and then made a disastrous new marriage. It appeared that he was incapable of effective decision-making. This was despite having an IQ of over 130 and performing well on a variety of tests including ones sensitive to prefrontal damage.

EVR provided the stimulus for the development of Damasio's (1996) *somatic marker* theory. The theory holds that making a complex decision involves many sub-decisions about smaller parts of the whole process, and that sub-decisions of parts of the whole are effectively summarised by an affective label (good, bad, etc)— the *somatic marker*. Without somatic markers there is no effective closure.[44]

Shallice and Burgess (1991), however, described patients with a similar syndrome to EVR but provided a different type of explanation. They described three frontal patients (AP, DN and FS) who were also grossly disorganised in everyday life but had intact performance on cognitive tasks sensitive to frontal lobe damage. It was, however, argued that the impairment was of a cognitive not an affective process. All three patients were grossly impaired in *multi-tasking,* where a number of subtasks need to be carried out with the patient obeying a small set of simple rules (see Figure 9.34). In multi-tasking, however, the subtasks have no relation to each other, and there is no cue as to when to switch from one subtask to another. It appeared that for the three patients the need to carry out a set of specific tasks did not lead to these tasks temporarily capturing control of ongoing behaviour as occurred in normal subjects. It was proposed that the patients had lost the ability to use *intentional markers*, held to be the cognitive vehicle for holding and realising intentions. They enable behaviour to be interrupted at some stage in the future so as to fulfil the one-off tasks that need to be carried out at that specific time, such as going to the post office on the way home.

---

[43] The subject is presented with the same set of items in an array on each trial, but in different spatial organisations. They must select one item from each array until all items have been selected once and once only across the set of trials.

[44] Somatic marker theory received strong support from the impaired performance of orbital frontal patients on the so-called Iowa Gambling Task (Becheara et al., 1997). However more recent studies on both normals and patients have cast doubt on the theory and/or on its neuropsychological support (see e.g. Manes et al., 2002; Fellows & Farah, 2005; Maia & McClelland, 2004).

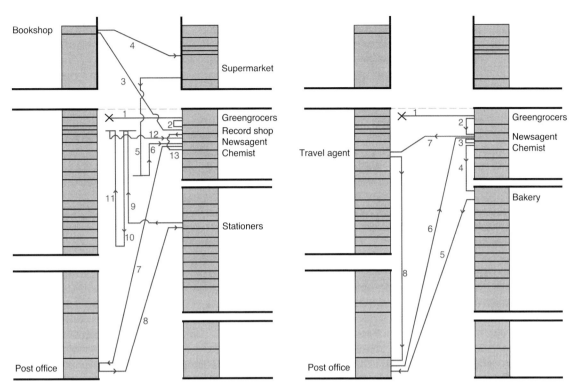

Fig. 9.34 Paths of a motivated high-IQ patient of Shallice and Burgess (1991) with a frontopolar lobe lesion (left) and a control adult (right) in carrying out a simple real-word planning task in a shopping precinct. (After Burgess and Alderman, 2004.)

AP had the best localised lesion of the three patients, it affected the frontopolar regions bilaterally—Brodmann areas 10 and 11 (see Figure 9.35). A later group study of Burgess et al. (2000) used another multi-tasking experiment with three unrelated subtasks carried out in the lab. Patients with left anterior prefrontal lesions had no difficulty with many aspects of the experiment. They learned the task rules normally, remembered them afterwards, developed an appropriate strategy, and remembered what they had done when asked later. However this group of patients scored very poorly on the test as a whole. They did not switch tasks efficiently and they also broke task rules; both of these processes involve the use of intentional markers.

In an attempt to localise the *intentional marker* component with fMRI, P. Burgess et al. (2001a) used the design discussed in Section 5.7. There were two types of task— *ongoing* tasks where the subject had to respond to every stimulus, and *intention* tasks where the subject was instructed to respond in a certain fashion if and only if a particular stimulus occurred. On some runs the stimulus did occur but on others it did not. The elegance of the design was that, as discussed in Chapter 5, Burgess et al. used the Price–Friston conjunction analysis procedure. Four different pairs of on-going and intention tasks were employed. Setting up and holding an intention even when it is never realised when compared with

carrying out the on-going task alone led to activation of the right dorsolateral prefrontal region. This fits with an active monitoring process being involved in waiting for the critical stimuli to activate the intention. More important for the present concerns it also led to activation of the left and right frontal pole (Figure 2.3).

The study of P. Burgess et al. (2001) is one of a number of studies pointing to a similar conclusion. Another had been carried out by Koechlin et al. (1999). Subjects were presented with a string of letters such as A...B...L...t... e...a, in one task. They have to determine whether successively presented upper-case letters occurred one after the other in the word *TABLET*. A second task also applied, but *only* at the point where there was a change from upper case to lower case. Subjects had then to decide if the letter after the change was a 't'. Koechlin et al. called their critical condition 'branching'. This is when the subject must return to either task in the appropriate place in the letter string after some letters have been processed on the other task. This requires picking up the letter string where it had been left off. The term emphasises the need to return to a main task after carrying out a subroutine.

The region activated in these critical comparisons in the Burgess et al. study, particularly for the left frontopolar region (−30, 62, −6), is virtually identically to that activated in the critical condition in the

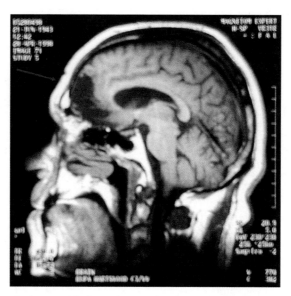

Fig. 9.35 The location of the lesion of patient AP of Shallice and Burgess (1991). Reproduced with permission from Shallice, T. (2004). The fractionation of supervisory control. In M. S. Gazzaniga (Ed.) *The Cognitive Neurosciences III* (pp. 943–956). Cambridge, MA: The MIT Press. (Figure 68.8, p. 953.)

Koechlin et al. one (–36, 57, 9). In addition both are similar to regions activated in related studies of Okuda et al. (1998) and Burgess et al. (2003).[45] Burgess et al. prefer instead of branching the concept of *anticipatory processing* of McCarthy and Warrington (1990a), relating it to the views of the Gestalt psychologist, Lewin (1935), on *goal tension*, which are in turn related to the ideas of Ach (1905) on the *determining tendency* to be discussed in Section 10.9. Lewin held that when a task remained uncompleted there remained an underlying psychological 'tension' which was only discharged when the goal was achieved. The perspective held by P. Burgess et al. (2001) was that the frontopolar cortex was the location of the system that implemented this process. There is clearly a family resemblance between these processes and that required to implement the sustained processing that Braver et al. attributed to frontopolar cortex (see Section 9.5).

More recently Burgess and his collaborators Dumontheil and Gilbert (Burgess et al., 2007) have put forward a more general view on the functions of the frontopolar cortex, which could include their earlier hypothesis as a special case. Intention realisation is a particular example of a stimulus-independent cognitive process like day-dreaming or insight in abstract problem-solving. They contrasted such *stimulus-independent* thought processes with processes dependent upon perception—*stimulus-dependent* processes. In an empirical

realisation of the contrast Gilbert et al. (2005) used an fMRI conjunction design in a somewhat analogous style to that of the P. Burgess et al. (2001) study. Figure 9.36a illustrates the experimental design. Consider *one* of the three basic tasks—the so-called Brooks (1968) task. Subjects must go round the figure saying whether each successive corner is a left or right turn. The critical point is that for part of the time the figure disappears—and is replaced by a cloud shape and the subject must continue the task using a mental image. When *external* phases are compared with *internal* phases then for all three basic tasks there are consistent results. The medial frontopolar cortex was the region showing most sustained activity in the external phase. By contrast more lateral parts of the frontopolar cortex showed transient activation at the time of the switch from the external to the internal phase (see Figure 9.36b).[46] No region showed more sustained activity in the internal than the external phase. This finding is the opposite of what might be expected on a task difficulty or a working memory account. That the lateral frontopolar cortex is more associated with internal processing was also supported by a meta-analysis of Gilbert et al. (2006). A wide variety of experimental paradigms were included that produced activation of area 10 (frontopolar cortex). The condition that produced the more lateral activation gave rise to significantly longer reaction times than

---

[45] We will also see this region discussed in Section 12.3 with respect to Christoff's concept of relational integration in thinking.

[46] There was also more activity in the right dorsolateral region as would be expected on the active monitoring hypothesis discussed in Section 9.10.

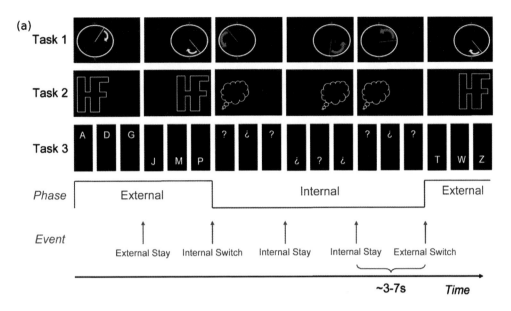

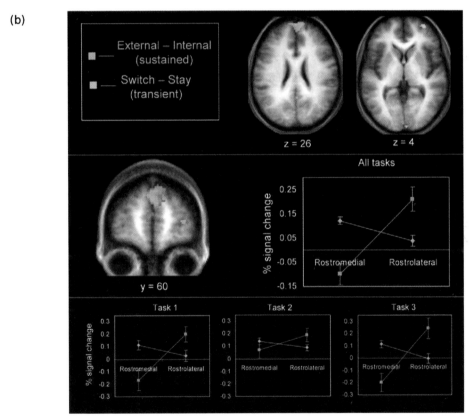

Fig. 9.36 The design and results of the study of Gilbert et al. (2005). (a) A schematic representation of the three tasks, each with external and internal phrases. In task 1 (the Brooks task) subjects were required to press a button whenever the rotating clock hand passed a red mark. The clock hand was not shown during internal phases. In task 2 subjects pressed buttons to indicate left or right turns as they imagined moving around the complex figure. During the internal phase the figure was not shown. In task 3 subjects classified letters as consisting of straight lines, curves, or both. Letters followed a regular sequence. In internal phases letters were not shown and subjects had to generate the letters according to that sequence. (b) Medial frontopolar cortex showed sustained activity in the external phases of all tasks, while lateral parts of the frontopolar cortex showed transient activation at the time of the switch from the external to the internal phases. Reprinted from S.J. Gilbert, C.D. Frith and P.W. Burgess, 2005, Involvement of rostral prefrontal cortex in selection between stimulus-oriented and stimulus-independent thought, *European Journal of Neuroscience*, 21(5), 1423–1431. Copyright © 2005, John Wiley and Sons.

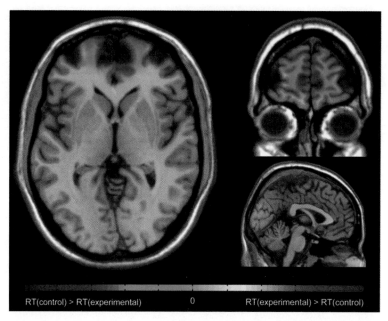

RT(control) > RT(experimental)   0   RT(experimental) > RT(control)

Fig. 9.37 Results of the meta-analysis of Gilbert et al. (2006) of reaction time studies reporting frontopolar activation. Studies in which the control condition was performed more quickly than the experimental condition tended to activate medial areas, while lateral activation was associated with slower experimental RTs. Reprinted from S.J. Gilbert, S. Spengler, J.S. Simons, C.D. Frith and P.W. Burgess, Differential functions of lateral and medial rostral prefrontal cortex (area 10) revealed by brain–behavior associations. *Cerebral Cortex*, 2006, *16*(12), pp. 1783–1789, by permission of Oxford University Press.

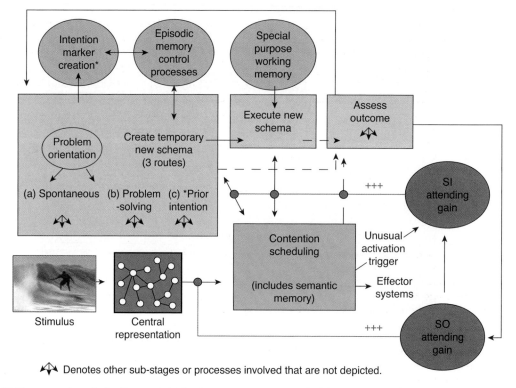

⤧ Denotes other sub-stages or processes involved that are not depicted.

Fig. 9.38 The gateway hypothesis of Burgess and colleagues. Input to contention scheduling comes either from perceptual systems (in stimulus oriented processing (from the left in the figure)) or the supervisory system (in stimulus independent processing (from the top)). Reprinted from *Trends in Cognitive Sciences*, *11*(7), P.W. Burgess, I. Dumontheil and S.J. Gilbert, The gateway hypothesis of rostral prefrontal cortex (area 10) function, pp. 290–298. Copyright (2007) with permission from Elsevier.

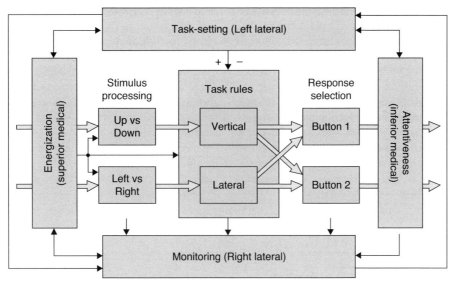

Fig. 9.39 The heterarchical structure of the supervisory system (in blue) proposed by Shallice et al. (2008c), in the context of their task switching experiment. Processes in contention scheduling are indicated in green and yellow. Reprinted from T. Shallice, D.T. Stuss, T.W. Picton, M.P. Alexander and S. Gillingham (2008), Mapping task switching in frontal cortex through neuropsychological group studies. *Frontiers in Human Neuroscience*, 2(1), 1–12. Copyright (2008), the authors.

their corresponding control conditions across a variety of tasks (see Figure 9.37).

The *gateway hypothesis* put forward by Burgess et al. (2007) using a supervisory system framework is shown in Figure 9.38. It is held that there are a competing pair of systems—*stimulus orienting (SO)* (in medial frontopolar cortex) and *stimulus independent (SI)* (in lateral frontopolar cortex). These systems control whether input to contention scheduling comes from perceptual systems or from the supervisory system—that is whether processing systems are responding to perceptions or thoughts respectively. For stimulus-orientated tasks, such as reaction time, the medial system is critical. This fits with the energisation deficits found with superior medial lesions.[47] By contrast, when there must be a switch to an internal cognitive source the lateral system is critical.[48]

As we will see in the next chapter one type of task that activates area 10 is retrieval from episodic memory. One hypothesis we will discuss in that chapter to explain this activity in such a task—far from the classical medial temporal regions associated with episodic memory—is that it involves what Tulving (1983) called *retrieval mode*, the state that facilitates the occurrence of what Tulving called *ecphory*, the process by which an episodic memory is retrieved. The processes held to be in competition in the gateway hypothesis are of a similar conceptual level to *retrieval mode*. They are states which facilitate certain very general classes of cognitive operation. One possibility is to see the variety of different types of general cognitive process that exist—reacting to or attending to perceptions, having abstract thoughts, thinking of others' mental states, episodic retrieval, performing routine internal operations (as in say mental arithmetic) and so on, as each being under the control of a different general cognitive mode. Which mode or modes is in operation would be the responsibility of area 10. Only humans would have such a variety of cognitive modes and only humans have a large area 10. But at present this remains only a rather wild speculation!

Overall in the second part of this chapter we have argued that a supervisory system needs to be internally composed of a set of systems, each of which has an abstract cognitive function different from but complementary to that of the others. We have used the Das and Fox framework as an intellectual justification for the existence of such a set of complementary systems with different high-level abstract functions, without

[47] Whether the superior medial reaction time slowing described in the discussion of energisation earlier in this chapter should be attributed specifically to medial frontopolar cortex and not, say, to the anterior cingulate and the pre-SMA remains to be determined. Nor are the two hypotheses presented about the functional processes involved equivalent!

[48] In the critical condition of P. Burgess et al. (2001) discussed earlier in this section, lateral area 10 activation occurred when an intention was merely being held not when it was realised—the 'Expectation' condition. To explain this on the Burgess et al. (2007) account one might have to presuppose that the subjects needed to refresh their intention to be able to act appropriately in the Expectation condition if the intention were to need to be realised.

wishing to suggest that their set of high-level abstract functions is necessarily the one implemented in the human brain. We have also argued that the computational specificity of each of these high-level cognitive functions, together with the frequency with which each of the individual functions, must be realised by an adult human, means that it is evolutiondarily efficient for the brain to realise them at least in part in different anatomical structures. Moreover, we have claimed that this qualitative difference between the computational

functions of the systems implies a heterarchical structure orthogonal to the hierarchical one which is currently so fashionable for characterising prefrontal cortex (see Figure 9.39). In this chapter we have reviewed cognitive neuroscience experiments mainly involving fairly simple tasks which provide support for these theses. In Chapters 10 and 12, on episodic memory and thinking respectively, we aim to provide further support for these positions.

CHAPTER 10

Higher Level Modulatory Processes: Episodic Memory

10.1 Towards the Modal Episodic Memory Model

To know how and why language is used one can tape social interactions. Indeed many hours of tape exist, for instance, on parent–baby interactions, and from these one can discover important quantitative and qualitative aspects of language use. Memory of one's past is not like that. If an autobiographical memory is retrieved in reverie, in the course of problem-solving, in planning a trip, in reading a book or watching a film or listening to other people, there is no necessary behavioural or simple physiological sign. It is a mysterious process very difficult to study.

The greatest advance in the history of research on memory was to enable an abstraction of this process to be studied quantitatively. Ebbinghaus in 1885, who made the advance, realised that memory could be studied by breaking it down into roughly equivalent elements with the retention of individual elements assessed quantitatively. He did not take a complex fairly open-ended situation lasting a few minutes to study. He abstracted from it something like the memory experiment we have today where lists of fairly rapidly presented items are presented to be later recalled or recognised.

Ebbinghaus also, though, thought that we should remove past knowledge from the memory elements, a hopeless task and one that mainly loses the basis of the phenomenon to be studied, and so he invented the nonsense syllable, e.g. *baff* as an ideal memory element. This proved a blind alley. However his legacy remains in experimental paradigms—such as free recall of lists of items, recognition[1] of different types of item and a host of others—that we now use to study memory quantitatively. Maybe this typical type of memory experiment captures the essence of the cognitive processes underlying remembering specific events in one's past. Maybe, as some so-called autobiographical memory theorists (Neisser, 1976) once argued, it captures little or nothing of importance about memory. Or maybe, as we will argue later, the truth, as usual, lies somewhere between the two.

This chapter will reflect the somewhat schizoid character of research in the area. The first part will be concerned with what we will call core memory processes, studied using behavioural methods coming from the Ebbinghaus tradition. The second part will be concerned with how and when autobiographical memory experiences relate to the ever-changing flux of thought. The hinge is represented by inclusion of memory procedures that stem indirectly from the loosening up of memory research that come from the work of autobiographical memory theorists such as Neisser, but considered in a cognitive neuroscience rather than a purely psychological context.

We will start with the post-Ebbinghaus approach, because these procedures work. As an example that they work, consider the second great advance in the study of memory—that memory can be dramatically and selectively lost after organic damage to particular parts of the brain. This can occur following surgery, as in the classic case of HM of Scoville and Milner (1957), discussed in Section 1.3, but also following herpes-simplex encephalitis (e.g. Parkin & Leng, 1988), bilateral vascular lesions of the posterior cerebral arteries (e.g. Benson et al., 1974) or Alzheimer's disease (Gainotti et al., 1998). A severe classical amnesic will have a gross permanent loss of the ability to remember new events (anterograde amnesia). For instance such patients may tell the same story many times in the same testing session not realising that they have told it before. Yet perceptual, language and cognitive skills and also short-term storage ability can be unimpaired. The patient will score at or near chance, and far below the normal range on recognition of words or faces.[2] The serial position curve of successful memory retrievals in his or her attempts to recall of a word list (see Section 1.4 and Figure 1.7) will show a normal recency effect but a gross reduction in the earlier part of the curve (Baddeley & Warrington, 1970). The simple artificial experiment using lists faithfully reflects the gross everyday life memory impairment. At the same time many other aspects of cognition can be quantitatively quite normal.[3]

The third great advance in the study of memory was the realisation in the 1960s and 1970s, that there is not just a single memory system in the human brain but a number of them. In part this was due to the advances connected with short-term buffer memory involving models of that time which demonstrated that these systems were quite separate from long-term memory ones (see Chapters 1 and 7 and FNMS Section 2.3). However, the core of the field of memory is the experience of remembering an event from one's own past. This gives rise to a distinct type of experience where one can resurrect after a fashion being in another time or place, which the Estonian-Canadian psychologist Endel

---

[1] The English word 'recognition' is unfortunately used in two quite different senses in cognitive neuroscience. In object or word recognition it relates to a process in the higher levels of perception, placing the stimulus in a particular known class or category of potential inputs (see Chapter 6). In memory experiments it relates to the ability to determine whether a particular item has been presented before over a period or in a place specified in the experimental procedure.

[2] There is a dispute as to whether this applies to pure hippocampal amnesics (see Section 10.5).

[3] For much more detail see FNMS Chapters 3, 4 and 15.

Tulving (1985) calls autonoetic consciousness. If one contrasts this experience with how one remembers facts or the meaning of words, then a key idea is the separation, discussed in Section 2.2, of episodic memory from semantic memory, first enunciated by Tulving and Donaldson (1972). Episodic memory is held to be intimately linked to our experience of our past. Semantic memory—the underpinnings of knowledge, as discussed in Chapter 6—has no such link. You generally know the meaning of a word with no knowledge of where you acquired it.

Within three years the neurologist Marcel Kinsbourne working with Frank Wood (1975) linked episodic memory to the second great advance by pointing out that a selective impairment of an episodic memory system was a far more apt characterisation of selective organic amnesia than any preceding one. Moreover, with the work of Elizabeth Warrington and Larry Weiskrantz, in patients, it soon became clear that semantic memory impairments can doubly dissociate from episodic memory ones and that priming, say, can be intact in a severely amnesic patient (see e.g. Warrington & Weiskrantz, 1968, 1970, 1978).[4] This set the way for the 'multiple memory model' in which there are held to be a variety of different memory systems. In this context, Schacter and Tulving (1994) produced three criteria for a memory system:

1 It should be required of a large class of tasks that have the same functional features.

2 It should exhibit unique functional features—so short-term memory systems typically involve representations that have not been deeply analysed (see Chapter 7).

3 There should be a consistent pattern of dissociations across patients between tasks according to the particular set of systems they require.[5]

Schacter and Tulving also produced a set of putative systems (see Table 10.1), which in general fit well with ones discussed in this book. On the neurobiological level, by the 1970s and 1980s it was becoming clear that, as Scoville and Milner have argued (see also Milner, 1972), the hippocampus was a key structure in amnesia, and hence a key structure in episodic memory. This contrasts

with the perirhinal cortex, which in Section 6.7 was argued to be the locus of the semantic memory hub. Moreover, particular approaches to understanding the functions of the hippocampus seemed to fit nicely with its playing a key role in episodic memory (see Section 2.2). For instance, Teyler and Di Scenna (1986) proposed that the hippocampus acts as an index for the whole complex of a memory which consists otherwise of elements stored cortically. Retrieval of the memory could only or best be done by accessing the index. This was the biological analogue of the so-called headed records processing model of memory developed by Morton et al. (1985).[6]

This rather loosely sketched position was widely held at the psychological level by the late 1970s, at least in Europe and Canada, as Tulving's and Donaldson's concept was found to fit neuropsychological evidence so well. The anatomical aspects, particularly the link with the hippocampus, were also part of the Zeitgeist. Indeed David Marr's model of the hippocampus as a memory store had been published as early as 1971, although this anatomical position did not become dominant until about 1990. By this time, however, the cognitive level model, which we will call the *modal episodic memory model* in the spirit of the modal memory model of the 1970s (see Section 7.1), had itself come under challenge.

10.2 Declarative Memory, Catastrophic Interference and Possible Problems with the Modal Episodic Memory Model

Beginning in the 1980s, a series of issues were raised which produced difficulties for the modal episodic memory model—some very directly and others almost implicitly. The most basic issue is that if semantic memory and episodic memory are functionally and anatomically separable systems, what is the relation between them? One way of thinking about the modal episodic memory model is as follows: 'It is possible […] that autobiographical memory is also neurally segregated from our semantic knowledge of the world, to the extent that knowledge about objects and animals, such as a dog, is stored separately from personal experience related to dogs' (Hodges & Graham, 2001, p. 1426). The authors argue that this position does not fit the neuropsychological facts. However given that 'personal experiences related to dogs' involve knowing what dogs are, it would be most surprising if neural segregation were the case.

---

[4] For discussion of the preservation of priming in amnesia see FNMS Chapter 15; Moscovitch et al. (1993) and Schacter et al. (1993). For a dissenting voice see Kinder and Shanks (2003). However, single-system accounts which reject the dissociation such as that of Kinder and Shanks would require priming to involve specifically the hippocampus or the medial temporal lobe. This is not the case (see Section 7.2).

[5] And one could now add consistently different patterns of activation in fMRI experiments.

---

[6] A related idea was McNaughton's (1989) view of the hippocampus providing a 'summary sketch' of a fuller neocortical representation.

TABLE 10.1 An up-dated and revised version of the memory system taxonomy of Schacter and Tulving (1994)

Memory Type	Other Terms	Subsystems	Retrieval
Priming		Visual word-form Phonological word-form Etc.	Implicit
Procedural	Non-declarative	Motor skills Cognitive skills Simple conditioning Simple associative learning	Implicit
Semantic (see Chapter 6)	Generic Factual Knowledge	Spatial Relational	Implicit
Short-term buffers (see Chapter 7)	Working Primary	Visuo-spatial short-term storage network Phonological Input Buffer Phonological Output Buffer Graphemic Output Buffer Unification Space (see Chapter 8) Episodic Buffer (?)	Explicit and Implicit
Episodic	Personal Autobiographical Event memory		Explicit

However, Alan Baddeley in England and Gus Craik and Bob Lockhart in Canada had discovered in the late 1960s and early 1970s that much of what we retain over a long time about an individual event is semantically encoded. Thus Baddeley (1966a, 1966b) showed that in retaining word lists over shorter intervals, phonological similarities affect later retrieval but over longer intervals it is semantic similarity. Experiences encoded with shallower types of representation than semantic ones, such as phonological ones, typically have much shorter half-lives (Craik & Lockhart, 1972). There are, though, striking exceptions to this general levels-of-processing type rule, as in recognition memory of scenes for which humans have a remarkably large capacity (Standing, 1973). It is unlikely that the core of this exceptional capacity is purely semantic. Thus semantic dementia patients, discussed in Chapters 4 and 6, can have nearly normal recognition memory of coloured pictures of familiar objects, while they are greatly impaired if the recognition examples are of the same type of object but perceptually very different (Graham et al., 2000) (see Figure 10.1). By contrast normal controls and Alzheimer's patients showed a comparable level of performance across the two conditions.[7] It is clear that episodic memory does not code semantic information alone.

Putting this complication on one side, the basic issue of the relation between semantic and episodic memory divides into two specific questions. The first is why is episodic memory so much dependent upon semantic encoding if the two systems are separable? A second question is how does material get into semantic memory? Does it first have to be stored in episodic memory? Given that these two issues are complex would it not be simpler to view memory for personal events and memory for facts as two parallel aspects of so-called 'declarative memory', to use the concept first developed by Cohen and Squire (1980)?

This newer 'standard' declarative memory position has its neurobiological side too. The hippocampus began to be treated by some as a somewhat less special structure, as part of an overall 'medial temporal lobe' system which also incorporates the entorhinal cortex and perirhinal cortex too (Squire & Zola, 1996) (see Figure 2.4). While the conclusion of Milner and her collaborators had been that the hippocampus is the key structure for producing the classical amnesic syndrome, the surgical operations of her time that led to severe amnesia typically involved the amygdala and other medial temporal systems too. While lesions to the amygdala do not produce episodic memory problems (Zola-Morgan et al., 1989), on Squire and Zola's perspective there is a global declarative memory system involving medial temporal structures, as well as the hippocampus, which in some sense acts as a single resource with the degree of deficit corresponding to the amount of loss of the resource.

---

[7] Technically the control group results could result from a ceiling effect. More detailed analyses indicate that this did not bias the interpretation of the finding.

(a)

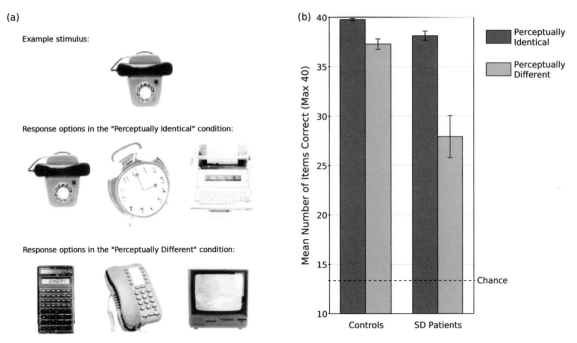

Fig. 10.1 Performance of semantic dementia patients on recognition of familiar objects (from Graham et al., 2000). (a) An example stimulus presented in the first phase of the study (top: a telephone) plus the alternatives for recognition in the perceptually identical condition (middle) and the perceptually different condition (bottom). (b) Accuracy for controls and semantic dementia patients on the Perceptual Identical and Perceptually Different conditions. Adapted from *Neuropsychologia, 38*(3), K.S. Graham, J.S. Simons, K.H. Pratt, K. Patterson and J.R. Hodges, Insights from semantic dementia on the relationship between episodic and semantic memory, 313–324. Copyright (2000), with permission from Elsevier.

Squire and Zola modify the impression of their declarative memory system being a single resource by arguing that lesion size may not be the only determinant of memory impairment in the medial temporal lobe system. However the example they give is simply that different modalities of input to the system may be preferentially represented in certain regions; thus perirhinal cortex receives stronger projections from unimodal visual areas than does the parahippocampal cortex and for spatial inputs the opposite is true. Squire and Zola provide no argument for a qualitative difference in subprocesses as discussed in Chapter 2.

The primary evidence for their single system approach is that in monkeys lesions to the perirhinal and parahippocampal cortices also severely impair memory performance, say on a delayed non matching-to-sample task (Zola-Morgan et al., 1993). In this task the monkey is presented with a sample object. Ten minutes later the animal sees the object together with a novel object, and must select the novel object to obtain a reward. However this is hardly a surprising finding if one considers the diagram of Figure 2.4 where these structures are on the key input and output pathways to the hippocampus.

There is however a second string to the argument. It is held that while damage limited to the hippocampus produces a significant memory impairment, this is less

severe than if the entorhinal and parahippocampal cortices are also involved. Thus Squire and Zola say 'the possibility must be kept in mind that the several components of the medial temporal lobe memory system all contribute similarly to behaviour' (Squire & Zola, 1996, p. 13521). This is suggested to be an anatomical analogue to an inclusive declarative memory system.

But why did the declarative memory view seem attractive? This relates to another aspect of the position, namely that the hippocampus and related structures collectively act as a system which holds new information while it consolidates in cortex (e.g. Squire & Alvarez, 1995; Murre, 1997). This in turn relates to the evolutionary function of episodic memory. Why do humans have such a system? This is an issue which has been made much more salient by a dramatic computational proposal of McClelland, McNaughton and O'Reilly (1995) that the function of the hippocampus is to overcome a major problem for the learning of new information in connectionist networks. On this approach the function of the hippocampus is to hold new information which is in conflict with existing associations and to drip feed this information to the cortex so as to overcome the so-called catastrophic interference effects on existing knowledge that can occur when new material is learned in connectionist networks.

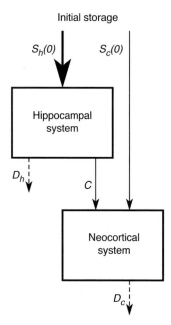

Initial storage

$S_h(0)$ $S_c(0)$

Hippocampal system

D_h C

Neocortical system

D_c

Fig. 10.2 Schematic illustration of the functional role of the hippocampal system according to the hypothesis of McClelland et al. (1995). Arrows are labelled with the parameters of the model: $S_h(0)$ and $S_c(0)$ refer to the strength of the hippocampal and neocortical traces resulting from the initial exposure to the event; D_h and D_c refer to the rate of decay from the hippocampal system and the neocortical system, respectively, and C refers to the rate of consolidation within the neocortex. Copyright © 1995 by the American Psychological Association. Adapted with permission. J.L. McClelland, B.L. McNaughton, R.C. O'Reilly (1995), Why there are complementary learning systems in the hippocampus and neocortex: Insights from the successes and failures of connectionist models of learning and memory. *Psychological Review, 102*(3), 419–457. The use of APA information does not imply endorsement by APA.

What though is catastrophic interference? In 1989 McCloskey and Cohen discovered that if a standard feed-forward connectionist network had been trained successfully on a certain set of input–output mappings, e.g. A → B, say using back propagation, and was then trained on a new set of input–output mappings which were in conflict with the first set, e.g. A → C, then it forgot the earlier associations almost completely. For instance, in one experiment a standard 3-layer net (see Section 1.7) was first taught 17 addition facts concerning 1, from 1+1=2 to 9+1=10 and from 1+2=3 up to 1+9=10, and could instantiate them with a very low error rate. It was then taught the equivalent 17 additional facts concerning 2, two of which it already knew. After a mere five learning trials with the set of 2s, the net's ability to retrieve the additional facts concerning 1s dropped from 100% to 20%. In five more trials recall of the older facts had fallen to 1%.

Classic experiments such as that of Barnes and Underwood (1959) have demonstrated so-called *proactive interference* where learning, say, a list of paired associates such as A → C affects remembering of an earlier list A → B. However, while humans are also susceptible to its effects, this is to a far lesser extent than for back propagation networks. A variety of procedures are available for alleviating this computational problem of the devastating effects of new learning on old (see French, 1999, for a review); for instance reducing representational overlap by using sparsely distributed representations does so (Kanerva, 1989). The idea of McClelland et al. was that if the cortex is viewed as a distributed net then learning could take place there through a slow drip-feed process coming from the hippocampus that retains information about individual new learning trials. The idea is that spreading the new learning process in the cortex out over time would allow the on-going day-to-day gentle rehearsal of old knowledge and this would be sufficient to prevent the new knowledge devastating the old.

McClelland et al. take a neural net for semantic processing which is a feed-forward predecessor of that considered in Chapter 6 (see Figure 6.6). The underlying principle of the position developed by McClelland and his colleagues is that such a connectionist net learns the structure of its world—the complex statistics of its environment. But to do so requires slow learning. If you allow the effect of any given input to be large the learning process is liable to be sent off course, the net arrives in a spurious local energy minimum and the retrieved outputs provide only a crude representation of the statistics of the input space. However, so-called gradient descent procedures (see Section 1.7) are guaranteed to lead to an improvement in how the network represents the input space, but only if infinitesimally small adjustments are made to the connection weights at each step.[8] A situation in which there is extensive new learning in a massed fashion produces a sudden discontinuity in the pattern of the input–output mapping. This violates the requirement for slow, gradual, acquisition of the appropriate weights, and the old learning is lost. If, however, one interleaves two different sets of stimulus–response (S–R) pairings in learning, then connectionist models do much better (McCloskey & Cohen, 1989).

To create this interleaving, McClelland and his colleagues add a second system that is intended to mimic the hippocampus (see Figure 10.2). They make no attempt to simulate the hippocampus. Instead they assume that the hippocampal system is used as a source of training data for the neocortical network. As far as

---

[8] See White (1989) for a technical discussion of this point.

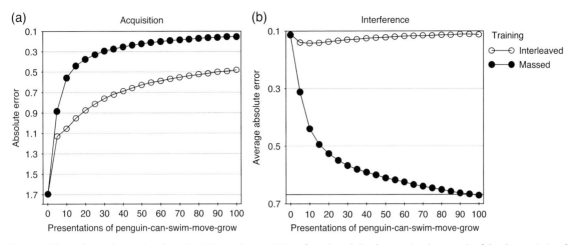

Fig. 10.3 Effects of massed versus interleaved training on the acquisition of new knowledge (concerning the example of the characteristics of penguins) in the semantic network model of Rumelhart (1990). Interleaved training results in (a) faster learning (with less absolute error over items during acquisition) and (b) less interference with existing knowledge (as measured by the average absolute error across similar items). Copyright © 1995 by the American Psychological Association. Adapted with permission. J.L. McClelland, B.L. McNaughton, R.C. O'Reilly (1995), Why there are complementary learning systems in the hippocampus and neocortex: Insights from the successes and failures of connectionist models of learning and memory. *Psychological Review, 102*(3), 419–457. The use of APA information does not imply endorsement by APA.

the cortical network is concerned it spreads the effect of a new experience out over time. Thus the training process in the cortex of a new conflicting set of S–R links would be interleaved with the after-effects of earlier experiences reflecting the older S–R relationship. With the two types of experience being interleaved, the capacity to produce either type of response becomes available given the appropriate information as to which of the two S–R domains one is in when a specific stimulus arrives. In simulations it is shown that catastrophic interference does not occur (see Figure 10.3).

The simulations of McClelland et al. and their theory of the function of the hippocampus support the idea that traces in the hippocampus are useful for only a limited time. This fits with the overall Squire and Zola approach and leads to that position now being viewed as the 'standard consolidation model'. This is aesthetically a very pleasing theory. It provides a clear computational function for an obscure structure—the hippocampus—and it saves the obvious type of model of how the cortex learns from a simple computational refutation. But is it true? McClelland and his colleagues test the model on one of the most famous and oldest established phenomena of neuropsychology. Ribot, in 1882, proposed that the longer a memory trace has been held the less it is subject to disruption by a subsequent cerebral insult. This is the so-called gradient of retrograde amnesia.

McClelland and his colleagues, however, did not just rely on clinical phenomena. They used analogues of it in animals. For instance, they discussed an experiment in which Zola-Morgan and Squire (1990) trained mon-

keys on a set of 100 pairs of junk objects. For each pair one was reinforced and the other not. The training of each pair was for 10 days; but this training period could end 1, 3, 7, 11 or 15 weeks before surgery. The surgery involved removing the hippocampus bilaterally. Two weeks later the animals were tested on how well they remembered which item of a pair had been reinforced. The results and how well the model of McClelland et al. simulated them are shown in Figure 10.4. Clearly a very good fit has been obtained. McClelland et al. also simulated studies by Kim and Faneslow (1992) of removal of the hippocampus in rats. They then developed equations that mimicked their simulations and showed they fitted findings of Winocur (1990) on rats and of Squire and Cohen (1979) on the effect of ECT on humans. This provides strong support for one aspect of the declarative memory positions that medial temporal structures hold information for a period of time sufficient to allow consolidation to occur in cortex.

10.3 Developments of the Modal Episodic Memory Model: Remote Long-term Memories and Recognition

Episodic memory was not, though, dead. In contrast to the views of Squire and Zola rejecting core assumptions of the modal episodic memory model, two other pairs of theorists have produced important elaborations of the earlier model. Both pairs oppose the idea that there is a unitary system and support the idea of a separable episodic memory system in the hippocampus.

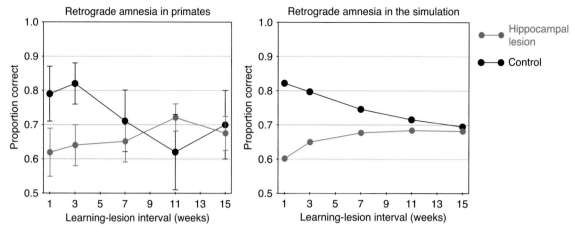

Fig. 10.4 The fit of the model of McClelland et al. (1995) to the primate lesion data of Zola-Morgan and Squire (1990). (a) Primate data derived from retention of 100 object discrimination problems learned between 1 and 15 weeks prior to hippocampal surgery. (b) Model data are based on a simulation involving both target discrimination problems and background training exemplars. Lesioning was simulated by disabling the drip-feed function of the model hippocampus. Further background exemplars were then presented for a number of simulated weeks prior to network testing. Critically, performance of control and lesioned systems (primates and models) converges if the period between learning and lesioning is greater than approximately 11 weeks. Copyright © 1995 by the American Psychological Association. Adapted with permission. J.L. McClelland, B.L. McNaughton, R.C. O'Reilly (1995), Why there are complementary learning systems in the hippocampus and neocortex: Insights from the successes and failures of connectionist models of learning and memory. *Psychological Review*, 102(3), 419–457. The use of APA information does not imply endorsement by APA.

The standard consolidation view fits with Ribot's classic lore about human amnesia. But is Ribot's lore a law? Some cognitive neuropsychologists have long doubted it. Among them were Nadel and Moscovitch (1997) (see also Moscovitch et al., 2006) who put forward their *multiple trace theory*. This theory makes a number of assumptions, of which the last is the most distinctive:

1 The retrieval of autobiographical episodes, through the use of episodic memeory, however old the memory might be, is always dependent on the hippocampal complex, namely the hippocampus and related medial temporal lobe structures.

2 Information held by the trace is sparsely encoded in a distributed fashion.

3 Following Teylor and Di Scenna (1986) this trace acts as an index or pointer to disparate cortical representations and so binds them together.

4 Each re-activation of the trace at retrieval creates a new experience and a new trace, which shares some features with the preceding traces of the episode.

5 The creation of multiple overlapping traces helps to facilitate the formation of semantic representations.

6 Retrieval of the spatial and temporal context information that carries the episodic quality of the memory depends upon the continuing involvement of the hippocampus (for spatial context) and the frontal cortex (for temporal context), and critically contra-Ribot,

these structures continue to be required however old the memory.

Many aspects of this position are not that original. Nearly all of the assumptions are also held, for instance, by the Rolls–Treves model discussed in Section 2.2, which uses a more elegant attractor framework that potentially provides a more powerful implementation of assumption 5. Finally, as we will discuss later in the chapter, the sixth assumption concerning the hippocampus stresses its role as the provision of a spatial context, which clearly relates to the spatial navigation functions of the hippocampus discussed in Section 2.2. It may also be critical in the rapid retrieval of different parts of the many-faceted whole that comprise what one can retrieve of a single incident. What, though, sharply distinguishes this position from the declarative memory position is the assumption that retrieval using the system located in the hippocampus can be useful however old the memory.

Another aspect of the declarative memory position has also been challenged, namely that the hippocampus and other parts of the medial temporal cortex should be viewed from the autobiographical memory perspective as a single resource. This relates specifically to the process of recognition. Since the work of George Mandler (1980) the most influential theory of recognition memory has been that recognition can occur by two processes—recollection or familiarity. Moreover recollection, as it involves conscious remembering of the episode, soon became specifically associated with episodic memory (Gardiner, 1988). Familiarity, however, could just be based on the degree of activation of semantic memory representations.

The two-process model of recollection remains controversial even within the cognitive science of memory (e.g. Wixted, 2007). However, two different groups have argued forcefully that recognition does depend on two processes and, moreover, that they have different neurobiological underpinnings—the hippocampus for recollection and the perirhinal cortex for familiarity (Brown & Aggleton, 2001; Eichenbaum et al., 2007).[9]

The fight-back by adherents of the modal episodic memory model to the claims of the standard consolidation model raises many complex empirical questions. We will consider a number of specific topics and then provide an overall review of the theories just considered. The standard consolidation model views the role of the hippocampal complex as being fairly limited in time. We will start therefore by discussing a key much contested issue, namely the status of very long-term memory in amnesia.[10]

We begin with the acquisition of new semantic memories and the relation to episodic memory. In classical amnesia, semantic memory is standardly accepted to be spared, given that the knowledge has been acquired very well before the lesion.[11] Both the standard declarative memory model with consolidation and the multiple traces theory, though, would expect this pattern. Then consider the period affected by a retrograde amnesia—the period prior to the onset of the amnesia for which autobiographical events can no longer be recalled. As we will see in the next section, this can be a very lengthy period of many years. Take knowledge of new words coming into the language, as an example of acquisition of a new semantic memory. For instance in Europe the word *euro*, which everyone now knows, was unknown before the turn of the century. Again it is generally accepted that acquisition of the meaning of such new words can be excellently preserved for periods that are well within the time period affected by a severe retrograde amnesia (e.g. Warrington & McCarthy,

1988; Barr et al., 1990; Verfaillie et al., 1995a; Moscovitch et al., 2005).

What about knowledge acquired since the onset of the brain damage? Unfortunately, the ability of amnesic patients to acquire new knowledge after their lesions, where it has been intensively studied, turns out to vary widely from one patient to another. The most consistently used procedure has been the acquisition of new vocabulary after the onset of a severe amnesic problem. Some severely amnesic patients, such as SS (Verfaillie et al., 1995b) and VC (Cipolotti et al., 2001) have very poor acquisition of such new words after they have become amnesic. Other patients, e.g. PS3 (Verfaellie et al., 2000), by contrast, show considerable learning but are still well below the normal range (see Table 10.2). Indeed at least one patient—AC (Van der Linden et al., 2001)—has been described with normal word acquisition following the lesion. In addition, patients, such as Jon of Vargha-Khadem et al. (1997) with selective bilateral hippocampal lesions induced by vascular hypoxia episodes occurring before birth, have also been described with intact semantic but impaired episodic memory. In general in this book we have not discussed the effects of lesions of early onset as such lesions are very likely to severely affect the developmental process itself (see, e.g. Thomas & Karmiloff-Smith, 2002). But, the hippocampus has a highly specific architecture (see Chapter 2) and, therefore, its functions are unlikely to be replaced in the developmental process by other tissue, for instance in the cortex. However, many amnesics will lead lives where they are not exposed to, say, new political vocabulary; they do not have a normal environment. Moreover, we have the problem that the wide range of semantic memory abilities in the normal population means that, as discussed in Chapter 4, it would be dangerous to put too much weight on apparently preserved performance in a small number of single cases who are not part of an unselected series.

Thus given the information currently available it is not possible to argue convincingly that semantic memory can or that it cannot be effectively increased following lesions to the hippocampus which produce severe episodic memory loss. Neither type of theory gains much strength from this evidence. The evidence relating to the temporal discrepancy between the extent of retrograde amnesia and new word learning has, though, been held by Nadel and Moscovitch (1997) to be somewhat problematic for the standard consolidation model. However, McClelland and his colleagues could retort that knowledge of the meaning of new words to which the patient is exposed occurs in a distributed rather than a massed fashion and so may not require hippocampal drip-feeding of cortex or induce catastrophic interference. Much more important, though, has been

---

[9] On this perspective a monkey in a non-matching-to-sample task, on which the Squire and Zola's general medial temporal lobe view is based (see e.g. Broadbent et al., 2002), could use either recognition process. Thus this empirical paradigm is insufficiently refined for the theoretical load it has had to carry.

[10] Issues that are central to Tulving's theory of episodic memory but relate to what he calls autonoetic awareness, the phenomenological immediacy and vividness of autobiographical recall which is held to be mediated by episodic memory, will be discussed in Chapter 11.

[11] This is reviewed in FNMS Sections 2.3 and 15.2. See also Parkin (1997).

TABLE 10.2 Performance of three amnesic patients and matched controls on word definition tasks for words which had entered the language at different times with respect to the onset of the patient's amnesia. All figures are percentage correct. Acquisition of new vocabulary by SS is near floor, in contrast, PS3 shows modest learning while AC's acquisition is low but within the normal range.

	Period 1	Period 2	Period 3
Period	1985–89	1980–84	1975–79
SS (onset 1971)	0	4.2	29.2
Controls	78.3 (17.2)	83.3 (16.0)	92.3 (13.0)
Period	1990–94	1985–90	1980–84
PS3 (onset 1981)	5	25	41.7
Controls	62 (22)	64 (27)	81 (12.4)
Period	1987–00	1965–85	Before 1920
AC (onset 1987)	55.8	78.8	79.4
Controls	70.0 (9.1)	76.9 (6.3)	75.0 (10.3)

Data for SS and PS3 from Verfaellie et al. (2000); data for AC from van der Linden et al. (2001).

the issue of long-duration autobiographical memories to which we now turn.

10.4 Very Long-term Retrograde Amnesia

Memory can be studied quantitatively in the laboratory using lists of words or pictures, but as was discussed at the beginning of this chapter, it can also be studied quantitatively in a somewhat less controlled way using naturally occurring events. The first to do so effectively, as far as amnesia is concerned, were Sanders and Warrington (1971) in a study that, though done long before, used an analogue in humans of the Zola–Morgan and Squire experiment discussed in Section 10.2. There were two major differences—the events being remembered were public events, and the time interval over which retention was being assessed was 30 years or so. Where the experiment was beautifully analogous to the later one done in monkeys is that the input experiences were matched in strength of encoding. Sanders and Warrington examined both memory for events and memory for faces. If we consider memory for events, they ensure equivalent memorability of individual events by taking accounts from year-books, which listed them in terms of salience. They made one type of exception. All events that had entered general knowledge in the culture were eliminated. So a drama at sea in 1953, famous at the time, when a ship's captain single-handedly stayed with

his ship while it was towed 1000 miles through Atlantic gales, was included. The assassination of John Kennedy was excluded.

The rationale for this was rather strange. One year before Tulving made his distinction between episodic and semantic memory, Sanders and Warrington wanted to get rid of the contribution of what was later to be called semantic memory. They developed a clever way of checking that questions such as 'What happened to the ship, the Flying Enterprise?' were not part of general knowledge in the culture.[12] They tested that their questions could not be answered by intelligent children of 16–18, who could, one hopes, at least in the late 1960s, answer the question 'What happened to John Kennedy in Dallas, Texas?'[13]

The results were striking (see Figure 10.5). The group of severe classically amnesic patients with highly selective impairments remembered virtually nothing about these unique public events from 35 years before. Their so-called gradients of retrograde amnesia were flat.

A paper with such a dramatic result quite contrary to Ribot's Lore with such an elegant control would of course surely become a key paper in all later discussions of retrograde amnesia. That is not how science works. Shortly thereafter, at least at the speed that science in the area operated at the time, Albert, Butters and Levin (1979), in a study of Korsakoff patients with very long-lasting retrograde amnesias, of up to 30 years or so, found decreasing deficit the further back one went (see Figure 10.6)—a so-called temporal gradient. In other words, Albert et al. obtained results with qualitative similarity to those quoted by McClelland et al., although the disorder for retrograde amnesia was much longer. However, there were subtle methodological differences between the two studies. Sanders and Warrington matched events according to their potential memorability at the time they occurred. Albert et al. matched memories of different ages so that at recall controls performed at an equivalent level for memories of different ages.[14]

After the work of Albert et al., it was widely believed that very long-lasting retrograde amnesia shows a temporal gradient and is a result of impairments to both semantic and episodic memory, or declarative memory for short (e.g. Kapur, 1993; Verfaellie et al., 1995b). This perspective, however, was challenged by Lynn Nadel

---

[12] This is only likely to be answerable by British readers over the age of 75, but probably by a fair percentage of these!

[13] The issue of whether knowledge of an event extensively discussed over a period and then never mentioned should be treated as semantic or episodic is very tricky. At present we will assume the trace to be primarily episodic.

[14] These results and the methodological differences are discussed in more detail in FNMS section 15.4.

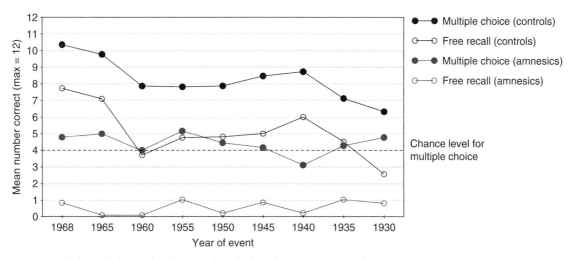

Fig. 10.5 Recall of controls (N = 200) and amnesics (N = 5) of significant events over the forty years prior to testing. The temporal gradient of retrograde amnesia for the amnesics is flat, for both multiple choice and free recall. Note that the controls perform more poorly the older the memory. Reprinted from H.I. Sanders & E.K. Warrington, Memory for remote events in amnesic patients, *Brain*, 1971, *94*(4), 661–668, by permission of Oxford University Press.

and Morris Moscovitch in 1997 in the development of their multiple-trace theory. They reviewed 12 studies reported to 1997, where retrograde amnesia was assessed in patients who also had an anterograde amnesia and in whom 'the major lesion included bilateral damage to the hippocampal complex …. In some cases damage extended beyond the medial temporal lobe' (p. 219). The typical pattern was 'flat loss', that is the pattern first described qualitatively by Sanders and Warrington with time spans of '30–40 years', 'at least 20 years' and in one case 'for 15 years' or minimally, but with very little information 'over one to ten years'. There was one exception, patient GD (Rempel-Clower et al., 1996) with 'no discernible loss'.

In a second review carried out nine years later by Moscovitch et al. (2006) of amnesic patients with lesions involving the entire hippocampus or the adjacent hippocampal complex, the summary is more complicated. They argue that if the lesion is restricted primarily to the hippocampus, then retrograde amnesia is limited to a few years at most. If, however, the lesion extends to 'the adjacent regions of the medial temporal lobe (the hippocampal complex)' (p. 82) then two different patterns emerge. One is a long-standing essentially ungraded retrograde amnesia (e.g. Steinvorth et al., 2005; Viskontas et al., 2000) but the other shows a temporal gradient (patients EP and GP of Bayley et al., 2003, 2005). Thus patient EP is held to have intact childhood

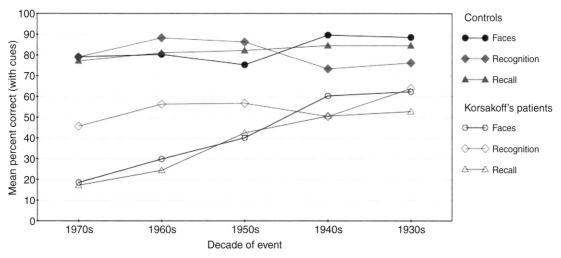

Fig. 10.6 Performance of Korsakoff patients and normal controls on recall and recognition of memories of different ages. Note that control performance is as good for very old memories as for more recent ones. Data from Albert et al., (1979).

memories, to be below normal for memories of young adulthood, and to be at floor for recent memories.

Much of the evidence reviewed by Moscovitch et al. in fact uses a technique, which is sometimes called the 'Galton-Crovitz' autobiographical memory procedure, in which subjects are given a word (e.g. holiday) and asked to generate a memory in a specific time period related to the word (e.g. up until age 18).[15] Such memories can be rated for vividness and the number of details produced.

Nadel and Moscovitch argue that the standard consolidation theory 'cannot readily account for evidence of very extensive and often flat RA [retrograde amnesia] temporal gradients, especially for autobiographical memory' (p. 24). In fact in their 1995 paper, McClelland et al. have a long but entirely speculative discussion about why the gradients of retrograde amnesia in humans may be so much flatter than for animals. One suggestion is that it might be due to the generally slower learning rates for humans, as they have so much more to learn. Alternatively there may be slowing of learning rate with age; humans being generally much older when suffering amnesia than are other animals when tested.[16]

Neither side in the dispute appears to be aware that the existence of temporal gradients in severe amnesics may arise simply due to a failure to match the strengths of the trace at encoding (Shallice, 1988; McCarthy & Warrington, 1990b). Indeed that the standard procedure is to match items so that controls have good memory performance for items of different age, indicates why this might be the case. Thus Bahrick (1984), in a study of what one knows of a language not spoken for many years, has argued that semantic memory is very durable. Assume then that semantic memories generally decrease more slowly in strength than episodic ones. It is then simple to prove that if one matches memories for the probability of recall, then the older the trace the greater the probability that it is retrieved from semantic rather than episodic memory.[17] This assumption also implies that with the Galton-Crovitz technique, the earlier the event occurs, the more likely it is to be recalled from semantic memory. Thus an Albert at al. type of temporal gradient obtained using these techniques does not necessarily mean that retrieval restricted to episodic memories shows a temporal gradient. Taking account of this methodological flaw in many of the studies strengthens the force of the Nadel and Moscovitch critique.

Kapur (1999) in a generally very useful review of retrograde amnesia argues against this conclusion on the grounds of two studies where salience was matched at encoding. One was a study of Squire et al. (1975) who examined memories for TV series shown in only a single year. They found that controls retrieved programmes from 1–2 years ago better than those from the 9–16 years before. Patients who had had ECT for depression showed the opposite pattern. A similar pattern was found for two Korsakoff patients in a study of Mayes et al. (1988) of memory for news events in which the events were matched for salience at encoding. However Kapur himself objected to the use of Korsakoff patients, as this condition usually derives from alcoholism and their drinking habits may preclude their following current affairs. The same could be said for depressives. So these two studies are not convincing.

Much more compelling is the study of Graham and Hodges (1997). They used two procedures. One was the Galton–Crovitz method used with just a single subject, a semantic dementia patient AM2, and controls. The results are shown in Figure 10.7. AM2 was significantly better at producing autobiographical memories from the most recent five years than from earlier periods in his life. By contrast, normal control subjects were equally good at providing similarly detailed memories across all time periods back to childhood. Graham and Hodges also employed the Autobiographical Memory Inventory, which requires a subject to produce three specific life events from each of three periods: childhood, early adulthood and the most recent five years. For example, the subject would be asked to recall an event that occurred while they were at secondary school (i.e. between age 11 and 18). In this part of their study they tested two groups of patients—six with early Alzheimer's disease and six with semantic dementia. The two groups of patients produced a strong double dissociation, with the Alzheimer's patients being much worse on recent events, showing the temporal gradient typical of retrograde amnesia (see Figure 10.8). By contrast the semantic dementia patients showed a 'reversed temporal gradient', corroborating the effects found for AM2 using the Galton–Crovitz procedure. A similar gradient was also found in studies using the more clinical procedure—the Autobiographical Memory Inventory—in two groups of semantic dementia patients in a study of Snowden, Griffiths and Neary (1996).[18]

---

[15] This procedure has many names. In FNMS it was called the Robinson procedure as it was used by Robinson (1976). Reed and Squire (1998) call it the 'word association test of autobiographical memory', which is too long-winded. As the first modern exponents were Crovitz and Schiffman (1974), we will follow the terminology of Graham and Hodges.

[16] Nadel and Moscovitch also review the animal literature and argue that flat retrograde amnesia is common in those studies too.

[17] See FNMS appendix to Chapter 15.

---

[18] A rather similar reverse temporal gradient has also been reported in a patient with bilateral temporal lobe pathology sparing the hippocampus (Kapur et al., 1994).

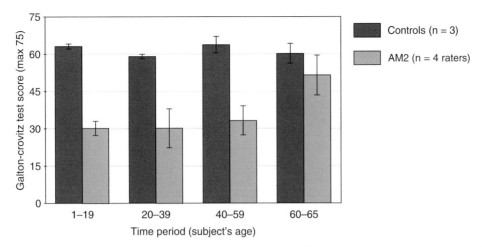

Fig. 10.7 Performance of controls and the semantic dementia patient AM2 on recall of events from different periods of the subject's life. AM2's recall is significantly better for the most recent five years than for earlier periods. Copyright © 1997 by the American Psychological Association. Adapted with permission. K.S. Graham and J.R. Hodges (1997) Differentiating the roles of the hippocampus complex and the neocortex in long-term memory storage: Evidence from the study of semantic dementia and Alzheimer's disease. *Neuropsychology, 11*(1), 77–89. The use of APA information does not imply endorsement by APA.

The Graham and Hodges pattern of findings has been the basis of a powerful objection made by Graham (1999) to the Nadel and Moscovitch position. She argues that this 'reverse temporal gradient' is not really a gradient at all but a 'step' with performance over the last few years preserved and that the findings strongly support the aspect of the standard consolidation model in which the hippocampus complex plays a time-limited role in the acquisition and storage of episodic and semantic memories.

There are a number of problems with Graham's argument. First, as Moscovitch and Nadel (1999) point out, why is the retention of the semantic dementia patients—a few years—so much shorter than the duration of retrograde amnesia revealed by their review of retrograde amnesia following lesions to the hippocampal complex? A second point is that the Galton–Crovitz procedure used by Graham and Hodges (1997) is very complex. Thus the control subjects of Reed and Squire (1998), who are admittedly of average age 74, took about a minute on average to begin to produce 'a well formed autobiographical recollection'. What is going on during this minute? For instance, using one of the stimuli of Graham and Hodges, parties, for the time period 19–39, the older author came up eventually (!) with a splendid party held by Lars-Goran Nilsson to celebrate the summer solstice at the Uppsala Memory conference in 1977.[19]. The process involved finding some retrieval cue to trigger *party*, which required

using knowledge of the organisation of one's life at that time—what Conway (1996) calls autobiographical memory knowledge. This would be a much more difficult process with a much reduced 'personal' as well as general semantic memory.[20] By contrast given the task of remembering a party in the last five years, a somewhat less memorable party held a few days before came immediately to mind without a search based on personal semantics.

Thus we would argue that the pattern obtained by Graham and Hodges on the Galton–Crovitz test arose because of the need to use a personal semantic memory to produce a means of cueing a memory. This need will be much greater for older memories than for those in the recent past.[21]

The potential role of semantic memory is even clearer for another finding of Graham and Hodges on the Autobiographical Memory Inventory. Here it should be noted, as for the Galton–Crovitz technique, that the scores obtained by controls for childhood are as good as for the last five years. This is very different from the pattern shown in the Sanders and Warrington findings,

---

[19] This party should be even more memorable to Michael Turvey.

[20] The concept of personal semantics was developed by Cermak and O'Connor (1983) to characterise the knowledge base from which the severe amnesic patient SS retrieved autobiographical incidents; he could never elaborate or describe them in detail. See FNMS Chapter 15.

[21] Hodges and Graham (2001) argue that poor strategic retrieval is unlikely to be the cause of the pattern they found. It should be noted that the proposal above is not of impairment to the control processes, but to the knowledge-base these control processes should use.

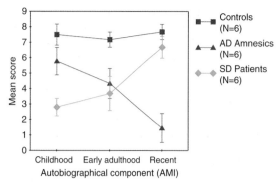

Fig. 10.8 Performance of controls and two patient groups (Alzheimer's Disease and Semantic Dementia patients) on the Autobiographical Memory Inventory. AD patients show the standard temporal gradient effect, while SD patients show a reversed temporal gradient similar to AM2. Copyright © 1997 by the American Psychological Association. Adapted with permission. K.S. Graham and J.R. Hodges (1997) Differentiating the roles of the hippocampus complex and the neocortex in long-term memory storage: Evidence from the study of semantic dementia and Alzheimer's disease. *Neuropsychology, 11*(1), 77–89. The use of APA information does not imply endorsement by APA.

where recall from episodic memory can be inferred, and suggests that semantic memory makes a very marked contribution for recall of childhood events. These events must have been very strongly laid down and are likely to have been frequently recalled. Take the childhood memory of one of our wives of gazing at beautiful balls falling from the sky while her family, knowing they were bombs, desperately tried to find her. In striking contrast is the pattern of performance for the Alzheimer's patients who would be expected to have primarily episodic memory loss, which on the argument of this section would lead to relative preservation of childhood memories. This is indeed what was found. Thus the reverse gradient of the semantic dementia patients can plausibly be attributed directly to their semantic memory impairment. Overall, the findings of Graham and Hodges are entirely compatible with the multiple memory trace position.

Does this mean that episodic memory is playing no role in recall from, say, childhood? Such a position would have difficulty explaining the very poor autobiographical recall of the childhood of patients whose general semantic memory was more intact than for other comparably amnesic patients, e.g. SS (Cermak & O'Connor, 1983), EA2 (Mair et al., 1979) and VQ (Cipolotti et al., 2001). More recently better controlled procedures for testing autobiographical memory have been developed by Levine et al. (2002). With them, a number of amnesic patients have been shown to be equally impaired at all time intervals, e.g. KC (Rosenbaum et al., 2004), SJ (Rosenbaum et al., 2008) and, for all except

one time period, the classic amnesic patient HM (Steinvorth et al., 2005).[22]

It would be foolish to assume that the last word has been said on the theoretical issues addressed in this section. The study of autobiographical memory does not allow for perfect control. No current technique can match the strength at encoding of traces of, say, childhood and adult events. If we accept the multiple memory trace position, then the most plausible account at present is that semantic and episodic memories are dependent on different but interacting systems with different half-lives and which can be separately damaged. In the next section we consider the anatomical loci of the two systems. In a later section (Section 10.9) we return to the function of episodic memory, as the computational idea that its function is to drip-feed new information to the cortex so as to avoid catastrophic interference seems at best incomplete; if its function were just that, episodic memories would have a much shorter half-life.

10.5 Episodic Memory: the Selective Loss of the Hippocampus

Isolated loss of the hippocampus is a rare condition, and one for which the selectivity of the localisation of damage is often much disputed. It is often claimed that there could be other damage which is silent on the scan, say after an anoxic episode. Thus there is much to recommend the approach advocated by Maguire, Nannery and Spiers (2006a) 'When attempting to deduce the functions of a particular brain area, ideally the patient's damage should be selective to that brain region. However, even exacting measurements for tissue volumes from patients' MRI scans cannot provide a definitive answer as to whether, in vivo, that tissue is functioning or not.' (p. 2896). They argue that the neurological evidence should be used as evidence as to whether a patient's 'lesions appear to implicate primarily' (p. 2896) a particular structure, such as the hippocampus.

On this approach there are a number of cases that have been reported over the last twenty years with lesions primarily implicating the hippocampus: NT (Warrington & Duchen, 1992; Chan et al., 2002), VC (Kartsounis et al., 1995; Cipolotti et al., 2001), GD (Reed & Squire, 1997), LJ (Reed & Squire, 1998), Jon (Vargha-Khadem et al., 1997),[23] AC (van der Linden et al., 2001),

---

[22] Interestingly the relatively preserved periods in the cases of SS and HM are the teenage years, which are known to be subject to a so-called reminiscence bump in normal controls (Rubin & Schulkind, 1997).

[23] As discussed earlier, Jon and other patients described by Vargha-Khadem et al. have a developmental disorder. Thus

YK (Hirano et al., 2002), YR (Mayes et al., 2002), AB3, MJ, LJ (Bayley et al., 2005), TT (Maguire et al., 2006a), FG (Hepner et al., 2007), SJ (Rosenbaum et al., 2008). There is complete agreement that patients with severe hippocampal damage perform very poorly in recall using episodic memory. Take Patient YR who had lost nearly 50% of her hippocampus, but was otherwise apparently neurologically intact. She performed on average 3.6 standard deviations below the level of matched controls on 34 tests of free recall. In this respect these later single case studies amply support the older group studies discussed in Chapter 2.

However, as far as other aspects of their memory is concerned there are profound disagreements. Thus as far as remote autobiographical memory is concerned, in nearly all the cases where there is severe damage that implicates primarily the hippocampus, there is a very long duration retrograde amnesia. Take patient NT (Warrington & Duchen, 1992) who had a right temporal lobectomy carried out in 1961 to reduce the severity of her epileptic seizures which resulted from an anterior right temporal lobe abnormality. The excision, typical of the time, removed the hippocampus and amygdala. Most unusually for patients who had a unilateral temporal lobectomy (see e.g. Milner, 1966), NT became severely amnesic. Twenty-five years later when she died, post-mortem revealed why. Blocks were taken from many regions of the two hemispheres, but apart from the obvious surgical lesion in the right temporal lobe, there were no changes observed other than several small scattered infarctions of fairly recent origin. The dramatic exception was in the left hippocampus, which was very abnormal at all four levels examined. The granule cells of the dentate gyrus, and CA1, CA3 and CA4 cells were all much reduced or drastically depleted in number[24] (Chan et al., 2002). However, no lesions were identified in the left temporal lobe. In particular there was no significant pathology involving the entorhinal cortex, perirhinal cortex or more lateral temporal regions. Apart from autobiographical memory, NT's cognitive capacities were essentially unaffected by the lesion. Her average verbal IQ was 101, the same as when tested a month before the operation and her average performance IQ was 93 compared to 99 just before (Warrington & Duchen, 1992).

On clinical tests, NT was found to be severely amnesic. Most critically she had a severe long-lasting retrograde amnesia. Her recall of public events in the 20-year period 1930 to 1950, as probed by Sanders and Warrington, was 0 (controls 18.5) and on the recognition version she was also close to chance. Thus she was very unclear what she had done in the war years, even though she had lived in London during 1940 when thousands died in bombing raids. She was then in her 30s. Recall of people who had stopped being famous at a particular time was also chance. Despite this, semantic memory was normal; for instance her scaled score on the Vocabulary Subtest of the WAIS was 10, the same level as her average verbal IQ. Yet in other patients with apparently the same type of damage, the retrograde amnesia is much less long-lasting.[25]

How can the discrepancy be resolved? We return again to the vexed issue of personal semantics and the quality of episodic recall. Thus, in Bayley et al.'s (2003) study where the hippocampal patients appeared normal as far as long-term autobiographical memory was concerned, the controls averaged only 18 details per memory, while in Moscovitch et al.'s (1999) study they averaged 100 (see Moscovitch et al., 2005).

Consider in this context the following protocol given by Bayley et al. (2003) as an example of the claimed preservation of episodic memory of childhood in amnesic patients, in their case EP. They categorized elements of the retrieved memory as either semantic (Sem) or episodic (Epi). So in response to the word fire, part of his protocol was 'Dad had 3½ acres of property (Sem) … and the back property would just grow (Sem) and would be dry (Sem) … the next thing we knew is that it was starting to burn (Epi). I told dad (Epi) and he called the Castro Valley fire department (Epi). They came up (Epi) and they got it out real quick (Epi)' (p. 139) The events categorised as episodic could well have been extensively rehearsed in the intervening 50 or so years since it was a dramatic event that directly affected the family. Indeed, Bayley et al. make a related point themselves. Thus they could be part of personal semantics.

However such an assertion needs to be directly tested. More convincing are direct comparisons between patients with differing degrees of damage to the hippocampus compared to other parts of the medial temporal cortex. Thus Rosenbaum et al. (2008) compared four patients with damage to the medial temporal cortex. In one, SJ, the damage was primarily bilateral hippocampal. The other three had varying degrees of hippocampal damage, but in all cases this was less than that of SJ, and two of the other three had considerably greater damage to the medial temporal structures (see Figure 10.9). SJ was generally worse than the other patients when his autobiographical memory was probed, but his deficit was, if anything, even more the case for earlier time periods. There was no suggestion

---

reorganisation of function may have taken place. This is unlikely, though, to result in loss of an ability.

[24] CA2 was relatively normal.

---

[25] These are primarily from Squire's laboratory (e.g. Bayley et al., 2003) but not all (see e.g. Hepner et al., 2007).

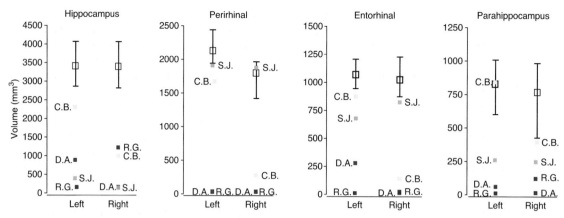

Fig. 10.9 Gray matter volumes for medial temporal lobe regions for four amnesic patients (SJ, with bilateral hippocampal damage, RG, CB, and DA) in comparison to the control distributions. Redrawn with permission from R.S. Rosenbaum et al., 2008, Patterns of Autobiographical Memory Loss in Medial-Temporal Lobe Amnesic Patients, *Journal of Cognitive Neuroscience*, 20(8), 1490–1506. Copyright © 2008, MIT Press Journals.

of a standard temporal gradient (see Figure 10.10). Indeed when specific probing of the details of memories was carried out, SJ was generally bad but especially so for events retrieved from the 0–11 year age period. This fits with the idea that the hippocampus is the critical structure in humans for the index-type storage for episodic memory traces of whatever duration.

10.6 Functional Imaging of Memory: the Hippocampus

The hypotheses being discussed so far in this chapter are rather different from those say in classical cognitive neuropsychology. We are not just considering whether particular neuropsychological dissociations exist but

also how they are linked to particular anatomical structures. The discussion has been much more messy as a result. Single-case study methodology in general is more effective in demonstrating strong dissociations. Single-case studies, though, are feeble vehicles on which to rest a case about localisation. This makes it evident that in this area we should pay greater attention to functional imaging evidence.

As far as the hippocampus was concerned, at least until some years ago, such an argument would be wishful thinking. Functional imaging of experimental paradigms relevant to episodic memory first began in about 1992. Activation of the hippocampus was more often not seen in an episodic memory paradigm than seen. Thus Lepage, Habib and Tulving (1998) in a meta-analysis

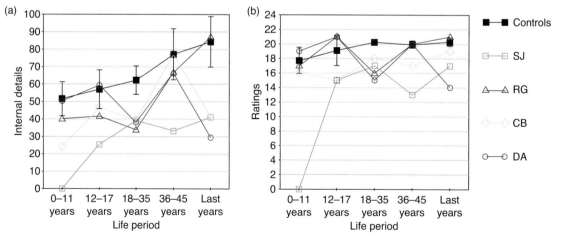

Fig. 10.10 Autobiographical recall for the controls and the patients shown in Figure 10.9 across five life periods after specific probing. (a) Total number of internal (i.e. episodic) details retrieved, (b) qualitative ratings of the richness of the internal details retrieved. All time periods correspond to memories formed premorbidly, with the exception of the two most recent time periods for DA and the most recent time period for the other patients. Redrawn with permission from R.S. Rosenbaum et al., 2008, Patterns of Autobiographical Memory Loss in Medial-Temporal Lobe Amnesic Patients, *Journal of Cognitive Neuroscience*, 20(8), 1490–1506. Copyright © 2008, MIT Press Journals.

examined 52 PET studies which involved encoding or retrieval of an episodic memory contrasted with a control condition. From the 52 studies they found that 13 task comparisons from 8 studies gave activation of the hippocampus at encoding. Nineteen task comparisons from 13 different studies gave retrieval activations. Thus less than half the studies gave significant activation of the structure.

One possibility, though, is that PET is just insensitive. In addition PET studies by necessity use blocked designs where all the activations induced by all trials in a 30–45-sec period are lumped together. Event-related fMRI should provide a much more sensitive procedure and one less contaminated by overall expectancy and strategic artefacts to which PET is liable. However, we will see in the next section that similar results occur with fMRI too.

We begin though by considering retrieval of remote autobiographical memories, to complement the discussion of its neuropsychology. A considerable number of functional imaging studies of the recall of remote autobiographical memories have now been carried out (see Maguire, 2001; Moscovitch et al., 2006, for reviews). They vary in the procedures used to retrieve the events, including the presentation of sentences that describe the event, using cue words as in the Galton–Crovitz technique and the use of family photographs. Many structures tend to be activated including the medial and ventrolateral prefrontal cortex, the medial and lateral temporal cortices, the temporo-parietal junction, the retrosplenial and the posterior cingulate cortices, the cerebellum and the thalamus. The complexity of the network and the potential lack of transparency of functional imaging data is such that Moscovitch et al. in a review of the remote memory studies merely say of these regions 'we do not speculate about their function here' (p. 185)!

Moscovitch et al. were probably wise to be cautious as we will see in the next section. The exception where their theorising was bold concerned, of course, the hippocampus, which unlike for the Ebbinghaus-type studies is consistently activated in fMRI studies of autobiographical memories—5/5 studies in the review of Maguire (2001).[26] Moreover hippocampal activation is greater when temporally specific events, e.g. *my brother's wedding*, are being recalled compared with autobiographical facts—personal semantics (e.g. *my brother's birthday*) (Maguire & Mummery, 1999), supporting a link with the retrieval of specifically episodic memories. In addition, if subjects are presented with cue words using the Galton–Crovitz technique in order to elicit a memory and then 24 sec later required to

start rating various aspects of the memory, hippocampal activation occurs early (Daselaar et al., 2008) (see Figure 10.11).[27] The early hippocampal activation fits with the hippocampus being critically involved in core episodic memory retrieval rather than in thinking about it.

Is the activation of the hippocampus the same for recent and remote autobiographical memories? Here the evidence is minimal. Thus Maguire et al. (2001) studied autobiographical memories of different ages and found no consistent effect of age of memory for the hippocampus. In this study the memories were elicited by the subjects having to decide whether sentences they heard did or did not correspond to aspects of real events they had experienced. The personal histories of the subjects were known from questionnaires which they had completed together with an interview several weeks before scanning.

A similar lack of effect of the age of the memory on hippocampal activation when comparing recent and remote autobiographical memories was found by Ryan et al. (2001) (see Figure 10.12). Here, cues were standard life events like an important career event or your wedding day. Critically there were no differences between recent and remote events in their importance, the arousal induced, or their emotional value when these were rated outside the scanner. However, unlike the two studies just discussed, Addis et al. (2004) did find that retrieving recent events gave stronger hippocampal activation than retrieving remote events. Yet the effect disappeared from the left hippocampus if ratings of the amount of detail retrievable or the personal significance or emotionality of the memory was partialled out. For the right hippocampus the effect also disappeared if ratings of personal significance were partialled out. Personal significance and amount of detail retrievable both in turn correlated with hippocampal activity, as we would expect if the structure is critical for retrieval of episodic memories.[28] Overall it appears that even if remote autobiographical memories are being retrieved, the hippocampus is as activated as much as it is for more recent events, if other factors are controlled. Functional imaging findings thus mesh with those from neuropsychology as far as the role of the hippocampus in autobiographical recall is concerned.

---

[26] For similar later findings, see Moscovitch et al. (2006).

[27] Along with activation of the retrosplenial and right prefrontal cortex at that time and other structures such as the left prefrontal cortex when subjects rate the memory.

[28] See Gilboa et al. (2004) for similar findings. Maguire and Frith (2003) have also found subtly different effects for activation of the left and right hippocampi in autobiographical memory.

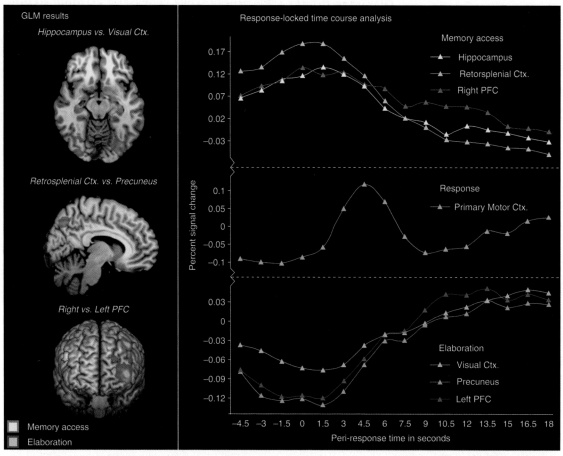

Fig. 10.11 BOLD response to regions associated with memory access and elaboration during the study of Daselaar et al. (2008). During memory access, the hippocampus, retrosplenial cortex, and right PFC showed greater activity, whereas visual cortex, precuneus, and left PFC showed greater activity during the elaboration period. Regions associated with retrieval showed a descending slope at the time the memory was accessed (top panel), whereas regions associated with elaboration showed an ascending slope (bottom panel). Plots on the right are the average of the cluster. Response-related activity in the motor cortex is displayed as a reference (middle panel). Reproduced from S.M. Daselaar, H.J. Rice, D.L. Greenberg, R. Cabeza, K.S. LaBar and D.C. Rubin, The Spatiotemporal Dynamics of Autobiographical Memory: Neural Correlates of Recall, Emotional Intensity, and Reliving, *Cerebral Cortex*, 2008, *18*(1), 217–229, by permission of Oxford University Press.

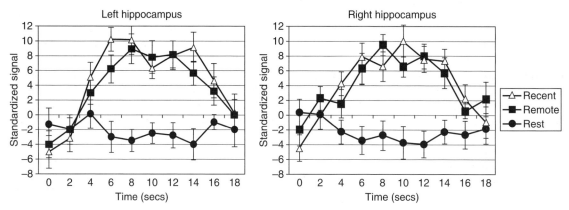

Fig. 10.12 Mean activations in left and right hippocampus for recollection of recent events, remote events, and rest. Subjects were three controls who had no prior knowledge of the event cues that were to be presented in the scanner. Note that for both left and right hippocampi there was no difference in activation between recent and remote events. From L. Ryan, L. Nadel, K. Keil, K. Putnam, D. Schnyer, T. Trouard, and M. Moscovitch, 2001, Hippocampal Complex and retrieval of recent and very remote autobiographical memories: Evidence from functional Magnetic Resonance Imaging in neurologically intact people, *Hippocampus*, *11*(6), 707–714. Copyright (2001) Wiley-Liss, Inc.; Reprinted with permission of John Wiley & Sons, Inc.

10.7 Episodic Memory and the Lateral Parietal Cortex

Maybe the reader thinks this discussion of findings from both neuropsychology and functional imaging is unnecessary overkill. It is not. Take the parietal cortex. A number of parietal regions are frequently activated in autobiographical memory studies. These include the retrosplenial cortex, a medial parietal region that is anatomically closely linked to the medial temporal cortex. Lesions in this region have often been held to give rise to amnesia because of the connections the region has with the medial temporal lobe (Valenstein et al., 1987; Rudge & Warrington, 1991; Cavanna & Trimble, 2006). A second medial parietal region activated is more superior and posterior—the precuneus. There has been speculation that its activation in episodic memory retrieval relates to the use of visual imagery (Fletcher et al., 1995; Roland & Gulyás, 1995; Cavanna & Trimble, 2006).

However a more surprising finding is that in retrieval from autobiographical memory there is frequently activation of lateral parietal areas, in particular inferior parietal cortex (e.g. Fink et al., 1996; Conway et al., 1999; Maguire & Mummery, 1999; Ryan et al., 2001). It does not occur in all autobiographical retrieval studies (e.g. Maguire & Frith, 2003). Some find it in 'suspicious' parts of the overall process; thus in the Daselaar et al. (2008) study where memories had to be rated, the left and right inferior parietal areas were activated in the rating phase rather than in basic autobiographical memory retrieval.

The inferior parietal regions are, though, frequently activated in other types of episodic memory studies too (Fletcher, Frith & Rugg, 1997; Wagner et al., 2005). Indeed, consider a task which is frequently used as a signature of episodic memory—the so-called remember-know task.[29] This is a modification of the recognition memory task in which subjects have to make an additional decision for words they recognise as having been presented earlier. They have to inspect their own thought processes and decide whether they recollect the word when it was initially presented or whether they merely know it had been presented without any conscious memory of the event itself. The utility of findings obtained from the task would appear to depend on the validity of the concept of episodic memory itself. It is very much a theory-laden experimental procedure. Indeed, as we will see shortly, there have been frequent challenges to its appropriateness (e.g. Wixted, 2007).

However, such challenges have not reduced its attraction to experimenters!

A typical move in functional imaging of memory is to contrast either at encoding or retrieval events given the recollection label with events given the know label (e.g. Henson et al., 1999). Whether an event is of the recollection or know type is decided post hoc by the subject's on-line introspection after they have retrieved the item. Then in later analyses items are grouped according to whether they are rated *Recollected*, *Known* or *New* at retrieval. Simons et al. (2008) carried out a meta-analysis of such studies.[30] When the contrast of recollection against known or non-recollective baseline conditions was made, various regions of prefrontal cortex were activated, each in roughly 50–60% of studies. The medial temporal cortex, which presumably included the hippocampus—although this is not stated—did worse with less than 40% of studies[31] However the lateral parietal cortex was activated in over 90% studies! In their thorough meta-analysis, Skinner and Fernandes (2007) found both lateral parietal and medial-temporal regions activated in 83% of 'recollectively-based' response conditions. The contrast claimed by Simons et al. is therefore probably a little exaggerated. However, lateral parietal activations frequently occur in recollection conditions. If any region is the signature region for recollective experience it might appear that the lateral parietal cortices have a strong claim!

Simons et al., however, compared their meta-analysis with a neuropsychological study. For this they used a slightly different procedure to the standard remember–know paradigm. At encoding subjects had to carry out one of two tasks—they had to decide whether the stimulus was related more to *entertainment* or to *politics*, or they had to decide whether the stimulus was *pleasant* or *unpleasant*. At retrieval, after a stimulus had been recognised as having occurred at encoding, the subjects had to decide which of the two tasks had been applied to that item. This is known as a source judgement, as it concerns the overall situation at the time of encoding. Stimuli could be of two types—famous faces or words. Performance was not particularly good, even for normal controls. However patients with left or right parietal lesions were collectively unimpaired in the task (see Figure 10.13). In addition, their lesions involved the

---

[29] This is the task that we discussed in Section 2.3 as an example of a procedure that raises deep philosophical cum methodological issues for cognitive neuroscience.

[30] Unfortunately no details are given of which studies were included, of the search procedure for studies, or even of how many were included. There are now a number of meta-analyses of recollection and familiarity. Technically the most thorough is that of Skinner and Fernandes (2007).

[31] This is surprisingly low given the meta-analysis of Diana et al. (2007) to be discussed in the next section, but reminds one of the Lepage et al. (1998) meta-analysis of PET studies discussed in Section 10.6.

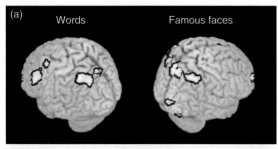

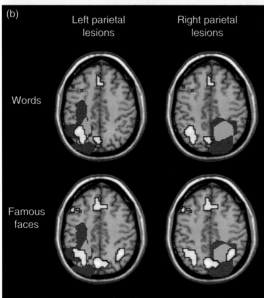

Fig. 10.13 (a) Brain regions consistently associated with source recollection across two separate fMRI experiments involving healthy volunteers. Regions include left lateral parietal cortex for words and bilateral lateral parietal cortex for famous faces, among other areas. (b) Lesion overlay diagrams (green > purple) illustrating the close correspondence between the location of Simons et al.'s patients' parietal lobe lesions and the areas of fMRI activation identified in the healthy volunteers. The patients were unimpaired on source judgements. Reprinted from *Neuropsychologia*, 46(4), J.S. Simons, P.V. Peers, D.Y. Hwang, B.A. Ally, P.C. Fletcher and A.E. Budson, Is the parietal lobe necessary for recollection in humans?, 1185–1191, Copyright (2008), with permission from Elsevier.

areas activated when normal subjects carried out the same task, when that is contrasted to the activation corresponding to 'baseline' stimuli unrelated to either entertainment or politics.[32]

If the inferior parietal activation is not a signature of core episodic memory retrieval when subjects are making remember–know judgement, why does it occur?[33] Vilberg and Rugg (2008) in a detailed review say 'There is no shortage of potential functions to choose from .... Among the more prominent are control of visuo-spatial attention, attention switching, the temporary storage of phonological and visual information, organisation of action sequences, and top-down control of working memory' (p. 1794) Yet another possibility they consider is that the inferior lateral parietal cortex contains a modality-independent 'attentional circuit-breaker' (Astafiev et al., 2006), assuming that recollection is an 'attention-grabbing internal event'. Yet another is that it is the locus of systems that support sustained focussing of attention on the contents of working memory (Ravizza et al., 2004). Finally the alternative they prefer is that the region 'supports' another type of memory system—the 'episodic buffer', a concept developed by Alan Baddeley (2000, 2007), which we discussed in Section 7.8.

We will not review the arguments put forward by Vilberg and Rugg against the other seven alternatives. Their arguments are highly cogent if one accepts one premise. This is that only one of the seven hypothetical processes is involved in a recollection judgement. Then the results of at least one of the sixteen experiments reviewed can be used to make each of the alternative hypotheses implausible. But why accept the premise? The regions involved for the right inferior parietal cortex stretch over 4.5 cm. There is ample possibility of the analogue of what would be called 'associated deficits' if an inference were being made from neuropsychological findings. Indeed one's experience of recognising an item is a complex process probably involving many subprocesses. More than one could be located in the inferior parietal cortex.

We would draw a different conclusion, more akin—but not identical—to the positions of Harley and Coltheart discussed in Chapter 5. However well-studied the task, if it involves a complex set of central processes, then given the weak power of behavioural data, conclusive interpretation of functional imaging

---

[32] In fact one left parietal patient, LI, showed a significant impairment on source judgements for famous faces, but the authors point out he was the only patient to score 2 SDs below controls on a measure of premorbid IQ and on copying the Rey figure—a complex line drawing composed of many rectangles, triangles, circles and so on. This means that his impairment on the experimental task may be due to more basic cognitive impairments.

[33] Simons et al. raise the possibility that the inferior parietal region could bilaterally carry out a recollection-related process, and indeed bilateral lateral parietal lesions which do not involve other cortex are rare in most acute neurological conditions. However parietal cortical functions tend to be strongly lateralised in humans, as we saw in the discussion of apraxia in Chapter 8; see also FNMS Chapter 8. Moreover Benson, Davis and Snyder (1988) report that posterior cortical atrophy, which is more often bilateral, produces fewer memory problems than Alzheimer's disease which affects the medial temporal lobe.

TABLE 10.3 Number of significant activation contrasts in the metaanalysis of Diana et al (2007) as a proportion of the number of comparisons.

	Hippocampal Activation	Anterior Parahippocampal Gyrus Activation
Recollection minus Control	21/26	4/26
Familiarity minus Control	3/14	13/14

Note: The perirhinal cortex is in the anterior part of the parahippocampal gyrus.

findings requires parallel neuropsychological findings to be persuasive.[34]

10.8 Recollection and the Hippocampus

It is unfair to judge the remember–know task by what it tells us about the parietal cortex. It attempts to operationalise the experience of consciously remembering the past, the essence of the theoretical concept of episodic memory. And most investigators[35] associate the medial temporal cortex, or for some the hippocampus alone, with the core recollection process named by Tulving (1983) *ecphory*, the initial process in the retrieval of an episodic memory and producing the task-relevant response.

How does the hippocampus fare in the functional imaging of this task? Diana et al. (2007) provide a meta-analysis. They combine remember–know judgements with source judgements and experiments where subjects give confidence ratings for their responses. If we limit ourselves to the first of these, then Table 10.3 shows the result. The hippocampus, and also probably the posterior parahippocampal gyrus, shows a stronger activation, both at encoding and at retrieval, for memories that are judged to be recollected; or in the case of encoding could later be so. The anterior parahippocampal gyrus, the seat of perirhinal cortex, is by contrast virtually silent. The opposite occurs when the know response is the key one, with now the anterior parahippocampal gyrus being the active area. Broadly speaking the source judgements reviewed show the same crossover pattern. In addition where cross-item associations

have to be formed the hippocampus is consistently involved.

The reader should, however, be warned. There is now a somewhat bewildering set of paradigms that relate to the recollection–familiarity contrast. The most popular alternative to the remember–know paradigm is the giving of confidence ratings, typically on a six-point scale as to whether a stimulus in a recognition task had or had not been presented before. Various models can then be used to fit the findings (Yonelinas et al., 1998; Wixted, 2007). The mapping of imaging of this task onto the recollection–familiarity contrast is broadly consistent with that of the remember–know one, but there are obscure complications. Thus a linear increase in activation with higher confidence is found in the anterior parahippocampal gyrus in two studies (Ranganath et al., 2004; Daselaar et al., 2006a), while a linear decrease is found in the same region with two others (Montaldi et al., 2006; Daselaar et al., 2006b) (see Diana et al, 2007)!

To complicate matters further, the set of paradigms that reviewers survey is subtly different. Thus in a less systematic review paper, Squire, Wixted and Clark (2007), echoing the position of this school of investigators on retrograde amnesia, argue that there is no qualitative difference within the medial temporal lobe in whether activation is linked to recollection or familiarity. Indeed they deny the existence of such qualitative differences in general, claiming that they are merely a reflection of differences in memory strength. So for them, what a devotee of 'autonoetic' awareness would call a recollection is merely a consequence of the rapidity and compellingness with which a strong memory trace is brought to mind. A memory which is 'familiar' or 'known'—and hence by followers of episodic memory held to lack 'recollective' experience—is merely for them a reflection on retrieving a weak memory trace.[36]

What is critical for rejecting this simple interpretation is the reverse pattern of familiarity but not recollection being associated with activation of the anterior parahippocampal gyrus and in particular the perirhinal cortex (see Table 10.3). Squire et al. explain this in terms of non-linearities in the relation between the BOLD responses of parts of the medial temporal lobe to memory strength, and to differences in this function between the different parts. Their argument has a family resemblance to the one we put forward about the Badre and D'Esposito study in Section 5.6. In particular Squire et al. argue that activation in the perirhinal

---

[34] A striking study that supports a position related to that of Astafiev et al.—that of Ciaramelli et al. (2010)—in fact uses precisely this dual methodology. These authors treat attention to memories by analogy to the endogenous versus exogenous contrast in attention to percepts discussed in Chapter 9.

[35] See Gaffan et al. (2001) for alternative perspectives.

---

[36] Whittlesea (1993) has particularly championed the view that the fluency with which an idea comes to mind increases one's confidence in it.

cortex can be assumed to be relatively insensitive to variations among traces which are strong, while activation in the hippocampus is relatively insensitive to differences in strength between traces that are weak. The BOLD to memory strength functions they assume are, however, ad hoc.[37] So while in principle the account is a possible hypothesis it is much weaker than the Aggleton–Brown–Diana et al. one on the *simplicity and falsifiability* criterion of Jacobs and Grainger discussed in Section 4.8. Apart from making their position operationally very similar to the two-process position by this assumption, the approach of Squire et al. does not explain why the perirhinal cortex often gives its strongest response to items with a weaker trace rather than to stronger trace ones, or to their equivalents in other paradigms (e.g. Henson et al., 1999; Gonsalves et al., 2005; Daselaar et al., 2006a; Montaldi et al., 2006).

In support of the idea that perirhinal cortex might be a vehicle for the familiarity component of recognition, Brown and Xiang (1998) have shown, using microelectrode recording in the monkey, that a class of neurons in perirhinal cortex exists which show responses specific to particular objects. These neurons can show a selective repetition-related decrease for 24 hours in responding of the sort discussed for the fusiform cortex in the context of priming (see Section 7.2). They could be the basis for familiarity judgments, which would make such judgements parasitic on the identification processes of semantic memory (see e.g. Buckley & Gaffan, 2006; Section 6.9). Recollection would then be a different process altogether.

The assignment of these two processes (identification/familiarity and recollection) to the perirhinal cortex and the hippocampus, respectively, was first proposed by Aggleton and Brown (1999) (see also Eichenbaum et al., 2007) on the basis of this type of neurophysiological finding but also on neuropsychological data. The neuropsychological evidence essentially related to patients with primarily selective damage to the hippocampus. If, however, the neuroimaging evidence was not exactly crystal clear, the neuropsychological evidence is distinctly murky. We will discuss not only paradigms held to be directly linked to the recollection-familiarity contrast but also recognition, which is held by the two-process theorists to involve both processes, and compare them to recall.

There is an inconsistent pattern of results. Strong support for the Aggleton-Brown position is provided by the extensive investigations of the recognition memory capacities of YR, a patient with selective hippocampal damage as assessed by MRI. The extraordinary number of 43 item recognition tasks were carried out by Mayes et al. (2002) on the patient, 19 being verbal and 24 visual. Both Yes/No (*n*=16) and forced-choice (*n*=27) designs were used. On average, the patient scored 0.5 SDs below the normal mean on these tasks, far better than the 3.6 SDs below the normal mean found for free recall tasks.[38]

The distinction between recall and item recognition performance is very clear in YR. It provides support for the Aggleton-Brown position. It should be noted, in particular, that the finding of relative sparing of a function—recognition by comparison with recall—cannot be explained by 'hidden' lesions producing undetected damage outside the hippocampus. A similar effect of intact familiarity and impaired recollection has been noted in a number of other primarily hippocampal patients (e.g. Hirano et al., 2002; Bastin et al., 2004; Aggleton et al., 2005; Barbeau et al., 2005; Wais et al., 2006).

However in other patients a different pattern has been found. Thus Manns and Squire (1999) used the *Doors ad People* test—a test of Baddeley, Emslie and Nimmo-Smith (1994) that provides standardised scores of recall and recognition for both verbal information and visual information; thus visual recognition is of a set of *doors*. Manns and Squire describe the performance of three classical amnesic patients, AB3, PH and LJ, held to have selective hippocampal lesions. Their scaled scores on *Doors and People*, corrected for age, were at worse than the 1st percentile for recall and at the 1st, 1st and 2nd percentiles, respectively, for recognition. In fact, though, they were somewhat above chance level, roughly half way between the normal control mean and chance for verbal recognition and 40% of the way for visual recognition. Technically, as no estimate was provided on the familiarity and recollection components of the task, no theoretical conclusions can be drawn from this evidence with respect to the Aggleton-Brown hypothesis. However their pattern of performance was quite different from that of YR, who was at the 1st percentile for recall and at the 84th for recognition.

Use of confidence ratings in certain other selective hippocampal patients has tended to support the conclusions of Manns and Squire. Thus VC (Cipolotti et al.,

---

[37] In addition they assume different functions for perirhinal cortex at encoding and at retrieval.

[38] This contrast is especially impressive as recall tends to be less sensitive to impairment as the range of performance (relative to 0) in normal controls is typically greater than for recognition. Baddeley (2002) raises the problem with the developmental amnesic patient Jon (Vargha-Khadem et al., 1997) as to how he can be so good at recognition—equivalent, like YR, to the normal mean—if he has only one of two processes available. However he might have been above the normal mean if he had not had his lesion, so the conundrum is not quite so problematic. However it illustrates the danger of assuming normality from performance in the normal range when that range is large.

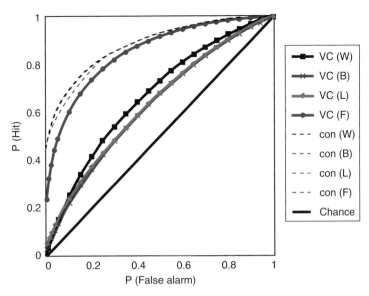

Fig. 10.14 Performance of a hippocampal amnesic (VC) and controls on four recognition memory tests of Cipolotti et al. (2006) plotted as Receiver Operating Characteristic (ROC) curves. ROC curves show the relationship between hits and false alarms as confidence changes. These curves derive from a signal detection approach to recognition. The subject gives a confidence rating for each item as to whether it is old or new. The curves plot the cumulative values for presented items (hits) and new items (false alarms), as confidence is decreased in steps from a high value of 6 to a low value of 1. (W: Words; B: Buildings; L: Landscapes; F: Faces.) Reprinted from *Neuropsychologia, 44*(3), L. Cipolotti, C. Bird, T. Good, D. Macmanus, P. Rudge and T. Shallice, Recollection and familiarity in dense hippocampal amnesia: A case study, 489–506, Copyright (2006), with permission from Elsevier.

2006) and RH and JC (Bird et al., 2007a) both showed a pattern of impairment for both recollection and familiarity, with the former deficit being apparently worse.

Why should there be this difference in pattern of performance on the task across patients? There may be subtle organic differences between patients, possibly in post-lesion recovery processes. Thus Holdstock et al. (2008) described a fairly young patient PR who lost roughly 50% of both hippocampi by volume after an anoxic episode and yet performed close to the normal mean on both recall and recognition.

Probably more important, though, is that we lack good task analyses for these paradigms. Take the confidence judgement paradigm, which is simpler than the remember–know one. Cipolotti, Bird and their colleagues have raised a major difficulty in the interpretation of this type of task in amnesic patients. In addition to the core memory retrieval process, the item must itself be held in working memory and compared to some standard types of retrieval which themselves need to be stored in memory, using presumably a mix of semantic memory—what it is like to have a strong and clear memory of an event—and episodic memory of recently preceding trials. These memories are not, though, nicely labelled by the mind with the ratings 1 to 6, so maybe the rating given in an earlier trial, say, was too low or too high; a complex assessment needs to be made requiring judgements as well as abstract comparisons with earlier retrievals; whatever in processing

terms this might be![39] And this does not take into account the variety of processes that have been proposed to be responsible for inferior parietal activations in recollection!

Now consider an amnesic. One thing that most amnesics always remember about their memory is that it is very bad. Are they likely, therefore to be able to assign a high confidence rating? Maybe they could overcome this and make even finer discriminations than others need to do among their retrieved memories. If not, and they virtually never use the maximum rating of 6, this will have the effect of reducing their recollection measure much more than their familiarity one. Technically this is because their so-called Receiver Operating Characteristic (ROC) curves will tend to have a point near (0,0) (see Figure 10.14). So an advocate of the single-memory trace position could argue that the apparent lack of recollection in amnesics is just a consequence of their strategy in tackling the task. Even considering normal subjects, the two process theory assumes that ratings of 5 and 4 differ only in the strength of the sense of familiarity. On giving a rating of 5 rather than 4 (out of 6) does a normal subject do this because they have a flicker of a recollective experience in one case but not the other? We do not know. We lack an

---

[39] These problems are related to those occurring with range-effects generally in within-subject designs (e.g. Poulton, 1973).

adequate phenomenological investigation of the use of confidence ratings in normal subjects, let alone in amnesics.

At this stage it is necessary to take stock. We have descended deep into the entrails of memory research. What is critical is that in both the more non-ecological of paradigms which we have just discussed and the more ecological ones which we discussed a little earlier there is support for a special system—that underlying recollection for memories of any age—sited in the hippocampus. The evidence is relatively good from neuropsychology for both types of paradigm and from functional imaging for the more ecological one. The neuropsychological literature, with the very occasional exception (Holdstock et al., 2008), also supports the claim that the hippocampus is critical for recollection; after all recall is typically gravely impaired following damage to the structure. For the more complex and artificial paradigms related to recollection and familiarity the functional imaging literature fits fairly well, but the neuropsychological literature is unclear. However, for the remember–know and similar tasks, which rely on complex introspection, and are dependent upon the subtle interpretation of instructions, both of which may well be undermined by an amnesic problem, functional imaging of young highly intelligent adults seems the preferable method. However, we will argue in Section 11.6 that these methods have been inadequately investigated from a methodological perspective.

10.9 Events and the Function of Episodic Memory

Given the discussion of judgemental processes at the end of the previous section it is not surprising that paradigms aiming to differentiate recollection and familiarity lead to extensive prefrontal activations (Skinner & Fernandez, 2007). What is much more surprising is that when much simpler episodic memory tasks were first carried out in the scanner, prefrontal activations occurred (Grasby et al., 1993; Shallice et al., 1994; Tulving et al., 1994b; see for review Fletcher & Henson, 2001). Yet the standard neuropsychological line at the time was that lesions to prefrontal cortex, just like lesions to parietal cortex, did not lead to a major memory disorder.[40] Why then should the prefrontal activation occur?

It is necessary to step back away from the standard experimental designs of the memory literature that derived very distantly from the methods of Ebbinghaus. We need to consider two issues. The first is what key biological functions does episodic memory serve in the human. The second is how events are structured in memory.

In Sections 10.2 and 10.4 of this chapter we considered the position that the biological function of episodic memory in humans was to allow traces to be laid down in semantic memory without suffering from catastrophic interference. However given the discussion in Section 10.4 it seems that episodic memory can last for many years, too long for this to be its sole function. Lengyel and Dayan (2008) consider a different type of biological function by posing the question of why an organism should act on the basis of its knowledge of single events—episodic memory—rather than the accumulated statistics from all the events it has experienced—semantic memory. Lengyel and Dayan consider an agent which, to obtain a reward, has to make two levels of decision, for each of which they choose between four alternative actions, which in turn result in one of three states of affairs. The link between the action selected and the state of affairs that follows is stochastic. Thus, which second decision is required is determined probabilistically from the action selected at the first level, and the reward received is determined probabilistically from the action selected at the second level (see Figure 10.15).

Lengyel and Dayan first investigate how an agent could learn to optimise its behaviour to maximise its reward using its 'knowledge'—a statistical model that averages over past events and outcomes which they equate with semantic memory. Then two additional factors are considered. The first is to assume a non-perfect semantic memory; the agent is assumed to have access to only a 'noisy' record of the average effect of its actions and their consequences. The second is to assume that the agent has only limited experience of its environment to form its semantic memory. Lengyel and Dayan show that these two factors can interact to cripple the effectiveness of using semantic memory alone to control the selection of actions when the domain is as complex as this one and not well learned.[41]

Instead Lengyel and Dayan consider an agent that stores exactly what has happened; that is the specific sequence of state–action pairs leading to a reward, when it obtains a reward it considers larger than expected. Then if it happens to find itself in one of these episodic states, it follows the sequence, particularly if that led to the best result when more than one 'good' sequence has occurred. In complicated environments that are not overlearned, this 'episodic memory' based agent performs better than the semantic memory

---

[40] There is one very important exception to which we will return in Section 10.12—confabulation.

[41] Daw et al. (2005) show that a purely habit-based controller performs even worse if environments are subject to change.

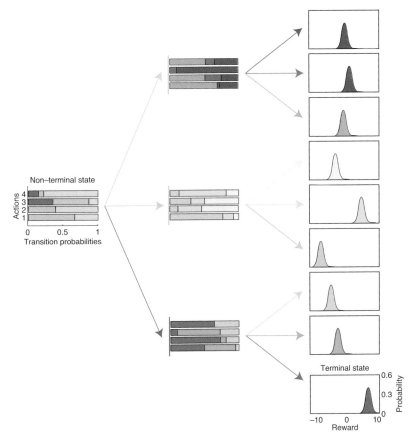

Fig. 10.15 An example of a tree-structured Markov decision process with depth 2, branching factor 3, and 4 actions available in each non-terminal state. The horizontal stacked bars in the boxes of the left and middle column show the transition probabilities for different actions at the non-terminal states, with colour coding indicating the successor states to which they lead. Reproduced with permission of the authors from M. Lengyel and P. Dayan (2008), Hippocampal contributions to control: The third way, *Advances in Neural Information Processing Systems, 20,* 889–896; Figure 1a.

based one, provided that the semantic memory is not perfect.

A similar conclusion that episodic memory may be critical in ill-learned complicated environments can be derived from so-called E-MOP (Episodic-Memory Organisation Packet) theory in symbolic artificial intelligence. Schank (1982) and Kolodner (1985) have argued that in confronting a novel situation vital raw materials for the reasoning process are provided by records of what happened in somewhat similar situations.[42] Unlike in the Lengyel–Dayan approach, the episodic record is not slavishly followed by the agent; instead it enters into a case-based reasoning process. Both approaches, however, argue for an intimate link between using episodic records of similar events and how an agent should act in ill-learned complex situations. They imply a strong link between the systems controlling novel actions—the Supervisory System—and the episodic store.

There is, though, another type of reason for assuming a close link—the nature of events that need to be stored in episodic memory. Consider the following memory: 'My own memory of the declaration of the Second World War, from September 1939, occurred when I was aged six... I have a clear image of my father standing on the rockery of the front garden of our house waving a bamboo garden stake like a pendulum in time with the clock chimes heard on the radio which heralded the announcement. More hazily, I have an impression that neighbours were also out in the adjoining gardens listening to the radio and, although my father was fooling around, the feeling of the memory is one of deep foreboding and anxiety. I have ... very rarely thought about it.' This memory from the British psychologist Gillian Cohen is quoted by Conway and Pleydell-Pearce (2000) in a major article on autobiographical memory. Like most if not all memories, it is of an event. It contains a clear structure. Thus it contains

---

[42] See FNMS Chapter 15 for further discussion.

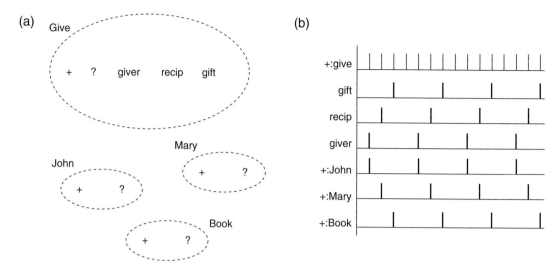

Fig. 10.16 Shastri's (2002) account of the structure of stored events. (a) Each element of an event is represented by a 'focal cluster', indicated in the figure as an ellipse. Relations such as *give* contain argument roles which correspond to cell ensembles within the focal cluster, and which must be bound to representations of the actors or objects that make up the event. The 'A' and '?' notation indicates that focal clusters may be accessed in two ways: via affirmation (+) or via a query (?). (b) The activity-based encoding of the event *John gives the book to Mary*, where the horizontal axis depicts time. Binding of arguments to argument roles is achieved through temporal synchrony (see text). Note that *giver* and *John* fire in synchrony, as do *recipient* and *Mary*, and *gift* and *Book*. Reprinted from *Trends in Cognitive Sciences, 6*(4), L. Shastri, Episodic memory and cortico-hippocampal interactions, 162–168. Copyright (2002), with permission from Elsevier.

elements which have been processed by different processing systems—visual and auditory perceptual, cognitive and emotional. There is a general event-type from the period (*playing in the garden*). There are elements which are what Conway and Pleydell-Pearce call event-specific knowledge (*the swinging bamboo stake, clock chimes*), details specific to that individual event. As the elements can come from a variety of different cognitive domains, so they need a system which receives input from virtually all parts of the cortex if they are to be retained by a single system. The hippocampus is well suited to this role. Moreover as Shastri (2002) has pointed out a system encoding events has to do more than integrate information of very many different types. Entities taking part in events, just like components in action and language discussed in Chapter 8, have functional roles. Indeed that entities in events have functional roles is why when language is used to describe events the lexical items have functional roles.

Shastri argues that any store of specific events must encode the bindings between contents and roles. He too adopts the schema as a conceptual basis. This is illustrated in Figure 10.16 in which a concept 'give' is shown with its three associated roles—the *giver*, the *recipient* and the *gift*. A particular role, say, give-(recipient), is held to be carried by an ensemble of cells with another ensemble representing a specific individual, say, John, somewhat analogous to the Competitive Queuing models discussed in Chapter 7. Binding is held to be the formation of specific connections between

these two sets of representations.[43] Shastri assumes that a trace of an event—the set of temporarily activated bindings within the schema—is laid down in the hippocampus; and this is the process of episodic memory encoding. Moreover as Barsalou (1988) has shown event memories can be retrieved by a variety of different types of cues. Retrieval requires parallel addressing. On a model such as that of Treves and Rolls discussed in Section 2.2, the collection of cognitive elements, linked to roles, will form an attractor. We will call each of these an *episodic memory complex*.

In addition, though, events have a temporal and semantic structure. In the example discussed by Conway and Pleydell-Pearce above, the narrator begins by referring to a lifetime period (*when I was six; 1939*), and details characteristics of the period (*father,*

---

[43] Shastri assumes that the specific associations are created by synchronous firing when many representations are being simultaneously elicited. The proposed mechanism of temporal binding (von der Malsburg, 1981) is normally invoked for binding together features of an object within perceptual experience (e.g. Engel & Singer, 2001) or of subsystems carrying out one temporally specified part of a more complex process (Gross et al., 2004). It remains contentious, largely due to intrinsic computational difficulties in maintaining and discriminating synchronous neural firing (e.g. Shadlen & Movshon, 1999; O'Reilly et al., 2003; LaRock, 2007). However a more serial process where specific associations are formed by short-term weights as discussed in Chapter 7 would also be a possible binding mechanism.

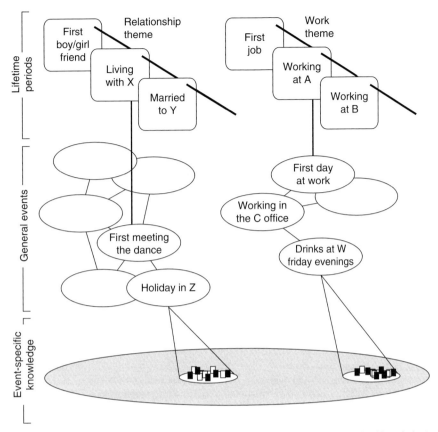

Fig. 10.17 Part of the *autobiographical knowledge base* of Conway & Pleydell-Pearce (2000). Autobiographical knowledge is characterised in terms of lifetime periods, general events and event-specific knowledge. Event-specific knowledge is activated by cues at the general event level, while gross temporal structure is provided by the lifetime period level. Copyright © 2000 by the American Psychological Association. Adapted with permission. M.A. Conway and C.W. Pleydell-Pearce (2000), The construction of autobiographical memories in the self-memory system, *Psychological Review*, 107(2), 261–288. The use of APA information does not imply endorsement by APA.

neighbour, radio). This is linked to a general event type (*playing in the garden*). These are all part of what Conway and Pleydell-Pearce call the *autobiographical knowledge base* (see Figure 10.17), which is temporally organised. We will assume that this corresponds to part of what Cermak and O'Connor called *personal semantics* (see Section 10.4), namely what you know about your life in a roughly analogous fashion to what you know about events in which you did not participate.

But events too have a finer temporal structure; they are themselves composed of sub-events in a multi-level fashion. Moreover the recall of the memory blends elements from those different levels. The narrator's father's waving of the bamboo-stick could not have taken more than a few seconds. Yet the neighbours' listening to the radio could well have lasted fifteen minutes or so. The structure laid down must be more complex than just a set of bound cognitive elements, each based on the firing of an attractor at the lowest of the multiple levels, say, one for each second. Thus there must be extensive indexing of the episodic memory

complex internal to the event as a whole, as well as from the autobiographical knowledge base.

How are such episodic memory complexes which form the basis of an event retrieved? The simple answer (Tulving, 1983) is by the subject being in *retrieval mode*, that is having the conscious intention to try to remember, and also by retrieval cues being present to reactivate part of the complex. The complex as a whole is then retrieved by the process Tulving calls *ecphory*. Computationally this can be closely approximated by the accessing of the corresponding attractor given partial retrieval cues. This appears to work fine for retrieval of word lists and the like of the typical psychological memory experiment. However even here the retrieval task is assumed. If you hear a word list and then are presented with a single word, then you could be required to do any of recognition, so-called part-list cueing—remember the rest of the list in any order given a selection of the words in the list—deciding which list the word came in, or serial recall—remember the next word—and so on. In other words the relation

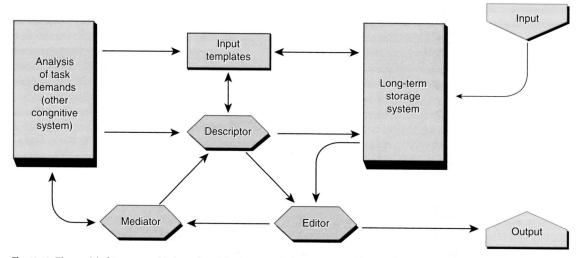

Fig. 10.18 The model of Norman and Bobrow (1979) for the control of memory retrieval. Derived from Burgess and Shallice (1996b).

between the retrieval cue and the relevant part of the memory, the relevant episodic memory complexes, needs to be specified. It is not specified sufficiently well either in the general intention to remember or in the retrieval cue.

In the typical use of autobiographical memory in conversation the relation between the retrieval task and the memory base is more complex still. Consider having a conversation with a colleague for half an hour or so. Just afterwards someone else may ask 'How did she seem?' What episodic memory complex has to be accessed? Leave aside the pragmatics of the question— had she recently been ill, had a member of her family died—and assume that the person had recently joined your department. Let's assume that you had been setting exam questions, then what would be relevant? Presumably competence, intellectual liveliness, interesting news different from the norm, jokes, warmth— or their absence—could all be relevant but all regulated by the social, interpersonal and intellectual context. Thus what might be memorable if uttered by a new colleague would not be memorable if said by an old friend in a pub.

Norman and Bobrow (1979) argued that accessing memories, which they call memory records and what we are calling episodic memory complexes, appropriate to the task in hand, requires a system which produces appropriate *descriptors* with which to search the episodic memory store.[44] Moreover Norman and Bobrow argued that because of the complex relation between the retrieval task and the memory records (in

their terminology) that there will inevitably be false positives. So there needs to be an editor system which verifies that retrieved memories are internally consistent and appropriate to the retrieval task. The overall system is presented in Figure 10.18.[45]

Thus encoding a memory so that it can be appropriately retrieved necessarily involves its placing in two levels of temporal structure of the person's life. First it requires it to be situated at the level of the temporal episodes and associated event schemas of Conway and Pleydell-Pearce's autobiographical knowledge base. In addition, how it is part of a larger event-unit needs to be specified.[46] The processes seem of a different type, involving abstraction and temporal structures, to any of those discussed previously in this chapter. In the light of the previous chapter these processes would appear to relate to the functions of the prefrontal cortex. How then are these structures involved in episodic memory?

10.10 Prefrontal Cortex: the Relation Between Encoding and Retrieval

With one important type of exception to be discussed in the last section of this chapter, patients with purely prefrontal lesions are not amnesic (Jetter et al., 1986; Janovsky et al., 1989). The lack of a major memory

---

[44] The descriptor can be thought of as analogous in the area of memory retrieval to the *determining* tendency of Ach (1905) in thinking discussed in Section 9.5.

[45] The approach has been developed by Morton and Bekerian (1986), Burgess and Shallice (1996b) and Conway and Pleydell-Pearce (2000).

[46] Almost by definition, both these processes need to be carried out after the initial encoding. Also in some situations there can be two different events occurring at the same time—like having a conversation and driving a particular route—so the assignment of content to an event is far from straightforward. We know of no models concerning either of these points!

problem is particularly clear when, as for instance in cued recall (Jetter et al., 1986; Janovsky et al., 1989) or in recognition (Jetter et al. 1986), the complex aspects of encoding and recall discussed in the last section do not play a major role in performance; in such situations groups of frontal patients can perform at close to normal levels. It was therefore a considerable surprise when initial functional imaging studies of episodic memory began to show extensive prefrontal activation (e.g. Grasby et al., 1993).

The conceptual frameworks used in Ebbinghaus-style memory research with respect to the role that the prefrontal cortex plays in memory encoding have been much simpler than the account presented in the preceding section. Three guiding themes are apparent in the psychological literature. A major conception has been the levels-of-processing approach, which holds that the 'deeper' an input is processed the stronger and more persistent is the storage of the memory trace (Craik & Lockhart, 1972). The idea, which is of course neuroscientifically now a truism, is that those are levels of analysis running from early sensory processing to much 'deeper' levels of semantic processing. In one version of the theory—that of Lockhart, Craik and Jacoby (1976)—there are held to be qualitatively different domains of processing—visual, orthographic (for print), articulatory, phonological, lexical and semantic—which reduces the theory to one similar to the early modal models discussed in Section 7.1. However in a more specific development, it is argued that 'deeper' also has relevance within a domain such as the semantic one (Craik & Tulving, 1975).

This psychological thesis relates very directly to an influential functional imaging experiment of Wagner et al. (1998). These authors used the clever technique of categorising the BOLD response in trials in one part of a recognition memory experiment—the encoding stage—according to performance on the corresponding items in another part—retrieval. Then, using an event-related design, they contrasted encoding trials in which the item was recognised correctly with high confidence later with trials where it was not recognised at all then. Wagner et al. found a so-called subsequent memory effect; a number of regions in which items were more activated at encoding when they were later recognised with high confidence than when they were later not recognised at all (see Figure 10.19). These included the fusiform gyrus, the parahippocampal gyrus, the frontal operculum and posterior and anterior parts of the inferior frontal gyrus (LIFC), all in the left hemisphere. Thus for a variety of subsystems involved in processing a stimulus, increased employment of resources led to increased probability of the later recognition of the item. Many other studies have produced similar conclusions (see Gabrieli, 2001). These effects are interpreted

by Wagner et al. as suggesting that 'Verbal experiences may be more memorable when semantic and phonological attributes of the experience are processed via the left prefrontal regions' (p. 1190). Whether the more 'extensive' processing proposed is the same or different to the within-domain 'deeper' processing of Craik and Tulving is not discussed by the authors!

There is unfortunately a rather severe possible confound in this study. The semantic task involved a concrete/abstract decision and the stimuli were composed of an equal number of abstract and concrete words. Any difference in performance on the two types of word—and one would expect better performance on concrete words—would lead to an unequal number of the two types of word being represented in the two word pools remembered and forgotten that were being contrasted. Thus any qualitative difference in word processing due to differences in word meaning on the abstract-concrete dimensions could lead to the quantitative activation differences; interpretation in terms of the 'extent' or 'depth' of processing within the same cognitive processing domain may not be warranted.[47]

A similar type of potential problem occurs for the interpretation of later studies using this type of paradigm. However they also show that an account of the result of the type put forward by Wagner et al. is at best insufficient. Thus Uncapher and Rugg (2008) had subjects make an animacy judgement on each of a series of concrete nouns presented visually. At the same time subjects had one of three possible auditory tasks (see Figure 10.20). At retrieval, subjects made remember-know judgements. Presentation rates at encoding were rather slow so performance on the secondary tasks remained reasonably good in all conditions (81–87%). Similar levels of the three kinds of subjective judgement were also obtained in the test phase, with 31–36% remember judgements, 27–28% know judgements and 25–28% misses. A variety of subsequent memory analyses of the Wagner et al. type were carried out. Some results were fairly straightforward. Thus in the left posterior hippocampus the subsequent memory effect was almost completely eliminated in both of the experimental dual-task conditions even though it did occur in the encoding control condition. This fits with the basic

---

[47] As the processing in comprehension of abstract words may involve left prefrontal cortex more than the analogous processing of concrete words (see Section 6.13) and as abstract words are likely to be recognised more poorly than concrete words—and no information is provided by Wagner et al. on this point—this particular explanation is not in fact that likely an account of the left inferior frontal gyrus activations. However no argument is presented in the paper against the idea that the encoding of recognised words involves at least in part qualitatively different cognitive domains from that of those not recognised.

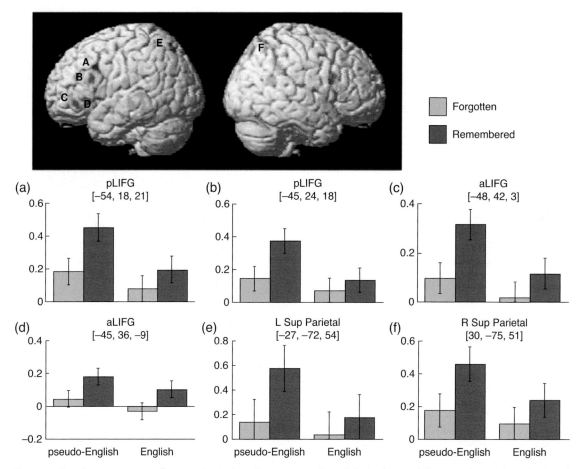

Fig. 10.19 The *subsequent memory effect*, occurring in the regions represented in red obtained in two different conditions of a study of novel word learning by Clark and Wagner (2003). The red columns correspond to the activation at encoding for items that were later remembered. The green columns show the corresponding activations for items that were forgotten. LIFG = Left Inferior Frontal Gyrus. Reprinted from *Neuropsychologia, 41*(3), D. Clark and A.D. Wagner, Assembling and encoding word representations: fMRI subsequent memory effects implicate a role for phonological control. 304–317. Copyright 2003, with permission from Elsevier.

memory trace being weakened by the subject having to carry out a demanding secondary task at encoding (Baddeley et al., 1984; Craik et al., 1996). However there were also complex qualitatively different effects. Three different regions of the left inferior frontal gyrus showed different task-selective subsequent memory effects (see Figure 10.21). Thus it was inferred that successful encoding involves qualitatively different, and not just quantitatively different, processing across conditions. The processes occurring at encoding are not simply captured by the concept of a greater 'depth' or 'extent' of processing in one condition than another (see Craik, 2002, for related considerations).[48]

Unccapher and Rugg do not give a detailed account of the pattern of frontal regions involved in the different subsequent memory effects. However, that different regions should be involved in encoding different types of material, at this level of processing, is hardly surprising given what we know of the relative specialisation of processing for different aspects of semantic memory. It can though be viewed as linked to a second psychological theme that permeates work on memory and prefrontal cortex, that different retrieval schemas are differentially effective in retrieving different types of material. One example of this is so-called transfer appropriate processing (Morris et al., 1977). This is that

---

[48] For the medial temporal lobe such a qualitative difference in the structures involved in memory encoding is now clear from patient data. Patients with bilateral hippocampal lesions who consequently have severe deficits on verbal or scene recognition memory tasks have been tested using the same type of task

(Warrington's (1984) Recognition Memory test) with different sorts of material. They can perform at a normal level on recognition memory for faces (e.g. Cipolotti et al., 2006) or perform much better on faces than on stimuli such as words or scenes (Bird et al., 2007a, 2007b; see also Carlesimo et al., 2001a).

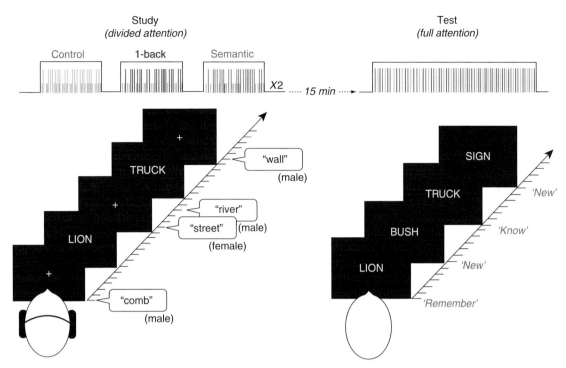

Fig. 10.20 The experimental design of Uncapher and Rugg (2008). In the study phase subjects made animacy judgements to visually presented words while concurrently performing one of three secondary tasks on auditory presented words - an encoding control condition (judging the sex of the voice), the one-back condition (indicating when the sex of the voice repeated across consecutive trials), and a semantic condition (indicating whether the spoken items were likely to be found outdoors). In the test phase subjects categorised the visually presented words as remembered, known, or new. Reproduced with permission from M.R. Uncapher and M.D. Rugg, 2008, Fractionation of the Component Processes Underlying Successful Episodic Encoding: A Combined fMRI and Divided-attention Study. *Journal of Cognitive Neuroscience*, 20(2), 240–254. Copyright © 2008, MIT Press Journals.

retrieval does not just depend on depth-of-processing, but on how closely the processing at input matches (in some sense) that at retrieval. In other words the probability of successful memory retrieval depends on the closeness of the relation between the thought schemas in operation at encoding and retrieval. For instance, if one is presented with words within a task which orients one to their meaning or a task orienting one to their rhyme and is later asked if another word rhymes with one of the presented words then one does better if it was initially presented in the rhyming context.

One example of the relevance of the second psychological theme comes from a study of Dobbins and Wagner (2005). Subjects had to remember either perceptual or conceptual information about an object. The perceptual information was how large physically the object was when presented. The conceptual information concerned the task they had had at encoding, whether they had been required to classify the object at study as pleasant or unpleasant or as living or non-living. A number of regions, including frontopolar cortex, to be discussed in the next section, were activated at retrieval, by comparison with a novelty detection condition, whatever the retrieval task. When

subjects recalled the appropriate sort of information the anterior ventrolateral PFC showed strong lateralisation effects dependent on the task—left for the conceptual task and right for the perceptual (see Figure 10.22). Moreover the activation in these regions correlated with specific posterior regions (left temporal for conceptual and bilateral lateral occipito-temporal for perceptual) suggesting that the anterior ventrolateral regions were involved in controlled retrieval of posteriorly located traces. By contrast the left mid-ventrolateral region is held to play a part in selection processes involved in retrieval that is somewhat analogous to the semantic selection processes of the type investigated by Thompson-Schill et al. (1997) and discussed in Chapter 9. However, so far computational formalisms reflecting this second psychological theme do not seem to exist. Indeed the processes of encoding in episodic memory, and particularly their 'control' aspects, remain psychologically somewhat mysterious. Moreover, adequate links to the event framework discussed in Section 10.9 do not yet seem to have been made. It may well be that only after we understand the functions of these subregions of the left inferior frontal gyrus, for instance, outside the episodic memory context, that we will have

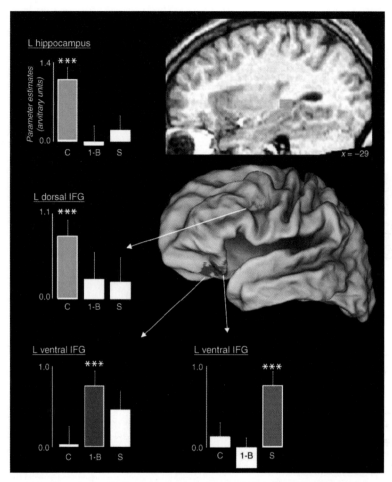

Fig. 10.21 Subsequent memory effects obtained by Uncapher and Rugg (2008), which varied as a function of the secondary task at encoding. Effects arising during the encoding control condition are shown in green. Effects arising during the one-back task are shown in blue. Effects arising during the semantic task are shown in red. IFG = Inferior Frontal Gyrus. Reproduced with permission from M.R. Uncapher and M.D. Rugg, 2008, Fractionation of the Component Processes Underlying Successful Episodic Encoding: A Combined fMRI and Divided-attention Study. *Journal of Cognitive Neuroscience*, 20(2), 240–254. Copyright © 2008, MIT Press Journals.

the conceptual framework available to understand their roles within episodic memory.

These effects, which we have grouped under the second psychological theme, all relate to how individual items are processed and transfer appropriate processing relates to the similarity of the induced tasks at encoding and retrieval. Clearer and simpler, but equally important in practice, is another higher level encoding process which constitutes our third psychological theme. It has been known since the work of Katona (1940) that the way material is organised as a whole is critical to how well each part of it is recalled. Thus if a subject organises a set of words semantically, this can lead to a dramatic increase in the amount recalled (Mandler, 1967). This effect has a clear brain basis. Using PET Fletcher et al. (1998a) presented subjects with lists containing 16 words for later recall outside the scanner. Each list contained a set of related words, for instance

in one they were all foods but in four subsets—four *fruit*, four *breads*, four *meats* and four *fish*. The lists were presented in one of three conditions—they were presented with the four subsets blocked in groups of four, or randomly but with the subcategories already known or, much the most difficult condition, randomly without the subject knowing the subcategories in advance. In addition as a further complication, as in some of the experiments previously described, subjects had to carry out at the same time an easy or difficult sensory-motor task. They had to press one of four buttons at a rate of one per second according to which light directly above each button was illuminated and to do this with the illuminated lights occurring in sequence (easy condition) or jumping about randomly (difficult condition).

Subjects performed roughly equally well in all conditions except for the Random-Categories Unknown condition as shown in Figure 10.23a. It is clear that the

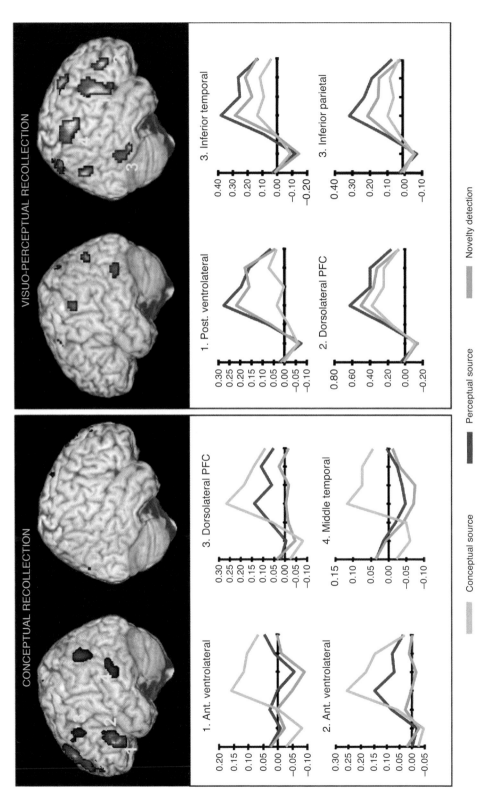

Fig. 10.22 Areas activated in the study of Dobbins and Wagner (2005) when recalling conceptual (left) and perceptual (right) information about a stimulus. The graphs show haemodynamic response functions for selected regions of interest for the three retrieval conditions (conceptual source, perceptual source, novel).Reprinted from I.G. Dobbins and A.D. Wagner, Domain-general and Domain-sensitive Prefrontal Mechanisms for Recollecting Events and Detecting Novelty, *Cerebral Cortex*, 2005, *15*(11), 1768–1778, by permission of Oxford University Press.

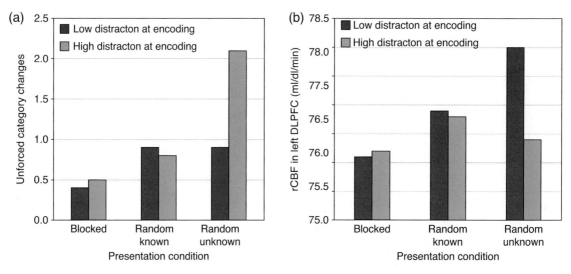

Fig. 10.23 (a) Mean excess category changes during recall, indicating inadequate organisation at encoding, as a function of presentation condition in the study of Fletcher et al. (1988a). (b) rCBF in left lateral PFC for each condition. Data from Fletcher et al. (1998a).

Random-Categories Unknown condition required subjects to actively organise the incoming words. With the easy sensory-motor task they could do this; their performance was fully comparable to the Blocked and Random-Categories Known conditions. When, however, they had the more difficult sensory-motor task, not only was their overall level of performance down but there was a considerable increase in unforced category changes at retrieval showing that they had failed to organise the material optimally.

One region of cortex showed an interaction of condition by sensory-motor task (see Figure 10.23b). This was the left mid-dorsolateral region (–36, 22, 28). This is an area 2–3 cm above the anterior ventrolateral PFC region involved in encoding specificity effects and 1–2 cm anterior of the mid-ventrolateral region so involved (see Badre & Wagner, 2007).[49] The left mid-dorsolateral region is a strong candidate for the key region involved in the early stages of task setting, namely the creation of an appropriate schema for tackling a novel task (see Sections 9.11 and 9.12). Thus both the analyses induced by deeper levels of processing and subjective organisation, at least of verbal material, seem to involve different groups of processes in the left prefrontal cortex, in ventrolateral and mid-dorsolateral cortex, respectively.

10.11 Retrieval Monitoring and Right Lateral Prefrontal Cortex

When prefrontal activation unexpectedly first began to be observed in episodic memory paradigms, it was even

more surprising that verbal material seemed to indicate that encoding into episodic memory and retrieval from episodic memory seemed to involve different prefrontal cortices, the left and the right respectively (Kapur et al., 1994; Shallice et al., 1994; Tulving et al., 1994a, 1994b). This effect, given the name of the Greek Goddess HERA (hemispheric encoding and retrieval asymmetry) (Tulving et al., 1994a), may well have been, at least in part, a consequence of the relative insensitivity of early PET studies which failed to show significant activation in the other hemisphere.

Very soon, however, other phenomena were described either overlaid on HERA or apparently in conflict with it. Thus complex memory tasks (e.g. Nolde et al., 1998) and autobiographical memory tasks (Maguire, 2001) frequently involve the left prefrontal cortex even at retrieval. Then, the nature of the material matters; when different types of material are used they may lateralise differently from each other both at encoding and at retrieval (Wagner et al., 1998). As a result HERA has gone out of fashion.

In fact, an exhaustive review paper by Fletcher and Henson (2001) of the rather heterogeneous set of episodic memory studies carried out up to that time using the same sort of material at encoding and retrieval supported the HERA principle for the ventrolateral prefrontal cortex and the dorsolateral prefrontal cortex but not for the anterior prefrontal cortex (see Table 10.4). However a later review of Gilboa (2004), which was less exhaustive but was able to use more studies, gave similar results to the Fletcher-Henson one for the dorsolateral and anterior prefrontal regions but not for the ventrolateral. Thus the HERA concept does seem reasonably solid, but only for the dorsolateral prefrontal cortex.

---

[49] In working memory analogous effects of organising material occur see, e.g. Bor et al. (2003).

| **TABLE 10.4** Number of significant activation contrasts in the metaanalysis of Fletcher and Henson (2001) as a proportion of the number of comparisons | | | | | | |

	VLPFC		DLPFC		Anterior PFC	
	Left	Right	Left	Right	Left	Right
Encoding	22/29	4/29	12/30	4/30	1/29	1/29
Retrieval	7/34	11/34	8/34	17/34	13/34	13/34

When the initial findings were made of specifically right frontal involvement in retrieval in verbal episodic memory two alternative perspectives were put forward. The Toronto group of Tulving et al. (1994a) suggested that the right anterior (BA 10) activations that they found in a recognition memory task should be attributed to the subjects being in what Tulving (1983) had proposed was a critical stage in memory retrieval, namely the subject being in retrieval mode. By contrast the London group (Shallice et al., 1994) found right mid-dorsolateral prefrontal (BA 9/46) activation when subjects were retrieving word lists in free recall (see also Fletcher et al., 1998b). They attributed the effect to subjects monitoring that they were not repeating words or incorporating associated but incorrect words into their output.[50] The rationale was that free recall of a list of words can take a minute or so. A study of frontal patients carried out at much the same time had shown that the patients with right frontal lesions produced over twice as many intralist repetitions as did normal controls suggesting that they did not monitor their own output (Stuss et al., 1994).[51]

The different patterns of lateralisation for the dorsolateral and anterior prefrontal regions in episodic memory retrieval studies discussed in the previous section support the idea that they may be the location of qualitatively different processes involved in retrieval. Both hypotheses have gained considerable further support. As far as the anterior prefrontal cortex is concerned, the original retrieval mode hypothesis of Tulving et al. (1994) is broadly in accordance with the position on anterior prefrontal cortex taken in Section 9.14.

More concretely, Duzel et al. (1999) tried to distinguish between task-related and item-related processes at retrieval. Their study was rather analogous in the memory domain to the Braver et al. (2003) study of task-setting discussed in the previous chapter. Subjects were presented with a series of words and for each word had to carry out one or two tasks according to an instruction on the screen. The task could be either an 'episodic' task—whether the word had been presented in an earlier list or not—or a 'semantic' task—whether it represented a living or non-living thing. The task-related difference in activation occurred in two right hemisphere sites—anterior prefrontal (BA 10) and right posterior cingulate cortex. This type of right anterior prefrontal locus occurs quite frequently in a meta-analysis by Lepage et al. (2000), although left anterior prefrontal loci also occur.[52] The identification of retrieval tasks—and retrieval mode—as a process involving right lateral area 10 would fit well with the functional characterisation of area 10 given in the last chapter. However the formulation of a description is also likely to involve ventrolateral prefrontal cortices. Indeed, bearing in mind the Dobbins and Wagner findings on domain-sensitive retrieval just discussed, it could be suggested that there is a hierarchical tree of areas producing increasingly precise memory descriptions with the most general—retrieval mode—being the most anterior. This would be another example of the hierarchical organisation of prefrontal functions discussed in Section 9.6.

As briefly discussed above, instead of retrieval mode, the London group preferred a different hypothesis and one that fits with another aspect of prefrontal functioning discussed in the last chapter. This was that retrieval from episodic memory required more active monitoring or checking than retrieval from semantic memory (the control condition). If one has to generate a novelist from knowledge and the word Dickens comes to mind, one hardly needs to check it (at least if one is English speaking!). On the other hand if Dickens had been one of four novelists in a list then when Dickens comes to mind at recall one needs to carry out a check of one's episodic memory that it really was in list and also that one has not already said it.

This initially rather flaky hypothesis has since been widely supported (e.g. Schacter et al., 1996; Rugg et al., 1998; Cabeza et al., 2003). Stronger support came from a later PET study of retrieval of organised material from a list just presented between the scans (Fletcher et al., 1998b). This was a complementary study to the one of episodic encoding of the same material, sixteen words

---

[50] Wilding and Rugg (1996), came to a similar position from quite different evidence.

[51] In a later study Alexander et al. (2003) found a similar doubling of intralist repetitions in free recall in both a posterior right dorsolateral and an anterior left dorsolateral group compared with controls but in neither case with very small ns was the effect significant.

[52] A later meta-analysis of 104 studies, which activated area 10 (Gilbert et al., 2006), found episodic memory tasks activated lateral area 10 bilaterally, in contrast to multi-tasking discussed in the last chapter, which was more anterior and medial in area 10. However tasks were not divided into retrieval and encoding.

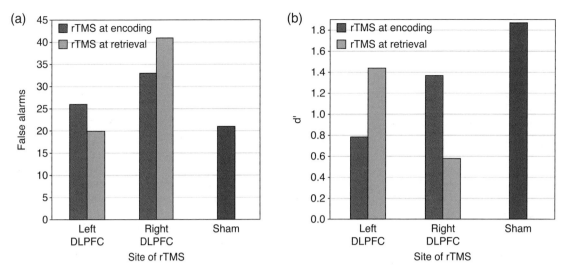

Fig. 10.24 Effects of rTMS to different sites at encoding and retrieval. Subjects had 8 blocks of 16 scenes, presented for 2 secs each. One hour later they were presented with blocks of 8 old and 8 new scenes and were required to discriminate between old and new scenes. rTMS was applied to left or right DLPFC at either encoding or retrieval. At retrieval, rTMS to right DLPFC led to (a) higher rates of false alarms than for left DLPFC, as well as (b) a lower d'. Data from Rossi et al. (2001).

forming four subcategories of a macro-category (e.g. four *breads*, four *edible fruits*, four *meats* and four *drinks*), discussed in Section 10.10 (Fletcher et al., 1998a). As far as prefrontal cortex is concerned, retrieval of an organised list involved greater activation of right mid-dorsolateral prefrontal cortex than did retrieval of an equally difficult set of paired associates (e.g. *bread-baguette*). The explanation given was that there were no competing possibilities (e.g. *croissant*) also occurring in the paired-associate list, and so no close checking was required. However with the organised list the subject had to ensure that each word was produced only once, which required active monitoring.

The assumption that in memory retrieval the dorsolateral prefrontal cortex, particularly on the right, is involved in monitoring of memory output clearly fits the position taken on active monitoring and checking in Section 9.10. If it is correct then right dorsolateral prefrontal effects should have a number of properties. Activation should occur after a possible response has come to mind. It should be more manifest when there are plausible alternatives. Impairments of the system should lead to false-positive responding.

All these properties hold. Thus Wilding and Rugg (1996), who used evoked response methods, found there was a late wave over prefrontal electrodes in memory retrieval that was stronger on the right than on the left, but only 1400 msec after the retrieval cue.[53] Sensitivity to the existence of plausible alternatives fits

the electrophysiological findings of Uhl, Podrecka and Deeke (1994) that the right prefrontal potential shift found with evoked responses is greater with high degrees of proactive interference.[54]

Most directly, Cabeza et al. (2003) compared regions activated in a word recognition memory task with those active during the task of monitoring over the same period whether a symbol on the screen blipped once, twice or never. Right dorsolateral, ventrolateral and dorsomedial prefrontal cortex showed a very similar and generally rising time course of activation through the 24 sec of a trial.

What results come from the selective impairment of right dorsolateral prefrontal cortex? One line of investigation, that of Rossi et al. (2001, 2006), fits the monitoring hypothesis well. Subjects received rTMS over one of a number of brain regions either while encoding six blocks of stimuli each consisting of a series of scenes, or an hour later when attempting to recognise the scenes in the context of an equal number of similar lures. The results are shown in Figure 10.24. HERA is strongly supported, as it is rTMS on left lateral PFC which impairs encoding and to the right which impairs retrieval. In addition there is a strong tendency to produce false-positive responses when rTMS is given at retrieval to the right lateral prefrontal cortex.

A neuropsychological study of Turner et al. (2007) gave a related but more complex pattern of results. In a free recall experiment using categorised lists, patients

---

[53] No one to our knowledge has used source analysis to localise the source of this wave more solidly.

[54] .Related fMRI evidence is also provided by Henson et al. (2002).

with right lateral prefrontal lesions produced fewer words than controls on their initial recall. However later, they gave more words than controls, but also showed a tendency to produce more so-called proactive interference intrusions from words of the same category presented in a previous list. Yet, they did this only when retrieval was specifically probed with a category cue after the patients had finished producing all they could spontaneously recall. In this situation, patients with orbital and medial lesions produce a large number of extra-list intrusions of words in the same category which had not been presented. The right lateral prefrontal patients do not do this. Thus their problem is only manifest when the situation strongly potentiates an intrusion response. It should be noted that Koriat and Goldsmith (1996) provide evidence that subjects use confidence judgements to make decisions about when to end recall in memory paradigms such as free recall. Thus, that right DLPFC patients produce too few word in their initial recall but then more than controls when prompted and in addition make proactive interference errors, fits with their not being able to monitor their own recall output properly.

Overall the idea that the right dorsolateral prefrontal cortex is involved in active monitoring and checking is also supported by memory experiments. There is, however, a rather awkward problem for the hypothesis. The review of retrieval from episodic memory of Gilboa (2004) discussed above was carried out in order to compare autobiographical and episodic memory. Protocol analysis of the retrieval of autobiographical memories in everyday memory situations, such as when you last cleaned your car (Burgess & Shallice, 1996b), shows that checking corrections frequently occur. Yet Gilboa found that the right dorsolateral activations frequent in Ebbinghaus-type episodic memory experiments do not generally occur when retrieval from autobiographical memory is being tested; virtually none of the 14 studies he reviewed showed activation in right area 9 or 46. To find out why this might be the case we need to move to a very different type of memory phenomenon, confabulation.

10.12 Confabulation

In the previous sections readers may have found themselves somewhat mired in complex paradigm-dependent effects. This section brings us back to the natural history of autobiographical memory and considers one of its most remarkable phenomena—confabulation. The young patient sits in front of you. You ask him where he is. He replies that he is at college. You ask him why then he is wearing pyjamas. With hardly a pause he starts to tell you a long rambling story of a night's carousing, having to stay at a friend's place and not being able to find his clothes in the morning.

Needless to say the story is false. The patient was in hospital where having a party, at least in those days, was frowned upon. But the patient believes it to be true. He has no intention to deceive.[55]

What is neurologically striking about confabulation is that it is closely linked to two neurological conditions. One involves the Circle of Willis, an arterial system that allows blood to circulate beneath the cortex and from which the three main cortical arteries—middle, posterior and anterior—stem. The anterior communicating artery is a short artery, which joins the left and right hemisphere parts of the Circle of Willis. It is one of the most common sites for aneurysms, which can rupture and produce a strong tendency to confabulate in the patient (Stuss et al., 1978).[56]

Confabulation can be provoked, as in the example just given, or spontaneously produced by the patient. The association of the syndrome with a lesion with a particular location suggests that it is anatomically fairly specific. Indeed Gilboa and Moscovitch (2002) reviewed 33 studies where severe confabulations were described, and argued that damage to the medial prefrontal cortex may be crucial in the production of confabulations and more specifically that 'lesions of the ventromedial aspect of the frontal lobes are sufficient even when damage to other regions is minimal or absent' (p. 323). Unselected case series of amnesics (Schnider et al., 1996) and of patients with focal frontal lobe lesions (Turner et al., 2008) confirm these conclusions (see e.g. Figure 10.25).

What might cause these confabulations? It is not necessary that there is a single cause, but at least three types of candidate explanation exist. The simplest is based on the way that, as we discussed in the section before last, normal episodic memory recall of routine one-off events, such as when you last cleaned your car, are full of errors. Thus in a protocol study of retrieving such everyday memories, Burgess and Shallice (1996b) found that recall of roughly one in three events contained an error which was admitted at later debriefing. Adopting the Norman and Bobrow model of the retrieval of event memories discussed in Section 10.9 (see Figure 10.18), it was argued that confabulations may arise from failures to either the Descriptor or the Editor. Strong support for an impairment of the Editor was produced in a study by Mercer et al. (1977) who tested 11 patients with memory problems, of whom two showed a severe confabulatory disorder and four showed it in a mild form. These patients were asked a

---

[55] This patient did not act on this confabulation, but he did on others.

[56] The second neurological condition is Korsakoff's syndrome following acute alcoholism, which is fortunately a much rarer condition than it used to be in OECD countries.

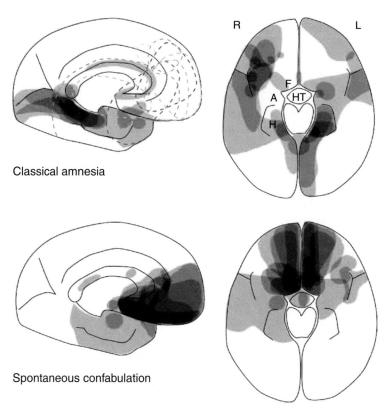

Fig. 10.25 Lesion overlap of patients from various studies by Schnider and colleagues. The shaded regions on the saggital views represent medial lesions, while the dashed lines show lateral lesions. Note that frontopolar cortex is spared in patients with classical amnesia but not in spontaneous confabulators. (A: amygdala; H: hippocampus, HT: hypothalamus, F: basal forebrain). Reprinted by permission from Macmillan Publishers Ltd: A. Schnider (2003) Spontaneous confabulation and the adaptation of thought to ongoing reality. *Nature Reviews Neuroscience*, 4, 662–671. Copyright (2003).

series of questions on their recent and remote memories. Mercer et al. found that the confabulators paused an only 10% of trials by comparison with 59% for the non-confabulating patients.[57] No similarly compelling evidence is available as far as failures of the Descriptor are concerned.

Burgess and Shallice proposed that the Editor system was the right dorsolateral active monitoring system discussed in Chapter 9. Yet more recent localisation evidence does not support this identification (Turner et al., 2008). Right dorsolateral patients do not generally confabulate. Instead the evidence favours Moscovitch's (1995) position that 'deficient strategic retrieval processes ... involved in monitoring, evaluating and verifying recovered memory traces, and placing these in their proper historical context' (p. 247) can be localised to the

ventromedial prefrontal cortex and related structures such as the basal forebrain.[58]

A second type of explanation is contained in an important refinement to Moscovitch's approach, which is present in a more recent and more elaborate model from his group (Gilboa et al., 2006) (see Figure 10.26). On this model the ventromedial prefrontal region is held to contain a system which is involved in setting the criterion for a preconscious 'feeling of rightness'. Confabulators, they show, tend to have very high confidence in their confabulations (see also Delbecq-Derouesné et al., 1990). It is held by Gilboa et al. that 'autobiographical memories evoke an extraordinary sense of confidence in their veracity (Brewer, 1986)' (p. 1412). The system in the ventromedial prefrontal cortex sets the criterion for this feeling of rightness and when it is damaged excessive confidence is the result.

It is rather mysterious on this account why there should be this very high confidence in autobiographical

---

[57] Confabulatory disorders are one of the few neuropsychological disorders on which a really definitive book has been written, in this case by Schnider (2008). It would appear from Schnider's exhaustive account that these critical early findings have never been replicated.

[58] This impaired process could be related to the lack of care found with patients in the inferior medial group in experiments such as task switching (see Section 9.11).

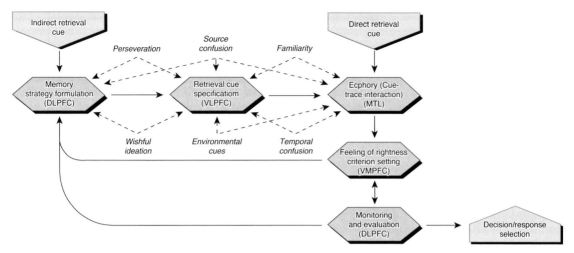

Fig. 10.26 The memory control model of Gilboa and colleagues (2006). Text in italics shows various kinds of influence, interference, or error to which the main processes are subject. Thus perseveration may affect both *memory strategy formulation* and *retrieval cue specification*. Based on Gilboa et al. (2006); Figure 12.

memory when the ventromedial prefrontal system is not working. However, if one accepts the hypothesis, it provides one way of dealing with the difference between typical autobiographical memories and episodic memories as far as activation of the right dorsolateral prefrontal cortex is concerned, which caused problems for the argument in the last section. The typical autobiographical memory when tested in a functional imaging study would not be of the word 'tractor' appearing in the last list or of when you last cleaned your car but, as in the example given earlier, of something much more memorable like a party. It is with respect to such memories, presumably, and not the other more prosaic ones, to which are attached 'the extraordinary sense of confidence' that Gilboa et al. hypothesise. So for these vivid memories the right dorsolateral checking system would not usually come into play.

The idea of a rapid reality check in the model of Gilboa et al. derives from a series of studies by Schnider and colleagues in Geneva. In an early study (Schnider et al., 1996) this group found that spontaneous confabulators had great difficulty with a continuous recognition task where they had to decide whether a picture had occurred before in the same run of pictures. Subjects had a number of runs with 80 pictures in each. The confabulators made many false positives when an item that had occurred in an earlier run occurred in a later run, as for the goat, aeroplane and trumpet stimuli in Figure 10.27. Moreover in an fMRI study using a related but more difficult paradigm (Schnider et al., 2000) it was found that in these later runs the posterior orbitofrontal cortex was activated. It was argued that temporal context confusion can lead to the conflating of memories from different time periods or the inability to suppress currently irrelevant memories. However, in their

2006 study Gilboa et al. showed that confabulators perform just as poorly on a task where they have to detect exactly the same items if they are repeated; here, though, the lures consisted of different examples from the same category, such as other dogs, and not the same item from an earlier run. Here temporal confusion is not the issue, but merely an inability to reject a similar but inappropriate candidate.

A follow-up evoked potential study in normal subjects by Schnider et al. (2002) using their temporal context confusion paradigm found that the main difference between targets and the critical lures such as the first two stimuli in run 2 in Figure 10.27 was over frontal electrodes and occurred only 200–300 msec after stimulus onset with a second deviation at 400–500 msec (see also Schnider, 2003). Schnider and colleagues argue that the early effect is a signature of a preconscious reality checking filter.

Is it plausible that a memory be accessed and reality checked a mere 220 msec after stimulus onset? Either way, there is another problem with this position. Where does the confabulatory content come from? Where for instance in one of Kraepelin's (1910) syphilitic encephalopathy patients did the idea come from that he had 28 first names, or for a vascular patient of Gentilini et al. (1987) that he lived with his wife's sister (who did not exist)[59] or in one of Turner et al.'s (in press) patients that he had met a woman at a party, who had the head of a bee. Of course there is nothing to show that these are not remembered fantasies of the patients which fail a reality check. Maybe many patients

---

[59] Both quoted by Schnider, 2008.

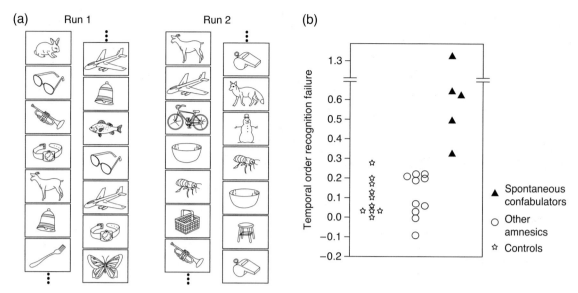

Fig. 10.27 (a) The procedure used by Schnider and colleagues. In each run, subjects were presented with a sequence of stimuli and asked to indicate when a stimulus had occurred earlier in that specific sequence. Run 2 was presented one hour after run 1. Subjects were instructed to forget about the first run and respond as if it had not occurred. (b) Temporal order recognition failures for three groups: spontaneous confabulators, other amnesiacs, and controls. Temporal order recognition failures are defined as the difference between the ratio of false positives to hits in run 1 and run 2. Right panel reprinted from A. Schnider, C. von Däniken and K. Gutbrod, The mechanisms of spontaneous and provoked confabulations, *Brain*, 1996, *119*(4), 1365–1375, by permission of Oxford University Press.

have a much richer fantasy life than that of these academic authors!

But there is another possibility. Take Damasio et al.'s (1985) anterior communicating artery aneurysm patient who believed he was a pirate and commanded a space ship. Damasio et al. gave the following account. They argued that the fabricated episodes were composed of unrelated events, some of which corresponded to real experiences and some of which were acquired through reading, conversation, television and even dreaming. To our knowledge no solid empirical evidence exists that in confabulations more than one episodic memory is conflated. However it is commonly believed.[60]

Earlier in the book—in Sections 2.2 and in 10.9—we discussed the Treves–Rolls model in which what we would now call episodic memories are carried by attractor nets in the CA1 and CA3 regions of the hippocampus. Assume episodic memories are indeed being carried by attractors located there with each attractor corresponding to an episodic memory complex. To lay down a new episodic memory and to retrieve an old one are computationally very different types of task. The system would seem to need to be in a different state to carry out one rather than the other. It has been argued by Hasselmo et al. (1996) that the neurotransmitter acetylcholine acts as the control switch for moving the hippocampus

between an encoding/new learning mode and a retrieval mode.[61] Thus it is argued by Giocomo and Hasselmo (2007) that with high levels of acetylcholine there is strong potentiation of input to the hippocampus. Encoding is facilitated. However in retrieval mode low levels of acetylcholine lead to a reduced impact of input from other systems, and instead a strong facilitation of recurrent connections within the CA3 system, making accessing of already formed attractors easier. But what happens if acetylcholine goes even lower. As we will see in Section 12.8 when their internal connectivity becomes high, attractor networks can go into a state called latching (Treves, 2005) where the system does not just settle into a single attractor basin given a single input but instead continues to hop from one attractor to the next for two or even more attractors. Phenomenally if this occurs in memory retrieval it would be experienced as a conflation of more than one episodic memory complex.

This is, of course, a completely speculative account. But why should it have any plausibility at all? The reason is because anatomically it fits with the hypothesis of Damasio et al. (1985) for the memory problems of their space pilot patient. 'It is our hypothesis that the amnesia results from interference with medial temporal function

[60] For a single example where two different events are clearly conflated see Delbecq-Derouesné et al., 1990.

[61] The computational functions of the different neurotransmitter systems are not discussed in this book. There has been much advance in the area in the last decade (see Levin, 2006).

in the hippocampus formation proper ... Damage to the basal forebrain could lead to significant reduction of cholinergic input to temporal lobe structures ...' (p. 270). The basal forebrain, a structure deep in the posterior part of the medial frontal lobes is a structure which houses the system that activates the cholinergic input to the medial temporal lobes including the hippocampus. It has often been considered a key structure for producing amnesia remotely through its effects on the hippocampus and is also a key location for confabulatory disorders, although this precise anatomical correspondence remains controversial (see, e.g. Irle et al., 1992; Morris et al., 1992; Hashimoto et al., 2000; see Schnider, 2008, for review). Thus we have a possible mechanism—latching—and a possible material cause—loss of the cholinergic input to the hippocampus—for the occurrence of conflations between memories.

We have given four possible hypotheses for the origins of confabulation—damage to Memory Descriptor and Editor systems, the inadequate setting of a criterion for feeling of rightness of a memory, the loss of a reality check system, and the loss of control over the potential for latching of memories. It remains to be established which if any or even all of these hypotheses for the functional origin of the confabulatory syndrome is correct. However the last three of the hypotheses postulate mechanisms within the memory system which had not previously been put forward. They are testament to the theoretical richness of neuropsychological evidence, particularly in the context of the much greater anatomical specificity that functional and structural imaging provide.

There is a second general point one can make about the discussion in this chapter. The reader may have found the discussion looser than in preceding chapters, and in particular with respect to the interpretation of functional imaging evidence. We believe this relates to a general problem to which we referred briefly in Chapter 4. The cognitive correspondence for the processing occurring in a localised brain region, whether assessed through imaging or through its malfunction due to a lesion, is, in the Marr approach, a specific computational process producing a type of output, Y, given a type of input, X. This is the type of conceptual entity that information-processing models in the box-and-arrow tradition represent. The history of research on the experimental psychology of episodic memory uses a looser conceptual framework that does not fit well into the traditional box-and-arrow approach. But boxes represent what goes on in a brain region. We dismiss them as an outdated legacy of the middle of the twentieth century at our peril.

Consciousness

11.1 **Introduction**

In 1989 one of the last iconoclasts of British science—Stuart Sutherland—wrote in *The International Dictionary of Psychology* 'Consciousness: the having of perceptions, thought and feeling: awareness'. The term is impossible to define except in terms that are unintelligible without a grasp of what consciousness means. Many fall into the trap of equating consciousness with self-consciousness—to be conscious it is only necessary to be aware of the external world. Consciousness is a fascinating but elusive phenomenon; it is impossible to specify what it is, what it does or why it evolved. Nothing worth reading has been written on it' (p. 90).

Can a cognitive-neuroscience approach dispel something of Sutherland's negativism? Let us approach the topic initially tangentially. The conceptual framework which we use to know about our minds is very different from that which we use to know about the interactions of objects in the physical world. It is the province of what we now call *theory of mind*—the concepts we use to understand how we and others are currently thinking, experiencing and feeling. These concepts have always seemed rather foreign to science. Indeed, the philosopher-of-science Patricia Churchland (1986) argued that a future science would cast such 'folk psychological' terms on the bonfire of failed ideas like 'phlogiston', 'epicycles' and the like.

Why should they be so alien to the scientific mind? In 1978 the American primatologists David Premack and Guy Woodruff considered the question of whether chimpanzees might have the ability to theorise about another's states of mind. They found that chimpanzees appeared to be capable of imputing intentions and desires to a human actor who was faced with various goal-directed problems. Thus, Premack and Woodruff showed that chimpanzees were able to reliably indicate, using a forced-choice paradigm, which of two tools the human actor should use to obtain food that was out of reach. However, evidence for a more complex theory of mind, where the chimpanzee was required to impute specific knowledge to the human actor (e.g. that an adult would have knowledge that a child would not) was weak.[1] Premack and Woodruff speculated that young children and those with some developmental cognitive impairments might fail on their tests of theory of mind. Subsequently, the Austrian psychologists Hans Wimmer and Josef Perner (1983)

developed the false-belief task in which subjects observe an object being hidden by actor A and then, in the absence of actor A, moved by actor B to another location. Subjects are required to indicate where actor A will look for the object when he/she returns. Wimmer and Perner found that 3–4-year-olds typically chose, incorrectly, the location where B had hidden the object, while 6–9-year-olds typically chose, correctly, the original location where A had hidden the object. The younger children appeared to be unable to represent the beliefs of actor A as distinct from reality.

Shortly thereafter Simon Baron-Cohen, Alan Leslie and Uta Frith (1985) in London showed that such abilities may not be available in others over 4. They discovered that autistic children had particular difficulty in carrying out operations dependent upon theory-of-mind concepts, even though they could be quite normal at carrying out cognitive operations in other domains. Moreover they had normal representations of other types of concept.[2]

Baron-Cohen and colleagues were studying a developmental abnormality. Analysis of developmental neuropsychological phenomena introduces an extra level of complexity by comparison with the analysis of adult neuropsychological phenomena. If atypical development is the product of normal developmental process operating upon an abnormal initial state, then it can be very difficult to reverse or decompose conceptually the resultant atypical adult state into its predisposing developmental causes (Thomas & Karmiloff-Smith, 2002). In certain cases, however, the abnormal developmental condition is appropriately interpretable in terms of damage to innately specified subsystems. Autism appears to be such a case (Frith & Frith, 1999, 2001) with particular types of operations—those that depend upon experiential concepts and that are collectively referred to as *mentalising* (Frith et al., 1991)—being especially vulnerable.

In adults theory-of-mind-type operations are selectively impaired by medial frontal lesions. Thus, Stuss et al. (2001), found that patients with bilateral frontal lesions were significantly worse than unilateral frontal and non-frontal patients on a task in which successful performance required that the patients understood that a third party was attempting to deceive them. The common lesion site of the impaired patients was in the

---

[1] Call and Tomasello (2008) revisit the question of theory of mind in the chimpanzee. They argue that 30 years of research has provided strong support for the idea that chimpanzees are able to understand the goals and intentions of others, but that the evidence for a fully-fledged theory of mind in terms of understanding another's beliefs remains less convincing.

[2] Consider what semantic features would be contained within the representation of say *ponder*, *disinclination* or *dismay*. They have virtually nothing in common with many concrete concepts such as *squirrel* or *mountain* or *foam* say. Even in self-organising connectionist systems, the representations would be in different regions of semantic space. See the discussion of concrete, abstract, and *pathic* or experiential concepts in Section 6.13.

medial prefrontal cortex. This region is also activated in theory-of-mind tasks (Frith & Frith, 2001). Moreover in a meta-analysis of 104 neuroimaging studies that reported selective activation of anterior prefrontal cortex (BA 10), Gilbert et al. (2006) found reliable involvement of medial (as opposed to lateral) regions in tasks held to involve mentalising. Such operations therefore appear to involve a separable subsystem.

The use of mental state, mental process and mental event terms such as *hear* and *think,* when we use them about ourselves, are all dependent upon our ability to reflect on our own mental processes and have as their common denominator conscious experience. Moreover when we use them about others we implicitly attribute consciousness to them. The semantic base of the concept of consciousness will therefore be very different from other scientific concepts that have their roots in the representations and operations we have for material objects. Thus the abstraction that we have for the two types of entity—conscious experience and matter—will have few if any properties in common. They will involve representations and operations in different cognitive systems. 'Dualism' is therefore a very natural abstraction with which to characterise the mind.[3]

Moreover if one reflects on one's mental life without any scientific guidance, 'dualism' appears to be corroborated. Dreams, visions under the effect of illness, drugs, or sensory or social deprivations and psychotic episodes are phenomena known to all cultures. In the absence of a scientific framework they are most easily explained by assuming that the body and the soul or mind are distinct entities, able at times to exist separately from each other. The normal primary Self leaves the body or the body becomes inhabited by an alien spirit.

Classical philosophers such as Locke and Kant made enormous contributions to our understanding of how the mind works. Yet they were essentially dualists, accepting (or not seriously challenging) Descartes' position on the essential separability of the mind and the body. The first proper articulation of an alternative—a materialist perspective on the body-mind relation—is held to be by the relatively obscure French thinker, La Mettrie, in the eighteenth century. However it was not until the nineteenth century that such perspectives became widely held. Complex machines were by then an only too obvious a part of urban life. Embryonic sciences such as physiology were beginning to treat the body as a machine, and even social entities such as a factory had many aspects of their organisation in common with the machines they contained. So to view the human mind as nothing but a very complex machine became a slightly less enormous leap of imagination.

However the clear articulation of a consistent and detailed position which directly confronted the philosophical paradoxes that a materialist theory of the mind would face had to wait until the period when the elements of cognitive neuroscience were being born, namely the 1950s and 1960s. It was in this period that a number of philosophers, principally the British Ullin T. Place (1956) and the Australians J.J.C. Smart (1959) and David Armstrong (1968) put forward the mind-brain identity theory, according to which 'any given mental state is, roughly, a brain state, brain processes, or feature of process in the central nervous system' (Borst, 1970, p. 13). The mental states of mind-brain identity theory were those postulated by psychologists in the post-behaviourist era. These were held to be causally interrelated, mirroring the causal relations between brain states.

The mind-brain identity theorists were what is now known in philosophy-of-mind as 'internalists'. If two creatures were to have the same brain organisation, down to some variously specified level of detail and to have the same sensory input their conscious experience would be the same. Conscious experience then depended upon what was going on in the brain *and nothing else*.[4]

Most of the brain-mind identity theorists were also functionalists. They saw consciousness as being a property of the system-level organisation of the mind. Even though they were in very general terms 'materialist', the actual stuff of which the brain was composed, as for instance its physical composition, was essentially irrelevant. Functionalism when initially developed was often linked to the idea that all that was critical for understanding the mind was the series of symbolic representations and operations which composed the program that underlay behaviour. This was the time of the research project of 'strong AI' which held that all that was required to understand behaviour was a specification of the program, which when run on any machine, would simulate it. Strong AI was not very successful as a research program for explaining thought.[5] Dan Dennett (2001), however, is particularly cogent on why its failure does not undermine functionalism as a more general approach to understanding consciousness. He writes 'The recent history of neuroscience can be seen

---

[3] This argument is developed from one presented in Jack and Shallice (2001).

[4] Theorists who rejected internalism and instead held a form of panpsychism—that consciousness like love permeated the universe—were common in the immediately post-hippy period of the 1970s (Clarke, 2004). More modern externalists (e.g. Dretske, 1995) are much drier and more abstract. However we see no evidence for the idea that consciousness involves any entities other than ones own cognitive system.

[5] See especially Section 1.7 but also Chapters 9 and 12.

as a series of triumphs for lovers of detail. Yes, the specific geometry of the connectivity matters; yes, the location of specific neuromodulators and their effects matter; yes, the architecture matters; yes, the fine temporal rhythms of the spiking patterns matter, and so on. Many of the fond hopes of opportunistic minimalists[6] have been dashed .... This has left the mistaken impression in some quarters that the underlying idea of functionalism has been taking its lumps. Far from it. On the contrary, the reasons for accepting the new claims are precisely the reasons of functionalism' (pp. 234–235). Neurochemistry matters because it is important for understanding cognition in general.[7] Therefore it is relevant for understanding consciousness. Put more abstractly, whatever levels of analysis are necessary for understanding cognition in general are also relevant for understanding consciousness.

Since the identity theorists, research on what consciousness might be has split into at least four strands. One strand consists of the philosophers who have remained true to the essence of the identity theory/ functionalist approach, and have tried to develop it synergistically with advances in the brain and cognitive sciences. Principal amongst them as the above quote indicates has been Dennett (1969, 1978, 1991, 2001, 2005) who for forty years has articulated a series of basically functionalist positions influenced by current cognitive and brain sciences. He has also continually attempted to cull the bizarre creatures that increasingly populate modern philosophical discussion of mind.[8]

A second strand comprises alternatives to functionalism which have become increasingly popular among philosophers for a number of reasons. Thus, functionalism is now an old, staid theory, and one does not easily make a career by supporting an old theory. And, a list of creatures that pose theoretical questions for functionalism now populate the conceptual world of modern, philosophers-of-mind: bats (the most reasonable, Nagel, 1974); the population of China somehow organised into a complex flag-waving exercise (Block, 1978); scribes writing meaningless texts in Chinese rooms (Searle, 1980); Mary, a scientist living in a black and white room who knows all there is to know about colour, but has never seen colours (Jackson, 1986); duplicates who are identical to you and have your history and yet

are held to have no conscious experience (Stich, 1983); Swampman, a being with no history but composed of molecules arranged randomly by a lightening bolt that, coincidently, take on exactly the same form as a recently deceased individual (Davidson, 1987); people who experience blue when you experience green and vice versa (Locke, 1690); Twin Tercel, a lorry that was not built but materialized spontaneously but with a gas gauge that does not work (Dretske, 1995).[9] Many of these are entities that do not, and could not, exist. They are designed as 'intuition pumps' to improve one's understanding. There is the danger though, that in some cases, the intuition pump may produce mainly hot air!

A further reason for the decline in popularity of functionalism is the intuition that there are aspects of phenomenal experience that are very difficult or even in principle incapable of being captured by current brain and cognitive science. This intuition has acted as the motor for a concept that was originally given the evocative name of *raw feels* but now has been bowdlerized in the philosophical and scientific literature into *qualia*. Consider one of us (TS) sitting here writing this. I am sitting on an old stone school terrace looking through the geraniums and prickly pears down to what the Italians call the 'turchino' blue of the sea far below, separated from the azure sky by the steep volcanic hills of the bigger outer Aeolian islands. The objective description does not capture the subjective quality of the experience—what it is like *to me* at this point in time. The relation between the mind known through the brain and cognitive science on the one hand and the domain of qualia on the other is widely held to be so wide that no currently conceivable scientific theory could possible account for it. How the relation should be explained is, according to a very influential position of David Chalmers (1996), the *Hard Problem*. This he argues will require a new sort of language to be developed, one which captures our 'first person' experience.

Scientists however have been more optimistic. In the 1990s for rather unfathomable reasons consciousness became a highly fashionable topic in a large set of the scientific community. Grand theories were developed which concentrated on one aspect of consciousness to the virtual exclusion of all other aspects of the topic. This represents a contemporary third strand of consciousness research. An early paradigmatic example was Penrose's (1989) theory, which attempted to solve the Hard Problem by linking it to the gap between

---

[6] This was an orientation within functionalism of which strong AI is the paradigm case where it is assumed that particular conceptual grains, e.g. all below the algorithmic level, are irrelevant.

[7] See, e.g. Miller and Cohen's (2001) speculations on the role of neuromodulatory systems in providing reinforcement signals during tasks requiring cognitive control.

[8] Other philosophers who have developed the identity theory approach have included Van Gulick (1994) and Papineau (2002).

---

[9] One of us must admit to adding an extra species to the menagerie—Rene—in collaboration with Tony Jack (Jack & Shallice, 2001). Rene is a being whose understanding of itself and its conspecifies is totally separate from its understanding of the material world. Rene is almost inevitably a dualist.

classical Newtonian physics and quantum mechanics—technically the so called collapsing of the Schrödinger wave equation. Somewhat disappointingly the material realisation of this great metaphysical design is held to be in a rather uninteresting part of the neuron—the so-called microtubials (Hameroff and Penrose, 1996).

Much more important, if less ambitious, is however the fourth strand, which this chapter adopts. This strand has the potential to flesh out the gaunt spectre of functionalism into a theory which like any good scientific theory relates to a wide variety of empirical phenomena with an experiential aspect and in addition is realised in a range of more local theories oriented towards these micro-experiential phenomena. On this approach the Hard Problem is either explicitly rejected as currently irrelevant (Shallice, 1988) or a conceptual illusion (Dennett, 1991) or more typically just ignored. Using a variety of methods related to ones we have previously discussed, a range of empirical phenomena related to conscious experience have been described over the last thirty years. A theory of consciousness can now chose to confront a complex range of empirical facts established in standard scientific fashion as well as, or even in part instead of, contorting itself through the range of bizarre conceptual hoops that modern philosophy-of-mind provides.

11.2 Non-conscious Processes

Up until 1974, experimental investigations into unconscious processes could be dismissed as probably empirically unsound (e.g. Eriksen, 1960). In 1974 that belief collapsed. The previous year, Pöppel, Held and Frost (1973) at the MIT had worked with patients with long-standing traumatic injuries, which had left them with unusual visual field defects—they were effectively blind in one region of their visual field. A spot of light was flashed at a point in the blind field, with the position of the spot varying across trials. Patients were asked to move their eyes to the position of the light they could not see—instructions they found rather odd! Nevertheless, there was a rather weak but significant tendency to move towards the correct position.

The following year Larry Weiskrantz, Elizabeth Warrington (1974) and their colleagues in London were working with a patient, DB, who had a large defect of the lower left visual field. They tested DB with an analogue of a test used successfully by Nick Humphrey (1970) on a monkey, Helen, who had had her visual cortex removed. DB was asked to point to the position of a spot of light, which varied randomly over trials but remained within the blind field of the subject by remaining on a given radius in the field of vision. As the subject could not see the light he was asked to guess. He was remarkably accurate—both considering

the mean and the standard deviation of a group of trials at the same position. Yet in most experiments DB said that he was just guessing and performing at chance. The same type of result came if he was given other types of test in the blind field such as orientation discrimination (see Weiskrantz, 1986a).

The interpretation of DB offered by Weiskrantz and colleagues was that DB had one particular set of visual processes left relatively undamaged by the lesion. However these processes were distinct from those supporting conscious vision and did not themselves give rise to conscious vision. A variety of alternative interpretations were put forward by critics but these were convincingly refuted by further experimentation (see Weiskrantz, 1986a, 1997).[10]

More recently two additional objections have been made. One relates to a suggestion made by Fendrich et al. (1992) is that blindsight might arise from tiny islands of intact function in an otherwise blind hemifield. They found this situation in patient CLT, who had an occipital lobe lesion. This possibility has been investigated in a second putative blindsight patient, GY, who has been very intensively studied (e.g. Barbur et al., 1980; Blythe et al., 1987; Finlay et al., 1997). The idea has been rejected for GY by Weiskrantz (1997) in an extensive review of blindsight for a range of reasons. For example, PET and fMRI studies of GY show no sign of activity in V1 (see Barbur et al., 1993; Sahraie et al., 1997, respectively). More critically Kentridge et al. (1997) have repeated with GY exactly the same experiment used by Fendrich et al. with CLT. No isolated islands of vision were found.

More important, however, is a second problem concerning the reproducibility of blindsight in other patients. Only a minority of patients with visual cortex lesions have shown evidence of blindsight according to Weiskrantz (1997) and it is probably a small minority. It is not known why, although Weiskrantz speculates that it is because most naturally occurring lesions affecting V1 also affect other regions in addition to V1.

The condition also appears to be very sensitive in an unknown fashion to stimulus parameters. Thus, Hess and Pointer (1989) retested GY thoroughly and argued that he had no ability to respond to stimuli he could not see but Weiskrantz et al. (1991) showed that with a slight increase in the slope of the temporal onset of the stimulus the blindsight capacities reappeared. From the

---

[10] These alternative accounts involved the possibilities that a) light from the target might have been scattered by or reflected off other objects or the eye itself into regions of the retina that were not affected by the field deficit, and b) blindsight may have been a result of the visual cortex operating in an abnormal fashion, rather than simply not operating at all (see Campion et al., 1983). They are extensively reviewed in FNMS Chapter 16.

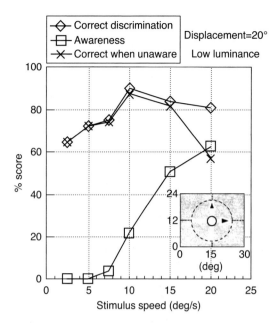

Figure 11.1 Performance of the blindsight patient GY on detection and awareness of the direction of movement of a horizontally or vertically moving stimulus as a function of stimulus speed. Note that his guessing performance (correct when unaware) was virtually unaffected by stimulus velocity. Reprinted with permission from L. Weiskrantz, J.L. Barbur and A. Sahraie, 1995, Parameters affecting conscious versus unconscious visual discrimination with damage to the visual cortex (V1). *Proceedings of the National Academy of Sciences, USA, 92,* 6122–6126. Copyright (1995) National Academy of Sciences, USA.

complementary perspective, in a PET study the patient was reported as showing 'conscious awareness of having seen the particular stimulus' (Barbur et al., 1993).[11]

More intensive investigation of the state of awareness of this patient again showed that in GY, like DB, there is a complex relation between when he was aware of the stimulus and performance. Thus in GY's case he could *see* the moving stimuli *only* when they moved very rapidly (greater than 15°/sec at low luminescence) but his guessing performance on whether movement was occurring was virtually unaffected by stimulus velocity (see Weiskrantz et al., 1995)—see Figure 11.1. Similarly for higher velocity if the background luminescence was increased he ceased to be aware of the direction of movement but could still guess correctly on 90% of occasions.[12]

Weiskrantz (1997) concludes from these studies, and the work on GY in particular, that the one type of stimulus presented in the area of the visual field deficits that can produce a conscious percept for him is a transient one. Indeed in GY the movement centre, V5, discussed in Chapter 2, can be activated without primary visual cortex also being activated (Barbur et al., 1993). Weiskrantz therefore argues that for non-transient visual stimuli, the primary visual cortex is essential for experiences. What, however, this pattern of findings also suggests is that the primary visual cortex is only essential for certain types of processing of stimuli, and that the actual experience of such stimuli depends on quite different later structures, a view championed by Crick and Koch (1995).

More basically Weiskrantz and his collaborators argue that blindsight involves a dissociation between the occurrence of certain types of cognitive process—say those involved in making a forced choice orientation, movement or colour judgement and those involved in the conscious experience of the stimulus—that would normally be present in control subjects carrying out the same sort of experiments. It strongly suggests that these same processes are not what make the normal subject conscious of the stimulus in these experiments.

Accepting Weiskrantz's explanation, it is still clear that blindsight is extremely hard to investigate in humans as the precise conditions under which it arises are not known. It is therefore important that Cowey and Stoerig (1995) have been able to reproduce blindsight in three monkeys with left visual cortex lesions. The animals were trained to maintain fixation on point F (see Figure 11.2, top panels). In the lower left panel is shown how the three monkeys (plus one control, 'Rosie') performed when trained to touch any of the small squares which are briefly lit. Performance can be seen to be very satisfactory. But the critical issue is to assess whether the monkeys are aware of the stimulus. The lower right panel shows performance in a subtly different situation. The animal is now trained to touch one of four small squares if it is lit but also to touch the large rectangle if no light occurs. When the probe light on the right was presented, the monkeys, other than Rosie, nearly always touched the rectangle indicating that they were not conscious of the probe. They treat a brief flash of a light on the right as equivalent to no light. Thus a clear analogue of blindsight appears to be obtained in the monkey, given that the 'no light' response be treated as a phenomenal report (which seems entirely appropriate).

The experiment of Cowey and Stoerig (1995) means that the difficulty in reproducing blindsight in humans is less critical. Nevertheless, it remains vital that any empirical generalisation, such as that of Weizkrantz, should be supported by evidence from other syndromes. Fortunately a number of other syndromes have since

---

[11] Weiskrantz (1997) attempts to argue that the perceptual experiences of GY in this experiment were abnormal. However an interview *a few months later* cannot be used to provide a phenomenal report.

[12] For discussion of replications of this phenomenon see the appendix to Weiskrantz (1997).

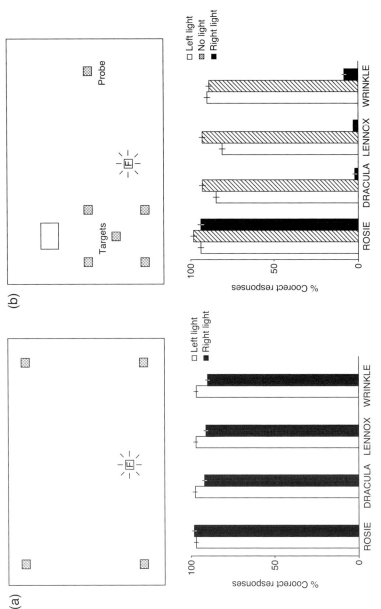

Fig. 11.2 The design and results of the Cowey and Stoerig (1995) study of blindsight in three monkeys with unilateral visual cortex lesions (Dracula, Lennox and Wrinkle). Rosie was a control monkey with no lesion. (a) In the control condition the monkey was required to fixate on and touch the square marked 'F'. One of the other target squares was then briefly lit and the monkey was required to touch it. Performance was good regardless of the position of the lit square. (b) In the experimental condition the monkey was required to touch the target square that was lit or the large white rectangle if no target was lit. Dracula, Lennox and Wrinkle generally failed to detect targets on the right. For the use of the probe, see the text. Adapted by permission from Macmillan Publishers Ltd: *Nature* (A. Cowey and P. Stoerig (1995) Blindsight in monkeys. *Nature, 373,* 247–249), copyright (1995).

been described in which a dissociation exists between the preserved operation of a process and the subject's lack of any experience related to the process. The patient while performing correctly believes him or herself to be guessing.

11.3 Unconscious Specific Effects of Insufficiently Specific Experiences

Phenomena of the sort alluded to in the last paragraph are of two types. In the first type, the subject does perceive something, but there is no experience related to a particular type of process that can be carried out. We will call this the phenomenon of *insufficiently specific experience*. There are two well-known examples. One is the preserved ability in semantic access dyslexia to judge the semantic category of a word of which the patient claims not to know the meaning (Shallice & Saffran, 1986; Coslett & Saffran, 1989; Coslett et al., 1993). A second relates to interference effects to related faces that occur in prosopagnosia—the inability to recognise faces—produced by faces, which the prosopagnosic cannot recognise (De Haan et al., 1987).[13]

The first has been well-established as a phenomenon in a number of patients, given that they adopted the appropriate strategy (see Chapter 6). In this syndrome when the patient is presented with a word for a short interval, such as 250 msec in some patients (e.g. JG, JC and AF: Coslett & Saffran, 1989), it can be shown by various means that the patient does not know the meaning of the word, yet they can carry out a forced-choice discrimination on the category of the word very effectively (see Table 11.1).

In this case, however, the dissociation can be simply explained. Take the attractor network model of reading by the semantic route shown in Figure 4.21(a). We considered there the effect of quantitatively relatively small lesions to connections or sets of hidden units in the model. The behaviour of the system corresponded to deep dyslexia. If however the lesions are more severe, one obtains behaviour corresponding to that which occurs in semantic access dyslexia. Hinton and Shallice (1991) analysed the network's output when the connections from semantic to the clean up units were fully lesioned (depressing correct specific mapping from orthographic to semantic units to 40%) and when the return connections from clean up to semantic units were 40% lesioned (depressing the accuracy to 24.5%).

Words from five different semantic categories were used in training and testing the network. The forced-choice discrimination task of patients was mimicked by

| **TABLE 11.1** | Forced-choice accuracy (% correct) of four pure alexic patients in categorising words as animal names or not. For the foils a no response must be given. Visual foils share at least the first two letters with an animal name, so a letter-by-letter strategy typical of pure alexic patients would not be sufficient given the brief presentation time used. Subjects were asked to say if they knew the word. The final column gives the percent of correct explicit naming responses produced. |

Patient	Exposure	Animal	Visual Foil	Unrelated Foil	Explicit reading of Word
JG	250 msec	80	72	72	1
TL	100 msec	96	52	60	2
JC	250 msec	68	92	96	7
AF	250 msec	80	60	72	0

Data from Coslett and Saffran (1989).

comparing, for each input word, the pattern at the semantic units of the lesioned networks with the centroids of the semantic patterns for the five categories of stimulus in the unlesioned network, and choosing as the response category that whose centroid was closest. It was found that the input word's category was correct on 92% and 74% of trials, respectively, both well above chance. Thus, while it was frequently not possible to extract the precise semantic representation of the input word from the lesioned network, extraction of the category of that word from the degraded semantic representation generally remained possible. Thus, in a complex hierarchically organised set of attractor systems, an input to the attractor level of the system which is insufficient for a specific attractor to be accessed may still be sufficient to allow a wider attractor to be accessed.[14]

A similar explanation together with simulations has been provided by Farah et al. (1993) for an analogous phenomenon in prosopagnosic patients. Thus De Haan et al. (1987) showed that a face, which a patient could no longer recognize, still had the power to produce interference when a different but related response was required. The task of the subject was to categorise a

---

[13] These dissociations are discussed in FNMS: (i) Section 12.6 (ii) Section 16.3.

[14] Indeed it has been argued that it is the movement within the state space of a system into an attractor basin that corresponds to accessing a conscious representation (e.g. Mathis & Mozer, 1996). This may be seen as a connectionist version of Dretske's (1995) representational theory of consciousness, in which to represent a property is to be conscious of that property, though the Mathis–Mozer position is an internalist perspective unlike the 'externalist' one underlying Dretske's approach.

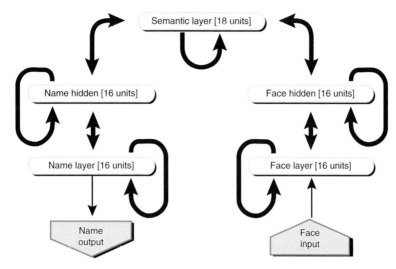

Fig. 11.3 The network architecture used by Farah et al. (1993) to illustrate a dissociation between overt and covert face recognition. Included in the semantic layer are units that represent, amongst other things, the occupation associated with a name/face.

male name as that of either a politician or a sportsman. The name was superimposed on a face. If the face belonged to a politician and the name belonged to a sportsman, for example, then a normal subject would be slowed in categorizing the name. A head-injury patient suffering from prosopagnosia, PH, who was at chance on the face categorisation task, still showed the normal interference effect.[15] Farah et al.'s connectionist model (see Figure 11.3) showed many effects of this type. Thus when the damaged network is primed by presenting it with the face associated with one occupation, it is slower to produce the occupation of a second name if it is different. For example, when 75% of the face hidden units are lesioned, and so the network is performing at only 15% correct in a 10-alternative forced-choice recognition task for faces, it is over 30% slower to give the correct occupation to a name that is paired with a face distractor (see Figure 11.4).

These phenomena, involving specific effects in behaviour of a less specific experience, then appear capable of being explained by a relatively simple account of consciousness in terms of the degree of detail required of the signal to activate later situations. Representations in connectionist networks are not activated in an all or none fashion; they can be graded. Explanations of dissociations between lack of awareness and behavioural effects can therefore be explained in this way. This type of explanation is called by Farah (1994) the 'quality of representation' account. One form of this

type of hypothesis is Mozer's 'attractor' approach to consciousness referred to earlier. Another is that the greater the degree of activation of a representation the more strongly is there awareness of the representation (Baars, 1988). This possibility is called by Kanwisher (2001) 'the activation strength hypothesis'.

11.4 **Completely Unconscious Specific Effects**

More dramatic are effects in which the stimulus gives rise to a change in behaviour that appears to require explicit identification of the stimulus but the patient experiences nothing. In addition to blindsight such effects have been found in extinction, a phenomenon related to unilateral neglect, discussed in Chapter 1.

In standard tests of extinction stimuli are presented in two positions symmetrically organised with respect to the vertical meridian in the visual field. Sometimes one stimulus is presented either to the patient's left or to their right and sometimes two stimuli. A patient showing extinction will report the presence of one stimulus wherever it is presented, but frequently will fail to report the left one when two are shown. Many studies have shown that an extinguished stimulus that the patient does not detect can have an effect on other processing. Thus Audet, Bub and Lecours (1991) used the *Eriksen flanker* procedure; the subject has to respond to a central letter flanked by irrelevant letters (see Figure 9.8). The flankers can be compatible or incompatible as far as any decision being made on the central letter is concerned. Thus the flankers could, if relevant, lead to the same response as the actual target or to a different one. Audet et al. found that compatible but extinguished flankers helped to speed target detection.

---

[15] See Young, Hellawell and De Haan (1988) for a related phenomenon. Somewhat similar inhibitory effects in the absence of awareness have been found in normal subjects by Vorberg et al. (2003) using a perceptual effect called metacontrast masking.

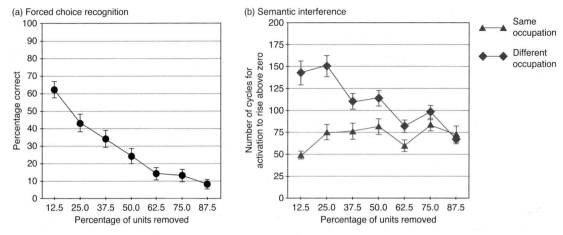

Fig. 11.4 Results from the simulation studies of Farah, O'Reilly & Vecera (1993). (a) Accuracy in a 10-alternative forced choice recognition task as a function of severity of lesion made to the face hidden units. (b) Semantic interference as illustrated by the number of cycles for the correct occupation unit to rise above zero when the network was primed with a face of the same or a different occupation, again as a function of severity of damage to the face hidden units. Copyright © 1993 by the American Psychological Association. Adapted with permission. M.J. Farah, R.C. O'Reilly, and S.P. Vecera (1993). Dissociated overt and covert recognition as an emergent property of a lesioned neural network. *Psychological Review, 100*(4), 571–568. The use of APA information does not imply endorsement by APA.

Similarly Berti and Rizzolatti (1992) found that neglect patients responded faster in judging category membership when the extinguished item was a member of the same category.

In some of these studies the trials compared are trials of different structure, and this can lead to a potential artefact. For instance, McGlinchey-Berroth et al. (1993) used trials where words had to be identified to establish that conscious recognition was not occurring, i.e. that the patient had neglect. To establish the existence of 'unconscious' priming, they used a different task—priming of lexical decision by objects by pictures of objects. There is a major problem with this type of design. The attentional field of the neglect patient can vary with the task. For instance, Làdavas, Shallice and Zanella (1997a) and Làdavas, Umiltà and Mapelli (1997b) showed that neglect patients have a wider attentional focus when making a semantic judgement on a word than when naming it.[16] Thus in the McGlinchy-Berroth et al. experiment the subject's attentional field in the priming condition where the semantic association is relevant may be wider than when object naming is required. This means the subject may be conscious of the priming item on some trials in the priming condition.

Very clear effects of preserved processing can, though, be found when the neglect or extinction on the one hand and the preserved processing on the other are measured on the same trial. Thus Rees et al. (2000) used the category-specific effects, discussed in Chapter 6, that occur when houses or faces are presented in a functional imaging experiment. They presented pictures of houses and faces in a standard *extinction* design to a neglect patient GK with a relatively small right parietal lesion, and whose extinction affected the left (see Figure 11.5). On each trial GK had to indicate by pressing one of three buttons whether the stimulus had occurred on the left, the right, or on both sides of the display. He detected only 2/60 stimuli in the left visual field when two stimuli were presented, but 58/60 when one was presented in the left visual field only. Yet when GK's fMRI activation on the extinction trials was compared to that on purely unilateral *right* trials there were significant responses in primary visual cortex and early extrastriate cortex (see Figure 11.6). Moreover the response to faces and houses in the right visual cortex for the extinction situation can be compared by using the situation when unilateral right visual field stimuli are presented as a control. Here weak but significant activation was obtained for extinguished faces in the right-hemisphere fusiform face region of Kanwisher et al. (1997), a region that is primarily specialised for face processing.[17] Thus, if the arguments of Chapter 6

---

[16] A related problem occurs for a phenomenon discussed by Vuilleumier and Rafal (1999). Patients extinguished stimuli briefly flashed to the left side. However, when asked how many stimuli there were, could correctly say 2, 3, or 4. They were presumably then using a so-called subitising procedure, based on parallel processing of the stimuli (Mandler & Shebo, 1982).

[17] There has been a long dispute on how specialised the region is for face processing rather similar to the one discussed in Chapter 5 regarding the selectivity of the visual-word form area

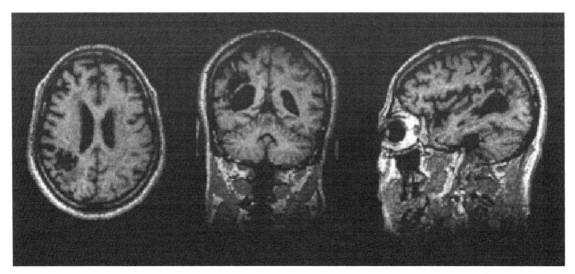

Fig. 11.5 The location of the lesion of patient GK who showed extinction of the left visual field. The lesion affects the right inferior parietal lobule, sparing visual cortex. Reprinted from G. Rees, E. Wojciulik, K. Clarke, M. Husain, C. Frith and J. Driver, Unconscious activation of visual cortex in the damaged right hemisphere of a parietal patient with extinction, *Brain*, 2000, *123*(8), 1624–1633, by permission of Oxford University Press.

are correct and the Bruce–Young model (see Figure 6.3) applies, then analysis of the stimulus up to the face identity unit level is occurring.[18]

The existence of 'unconscious' effects of neglect depends critically on the place of the lesion. Mattingley, Davis and Driver (1997) used the figures named after the Trieste psychologist, Gaetano Kanizsa. In the Kanizsa figure (see Figure 11.7c), an illusory square is seen floating in front of the four three-quarter disks. Such a square is not seen in the control figures, which in this experiment were produced by filling in the circumference of the disks (Figure 11.7b, d). In one condition of the Mattingley et al. study, either all four of the quarter-squares were briefly removed or just two (the left pair or the right pair; Figure 11.7a). A patient, VR, with extinction following right-hemisphere damage showed fairly severe extinction when the non-Kanizsa figures were used but very little with the Kanizsa figures (see Figure 11.7e). Similar results were obtained in other conditions with equivalent manipulations. These result suggests that extinction occurs relatively late in visual processing, after the point giving rise to the Kanizsa illusion.

Vuilleumier et al. (2001) used a closely related procedure with 12 patients who showed unilateral left

neglect. Six of these showed the same effect as in patient VR, but six did not extinguish either type of stimulus. This difference could not be explained by differential sensitivity to neglect as the two types of patient did not differ in the magnitude of neglect on standard clinical tests. However there were marked anatomical differences between the two groups. Both groups had damage to the right inferior posterior parietal area (Brodmann's area 40), long known to be a key area for neglect (see Driver et al., 2004, for review). Those who did not show the VR-type effects also had lesions extending into the lateral occipital lobe which could damage early visual processing such as in area V2.

It is now clear from many studies that there is some preserved processing in the occipito-temporal ventral pathway in subjects who show extinction but in whom the pathway is undamaged. However, as Driver and Vuilleumier (2001) say in their detailed review of their studies: 'It remains to be determined exactly how comparable the residual occipito-temporal processing is for extinguished stimuli versus consciously seen stimuli' (p. 66). Indeed, with a model of neglect such as that of Mozer and Behrmann (1990), Pouget and Sejnowski (2001) found that the effect of neglect could lead to a reduction in the normal level of activation in the ventral route (see Section 3.7). Thus it may after all be possible to provide a similar type of activation strength explanation for unconscious processing as was given for the semantic access dyslexia and prosopagnosia phenomena in the previous section.

A similar possibility also exists for studies on normal subjects. Studies of subliminal processing have been taking place in normal subjects since the nineteenth

---

for reading. The alternative is that it is specialised for visual stimuli of any sort in which one becomes expert (Tarr & Gauthier, 2000). In our view the evidence supports the Kanwisher specificity position (see e.g. Grill-Spector et al, 2004).

[18] A study by Vuilleumier et al. (2001) on another right parietal patient suffering from neglect gave very similar results.

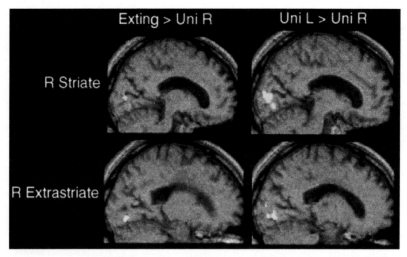

Fig. 11.6 The fMRI results of presenting either unilateral or bilateral visual stimuli to patient GK (see Figure 11.5). The scans show (left) areas activated by extinguished left visual stimuli and (right) by consciously seen unilateral stimuli in the left visual field, in both cases compared with the effects of unilaterally presented stimuli in the right visual field. Reprinted from G. Rees, E. Wojciulik, K. Clarke, M. Husain, C. Frith and J. Driver, Unconscious activation of visual cortex in the damaged right hemisphere of a parietal patient with extinction, *Brain*, 2000, *123*(8), 1624–1633, by permission of Oxford University Press.

century (see Merikle et al., 2001 for review). They have had a very chequered history, as the issue was associated in the minds of experimental psychologists with research on psychoanalysis—long viewed by many as not satisfying Popperian criteria, which were then high intellectual fashion, for what counts as a science.[19] Major hostile reviews were produced 25 years apart (Eriksen, 1960; Holender, 1986). However recently a spate of studies has supported the existence of subliminal perception. Possibly the most powerful are those that use the design developed by Debner and Jacoby (1994). A target word is presented preceded and followed by unrelated words, which act as forward and backward masks. If the target word is presented for a very short time, say 50 msec, typically only the masks are seen. The clever methodological development of Debner and Jacoby was to give the subjects instructions that said what they were *not* to do if they perceived the word.[20] In this case after being presented with the masked target the subject is presented with a completion cue, the first three letters of the target word (e.g. *tab* for *table*). The instructions had been to give any word beginning with these three letters *other* than the word presented before the mask. The results are shown in Figure 11.8.[21] When the stimulus is exposed for long enough to be clearly perceived—150 msec—the subjects obey instructions. The presented stimulus is given in the response much less frequently than if no stimulus at all had been presented. However for a 50-msec exposure a very different pattern of results was obtained. Now subjects gave the presented word more frequently than if no word had been presented.

In normal subjects subliminal perception can have effects at higher levels than the simple representation of the stimuli from processing at the early levels of the visual processing system. For instance, semantic processing can also occur from a word masked so that it cannot be seen. This was originally shown in classic experiments of Marcel (1983b) (see also Greenwald & Draine, 1997). However dramatic corroboration of Marcel's early experiments was made by Dehaene et al. (1998b) using fMRI. In this study subjects had to report whether a target number was larger or smaller than 5. The target was preceded by a masked prime, also a number, which was presented for 43 msec. Subjects were unable to reliably report the presence or absence of the prime, or its value. Even so, a priming effect was obtained on congruent trials compared with incongruent trials.[22] When the prime and target where either both greater than 5 or both less than 5, subjects were

---

[19] The association was not unjustified. If unconscious influences exist they can clearly be affected by affective processing (see Morris et al., 1998).

[20] This is an example of the general and very powerful process-dissociation methodology widely used by Jacoby and his collaborators. It is called the *exclusion task* procedure.

[21] Somewhat analogous results were found in a study of Rock et al. (1992) in which attention was directed away from the stimulus; a mask was not used.

[22] See Section 7.2 for discussion of processes that might underlie priming.

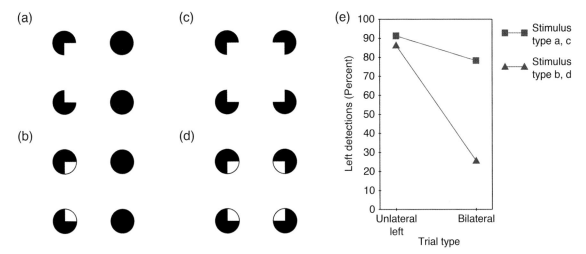

Fig. 11.7 Kanizsa-type stimuli and results from the study by Mattingley et al. (1997) of the left-side extinction patient VR. Each trial began with VR fixating on 4 black disks. After 2 sec, the display changed to briefly show one of the figures a, b, c or d. (Catch trials with no change and unilateral right trials consisting of reflections about the vertical axis of figures a and b were also used). VR was required to indicate which the side or sides of the figure, if any, changed. Results of the study are shown in figure e. VR was generally correct at detecting changes on the left with standard Kanizsa-type stimuli (as in c), but tended to miss such changes when the stimuli were of the minimally different form shown in a. VR made no misses or false alarms for right detections. Data from Mattingley et al. (1997).

on average 24 msec faster at responding than when one number was greater than 5 and the other was less than 5. This was true regardless of whether the stimuli were presented as digits (e.g. '1') or words (e.g. *one*). Moreover, on incongruent trials ERP measurements of the lateralised readiness potential, held to measure covert response activation in the motor cortex, revealed preparation of the (incorrect) primed response, which was quickly suppressed as the target was processed. A follow-up fMRI study confirmed that the locus of the ERP signals was the left and right motor cortices. Related findings have been obtained by Neumann and Klotz (1994) and Eimer and Schlaghecken (1998), amongst others.

One possibly interpretation of the Dehaene et al. result, given the discussion of priming in Section 7.2, is that priming on congruent trials reflects learned stimulus–response mappings rather than semantic processing of the stimulus. The experiment involved just eight stimuli (1, 4, 6, 9 in digit and word form, acting both as primes and targets). With a minimum of 16 practice trials in each block, each target will have been responded to at least twice during practice. In a modified design, Abrams, Klinger and Greenwald (2002) demonstrated that semantic processing of the subliminally presented primes does occur. Words (such as *happy*, *warm*, *scum* and *kill*) were classified as pleasant or unpleasant during practice. These words were then presented subliminally (with new targets) in the test phase. For half of the participants, response keys were reversed between the practice and test phases. Similar levels of priming were

found regardless of this reversal, indicating that semantic processing of the primes was occurring.

The study of Abrams et al. (2002) was purely behavioural. Using fMRI, Diaz and McCarthy (2007) found activation of left-hemisphere language regions, including

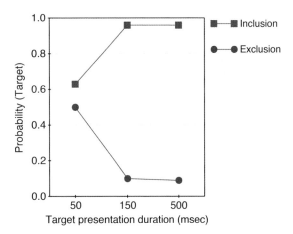

Fig. 11.8 Results from a study of subliminal perception. Debner and Jacoby (1994) presented a target word sandwiched between two masks, with target presentation ranging from 50 msec to 500 msec. Subjects were then required to complete a three-letter stem. In the *inclusion* condition they were required to complete the stem with the target. In the *exclusion* condition they were required to complete the stem with some other word. When the target presentation duration was short (50 msec) subjects tended to incorrectly produce the target as a completion in the exclusion condition. Data from experiment 1 and the full attention condition of experiment 2 of Debner and Jacoby (1994).

left inferior frontal and inferior temporal gyri, when masked words as opposed to masked non-words were presented incidentally in a target detection task, suggesting lexical semantic processing of the subliminal word stimuli. Almost ten years earlier, Morris et al. (1998) had been the first to show subliminal effects using functional imaging. They however had used not words but learned valence associations for faces. In pre-training, subjects were classically conditioned to associate one of two angry faces with a burst of white noise. Subsequently, in the MRI scanner the faces were briefly presented followed by a mask (a neutral face). Greater activity was found in the right amygdala for the negatively conditioned masked faces than for the unconditioned masked faces. In contrast, when the angry faces were presented in an unmasked condition, the negatively conditioned face led to greater activity in the left amygdala. It therefore appears that, while the amygdala responds to aversively conditioned stimuli, that response is lateralised depending on awareness of the stimulus.

Non-conscious processing of aversive stimuli is not unexpected given the amygdala's role at the interface of cognition and emotion (but see Pessoa et al., 2005). However, in studies involving semantic categorisation, two factors appear to be critical for obtaining priming effects: practice with the stimuli and the subjects' intentions. Using the same type of word classification task as in their earlier work, Abrams and Grinspan (2007) found priming only for those stimuli which were in the practice set, and not for additional pleasant or unpleasant words which their subjects had not seen. Enns and Oriet (2007), on the other hand, used multi-dimensional stimuli in two visual classification tasks. Subjects were required to classify stimuli according to one dimension, ignoring the other two. Priming was possible along any of three stimulus dimensions, but it was only found for the dimension that was critical to the classification task.

It is clear from the above that extensive cognitive processing of stimuli can occur in the absence of awareness of those stimuli. This processing is at least in part determined by one's intentions. For verbal stimuli, it may include semantic classification and for face stimuli, classification of emotion. This processing, though, relates to stimuli that are not consciously perceived. Consider though the situation for those stimuli of which we are conscious. Are there systematic relations between brain processes and conscious awareness? Clearly, on the basis of the functional imaging studies of subliminal processing, activity in the amygdala, the motor cortices, and the left hemisphere language regions, as activated in the study of Diaz and McCarthy (2007), are probably not sufficient for conscious experience. But might there be other neural regions in which activity is necessary and sufficient for conscious experience? It is to this question that we now turn.

11.5 Neural Correlates of Conscious Experience

The study of Cowey and Stoerig (1995) on monkeys discussed earlier used a clever procedure in one condition of training the monkey to distinguish between light and no light as a means of obtaining an analogue of a phenomenal report in a monkey. This is a development of an idea first realised by Nikos Logothetis and his colleagues in a classic series of experiments (Logothetis and Schall, 1989; Leopold and Logothetis, 1996; Sheinberg and Logothetis, 1997; Logothetis, 1998). Monkeys were trained to discriminate between two stimuli which in humans produce the phenomenon of binocular rivalry. This occurs when the two stimuli are presented, one to each eye, in the same part of the visual field. One experiences the rapid fluctuations of the two possible percepts and not the suppression of one or their blending.

The monkeys were initially trained to respond to a sequence of two alternating stimuli by pulling a lever associated with each stimulus when that stimulus was present. They were then presented with the rivalry condition, where both stimuli were present. The monkey shows the same pattern of responding as in human binocular rivalry. It is very plausible that the experience of the monkey is the same as that of a human. If so, the responses of the monkey can be used to track their phenomenal states, or to provide what Weiskrantz (1997) calls a *commentary response*. Logothetis and his colleagues then examined the neural responses of cells at different levels of the ventral visual system. Relatively few neurons in early visual response areas showed a close correspondence with the commentary response—less than 20% in V1 and V2 and less then 40% in V4 and V5/MT. A much higher number (90% or so) did in inferotemporal cortex and the superior temporal sulcus. Thus, as discussed earlier, the correspondence with the conscious percept only seemed a characteristic of cells higher in the visual system and not in early visual cortex.

Virtually the same experiment was done in humans using fMRI by Tong et al. (1998). During a scan the subject would see a single face-house pair with one of the pair presented to one eye and the other to the equivalent position of the other eye. The stimuli flipped perceptually for each subject every few seconds in the standard fashion for binocular rivalry. Each subject had to report, using a button press, when the switch occurred. In the analysis the MR responses were time locked to perceptual change in the stimulus. As discussed above and in Section 6.3 (see Figure 6.4), the fusiform face area (FFA) responds more strongly to faces than to non-face visual stimuli such as houses. Another region—the parahippocampal place area (PPA)—responds to images of places including houses but virtually not at all to faces. In the rivalry situation the FFA

(a) 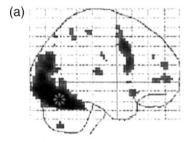 (b) 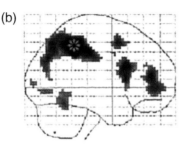 (c)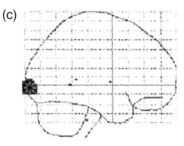

Fig. 11.9 Coactivation maps during binocular rivalry in the study of Lumer and Rees (1999). The marker on each image shows the locus of activity used as the regressor. (a) Areas where activity was significantly correlated with that in the posterior fusiform gyrus. (b) Areas where activity was significantly correlated with that in superior parietal cortex. (c) Areas where activity was significantly correlated with that in V1. All images reprinted with permission from E.D. Lumer and G. Rees, 1999, Covariation of activity in visual and prefrontal cortex associated with subjective visual perception. *Proceedings of the National Academy of Sciences, USA*, 96, 1669–1673. Copyright (1999) National Academy of Sciences, USA.

and PPA regions were activated appropriately when the subject began to perceive the corresponding stimuli. In complementary fashion when the subject stopped seeing the stimulus the activation in the corresponding region decreased. Thus the pattern of activation in the two regions tracked the awareness of the subject. Even more striking was the result of a control condition in which a single stimulus was presented to both eyes but it changed in a way that reproduced the experience of the same subject in an earlier scan (face → house → face, etc.). The fMRI results were indistinguishable for the FFA and PPA regions from that of the rivalry condition.[23]

Now activation of these temporal lobe regions in the above experiments does not necessarily mean that they have any specific relations to consciousness. Indeed V1 is activated in many studies and yet the evidence of the studies of Logothetis and collaborators strongly suggests that activation there is not closely related to consciousness. (See also Crick & Koch, 1995.)

In a related study, Lumer, Friston and Rees (1998) pushed the analysis further. They presented a red grating to one eye and a green face to the equivalent position of the other eye. Rivalry occurs between the perception of the two stimuli and subjects must respond with a key press when it occurs. In a control (replay) condition each stimulus is presented alone to its eye with the equivalent timing for switches. They found that when a given image becomes perceptually dominant this is characterised by a change of activation in many regions including parietal, prefrontal and anterior cingulate cortices. This was not the case for the occipital

lobe.[24] Moreover the change of image effect is greater for rivalry than for replay in the parietal and inferior frontal regions. Similar effects have been found in many other studies (see Rees, 2007).

In a later fMRI study using the same stimulus situation, Lumer and Rees (1999) found increases in the inter-correlations between regions (see Figure 11.9). Activation in many regions (a, b) is correlated with each other, but this does not include V1 (c); as for the effects found in the monkey, activation in V1 does not appear to be linked to that in fronto-parietal areas, held to be in turn linked to conscious perception.

11.6 On Phenomenology

So far we have discussed the negative aspects of consciousness, its absence when on other grounds such as behaviour, one might expect it to be present. But, can one say anything about the nature of conscious experience itself? As Sutherland's (1989) acerbic dictionary entry with which this chapter began indicates, consciousness is a concept we derive from reflection on our own experience and from that alone. It is therefore striking that most discussions of the relation between consciousness and the brain essentially take little interest in whether we can refine further our notions about consciousness. If one is to produce an explanation of consciousness in terms of brain or system level processes would it not be advisable to specify better with what the correspondence is being made? In fact both philosophers and psychologists have attempted to do just this. There is a quite different type of 'intuition pump' in philosophical discussions of consciousness from the postulating of bizarre entities which are intuitively endorsed or not attributed with consciousness by the reader. This is the use of experiential accounts of typical

---

[23] Technically this result should be treated with a little suspicion as in this design there is inevitably no control for the time during scanning that a stimulus is presented. The authors note, however, that for each subject the mean duration of the two percepts was similar, ranging across subjects from 2.5 sec to 5.5 sec.

[24] But see Haynes and Rees (2005) for discussion of certain later studies where this simple conclusion does not hold.

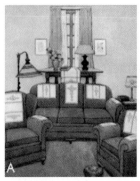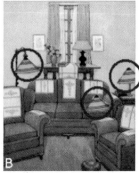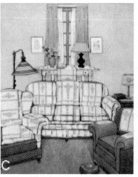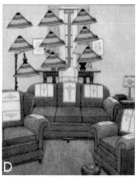

Fig. 11.10 The palinopsias. (a) A room as correctly observed. (b) Perseveration of the image of the lampshade at successive fixation points. (c) Illusory visual spread, where a pattern on one object has spread to other objects. (d) Polyopia, where the image of an object is repeated in rows and columns. Reprinted from D.G. ffytche and R.J. Howard, The perceptual consequences of visual loss: 'positive' pathologies of vision, *Brain*, 1999, *122*(7), 1274–1260, by permission of Oxford University Press.

situations which allow the reader to understand some characteristic experience that they have in common with the writer and on which an argument can be based. This is the phenomenological approach.[25]

In the early years of the last century there was a dispute between the so-called Wurzberg school from Germany and the American psychologist Titchener, who both used the introspective method to analyse thought processes but got different results. In psychology it became widely accepted that the appropriate conclusion from the dispute was that it demonstrated that the introspection was useless. The introspective approach to psychology was replaced by behaviourism, and phenomenal reports held to be inherently unsuitable as scientific evidence. However this is the history of the time as seen through the perspective of the behaviourists who subsequently became the dominant movement academically in the USA. In fact scholarly analysis showed the Wurzberg school's more constrained introspective method to be inherently the more reliable (see Humphrey, 1951, for a highly sophisticated discussion). However, the anti-introspectionist position remained very strong (e.g. Nisbett & Wilson, 1977).

In fact there are many areas where phenomenal reports are invaluable. Thus the so-called think-aloud protocol procedures, where subjects give a *limited* verbal account of salient aspects of their thought processes while solving problems, have been extensively used in the study of thinking and proved a reliable source of evidence if appropriate precautions are taken (Ericsson & Simon, 1993). Thus most production system models

of thinking (see Newell & Simon, 1972; Newell, 1990 see Chapters 1, 3 and 12) are heavily reliant on evidence obtained from such think-aloud procedures.

Just as critically, our clinical knowledge of unusual thought processes in a range of areas is heavily dependent upon the description by the experiencer. These include certain unusual effects of disease, such as on perception. Thus ffytche and Howard (1999) show that a common pattern of visual hallucinations occurs after neurological disease, migraine and eye disease, through sensory deprivation, and from taking mescaline. These include three forms of palinopsia (see Figure 11.10)—perseveration, polyopia and illusory visual spread[26]—and tessellopsia, where the visual field contains lines creating a lattice or grid pattern, often on diagonals. Another even more common source is in psychiatric illness where the symptomology of even such a key condition as schizophrenia is heavily dependent upon self reports of patients; consider, for instance, the importance of auditory hallucinations and delusions in the diagnostic process.

Third, there are the types of experience had by only a limited subset of the population. Thus over the last decade many fascinating accounts have been given of the experience of synaesthesia—where a person reliably experiences sensations linked to one modality or dimension when presented with stimuli in another. For instance, a grapheme-colour synaesthete experiences written letters as having their own colours, such as *A* tending to be seen as red; these phenomenological reports have become the bases for complex experimental analyses (see Ward & Mattingley, 2006). Roughly 4% of the population report such experiences (Simner et al., 2006) and they are clearly genuine as the rate of making the identical voluntary cross-sense associations

[25] In the early part of the last century the German philosopher Husserl put the term *phenomenology* into something of a conceptual strait-jacket. The term is not used in Husserl's sense here but means the analysis of empirical generalizations about the nature of consciousness and experience from the perspective of the experiencing subject.

[26] Illusory visual spread is not reported in sensory deprivation or after taking mescaline.

of the appropriate type after a month is much higher than in non-synaesthetes (Baron-Cohen et al., 1996).

Empirical examples such as the use of think-aloud protocols in problem-solving or theoretically the development of a theory of schizophrenia such as that of Frith (1992), in part based on patient's accounts of their experience, indicate that in science it can be useful to go beyond the mere existence of consciousness and to attempt to document and classify conscious experience. However, Jack (1998) makes the strong argument that any type of phenomenal report is potentially unreliable if the conceptual structure used to characterize the reports is unsatisfactory. He takes as an example the search for basic psychophysical laws such as the so-called Stevens (1957) power law, which claims that absolute judgements of sensory magnitudes obey a power law; thus if E is the experience and I is a measure of the physical stimulus then:

$$E = kI^a,$$

where k and a are constants. Exponents were held to range from 0.42 for viscosity to 3.5 for electric shock. One method that Stevens used was magnitude estimation where subjects are first given a standard stimulus with a number assigned to it. They must then produce numbers when a series of stimuli differing in magnitude are presented.

Laming (1997), in a book reviewing the history of the power law, argues cogently that Fechner, who originated the search for such psychophysical laws in the nineteenth century, was wrong 'in the implicit assumption that sensation admitted measurement on any kind of continuum at all .... The evidence so far to hand does not support any intermediate continuum at the psychological level which might reasonably be labelled "sensation" ... essentially because there is no corresponding psychological entity .... Experiments by different investigators, seeking to measure the perception of neural activity as a sensation by different methods have found no basis for agreement'.[27] The critical point is that even if a procedure based on introspective reports produces replicable results this does not mean that the results are scientifically meaningful.

We may draw two conclusions from these caveats. The first is that phenomenal reports necessarily involve a conceptual framework for making the reports. This can be simple, as when the patient describes a palinopsic hallucination. It can be complex, as when a subject makes a remember–know judgement or assigns a confidence judgement on whether a memory is accurate or not (see Chapter 10). The second is that the judgement must reflect the natural history of experience, namely that it has what we call *experiential validity*. Instead it can be more or less illusorily constructed by experimental instructions, as, if Laming's analysis is accepted, by the instruction to assign a number to the magnitude of a perceived stimulus.

Thus for greater reliability, the use of any particular type of phenomenal report produced in a given type of experimental paradigm needs to be first confirmed by more open-ended, phenomenal reports, not prefigured by the theoretical interpretation to be used.[28] Secondly the phenomenal reports need to be correlated with cognitive neuroscience evidence.

If we take episodic memory as an example there have been a few phenomenological investigations of traditional paradigms, such as free recall (Koriat & Goldsmith, 1996) and autobiographical recall (Burgess & Shallice, 1996b), but there are none to our knowledge of the much more contentious procedures such as the use of confidence judgements and, more particularly, remember-know judgements discussed in Section 10.8. Such methods are used on the assumption that they reflect the natural history of our experience of remembering but there is little direct phenomenological evidence that they do. To make matters worse we have argued in the previous chapter that these experiential report paradigms on remembering may be differentially appropriate for different types of subjects. This is a major lacuna in current cognitive neuroscience approaches to memory. For other areas the situation is better. For instance, the think-aloud procedures used to provide empirical evidence relating to production system approaches to problem-solving have been most appropriately investigated (Ericsson & Simon, 1993).

We will examine in detail an experimental paradigm directly related to claims about consciousness. In the 1980s the neurologist Benjamin Libet put forward the idea that time as it is experienced is off-set by a few hundred milliseconds from the physical time of brain processes. This rather strange idea was proposed on the basis of the results of two experimental paradigms—one involving perception and the other willed action (see Libet, 1985). We will consider the second of these, which has been the one examined in more detail

---

[27] See also Poulton (1979) for classic methodological objections to the procedures used by Stevens—principally that the ratings given by a subject to successive stimuli are far from independent—and Zimmer (2005) and Steingrimsson and Luce (2006) for more positive views of the method.

[28] To make matters yet more complex, the Wurzberg School argued that in making introspections on the thought processes expert subjects were required, and their conclusions have in general stood the test of time (see Humphrey, 1951). We would argue that the ideal degree of expertise of the subjects in phenomenological investigations should depend on the type of task.

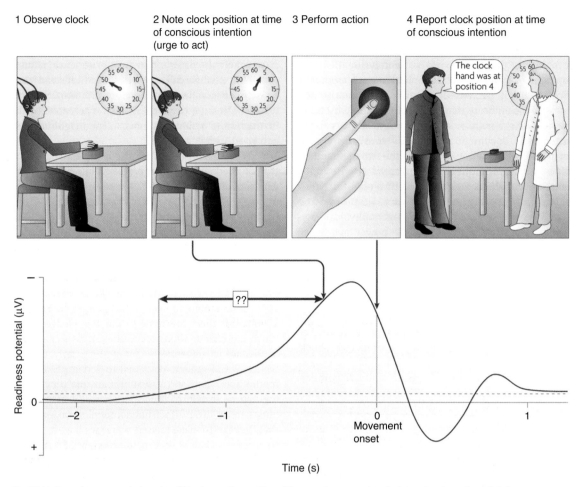

1 Observe clock 2 Note clock position at time of conscious intention (urge to act) 3 Perform action 4 Report clock position at time of conscious intention

Fig. 11.11 Procedure and typical results of Libet's experiment. The subject watches a rotating clock hand and at a time of their own choosing presses a button. The subject is asked to report the position of the clock hand when they first 'felt the urge' to move their hand. Typically subjects report the urge to have occurred approximately 200 ms before the movement onset. However, simultaneous ERP recordings (illustrated by the schematic readiness potential) reveal brain activity relating to the button press up to 1 s before the movement onset. Reprinted by permission from Macmillan Publishers Ltd: *Nature Reviews Neuroscience* (P. Haggard (2008) Human volition: towards a neuroscience of will. *Nature Reviews Neuroscience, 9*, 934–946), copyright (2008).

experimentally (see Haggard, 2008). In the willed-action paradigm subjects had to move their right hand at some moment during a prespecified interval, with the precise timing of the movement being for them to freely decide. They carried out this simple task while looking at a clock. After moving they had to say where the clock hand had been when they decided to move. On average subjects said they experienced the will to move about 200 msec before the actual movement. Brain activity began, however roughly 1 sec before the movement (see Figure 11.11). This was the paradox that led Libet to make his counter-intuitive proposal.

In the light of our earlier discussion we can ask two questions about this report of experience—is it experientially valid and does it have any cognitive neuroscience support? The will has had a bad name for the last sixty years because of its association with Nazi ideology. However anyone who has had to ford a swollen river knows the concept is not completely spurious. Yet, there is a long way from fording a swollen river to the Libet paradigm. Is *an act of will* experientially valid there? Consider Wittgenstein's comment in the Philosophical Investigations 'What is left when I subtract the fact that my arm goes up from the fact that I raise my arm?'. More recently Wegner (2003) has answered Wittgenstein's rhetorical question by arguing that the experience of will is a *post hoc* reconstruction. Haggard (2008) has, though, pointed out that epileptic patients reported a strong urge to move a limb when their brain was stimulated in the pre-SMA, an area in the medial premotor cortex, during neurosurgical operations of Fried et al. (1991).[29] An urge to move a part of the body thus can have experiential validity.

From a cognitive neuroscience perspective, in a modification of the Libet paradigm, Haggard and Eimer (1999) asked subjects to make a free movement using either the left or the right hand. Across trials they showed that with respect to the actual time of movement the reported time of the urge to move correlated with respect to one particular EEG wave—the lateralised readiness potential in which brain activity is linked to the contralateral hemisphere to the hand selected—and not with other waves.[30] Moreover in an fMRI study using a similar task, Soon et al. (2008) found that the free choice of hands was linked to activation of the pre-SMA. In addition the pre-SMA was one of the structures more activated—along with the dorsolateral prefrontal cortex and the anterior cingulate—in internally generated finger movements by contrast with visually cued ones (Deiber et al., 1996). From a clinical perspective incidental utilisation behaviour (see Section 9.2) has been described with specifically pre-SMA lesions (Boccardi et al., 2002). We therefore see the pre-SMA as a key structure in the top-down activation of contention scheduling in motor tasks.[31]

The pre-SMA is not the only system involved in the experience of will. In an early PET experiment, Frith et al. (1991), in a Libet-like task but without the subjective timing aspect, found that spontaneous generation of a tap activated lateral prefrontal cortex. We see this region as the outflow from the Supervisory System in this task and the pre-SMA as the input into contention scheduling. Thus the experience of *willed action* seems to pass, if a little shakily, the criteria specified above. Does that mean that we should accept Libet's dualistic ideas about time? It has been argued by Dennett and Kinsbourne (1992) that Libet's dualist conclusions do not follow, because the temporal grain of experiences is not fine enough to produce contradictions with the specific timing of processes in the brain. Whether this argument applies depends on the theory of consciousness one holds, so we will come back to this later. However, this discussion of consciousness is becoming rather rarefied. Does such discussion have any applications?

11.7 Potential applications of a theory of consciousness: Vegetative State

From a philosophical perspective, consciousness does not just pose profound questions concerning the nature of mind. It is also deeply involved in issues of morality and law. Thus we are generally held responsible for our actions, which we in some sense willed, and our feelings of empathy toward another creature are intimately linked to their being conscious, or at least capable of consciousness. The arcane complexities of philosophical debate need moreover to confront the brutal medical realities of a condition like *vegetative state*.

After traumatic brain injury a number of related conditions can result—coma, vegetative state, minimally conscious state and locked-in syndrome. In vegetative state the diagnosis differs from coma in that the patient is viewed as showing wakefulness, as indicated by eye opening. However as in coma, the patient shows no evidence of awareness, and as such, if the condition is persistent he or she becomes a potential candidate to be withdrawn from life support. Diagnosis is typically made on the basis of the clinical history together with behavioural observations (Owen & Coleman, 2008) with the internationally accepted criteria emphasising the importance of there being 'no evidence of awareness of environment or self' but without specifying how such awareness is to be established.

Owen et al. (2006) have recently developed a functional imaging method that they hold strongly suggests that a patient diagnosed as vegetative state on behavioural grounds was indeed conscious at least for auditory input. The study is based on the principle that imagining something tends to activate the same structures, if at reduced level, as those involved in carrying it out (Jeannerod & Frak, 1999). More specifically it is based on an experiment in which 12 normal volunteers carried out four tasks repeatedly in the scanner (Boly et al., 2007). One of the tasks (motor imagery) was to imagine playing tennis, concentrating on hitting the ball very hard as though in a match. A second (spatial imagery) was to imagine visiting all the rooms of one's house, starting from the front door and noting all the details in each room. Instructions such as 'play tennis' are given once every 30 sec. For all tasks all subjects activated the pre-SMA, discussed above, more than if they were instructed to rest. More specifically, all subjects activated the medial posterior parietal cortex and the retrosplenial cortex significantly more in the spatial imagery task than in the motor task and all bar one showed the opposite pattern for the inferior parietal lobules and the supplementary motor area. Activation of task-appropriate regions was highly consistent.

In Owen et al. (2006) a patient diagnosed as a vegetative state patient carried out the same pair of tasks with the same type of instructions and a basically similar

---

[29] See the discussion of Kennerley et al. (2004) in Section 9.9.

[30] The lateralised readiness potential is a component of the EEG wave that is generally taken to be an indicator of activation of a motor response. Physiological studies have shown that the wave is generated in the contralateral motor cortex and pre-SMA (see Eimer, 1998).

[31] See Haggard (2008) for extensive discussion.

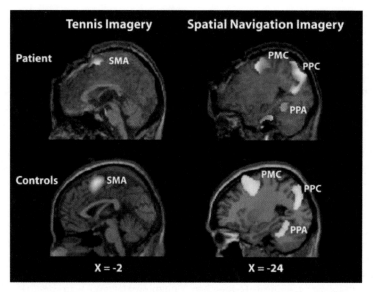

Fig. 11.12 BOLD activity in a vegetative state patient and controls when given instructions to produce tennis imagery compared with ones concerning spatial navigation imagery. The supplementary motor area (SMA) was active in both the patient and controls during tennis imagery. The parahippocampal gyrus (PPA), posterior parietal-lobe (PPC), and lateral premotor cortex (PMC) were active in both the patient and controls during spatial navigation imagery. From A.M. Owen, M.R. Coleman, M. Boley, M.H. Davis, S. Laureys & J.D. Pickard, 2006, Detecting awareness in the vegetative state. *Science, 313*(5792), 1402. Reprinted with permission from AAAS.

pattern of findings (see Figure 11.12). Owen et al. interpreted the results as an indication of conscious awareness in the patient. Others, however, have criticised the conclusion arguing, for instance, that the results may just reflect an 'implicit preconscious neural response' (Greenberg, 2007; Nachev & Husain, 2007).[32] However as Owen and Coleman (2008) point out, this presupposes that a word like 'house' can be unconsciously learned to stand for a sentence, that the sentence can be understood and interpreted unconsciously and that any activation so produced would last for 30 sec and immediately end when another instruction like 'rest' occurs. This all seems implausible. Moreover it should be remembered that the preconscious activations observed, say in Dehaene et al. (2001) with masked stimuli, are much weaker than their conscious equivalents. There is no suggestion of such a quantitative difference in the present situation. One cannot rule out the possibility that the patient showed an implicit preconscious neural response but it is more plausible that she was conscious. Moreover she is not unique; in another type of speech comprehension test two vegetative state patients demonstrated high-level fMRI speech activations (Coleman et al., 2009). So what is it that a conscious patient has that a patient in a non-conscious vegetative state does not?

---

[32] The situation would then be analogous to that of the preconscious state on the Dehaene–Changeux theory to be discussed in Section 11.11.

11.8 What a Theory of Consciousness Must Explain

We have so far in this chapter shown that consciousness is something that cannot be ignored in science. It is too closely associated with many fascinating phenomena. It is intimately associated too with major clinical and ethical issues. We can also develop a valid language in which to characterise it. But what is it as a scientific object? Before discussing this we need to consider what a theory of consciousness would need to explain.

Where cognitive neuroscience has been most effective is in providing a range of situations where the conscious-to-non-conscious contrast can be mapped onto ranges of experimental dependent variables or with respect to types of clinical condition. Section 11.6 has indicated that a theory of consciousness can be required to explain how a conscious state can be characterised. Language, indeed, has a plethora of words for categorising experiences—what one sees or hears or feels or imagines or remembers and so on, and also for their aspects—so for seeing colour, shape, scenes among many other aspects of visual experience—but also for the objects of our mental operations—to guess X, to imagine Y, to dream Z. There are also conscious states of mind without low-level conscious contents like *tip-of-the tongue* states or the Wurzberg School's *Bewusstseinslagen* (imageless thought) (see Humphrey, 1951). Moreover in Section 11.6 we have seen how ways of categorising different types of experience can be validated against experimental findings as was done for *will*.

A scientific theory of consciousness, however, needs to do more than underpin a sort of validated Mendeleev's table of normal and disturbed types of experience. As the philosopher-of-mind Alan Thomas (2003) expresses it 'We apply the term 'conscious' both as a person level predicate applied to whole people or other animals' (p. 176), as well as to states of such organisms. He continues in an understated fashion 'the relation between 'creature consciousness' and 'state consciousness' is not, itself, a straightforward one'. And then, lucidly summarising the position of an obscure philosopher Brian O'Shaughnessy (2000), he says 'We implicitly define what it is to be a conscious subject by considering the role that consciousness plays in the global mental economy of the agent, where it seems to contribute to the co-ordination and focusing of the rational powers of the agent'. In other words consciousness should not be viewed as an inner theatre of the contents of experience. Instead it has the biological function of enabling bodily and mental actions and *its properties reflect this*. However, the way one should characterise the creature-level properties of waking consciousness is subject to much abstruse philosophical debate, and probably we will only be able to capture them adequately when we have a satisfactory scientific theory of consciousness. At the very least, though, the following characteristics are among the properties of creature-level consciousness that need to be addressed by a scientific theory of consciousness:[33]

1 *Experiences are continually occurring when one is conscious.* One cannot be conscious and experience nothing.

2 *When awake and conscious the conscious subject is typically mentally active.*[34] Consciousness is assumed to exist to enable this activity.

3 *Experiences are directly known to self-conscious subjects as occurring 'now'.* Also this time is directly known to relate to neighbouring times—this is linked to William James's (1890) metaphor of the 'stream of consciousness'.

4 *In normal waking consciousness the subject has the sense of knowing directly what he/she is doing and why.*[35]

5 *Conscious experience of a state of affairs is necessary for intentional action.* This is a critical property widely discussed in the philosophical literature. For instance,

Armstrong (1968) held that consciousness is 'a mental state of a person apt for bringing about a certain sort of behaviour' (p. 82). Similarly, the philosopher-of-mind van Gulick (1994) argues that 'Information needs to be presented to us phenomenally for it to play a role in the choice, initiation or direction of the intentional action' (p. 33). This property is the bedrock of the legal concept of responsibility.

6 Following William James (1890), *consciousness is held to have a foreground and background, but the degree to which it has a foreground varies.* Thus William James contrasts concentration or focal awareness with what he calls distraction 'The eyes are fixed on vacancy, the sounds of the world melt into confused unity, the attention is dispersed … and the foreground of consciousness is filled, if by anything, by a sort of solemn sense of the passage of time' (p. 404).

7 *The foreground of consciousness is very limited in capacity* compared with the myriad experiences one could potentially be having given your circumstances at a given time.

8 *The primary structuring feature of consciousness—* attention—can, again following William James— be passive, automatically drawn, non-voluntary or effortless on the one hand or active or voluntary on the other.

9 *To produce a novel sentence-length utterance about something requires that one is aware of it,* and to understand a novel sentence also requires awareness; this relates to Weiskrantz's ideas on *commentary processes* discussed earlier.

These characteristics of creature consciousness are hardly precise. However they at least provide us with some criteria by which to evaluate possible scientific accounts of consciousness. We begin with the simplest type of position.

11.9 The Activation Strength/Quality of the Representation and Related Theories of Consciousness

In Section 11.3 we referred to Farah's (1994) 'quality of representation' theory and the activation strength theories of the difference between conscious and unconscious experiences. Theories of this type hold that awareness derives in some way from processing in the individual subsystems being activated.[36] Consider a subsystem, i. When it is activated in one of states $a_{1i} \ldots a_{ni}$ at time t_i then assume that the subsystem contributes

---

[33] Properties 1–4 come from O'Shaughnessy (2000).

[34] O'Shaughnessy, says 'continually' which is an academic's characterisation of consciousness. Consider the counter-example of sunbathing (Evans, 1970).

[35] This does not apply to dreams or altered states of consciousness.

---

[36] They are compatible with the philosophical position taken by Dretske (1995) except that they are typically 'internalist'.

a conscious experience c_i to the overall state of consciousness at t_i.[37] However when it is activated in one of states $b_{1i} \ldots b_{mi}$ at time t_i then assume it makes no contributions to the overall conscious experience. The overall conscious experience of a person at time t_i would then be the simple sum of the conscious experiences derived for each of the subsystems a_{ji}. One could formalise the activation strength theory, by assuming that if there exists a function f such that for all p, q:

$$f(a_{pi}) > K > f(b_{qi}),$$

then the function $f(\ldots)$ is critical for mapping from the material state of the system to the experience of the person. For instance f could correspond to some sum across all the neurons of a particular type of a monotonic function of their firing rate. Plausibly the monotonic function might be strongly accelerating with increasing firing rate.

This theory is extremely simplistic. It is, however, the obvious realisation of a reductionist approach to consciousness with the 'experience' of each subsystem being viewed as the collective 'experience' of each of its cells. This type of assumption has been called *microconsciousness* by Zeki and Bartels (1999). Moreover it would be compatible with many of the findings already discussed such as those on prosopagnosia and neglect. The idea has, however, a number of problems.

1. *Activation Strength.* As Kanwisher (2001) notes, at least two studies—those of Luck et al. (1996), using EEG, and Rees et al. (2000), using fMRI—contain comparisons in which the brain activations in the non-conscious and conscious conditions are roughly equal in strength. However, even if the activations are globally of roughly the same strength, this does not mean that there may not be important differences at a more micro-level, although then the need for some alternative to the simplistic account given above becomes even more pressing. There are, though, a number of other reasons why the approach is implausible.

2. *There is an explanatory gap.* What grounds are there for assuming a threshold relation between degrees of activation and contributions to experience and how could this be made in some way independent of what system was being activated? One possible candidate is related to Mozer's idea that conscious experience may correspond to the state-space of a system moving into an attractor basin. However there is a critical problem with this solution. If the state of a system, which leads to its content being in some sense conscious, can be described in terms of the subsystem operating in such a

way as to allow consistent transmission of information from that subsystem to other systems, what grounds are there for preferring the activation strength hypothesis to an account of consciousness which relates to the existence of effective transmission of information *between* subsystems? For this is also a consequence of the accessing of an attractor basin.

3. *Non-conscious systems.* There are systems where activity does not appear to be related to conscious experience. The obvious example is V1 given the findings, just discussed, of Logothetis and of Lumer and Rees (see also the arguments of Crick & Koch, 1995). A second would be the superior colliculus, if Weiskrantz's position is correct that blindsight depends upon the use of the visual pathway to the superior colliculus.[38] If consciousness is intrinsic to a given subsystem as this set of hypotheses hold then one needs an explanation of why activity in some subsystems does not seem to produce it.

4. *Consciousness and bodies.* If consciousness is a property of individual subsystems in the brain, and more than one of them can contribute at any given time, then why is consciousness limited to individual persons? Why does consciousness not fuse or conflate across subsystems in different people when two people's heads are close? In other words why should consciousness conflate across subsystems in the same brain and not across subsystems in nearby regions of space? What must be critical is that the subsystems are part of the same overall system, rather than consciousness corresponding to any collective 'experience' at the neuronal level. Moreover if one accepts that a person with lesions to the corpus callosum and anterior commissure producing disconnections of the two hemispheres—the split-brain patient—can have a different conscious experience in the two hemispheres,[39] then what is critical is the system-level of operation, as a functionalist would expect, and not anything about the uniqueness of the biological stuff in which it is implemented.

As yet there are in our view no strong empirical reasons for rejecting this type of theory. However the conceptual problems associated with it seem severe.

11.10 Type C processes

Can one improve the database against which to assess theories of consciousness? One way to do this is to presuppose that what is critical for whether one is conscious of a representation or not is the nature of the cognitive process or processes which operate upon it.

---

[37] This contribution could potentially vary across the a_{ji}, to produce contributions of different strength.

[38] This interpretation of blindsight is supported by the fMRI results of Sahraie et al. (1997) on the patient GY.

[39] This is Sperry's (1984) position. The issue is discussed at length in FNMS Section 16.4.

It is not the nature of a representation that is critical in determining whether it is conscious but the nature of the cognitive process. This is the approach implicitly adopted by Owen and his colleagues in their work on the vegetative state discussed in Section 11.7.

A position developed by Tony Jack and one of us (Jack & Shallice, 2001) divides processes into two types. For instances of one type, in line with principle 4 of Section 11.8, one would always be conscious of carrying out the process whenever it was carried out. These are *conscious-type processes* (C-processes).[40] By contrast, any process which is not *always* accompanied by the conscious knowledge it is occurring and giving rise to an experience of the relevant representations is a *non-conscious type process* (*non-C-process*). It is assumed that if one is conscious on one occasion when a putatively *non-C-process* is being carried out then this is because some other process such as monitoring is also operative at the same time and it is this second process which is crucial for giving rise to the conscious experience.

Jack and Shallice approached C-processes in two steps. First, they consider processes that are either phenomenally characterisable, using a particular mental state term, or operationally chacterisable, in terms of the carrying out of specific tasks. They ask whether they are ones that are always associated with a particular conscious experience. For instance, it would be argued that the task of imagining playing tennis for 30 sec would be a process of this type. Second, as we will discuss later, they asked to what theoretically defined computational process do the empirically characterised C-processes correspond? As far as the first step is concerned, they produced a number of putative empirical generalisations about situations where appropriate responding entails C-processes. Such empirical generalisations can in principle provide a more adequate data-base for theorising about consciousness.

On this approach the empirically characterisable types of situations, where C-processes are held to occur, can be divided into three sub-types:

1 Pre-experimentally characterised type-C processes. These include:

  C1 *Conscious reflection.* Experimentally this underlies the ability to make judgements based on aspects of an experience such as making confidence judgements, judgements of familiarity or of perceptual clarity (e.g. Whittlesea et al., 1990).

  C2 *A process that depends on its object being conscious.* One example would be reporting of the identity of an unanticipated but previously known stimulus, such as underlies the experience of spontaneously recognizing or 'noticing' (Bowers, 1984) a stimulus. This is a process which can be contrasted with 'unconscious' perceptual effects like priming. Another example is given by Alan Leslie (personal communication), who pointed out that there are non-routine 'decoupled' operations like pretending which can only be carried out on objects of which we are conscious.

2 Semi-experimentally characterised c-processes. There are the processes that are pre-experimentally associated with the occurrence of conscious experience but also have been intensively experimentally investigated. We will consider specifically the domain of memory. These include:

  C3 *The process of remembering a past event.* This is Tulving's (1983) 'autonoetic consciousness', which he holds to involve the process of 'ecphory', retrieval from episodic memory, discussed in Sections 10.1 and 10.8.[41] That this is a specifically conscious process has been the basis for the development of remember-know judgements extensively discussed in this chapter and the previous one.

  C4 *The encoding of information into episodic memory.* One of the standard ways of assessing whether something has been perceived is to test after list presentation whether a stimulus can be recalled (e.g. Dehaene et al., 2001). This presupposes that encoding into episodic memory involves awareness.

3 Experimentally characterised type-C processes. There are processes that are well captured in specific experimental paradigms, such as:

  C5 *The so-called Exclusion process developed by Jacoby (1991),* discussed in Section 4 of this chapter, in which subjects must select a response which does *not* correspond to the stimulus of which they are aware.

  C6 *The process involved in adding a stimulus to a discrimination response set.* Jack (1998) investigated a situation in which a letter was flashed to the subject for a brief exposure. The subject was told that

---

[40] As far as the terminology used so far in this book is concerned, the term *process* can relate to one or more combinations of *operations, accessing a representation, encoding, rehearsing or retrieving from a buffer,* the analogous processes related to *episodic memory* or to any of the Supervisory System processes discussed in Chapter 9.

[41] It is presupposed that the use of 'personal semantics', knowledge of one's past such as the day on which you were born (see Section 10.4 and FNMS chapter 15), does not qualify.

four different letters could occur but knew the identity of only three of these. Initially the stimuli were all heavily masked. Subjects were able to perform well above chance for the three known letters but were at chance for the fourth. Later in the experiment lighter masking was also used. If the fourth letter was then able to be identified under the lighter masking, it later became detectable under heavy masking at the same level as the three known letters.

This is of course a list that could potentially be greatly extended. Such generalizations provide a potentially more solid data base than that of a Mendeleev-table analogue of types of experience and philosophical characterisations of creature consciousness given in Section 11.8. Having a means of increasing the solidity of the database is important in the consciousness domain as otherwise the development of theory is grossly under-constrained. Thus returning to the Activation Strength theory, it becomes implausible as it has the problem that there is no apparent explanation as to why consciousness should have such properties.

We come now however to a theory of consciousness, which can address these properties better. There are many theories of consciousness which attempt to base it on neuroscientific concepts, but these concepts have been very diverse. They include for sensory awareness, gamma band oscillations (Crick & Koch, 1995), with its claimed role in the temporal binding together of the attributes of an experience (Engel & Singer, 2001), sustained activity in primary sensory areas such as visual area V1 (Lamme & Roelfsema, 2000), and the so-called P300 waveform (Vogel, Luck & Shapiro, 1998). However, as discussed in Section 11.5, another group of investigators have linked conscious experience to processing in parietal, cingulate and frontal cortices (e.g. Lumer & Rees, 1999; Kleinschmidt et al., 2002). This type of neuroscientific basis seems to have more promise in that it is potentially able to produce a link with functional or information-processing accounts which have a wider scope than being just concerned with perception. They may therefore address better the properties of creature consciousness considered in Section 11.8 and this section. The other approaches, by contrast, tend to be too oriented towards perceptual awareness alone. It is then to a theory relating to these last type of correspondences that we now turn.

11.11 The Global Workspace Approach

In the 1980s the American psychologist Bernie Baars developed the idea that consciousness should be conceived of as resulting from the operation of a *global workspace* or *blackboard* through which a very large number of otherwise autonomous specialised processors

communicate and collaborate with each other when tasks too complex for individual processors need to be carried out (see e.g. Baars, 1988; Baars et al., 1997).[42] And these specialised processors may display their output in the global workspace 'like actors who can appear on stage' (Baars et al., 1997, p. 430). Messages in the global workspace correspond to conscious contents. On this view consciousness is seen as creating 'global access' but having limited capacity, as only a restricted amount of information created by a small number of compatible processors can have effective access to the global workspace at any one time. It is, of course, a system-level theory of consciousness.

In its original form the global workspace approach to consciousness operated, however, as a rather loose AI analogy not closely linked to particular scientific paradigms. More recently, Stan Dehaene, Jean-Pierre Changeux and colleagues in Paris (Dehaene et al., 1998a; Dehaene & Naccache, 2001, Dehaene & Changeux, 2005; Dehaene et al., 2003, 2006) have presented a related idea in a more neuroscientific form, and critically through simulations and functional imaging experiments have linked the idea more directly to empirical evidence. Like Baars, they argue that the human brain contains, in addition to a large number of processing modules, a distributed system through which the large variety of specialist processors communicate. The communication medium is held to be a system of 'workspace' neurons, spread throughout the cortex but with long distance connections existing between them. They are thought to be particularly densely located in dorsolateral prefrontal cortex and the anterior cingulate which confers on these structures a major but not exclusive role in the operation of the workspace.

Dehaene and Naccache argue 'Through the workspace, modular systems that do not directly exchange information in an automatic mode can nevertheless gain access to each other's content' (p. 13) (see Figure 11.13). Unfortunately no example is given of this. Many modular processors, say, those used in syntactic processing and in making a visual transformation of a figure (say by rotation), would seem to have little useful to say to each other. Nor indeed would they operate on sets of compatible representations. The situation with systems not accessible to the workspace is clearer. Operations carried out by modular processors that are not directly connected to the workspace are never available as conscious contents. One simple example would be the

---

[42] The concept of a *blackboard* derives from early AI programs such as the *Hearsay* program for language comprehension (Erman et al., 1980) where specialised processors can exchange information by putting it on a blackboard.

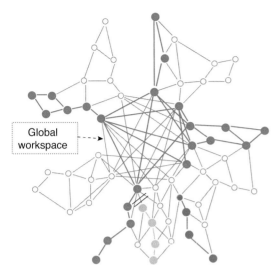

Fig. 11.13 The global workspace model of Dehaene and colleagues. The green lines represent connections between peripheral systems that are currently occupying the workspace. This prevents access to it by other peripheral processing systems (brown, red lines). Reprinted from *Trends in Cognitive Sciences, 10*(5), S. Dehaene, J.-P. Changeux, L. Naccache, J. Sackur and C. Sergent, Conscious, preconscious, and subliminal processing: a testable taxonomy, pp. 204–211. Copyright (2006) with permission from Elsevier.

superior colliculus circuitry for gaze control, which may well mediate the operations utilised in blindsight, as discussed in Sections 11.2 and 11.9.

Overall Dehaene and colleagues argue that five main systems participate in the workspace—perceptual circuits, motor circuits that allow controlled execution of action, long-term memory circuits, attentional top-down circuits and 'evaluation circuits' that attribute a valence to a previous experience. In addition it is suggested that 'top-down attentional amplification is the mechanism by which modular processes become temporally mobilized and made available to the global workspace' (Dehaene & Naccache, 2001, p. 14). Without this dynamic mobilization a process may contribute to cognitive performance but only unconsciously.

Figure 11.14 shows a neural network that provides a reductionist model for the basic idea. At the more macro-level it is assumed that a set of cell assemblies are organised in a feed-forward cascading fashion through four hierarchical levels of processing. Two of the levels (A and B) are specific to one input stream and two (C and D) correspond to the core of the global workspace, which rival inputs compete to claim.[43] At the more micro-level each assembly is represented as a

thalamo-cortical column composed of 80 excitatory and 40 inhibitory neurons organised in three layers. Neurons are modelled as so-called integrate-and-fire units.

If a short input burst is allowed to propagate through the feed-forward processors, each is activated to a relatively weak level of activation and then rapidly declines (see the white curves in Figure 11.15). This is held to correspond to the processing of a masked prime. Once, however, the input is above a certain strength, the *global neuronal workspace* network clicks in and sustained activity then follows both at all levels of the cascade at or above the assemblies that have top-down connections to the workspace and in the workspace itself (see the grey curves in Figure 11.15a). This *ignition* phenomenon corresponds to the transition from the white to the grey curve and can only occur for a single related complex of information at a time.

Since the 1950s it has been hypothesised that key central processes can only operate in an essentially serial fashion. Empirically phenomena such as the *psychological refractory period* have been described (Welford, 1952). This occurs when two signals, to each of which there is a well-learned response, are presented very close to each other in time. Then the response to the second is delayed by a time dependent on the interval between the stimuli. Welford held there was a processing bottleneck and the second stimulus must wait until the processing of the first stimulus was over (see also Pashler, 1998). Broadbent took over essentially the same idea in his single-channel hypothesis (see Figure 1.23).

An ignition process available to only a single line of thought at a time can be a computational neuroscience implementation of this idea. Dehaene and colleagues applied their model to a phenomenon quite closely related to the psychological refractory period—the so-called *attentional blink* phenomenon (Raymond et al., 1992). This involves the *rapid serial visual presentation (RSVP)* paradigm in which items in the same category, say letters or words or pictures, are presented one at a time at a rapid rate such as ten per second. One or more targets are distinguished in some way, say by being in a different colour from the other stimuli. The attentional blink refers to the way that detection of a target greatly impairs detection of a second target or other probe for a few hundred milliseconds starting very shortly after the target presentation. On the simulation of Dehaene et al. (2003), if levels C and D are occupied by detection of the first target, then ignition cannot occur in the processing of a second target presented shortly after (see Figure 11.16). Thus the theory predicts the existence of an attentional blink.[44]

---

[43] Levels A and B correspond to areas such as V1 or the frontal eye fields that are rapidly activated bottom-up; areas C and D would correspond to higher temporal, parietal, cingulate and frontal areas.

---

[44] The theory provides essentially the same explanation for the attentional blink and for the psychological refractory period.

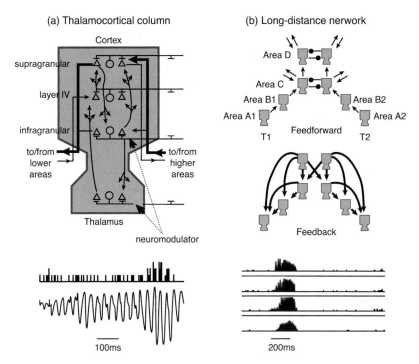

Fig. 11.14 (a) The structure of a single cell-assembly (a thalamocortical column) used in the simulations of Dehaene and colleagues, and the typical EEG-like oscillatory activity produced. (b) The overall organisation of such columns in the complete simulation, which shows firing activity corresponding to stable global states. Adapted from S. Dehaene and J.-P. Changeux, 2005, Ongoing spontaneous activity controls access to consciousness: a neuronal model for inattentional blindness. *PLoS Biology*, 3(5), 910–927.

Dehaene et al. (2006) distinguish three qualitatively different situations with respect to consciousness for processing of stimuli on any input stream. They echo Freud's terminology in calling them *subliminal, preconscious* and *conscious* (see Figure 11.17). Their functional imaging studies broadly support these distinctions. Thus in one condition of an fMRI study, Dehaene et al. (2001) presented words for 29 msec embedded in a stimulus stream in which the 71 msec that preceded and followed them were filled with a visually confusing mask. In a second condition these intervals were left blank. In the latter case—as tested by a variety of means—the words were generally seen, in the former case they were not. Thus in a subsidiary study the words were presented in the same way but subjects now had to say when they saw a word and if so to read it; they said they saw 90% of the non-masked words but only 1% of the masked ones. By comparison with otherwise identical trials, where no word was presented, masked

words led to activation of a sizeable part of the posterior left fusiform region including the visual word-form area discussed in Chapter 5.[45] By contrast in the supraliminal (second) condition many other areas of the prefrontal, cingulate and parietal cortices are activated (see Figure 11.18). This fits nicely with the findings of Rees and Lumer on rivalry discussed earlier.

This theory is the first real cognitive neuroscience theory of consciousness. It is well linked through simulations to empirical paradigms, such as the attentional blink. It is broadly supported by neuroscientific evidence, in particular functional imaging. Thus the findings of Dehaene et al. (2001) and related ones of Kouider et al. (2007) give broad support for the anatomical aspects of the global neuronal workspace theory. However, empirically the functional imaging findings are not completely compelling. They are also compatible with the activation strength position. In both conditions in the Dehaene et al. study, the activation in the left fusiform is the largest activation cluster and the most significant. Even in this area, though, the activation is much reduced when comparing the subliminal to the

---

Yet some have suggested that the capacity limitations of the two processes are at least in part different (e.g. Luck & Vogel, 2001). Thus meta-analyses of Marois and Ivanoff (2005) indicate that in the frontal cortex the attentional blink primarily involves lateral prefrontal cortex (see their figure 4) but the psychological refractory period involves the dorsal premotor cortex too, which is compatible with a motor execution component to its bottleneck.

---

[45] And also a region of the left precentral sulcus, for reasons that are unclear.

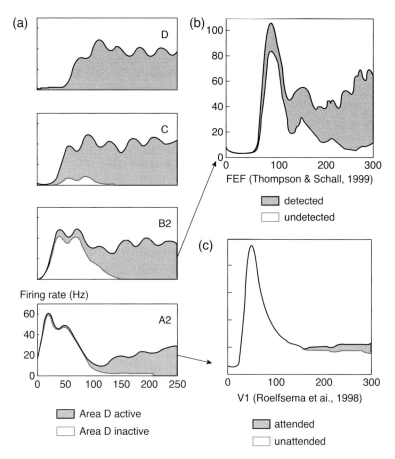

Fig. 11.15 Neural activity evoked by seen and unseen T2 targets in (a) the simulations of Dehaene and colleagues and neurophysiological records in monkey of (b) frontal eye fields with visual masking (Thompson and Schall, 1999) and (c) V1 with an attentional paradigm (Roelfsema et al, 1998). Trials in which area D (part of the global workspace) becomes active are characterised by long-lasting amplification in area C and, to a lesser extent, area B2. (See also Figure 11.14.) Reprinted with permission from S. Dehaene, C. Sergent and J.-P. Changeux, 2003, A neuronal network model linking subjective reports and objective physiological data during conscious perception. *Proceedings of the National Academy of Sciences, USA, 100*, 8520–8525. Copyright (2003) National Academy of Sciences, USA.

supraliminal condition (see Figure 11.18) and this is also so in the Kouider et al. (2007) study.[46]

At the same time the global neuronal workspace is conceptually much superior to the Activation Strength theory. It has an answer for all of the three major difficulties we raised with the Activation Strength type model. The threshold characteristics flow directly from the simulation which the theory includes. That activation in some structures does not produce any conscious correlates is simply explained in terms of accessibility to the global workspace. Also consciousness is *not* a property of particular individual subsystems but of a type of cross-system-level process that can occur in how a critical set of cognitive subsystems interact. It is not to be understood at the simple physical level where properties like physical proximity apply; so the third objection concerning nearby brains fails.

These functional reasons for preferring the global neuronal workspace theory to the more simple-minded Activation Strength approach are however, very general. Can the functioning of the global neuronal workspace be characterised more tightly?

11.12 The Functional Role of Consciousness

Consider first the anatomical basis of the global neuronal workspace. Why are the dorsolateral prefrontal cortex and anterior cingulate held to be critical brain regions for the global workspace? Anatomically it is

---

[46] The model needs some elaboration. The purely bottom-up relation between level A, level B and the higher levels in the feed-forward phase is probably over-simple in the light of evidence for the importance of recurrent activation down to area V1 (corresponding to level A) for conscious perception (Lamme, 2006). Thus Silvanto et al. (2005) showed that detection of motion in a briefly exposed array was disrupted by TMS over V5 about 120 msec post-stimulus onset, but later—at about 140 msec post-stimulus onset—by TMS over V1!

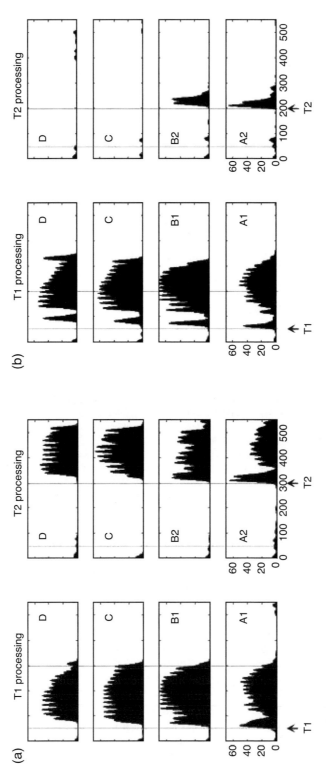

Fig. 11.16 Results of simulations by Dehaene et al. (2003) of two trials of the attentional blink task. The boxes represent activity of simulated neurons in different regions of the model, with the lower boxes (A1, B1, A2, B2) corresponding to neurons outside of the global workspace and the upper boxes (C, D) corresponding to neurons within the global workspace. (a) A 'seen' trial, where the interval between targets is long (250ms). (b) A 'blinked' trial, where the interval between targets is short and T2 activity fails to progress into the global workspace due to occupation of the workspace by T1. Reprinted with permission from S. Dehaene, C. Sergent and J.-P. Changeux, 2003, A neuronal network model linking subjective reports and objective physiological data during conscious perception. *Proceedings of the National Academy of Sciences, USA, 100*, 8520–8525. Copyright (2003) National Academy of Sciences, USA.

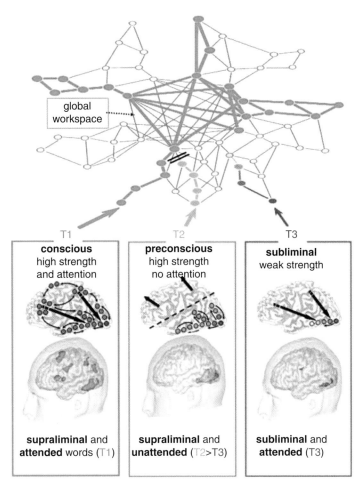

Fig. 11.17 A taxonomy of processing types within the global workspace model of Dehaene and colleagues. In conscious processing (green) the global workspace is invaded by content originating in a peripheral processor. Preconscious processing (yellow) occurs when peripheral processors are not attended. In subliminal processing (red) peripheral processors can affect processing in the global workspace (e.g. by priming) but the workspace is not taken over by the outputs of the peripheral processors. Reprinted with permission from S. Kouider and S. Dehaene, 2007, Levels of processing during non-conscious perception: a critical review of visual masking. *Philosophical Transactions of the Royal Society, B, 362*, 857–875; figure 3, p. 870.

stated that the global neuronal workspace is mediated by long-range connectivity, and Dehaene et al. (1998a) hold that long-range cortico-cortico connections mostly arise from layers 2 and 3 of the 6-layer cortical sheath. These layers, they argue, although present throughout the cortex are particularly thick in the prefrontal cortex and inferior parietal cortical structures. A second anatomical reason is to follow Goldman-Rakic (1987) who pointed out that dorsolateral prefrontal cortex—or more specifically area 46—was a major component of a network of connections involving the anterior cingulate and part of the posterior parietal cortex, amongst other areas.[47]

But why functionally might such regions be critical for consciousness? Dehaene and Naccache (2001) argue that they 'do not seem to be needed for automatised tasks but appear suddenly when an automatised task calls for conscious control' (p. 24). More specifically three types of process are considered—post-buffer retention of information in working memory, the producing of novel combinations of operations and intentional, that is non-automatic, behaviour. This approach identifies conscious processes with those responsible for cognitive control. This idea has a long history in modern human experimental psychology being expressed using different conceptual frameworks by Mandler (1975), Posner (1978) and Umiltà (1988) among others.

In the conceptual framework being articulated in this book, it corresponds to a possible link between

---

[47] The other regions in the circuit were the superior temporal sulcus, the parahippocampal gyrus, the posterior cingulate and a superior posterior medial parietal area.

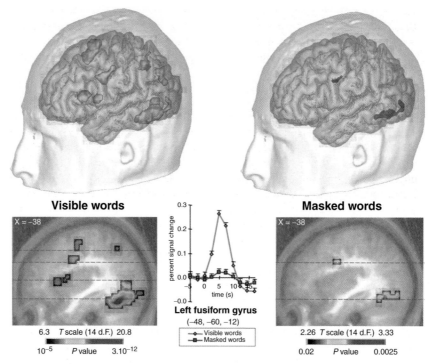

Fig. 11.18 Results of the fMRI study of word identification of Dehaene et al. (2001). When words were masked activation was seen in the fusiform word form area (and the precentral sulcus), relative to a no-word condition. When words were visible there was additional activation in prefrontal, cingulate and parietal regions. Note the difference in activation strength between masked and unmasked conditions in the left fusiform gyrus. Reprinted by permission from Macmillan Publishers Ltd: *Nature Neuroscience* (S. Dehaene, L. Naccache, L. Cohen, D.L. Bihan, J.-F. Mangin, 2001, Cerebral mechanisms of word masking and unconscious repetition priming. *Nature Neuroscience*, 4(7), 752–758), copyright (2001).

conscious processes and Supervisory System processes. Jack and Shallice (2001) develop a position of this type. More specifically they argue that a type-C process is a process with two properties:

1 It involves the Supervisory System, and in particular outputs from the energising and/or task-setting systems.[48]

2 These outputs from the Supervisory System lead directly to the selection in contention scheduling of an action or thought schema together with the setting of its arguments. This selection in turn leads to action and/or to qualitative change in the operation of a lower-level special-purpose processing system or systems.[49]

Crucially, and in common with the global workspace theory, consciousness relates to the collective effect of supervisory subprocesses on the other processing systems. Such outputs can alter the long-term operation of the cognitive system much more widely than the outputs of other informationally encapsulated systems. Thus if the system can reflect on its own operation—which it can—it would be valuable to have a special concept to characterise such outputs of the Supervisory System. This special concept is held to be *consciousness*. This breadth of effects is a similar property to that held to hold for the global workspace on the Dehaene–Changeux theory. By contrast a process that does not involve output from the Supervisory System would not give rise to a conscious experience. Moreover this would apply to a process purely internal to the Supervisory System which did not lead to a major change in its output. Thus the theory developed in Chapter 9 holds that when any non-overlearned action is being executed, and also for routine actions when the situation is more critical than usual, the environment and the progress

---

[48] It is presupposed that sentence comprehension requires mediation via the Supervisory System so that a novel sentence could not be comprehended without awareness. See creature consciousness property 9.

[49] This would be a relatively slow serial process thus supporting the criticism made by Dennett and Kinsbourne (1992) of Libet's arguments, discussed in Section 11.6. From the localisationist perspective, the Supervisory System outputs would be from lateral prefrontal cortex, the inputs to the contention

scheduling system in premotor cortex and the SMA, as discussed in Chapter 9.

of the operations are being monitored on many levels. The effects of this monitoring will however only become conscious when the monitoring system detects that something is not as it should be and so interrupts on-going action.

As we have seen in Chapter 9, supervisory processes may be identified with prefrontal processes with some caveats. A conscious act should therefore activate lateral prefrontal cortex or the anterior cingulate.[50] If one takes the properties of consciousness considered in Section 11.10, of the ones that can be immediately related to experimental paradigms—in other words— the semi-experimental and experimental type C-processes, they involve prefrontal processes extensively. Thus the role of prefrontal cortex in encoding and retrieval of episodic memory was extensively discussed in Chapter 10. The Jacoby exclusion task is conceptually similar to the Hayling B Sentence Completion task, which has a strong prefrontal involvement, as discussed in Section 9.12. Adding a stimulus to a discriminating response set is setting up 'target specification', widely held to be a prefrontal characteristic (e.g. Houghton & Tipper, 1996).

But, a sceptic might say, you have selected the empirical criteria for creature consciousness to fit the theoretical framework. For instance, this type of position on consciousness has been characterised by the philosopher-of-mind Ned Block as being of reflexive consciousness only. It is not. Consider a climber trying to move up a rock face. He or she is intimately aware of all sorts of cracks and lips in the rock, of other possible holds, of the difficulties in making particular sorts of movement, of the space below. Supervisory System processes are strongly involved in this type of visuo-spatial problemsolving. But unless the climber becomes very afraid, he or she is not reflexively conscious of the thought processes. The mind is filled by the immediate practical difficulties.

Recently there have been suggestions that the prefrontal cortex, and in particular its output, does not have a special relation to consciousness. Thus van Gaal et al. (2008) write 'complex behaviors are often thought to result from conscious cognitive control .... Inhibitory control, the ability to cancel a planned or already initiated action, is an extreme form of cognitive control, in larger part relying on the prefrontal cortex ... and associated exclusively with consciousness. A crucial issue is

whether such high-level cognitive (control) processes are evident in the absence of consciousness' (p. 8053). They explored a go/no-go task in which the subject has to make a response given one type of stimulus but to withhold it given another stimulus. Patients with frontal lobe lesions, particularly to area 6 and area 46, make an excessive number of false alarms. They fail to withhold responses when they should (Drewe, 1975; Picton et al., 2007). Van Gaal et al. used so-called metacontrast (Figure 11.19), a masking procedure in which a grey circle presented for 17 msec is followed by a black ring. The grey circle fits exactly inside the black ring. When the gap between the two is a mere 17 msec the grey circle is not seen; in another condition it is 83 ms and in that case the grey circle is typically seen. The subject's task is to respond to the black ring except if a grey circle occurs first.

Van Gaal et al. found that even when the grey ring was not seen the response was delayed, and they provide ERP evidence that prefrontal cortex was activated. However there is no evidence that outputs from the Supervisory System occur sufficient to dominate the operation of contention scheduling (C-processes). Thus the rate of correctly inhibiting a triggered response only went up from 1% of trials for a control condition to 2.25% in the experimental condition. This compares with 61% for the conscious inhibition condition.[51] Moreover the RT for the unconscious no-go condition was identical to that in the go condition. There is no evidence that strong outputs from the Supervisory System occurred, and so this study presents no problem for the presented theoretical framework.

Much the same group of investigators carried out a second study (van Gaal et al., 2009) using a related task—the stop signal task—where the signal to inhibit the response occurs after the stimulus. This study uses the same procedure except now the grey circle and black ring occur after the go-stimulus on which the subject must begin the response process. The go-stimulus required a tricky blue–green discrimination, which led to go-response RTs of about 620 msec. On every trial a black ring occurs and on some there is also a briefly presented grey circle. This can occur immediately before the black ring (*short-stop trials*) or at least 100 msec before (*long-stop trials*). In the latter case, but not the former, the grey circle is typically seen. If, however, the grey circle is seen, the response must be stopped in its tracks. Subjects could do this if the grey circle occurred no more than 320 msec after the onset of the go-stimulus.

---

[50] This may not be easily detectable in some situations, especially with subtraction designs as they would require the subject not to be similarly conscious in control conditions too. Thus in Boly et al.'s background studies for the investigation of the vegetative state, where prefrontal activation is generally not found the comparison is with rest, but subjects are conscious during rest.

[51] A non-significant rise from 0.8% to 2.0% was also obtained on unconscious no-go trials when subjects were asked to explicitly discriminate go from no-go trials.

(a) Masked Go/No-Go task

(b) Control experiment

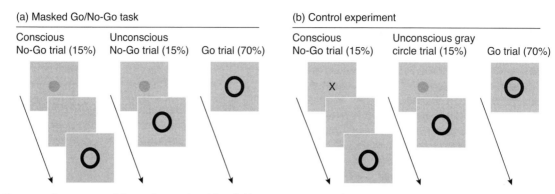

Fig. 11.19 The experimental design of van Gaal et al. (2008). (a) The go/no-go task. Subjects were required to respond to the black circle, unless it is preceded by a gray disk. In no-go trials the no-go stimulus appeared for 16.7 msec. It was followed either immediately or after a short interval (83.3 msec) by the black circle. (b) The control task. Here the no-go stimulus was a black cross, and the gray circle was irrelevant. Reprinted with permission from S. van Gaal, K.R. Ridderinkhof, J.J. Fahrenfort, H.S. Scholte and V.A.F. Lamme, 2008, Frontal cortex mediates unconsciously triggered inhibitory control. *The Journal of Neuroscience, 28*(32), 8053–8062.

Again we are concerned with what happens if the grey circle is present but not seen. There was a small but clear slowing effect on unconscious short-stop trials, which was related to how good the subject was at the task (see Figure 11.20). However this effect only occurred by possibly the second and more convincingly third session of testing, and subjects were performing nearly 1000 trials in each session. By this time one would expect schemas and trigger functions to be developing in contention scheduling, so inhibition effects could well be occurring at that level even in the absence of top-down signals from prefrontal cortex as would be assumed on the current approach if there is no conscious perception of a stop signal. Again the study presents no problem for the presented theoretical framework.[52]

A final study that appears to present difficulties is that of Lau and Passingham (2007). They too used meta-contrast. In this case an instruction stimulus of 50ms which could be a square or a diamond was followed after 100 msec by a word that lasted 300 msec. The instruction stimulus specified which task was to be carried out with the word. If it was a square, the subject's task was phonological: they had to decide whether the word contained two syllables or not. Instead if it was a

diamond, subjects had a semantic task: they had to decide if the word was a concrete object. The instruction stimuli were cleverly designed so that they each masked a smaller square or diamond (the prime) presented for 33 msec, if they occurred at the appropriate time before (see Figure 11.21).

There were two possible intervals between the prime and the instruction stimulus—a short one, i.e. 16 msec, and a long one, i.e. 83 msec. The behavioural results echoed earlier findings of Vorberg et al. (2003) in showing poorer performance in the long interval condition only in the incongruent condition—if the prime was different from the instruction stimulus i.e. a square preceding a diamond. The theoretically critical findings in this study were functional imaging ones. Lau and Passingham specified two regions determined on the basis of experiments related to those of Sakai and Passingham (2003), discussed in Section 9.5 as ones which would be activated at schema level for the phonological and semantic tasks. For the long interval condition, but not the short interval one, the degree of activation in these regions was affected by whether the primes were congruent or not. Finally, and most critically, in the long interval condition, but that alone, there was increased activation in left mid-dorsolateral regions for incongruent but not congruent primes, again in the long interval condition (see Figure 11.22).

Lau and Passingham argue their results refute the claim that 'mid-DLPFC is exclusive to conscious processing' (p. 5810), but the result is only critical for the present approach if two different things hold, and neither is shown. First, the mid-dorsolateral activation must be part of the causal chain leading to a slow response. Second, there must be lack of awareness not only of the stimuli but also of, say, whether the subject is sure of the response. Yet, if the incongruent long interval condition leads to slower coding of the instruction

---

[52] The idea that automatic inhibitory processes may be mediated at the contention scheduling level is derived from Sumner and Husain (2008). They use the framework to account for a variety of phenomena including utilisation behaviour (see Section 9.2) and the so-called negative compatibility effect (Schlaghecken & Eimer, 2006) in which an unseen masked prime has a facilitatory effect if it precedes a stimulus by 0–60 msec but an inhibitory effect if it occurs 100–200 msec beforehand. The possible automatisation of response inhibition in the stop signal paradigm is discussed by Verbruggen and Logan (2008).

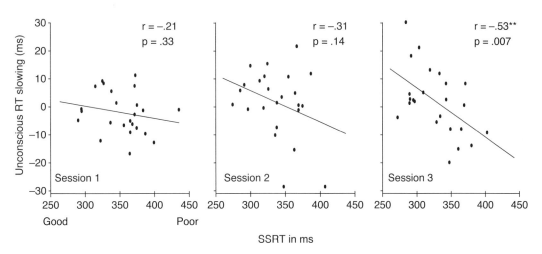

Fig. 11.20 Scatter plots showing the correlation between unconscious RT slowing (i.e. the difference in mean RT on short-stop trials versus short-go trials) and stop-signal RT across the three sessions of the study of van Gaal et al. (2009). Copyright © 2009 by the American Psychological Association. Reproduced with permission. S. van Gaal, K.R. Ridderinkhof, W.P.M. van den Wildenberg and V.A.F. Lamme, 2009, Dissociating consciousness from inhibitory control: Evidence for unconsciously triggered response inhibition in the stop-signal task, *Journal of Experimental Psychology: Human Perception and Performance, 35*(4), 1129–1139. The use of APA information does not imply endorsement by APA.

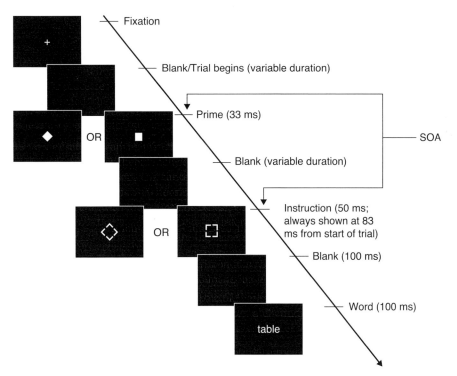

Fig. 11.21 The experimental design of Lau and Passingham (2007). The briefly presented prime (small diamond or small square) was followed by a symbolic instruction which indicated the task to be carried out on the following word, which either involved a semantic (diamond) or phonological (square) decision. The interval between the prime and the instruction was either short (16 msec) or long (83 msec), and the prime could be either congruent or incongruent with the instruction. Reprinted with permission from H.C. Lau and R.E. Passingham, 2007, Unconscious activation of the cognitive control system in the human prefrontal cortex. *The Journal of Neuroscience, 27*(21), 5805–5811.

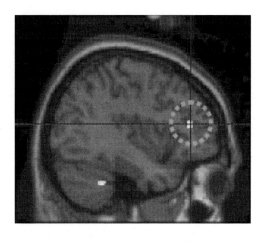
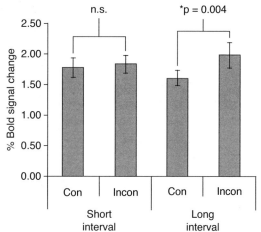

Fig. 11.22 Greater activation in left mid-dorsolateral area in the long interval condition for incongruent rather than congruent stimuli. A similar effect is not found for the short interval condition. Reprinted with permission from H.C. Lau and R.E. Passingham, 2007, Unconscious activation of the cognitive control system in the human prefrontal cortex. *The Journal of Neuroscience, 27*(21), 5805–5811.

stimulus, as it may well do given the related findings of Vorberg et al., then the processing of the instruction stimulus and of the word itself—very briefly presented a mere 100 msec later—will become dreadfully entangled; it would not be surprising if the dorsolateral PFC needed to become involved. Such a speculation remains to be tested. However, as Kouhou (personal communication) points out, one would have in this condition a cognitive analogue of the psychological refractory period and the lateral prefrontal cortex is known to be activated in this type of paradigm (Marois and Ivanoff, 2005). Thus awareness of the prime—or lack of it—may not be the critical factor in the prefrontal activation obtained.

But is this emphasis on prefrontal cortex with respect to consciousness overdone? Thus it is often argued that patients with extensive bilateral prefrontal lesions remain fully conscious (Pollen, 2008).[53] Take the philosopher O'Shaughnessy's perspective. His position on consciousness has one important aspect we have yet to discuss. Of the different types of experience he holds one to be special—perception. 'Even though perception does not actually fill the conscious mind, it is an overwhelming presence, especially the visual variety. We wake to consciousness every morning and light floods in upon as we do, and so long as consciousness endures our surroundings steadily impinge upon

us in this concrete sensuous fashion, also absorbing much of our attention at the time!' (pp. 6–7). However it is not for him just a question of quantity which marks perception out from all other forms of experience. He argues it is the one type of experience that it is inconceivable that a conscious mind could lack the power to have.

Is the view that perceptual experiences have a special place in consciousness by contrast to other types of experience compatible with the information-processing types of theory discussed above? Driver and Vuilleumier (2001) have argued that the spatial functions of the inferior parietal cortex may be intimately linked with visual experience. Referring to unilateral neglect, where the patient loses all awareness of half of space (see Section 1.8), they say 'We would not suggest that perceptual awareness resides exclusively in the parietal lobe and those interconnected brain structures which are also implicated in neglect. But we would be amazed if these brain areas do not turn out to play a very major role' (p. 78). They argue that the inferior parietal lobe is critical for computing stable representations of the location of external stimuli relative to the observer. Moreover they echo Treisman (1998) in arguing that visual awareness may depend upon binding of many types of visual property; they suggest that the inferior parietal cortex may be critical here too.[54]

Most critically they point out that when the neglect patient loses information about the left part of space, what is lost is not just spatial information but also all

[53] We know of no convincing reports on the cognitive effects of complete bilateral prefrontal lesions. Prefrontal leucotomy certainly does not generally produce this result (Meyer, Beck & McLardy, 1947). Indeed, Gazzaniga (1966) described lesions in two split-brain monkeys beginning at the frontal pole and extending slightly outside the isolated full frontal lobe as apparently producing functional blindness in the relevant hemisphere.

[54] But see the discussion of attentional dyslexia in FNMS Chapter 11, which suggests that the left pulvinar may also be important in this respect.

other aspects of perceptual experience. By contrast a prosopagnosic patient who is no longer able to recognise faces or an achromatoposic patient who no longer sees colour can have access to all other types of information about the object. Driver and Vuilleumier therefore argue that 'our internal representations of external space (at the level of multi-modal sensorimotor interfaces) provided the basic medium for perceptual experience .... From a philosophical perspective this may in part reflect a special role for location in the mental representation of "out there"' (pp. 74–75).

Returning to the perspective previously developed of the link between Supervisory System outputs and conscious experience, it does not seem likely that the experience of the visual field is explicable in terms of the two properties concerning the Supervisory System outputs that were linked to conscious experience earlier in the section. Moreover, although, it has not yet been discussed, one of the properties of creature consciousness also does not fit well with the Supervisory System approach to consciousness previously being considered. This is the contrast between the foreground and background of consciousness. It seems appropriate to modify the mapping of the two Supervisory System properties into phenomenology made earlier in this section and say they provide a processing correspondence for the foreground of consciousness. The background of consciousness corresponds to representations that can be very rapidly brought to the foreground. In other words it corresponds to representations that can be accessed by means of the inferior parietal visuo-spatial attention system.

This distinction relates to one drawn by Lambie and Marcel (2002) who argue for a distinction between *phenomenology*—what something is like—and *awareness*—a kind of knowing (see also Block, 1995). They give the example of Anton's syndrome where the cortically blind patient denies being blind, which they interpret

as phenomenology without awareness. In the current framework it would correspond to the failure of the visuo-spatial attentional control systems to bring any part of the visual field to the focus of attention. However, one potential difficulty for this way of producing different types of phenomenological correspondence for the prefrontal and parietal activations is provided by Kinsbourne's (1988) example of admiring a view. Here we may assume that a particular set of visual attentional routines (or schemas) are selected so that the spatial focus of attention is not limited to an individual object. Instead it is spread over a wide section of the visual field. However, at the same time the function is not apparently to aid an attentional shift to a different representation. Undoubtedly to adequately account for this situation, one will need a theory of aesthetics, which is well outside the scope of this book!

In the light then of the arguments presented by Driver and Vuilleumier one may add a second system in addition to the Supervisory System to those related to consciousness, namely the spatial attention systems of the inferior parietal cortex.[55] They may be seen as the location of the pointers to the elements of perceptual representations that are available for triggering schema selection and forming their arguments. They correspond phenomenologically to the *background of consciousness* (see point 6 of Section 11.8). It should be noted, however, that if O'Shaughnessy is correct, there will be no further systems to be added to the list of those critical for consciousness. Perceptual experience is held to be special.[56]

The last decade has seen a great advance in the study of consciousness. A plausible model—the global neuronal workspace—has been developed and a rich set of experimental studies are producing critical findings. It should not be too long before a definitive theory is developed.

---

[55] They are part of the global workspace.

[56] An interesting other possibility relates to emotion. As Lambie (2009; see also Lambie & Marcel, 2002) says about, at least, one form of experience—emotion experience—that it can 'only play a part in rational action if one is appropriately (i.e. reflectively) aware of it' (p. 272), but emotional phenomenology—in their terminology—would not require it. However, emotion is not addressed in this book.

Thinking

12.1 Introduction

Thinking, like consciousness, is one of the most central yet mysterious aspects of the mind. Can a cognitive neuroscience approach improve our understanding of it? It was argued in Chapter 9 that supervisory processes, such as task setting, energisation and monitoring, modulate the basic operation of contention scheduling in non-routine or novel situations. Moreover, it was argued that these are separable processes with frontal localisations that differ (left lateral, superior medial and right lateral, respectively). These 'elementary' executive functions are held to play key roles in the control of non-routine behaviour, but they are insufficiently specified to account for the generation of most complex intelligent behaviours. Consider the processes involved in solving a Sudoku puzzle, or those required in planning a holiday (arranging transport and accommodation subject to numerous constraints), or more generally the process or processes loosely characterised as *thinking*. Thus, the conceptual framework developed so far in this book needs refinement.

Within cognitive psychology, discussion of thinking is standardly organised around specific types, such as problem-solving, reasoning, decision-making and so on. One difficulty with this approach is that it implicitly endorses the view that each form of thinking is self-contained, not just with respect to the findings of interest but even in the cognitive processes involved. This is reinforced by the way that each form of thinking has also spawned a different set of tasks for its study. Thus, within the reasoning literature the primary tasks of choice have been variations of syllogistic reasoning (Johnson-Laird & Steedman, 1978) and the Wason card-selection task (Wason, 1968). In the former, subjects are required to deduce the relation between categories A and C from one statement that expresses a relation between categories A and B and another that expresses a relation between categories B and C. In the latter, subjects are required to indicate what information is needed to verify a simple rule of the form 'if A then B'. The key debates have then concerned whether thinking is based on the construction of 'mental models' (Johnson-Laird, 1983, 2006), the application of formal rules of inference (i.e. the 'mental logic' of Rips, 1994, and Braine & O'Brien, 1998) or Bayesian inference (Oaksford & Chater, 1994, 2007).

In contrast to the reasoning literature, within the problem-solving literature researchers have distinguished between well-defined and ill-defined problems, focussing in the former case on tasks such as game playing (e.g. chess, draughts, etc.), puzzles involving the movement or rearrangement of pieces (such as the Tower of Hanoi and the Tower of London problems discussed at length in Section 12.5), and number puzzles (e.g. cryptarithmetic: Newell & Simon, 1972; see Figure 1.20). For ill-defined problems the focus has often been on so-called *insight problems* where the approach to the problem is not obvious and where the solution is accompanied by a sudden phenomenological experience of insight.[1] The conception of thinking that has emerged from the study of well-defined problems has been as search in a space of *problem states* for one or more goal states (Newell & Simon, 1972), with legitimate moves in the game or puzzle corresponding to transitions between problem states. The key issue has then been to specify search heuristics (such as hill-climbing, means-ends analysis and limited look-ahead) and their conditions of use. By contrast, ill-defined problem-solving research has mainly focussed on the characteristics of a problem that block problem-solving and how such blockages may be overcome.

The third major subdivision of thinking research, decision-making, has employed yet another set of canonical tasks—tasks involving selecting the best from a set of alternatives that vary on a range of dimensions, including tasks where information on some dimensions is uncertain or unavailable. This has led to a view of thinking as involving the application of either economic utility theory subject to cognitive biases (Kahneman & Tversky, 1973; Tversky & Kahneman, 1974), or simple resource-bound choice heuristics (Gigerenzer et al., 1999).

The existence of such different conceptions of thinking may just reflect the flexibility of thought processes, which can be directed towards a range of apparently distinct situations. Indeed, the wide divergence in theoretical approaches should, if the overall approach of this book is correct, make thinking a prime candidate for the fruitful application of the methods of cognitive neuroscience. Yet it is not clear that the topic of thinking is amenable in principle to the methods of cognitive neuroscience. As discussed in Chapter 3, Fodor (1983) famously argued that central processes were non-modular. If this were the case, one would expect a cognitive neuroscience approach to thinking to flounder. In practice, however, research on thinking has ignored Fodor by extensively applying the methods of cognitive neuroscience. In this chapter we will therefore address whether, given this work, the rejection of Fodor's pessimism in his core domain of thinking has been justified. We begin by considering one of the simplest forms of thinking, namely reasoning with relations.

12.2 Reasoning with Relations

Consider first reasoning with relations such as *bigger* or *taller*, where the things being related may be mapped to a dimension (*size* or *height* in these examples) and where, if the relation holds between A and B and between B and C, then it may be inferred that the relation must also hold between A and C. This most basic form of reasoning with relational information is known as transitive inference. Transitive inference has been reported in animal species ranging from pigeons (Delius & Siemann, 1998) to squirrel monkeys (McGonigle & Chalmers, 1992), as well as in children as young as 3 to 4 years of age (Goswami, 1995).

In animal studies, animals are typically trained to prefer one of a pair of stimuli. Transitive inference is shown when an animal that has been trained to prefer A to B and B to C spontaneously prefers A to C. Acuna et al. (2002) applied this methodology to human subjects using a set of eleven arbitrarily ordered shapes of various sizes and colours (see Figure 12.1). Subjects were presented with pairs of figures that, they were told, were adjacent items in a sequence and asked to select the figure closest to a given end figure. Initially subjects had no reason for selecting either figure, but they were provided with feedback after each trial. It was argued that this would allow them to learn the linear order of the entire sequence, as in the animal studies.[2] Once subjects had learned the sequence (as indicated by greater than 90% accuracy on forced choice), they were scanned

---

[1] Insight can also occur in well-defined problems such as chess and may well be a major reason they are so addictive. However it has been less studied there.

[2] The task bears a family resemblance to ones used in the literature concerning whether an internal number line is a basis for arithmetic processing (see Fias & Fischer, 2005).

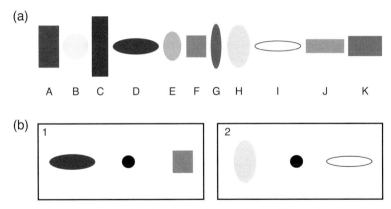

Fig. 12.1 The transitive inference task of Acuna et al. (2002). With stimuli such as those in (b), the subject must decide which of the two figures is closest to the right hand end of the sequence shown in (a). The stimulus set for the transitive inference sequence consisted of eleven stimuli of different shapes and hues. The entire sequence was never seen. Instead, stimuli were shown in pairs during both learning and testing phases. The letters below each shape are presented in the figure for explanatory purposes—they were not presented to subjects. For any given pair of stimuli, the correct choice was always the stimulus closest to K. (b) Display configuration of stimuli in the MR scanner. The circle in the centre served as the fixation point and the flanking stimuli were items from the sequence. Scans contrasted neural activity during transitive inference and a height comparison control task that used the same stimuli. Reproduced from B.T Acuna, J.C. Eliassen, J.P. Donoghue and J.N. Sanes, Frontal and parietal lobe activation during transitive inference in humans, *Cerebral Cortex*, 2002, *12*(12), 1312–1321, by permission of Oxford University Press.

using fMRI while (a) applying their acquired knowledge of the sequence to non-adjacent stimulus pairs, and (b) performing a perceptual comparison task with similar stimuli. In the former condition, subjects were faster and more accurate on non-adjacent items when there were many intervening items than when there were few intervening items. Acuna et al. argue from this behavioural evidence that transitive inference involves 'actively searching a unified mental model, similar to … mentally visualizing a map' (p. 1317).[3] Comparison of the BOLD responses in the two conditions revealed significantly greater bilateral activation in a network of areas, including the middle and superior frontal gyri (including BA 9 and 46), insula, and extensive regions of the posterior parietal cortices (BA 7, 39 and 40). The authors interpret this activity in terms of search of a spatial representation, attributing dorsolateral frontal activation to a process of 'manipulating relations among visual shapes' (p. 1317) and parietal cortical activation to 'spatial-like operations' (p. 1318).

The interpretation of parietal activity given by Acuna et al. shows the beguiling but potentially misleading nature of imaging data in the field of higher cognitive functions. The difficulty stems from the great extent of the parietal activity, the wide variety of different functions supported by the parietal cortices (see Section 10.7), and the lack of a clearly specified model of performance on the task. Thus, if search of a spatial representation is

involved, how does this relate to processes of 'manipulating relations among visual shapes' and 'spatial-like operations'?

A second concern with the study of Acuna and colleagues relates to whether performance during the transitive inference condition actually involves transitive inference. Cognitive studies of inference treat the integration of two (or more) premises to be the critical process in inference. However, the behavioural data, and also Acuna et al.'s interpretation, suggest that this integration is done during the learning phase of their experiment, and not while subjects were being scanned.

Consider then a second study. Vinod Goel and colleagues (2007) explored transitive inference in three groups of subjects: 9 left prefrontal patients, 9 right prefrontal patients, and 22 age- and education-matched controls. The authors were specifically interested in the difference between reasoning in determinate situations, where two transitive premises fully specify the order of the three objects (e.g. A > B, B > C), and indeterminate situations, where the two premises specify only a partial order over the three objects (e.g. A > B, A > C). Prior to testing, the concept of logical validity was explained to all subjects. They then worked through 102 problems, each consisting of three statements such as 'Mary is smarter than John. Michael is smarter than John. Mary is smarter than Michael'. Their task was to evaluate whether the third statement followed logically from the first two. Control subjects performed at similar levels on determinate and indeterminate problems (see Figure 12.2). Left-frontal patients were impaired relative to controls on both problem types, while right-frontal patients were specifically impaired on indeterminate

---

[3] In the literature there is a contrast between spatial and non-spatial means of tackling, say, 3-term series problems, which goes back to Huttenlocher (1968).

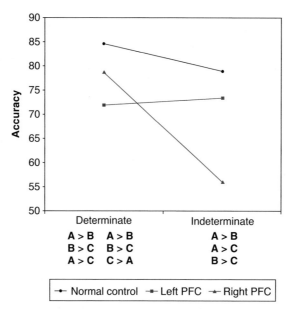

Fig. 12.2 Accuracy in verifying the logical validity of three-term transitive inference problems involving determinate and indeterminate premises in the study of Goel et al. (2007). Left frontal patients showed a general impairment across all problem types. Right frontal patients were specifically impaired on problems involving indeterminate premises.Reproduced from V. Goel, M. Tierney, L. Sheesley, A. Bartolo, O. Vartanian and J. Grafman. Hemispheric specialization in human prefrontal cortex for resolving certain and uncertain inferences, *Cerebral Cortex*, 2007, *17*(10), 2245–2250, by permission of Oxford University Press.

problems. Goel and colleagues argue that the deficit of right-frontal patients lies in an inability to maintain an ambiguous representation, as required by indeterminate problems. What this amounts to in computational terms is unclear. One possibility, consistent with a model-based approach to reasoning, is that right-frontal patients fail to generate or maintain more than one model that is consistent with a set of premises. Alternatively, the difficulties of right-frontal patients with indeterminate problems may be due to faulty active monitoring. To correctly reject an indeterminate problem as logically invalid, one must detect not only that the conclusion is consistent with the premises, but also that there is a second conclusion that is also valid. It probably requires an active checking process to see that a second valid conclusion exists.

A somewhat different interpretation of the key processes involved in transitive inference is held to follow from a second patient study, that of Waltz and colleagues (1999). This study investigated the reasoning abilities, episodic memory and semantic knowledge of a group of fronto-temporal dementia (FTD) patients, a disorder discussed in Section 6.3. The patients were divided into frontal-variant (*n* = 6) and temporal-variant (*n* = 5) FTD subgroups, the latter presumably having semantic dementia. Two reasoning tests were administered—a transitive inference test and an inductive reasoning test. Both tests required that subjects combine information from two binary relations to obtain their solutions. Thus, in the transitive inference test, patients

were presented with a series of statements of the form 'Sam is taller than Nate', 'Nate is taller than Roy'. Their task was to arrange the names given in those statements into a linear order (from tallest to shortest). In one condition, the statements introduced the names in height order, allowing subjects to use a simple chaining strategy linking one statement to the next. In the other condition, the order in which the statements were presented was scrambled, meaning that subjects had to consider simultaneously pairs of relations. Temporal-variant FTD patients performed as well as age and education-matched controls in both conditions. Frontal-variant FTD patients also performed well in the easier condition, but when two relations had to be combined they performed at chance levels. Similar results were found in the inductive reasoning test, which was based on *Progressive Matrices*:[4] the frontal-variant FTD patients were selectively impaired when multiple relations had to be integrated. In contrast, temporal-variant FTD patients were selectively impaired on the episodic and semantic memory tasks.

Waltz and colleagues explain the difficulties that frontal-variant FTD patients have in terms of a specific process of *relational integration* being necessary when

---

[4] 'Progressive Matrices' is often called 'Raven's'. It was invented by Penrose and Raven (1936). Lionel Penrose was the father of Roger Penrose, the mathematician and Jonathan Penrose, for many years British chess champion.

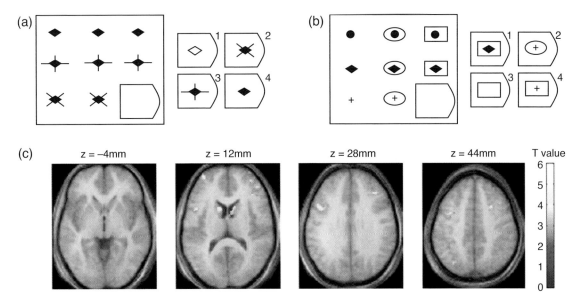

Fig. 12.3 Stimuli used and imaging results of the study of Christoff et al. (2001). (a) A progressive matrix problem in which the solution (item 2) does not require integration of information across rows or columns. (b) A progressive matrix problem in which the solution requires abstracting a common feature across rows and columns and combining this to produce the solution (item 4). (c) Brain regions more active for problems of type (b) than of type (a), as revealed by fMRI with RT-convolved heamodynamic response function. Reprinted from *NeuroImage, 14*(5), K. Christoff, V. Prabhakaran, J. Dorfman, Z. Zhao, J.K. Kroger, K.J. Holyoak and J.D.E. Gabrieli, Rostrolateral prefrontal cortex involvement in relational integration during reasoning, 1136–1149, Copyright (2001), with permission from Elsevier.

information concerning two or more relations must be integrated into a single representation, as required by both transitive and inductive inference tests. They hypothesise that this process is supported by the prefrontal cortex and moreover that an impairment of the process is responsible for the difficulties that frontal patients often have with other thinking tasks (as discussed in subsequent sections of this chapter).

Numerous studies support the claim that prefrontal processes are involved in both relational and inductive reasoning. It is less clear that the difficulties found in both tasks following prefrontal cortical damage are due to a functional impairment in relational integration, or that deficits of frontal patients in other thinking tasks should be attributed to such a functional impairment. Part of the difficulty with the interpretation of Waltz and colleagues lies in the nature of fronto-temporal dementia. It is characterised by relatively widespread cortical damage originating in either prefrontal or temporal regions. Thus, while impairments in transitive and inductive inference may be associated in the patients of Waltz and colleagues, it is possible that they may dissociate in patients with more localised lesions.

A second difficulty with the claim that transitive inference involves a general process of relational integration concerns the fit with the imaging results of Acuna et al. (2002) and the behavioural data from non-human and developmental studies. As discussed above,

Acuna et al. interpret their results in terms of the use by subjects of an acquired spatial representation of the stimuli, ordered, for example, from left to right. How then should the patient results of Waltz et al. be interpreted? In fact, there is converging evidence from fMRI studies that adds weight to the view of Waltz and colleagues that prefrontal cortex, and in particular lateral fronto-polar cortex, is involved in the integration of relational information. Kalina Christoff and colleagues (2001) scanned subjects while they completed induction problems similar to those investigated by Waltz et al. (1999). In all cases the problems, based on Progressive Matrices, required subjects to select from a set of four the figure that correctly completed a 3 by 3 array (see Figure 12.3a, b). Three levels of problem complexity were administered, but in only the most complex problems was it necessary to abstract and then combine information about changes to both horizontal and vertical dimensions of the arrays. This, it was held, involved integration of the two relations. Unsurprisingly, subjects took longer to respond in the most difficult condition, and produced more errors. However, when response time was controlled for, increased activation was found bilaterally in frontopolar cortex (BA 10) and the caudate, as well as in left inferior frontal gyrus (BA 6, 44) and right middle frontal gyrus (BA 9, 46) (see Figure 12.3c). It would appear from this study that these regions operate in concert to support complex relational reasoning.

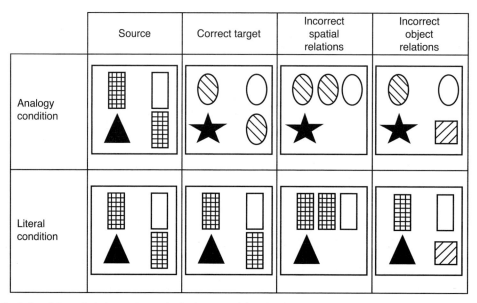

Fig. 12.4 The design of the analogical reasoning study of Wharton et al. (2000). Subjects were required to indicate whether a target 'matched' a source item which was presented 3 sec earlier. In the analogy condition, a target was correct if the objects differed from the source but shared both spatial and object relations. In the literal condition, a target was correct if it matched exactly with the source.Reprinted from *Cognitive Psychology*, *40*(3), C.M. Wharton, J. Grafman, S.S. Flitman, E.K. Hansen, J. Brauner, A. Marks and M. Honda, Toward Neuroanatomical Models of Analogy A Positron Emission Tomography Study of Analogical Mapping, 173–197.Copyright (2000), with permission from Elsevier.

Unlike the transitive inference problems of Acuna et al., the induction problems used in the study of Christoff and colleagues cannot be solved by reading off elements from an acquired spatially organised representation of the stimulus set. In solving induction problems, processes of abstraction and recombination would seem to be necessary. Christoff and colleagues argue that lateral frontopolar cortex is concerned not specifically with relational reasoning *per se*, but rather with the manipulation of 'self-generated information' (Christoff et al., 2001, p. 1146). Thus, in the difficult condition of the induction task, subjects are argued to generate for themselves the product of combining the two relations; unlike in the simpler induction conditions, the correct figure is not present in the original array. This manipulation of self-generated information is a common feature of complex relational reasoning, and the attribution of this function to lateral frontopolar cortex is consistent with both the gateway hypothesis of Burgess et al. (2007), discussed in Section 9.14, and imaging results concerning goal-directed problem-solving to be discussed below in Section 12.5. However the hypothesis should not be accepted too readily. It is possibly, for example, that subjects in Christoff et al.'s induction experiment do not use information abstracted from the stimulus array to generate the correct missing item. Subjects are required to select which of four possible missing items is correct. They may thus use a verification strategy of comparing each of the possible items to the stimulus array.

12.3 Reasoning by Analogy

Lateral frontopolar cortical activity, particularly on the left, has also been found in several studies of analogical reasoning (e.g. Wharton et al., 2000; Bunge et al., 2005; Green et al., 2006). Consider first the study of the use of spatial analogy by Wharton et al. (2000). Subjects were shown diagrams of two sets of geometrical figures with an intra-trial delay of 3 sec. In one condition (the literal match condition) they were required to determine merely if the diagrams were identical. In the other (the analogy condition) they were required to determine if the elements of the diagrams shared a common abstract spatial arrangement (see Figure 12.4). For this, it was necessary first for subjects to represent the spatial relationships between the elements of the diagrams, while abstracting from the specific features (e.g. shape, colour) of those elements, then to maintain those relations during the intra-trial interval, and finally to determine whether the spatial relationships in the second diagram matched those in the first. Subtracting the literal condition from the analogy condition revealed a left-lateralised network of regions implicated specifically in the analogy condition. This included regions typically associated with language (BA 44, 45),[5] as well as premotor (BA 6),

_____

[5] But see Section 9.5 for a discussion of processes other than language ones which involve this region.

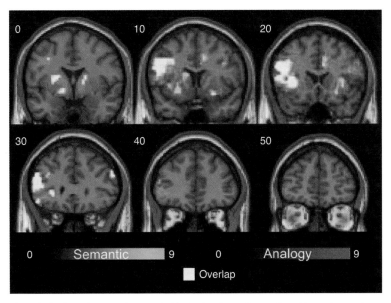

Fig. 12.5 Coronal slices through the frontal cortex of a canonical brain showing regions activated by analogy and semantic trials relative to fixation in the study of Bunge et al. (2005). The y coordinate of each slice is shown in the top left. Areas of overlap between the two contrast maps appear in yellow. Reprinted from S.A. Bunge, C. Wendelken, D. Badre and A.D. Wagner, Analogical Reasoning and Prefrontal Cortex Evidence for Separable Retrieval and Integration Mechanisms, *Cerebral Cortex*, 2005, 15(3), 239–249, by permission of Oxford University Press.

medial frontal (BA 8), inferior parietal (BA 40) and left lateral frontopolar (BA 46/10) cortices. With the notable exception of left lateral frontopolar cortex, this is largely consistent with the use of a verbal strategy in the analogy condition (e.g. in which spatial relations are rehearsed in verbal form during the intra-trial interval).[6] The left lateral frontopolar region active in the analogy condition matches closely the region claimed by Christoff et al. (2001) to be implicated in the manipulation of self-generated information.

Wharton et al.'s spatial analogy task contrasts with simple verbal analogical reasoning tasks, which generally take the form of '*A is to B as C is to what?*'. This kind of task is commonly argued to involve abstracting a relation that holds between two given terms (e.g. *cat* and *kitten*) and applying that relation to a third given term (e.g. *dog*) to infer a fourth term (in this case *puppy*) that lies in the same relation to the third term as the second does to the first. Silvia Bunge and colleagues (2005) used an event-related design to investigate neural activity during verbal analogical reasoning. Subjects were presented with a pair of semantically related words (e.g. *bouquet* and *flowers*), then a cue indicating which of two tasks

was to be performed (an analogy task or a semantic task), and finally a second pair of words (e.g. *chain* and *link*, or *rain* and *drought*). In the analogy task, subjects were required to indicate whether the words in the second pair were related in an analogical way to the words in the first pair. In the semantic task, they were required to indicate whether the words in the second pair were semantically related. The associative strength of the relationship between the first pair or words (high, medium, low) was also varied, so that effects of semantic relatedness could be disentangled from effects of analogical reasoning. The BOLD response of the two tasks relative to fixation is shown in Figure 12.5. Activity was observed in left frontopolar cortex, left inferior PFC and right dorsolateral PFC in both conditions (relative to rest), but more so in the analogy condition. Subsequent analyses examined the components of the tasks to which these regions were insensitive. Lateral frontopolar cortex was found to be active during the analogical task but not the semantic task, regardless of the associative strength of the initial word pairs. The authors interpret this as indicating that in the analogy task left lateral frontopolar cortex operates after semantic retrieval and 'plays a domain-general role in integrating across multiple relations in the service of analogical reasoning' (p. 246). We return to this conclusion below.

Conclusions were also drawn regarding other cortical areas differentially involved in the tasks. Thus, activity of left inferior PFC was sensitive to the associative strength of the terms in the cue phase, reflecting the semantic retrieval demands of the tasks. This is consistent with

---

[6] Wharton et al. (2000) attribute activity in BA 6 and BA 8 to the greater attentional demands of the analogy condition in comparison with the literal condition, and suggest that the left inferior parietal activity (BA40) reflects the identification by subjects of spatial relationships in the various diagrams. However, as discussed with respect to the Acuna et al. study, this last is a rather flaky attribution.

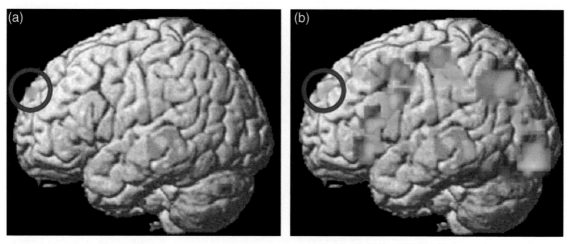

Fig. 12.6 Results of the study of analogical reasoning of Green et al. (2006). (a) The contrast between the analogy condition and the control non-analogy condition. The area in green was significantly more active in the analogy condition. The area in red was significantly more active in the non-analogy condition. (Threshold: $p < 0.0005$.) (b) Common areas recruited by the analogy (green) and non-analogy (red) tasks, both contrasted with the semantic task. The overlap between the tasks is shown in yellow. (Threshold: $p < 0.005$.) Reprinted from *Brain Research*, *1096*(1), A.E. Green, J.A. Fugelsang, D.J.M. Kraemer, N.A. Shamosh and K.N. Dunbar, Frontopolar cortex mediates abstract integration in analogy, 125–137. Copyright (2006), with permission from Elsevier.

the suggestion of Badre and Wagner (2002), discussed in Section 9.13, that this area is involved in controlled semantic retrieval. By contrast, right dorsolateral PFC activity was found to be insensitive to the associative strength, but significantly greater during rejection of invalid analogies. The authors interpret this finding in the context of the behavioural result that subjects showed a bias towards endorsing invalid analogies. They suggest that right dorsolateral PFC is involved in over-riding this bias, and further relate the function of right DLPFC to response selection. An alternative possibility, consistent with the position taken in Section 9.10, is that the right lateral activity reflects a monitoring or checking function.

Green and colleagues (2006) report a second event-related fMRI study of analogical reasoning that is often cited alongside the Bunge et al. (2005) study as evidence for the claim that lateral frontopolar areas are involved in relational integration. As in the Bunge study, Green and colleagues required subjects to determine whether four terms stood in an analogical or a semantic relationship. A third condition required subjects to determine whether the words stood in pair-wise, but not necessarily analogical, relationships. To clarify this odd concept of a pair-wise non-analogical relationship, consider the example of *cow / milk, duck / water*. Note that *cow* and *milk* are semantically related, and *duck* and *water* are also semantically related. However, while *cow* and *duck* are members of the same category, as are *milk* and *water*, the terms do not form an analogy: *cow is NOT to milk as duck is to water*. The critical fMRI contrasts are shown in Figure 12.6. In comparison to either of the other conditions, the analogy condition led to

significantly greater activation of an area of left frontopolar cortex. Green et al. conclude that this region is selectively active for 'the abstract relational integration component of analogical reasoning', claiming that other aspects of the reasoning tasks engage a common fronto-parietal network.

This final claim, that reasoning about analogical and other semantic relationships engages a common fronto-parietal network, is not well supported by the imaging results, since the yellow regions are small compared to the red and green ones in those cortices (see Figure 12.6). There are also a number of other reasons to be cautious about the results of Bunge et al. (2005) and Green et al. (2006). Thus, while both studies locate relational integration in left frontopolar PFC, and relate this to the position of Christoff et al. (2001), the two studies implicate quite distinct regions. The region identified by Green et al. is centred on (–8, 60, 26). This is several centimetres from the region identified by Bunge et al., centred on (–42, 48, –15). Neither region matches particularly well with the region identified by Christoff et al. (2001), namely (–34, 50, 9).

Perhaps more critically, the process of 'relational integration' is itself not well defined. In the Christoff et al. task, subjects were required to select the item that fitted within a progressive matrix. If we accept Christoff et al.'s assumptions on the strategy adopted by subjects in the task—an issue to which we return below—then left lateral frontopolar cortex was differentially activated when it was necessary to construct the solution by applying two rules, one relating to properties common to elements in the target column and one relating to properties common to elements in the target row. In the tasks

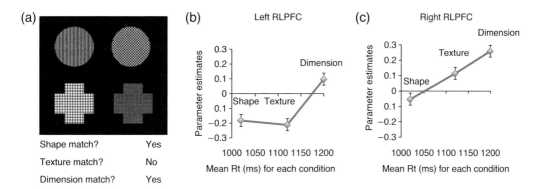

Fig. 12.7 (a) The design of the task used in the Bunge et al. (2009) study. In the *shape match* condition subjects must indicate whether two horizontally related figures match (regardless of their shading). In the *texture match* condition the question is whether the shading in either pair of horizontally related figures matches (regardless of their shape). In the *dimension match* condition the question is whether the upper two figures and lower two figures match on the same dimension. (b) BOLD activity in each condition (relative to a resting baseline) showed that left frontopolar cortex (RLPFC) was significantly more active in the dimension condition than in either of the other conditions. (c) In contrast, activity in right frontopolar cortex tracked task difficulty, as shown by mean RT on the horizontal axis. Reprinted from *NeuroImage*, *46*(1), S. Bunge, E.H. Helskog and C. Wendelken, Left, but not right, rostrolateral prefrontal cortex meets a stringent test of the relational integration hypothesis. 338–342. Copyright (2009), with permission from Elsevier.

of Bunge et al. (2005) and Green et al. (2006), subjects were required to judge the correctness of a possible analogy. These tasks require that subjects abstract relations between the various terms and then compare those relations. Relational integration as operationalised in the Christoff et al. study is *not* involved.

Moreover, a more recent study by Bunge's group (Wendelken et al., 2008) found bilateral frontopolar activity when subjects were required to determine whether a given verbal analogy was valid (e.g. *painter:brush::writer:pen*) but not when they were required to complete a partial verbal analogy (*painter:brush::writer:?*). On Wendelken et al.'s account, the former involves abstracting and comparing relations while the latter involves abstracting a relation between the first two given terms and then combining or integrating that relation and the third given term to complete an analogy. Wendelken and colleagues conclude that the involvement of lateral frontopolar cortex in analogical reasoning 'is linked specifically to the comparison of relational information, rather than relational integration' (Wendelken et al., 2008, p. 690), and furthermore that this comparison of relational information is fundamentally different from the process of relational integration involved in progressive matrices and as investigated by Christoff et al. (2001). While this interpretation could explain away any differences in localisation, it multiplies abstract functions. How might the two positions be resolved?

Note first that while the maxima of the frontopolar regions identified by the three groups (i.e. of Bunge/Wendelken, Wharton and Christoff) differ, there is some overlap in the activated regions. Moreover a more recent study by Bunge and her colleagues (Bunge et al., 2009) provides further support for the left frontopolar

localisation of a relational comparison process, and places it nearer to the original Christoff location. In this study, subjects completed a series of yes/no judgements on stimulus arrays consisting of four figures (Figure 12.7a). In the *shape match* condition subjects were required to indicate if the top or the bottom pair of shapes matched. In the *texture match* condition subjects were required to indicate if the shading matched in the top or the bottom pair of shapes. In the *dimension match* condition subjects were required to indicate if the top pair of shapes and the bottom pair of shapes matched on the same one of these two dimensions. Behavioural results indicated that the dimension match condition was the most difficult while the shape match was the easiest, and BOLD activity in right frontopolar cortex tracked this effect of difficulty (Figure 12.7c). BOLD activity in left frontopolar cortex, however, was greatest for the dimension match condition and did not differ for the other two conditions (Figure 12.7b). Bunge et al. (2009) report the maximum for this region to be (–36, 57, 9), which fits well with the region identified by Christoff et al. (2001). Indeed, in a subtle shift of their position, Bunge et al. identify the region with Christoff's relational integration function.

There would therefore seem to be a convergence of opinion on the functional role of lateral frontopolar cortex within complex relational reasoning tasks, namely, that the region supports *relational integration*. Two issues remain. First, most studies suggest a left lateralised location of function, though Bunge et al. (2009) also found right lateral activity in some experimental conditions. How might this be explained? Second, can we characterise relational integration more precisely in processing terms?

Consider first the issue of lateralisation. Two interpretations of the results are forthcoming. Bunge et al. (2009) suggest that relational integration might lateralise as a function of the materials, with right lateral frontopolar cortex specialised more for visuo-spatial relations and left lateral frontopolar cortex specialised more for verbal or semantic relations. This does not account for the tracking of task difficulty in Bunge et al.'s study by right lateral frontopolar cortex. An alternative interpretation is that the right lateral activation relates to a process such as monitoring which tracks task difficulty (see Section 9.10). In Section 12.6 we consider an alternative characterisation of left lateral frontal activity, namely that it reflects a process of *hypothesis generation* as required by rule induction tasks; this can be a subcomponent of the task-setting functions postulated for the left lateral prefrontal cortex in Chapter 9.

What though of the process of relational integration? What does it involve and how does it relate to analogical reasoning? Christoff et al.'s original concept was of the manipulation of self-generated information. This is sufficiently general to be consistent with the Bunge et al.'s (2009) study, since in the critical condition subjects must generate for themselves the relation, if any, that holds between the two pairs of items. Bunge et al. do not favour this interpretation. They suggest that it is not supported by the group's earlier work (Wendelken et al., 2008). Moreover it does not necessarily following from the original 2001 study of Christoff and colleagues or from subsequent imaging studies of analogical reasoning. Take the Christoff et al. (2001) task. Subjects were required to select one of four possible figures to complete each progressive matrix (recall Figure 12.3a, b). They may have achieved this by abstracting the common features across the rows and the columns of the matrix and combining these features to yield the result. This would require the subject to self-generate the relations and then to manipulate them to produce the solution. But subjects may instead have considered the four possible solutions in turn to see which fitted best. This latter strategy would convert the task into one of verification rather than completion, and hence be consistent with the proposal by Wendelken and colleagues that analogy completion (as opposed to analogy verification) does not require lateral frontopolar cortex. Similar comments apply to the other analogical tasks discussed above.

In fact, the possibility that analogical reasoning does not require lateral frontopolar cortex is also supported by developmental evidence. Simple analogies of the form *A is to B as C is to what?* can be solved by children as young as 3 to 4, provided they are familiar with the terms (i.e. *A, B, C*) and the relations between them (Goswami & Brown, 1990a; Ratterman & Gentner, 1998). Yet, at this age the frontopolar cortex is poorly developed. Working from this perspective, Leech et al.

(2008) propose a developmental and computational account of simple analogical reasoning in which analogy is achieved not by relational integration, but instead by a priming process: the priming is held to be of relations, which are themselves treated as uni-directional transformations. Thus, comprehension of a relation—an operation—is held to have a specific material basis and so the *A is to B* statement is held to result in priming not only of the concepts *A* and *B* but also of the operation of the relation that maps *A* to *B*. When this relation is primed and the *C* term is given, that term is mapped to an appropriately constrained solution term (i.e. a term *D* that is related to *C* in the same way that *B* is related to *A*). Leech et al. demonstrate using a connectionist implementation that the account is able to explain a range of developmental evidence, such as the correlation between relational knowledge and analogical ability, without explicit processes of relation abstraction or the integration of relational information.

That analogical reasoning need not involve frontopolar cortex leaves unexplained both the activity in this region observed in fMRI studies and the process of relational integration. Thus our conclusions so far concerning the cognitive neuroscience of relational reasoning are rather negative. Both transitive inference and analogical inference have been held to require a process of relational integration that has been localised to a left lateral region of frontopolar cortex, but as we have seen, both forms of inference are possible without the necessary involvement of this region and the referent of 'relational integration' remains poorly defined. Critically, in both cases there is more than one way to complete the reasoning task. A more adequate task analysis is therefore essential when attempting to interpret the imaging (and behavioural) results. One difficulty is that many reasoning tasks used in the imaging literature require subjects to verify a possible solution, rather than to generate one for themselves. Given this, it seems at present difficult to decide on whether activation of left lateral frontopolar cortex in analogical reasoning relates to the process of hypothesis generation or one of comparing different relations between objects.

12.4 Deductive Inference

Where does this leave the relational integration hypothesis and what is the involvement of left lateral frontopolar cortex in some relational and analogical reasoning tasks? Monti and colleagues (2007) report a particularly important and tightly controlled study, which was discussed from the perspective of its methodology in Section 5.7. They were concerned not with relational reasoning of the form discussed above but with deductive reasoning using the logical connectives *and*, *or*, *not* and *if/then*. In two event-related fMRI studies, subjects

TABLE 12.1 The design of the stimuli used in the two experiments of Monti et al (2007)

Experiment 1

Argument Status	Formal Arguments	Block Instantiation	Abstract Instantiation
Valid, Simple	$(P \lor Q) \Rightarrow \neg R$ P $\therefore \neg R$	If the block is either round or large then it is not blue. The block is round. $\therefore$ The block is not blue	If there is either sug or rop then there is no tuk. There is sug. $\therefore$ There is no tuk.
Valid, Complex	$(P \lor Q) \Rightarrow \neg R$ R $\therefore \neg P$	If the block is either red or square then it is not large. The block is large. $\therefore$ The block is not red.	If there is either bep or tuk then there is no gez. There is gez. $\therefore$ There is no bep.

Experiment 2

Argument Status	Formal Arguments	Face Instantiation	House Instantiation
Valid, Simple	$(P \lor Q) \Rightarrow \neg R$ P $\therefore \neg R$	If he has either open eyes or a smile then he doesn't have a long nose. He has open eyes. $\therefore$ He doesn't have a long nose.	If it has either a front stoop or a bay window then it has no garage. It has a front stoop. $\therefore$ It has no garage.
Valid, Complex	$(P \lor Q) \Rightarrow \neg R$ R $\therefore \neg P$	If he has either a small nose or closed eyes then he doesn't have a frown. He has a frown. $\therefore$ He doesn't have a small nose.	It if has either brick siding or a chimney then it has no tree in front. It has a tree in front. $\therefore$ It has no brick siding.

Reprinted from *NeuroImage*, *37*(3), M.M. Monti, D.N. Osherson, M.J. Martinez and L.M. Parsons, Functional neuroanatomy of deductive inference: a language-independent distributed network, 1005–1016. Copyright (2007), with permission from Elsevier.

were required to complete a series of inferences. Half of the inferences involved simple deductions based on the use of an *if/then* rule, while the other half involved more complex deductions in which the *if/then* rule had to be used in reverse (see Table 12.1). A second factorial condition varied the content of the problems (concrete versus abstract in experiment 1, and faces versus houses in experiment 2). Stimuli were carefully matched for linguistic complexity.

During both tasks, the first premise was presented for 3 sec prior to presentation of the second premise and a possible conclusion. Subjects were required to say whether the conclusion held by pressing a 'yes' or 'no' response key. A number of areas were active during presentation of the initial premise (in contrast to rest). These areas all corresponded to what would be expected from reading (i.e. visual attention and language areas; Figure 12.8, yellow areas). The key result, however, was the contrast between complex and simple deductions (Figure 12.8, green areas). This yielded a fronto-parietal network that was (a) almost entirely distinct from the network of regions involved in the reading part of the task, and (b) included left lateral frontopolar cortex (BA 10), as well as bi-lateral ventrolateral frontal (BA 47), medial frontal (BA 8), left premotor (BA 6) and left superior parietal (BA 7) cortices. In addition, some subregions of this network were found to be sensitive to the semantic content of the task. For example, in addition

to the basic network, activity in cingulate gyrus (BA 32 left, BA 24 right), left medial occipital and lingual gyri (BA 18) and right inferior parietal lobule (BA 40) was associated with the concrete materials used in one condition of experiment 1 (see Table 12.1, block instantiation), while the face instantiation condition of experiment 2 (see Table 12.1) resulted in additional activity in left inferior and superior temporal gyri (BA 20, BA 19/22) and right superior frontal gyrus (BA 11).

The results of Monti et al. (2007) provide support for four hypotheses: (1) that verbal reasoning is supported by a content-general left-lateralised fronto-parietal network; (2) that this network is predominantly not a network of language centres; (3) that supplementary neural areas may also be recruited in reasoning, depending on the semantic content; and (4) that the network may include left lateral fronto-polar cortex. Consider first hypothesis 4. Monti and colleagues provide a precise characterisation of the possible role of left lateral fronto-polar cortex in deductive inference: namely 'transforming logical structure by changing the polarity of variables (e.g. negating), displacing variables, and substituting or eliminating logical connectives' (pp. 1010–1011). Similar operations on structured propositional representations are required by the tasks of Wharton et al. (2000), Christoff et al. (2001) and the analogy verification condition of Wendelken et al. (2008), which were also found to activate this area.

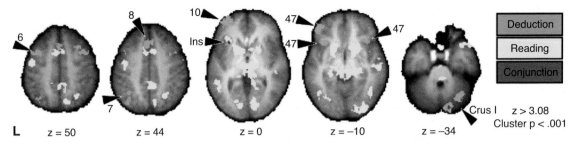

Fig. 12.8 Areas activated in the deductive reasoning study of Monti et al. (2007). Areas shown in yellow were active (relative to rest) during initial reading of the premises. Areas significantly activated by the complex minus simple reasoning contrast are shown in green (see Table 12.1). The overlap is shown in pink. Numbers beside arrow heads indicate Brodmann areas. Reprinted from *NeuroImage, 37*(3), M.M. Monti, D.N. Osherson, M.J. Martinez and L.M. Parsons, Functional neuroanatomy of deductive inference: a language-independent distributed network, 1005–1016, Copyright (2007), with permission from Elsevier.

Of the remaining hypotheses, hypothesis 1 and 3 are supported by a series of earlier imaging studies of syllogistic reasoning by Goel, Dolan and colleagues (Goel et al. 1998, 2000; Goel & Dolan 2003a, 2003b). Goel et al. (2000) explored the effect of material type on the neural processes underlying syllogistic reasoning using event-related fMRI. Subjects were required to determine whether a given conclusion was a logical consequence of the given premises for three types of syllogism. These were concrete syllogisms that fitted common experience (e.g. *All poodles are pets. All pets have names. Therefore all poodles have names.*), concrete but incongruent syllogisms (e.g. *All pets are poodles. All poodles are vicious. Therefore all pets are vicious.*), and abstract syllogisms (e.g. *All P are Q. All Q are R. Therefore all P are R.*) In all cases the materials were presented visually. Overlapping but distinct networks of cortical and subcortical regions were found to be active during concrete reasoning and abstract reasoning. In the concrete case (when contrasted with a condition in which verbally similar stimuli were presented and reasoning was not required), increased activity was observed bilaterally in the basal ganglia, left laterally in the middle/superior temporal lobe (BA 21/22) and inferior frontal lobe (BA 44), and right laterally in the cerebellum (see Figure 12.9b). Goel et al. interpret this as reflecting a linguistic network including both syntactic (BA 44) and semantic (BA 21/22) sites, suggesting that concrete reasoning is verbally mediated and subject to semantic influence.

The apparent involvement of a linguistic network in concrete reasoning directly contradicts the position of Monti and colleagues discussed earlier. The differences in activation are explicable in terms of the different baseline conditions used in the subtractions in each study and differences in difficulty between the reasoning tasks. Thus, Monti and colleagues used reading of the first premise to establish their baseline activation, and their *if/then* problems were relatively easy (with mean accuracy of approximately 94% across conditions). Here, any potential role of linguistic processing

regions would be subtracted out. Goel et al. also used reading of the premises as a baseline, but their syllogistic problems were more difficult (with mean accuracy of approximately 78% across conditions), and no evidence is presented to suggest that subjects had fully comprehended the premises during the baseline condition. Indeed if subjects wished to minimise cognitive effort then the experimental design of Goel et al. would allow them to scan the premises for nouns during the baseline condition, and then re-read and comprehend them during the reasoning condition.

A more recent study by Monti and colleagues (2009) provides further support for the existence of a language-independent component to logical deduction taking place in left frontopolar cortex. In this study, arguments involving logical connectives such as *if, then, either* and *not* are contrasted with purely linguistic arguments involving reversal of active and passive sentences. Both tasks recruited a network of areas, including left frontopolar cortex, but the region involved in logical inference was more anterior than that involved in linguistic inference.

Returning to syllogistic reasoning, and in particular abstract syllogistic problems, here Goel and colleagues found a pattern of activity that differed from that found with concrete syllogisms. When reasoning with abstract materials (see Figure 12.9c), activity was found bilaterally in the fusiform gyrus (BA 18), cerebellum and basal ganglia, left laterally in the superior parietal lobe (BA 7) and inferior frontal lobe (BA 44, 45), and right laterally in the inferior frontal lobe (BA 45). These regions, Goel and colleagues note, are similar to those reported to be involved in some spatial tasks (Kosslyn et al., 1989; Jonides et al., 1993; see Section 8.6), and the authors speculate that spatial processes may be invoked in solving abstract syllogisms, consistent with the mental model theory of Johnson-Laird (1983).[7]

---

[7] The involvement of spatial processes in the solution of abstract syllogisms is also consistent with other model-based

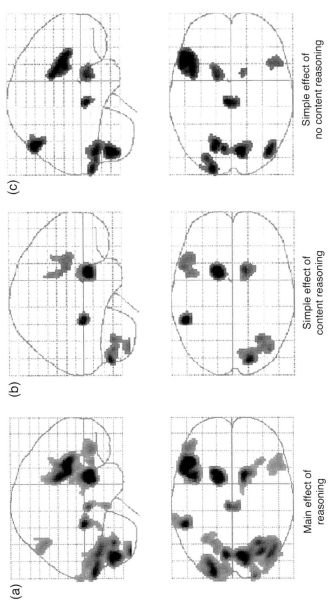

Fig. 12.9 Results from the syllogistic reasoning study of Goel et al. (2000). (a) The main effect of reasoning, regardless of content type (reasoning preparation). (b) The effect of reasoning with contentful material (content reasoning – content preparation). (c) The effect of reasoning without content (no-content reasoning no-content preparation). Reprinted from *NeuroImage, 12(5)*, V. Goel, C. Buchel, C. Frith and R.J. Dolan, Dissociation of mechanisms underlying syllogistic reasoning, 504–514. Copyright (2000), with permission from Elsevier.

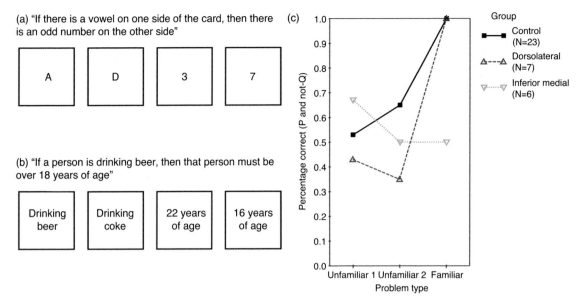

(a) "If there is a vowel on one side of the card, then there is an odd number on the other side"

| A | D | 3 | 7 |

(b) "If a person is drinking beer, then that person must be over 18 years of age"

| Drinking beer | Drinking coke | 22 years of age | 16 years of age |

Fig. 12.10 The Wason Four-Card Selection Task in (a) abstract and (b) concrete forms. In the abstract form, each card has a letter on one side and a number on the other. The subject's task is to select the card or cards needed to verify the rule: 'If there is a vowel on one side of the card, then there is an odd number on the other side'. The correct response is the card showing a vowel (the so-called *P* card), the card showing a number that is not odd (the so-called *not-Q* card), and no other cards. (c) Patient data from the study of Adolphs et al. (1996) for three variants of the task, two using unfamiliar materials and one using familiar materials.

If one accepts that the preparation conditions provide adequate baselines, then the critical comparisons for establishing whether abstract and concrete reasoning involve different neural processes are between the reasoning and preparation conditions of contentful versus abstract tasks (i.e. (concrete reasoning – concrete preparation) – (abstract reasoning – abstract preparation), and vice versa). These yielded increased activity in left superior temporal sulcus (STS; BA 21/22) for the concrete case and increased activity in the left superior parietal lobe (SPL; BA 7) for the abstract case. No frontal regions were implicated in either comparison. The left STS activity is not surprising given that the nouns involved in the concrete case will have had semantic content. The left SPL activity fits with recruitment of some form of spatial processing in the abstract case. However, the lack of frontal activity in either contrast undermines the argument that distinct frontal regions are involved in contentful versus abstract reasoning.

A further finding of Goel et al. (2000) concerned an effect of congruency. Increased activity was found in right dorsomedial (BA 8) and right dorsolateral (BA 46/45) prefrontal cortex when the conclusion was not congruent with common knowledge. The authors suggest that one or other (or both) of these regions may be involved in detecting and resolving the belief/logic

conflict that arises in the incongruent condition. These results are therefore also consistent with the active monitoring interpretation of right dorsolateral prefrontal cortex given in Section 9.10.

One apparent difficulty with Goel et al.'s results is that they appear to be at odds with another line of research, which locates belief-based reasoning in inferior medial PFC. Adolphs et al. (1996) compared the performance of three brain-lesioned patient groups, inferior medial frontal, dorsolateral frontal and nonfrontal, on the Wason card-selection task (Wason, 1968), a task first investigated neuropsychologically by Golding (1981). In the task, subjects are shown four cards each of which declares a property (*P* or *Q*) to be either true or false. They are told that the reverse side of each card provides information about the second of the properties (so if a card indicates *not Q* on one side, then it will give information about the truth *P* on the other side). Subjects are also given a rule of the form *if P then Q*. The subject is required to select the card or cards required to verify the rule. The task may be administered with either abstract or concrete materials. Control subjects are known to perform poorly on the task when the materials are abstract, as with the vowel/even number rule illustrated in Figure 12.10a, or unfamiliar. They typically select the two cards that confirm the rule, rather than cards that may potentially falsify it. The three patient groups of Adolphs et al. were no different in this respect. However, when the materials are concrete and/or the rule is familiar (as with the age-related

approaches to the task, such as the use of Euler circles (Stenning & Oberlander, 1995; Stenning & Yule, 1997).

(a) Correct inhibitory trails

(b) Incorrect inhibitory trails

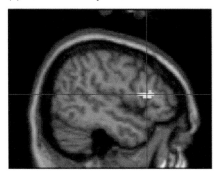 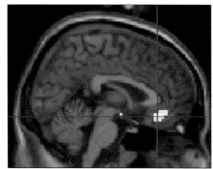

Fig. 12.11 BOLD activity arising during syllogistic reasoning with materials that contradict one's beliefs. (a) The comparison of correct versus incorrect trials revealed activation of right lateral PFC (BA45). (b) The reverse comparison revealed (bilateral) activation of inferior medial PFC. Reprinted from *Cognition*, 87(1), V. Goel and R.J. Dolan, Explaining modulation of reasoning by belief, B11–B22. Copyright (2003), with permission from Elsevier.

drinking rule; see Figure 12.10b), control subjects typically perform well (Johnson-Laird et al., 1972). Adolphs et al. also found this to be the case for their dorsolateral frontal and non-frontal patients. However, the inferior medial frontal group performed no better on familiar materials than on unfamiliar materials (see Figure 12.10c). The authors interpret these results as suggesting that subjects typically use existing knowledge to solve the Wason card-selection task, reasoning by analogy with previous experience. Inferior medial patients are held to have difficulty in accessing or appropriately using this knowledge in the service of the task.[8]

Two studies by Goel and Dolan (2003a; see also Goel & Dolan, 2003b) provide a potential resolution of the apparent conflict between the results of Adolphs et al. (1996) and those of Goel et al. (2000) concerning the localisation of belief-based reasoning. Goel and Dolan again used event-related fMRI and again contrasted congruent and incongruent syllogistic reasoning. The primary difference was in the analysis of incongruent trials, i.e. those trials in which the belief-laden response was in conflict with the logical response. Right dorsolateral prefrontal cortex was found to be activated more strongly in trials where subjects successfully overcame the tendency to respond according to their beliefs (see Figure 12.11a). This is again consistent with the role of right dorsolateral prefrontal cortex in active monitoring.

However, inferior medial prefrontal cortex was found to be preferentially active (bilaterally) when subjects responded incorrectly in accord with their beliefs on incongruent trials (see Figure 12.11b). This fits with the findings of Adolphs et al. (1996). Again, however, an alternative interpretation is also plausible. In a task in which subjects were required to guess the colour or suit of a standard playing card, Elliot et al. (1999) found inferior medial prefrontal activity to be greater during a guessing condition (where the front of the card was not shown) than in a reporting condition (where the front of the card was shown). Furthermore, this activity was greater when there were more alternatives (i.e. when guessing suit) than when there were fewer (when guessing colour). Thus, the inferior medial activity observed by Goel et al. may simply have reflected (incorrect) guessing.

How do the various imaging results discussed above relate to the key debate in the cognitive theory of reasoning, namely that between rule-based and model-based theories? Monti et al. (2007) suggest that the involvement of frontopolar cortex (and specifically the above interpretation of its function) argues for the rule-based approach, while the lack of involvement of right parietal cortex (as would be expected if spatial operations were involved; see Section 8.6) argues against the model-based approach. This second argument is based on a null result and is therefore somewhat weak. Monti et al. also provide no real explanation of the increased left superior parietal activity observed in their more difficult problems (and in the abstract problems of Goel et al., 2000). Other researchers have found bilateral parietal activity during reasoning tasks and interpreted this as evidence of model-based reasoning (e.g. Acuna et al., 2002; Goel & Dolan, 2003a), so the claim that human deductive reasoning does not involve mental models is premature. One possibility that is consistent with the data is that both model-based and rule-based

---

[8] There are substantial difficulties in interpreting the results of this study. Most seriously, the effect of theoretical interest is a null effect—inferior medial patients are poor with both unfamiliar and familiar versions of the selection task. In fact, the inferior medial patients of Adolphs et al. selected fewer cards on average over all versions of the selection task than dorsolateral or non-frontal control patients. Their poor performance on the task may therefore have been due to other factors (e.g. lack of motivation or of giving insufficient care to the task; see Section 9.11).

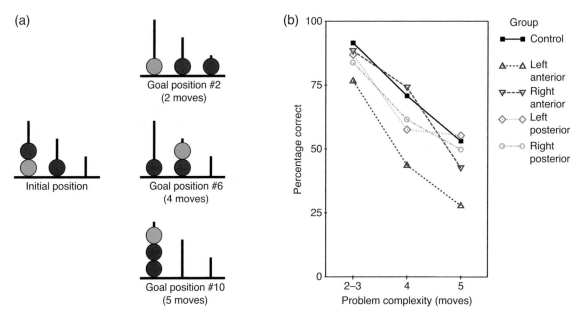

Fig. 12.12 (a) Three Tower of London problems. The same initial position is used for each problem. (b) Solution accuracy for controls and four patient groups on Tower of London problems of different complexity. Data from Shallice (1982).

processes may be called on, with the rule-based processes being specifically involved in manipulating propositions into a form that is compatible with a model-based representation.

12.5 Goal-directed Problem-solving

An appealing feature of a model-based approach to deductive inference is that it makes possible a link to a second area of thinking that, as described in the introduction, is normally seen as entirely distinct. This is goal-directed problem-solving. Standard theories in this area assume that thinking in these situations involves the representation and manipulation of an internal representation of a problem's state, i.e. a model.

It has long been known that goal-directed problem-solving may be impaired following frontal lesions (e.g. Luria, 1966). Can this general characterisation be made more precise, either at the cognitive level or the neurological level? Early evidence that the second part of this question may be answered positively was provided by a patient study by Shallice and McCarthy of the Tower of London task (Shallice, 1982). The task apparatus consists of three pegs of different heights and three different coloured wooden balls (see Figure 12.12a). Subjects are given the apparatus with the balls arranged in one position and required to rearrange the balls, moving one at a time, to attain a goal configuration. Control subjects and patients with unilateral lesions were required to complete a series of problems in the minimum number of moves. Right anterior, right posterior and left posterior patient groups performed as well as controls on the task,

but the left anterior group was impaired, even on simple two and three move problems (see Figure 12.12b).

Initial attempts to replicate the left anterior impairment on the Tower of London task supported the frontal effect but not its laterality. Thus, while Owen et al. (1990) found that a group of 26 frontal patients were impaired on the task, no reliable effects of laterality were observed. Similarly, using the closely related Tower of Hanoi task (see Figure 12.13), Goel and Grafman (1995) found that a group of 20 frontal patients were impaired relative to age-matched controls. Again though, no reliable difference was found between left and right frontal subgroups. However, evidence of a left-lateral bias was found in a SPECT study by Morris et al. (1993). Six healthy volunteers where scanned while they completed a set of 2- to 5-move Tower of London problems. In comparison to a control task with equivalent visual and motor characteristics, Tower of London problem-solving was associated with increased rCBF in the left-prefrontal cortex. Furthermore, rCBF in this region was positively correlated with planning time and negatively correlated with number of moves taken to solve the problems.[9]

The nature of the left frontal deficit was further clarified by Morris et al. (1997). The Tower of London was initially designed to require intermediate moves away from the eventual goal as this was a situation in which

---

[9] See Schall et al. (2003) for a replication of this left prefrontal localisation using both PET and fMRI with a modified version of the Tower of London.

(a) Four move congruent

(a) Four move conflict

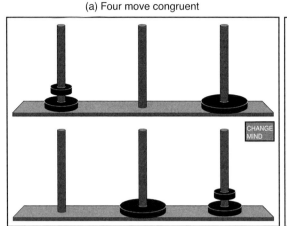
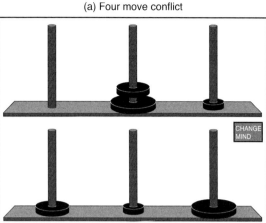

Fig. 12.13 Tower of Hanoi problems used in the study of Morris et al. (1997). In each case the aim is to move the disks in the bottom panel, one at a time, to match the goal state shown in the top panel subject to the constraint that a large disk may not be placed on a smaller disk. (a) A four move congruent problem. Each move involves moving a disk towards its desired state. (b) A four move conflict problem. In this case successful solution involves temporarily moving one disk (the smallest) in a direction opposite to its desired state (I.e., to the left). Reprinted from *Neuropsychologia*, 35(8), R.G. Morris, E.C. Miotto, J.C. Feigenbaum, P. Bullock and C.E. Polkey, The effect of goal–subgoal conflict on planning ability after frontal- and temporal-lobe lesions in humans, 1147–1157. Copyright (1997), with permission from Elsevier.

the artificial intelligence theorist Sussman (1975) had argued that novel planning was required; he was dealing with block-stacking problems in the so-called Blocks World, a programming environment that was used in a variety of applications at the time, including a famous language-comprehension program of Winograd (1972). Goel and Grafman (1995), too, had noted, in their patient study of the Tower of Hanoi, that successful solution of some problems requires making a counter-intuitive move in which a disk is moved to a position that appears to conflict with the overall problem goal. They referred to these problems as goal/subgoal conflict problems (see Figure 12.13b). Goel and Grafman found that frontal patients were significantly more impaired on these conflict problems than on problems not involving goal/subgoal conflict, and suggested that the frontal deficit concerned the resolution of such conflicts. Morris et al. (1997) followed up this hypothesis in a patient study in which four patient groups—left prefrontal, right prefrontal, left temporal and right temporal—and age-matched controls completed a number of Tower of Hanoi problems. Following Goel and Grafman's analysis, Morris and colleagues divided problems into those that did and those that did not involve goal/subgoal conflicts. It was found that for 4-move problems, which were tackled first, the left-frontal patients had severe difficulties on the goal/subgoal conflict problems but not on the non-conflict problems (see Figure 12.14). However when patients later tackled the apparently more difficult 5-move problems their difficulties had resolved. Practice had made perfect! In contrast, the other patient groups performed within the normal range on all problems, with the exception of right-temporal

patients who had difficulties with all problems. The difficulties of these patients did not diminish following practice.

At least three accounts of the difficulty of goal/subgoal conflict problems may be advanced. Goel and Grafman initially related the resolution of the conflict to response inhibition, noting the commonly reported finding that frontal patients can have difficulty inhibiting prepotent responses and arguing that correct resolution of the conflict requires inhibition of the goal-directed response in favour of the subgoal-directed response. The behavioural literature also suggests the involvement of response inhibition in tower-building tasks. Several individual-difference studies have examined correlations between performance on either the Tower of London or the Tower of Hanoi tasks and performance on a range of simpler tasks held to tap more elementary executive functions, such as set shifting, memory updating and response inhibition—functions at the level of those investigated in the ROBBIA studies by Stuss and colleagues and discussed in Chapter 9. In these studies measures of response inhibition have been found to be predictive of performance on the tower-building tasks (Miyake et al., 2000; Welsh et al., 1999; Bull et al., 2004).[10]

---

[10] Goel and Grafman (1995) state that the Tower of London does not 'require the counterintuitive backward move' (p. 634), implying that goal/subgoal conflicts are not possible within this task. This is not so. Goal/subgoal conflicts can occur in Tower of London problems. As noted above, the Tower of London was specifically designed to explore this kind of conflict, and in several Tower of London problems there are points in the solution

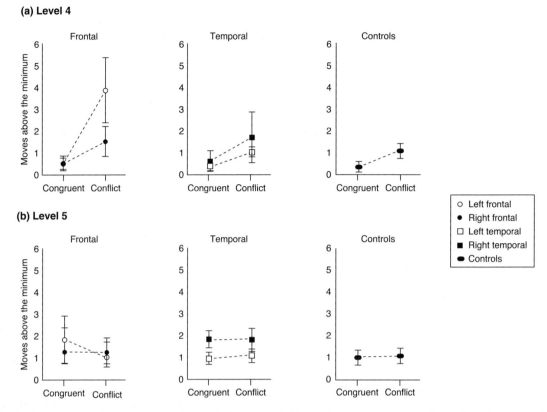

Fig. 12.14 Mean number of moves above the minimum for five groups of subjects on four move and five move Tower of Hanoi problems. Left frontal patients where impaired on four move conflict problems but showed no disproportionate difficulty later when solving five move problems. Reprinted from *Neuropsychologia, 35*(8), R.G. Morris, E.C. Miotto, J.C. Feigenbaum, P. Bullock and C.E. Polkey, The effect of goal–subgoal conflict on planning ability after frontal- and temporal-lobe lesions in humans, 1147–1157. Copyright (1997), with permission from Elsevier.

The need for response inhibition appears to be a possible factor in the behavioural difficulties arising from goal/subgoal conflicts because if one does not inhibit the most obvious move, then one does not plan ahead. However, Goel, Pullara and Grafman (2001) have proposed an alternative account. These authors developed a computational model of behaviour on the Tower of Hanoi within the 3CAPS production system architecture (see Section 3.8). Parameters within the model were calibrated using findings from the normal subjects reported in Goel and Grafman's (1995) study. The model then yielded good fits for the percentage of problems solved, the number of moves to solution and solution time for the nine problems used. The model was then 'lesioned' in two ways. First, to assess the effect of response inhibition (or more specifically response competition) on goal/subgoal conflict, Goel and colleagues manipulated the strategy used by their model for selecting the target peg

path where one has a choice of moving a ball either to its goal position or to some other position, but where moving the ball to its goal position leads to a dead end and is hence inappropriate. These moves involve goal/subgoal conflict.

for each move. This manipulation was not successful—increasing response competition led to an increase in the time and number of moves required to solve a problem, but it did not led to the critical effect observed in the frontal patients, namely a decrease in the percentage of problems solved. In contrast, all key aspects of the frontal impairment were found to arise following an alternative manipulation—simultaneously increasing both the rate of decay of working memory elements and the time required for each step of processing. On these grounds, Goel and colleagues revised their earlier account of the problem-solving deficit of frontal patients, arguing that a sufficient condition for the deficit is an increased rate of decay of working memory elements. Unfortunately Goel and Grafman did not report any assessment of the working memory abilities of their frontal patients, so it is not possible to determine whether their frontal patients were impaired specifically on tests of working memory, as would be predicted by this account.[11]

[11] There is evidence from behavioural studies with normal participants that working memory, at least with respect to spatial

The work of Goel et al. (2001) is valuable as it demonstrates the importance of developing a computationally complete account of the task. However, it leaves several issues unresolved. First, can the account of a working memory deficit be extrapolated to the performance of frontal patients on the Tower of London? We have considered the two tasks as if they have similar cognitive requirements, but there are substantial differences between them. Most notably, the Tower of Hanoi can be solved by the application of a recursive strategy that, once learned, requires no look-ahead; each move is cued by the current subgoal and the current perceptual representation of the task (Simon, 1975; Patsenko & Altmann, 2010). This is not the case for the Tower of London, which requires look-ahead for its solution.[12] Second, does the failure to replicate the frontal pattern of performance by manipulating response competition within the Goel et al. computational model rule out a response inhibition account of the frontal deficit? Goel and colleagues are clear that it does not. The modelling work shows that a working memory impairment is *sufficient* to reproduce frontal behaviour. It does not show that it is *necessary*.[13] An alternative implementation, perhaps involving different strategic components, may demonstrate that the frontal pattern of performance can be modelled in terms of a failure in response inhibition. Third, how does learning affect behaviour in the two tasks? The claims of Goel et al. (2001) are based on a model that does not learn, so behaviour on the ninth problem does not benefit from the experience gained on the previous eight. This may be justified for the Goel and Grafman (1995) behavioural study where the difficulties of frontal patients persisted over the entire experiment. Yet Morris et al. (1997) traced the frontal deficit on their modified version of the Tower of Hanoi to task novelty, with the experience of 4-move problems which produces goal/subgoal conflict being sufficient to resolve the difficulties of their frontal patients on 5-move problems of this type. Hence, the account of Goel and colleagues is not entirely satisfactory.

There is a third potential account of the difficulties of left-frontal patients on goal/subgoal conflict problems, namely that the difficulties arise not from response inhibition but from a difficulty in shifting between a goal and its subgoals. Thus, in a developmental study, Bull et al. (2004) found that set-shifting was a significant predictor of performance on goal/subgoal conflict problems in both tower-building tasks, and in Section 9.11 it was argued that task-setting, a closely related process, is a function of left prefrontal cortex.[14]

Can imaging studies shed light on the veracity of any of these hypotheses, or on the localisation of other processes supporting goal-directed problem-solving? While several imaging studies have explored brain activity during tower-building tasks, the critical study, comparing performance on otherwise matched goal/subgoal conflict and non-conflict problems, remains to be carried out. However, given the complex nature of goal-directed problem-solving it is not surprising that those studies that have been conducted have revealed that goal-directed problem-solving is subserved by a network of cortical regions and sub-cortical structures. Thus, in one of the earliest PET studies, Baker and colleagues (1996) compared activity during the solution of easy (2- or 3-move) and hard (4- or 5-move) Tower of London problems with that of a control task with matched visuo-motor requirements. For each problem subjects were presented with a diagram showing the initial and desired task state and asked to indicate the number of moves required to solve the problem. Task specific activity was observed bilaterally in many anterior regions—the premotor cortex, supplementary motor area, anterior cingulate gyrus, and dorsolateral prefrontal cortex (DLPFC), as well as in the right lateral frontopolar cortex (BA10). Bilateral parietal activation was also observed as one would expect from the spatial processing involved, as was activation in the left cerebellar hemisphere and the vermis. Critically, activity in right lateral frontopolor cortex and bilateral DLPFC was greater during the solution of hard problems than of easy problems. Consistent with studies cited earlier, the authors attribute DLPFC activity to 'active maintenance' of representations in working memory, arguing that the task has both spatial (right) and non-spatial

---

content, affects performance on tower building tasks (see Welsh et al., 1999). It is not clear, however, whether the effect relates specifically to conflict problems.

[12] This difference may account for the fact that in behavioural studies in which response inhibition has been related to performance on both the Tower of London and the Tower of Hanoi, the relation has been found to be stronger in the case of the Tower of London than the Tower of Hanoi (Welsh et al., 1999; Bull et al., 2004).

[13] Note that as far as the Tower of London is concerned, an increase in number of moves and time to solution, as produced by ineffective response competition in the Goel et al. simulation, would in fact lead to poorer performance since the Tower of London is a timed task and requires perfect solutions.

---

[14] Note, however, that some researchers are sceptical about the relationship between tower-building ability and executive functions, at least in children. Thus, in a developmental study of 238 children aged 7 to 15, Bishop et al. (2001) found no significant correlation between performance on a graded version of the Tower of Hanoi and measures of inhibition. Moreover, when children were retested on the Tower of Hanoi after one month, Bishop and colleagues found only moderate test/retest reliability ($r = 0.5$), suggesting that the task is not a good measure of executive function.

(left) aspects. It is speculated that (right) lateral frontopolar cortical activity reflects planning and the manipulation of items in working memory.

Several subsequent studies of planning have also found right lateral frontopolar activity (e.g. Dagher et al., 1999; Rowe et al., 2001), though the interpretation of this activity is a matter of debate. Recall that in Section 9.14 lateral frontopolar function was related to the setting of cognitive modes, with more lateral regions of BA10 being involved in so-called stimulus-independent processing including intention-realising, while medial regions were required for stimulus-directed processing. Complex planning (and more generally manipulation of items within working memory) is stimulus independent, so the gateway hypothesis of Burgess and colleagues discussed in Section 9.14 is also consistent with these imaging results. Chapter 9 also presented evidence for specific functions of two further cortical regions commonly found to be active during planning tasks, namely left and right DLPFC. The hypothesis that left DLPFC is related specifically to task setting is consistent both with the activation of this region in studies of planning and goal-directed problem-solving and with the third of the above hypotheses concerning the difficulties of left-frontal patients on goal/subgoal conflict problems, namely that their difficulties arise from problems in shifting set between tackling a subgoal and tackling the overall goal. The hypothesised role of right DLPFC in monitoring is also consistent with the activation of this area in planning studies, on the assumption that planning is also generally accompanied by active monitoring of the plan as it is generated.

The comparison of activity during the solution of easy and hard problems by Baker and colleagues is a potentially powerful technique for revealing the neural regions involved in planning. As a technique it is mirrored by the method used by Monti et al. (2007), discussed in Section 12.4, in the functional imaging of deductive inference. However the power of the Baker et al. study was limited as the authors considered only two levels of task difficulty. Several subsequent imaging studies of goal-directed problem-solving have therefore employed similar methods but with more levels of difficulty. For instance, Dagher and colleagues (1999) used 5 levels of task difficulty (corresponding to problems requiring 1 to 5 moves), while Newman et al. (2003) used 3 levels (corresponding to 1–2-move problems, 3–4-move problems and 5–6-move problems). The task in both of these studies was the Tower of London. Fincham et al. (2002) also investigated different levels of task difficulty, although in this case the task was 'the Grid of Pittsburgh', an isomorph of the Tower of Hanoi, while Schall et al. (2003) used both PET and fMRI to explore the effects of problem difficulty in a simplified version of the Tower of London.

Direct comparison of the various studies is made difficult by differences in the procedures used. Critical differences exist in the instructions given to subjects, the extent of training prior to scanning and the precise form of the task apparatus.[15] However, despite these differences, there is some consistency in the imaging results. For example, as in the Baker et al. study, Dagher et al. (1999) found certain regions to be active during problem solution regardless of problem difficulty. These included areas within striate cortex, extrastriate cortex and the inferior parietal lobe, which Dagher et al. relate to visual processing, but could well concern triggering of subgoals analogous to the triggering of actions discussed in Section 8.5, and also areas within the primary motor cortex, cerebellum and pre-supplementary motor area, which Dagher et al. relate to motor processing. Similar findings, taking into account differences in the required response and the control conditions, were obtained in the other imaging studies.

More interesting are those regions where activity correlates with task difficulty. Of the studies cited above, Dagher et al. (1999) used the most complex task and found the most extensive network of such regions, including lateral premotor cortex (BA 6 bilaterally), dorsolateral prefrontal cortex (left BA 9/46, right BA 9), anterior cingulate cortex (left BA 32, right BA 24), left precuneus (BA 7), left putamen, right frontopolar cortex (BA 10) and right caudate nucleus. Plots showing relative rCBF across conditions for some of these areas are shown in Figure 12.15. In contrast, Schall et al. (2003), who used a far simpler task, found more focussed difficulty-related activity, with the frontal

---

[15] Thus some studies required participants to produce a sequence of moves (Dagher et al., 1999; Fincham et al., 2002), while others required participants to indicate the number of moves required to solve a problem (Newman et al., 2003; Schall et al., 2003). Requiring subjects to indicate the number of moves puts them in a complex dual-task situation, so involving yet more component processes. Just as critically, Dagher et al. (1999) provided subjects with extensive practice prior to scanning, while Fincham and colleagues (2002) were concerned specifically with the processing of goals and subgoals, and so trained their subjects to use a specific strategy. Newman et al. (2003) were concerned specifically with expert performance and four main regions of interest (left and right DLPFC and SPL). Subjects were given extensive experience on the task prior to scanning and analysis was restricted to the prespecified regions of interest. Instead, Schall et al. (2003) were concerned primarily with the comparison of PET and fMRI. They used a modified version of the Tower of London where all pegs were of equal length. This eliminates important constraints on problems, effectively eliminating the need for look-ahead. Finally, only one study—that of Fincham et al. (2002)—considered the possibility that different problems may engage different cognitive, and hence different neural, processes.

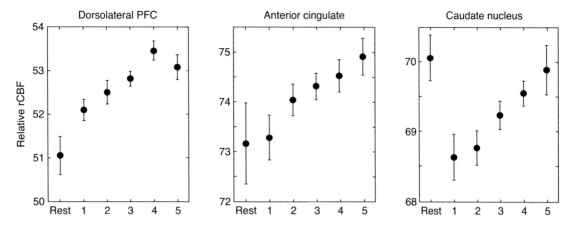

Fig. 12.15 Relative rCBF for two regions of the prefrontal cortex and the caudate nucleus as a function of problem complexity in the Tower of London study of Dagher et al. (1999). All three regions show a positive correlation with the number of moves required to solve the problem. All the regions shown are right hemisphere ones, but similar results were found for left dorsolateral PFC and anterior cingulate. Reprinted from A. Dagher, A.M. Owen, H. Boecker and D.J. Brooks, Mapping the network for planning: a correlational PET activation study with the Tower of London task, *Brain*, 1999, 122(10), 1973–1987, by permission of Oxford University Press.

contribution as shown by both PET and fMRI being limited to the left middle and superior frontal gyri.

Taken together, the imaging studies suggest that goal-directed problem-solving recruits a network of cortical regions that most commonly includes right frontopolar cortex (BA10), right dorsolateral prefrontal cortex (BA 9/46), left inferior/medial frontal gyrus (BA 44, 8), anterior cingulate cortex (BA 32, bilaterally), and the superior parietal lobule (BA 7, bilaterally), with many of these areas showing greater involvement with more difficult problems.

For the most part, imaging studies of goal-directed problem-solving have not contrasted conditions which differ in just one part of the hypothesised problem-solving process. Consequently any association of function to structure must be shakily based on converging evidence (such as that relating left inferior frontal gyrus to response selection; see Section 9.13). Indeed the very variety of regions activated makes a convincing account of the specific functions involved for each region especially difficult. Moreover this is one motivating factor for the types of investigations reported in Chapter 9.

One exception to this implicit dismissal is the PET study of Rowe et al. (2001), who compared neural activity during four goal-directed moves which were part of a solution attempt with activity during the generation of four connected but otherwise random moves. In both conditions subjects were presented with an initial Tower of London problem state. In the first condition they were also given a goal state which had to be obtained, while in the second they were asked to imagine manipulating the start state with any four valid moves in sequence. Subjects were given extensive practice on the task before scanning, and took roughly the same length of time in both conditions.

As would be expected from the previous discussion, prefrontal areas were activated in both conditions (including dorsolateral PFC, orbitofrontal PFC and anterior cingulate cortex, all bilaterally activated).[16] However, none of these areas survived the subtraction of conditions. The main areas found to be more active in the goal-directed condition than in the undirected condition were in prestriate cortex (BA 18, 19, bilaterally) and the lingual and right fusiform gyri (BA 37, bilaterally).[17] Rowe and colleagues argue that systems in prefrontal areas are involved in the generation and selection of moves, in mentally manipulating a representation of the task state according to the selected move, and in holding a sequence of selected moves in memory during the task, but that the evaluation of moves (through comparison of the imagined state with the goal state) occurs in systems in prestriate cortex or the lingual/fusiform gyri. The authors note that this is consistent with Kosslyn et al.'s (1997) localisation of a visual imagery buffer in prestriate cortex[18] and an inferior temporal subsystem

---

[16] Left lateral frontopolar cortical activation was also found in one analysis. Activity in this region was correlated with thinking time.

[17] Activation of right premotor and left intraparietal cortex also survived the subtraction.

[18] See Sections 7.4 and 8.6 for discussion of properties and possible localisations of visual short-term stores. Note in particular that a distinction must be drawn between categorical and metrical spatial encoding. The claimed localisation of Kosslyn's visual imagery buffer in early visual processing would suggest that it would not employ categorical coding. This, combined with the brain-imaging results, suggests that, on this approach, coding of intermediate and goal states would also not employ categorical coding. This seems implausible.

for matching object properties to visual memories. However, these findings could also be explained in terms of visual attention processes—in the plan conditions both displays are different and relevant, while in the control conditions the displays are identical.

It is clear from these studies that goal-directed problem-solving is not a unitary process. Given extensive practice of the domain, problem-solving must draw upon a set of subprocesses, potentially including those responsible for the generation, evaluation and selection of possible moves. This alone can differ from problem type to problem type as can the modality-specific working memories required for storing the representation of the current problem state and the sequence of moves held to be solving the problem. Even these processes, however, are insufficient to support thinking in all its forms. Indeed nearly all the functional imaging studies of tower-tasks involve extensive practice, which some of the neuropsychological studies deliberately avoided. Yet the findings of Morris et al. (1997) show how important that factor is. Indeed in Chapter 9 it was argued that a key aspect of prefrontal functions is to make the changes from novel to practiced state. Further afield, consider situations in which one abstracts a common feature from a set of premises. The processes required for this kind of thinking would appear to be highly relevant to goal-directed problem-solving in its most general form. Equally they would appear to be far removed from those involved in manipulating or searching a solution space. We therefore now turn to those processes.

12.6 Rule Induction

In Sections 12.2 and 12.3 we considered a key process required both for the solution of verbal or pictorial analogies and the solution of progressive matrices, namely the induction of a relation or rule that holds between the stimuli. In these tasks, the relation or rule is induced based on common features of two or three stimuli. Within experimental psychology there is a long history of studies within the general topic of *category learning* where subjects must induce or abstract the rule or common features that relate a large series of stimuli (e.g. Hull, 1920; Berg, 1948).

Essentially three positions have developed as to how induction might be achieved. All three assume that stimuli are preprocessed into a set of features, with category membership defined as a function of those features. According to the associationist view, features are associated with categories via weighted links. When an exemplar is discovered to belong to a category, the links between features possessed by the exemplar and the category are strengthened, while the links between features not possessed by the exemplar and the category are weakened. This view corresponds to the computational approach of connectionism. A second, Bayesian, view holds that subjects develop estimates for the probability of an exemplar belonging to a category given each cue. When given a novel exemplar, they implicitly apply Bayes' rule (see Section 5.5) to combine the information in the exemplar's features with their knowledge of the frequency of each category to determine the probability that the exemplar belongs to each category. The exemplar may then be categorised as belonging to the most likely category. The final view, that of hypothesis-testing, holds that subjects generate explicit hypotheses concerning category membership (e.g. 'if features X and Y are present and Z is absent then the exemplar belongs to category C'), testing and modifying those hypotheses when information about category membership becomes available.

The three accounts are difficult to distinguish behaviourally. Indeed, the theories can all be modified to include the modulation of behaviour by cognitive biases.[19] Each can then provide a plausible account of how normal subjects behave (Cooper et al., 2003). It is therefore natural to ask if cognitive neuroscience evidence might help discriminate between the approaches.

Perhaps the most widely used task within the cognitive neuropsychological literature with a rule-induction component is the Wisconsin card-sorting test (Milner, 1963; see Figure 12.16). Here, subjects are presented with a succession of cards showing; for example, two green triangles or four blue circles. Subjects are required to sort each card in turn according to a rule known only to the clinician (e.g. sort according to the colour of the figures on the card, ignoring the number or shape of the figures). They do this by matching the stimulus card with one of four target cards, where the target cards show one red triangle, two green stars, and so on. Feedback is given after each card is sorted, allowing the subject to infer the sorting rule, but after some number of correct sorts (six or ten, depending on the version of test being used) the administrator changes the sorting rule.[20] Frontal patients are frequently impaired on this test, with some producing high rates of perseverative errors, in which the subject appears to

---

[19] This could be by adding a bias in the prior probabilities of different features or categories within the Bayesian framework, by adjusting the learning rate within the associationist approach thus altering the relative weight of recent experience, or by a focus on confirmation rather than disconfirmation in the hypothesis-based approach.

[20] In the original versions of Grant and Berg (1948) and of Milner (1963) this is done without telling the subject; the subject must then realise from the feedback that his/her rule is incorrect, and discover the new rule. In Nelson's (1976) version the subject is told when but not how the rule changes.

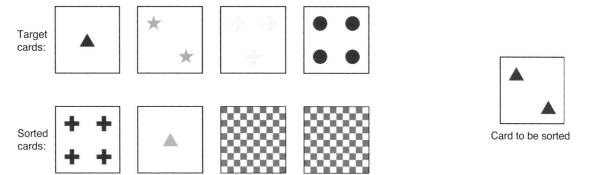

Fig. 12.16 The Wisconsin Card-Sorting Test. Four target cards, each showing from one to four figures of one to four different types in one of four different colours, are placed at the top of the table. The subject is then required to sort a succession of similar cards into piles beneath the target cards. The figure shows the situation after two cards have been sorted and as the subject is about to sort the third card, showing two blue triangles. Should it be placed under the red triangle (matching on shape), the two green stars (matching on number), or the four blue circles (matching on colour)?

ignore negative feedback and continue sorting with a previously correct rule.[21]

The diversity of effects found with different patient groups on the Wisconsin card-sorting task can be explained by the range of processes that must be involved in normal performance. These include processes that have generally been held to be frontally localised, such as generating a set of possible sorting rules, reasoning from feedback, following a rule once one has been determined to be plausible, maintaining this current sorting rule in working memory, switching between rules and avoiding impulsivity (see Reverberi et al., 2005b for discussion). In addition there are some that are presumably non-frontal (e.g. matching to a feature), and imaging studies have confirmed the involvement of temporal, parietal and cerebellar regions in the task (e.g. Berman et al., 1995; Nagahama et al., 1996). Its complexity means that the Wisconsin card-sorting test, while an excellent clinical instrument, is not ideal for investigating the cognitive and neural processes underlying rule induction.[22]

A more appropriate task for addressing rule induction is the Brixton Spatial Rule Attainment task (Burgess & Shallice, 1996a). In this task, subjects are presented with a series of cards showing 10 circles, with one filled circle on each card (see Figure 12.17a). The circle that is filled on successive cards follows a simple rule (e.g. alternating between two positions, or moving clockwise around the card). The subject's task is to indicate where they think the next filled circle will be. As in the Wisconsin

card-sorting task, the subject is not told the rule, but unlike the Wisconsin the rule changes without warning after 5–9 trials, regardless of how the subject responds.

The Brixton and Wisconsin tasks both require that subjects induce a rule based on a series of exemplars, but in the Brixton task responses are driven by applying a rule to a stimulus card, rather than by matching the stimulus card on some dimension with a response card. Thus, a perseverative error on the Brixton task is scored when the location indicated by a subject corresponds to that which would have resulted given the current stimulus location and the previous rule. In the original work with the Brixton task it was found that frontal patients did *not* produce more perseverative errors than nonfrontal patients. Rather, frontal patients were impaired at achieving and maintaining the correct rule.

There are several potential explanations of the frontal impairment on the Brixton task. It may, for example, stem from a working memory deficit. This could hinder both attainment of a rule (if the subject is unable to maintain sufficient exemplars from which to induce a rule) and maintenance of a rule (if the subject forgets the rule after it has been induced). Alternatively, it may result from, amongst others, a deficit in the induction process itself or a deficit in applying an induced rule. In order to evaluate different potential explanations of the frontal impairment on the task, and to further localise that impairment, Reverberi et al. (2005a) used a modified version of the Brixton task, together with the patient sub-classification developed by Stuss and colleagues in their ROBBIA studies (as discussed in Section 9.8). Altogether 40 frontal patients (10 left lateral, 10 right lateral, 11 inferior medial and 9 superior medial) and 43 age- and education-matched controls completed (a) a working memory test, (b) standard Progressive Matrices, and (c) a modified form of the Brixton test (see Figure 12.17b). The modified Brixton test began with

---

[21] Different subgroups of frontal patients show different patterns of deficits on the task (see Stuss et al. 2000), and some non-frontal patients also show impairments on the test (Anderson et al., 1991).

[22] It should be stressed that while the test has a rule-induction component, it is normally considered a test of set-shifting ability.

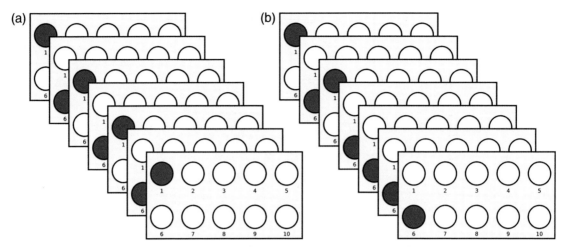

Fig. 12.17 (a) The Brixton Spatial Rule Attainment task of Burgess and Shallice (1996a). The subject is shown a series of cards, each with 10 circles one of which is coloured blue. For each card the subject is required to predict (by pointing) where they think the blue circle will appear next. (b) The modified Brixton task of Reverberi et al. (2005). Subjects completed the standard task except that for some cards the coloured circle was red. For such cards the subject was required to touch the red circle, but ignore it as far as the prediction task was concerned. When a card with the blue circle returned they must obey the 'blue' rule.

the standard presentation—on each card one circle was filled (in blue) and subjects were required to predict which circle would be filled on the next card. An interference procedure was introduced in the second half of the test. After sufficient blue cards had been presented for subjects to induce the rule, four cards with red filled circles were presented. Subjects were instructed that for these cards they should touch the red filled circle but that they were not relevant for the prediction task. Furthermore, they were instructed that when blue cards returned they should resume where they had left off with the prediction task.

Reverberi and colleagues replicated the principal finding of Burgess and Shallice (1996a): on the standard Brixton task; frontal patients produced significantly fewer correct responses than controls on abstracting rules with the blue cards. However the subclassification of the frontal patients into the four groups and the inclusion of a working memory task revealed a dissociation. First, only the left lateral and inferior medial groups were found to be impaired relative to controls on the standard Brixton task. Second, all four groups contained both patients who scored within the normal range on the working memory test and patients who scored below the normal range. For three of the four groups—right lateral, inferior medial and superior medial—an impairment on the Brixton task could be attributed to a working memory impairment. This was not the case for the left lateral group: The impairment of the left lateral patients was independent of any working memory deficit (see Figure 12.18a).

The inclusion of the interfering trials in the second half of the Brixton procedure revealed a second dissociation: right lateral patients were nearly three times

more likely than controls to produce a capture error to the first blue card after a sequence of red cards. They were significantly more likely to adhere to the rule governing the red cards on presentation of a subsequent blue card. This was not so for any of the three other patient groups (see Figure 12.18b). Note though that right lateral patients were able to correctly apply negative feedback when this occurred, recovering the old rule at a rate comparable to controls. In contrast, the recovery rate of left lateral patients following negative feedback was significantly below that of controls.

The results of Reverberi and colleagues argue against many potential explanations for the frontal impairment on the Brixton task, and furthermore support the claim that the superficially similar behavioural impairments of at least some of the frontal groups are a consequence of different functional impairments. First, there were no differences in response times for any of the groups. This argues against an explanation of impairment on the task as resulting from impulsivity. Second, an analysis of errors found that neither perseverations of the previous response nor perseverations of the previous rule were statistically more frequent in any of the patient groups than in the control group. This argues against a 'stuck-in-set' explanation of frontal performance on the Brixton task.[23] Third, in the case of the left lateral group, those who were not so impaired on the working memory task performed as poorly on the Brixton task as those who were really impaired.

---

[23] Further analyses suggest that perseverative responses on the task are more reasonably attributed to patients ignoring negative feedback.

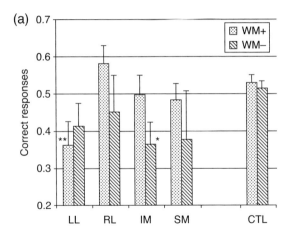 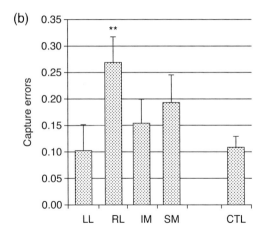

Fig. 12.18 (a) Performance of several patient groups on the standard Brixton task. All groups are divided into those with poor and good working memory as assessed by a separate working memory test. In the left lateral group (and only that group), participants with good working memory performed significantly below the control mean. (b) Capture errors for the various patient groups on the modified Brixton task (see Figure 12.17b). Right lateral patients were significantly more likely to produce such errors than any other patient group. (LL: Left lateral; RL: Right lateral; IM: Inferior medial; SM: Superior medial; CTL: Control.) Adapted from *Neuropsychologia, 43*(3), C. Reverberi, A. Lavaroni, G.L. Gigli, M. Skrap and T. Shallice, Specific impairments of rule induction in different frontal lobe subgroups, 460–472. Copyright (2005), with permission from Elsevier.

The difficulties that the left-lateral group have in abstracting rules in the task therefore cannot be attributed to a working memory impairment. Fourth, no group showed an elevated tendency to err after having obtained the rule. Reverberi et al. argue that this implies that the difficulty for patients is not in applying a known rule.[24] Fifth, while capture errors were more frequent in the right-lateral group during the second-half of the procedure, than in any other frontal group, right-lateral patients were not impaired on the standard Brixton task. This argues against an account of poor performance on the standard Brixton task as an impairment of monitoring or checking.[25]

How then is impaired performance on the Brixton task to be explained? While a working memory impairment may account for the performance of the inferior medial group, none of the above explanations can account for the performance of the left lateral group. Reverberi et al. argue instead that the left-lateral impairment reflects a specific deficit in rule induction.[26] This hypothesis has been refined by a second patient study of Reverberi and colleagues (Reverberi et al., 2005b). In the first phase of this study, further groups of frontal patients (and age- and education-matched controls) were given 10 min to generate and demonstrate as many potential rules for the Brixton task as they could. The left-lateral patients produced fewer rules than the right-lateral patients, and significantly fewer rules than the controls.[27] In the second phase of the study, the subjects completed another modified version of the Brixton test in which they were given, prior to the standard task, a training session featuring the types of rules to be used in the standard task. Testing with the standard task was only commenced when the patient had demonstrated, both on a sample Brixton card and verbally, that he/she understood the rule. On the subsequent standard test, patients, including those with left-lateral lesions and unimpaired working memory, performed on a par with controls. The implication of this study is that rule induction, at least as it pertains to the Brixton task, involves the generation and testing of hypotheses, and it is the generation of hypotheses on which left lateral patients are impaired.

Further support for the view of induction as a left-lateralised process comes from a study of split-brain and unilateral lesion patients by Wolford et al. (2000).

[24] This is in contrast to patient behaviour on the Wisconsin card-sorting test, where Stuss et al. (2000) showed that the IM group had a tendency to drift off correct applications of a rule they had attained.

[25] The data add further support, however, to the argument that monitoring and checking processes are right lateralised (see Section 9.10). On most trials, right-lateral patients were able to adjust their behaviour following external negative feedback, as indicated by their good recovery scores, but still failed to monitor or check their response prior to producing it on 30% of trials.

[26] Consistent with this interpretation, left-lateral patients also showed a trend towards an impairment on Progressive Matrices,

a task that depends heavily on induction as discussed in Section 12.2 (see also Carpenter et al., 1990; Verguts & De Boeck, 2002).

[27] In this study the inferior and superior medial patients were treated as a single group. This group also produced significantly fewer rules than control subjects.

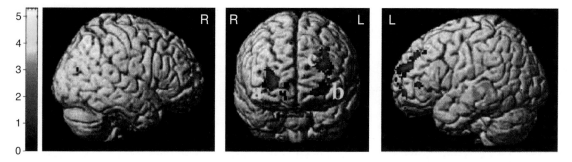

Fig. 12.19 The main effect of rule change in the rule induction task of Strange et al. (2001). Three activation difference peaks were found in frontopolar cortex associated with rule change trials versus non-rule change trials: (a) located at (30, 66, 4), (b) located at (−30, 58, −4) and (c) located at (−28, 60, 24). The coloured bar denotes the T value of the activation difference. Reprinted from B.A. Strange, R.N.A. Henson, K.J. Friston and R.J.Dolan, Anterior prefrontal cortex mediates rule learning in humans, *Cerebral Cortex*, 2001, *11*(11), 1040–1046, by permission of Oxford University Press.

When split-brain patients were required to predict a stimulus based on a preceding series which had been presented to their left hemisphere, they responded by probability matching (i.e. generating predictions with probabilities which matched the probabilities in the input). When, instead, the series was presented to their right hemisphere, they responded by maximising (i.e. generating the most frequent stimulus as their prediction). Similar results were obtained from the unilateral lesion patients. Wolford and colleagues interpret the finding as indicating that the left prefrontal cortex is involved in 'searching for patterns of events', i.e. in inductive hypothesis generation. This would be a key component in task-setting, the creating of a procedure to cope with a novel situation (see Section 9.11), which we also hold to be a left lateral prefrontal process.

If the left lateral prefrontal cortex is involved in the inductive generation of hypotheses then one would expect this area to be preferentially activated in relevant imaging studies. We have already seen that Christoff et al. (2001) found left frontal cortical activity in their complex Progressive Matrices condition (BA10 and BA 6/44), and several other studies of induction and rule learning have also found this to be the case (e.g. Berman et al., 1995; Goel et al., 1997; Osherson et al., 1998; Duncan et al., 2000; Parsons & Osherson, 2001; Strange et al., 2001; Seger & Cincotta, 2006). However, interpretation of the results must remain tentative given the large number of areas activated in most of these studies. Consider for example the areas activated in the study of Duncan et al. (2000), discussed in Section 9.4 (see Figure 9.9), which used an odd-one-out task, or the study of Strange et al. (2001). This used an event-related fMRI design. Subjects were scanned while they were presented with a series of 4 letter strings. Their task was to learn a categorisation rule for the strings based on feedback by following a trial-and-error strategy. Thus, after each trial, the subject attempted to categorise the string (using a yes/no push button response)

and was given feedback. The rule was periodically changed (as in the Wisconsin and Brixton tasks), but all subjects were able to use the feedback effectively to learn the changing rules. As shown in Figure 12.19, three cortical regions were found to be significantly more active in rule-change than in no-rule-change blocks, including left frontal polar cortex (BA 10) and left superior frontal sulcus (BA 9/10).

However a first major problem in interpreting these functional imaging studies of induction is that a variety of other regions have been found to be activated in other studies of rule induction, including right lateral prefrontal cortex (Goel & Dolan, 2000), bilateral frontopolar cortex (Strange et al., 2001; see Figure 12.19), and bilateral medial frontal cortex (BA 6 and 8: Seger & Cincotta, 2006), as well as numerous subcortical structures (e.g. the hippocampus and the caudate: Seger & Cincotta, 2006). Second, many rule induction studies are of only tangential relevance to localising the systems responsible for the form of induction analysed in the studies of the Brixton task. For example, the 'induction' condition of the study of Goel et al. (1997) involved plausibility judgements of arguments, rather than induction *per se*, while in the study of Seger and Cincotta (2006), stimuli consisted of pairs of letters that differed in font, colour and size. On each trial subjects were required to select one letter and given positive or negative feedback about whether the letter belonged to an unknown category. On the basis of this feedback, subjects were able to learn the category rule after 4 to 7 trials. In this task, however, subjects were told that the categorisation rule would always be based on one of the three features. The task is therefore more akin to that of Reverberi et al. (2005b), where subjects were primed with all possible rules and where left lateral patients were not impaired.

Regardless of these issues, the involvement of frontal processes in rule induction suggests that rule induction involves more than simple associationist or Bayesian computation. The positive arguments for a hypothesis

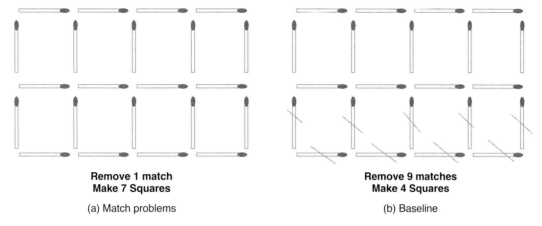

Remove 1 match
Make 7 Squares

(a) Match problems

Remove 9 matches
Make 4 Squares

(b) Baseline

Fig. 12.20 The matchstick tasks of counting small squares of Goel and Vartanian (2005). (a) In the experimental condition the subject was given a problem statement and required to indicate how many solutions where possible. (In this case 4.) (b) In the baseline condition the subject was required to verify whether a given solution attempt was correct. (In this case the answer is 'yes'.) Reprinted from V. Goel and O. Vartanian, Dissociating the roles of right ventral lateral and dorsal lateral prefrontal cortex in generation and maintenance of hypotheses in set-shift problems, *Cerebral Cortex*, 2005, *15*(8), 1170–1177, by permission of Oxford University Press.

testing approach though are not strong. In particular, it is unclear how the computational processes that might support hypothesis testing are related to other putative processes of the left prefrontal cortex.

12.7 Hypothesis Generation and Lateral Thinking

The view that we have presented of hypothesis generation as it occurs in rule induction tasks is that it is a left-lateralised process. However it is plausible that a range of different processes may result in the generation of a hypothesis. Rule induction is just one of these. Goel and colleagues (e.g. Goel & Grafman, 2000; Goel & Vartanian, 2005; Goel, 2009) have developed an alternative view of hypothesis generation related to what they term *lateral transformations* in thinking. These they see as a function of the right hemisphere, and in particular of right ventrolateral prefrontal cortex.

Goel and Vartanian define a lateral transformation as 'a movement from one state in a problem space to a horizontally displaced state rather than a more detailed version of the same state (i.e. vertically displaced)' (Goel & Vartanian, 2005, p. 1170). Consider a problem such as designing an artefact for a specified purpose. A vertically displaced state would be one in which an existing partial design is elaborated. A horizontally displaced one (i.e. a lateral transformation) would involve reversing or discarding or conceiving in a different fashion some previous design decisions.

In order to investigate the neural correlates of lateral transformations, Goel and Vartanian scanned 13 normal subjects while they attempted a series of matchstick problems. In these problems, subjects are presented

with an array of matchsticks (see Figure 12.20a) and asked, for example, how many ways one matchstick can be removed to leave seven small squares with each remaining match being part of a square. The authors argue that lateral transformations are required for successful solution of these problems. Subjects were given up to 15 sec to solve each problem, though one-third of the problems had no solutions. Subjects were also scanned in a baseline condition where their task was to verify whether a specific solution to a matchstick problem was correct (Figure 12.20b).

A direct comparison of activation during the matchstick problems with that during the baseline condition, controlling for problem difficulty, yielded two regions of prefrontal cortex that were more active in the former condition than the latter: one in left dorsolateral PFC (BA 46) and one in right ventrolateral PFC (BA 47). Goel and Vartanian argue that the difference between conditions is one of hypothesis generation, with both conditions requiring hypothesis checking.[28]

In a second analysis, Goel and Vartanian restricted their attention to matchstick problems with valid solutions. They compared neural activity when subjects found at least one solution to such problems with activity when they failed to find any solutions. Three frontal regions were implicated by this contrast: right ventrolateral PFC (BA 47), left middle frontal gyrus (BA 9) and left frontal pole (BA 10). On the basis of their finding that right ventrolateral PFC is the only region that is preferentially active, both when solving matchstick

---

[28] No regions of prefrontal cortex were found to be more active in the baseline condition than when completing matchstick problems.

problems and when generating non-null solutions to those problems, Goel and Vartanian argue that this region is critical to the production of lateral transformations in the generation of hypotheses, as required to solve the task. The implication is that left dorsolateral PFC is involved in the production of other kinds of hypothesis generation (i.e. those involving non-lateral transformations), which are subtracted out in this second analysis.

In a final analysis, Goel and Vartanian sought neural regions whose activity covaried with the proportion of solutions generated by each subject for each solvable problem. Only one area of prefrontal cortex showed such a covariation: right dorsolateral PFC (BA 46). Three possible roles of this region in the task are considered, with the most plausible, in our view, being the storage of successful solutions (i.e. a working memory maintenance function).

How does Goel and Vartanian's ascription of hypothesis generation to right VLPFC square with the findings from the Brixton task of Reverberi and colleagues discussed earlier? Three possibilities need to be considered. First, Goel and Vartanian make no attempt to interpret the left lateralised activations found in their second analysis. Perhaps hypothesis generation should be associated with these regions, and not right VLPFC. Second, the task analysis of Goel and Vartanian may be questioned. Their account of lateral and non-lateral transformations in the solution of their problems is not well-specified and the contrast made in their analysis between whether or not solutions were found does not necessarily correspond to a contrast in whether or not hypotheses were generated. A more plausible alternative is that subjects reported no solutions only after generating and then rejecting—possibly incorrectly—a series of hypotheses.[29] On this explanation, the right VLPFC activity could reflect monitoring and checking processes. Indeed, if one accepts the plausible assumption that the proportion of solutions found will co-vary with the number of hypotheses considered, then the authors' final analysis, in which right DLPFC was implicated, could equally be interpreted as evidence for the involvement of this region, rather than right VLPFC, in hypothesis generation. Finally, the form of hypothesis generation investigated in this study, i.e. what Goel and Vartanian refer to as lateral transformations, may be qualitatively different from that required by the Brixton

task. Moreover it may be more closely linked to perceptual processes than the Brixton task.

Goel and Vartanian (2005) do not explicitly consider any of these possibilities. They do, however, provide converging evidence to support their interpretation. They point to a patient study of Miller and Tippett (1996) in which subjects were required to solve a series of matchstick problems. Miller and Tippett divided patients with focal lesions into 6 groups: left frontal, left temporal/occipital, left central/parietal, and right frontal, right temporal/occipital, right central/parietal. They employed a task that was designed to induce a form of mental set, with the last problem in each group of four requiring the mental set to be broken. On the basis of an analysis of solutions and errors, Miller and Tippett conclude that 'patients with right frontal-lobe damage demonstrated a selective impairment in the ability to shift strategy' (Miller & Tippett, 1996, p 387). While this is consistent with Goel and Vartanian's position, Miller and Tippett's results are not strong. In comparison to age- and education-matched controls, their right-frontal patients were indeed significantly impaired on a measure of strategy shift (number of correct solutions for the final problem in each block). However, they were also significantly impaired on a measure of strategy application, namely the number of correct solutions for non-final problems in each block, where each problem requires an analogous strategy. The findings of the study do not allow independent assessments of strategy shift and strategy application to be made. Moreover, while the left-frontal group performed better than the right-frontal group on both measures (strategy shift and strategy application), the difference between groups was not statistically significant.

Two further studies have been taken to suggest right prefrontal cortical involvement in the hypothesis generation phase of thinking, namely those of Goel and Grafman (2000) and Vartanian and Goel (2005). In the former, patient PF, a trained architect with extensive right-frontal lesions (including right BA10), was asked to complete an architectural design task, which should have been relatively straightforward given his training and experience. While PF volunteered that it was 'a very simple problem', his performance in comparison to a second age- and education-matched architect was poor. PF devoted most of his time to the initial problem-structuring phase of the task. His preliminary designs were minimal and erratic, and there was no clear progression in the design fragments he produced. He observed that 'I seem to be doing several different thoughts on the same piece of paper in the same place, and it's confusing me ... instead of the one direction that I had at the beginning, I have three or four contradictory directions with not a kind of anchor to work from' (Goel & Grafman, 2000, p. 426). All these problems

---

[29] This account would be supported if subjects took longer on matchstick problems to which they responded 'no solutions' than on problems for which solutions were found. Unfortunately Goel and Vartanian do not report this comparison. It should also be noted that a more sensitive analysis would mask out the time after a solution is given, as activation during this period is likely just to be equivalent to that in a rest condition.

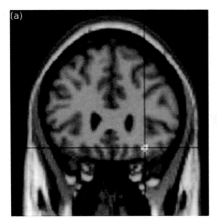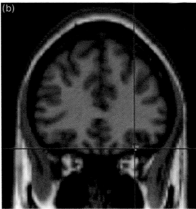

Fig. 12.21 (a) The comparison of match problems versus baseline problems in the study of Goel and Vartanian (2005) (see Figure 12.20). Differential activation is seen in right ventrolateral PFC (32, 28, −16). (b) The comparison of unconstrained versus semantically constrained anagram generation in the study of Vartanian and Goel (2005). Again, significantly greater activation is seen in right ventrolateral PFC (32, 34, −22) .Panel (a) reprinted from V. Goel and O. Vartanian, Dissociating the roles of right ventrolateral and dorsolateral prefrontal cortex in generation and maintenance of hypotheses in set-shift problems, *Cerebral Cortex*, 2005, 15(8), 1170–1177, by permission of Oxford University Press. Panel (b) reprinted from *Neurolmage*, 27(4), O. Vartanian and V. Goel, Task constraints modulate activation in right ventral lateral prefrontal cortex, 927–933, Copyright (2005), with permission from Elsevier.

occurred despite superior intelligence and memory as measured by standardised tests (the Wechsler Adult Intelligence Scale—Revised, and the Wechsler Memory Scale—Revised). Goel and Grafman interpret PF's deficit as an impairment in his ability to generate or execute lateral transformations, as required by so-called *ill-structured problems*—problems with vague or abstractly specified state transformations and goal states. This is plausible, but it relies on a subjective assessment of whether the transformations proposed by PF are in fact lateral. Moreover, it is unclear how it relates to the potential role of right prefrontal cortex in the matchstick problems of Goel and Vartanian (2005) or Miller and Tippett (1996). Those problems are well-structured, with concrete rules for transforming and assessing states (removing matchsticks and counting squares, respectively). PF's disorganisation and time-management was also not qualitatively dissimilar to that of the three frontal patients reported by Shallice and Burgess (1991) and discussed in Section 9.14. Thus, PF took more than an hour to generate his first design proposal, while the control architect did so within 20 min. Difficulties with time-management and task-shifting may well have limited PF's performance on the design task.

Vartanian and Goel (2005) report a further imaging study that suggests a role for right ventrolateral PFC in problem-solving. In this case, the task required subjects to solve anagrams presented in three different conditions. The first was an unconstrained condition, where no clue is given, such as: *Can you make a word from the letters VOED?* In a second semantically constrained condition, category information is given, e.g. *Can you make a type of bird with the letters VOED?* Finally there is a fully

constrained condition, where the full word is given, e.g. *Can you make the word DOVE with the letters VOED.* Right ventrolateral PFC was found to be preferentially activated in the unconstrained condition when compared with either of the other conditions.[30] Moreover, as shown in Figure 12.21, the identified region was almost the same as that found in the same authors' study of matchstick problems (Goel & Vartanian, 2005). Vartanian and Goel argue that it is the lack of constraints in the hypothesis generation phase of the task that engages right ventrolateral PFC.

Two caveats must be accepted if the position of Vartanian and Goel is to be accepted. First, the processing differences between the conditions are not well-understood. It is implausible that the only processing difference between the unconstrained and semantically constrained conditions is that hypothesis generation is more constrained in the latter condition. When category information is given, solution of the anagram is likely to involve a different, more semantically based strategy than when it is not given. For instance, enumerating exemplars from the category could be used in the former case instead of just permuting the letters as in the latter. Second, numerous other cortical areas were also preferentially activated in the unconstrained condition (including left superior frontal gyrus and

---

[30] As might be expected, response latency varied systematically across conditions reflecting differences in task difficulty. It was therefore entered as a covariate in the fMRI analysis. BOLD differences between conditions could therefore not be attributed to more time on task.

right orbitofrontal cortex). The functional roles of these areas as they relate to differences between the conditions are not well articulated.

Our assessment of a possible role for the right ventrolateral prefrontal cortex in lateral hypothesis generation has been largely negative. How should one understand the role of this area in thinking? Three alternatives seem worthy of consideration based on the tasks and imaging results of Goel and Vartanian (2005; Vartanian & Goel, 2005). The first possibility is that right VLPFC plays a critical role in strategy application (see also Burgess, 2000), and more specifically in the manipulation of the subject's representation of a problem's state, particularly when the space of such states is large. Thus, as discussed in Section 12.1 (see also Section 1.6), Newell and Simon (1972) argued that problem-solving can be understood as a process of finding a series of moves that transforms an initial state into a goal state. On this view, the subject must maintain and manipulate a representation of the problem state. Such manipulation is an essential component of the solution of matchstick problems, where a critical step is considering ways of removing matchsticks from the array. It is also essential in the solution of unconstrained anagrams, where ways of rearranging the given letters are required.[31]

A second possibility is that right VLPFC plays a critical role in the generation of novel hypotheses in insight problem-solving. Solving both matchstick problems and anagrams can be accompanied by the subjective 'Aha!' feeling associated with insight (see Katona, 1940 and Novick & Sherman, 2003, respectively), and right-frontal patients are also known to be impaired at humour appreciation (Shammi & Stuss, 1999)—an ability that has been claimed to relate to insight. Furthermore, it is conceivable that some form of insight is also associated with satisfactory architectural design as required of PF in Goel and Grafman's (2000) study, and the generation of insightful hypotheses is consistent with Goel's claims for a role of right VLPFC in supporting lateral transformations within a problem space (assuming that such transformations are considered to be 'insightful').

A third very different possibility which would fit with hypotheses of Petrides (1994) and of Fletcher et al. (1998b) on ventrolateral prefrontal cortex is that in this study the right ventrolateral region is involved in retrieval specification, in this case, of word-forms which could be made up of the relevant letters available. [32] There are too many options for the function being realised by systems

located in this area! Let us begin by considering just one: insight.

12.8 Insight and Restructuring

A distinction that is commonly made in the problem-solving literature is between problem-solving that does and problem-solving that does not involve *insight*. The precise nature of insight is unclear, but it is generally held to involve initially an impasse or block to problem-solving, where no solution is obvious, followed by a sudden and unanticipated realisation of the problem solution. This realisation is accompanied by a subjective feeling of understanding. Problem-solving that does not require insight is well-described within the information processing tradition by Newell and Simon's (1972) theory of problem spaces referred to in the previous section. A recurring question though is whether the solution of problems with and without insight involves qualitatively different processes.[33]

The dominant processing-level theory of insight problem-solving is representational change theory. This holds that impasses arise when the problem representation (or problem space, in Newell and Simon's terms) adopted by the problem solver does not support or facilitate the problem's solution (Ohlsson, 1992; Knoblich et al., 1999). The theory posits that insight involves representational change or *restructuring* of the problem. Once an appropriate structure has been found, problem-solving may proceed within the restructured problem space as Newell and Simon envisaged for non-insight problem-solving.[34]

Consideration of well-known insight problems provides intuitive support for representational change theory. Consider the mutilated checkerboard problem shown in Figure 12.22. Here one must determine if an 8 by 8 checkerboard with two diagonally opposite squares removed can be covered by 31 rectangular dominos, where each domino exactly covers two squares. Representing this problem as an array of squares that

---

[31] This form of manipulation of a problem state representation would also be required in Tower problems such as those discussed in Section 12.5. The key difference is that in those problems the state space is relatively constrained.

[32] The area is also close to one of Duncan and Owen's (2000) multiple demand regions (see Section 9.4).

---

[33] The question was posed in the Gestalt literature well before Newell and Simon's work, where a similar distinction was drawn between productive thinking and reproductive thinking (Wertheimer, 1920).

[34] Unfortunately representational change theory does not provide a general account of *how* restructuring might occur. An alternative view of insight problem-solving has been developed by MacGregor et al. (2001). The *criterion for satisfactory progress theory* argues that impasses are a consequence of inappropriate constraints on possible transformations within a problem space. In this case, insight involves relaxing constraints on possible problem space transformations, rather than restructuring of the problem space. As in representational change theory, once such constraints are relaxed, problem-solving may proceed as in non-insight problem-solving.

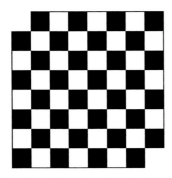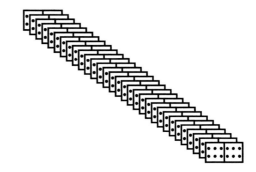

Fig. 12.22 The mutilated chequerboard problem. The chequerboard on the left is a standard 8 by 8 board with opposite corners removed. It therefore consists of 62 squares. Each domino on the right will exactly cover two squares of the board. Can 31 dominos be placed on the board to fully cover every square?

must be covered leads to a lengthy process of trial-and-error. In contrast, representing each domino as necessarily covering one black and one white square, and the board as an array specifically of black and white squares, in which the diagonally opposite corner squares are of the same colour, leads to the immediate realisation that on the mutilated board there are 32 squares of one colour but only 30 of the other. The problem therefore has no solution.

The group of Bowden, Jung-Beeman, Kounios and colleagues have conducted a series of behavioural, fMRI and EEG studies of insight in normals with the aim of clarifying whether insight problem-solving is qualitatively different from non-insight problem-solving and, if so, localising the processes that differ (see, e.g. Bowden & Jung-Beeman, 2003; Jung-Beeman et al., 2004; Bowden et al., 2005; Kounios et al., 2006). Their choice of task was the compound remote associates task, where subjects are given three words and required to produce a fourth that can form a compound word or phrase with each of the three stimulus words (e.g. given *crab*, *sauce* and *pine*, a correct response would be *apple*). An advantage of these problems is that they are relatively easy; generally being soluble within the time available for an experimental trial, yet their solution is frequently accompanied by the phenomenological experience of insight.

Using compound remote associates, Bowden and Jung-Beeman (2003) found evidence of hemispheric differences in the solution of insight problems. On each of 144 trials, subjects were presented with the three words that were to be linked. 7 sec after presentation, a target word was presented in either the subject's left or right visual field. On half of the trials the target word was the solution of the compound remote associate problem. Subjects were required to indicate (via a key-press) whether the target word was a solution (or not) as quickly as possible. Following this, they rated the problem as involving low or high insight. Response times for correct solution words were reliably shorter than for unrelated words. However, while the facilitation of

solution words presented to the right visual field was independent of the insight rating, facilitation of solution words presented to the left visual field was significantly greater for 'high insight' problems than 'low insight' problems. Bowden and Jung-Beeman argue therefore that a) the solutions of insight problems are weakly activated prior to the phenomenological feeling of insight, and b) this activation is supported by right hemisphere processing of the stimuli.

Further support for this position was obtained in a subsequent event-related fMRI study. Jung-Beeman et al. (2004) scanned 18 normal subjects, while they attempted to solve 124 compound remote associate problems. On each trial, subjects were presented with three words and asked to press a button when they had found an appropriate associate. Once they had done this, they verbalised their response and then indicated by another button press whether that response was associated with a phenomenological experience of insight. Trials were timed out after 30 sec, in which case subjects were required to respond with 'Don't know'. Since subjects verbalised their responses, the experimenters were able to verify that they were engaging in the task. Subjects solved 59% of problems, and claimed insight for 56% of those that they solved. The difference in solution time between insight and non-insight problems was not significant, with insight solutions being produced slightly more quickly on average (10.25 sec) than non-insight solutions (12.28 sec).

Figure 12.23 shows the difference in hemodynamic response when solving problems with claimed insight and without claimed insight. Neural activation was greater in right anterior superior temporal gyrus (STG) when insight was reported than when it was not. A further study using the same experimental design but with EEG linked the increased activation in correct insight trials to a burst of gamma-band activity at the right anterior temporal electrode site starting approximately 300 msec before subjects gave their response. Since problems that involved insight did not take longer

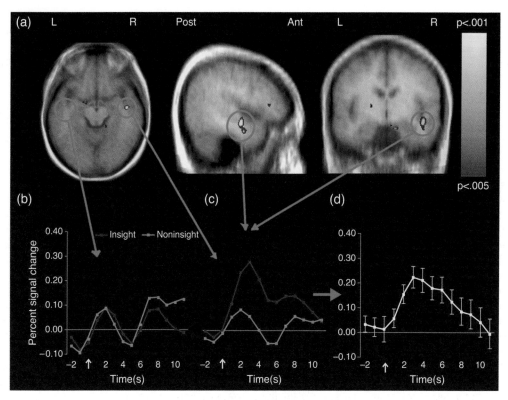

Fig. 12.23 Insight during the solution of compound remote associate problems. (a) Comparison of BOLD activity in insight minus non-insight trials. (b) Similar activity was observed in left anterior STG for trials associated with insight and without insight. (c) In contrast, right anterior STG showed reliably greater activation when the solution was associated with insight than when it was not. (d) The difference curve associated with the contrast in panel (c). Reprinted from M. Jung-Beeman, E.M. Bowden, J. Haberman, J.L. Frymiare, S. Arambel-Liu, R. Greenblatt, P.J. Reber and J. Kounios, 2004, Neural Activity When People Solve Verbal Problems with Insight. *PLoS Biology*, 2(4) e97. Copyright (2004) the authors.

to solve, the effect cannot be attributed to problem difficulty. Instead, Jung-Beeman and colleagues attribute the anterior STG activity to an insightful process involving the integration of 'distant or novel semantic relations' (Jung-Beeman et al., 2004, p. 505).

As Jung-Beeman and colleagues note, right anterior STG has been implicated in processing semantic relations related to language comprehension in a variety of earlier studies (e.g. Bottini et al., 1994; Stowe et al., 1999; Meyer et al., 2000; Humphries et al., 2001). The functional role that Jung-Beeman and colleagues associate with anterior STG in solving compound remote associate problems is therefore plausible. However, the region's relation to a general process of insight remains unsubstantiated. Indeed, its involvement in studies of language comprehension that do not involve insight argues against any role in insight per se. Critically, if right anterior STG is related to insight, then it is essential to show activity in this region across a range of insight problems, including non-verbal problems. As discussed below, this remains to be done.

A further requirement for demonstrating a relation between STG and insight is to show how this putative

functional role of right anterior STG relates to cognitive theories of insight. Bowden et al. (2005) attempt this by describing what they refer to as a 'neurological model' of insight problem-solving. The model holds that non-insight problem-solving involves many processes that are also involved in language comprehension, including the use of general knowledge to fill in missing information and the unconscious integration of information from a variety of sources into a coherent unit. These processes, it is assumed, are localised in the left hemisphere. Insight is held to occur in problem-solving when three conditions co-occur: (1) 'initial processing [...] produces strong activation [in the left hemisphere] of information that is not related to a solution and weak activation [in the right hemisphere] of information that is critical for solution'; (2) 'processing that leads to solution involves the integration of problem elements across relations or interpretations that are non-dominant for the individual or contextually non-biased'; and (3) 'the solver must switch the focus or processing to the unconscious activation and select it for consciousness and output' (p. 324). The claim is that the strong activation of the incorrect answer in the left hemisphere blocks the weaker activation of the correct answer in the right hemisphere. Bowden and colleagues make no comment on the mechanism of switching focus, though of the three putative processes this would seem to be the key element of any general mechanism of insight.

A second study that suggests a privileged role for the right hemisphere in insightful problem-solving is that of Sandkühler and Bhattacharya (2008), who repeated the EEG study of Jung-Beeman et al. (2004) using similar compound remote associate problems, but with two critical differences. First, if subjects judged they had reached an impasse, or if they failed to find a solution within the allotted time, there were able to request a hint. The hint consisted of up to 75% of the letters of the solution word, always including the first letter. Second, following each trial, subjects were asked to rate the degree of suddenness of the solution, the degree of restructuring involved (!) and their confidence in their solution. With regard to restructuring, subjects were instructed to rate the solution as follows: 'one finds a new function of use for a word [3 points]; … one rejects the use of a word and uses another meaning or application of that word which was not considered previously [2 points]; … one changes his/her problem representation' [1 point], or no restructuring [0 points] (Sandkühler & Bhattacharya, 2008, p. 1459). It is unclear how well subjects understood these distinctions, and due to differences in analysis it is not possible to directly compare the results of Jung-Beeman and colleagues with those of Sandkühler and Bhattacharya. However most comparisons in the latter study did associate insight processes with right hemisphere activity. Interestingly, in an analysis of their restructuring ratings, Sandkühler and Bhattacharya report decreased alpha-band activity in right prefrontal cortex prior to successful restructuring.[35] This decrease is held to reflect increased neural activity, which would be consistent with the function ascribed to right ventrolateral PFC by Goel as discussed in the previous section. However, the frontal localisation of insight is at odds with the temporal localisation claimed by Jung-Beeman et al., and the effect needs to be replicated by a different group working with different materials if it is to be accepted with confidence, particularly given the limitations of localisation from ERP.

Indeed, the most critical problem for the right STG hypothesis is that it has not been replicated with different classes of insight problem. Thus, a series of studies of insight problem-solving by Luo, Niki, Knoblich and colleagues using riddles (Luo & Niki, 2003; Mai et al., 2004), hard-to-comprehend sentences (Luo et al., 2004) and rearrangement of Chinese characters (Luo et al., 2006) has failed to show any relation between the phenomenological experience of insight and right anterior STG. This further supports the argument above that the relation, if any, between STG and insight is specific to tasks involving semantic associations. Consider the event-related fMRI study of Luo et al. (2004). Subjects were presented with sentences that were difficult to comprehend, such as: *His position went up because his partner's position went down.* They then read a cue (e.g. *see-saw*) which was designed to trigger an unusual interpretation of the sentence and allow subjects to comprehend it. On almost three-quarters of the trials in which subjects initially failed to understand the sentence, they attributed their failure to having thought about the sentence in the wrong way. Scanning during comprehension of the cue on these trials (which was assumed to involve insight) revealed increased activity in a number of left-lateralised regions, including the insula (BA 13), inferior, middle and superior frontal gyri (BA 6, 9, 8), as well as bilaterally in the cingulate gyrus, but not in right frontal cortex.

The discussion so far with respect to insight has been concerned purely with imaging studies. There are few patient studies that shed light on the underlying processes. One of potential relevance is the study of humour appreciation by Shammi and Stuss (1999) referred to earlier. As in the case of understanding riddles, understanding humour frequently involves perceiving the stimulus, whether it be a verbal joke or a carton, in two alternative ways. Consider one of the verbal jokes used by Shammi and Stuss, a sign in a Hong Kong tailor's shop which read 'Please have a fit upstairs'. To appreciate this as humorous requires understanding both the intended and actual meanings. Shammi and Stuss tested 21 patients and 10 sex-, age- and education-matched controls on three tests of humour appreciation: (a) humour ratings on a five-point scale for statements such as the above Hong Kong sign (including one in four neutral statements); (b) completion selection for verbal jokes given a set of four possible punch lines per joke; and (c) 'mirth' responses to a series of non-verbal cartoons. Patients were divided on the basis of their lesions into four groups: right frontal (8), other frontal (5), right posterior (5) and left posterior (3). As shown in Figure 12.24, the right-frontal patients were impaired relative to the other groups and controls on all tasks. These results sharpen those of previous related lesion studies (e.g. Wapner et al., 1981; Bihrle et al., 1986), which have found humour appreciation to be more severally impaired by right than left hemisphere damage.

---

[35] This localisation is based on source analysis—a technique that involves localising in three-dimensional space the source of a complex signal obtained from two-dimensional scalp recordings. The technique has inherent limitations, particular with respect to the localisation of temporally correlated sources, and as such the results of this analysis must be interpreted with caution.

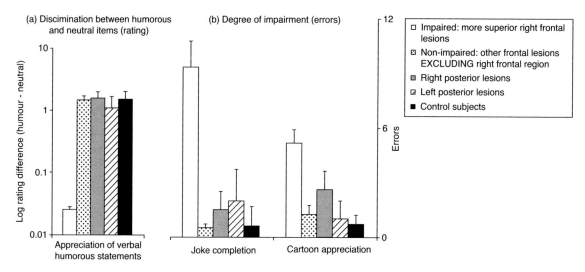

Fig. 12.24 Humour appreciation as a function of lesion site. (a) Right frontal patients were significantly worse at discriminating between humorous and neutral items. (b) They also made more errors in selecting joke punch lines and detecting 'mirth' in cartoons. Reprinted from P. Shammi and D.T.Stuss, Humour appreciation A role of the right frontal lobe, *Brain*, 1999, *122*(4), 657–666, by permission of Oxford University Press.

Three questions are raised by the above. What general computational processes are responsible for humour appreciation? How do these relate to the notion of representational change or restructuring associated with cognitive theories of insight? And why should such processes be right frontal? Shammi and Stuss (1999) provide two tentative arguments for the right lateralisation: first, that such appreciation requires retrieval from episodic memory and second, that it involves the integration or generation of an emotional response. Both of these processes have been argued to be right lateralised, though in both cases the evidence is currently weak.[36]

One highly speculative possibility is that, as noted above, humour appreciation requires simultaneously conceiving of the object of humour in two distinct ways. Insight likewise involves bringing together two ideas. Thus, in the case of the mutilated checkerboard (Figure 12.22), the insightful solution requires recognising both that each domino necessarily covers one white square and one black square, and that removal of the diagonally opposite corner squares leaves an imbalance in the number of black and white squares. Amati and Shallice (2007) speculate on the basis of anthropological evidence that this 'bringing together' requires a computational process that is unique to modern homonims. More specifically, they distinguish between *routine operations*, *supervisory operations*, and *fluent sequences* of supervisory operations. The latter are held to be required for bringing together distinct thoughts and

to be supported by a computational process, latching, that is only possible within a cortical network with sufficient connectivity. Treves (2005) has demonstrated that such latching behaviour can occur in networks of artificial neurons provided that the mean connectivity exceeds a critical limit, and Amati and Shallice suggest that connectivity of the modern homonim prefrontal cortex, and in particular of the frontopolar cortex, exceeds this limit and hence can support latching.

This position does not address the question of lateralisation. Many of the imaging studies discussed throughout this chapter, particularly those on analogy and induction which implicate frontopolar cortex (e.g. Wharton et al., 2000; Christoff et al., 2001), can be argued to require the subject to bring together two sources of information. These appear to suggest a left lateralisation for such processing. Consider though the study of Braver and Bongiolatti (2002). Here, subjects were scanned while they completed two versions of the AX-CPT task, a continuous performance task similar to the 12-AX task discussed in Section 7.9 in which subjects must monitor a stream of stimuli for two consecutive targets ('X' preceded by 'A') and respond when and only when they detect the consecutive targets. In one version (*word AX-CPT*) the targets were words ('LIME' preceded by 'FATE'). In the other version (*semantic AX-CPT*) a semantic classification was required. The targets were any concrete word preceded by any abstract word. Target trials were equally frequent in both conditions. As a control condition, subjects were also scanned while completing a semantic classification task with semantic demands similar to that of the semantic AX-CPT task. Figure 12.25a shows a horizontal brain section (z = –3)

---

[36] See Section 10.11 for a discussion of the possible right lateralisation of episodic memory retrieval.

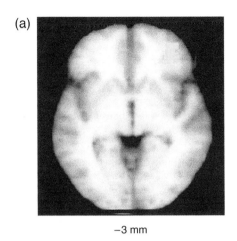
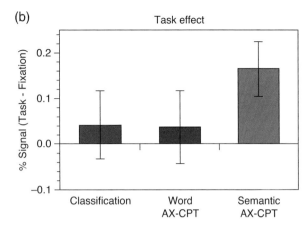

Fig. 12.25 Frontopolar activity observed in the study of Braver and Bongiolatti (2002). (a) Horizontal cross section at z = −3 showing the area engaged during the combined task (semantic AX-CPT) but not in either of the component tasks (semantic classification or word AX-CPT). (b) Percentage signal change in each task in comparison to fixation. See text for full details of the tasks. Reprinted from *NeuroImage*, *15*(3), T.S. Braver and S.R. Bongiolatti, The role of frontopolar cortex in subgoal processing during working memory, 523–536, Copyright (2002), with permission from Elsevier.

for the difference between the semantic AX-CPT and the semantic classification tasks. An area of right frontopolar cortex, centred on (35, 40, −2), was more active during the semantic AX-CPT than during the classification task. Figure 12.25b shows that this area was also not differentially active during the word version of the AX-CPT (in comparison to the classification task). Only when it was necessary to bring together both semantic classification and the requirements of the AX-CPT task did activity in the area increase. Right frontopolar cortex is therefore implicated in at least some tasks that require combining two sources of information.[37]

Despite these speculative proposals, the contribution of cognitive neuroscience methods to the understanding of insight problem-solving is currently unsatisfactory. Several hypotheses have been advanced, but each has only really received support from studies conducted by their originators. This may be because different groups have used different materials (compound remote associates, riddles and matchstick problems). With the exception of the fMRI and EEG studies of the Jung-Beeman and Bowden group, there is also a lack of converging evidence from differing methodologies.

This pessimism should be tempered, however, as the area remains under-explored. Relatively few studies have so far been conducted and more would seem to be necessary if the underlying processes are to be properly understood. At the same time, these studies must address a slue of methodological difficulties. Most critically, progress is limited by the difficulty in producing problems which reliably provoke insight and yet are suitable for laboratory or imaging studies (Bowden et al., 2005; Luo & Knoblich, 2007). Regardless of these concerns, the question with which we began this section, namely whether the functions ascribed by Goel to right ventrolateral PFC might be understood in terms of processes related to insight problem-solving, remains unresolved. There is some evidence which is suggestive of right frontal involvement in processes related to insight, but the precise nature of those processes, and whether they are necessary and sufficient for insight, remains a matter of speculation.

12.9 Towards a Unified Account of Thinking and Reasoning

In Chapter 3 we raised the issue of whether the more central cognitive processes have some degree of modularity or, as Fodor (1983) would have us believe, equipotentiality reigns. Both imaging and patient studies support a more modular view of the processes related to thinking. It is not the case that, for example, BOLD activity in all regions of the cortex (or even the prefrontal cortex) tracks behavioural measures of problem difficulty, as an equipotential view would suggest. Similarly, it is not the case that the deficits found in frontal patients are well-described by a single scalar variable (degree of

---

[37] Braver and Bongiolatti (2002) attribute right frontopolar activity to subgoaling, noting that semantic classification is a subgoal of the more general task goal in the semantic AX-CPT condition. However, this attribution does not tie in either with other findings on subgoaling in goal-directed problem-solving described in Section 12.5, where left prefrontal cortex appears to be most critical, or with Goel's position on the role of right prefrontal cortex in ill-defined problem-solving, where right prefrontal cortex is not specifically involved in well-defined problem-solving, as occurs in the semantic AX-CPT.

damage), as an equipotential view would require. The evidence thus points to some form of modular organisation of function. At the same time, the various studies reviewed in this chapter do not appear to present a coherent picture of the processes underlying complex thought. In our view this is not surprising, given that, as noted in the introduction, the picture derived from a purely cognitive psychological perspective also lacks coherence. Largely disjoint research traditions focus on reasoning, problem-solving and decision making, and while these disjoint research traditions have engaged with cognitive neuroscience evidence they have continued to function largely as disjoint entities.

Can we move towards a more unified account of thinking? Some computational approaches suggest that we can. Perhaps the most ambitious proposal was made by Newell (1990), who argued that (1) all thinking is goal-directed, (2) all goal-directed activity is problem-solving, and hence (3) all thinking is problem-solving. This allows reasoning and decision-making to be subsumed within problem-solving by seeing each as being directed towards a goal (e.g. the goal of selecting the best alternative in a decision-making problem, which in turn requires that each alternative is either evaluated or dismissed). Newell supports this view by pointing to computationally explicit accounts of various types of thinking expressed within the Soar cognitive architecture, a system in which all processing is goal-directed (see Sections 1.7 and 3.8). Thus Polk and Newell (1995) present a comprehensive account of deductive reasoning that was originally developed within Soar.

Newell's argument deserves closer inspection. There appear to be forms of thinking, such as associative thinking, which are not goal-directed. Equally, there appear to be forms of goal-directed activity which are not problem-solving, such as applying a learned sequence of actions to achieve a goal. Newell's argument does, however, allow us to enumerate a set of interacting subprocesses that may, in principle, support thinking. These subprocesses include the generation, comparison and selection of goals, problem spaces, and operators.[38] The subprocesses are broadly

equivalent to the subprocesses of the domino model discussed in Section 9.7. Newell's subprocesses are known collectively as the PSCM (Problem Space Computational Model). They derive from the GOMS (Goals, Operators, Methods and Selection Rules: Card et al., 1983) approach to the study of human-computer interaction, which also influenced the development of the domino model.[39] Sloman (2000) provides a more complex, but essentially compatible, view derived from an AI analysis of intelligence; namely that intelligent behaviour is supported by a multitude of special purpose but interacting processes.

An alternative way to unify thinking is to consider the various forms as involving the generation of some kind of internal representation (a 'mental model', in the broad sense of Gentner & Stevens, 1983) of a situation and the manipulation of that representation according to task-dependent rules—a process that may or may not be goal-directed. What this and the 'thinking as problem-solving' approach have in common is the requirement for some form of temporary storage system in which a potentially abstract, counterfactual or hypothetical task representation can be maintained and manipulated. Both approaches also require processes for proposing and selecting modifications to the representation (hypothesis generation and selection), as well as some kind of monitoring and evaluative mechanisms, and presumably mechanisms for drawing on previous experience. Throughout this and previous chapters (particularly Chapters 9 and 10) we have seen both cognitive and neural evidence for many of these processes.

How does this general view of thinking relate to the contention scheduling/supervisory system account of cognition? We conceive of thinking as the functioning of various supervisory processes, which modulate contention scheduling. A preliminary decomposition of those processes was provided by Shallice and Burgess (1996). Figures 12.26 and 12.27 present a refinement of that decomposition, based on the evidence discussed in this and previous chapters.

Consider first the top-level structure (Figure 12.26). Working from the left, *perceptual triggers and primed knowledge* can lead to the generation of a goal, the generation of what we have called a strategy (i.e. a temporary control structure; see Section 9.12), or the running of cognitive or action routines. *Goal generation* relates to

---

[38] Within the problem-solving literature an *operator* is a transformation of the problem state, which is consistent with the physics of the world and any constraints imposed by the problem. Conceptually, as transformations of representations, they are equivalent to the cognitive operations discussed in Chapter 8. A *problem space* consists of a representation of the initial and goal states of the problem, plus a set of operators and the states that may be generated from the initial state by application of some sequence of operators. Operators normally correspond to atomic transformations (e.g., the transformation in a chess problem representation that corresponds to moving a single piece), but they may also be defined to include learned sequences of transformations—*macro-operators*.

---

[39] A notable difference between Soar and other production system accounts of higher cognition such as ACT-R, EPIC, and 4-CAPS discussed in Section 3.8 is the lack in these other systems of anything equivalent to a PSCM level account of thinking. The difficulty is that, as discussed in Chapter 1, production systems can be used as general programming languages and hence can be applied to any Turing computable process. They therefore do not, in and of themselves, provide a decomposition of thinking into a set of supporting subprocesses.

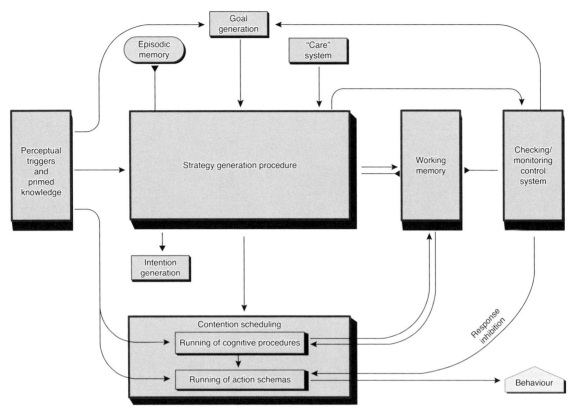

Fig. 12.26 The Supervisory System (Mark III) and contention scheduling.

the problem orientation phase of problem-solving, where an initial goal is set based on an analysis of the problem. The process may also be triggered by the *checking/monitoring control system*, if that system detects that progress towards the current goal is unsatisfactory. Checking/monitoring is, we assume, a process that operates in parallel with other cognitive processes and that we relate to right lateral PFC (see Section 9.10). Damage to this system results in a tendency to perseverate in the face of negative feedback, as demonstrated, for instance, by the right lateral patients in the ROBBIA studies.

The most complex element of the model is *strategy generation procedure*. The functioning of this system is described in more detail below, but its role is to produce a temporary structure for the control of thought or action, triggered either directly by perceptual input or in response to a specified goal. In generating a strategy, the system may draw upon *episodic memory* and the *care system*. The latter is assumed to be involved in keeping the system orientated towards the primary task and avoiding deflection onto other tasks or daydreaming. It has the complimentary function to checking, which blocks inappropriate continuation of the task. Damage to the care system results in higher error rates, particularly when responses potentiated in contention scheduling are inappropriately selected. These errors are characteristic of inferior medial patients (see Section 9.11).

Our account, therefore, of the difficulties of inferior medial patients on reasoning tasks (e.g. Adolphs et al., 1996) is that they arise from damage to this care system, and the subsequent generation of a suboptimal strategy for problem solution.

Within that part of the model related to contention scheduling we distinguish between two processes: *running of cognitive procedures* and *running of action schemas*. The former is assumed to potentially involve working memory, while the latter must interact directly with the systems controlling the three-dimensional interaction of the body with the physical world, as discussed in Sections 8.3 and 8.4. Moreover the inhibitory function of the checking/monitoring process is assumed to apply only to the running of action schemas (in the form of response inhibition), and not the running of cognitive procedures.

Figure 12.27 shows the processes held to be involved in strategy generation. As in previous versions of the model, there are three ways in which a strategy might be produced:

(1) by using or adapting a strategy previously applied in a similar situation (obtained from episodic memory);

(2) by procedures similar to those postulated by Newell and colleagues, involving model building and selective search of the problem's state space; or

(3) by realising a previously stored intention.

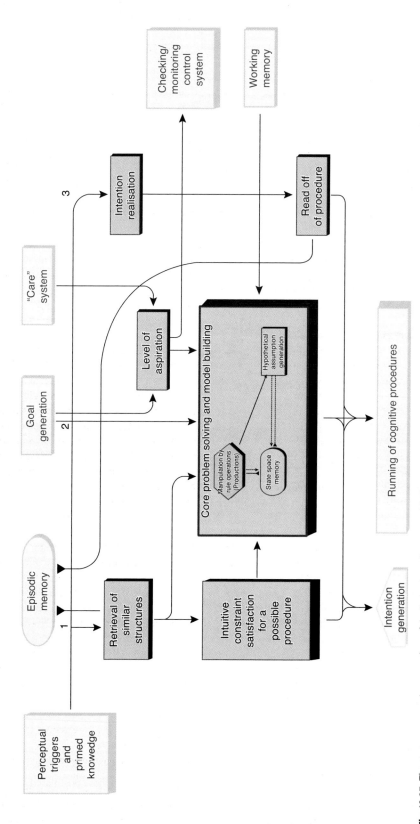

Fig. 12.27 The strategy generation procedure of the Supervisory System model. Three routes are proposed: through retrieval and adaptation of a previous strategy; through model-based problem solving; or through realisation of a previously generated intention. See Shallice and Burgess (1996).

The second of these processes involves the generation and manipulation of a representation of the problem state through a set of core problem-solving and model building procedures. These procedures are held to implement problem-solving through progressive deepening—the representation and serial manipulation of one problem state at a time (see De Groot, 1965). The *hypothetical assumption generation* component relates to the Soar procedure for dealing with an impasse, or blockage in problem-solving, by constructing a new problem space. The process will normally require abstraction over specific stimuli, and so is also linked to the ideas of Christoff et al. (2001) concerning relational integration.

It is assumed that *core problem-solving and model building* (and *checking/monitoring control system*) is affected by the *level of aspiration*. This derives from De Groot's (1965) classic studies of chess, and determines what counts as an adequate problem solution. It is set by the goal generation process and is a product of the general assessment of the problem-solving situation. Thus, in chess, if a player is in a strong position the level of aspiration will be high and the goal will be to force a win, while if the player is in a weak position the level of aspiration will be low and the goal will be to achieve a draw.

The distinction between routes 1 and 2 in *strategy generation procedure* is partly motivated by work on case-based reasoning, but it also relates to the dual-process theory of reasoning first proposed by Evans et al. (1983; see also Evans & Over 1996; Evans, 2006). Thus, Evans (2006) argues that reasoning may be effected by one of two systems, a fast, content-specific, associative system (route 1 in Figure 12.27) or a slower, content-free, analytic system (route 2 in Figure 12.27).

12.10 Conclusion

There is now a substantial body of evidence which, in contrast to Fodor's (1983) claims of the equipotentiality of central cognition, supports the view that thinking is effected by a complex set of separable subprocesses. However, we do not as yet have a clear picture of these processes. How are we to make sense of the neuroscience data relevant to thinking, particularly given the theories developed within cognitive psychology?

Goel (2007) is pessimistic. In an analysis of cognitive neuroscience evidence related to deductive reasoning, he argues that the functional imaging and patient data support three dissociations—between (1) 'systems for dealing with familiar and unfamiliar material', (2) 'systems for dealing with conflict and belief bias', and (3) 'systems for dealing with certain and uncertain information' (p. 439). He suggests, however, that 'these data [i.e. the functional imaging and patient data] are telling us that the brain is organised in ways not anticipated

by cognitive theory' (p. 440). Certainly there are many unresolved questions, and the neuroscience evidence does not support unequivocally one or other existing theory of, for example, deductive reasoning. However we do not believe that Goel's pessimism is warranted.

Consider first the dissociations claimed by Goel. The primary evidence for dissociations (1) and (2) are the studies of Goel et al. (2000) and Goel and Dolan (2003a, 2003b), discussed in Section 12.4. These studies have not been replicated with different materials and methods, and the study by Monti et al. (2007), also discussed in Section 12.4 casts doubt on some aspects of Goel's interpretation. Thus, while Monti and colleagues found support for Goel's claims of the involvement of content-specific cortical areas when reasoning with different content, they failed to find support for the claim that deductive reasoning recruits a network of linguistic regions. There are also difficulties with the interpretation of the results of Monti et al. However, their results are consistent with an approach to reasoning which recruits rule-based processes in the construction of model-based representations. Turning to dissociation (3), Goel's primary evidence here is his study of determinate and indeterminate transitive inference discussed in Section 12.2 (Goel et al., 2007). The claim that left-frontal patients tend to be impaired on determinate but not indeterminate problems is not clearly supported by the findings, while the impairment of right-frontal patients on indeterminate problems may be attributable, as discussed, to a failure of monitoring processes in detecting that multiple models are consistent with indeterminate premises. Thus, in our view Goel's dissociations, such as they are, support a progressive shift (in the Lakatosian sense) of theories developed in cognitive psychology, rather than their outright rejection.

In fact, if further support for dissociations (1) and (2) does emerge, then these dissociations would provide strong support not only for the distinction between the various routes within *strategy generation procedure* of Figure 12.27, but also for the dual-process theory of reasoning first proposed by Evans et al. (1983). That theory, at least in its original 1983 form, predates much of the cognitive neuroscience evidence and all of the imaging studies. Moreover, support for related dual-systems views has recently been adduced from a number of purely behavioural studies (e.g. see Stanovich & West, 2000; Barbey & Sloman, 2007). Again Goel's pessimism appears in our view to be a case of seeing the glass as half empty, rather than half full.

At the same time, the cognitive neuroscience evidence discussed in this chapter is less satisfactory than that discussed in earlier chapters. Few, if any, hypotheses are supported by converging evidence from computational, patient and functional imaging studies, and consequently the theoretical interpretation of several key results (e.g. the roles of left and right lateral frontopolar cortex) remains speculative. In part, this is a result of the complexity of thinking processes and the methodological difficulties raised by this complexity. How, for example, should one interpret the functional imaging evidence when the contrasts investigated in most thinking studies reveal networks consisting of numerous regions? And why do so many imaging studies implicate so many regions? Moreover, why are results often not replicated across studies which use different materials or different experimental paradigms? In our view, some of these questions arise from the use of inappropriate contrasts based on an inadequate understanding of both the cognitive processes underlying thinking and the range of strategies available to the subject in the typical thinking task.

How might this situation be addressed? First, many imaging studies of thinking lack comprehensive task analyses for the various experimental conditions. This is particularly evident in studies of insight, but task analysis is an informal exercise based on intuition, even in more standard deductive and inductive reasoning studies. Clearly such analyses are critical for understanding the processes required by a task and the processes revealed by the subtraction methodology which dominates neuroimaging studies of thinking. Second, while it is relatively straightforward to develop computational simulations of complex thinking tasks using production systems, there is a lack of simulation work that links more closely to known neural processes. The development of such simulations would, of course, go hand-in-hand with the construction of comprehensive task analyses. Together, they are likely to allow the methods of cognitive neuroscience to address the challenges of thinking.

In this chapter we have confronted one of the general questions we posed in the earlier part of the book, and in particular in Chapter 3, namely whether the central processes underlying thought are in some sense modular. We have argued that they are modular but also abstract. But there is a more basic question. Do we—for higher cognitive functions—yet have a set of experimental paradigms in each of the cognitive domains we have considered which are inferentially solid? This is in the sense that nearly all subjects make the same interpretation of the instructions and so realise an equivalent set of action and thought schemas for task performance as each other and so create qualitatively the same resource demands on the cognitive system. If this is not the case then theoretical interpretation of any average findings can only produce an intellectual mirage. That this is not necessarily a wild fear is shown by the discussion of the remember–know paradigm in Chapter 10. There is no agreed interpretation

across theorists of either the neuropsychological or the imaging evidence. Worse, we argued that at least one set of subjects interpret the instructions differently—amnesic patients.

But the possibility that subjects differ in how they interpret task instructions is only one of the many dangers of cognitive neuroscience methodology as far as developing theories of higher cognitive functions are concerned. In addition to the inherent difficulties of pinning down the processing components underlying task performance, not just the problem that they may differ across individuals and also possibly in the same individual with learning, there is the flakiness of the cognitive assumptions we need to make in order to make theoretical progress and the inherent lack of discriminatory power of the behavioural experiment whatever brain-related empirical method we use. We need therefore to consider whether we are making solid progress at all. Is the production line of the modern scientific experiment—with in many cases the great technical sophistication that is involved—beginning to produce a solid picture or are our theoretical constructions as far as higher cognitive processes are concerned to be as subject to the vagaries of intellectual fashion as their equivalents were in the past?

Our answer has been the traditional one going back to the converging operations approach of Garner, Hake and Eriksen (1956). We have argued that if one takes the two empirical methods of cognitive neuropsychology (broadly understood) and functional imaging, then to draw theoretical conclusions from either about cognition requires a range of assumptions. And these assumptions may in some experimental situations be basically correct, if rough-and-ready, in others somewhat dubious and in yet others essentially inadequate. Worse, we often have little idea in drawing theoretical conclusions in a particular experimental domain which of these three alternatives applies. But if we take the two broad cognitive neuroscience methods on which we have concentrated, the inferential assumptions made—in Chapters 4 and 5, respectively—are very different from each other. So if the same theoretical conclusions can be drawn from both methods it is reasonable to assume that real progress is being made. If there is a general convergence of theoretical conclusions across empirical methodologies this supports the plausibility of both sets of inferential assumptions as well as the specific theoretical conclusions drawn.

If we take many of the areas we have considered we need to distinguish between first-level theories of the gross modular organisation of the functional architecture and second-level computational theories of the respective domains. With possibly the solitary example of basic concrete word semantics we know of no higher-level cognitive area where a second-generation model, including its notational variants, is relatively unchallenged by competitors. Take for example the area of reading, which we considered in Chapters 4 and 5. As we showed there the assumption standard since the 1970s and 1980s of a word-form system and phonological and semantic routes is supported by both neuropsychological and functional imaging evidence. However the range of more specific computational models that claim precedence not only continues to grow but the hoary initial candidates continue to show life with respect to the adequacy of their accounts of the neuropsychological data, and as far as functional imaging is concerned there has not yet, to our knowledge, been a major attempt to assess their relative adequacy.

Essentially the same first generation theory has, however, been basically supported by both neuropsychological and functional imaging findings not only with respect to reading and core semantics but also with respect to category specificity, in aspects of attention, to phonological and visuo-spatial short-term memory, to generation of object-appropriate actions in left temporoparietal cortices, to externally-oriented spatial operations in right parietal cortex, to syntactic (or as we prefer unification) operations in left BA 44/45, to energisation of non-routine operations in medial prefrontal cortex, to novel schema construction (in left BA 9/46), to monitoring/checking (in right lateral prefrontal cortex), to intention generation and realisation (branching) in frontopolar cortex, to episodic memory storage and to inductive generation in left lateral prefrontal cortex. The list is long and far from complete. The widespread nature of theoretical convergence between the two methodologies provides support for the basic sets of inferential assumptions made.

As we saw in the last chapter there are even the beginnings of a scientific theory of consciousness, although it would be highly premature to consider it unchallenged. Moreover the overall organisation of the subsystems concerned with language and thought and their interrelations are still far from clear, so there is still much work to be done on the basic functional architecture. However eventual theoretical convergence seems very likely. Whether we will achieve a similar degree of relative closure concerning second-generation computational models remains, however, an open question. Success will need a much more sophisticated combination of cognitive theory and brain-related behavioural methods than has yet been achieved.

References

Abbot, L., Varela, J., Sen, K., & Nelson, S. (1997). Synaptic depression and cortical gain control. *Science*, *275*, 220–224.

Abrams, R. L. & Grinspan, J. (2007). Unconscious semantic priming in the absence of partial awareness. *Consciousness and Cognition*, *16*, 942–953.

Abrams, R. L., Klinger, M. R., & Greenwald, A. G. (2002). Subliminal words activate semantic categories (not automated motor responses). *Psychonomic Bulletin and Review*, *9*, 100–106.

Ach, N. (1905). *Über die Willenstätigkeit und das Denken.* Göttingen: Vandenhoeck & Ruprecht.

Acuna, B. D., Eliassen, J. C., Donoghue, J. P., & Sanes, J. N. (2002). Frontal and parietal lobe activation during transitive inference in humans. *Cerebral Cortex*, *12*, 1312–1321.

Addis, D. R., Moscovitch, M., Crawley, A. P., & McAndrews, M. P. (2004). Recollective qualities modulate hippocampal activation during autobiographical memory retrieval. *Hippocampus*, *14*, 752–762.

Adolphs, R., Tranel, D., Bechara, A., Damasio, H., & Damasio, A. (1996). Neuropsychological approaches to reasoning and decision-making. In Y.Christen, A. Damasio, & H. Damasio (Eds), *Neurobiology of decision-making* (pp. 157–179). Berlin: Springer.

Aggleton, J. P., & Brown, M. W. (1999). Episodic memory,amnesia, and the hippocampal-anterior thalamic axis. *Behavioral and Brain Sciences*, *22*(3), 425–444.

Aggleton, J. P., Vann, S. D., Denby, C., Dix, S., Mayes, A. R., Roberts, N. et al. (2005). Sparing of the familiarity component of recognition memory in a patient with hippocampal pathology. *Neuropsychologia*, *43*, 1810–1823.

Aguirre, G. K. & D'Esposito, M. (1999). Topographical disorientation: a synthesis and taxonomy. *Brain*, *122*(9), 1613–1628.

Akrami, A., Liu, Y., Treves, A., & Jagadeesh, B. (2009). Converging neuronal activity in inferior temporal cortex during the classification of morphed stimuli. *Cerebral Cortex*, *19*, 760–776.

Albanese, E., Capitani, E., Barbarotto, R., & Laiacona, M. (2000). Semantic category dissociations, familiarity and gender. *Cortex*, *36*, 733–746.

Albert, M. S., Butters, N., & Levin, J. (1979). Temporal gradients in the retrograde amnesia of patients with alcoholic Korsakoff's disease. *Archives of Neurology*, *36*, 211–216.

Alexander, G. E., DeLong, M. R., & Strick, P. L. (1986). Parallel organization of functionally segregated circuits linking basal ganglia and cortex. *Annual Review of Neuroscience*, *9*(1), 357–381.

Alexander, M., Hiltbrunner, B., & Fischer, R. (1989). Distributed anatomy of transcortical sensory aphasia. *Archives of Neurology*, *45*, 885–892.

Alexander, M. P., Stuss, D. T., & Fansabedian, N. (2003). California verbal learning test: performance by patients with focal frontal and non-frontal lesions. *Brain*, *126*, 1493–1503.

Alexander, M. P., Stuss, D. T., Shallice, T., Picton, T. W., & Gillingham, S. (2005). Impaired concentration due to frontal lobe damage from two distinct lesion sites. *Neurology*, *65*, 572–579.

Alexander, M. P., Stuss, D. T., Picton, T., Shallice, T., & Gillingham, S. (2007). Regional frontal injuries cause distinct impairments in cognitive control. *Neurology*, *68*, 1515–1523.

Allman, J. & Kaas, J. (1971). A representation of the visual field in the caudal third of the middle temporal gyrus of the owl monkey (Aotus trivirgutus). *Brain Research*, *31*, 85–105.

Allport, D. A. (1984). Auditory-verbal short-term memory and aphasia. In H.Bouma & D. Bouwhuis (Eds), *Attention and performance X: Control of language processes.* London: Lawrence Erlbaum Associates.

Allport, D. A. (1985). Distributed memory, modular subsystems and dyspahsia. In S. Eppstein (Ed.), *Current perspectives in dysphasia* (pp. 32-60). Churchill Livingstone.

Allport, D. A. (1988). What concept of consciousness. In A.J. Marcel & E. Bisiach (Eds), *Consciousness in contemporary science* (pp. 159-182). Oxford: Clarendon Press/Oxford University Press.

Allport, D. A. & Wiley, G. (2000). Task switching, stimulus-response bindings, and negative priming. In S.Monsell & J. Driver (Eds), *Attention and performance XVIII: Control of cognitive processes* (pp. 35-70). Cambridge, MA: MIT Press.

Allport, D. A., Antonis, B., & Reynolds, P. (1972). On the division of attention: A disproof of the single-channel hypothesis. *Quarterly Journal of Experimental Psychology*, 24, 225-235.

Allport, D. A., Styles, E., & Hsieh, S. (1994). Shifting intentional set: exploring the dynamic control of tasks. In C. Umiltà & M. Moscovitch (Eds), *Attention and performance XV* (pp. 421-452). Cambridge, MA: MIT Press.

Alstott, J., Breakspear, M., Hagmann, P., Cammoun, L., & Sporns, O. (2009). Modeling the impact of lesions in the human brain. *PLoS Computational Biology*, 5, e1000408.

Altmann, G. & Steedman, M. (1988). Interaction with context during human sentence processing. *Cognition*, 30, 191-238.

Altmann, G., Garnham, A., & Dennis, Y. (1992). Avoiding the garden path: eye movements in context. *Journal of Memory and Language*, 31, 685-712.

Alvarez, P., Carreiras, M., & Perea, M. (2004). Are syllables phonological units in visual word recognition? *Language and Cognitive Processes*, 19, 427-452.

Álvarez, C. & Squire, L. (1994). Memory consolidation and the medial temporal lobe: a simple network model. *Proceedings of the National Academy of Sciences*, 91, 7045.

Amit, D. (1989). *Modeling Brain Function - The world of attractor neural networks*. Cambridge, MA: Cambridge University Press.

Amati, D. & Shallice, T. (2007). On the emergence of modern humans. *Cognition*, 103, 358-385.

Andersen, R., Essick, G., & Siegel, R. (1985). Encoding of spatial location by posterior parietal neurons. *Science*, 230, 456-458.

Andersen, R. A., Meeker, D., Peseran, B., Breznen, B., Buneo, C. & Scherberger, H. (2004). Sensorimotor transformations in posterior parietal cortex. In M. S. Gazzaniga (Ed.), *The Cognitive Neurosciences III* (pp. 463-474). Cambridge, MA: MIT Press.

Anderson, J. R. (1983). *The architecture of cognition*. Cambridge, MA: Harvard University Press.

Anderson, J. R. (1990). *The adaptive character of thought*. Hillsdale, NJ: Erlbaum.

Anderson, J. R. (1993). *Rules of the mind*. Hillsdale, NJ: Erlbaum.

Anderson, J. R. (2005). Human symbol manipulation within an integrated cognitive architecture. *Cognitive Science*, 29(3), 313-341.

Anderson, J. R. (2007). *How can the human mind occur in the physical universe?* New York: Oxford University Press.

Anderson, J. R. & Bower, G. (1973). *Human associative memory*. Winston.

Anderson, J. R. & Douglass, S. (2001). Tower of Hanoi: Evidence for the cost of goal retrieval. *Journal of Experimental Psychology: Learning, Memory and Cognition*, 27, 1331-1346.

Anderson, J. R. & Lebière, C. (1998). *The atomic components of thought*. Hillsdale, NJ: Erlbaum.

Anderson, J. R., Bothell, D., Lebière, C., & Matessa, M. (1998). An integrated theory of list memory. *Journal of Memory and Language*, 38(4), 341-380.

Anderson, J. R., Bothell, D., Byrne, M., Douglass, S., Lebiere, C., & Qin, Y. (2004a). An integrated theory of the mind. *Psychological Review*, 111, 1036-1060.

Anderson, J. R., Qin, Y., Stenger, V. A., & Carter, C. S. (2004b). The relationship of three cortical regions to an information-processing model. *Journal of Cognitive Neuroscience*, 16, 637-653.

Anderson, J. R., Albert, M. V., & Fincham, J. M. (2005). Tracing problem solving in real time: fMRI analysis of the subject-paced Tower of Hanoi. *Journal of Cognitive Neuroscience*, 17, 1261-1274.

Anderson, J. R., Byrne, D., Fincham, J. M., & Gunn, P. (2008a). Role of prefrontal and parietal cortices in associative learning. *Cerebral Cortex*, 18, 904-914.

Anderson, J. R., Fincham, J. M., Qin, Y., & Stocco, A. (2008b). A central circuit of the mind. *Trends in Cognitive Sciences*, 12, 136-143.

Anderson, M. L. (2007). Evolution of cognitive function via redeployment of brain areas. *Neuroscientist*, 13, 13-21.

Anderson, S. W., Damasio, H., Jones, R. D., & Tranel, D. (1991). Wisconsin Card Sorting Test performance as a measure of frontal lobe damage. *Journal of Clinical and Experimental Neuropsychology*, 13, 909-922.

Annoni, J. M., Lemay, M. A., de Mattos Pimenta, M. A., & Lecours, A. R. (1998). The contribution of attentional mechanisms to an irregularity effect at the graphemic buffer level. *Brain and Language*, 63, 64-78.

Archambault, P. S., Caminiti, R., & Battaglia-Mayer, A. (2009). Cortical mechanisms for online control of hand movement trajectory: the role of the posterior parietal cortex. *Cerebral Cortex*, 19(12), 2848-2864.

Armstrong, D. (1968). *A Materialist Theory of the Mind*. London: Routledge.

Arnott, S., Kibble, T., & Shallice, T. (2006). Maurice Hugh Frederick Wilkins CBE: 15 December 1916–15 October 2004. *Biographical Memoirs of Fellows of the Royal Society*, 52, 455–478.

Aron, A. R., Monsell, S., Sahakian, B. J., & Robbins, T. W. (2004). A componential analysis of task-switching deficits associated with lesions of left and right frontal cortex. *Brain*, 127, 1561–1573.

Arrington, C. M., Carr, T. H., Mayer, A. R., & Rao, S. M. (2000). Neural mechanisms of visual attention: Object-based selection of a region in space. *Journal of Cognitive Neuroscience*, 12, 106–117.

Asaad, W. F., Rainer, G., & Miller, E. K. (1998). Neural activity in the primate prefrontal cortex during associative learning. *Neuron*, 21, 1399–1407.

Asaad, W. F., Rainer, G., & Miller, E. K. (2000). Task-specific neural activity in the primate prefrontal cortex. *Journal of Neurophysiology*, 84, 451–459.

Ashburner, J. & Friston, K. J. (2007). Spatial transformation of images. In K.J.Friston, J. Ashburner, S. Kiebel, T. Nichols, & W. Penny (Eds), *Statistical parametric mapping.* Academic Press.

Ashby, F. G. (1982). Deriving exact predictions from the cascade model. *Psychological Review*, 89, 599–607.

Astafiev, S. V., Shulman, G. L., & Corbetta, M. (2006). Visuospatial reorienting signals in the human temporo-parietal junction are independent of response selection. *European Journal of Neuroscience*, 23, 591–596.

Atkinson, R. & Shiffrin, R. (1968). Human memory: a proposed system and its control processes. In K.Spence & J. Spence (Eds), *The psychology of learning and motivation: advances in research and theory, vol. 2.* Academic Press.

Audet, T., Bub, D., & Lecours, A. R. (1991). Visual neglect and left-sided context effects. *Brain and Cognition*, 16, 11–28.

Averbeck, B. B., Chafee, M. V., Crowe, D. A., & Georgopoulos, A. P. (2002). Parallel processing of serial movements in prefrontal cortex. *Proceedings of the National Academy of Sciences, U S A*, 99, 13172–13177.

Awh, A., Jonides, J., Smith, E. E., Schumacher, E. H., Koeppe, R. A., & Katz, S. (1996). Dissociation of storage and rehearsal in verbal working memory: evidence from positron emission tomography. *Psychological Science*, 7, 31.

Baars, B. J. (1988). *A cognitive theory of consciousness.* Cambridge: CUP.

Baars, B. J., Fehling, M. R., LaPolla, M., & McGovern, K. (1997). Consciousness creates access: conscious goal images recruit unconscious action routines, but goal competition serves to 'liberate' such routines, causing predictable slips. In J. D. Cohen & J. W. Schooler (Eds), *Scientific approaches to consciousness* (pp. 423–444). Routledge.

Baayen, R., Feldman, L., & Schreuder, R. (2006). Morphological influences on the recognition of monosyllabic monomorphemic words. *Journal of Memory and Language*, 55, 290–313.

Baddeley, A. D. (1966a). Short-term memory for word sequences as a function of acoustic, semantic, and formal similarity. *Journal of Experimental Psychology*, 18, 334–336.

Baddeley, A. D. (1966b). The influence of acoustic and semantic similarity on long-term memory for word sequences. *Quarterly Journal of Experimental Psychology*, 18, 302–309.

Baddeley, A. D. (1968). How does acoustic similarity influence short-term memory? *Quarterly Journal of Experimental Psychology*, 20, 249–263.

Baddeley, A. D. (1986). *Working Memory.* London: Oxford University Press.

Baddeley, A. D. (2000). The episodic buffer: A new component of working memory? *Trends in Cognitive Sciences*, 4(11), 417–423.

Baddeley, A. D. (2002). Developmental amnesia. A challenge to current models? In L. R. Squire & D.L. Schacter (Eds). *Neuropsychology of Memory* (3rd edn), pp. 88–96. New York: Guilford Press.

Baddeley, A. D. (2003a). Working memory: looking back and looking forward. *Nature Reviews Neuroscience*, 4, 829–839.

Baddeley, A. D. (2003b). Working memory and language: an overview. *Journal of Communication Disorders*, 36, 189–208.

Baddeley, A. D. (2007). *Working Memory, Thought, and Action.* Oxford: OUP.

Baddeley, A. D. & Hitch, G. J. (1974). Working memory. In G. Bower (Ed.), *Recent Advances in Learning and Motivation* (pp. 47–89). New York: Academic.

Baddeley, A. D. & Hitch, G. J. (1977). Recency re-examined. In S. Dornick (Ed.), *Attention and performance VI* (pp. 647–667). Hillsdale, NJ: Erlbaum.

Baddeley, A. D. & Warrington, E. K. (1970). Amnesia and the distinction between long- and short-term memory. *Journal of Verbal Learning and Verbal Behavior*, 9, 176–189.

Baddeley, A. D. & Wilson, B. A. (2002). Prose recall and amnesia: implications for the structure of working memory. *Neuropsychologia*, 40, 1737–1743.

Baddeley, A. D., Thomson, N., & Buchanan, M. (1975). Word length and the structure of short-term memory. *Journal of Verbal Learning and Verbal Behavior*, 14, 575–589.

Baddeley, A. D., Lewis, V., Eldridge, M., & Thomson, N. (1984). Attention and retrieval from long-term memory. *Journal of Experimental Psychology: General*, 13, 518–540.

Baddeley, A. D., Vallar, G., & Wilson, B. (1987). Sentence comprehension and phonological memory:

some neuropsychological evidence. In M. Coltheart (Ed.), *Attention and performance XII: the psychology of reading* (pp. 509–529). Hove, UK: Lawrence Erlbaum Associates.

Baddeley, A. D., Papagno, C., & Vallar, C. (1988). When long-term learning depends on short-term storage. *Journal of Memory and Language*, *27*, 586–596.

Baddeley, A. D., Emslie, H., & Nimmo-Smith, I. (1994). *Doors and people: a test of visual and verbal recall and recognition*. Bury St Edmonds: Thames Valley.

Badre, D. (2008). Cognitive control, hierarchy, and the rostro-caudal organization of the frontal lobes. *Trends in Cognitive Science*, *12*, 193–200.

Badre, D. & D'Esposito, M. (2007). Functional magnetic resonance imaging evidence for a hierarchical organization of the prefrontal cortex. *Journal of Cognitive Neuroscience*, *19*, 2082–2099.

Badre, D. & Wagner, A. D. (2002). Semantic retrieval, mnemonic control, and prefrontal cortex. *Behavioral Cognitive Neuroscience Review*, *1*, 206–218.

Badre, D. & Wagner, A. D. (2005). Frontal lobe mechanisms that resolve proactive interference. *Cerebral Cortex*, *15*, 2003–2012.

Badre, D. & Wagner, A. D. (2007). Left ventrolateral prefrontal cortex and the cognitive control of memory. *Neuropsychologia*, *45*, 2883–2901.

Badre, D., Poldrack, R. A., Pare-Blagoev, E. J., Insler, R. Z., & Wagner, A. D. (2005). Dissociable controlled retrieval and generalized selection mechanisms in ventrolateral prefrontal cortex. *Neuron*, *47*, 907–918.

Badre, D., Hoffman, J., Cooney, J. W., & D'Esposito, M. (2009). Hierarchical cognitive control deficits following damage to the human frontal lobe. *Nature Neuroscience*, *12*, 515–522.

Bahrick, H. P. (1984). Semantic memory content in permastore: fifty years of memory for Spanish learned in school. *Journal of Experimental Psychology: General*, *113*, 1–29.

Baker, S. C., Rogers, R. D., Owen, A. M., Frith, C. D., Dolan, R. J., Frackowiak, R. S. et al. (1996). Neural systems engaged by planning: a PET study of the Tower of London task. *Neuropsychologia*, *34*, 515–526.

Baldo, J. V. & Dronkers, N. F. (2006). The role of inferior parietal and inferior frontal cortex in working memory. *Neuropsychology*, *20*, 529–538.

Barbarotto, R., Capitani, E., & Laiacona, M. (1996). Naming deficit in herpes simplex encephalitis. *Acta Neurologica Scandinavica*, *93*, 272–280.

Barbarotto, R., Laiacona, M., Macchi, V., & Capitani, E. (2002). Picture reality decision, semantic categories and gender. A new set of pictures, with norms and an experimental study. *Neuropsychologia*, *40*, 1637–1653.

Barbeau, E. J., Felician, O., Joubert, S., Sontheimer, A., Ceccaldi, M., & Poncet, M. (2005). Preserved visual recognition memory in an amnesic patient with hippocampal lesions. *Hippocampus*, *15*, 587–596.

Barber, H. & Carreiras, M. (2005). Grammatical gender and number agreement in Spanish: an ERP comparison. *Journal of Cognitive Neuroscience*, *17*, 137–153.

Barbey, A. K. & Sloman, S. A. (2007). Base-rate respect: from ecological rationality to dual processes. *Behavioral and Brain Sciences*, *30*, 241–254.

Barbur, J. L., Ruddock, K. H., & Waterfield, V. A. (1980). Human visual responses in the absence of the geniculo-calcarine projection. *Brain*, *103*, 905–928.

Barbur, J. L., Watson, J. D., Frackowiak, R. S., & Zeki, S. (1993). Conscious visual perception without V1. *Brain*, *116* (6), 1293–1302.

Barnes, J. M. & Underwood, B. J. (1959). Fate of first-list associations in transfer theory. *Journal of Experimental Psychology*, *58*, 97–105.

Baron-Cohen, S., Leslie, A. M., & Frith, U. (1985). Does the autistic child have a 'theory of mind'? *Cognition*, *21*, 37–46.

Baron-Cohen, S., Burt, L., Smith-Laittan, F., Harrison, J., & et al. (1996). Synaesthesia: prevalence and familiarity. *Perception*, *25*(9), 1073–1080.

Barr, W. B., Goldberg, E., Wasserstein, J., & Novelly, R. A. (1990). Retrograde amnesia following unilateral temporal lobectomy. *Neuropsychologia*, *28*, 243–255.

Barry, C. & Gerhand, S. (2003). Both concreteness and age-of-acquisition affect reading accuracy but only concreteness affects comprehension in a deep dyslexic patient. *Brain and Language*, *84*, 84–104.

Barry, C. & Richardson, J. (1988). Accounts of oral reading in deep dyslexia. In H.Whitaker (Ed.), *Phonological processes and brain mechanisms* (pp. 118–171). New York: Springer-Verlag.

Barsalou, L. (1988). The content and organization of autobiographical memories. In L. Barsalou, U. Neisser, & E. Winograd (Eds), *Remembering reconsidered: ecological and traditional approaches to the study of memory* (pp. 193–243). New York: CUP.

Barsalou, L., Simmons, W., Barbey, A., & Wilson, C. (2003). Grounding conceptual knowledge in modality specific systems. *Trends in Cognitive Science*, *7*, 84–91.

Bartlett, F. C. (1932). *Remembering: an experimental and social study*. Cambridge: CUP University.

Basso, A., Capitani, E., & Laiacona, M. (1988). Progressive language impairment without dementia: a case with isolated category specific semantic defect. *The Journal of Neurology, Neurosurgery, and Psychiatry*, *51*, 1201–1207.

Bastin, C., Van der Linden, M., Charnallet, A., Denby, C., Montaldi, D., Roberts, N., & Andrew, M. (2004). Dissociation between recall and recognition memory performance in an amnesic patient with hippocampal damage following carbon monoxide poisoning. *Neurocase*, *10*(4), 330–344.

Bates, E. & MacWhinney, B. (1989). Functionalism and the competition model. In E. Bates & B. MacWhinney (Eds), *The crosslinguistic study of sentence processing* (pp. 3–73). Cambridge: CUP.

Bates, E., Wilson, S. M., Saygin, A. P., Dick, F., Sereno, M. I., Knight, R. T., & Dronkers, N. F. (2003). Voxel-based lesion-symptom mapping. *Nature Neuroscience*, *6*(5), 448–450.

Bateson, G. (1972). *Steps to an Ecology of Mind*. New York: Ballantine.

Battaglia-Mayer, A. & Caminiti, R. (2002). Optic ataxia as a result of the breakdown of the global tuning fields of parietal neurones. *Brain*, *125*, 225–237.

Battaglia-Mayer, A., Mascaro, M., Brunamonti, E., & Caminiti, R. (2005). The over-representation of contralateral space in parietal cortex: a positive image of directional motor components of neglect? *Cerebral Cortex*, *15*, 514–525.

Batuev, A., Pirogov, A., & Orlov, A. (1979). Unit activity of the prefrontal cortex during delayed alternation performance in monkey. *Acta Physiologica Academiae Scientiarum Hungaricae*, *53*, 345–353.

Baxter, D. M. & Warrington, E. K. (1985). Category specific phonological dysgraphia. *Neuropsychologia*, *23*, 653–666.

Bay, E. (1953). Disturbances of visual perception and their examination. *Brain*, *76*, 515–550.

Bayley, P. J., Hopkins, R. O., & Squire, L. R. (2003). Successful recollection of remote autobiographical memories by amnesic patients with medial temporal lobe lesions. *Neuron*, *38*, 135–144.

Bayley, P. J., Gold, J. J., Hopkins, R. O., & Squire, L. R. (2005). The neuroanatomy of remote memory. *Neuron*, *46*, 799–810.

Bays, P. M. & Wolpert, D. M. (2007). Computational principles of sensorimotor control that minimize uncertainty and variability. *The Journal of Physiology*, *578*, 387–396.

Beauchamp, M. S., Lee, K. E., Haxby, J. V., & Martin, A. (2002). Parallel visual motion processing streams for manipulable objects and human movements. *Neuron*, *34*, 149–159.

Beauchamp, M. S., Lee, K. E., Haxby, J. V., & Martin, A. (2003). FMRI responses to video and point-light displays of moving humans and manipulable objects. *Journal of Cognitive Neuroscience*, *15*, 991–1001.

Beauvois, M.-F. (1982). Optic aphasia: a process of interaction between vision and language. *Proceedings of the Royal Society of London, Series B*, *298*, 35–47.

Beauvois, M.-F. & Derouesné, J. (1979). Phonological alexia: three dissociations. *The Journal of Neurology, Neurosurgery, and Psychiatry*, *42*, 1115–1124.

Beauvois, M.-F. & Saillant, B. (1985). Optic aphasia for colours and colour agnosia: a distinction between visual and visuo-verbal impairments in the processing of colours. *Cognitive Neuropsychology*, *2*, 1–48.

Bechara, A., Damasio, H., Tranel, D., & Damasio, A. R. (1997). Deciding advantageously before knowing the advantageous strategy. *Science*, *275*, 1293–1295.

Beck, J. & Ambler, B. (1973). The effects of concentrated and distributed attention on peripheral acuity. *Perception and Psychophysics*, *14*, 225–230.

Becker, J. T., MacAndrew, D., & Fiez, J. (1999). A Comment on the functional localisation of the phonological storage subsystem of working memory. *Brain and Cognition*, *41*, 27–38.

Behrmann, M. & Bub, D. (1992). Surface dyslexia and dysgraphia: dual routes, a single lexicon. *Cognitive Neuropsychology*, *9*, 209–258.

Behrmann, M., Nelson, J., & Sekuler, E. B. (1998a). Visual complexity in letter-by-letter reading: 'pure' alexia is not pure. *Neuropsychologia*, *36*, 1115–1132.

Behrmann, M., Plaut, D. C., & Nelson, J. (1998b). A literature review and new data supporting an interactive account of letter-by-letter reading. *Cognitive Neuropsychology*, *15*, 7–51.

Bell, B. D. (1994). Pantomime recognition impairment in aphasia: an analysis of error types. *Brain and Language*, *47*, 269–278.

Ben-Shachar, M., Dougherty, R. F., Deutsch, G. K., & Wandell, B. A. (2007). Differential sensitivity to words and shapes in ventral occipito-temporal cortex. *Cerebral Cortex*, *17*, 1604–1611.

Ben-Shachar, M., Palti, D., & Grodzinsky, Y. (2004). Neural correlates of syntactic movement: converging evidence from two fMRI experiments. *Neuroimage*, *21*, 1320–1336.

Benson, D. (1967). Fluency in aphasia. *Cortex*, *3*, 373–394.

Benson, D. F., Marsden, C. D., & Meadows, J. C. (1974). The amnesic syndrome of posterior cerebral artery occlusion. *Acta Neurologica Scandinavica*, *50*, 133–145.

Benson, D. F., Davis, R. J., Snyder, B. D. (1988). Posterior cortical atrophy. *Archives of Neurology*, *45*, 789–93.

Benton, A. L. (1968). Differential behavioral effects in frontal lobe disease. *Neuropsychologia*, *6*, 53–60.

Ben-Yishay, Y. & Diller, L. (1983). Cognitive deficits. In M.Rosenthal, E. Griffith, & M. Bond (Eds), *Rehabilitation of the head injured adult*. Philadelphia, PA: FA Davis Co.

Beretta, A., Campbell, C., Carr, T. H., Huang, J., Schmitt, L. M., Christianson, K. et al. (2003). An ER-fMRI investigation of morphological inflection in German reveals that the brain makes a distinction between regular and irregular forms. *Brain and Language*, *85*, 67–92.

Berg, E. (1948). A simple objective test for measuring flexibility of thinking. *Journal of General Psychology*, *39*, 15–22.

Berger, T., Yeckel, M., & Thiels, E. (1996). Network determinants of hippocampal synaptic plasticity. In M.Baudry & J. Davis (Eds), *Long-term potentiation*. Cambridge, MA: MIT Press.

Berman, K. F., Ostrem, J. L., Randolph, C., Gold, J., Goldberg, T. E., Coppola, R. et al. (1995). Physiological activation of a cortical network during performance of the Wisconsin Card Sorting Test: a positron emission tomography study. *Neuropsychologia*, *33*, 1027–1046.

Berndt, R. S. & Mitchum, C. C. (1990). Auditory and lexical information sources in immediate recall: Evidence from a patient with a deficit to the phonological short-term store. In G.Vallar & T. Shallice (Eds), *Neuropsychological impairments of short-term memory* (pp. 115–144). New York: CUP.

Berndt, R. S., Mitchum, C. C., & Haendiges, A. N. (1996). Comprehension of reversible sentences in 'agrammatism': a meta-analysis. *Cognition*, *58*, 289–308.

Berndt, R. S., Mitchum, C. C., & Wayland, S. (1997). Patterns of sentence comprehension in aphasia: a consideration of three hypotheses. *Brain and Language*, *60*, 197–221.

Berry, C. J., Shanks, D. R., & Henson, R. N. (2006). On the status of unconscious memory: Merikle and Reingold (1991) revisited. *Journal of Experimental Psychology: Learning, Memory and Cognition*, *32*, 925–934.

Berry, C. J., Shanks, D. R., & Henson, R. N. (2008). A unitary signal-detection model of implicit and explicit memory. *Trends in Cognitive Sciences*, *12*, 367–373.

Berti, A. & Rizzolatti, G. (1992). Visual processing without awareness: evidence from unilateral neglect. *Journal of Cognitive Neuroscience*, *4*, 345–351.

Bestmann, S., Ruff, C. C., Blankenburg, F., Weiskopf, N., Driver, J., & Rothwell, J. C. (2008). Mapping causal interregional influences with concurrent TMS-fMRI. *Experimental Brain Research*, *191*, 383–402.

Bianchi, L. (1922). *The mechanism of the brain and the function of the frontal lobes*. London: MacMillian.

Bienenstock, E., Cooper, L., & Munro, P. (1982). Theory for the development of neuron selectivity: Orientation specifity and binocular interaction in visual cortex. *Journal of Neuroscience*, *2*, 32–48.

Bihrle, A. M., Brownell, H. H., Powelson, J. A., & Gardner, H. (1986). Comprehension of humorous and nonhumorous materials by left and right brain-damaged patients. *Brain and Cognition*, *5*, 399–411.

Binder, J. R. & Mohr, J. P. (1992). The topography of callosal reading pathways. A case-control analysis. *Brain*, *115* (6), 1807–1826.

Binder, J. R. & Price, C. J. (2001). Functional neuroimaging of language. In R. Cabeza & A. Kingstone (Eds), *Handbook of Functional Neuroimaging* (pp. 187–251). Cambridge, MA: MIT Press.

Binder, J. R., Medler, D. A., Westbury, C. F., Liebenthal, E., & Buchanan, L. (2006). Tuning of the human left fusiform gyrus to sublexical orthographic structure. *Neuroimage*, *33*, 739–748.

Bird, C. M., Shallice, T., & Cipolotti, L. (2007a). Fractionation of memory in medial temporal lobe amnesia. *Neuropsychologia*, *45*, 1160–1171.

Bird, C. M., Vargha-Khadem, F., & Burgess, N. (2007b). Impaired memory for scenes but not faces in developmental hippocampal amnesia: a case study. *Neuropsychologia*, *46*, 1050–1059.

Bird, H., Lambon Ralph, M. A., Seidenberg, M. S., McClelland, J. L., & Patterson, K. (2003). Deficits in phonology and past-tense morphology: what's the connection? *Journal of Memory and Language*, *48*(3), 502–526.

Bishop, D. V., Aamodt-Leeper, G., Creswell, C., McGurk, R., & Skuse, D. H. (2001). Individual differences in cognitive planning on the Tower of Hanoi task: neuropsychological maturity or measurement error? *Journal of Child Psychology and Psychiatry*, *42*, 551–556.

Bisiacchi, P., Cipolotti, L., & Denes, G. (1989). Impairments in processing meaningless verbal material in several modalities: the relationship between shortterm memory and phonological skills. *Quarterly Journal of Experimental Psychology*, *41A*, 292–320.

Bjoertomt, O., Cowey, A., & Walsh, V. (2002). Spatial neglect in near and far space investigated by repetitive transcranial magnetic stimulation. *Brain*, *125*, 2012–2022.

Blackburn, P., de Rijke, M., & Venema, Y. (2001). Modal logic. *Cambridge Tracts in Theoretical Computer Science*, *53*.

Blamire, A. M., Ogawa, S., Ugurbil, K., Rothman, D., McCarthy, G., Ellermann, J. M. et al. (1992). Dynamic mapping of the human visual cortex by high-speed magnetic resonance imaging. *Proceedings of the National Academy of Sciences, USA*, *89*, 11069–11073.

Blank, S. C., Scott, S. K., Murphy, K., Warburton, E., & Wise, R. J. S. (2002). Speech production: Wernicke, Broca and beyond. *Brain*, *125*(8), 1829 –1838.

Blaxton, T. A., Bookheimer, S. Y., Zeffiro, T. A., Figlozzi, C. M., Gaillard, W. D., & Theodore, W. H. (1996). Functional mapping of human memory using PET: comparisons of conceptual and perceptual tasks. *Canadian Journal of Experimental Psychology*, *50*, 42–56.

Blazely, A., Coltheart, M., & Casey, B. (2005). Semantic impairment with and without surface dyslexia: Implications for models of reading. *Cognitive Neuropsychology*, *22*, 695–717.

Block, N. (1978). Troubles with functionalism. In C. W. Savage (Ed.), *Perception and cognition: issues in the foundations of psychology*, Minnesota Studies in the Philosophy of Science (Vol. 9, pp. 261–325). Minnesota: University of Minnesota Press.

Block, N. (1995). On a confusion about a function of consciousness. *Behavioral and Brain Sciences*, 18, 227–247.

Bloom, P. A. & Fischler, I. (1980). Completion norms for 329 sentence contexts. *Memory and Cognition*, 8, 631–642.

Blythe, I. M., Kennard, C., & Ruddock, K. H. (1987). Residual vision in patients with retrogeniculate lesions of the visual pathways. *Brain*, 110 (4), 887–905.

Boccardi, E., Della, S. S., Motto, C., & Spinnler, H. (2002). Utilisation behaviour consequent to bilateral SMA softening. *Cortex*, 38, 289–308.

Boden, M. (1977). *Artificial intelligence and natural man.* New York: Basic Books.

Boden, M. (1988). *Computer models of mind: computational approaches in theoretical psychology.* New York: CUP.

Boly, M., Coleman, M. R., Davis, M. H., Hampshire, A., Bor, D., Moonen, G. et al. (2007). When thoughts become action: an fMRI paradigm to study volitional brain activity in non-communicative brain injured patients. *Neuroimage*, 36, 979–992.

Bor, D., Duncan, J., Wiseman, R. J., & Owen, A. M. (2003). Encoding strategies dissociate prefrontal activity from working memory demand. *Neuron*, 37, 361–367.

Borgo, F. & Shallice, T. (2001). When living things and other 'sensory quality' categories behave in the same fashion: a novel category specificity effect. *Neurocase*, 7, 201–220.

Borgo, F. & Shallice, T. (2003). Category specificity and feature knowledge: Evidence from new sensory-quality categories. *Cognitive Neuropsychology*, 30, 327–353.

Borst, C. (1970). *The mind-brain identity theory.* London: Macmillan.

Bošković, Ž. & Lasnik, H. (Eds) (2007) *Minimalist syntax: the essential readings.* Blackwell Publishing Ltd., Malden, MA.

Bottini, G., Corcoran, R., Sterzi, R., Paulesu, E., Schenone, P., Scarpa, P. et al. (1994). The role of the right hemisphere in the interpretation of figurative aspects of language. A positron emission tomography activation study. *Brain*, 117 (6), 1241–1253.

Botvinick, M. M. & Bylsma, L. M. (2005). Regularization in short-term memory for serial order. *Journal of Experimental Psychology: Learning, Memory and Cognition*, 31, 351–358.

Botvinick, M. M. & Plaut, D. C. (2004). Doing without schema hierarchies: a recurrent connectionist approach to normal and impaired routine sequential action. *Psychological Review*, 111, 395–429.

Botvinick, M. M. & Plaut, D. C. (2006a). Short-term memory for serial order: a recurrent neural network model. *Psychological Review*, 113, 201–233.

Botvinick, M. M. & Plaut, D. C. (2006b). Such stuff as habits are made on: a reply to Cooper and Shallice (2006). *Psychological Review*, 113(4), 917–927.

Botvinick, M. M. & Watanabe, T. (2007). From numerosity to ordinal rank: a gain-field model of serial order representation in cortical working memory. *Journal of Neuroscience*, 27, 8636–8642.

Botvinick, M. M., Nystrom, L. E., Fissell, K., Carter, C. S., & Cohen, J. D. (1999). Conflict monitoring versus selection-for-action in anterior cingulate cortex. *Nature*, 402, 179–181.

Botvinick, M. M., Niv, Y. & Barto, A. C. (2009). Hierarchically organized behavior and its neural foundations: A reinforcement learning perspective. *Cognition*, 113(3), 262–280.

Bowden, E. M. & Jung-Beeman, M. (2003). Aha! Insight experience correlates with solution activation in the right hemisphere. *Psychonomic Bulletin and Review*, 10, 730–737.

Bowden, E. M., Jung-Beeman, M., Fleck, J., & Kounios, J. (2005). New approaches to demystifying insight. *Trends in Cognitive Sciences*, 9, 322–328.

Bowers, J. S. (2009). On the biological plausibility of grandmother cells: implications for neural network theories in psychology and neuroscience. *Psychological Review*, 116, 220–251.

Bowers, K. S. (1984). On being unconsciously influenced and informed. In K. S. Bowers & D. Meichenbaum (Eds), *The unconscious reconsidered* (pp. 227–272). Wiley.

Bozeat, S., Gregory, C. A., Ralph, M. A., & Hodges, J. R. (2000). Which neuropsychiatric and behavioural features distinguish frontal and temporal variants of frontotemporal dementia from Alzheimer's disease? *The Journal of Neurology, Neurosurgery, and Psychiatry*, 69, 178–186.

Braine, M. (1978). On the relation between the natural logic of reasoning and standard logic. *Psychological Review*, 85, 1–21.

Braine, M. & O'Brien, D. (1998). *Mental logic.* Erlbaum.

Braitenberg, V. & Schuz, A. (1991). *Anatomy of the cortex: statistics and geometry.* Berlin: Springer.

Brambati, S. M., Myers, D., Wilson, A., Rankin, K. P., Allison, S. C., Rosen, H. J. et al. (2006). The anatomy of category-specific object naming in neurodegenerative diseases. *Journal of Cognitive Neuroscience*, 18, 1644–1653.

Brass, M., Derrfuss, J., Forstmann, B., & von Cramon, D. Y. (2005). The role of the inferior frontal junction area in cognitive control. *Trends in Cognitive Sciences*, 9, 314–316.

Braver, T. S. & Bongiolatti, S. R. (2002). The role of frontopolar cortex in subgoal processing during working memory. *Neuroimage*, *15*, 523–536.

Braver, T. S., Reynolds, J. R., & Donaldson, D. I. (2003). Neural mechanisms of transient and sustained cognitive control during task switching. *Neuron*, *39*, 713–726.

Brazzelli, M. & Spinnler, H. (1998). An example of lack of frontal inhibition: the 'utilization behaviour'. *European Journal of Neurology*, *5*, 357–353.

Breedin, S. & Saffran, E. M. (1999). Sentence processing in the face of semantic loss: a case study. *Journal of Experimental Psychology: General*, *128*, 547–562.

Breedin, S., Saffran, E., & Coslett, H. (1994). Reversal of the concreteness effect in a patient with semantic dementia. *Cognitive Neuropsychology*, *11*, 617–660.

Bremmer, F., Schlack, A., Shah, N. J., Zafiris, O., Kubischik, M., Hoffmann, K. et al. (2001). Polymodal motion processing in posterior parietal and premotor cortex: a human fMRI study strongly implies equivalencies between humans and monkeys. *Neuron*, *29*, 287–296.

Bresnan, J. (2001). *Lexical-functional syntax*. Oxford: Blackwell.

Brewer, W. F. (1986). *What is autobiographical memory? In* D. C. Rubin (Ed.), *Autobiographical memory* (pp. 25–49). Cambridge, England: Cambridge University Press.

Bricolo, E., Shallice, T., Priftis, K., & Meneghello, F. (2000). Selective space transformation deficit in a patient with spatial agnosia. *Neurocase*, *6*, 307–319.

Britten, K. H., Shadlen, M. N., Newsome, W. T., & Movshon, J. A. (1992). The analysis of visual motion: a comparison of neuronal and psychophysical performance. *Journal of Neuroscience*, *12*, 4745–4765.

Britten, K. H., Shadlen, M. N., Newsome, W. T., & Movshon, J. A. (1993). Responses of neurons in macaque MT to stochastic motion signals. *Visual Neuroscience*, *10*, 1157–1169.

Broadbent, D. E. (1958). *Perception and communication*. Pergamon Press.

Broadbent, D. E. (1968). *Behaviour*. London: Methuen.

Broadbent, D. E. (1971). *Decision and stress*. Academic Press.

Broadbent, D. E. (1985). A question of levels: Comment on McClelland and Rumelhart. *Journal of Experimental Psychology: General*, *114*, 189–192.

Broadbent, N., Clark, R. E., Zola, S., & Squire, L. R. (2002). The medial temporal lobe and memory. In L. R. Squire & D. Schacter (Eds), *The neuropsychology of memory* (pp. 3–23). New York: Guilford.

Brodmann, K. (1909). *Vergleichende Lokalisation8lehre der Grosshirnrinde*. Leipzig: J. A. Barth.

Brooks, L. R. (1968). Spatial and verbal components of the act of recall. *Canadian Journal of Psychology*, *22*, 349–368.

Brooks, R. (1985). A robust layered control system for a robot. *MIT Artificial Intelligence Lab*. Memo, *864*

Brooks, R. (1991). Intelligence without reason. *Artificial Intelligence*, *47*, 139–159.

Brown, G. D. A., Preece, T., & Hulme, C. (2000). Oscillator-based memory for serial order. *Psychological Review*, *107*, 127–181.

Brown, G. D. A., Neath, I., & Chater, N. (2007). A temporal ratio model of memory. *Psychological Review*, *114*, 539–576.

Brown, M. W. & Aggleton, J. P. (2001). Recognition memory: what are the roles of the perirhinal cortex and hippocampus? *Nature Reviews Neuroscience*, *2*, 51–61.

Brown, M. W. & Xiang, J. Z. (1998). Recognition memory: neuronal substrates of the judgement of prior occurrence. *Progress in Neurobiology*, *55*, 149–189.

Bruce, V. & Young, A. (1986). Understanding face recognition. *British Journal of Psychology*, *77*, 305–327.

Bryson, A. E. & Ho, Y. C. (1969). *Applied optimal control*. Waltham, Massachusetts: Blaisdell.

Bub, D. (2000). Methodological issues confronting PET and fMRI studies of cognitive function. *Cognitive Neuropsychology*, *17*, 467–484.

Bub, D. & Kertesz, A. (1982). Evidence for lexicographic processing in a patient with preserved written over oral single word naming. *Brain*, *105*, 697–717.

Bub, D., Cancelliere, A., & Kertesz, A. (1985). Whole-word and analytic translation of spelling-to-sound in a non-semantic reader. In K. Patterson, M. Coltheart, & J. Marshall (Eds), *Surface dyslexia* (pp. 15–34). Hillsdale, NJ: Lawrence Erlbaum Associates.

Bub, D., Black, S. E., Howell, J., & Kertesz, A. (1987). Speech output processes and reading. In M.Coltheart, G. Sartori, & R. Job (Eds), *The Cognitive Neuropsychology of Language*. Hove, UK: Lawrence Erlbaum Associates Ltd.

Buccino, G., Binkofski, F., Fink, G. R., Fadiga, L., Fogassi, L., Gallese, V. et al. (2001). Action observation activates premotor and parietal areas in a somatotopic manner: an fMRI study. *European Journal of Neuroscience*, *13*, 400–404.

Buchsbaum, B. R. & D'Esposito, M. (2008). The search for the phonological store: from loop to convolution. *Journal of Cognitive Neuroscience*, *20*, 762–778.

Buckley, M. J. & Gaffan, D. (2006). Perirhinal cortical contributions to object perception. *Trends in Cognitive Sciences*, *10*, 100–107.

Buckley, M. J., Gaffan, D., & Murray, E. A. (1997). Functional double dissociation between two inferior temporal cortical areas: perirhinal cortex versus middle temporal gyrus. *Journal of Neurophysiology*, *77*, 587–598.

Buckner, R. L., Logan, J., Donaldson, D. I., & Wheeler, M. E. (2000). Cognitive neuroscience of episodic memory encoding. *Acta Psychologica (Amsterdam)*, *105*, 127–139.

Buiatti, T., Mussoni, A., Toraldo, A., Skrap, M., & Shallice, T. (In press). Two qualitatively different impairments in making rotation operations. *Cortex*.

Buiatti, T., Mussoni, A., Skrap, M., & Shallice, T. (in preparation). Localising phonological alexia in a tumour patient series.

Bull, R., Espy, K. A., & Senn, T. E. (2004). A comparison of performance on the Towers of London and Hanoi in young children. *Journal of Child Psychology and Psychiatry*, *45*, 743–754.

Bullinaria, J. (1994). Representation, learning, generalization and damage in neural network models of reading aloud. Edinburgh University Technical Report, 94/1.

Bullinaria, J. (2007). Understanding the emergence of modularity in neural systems. *Cognitive Science*, *31*, 673–695.

Bullinaria, J. (2009). The importance of neurophysiological constraints for modelling the emergence of modularity. In D. Heinke & E. Mavritsaki (Eds), *Computational modelling in behavioural neuroscience* (pp. 187–208). Hove: Psychology Press.

Bullinaria, J. & Chater, N. (1995). Connectionist modelling: implications for cognitive neuropsychology. *Language and Cognitive Processes*, *10*, 227–264.

Bunge, S. A. & Wallis, J. D. (Eds) (2008). *Neuroscience of rule-governed behavior*. Oxford, Oxford University Press.

Bunge, S. A., Wendelken, C., Badre, D., & Wagner, A. D. (2005). Analogical reasoning and prefrontal cortex: evidence for separable retrieval and integration mechanisms. *Cerebral Cortex*, *15*, 239–249.

Bunge, S. A., Helskog, E. H., & Wendelken, C. (2009). Left, but not right, rostrolateral prefrontal cortex meets a stringent test of the relational integration hypothesis. *NeuroImage*, *46*(1), 338–342.

Bunn, E., Tyler, L. K., & Moss, H. E. (1997). Patient JBR: The role of familiarity and property type in a selective deficit for living things. *Brain and Language*, *60*, 10–2.

Bunn, E., Tyler, L. K., & Moss, H. E. (1998). Category-specific semantic deficits: the role of familiarity and property type reexamined. *Neuropsychology*, *12*, 367–379.

Burani, C., Vallar, C., & Bottini, G. (1991). Articulatory coding and phonological judgments on written words and pictures. The role of the phonological output buffer. *European Journal of Cognitive Psychology*, *3*, 379–398.

Burgess, N. & Hitch, G. J. (1992). Towards a network model of the articulatory loop. *Journal of Memory and Language*, *31*, 429–460.

Burgess, N. & Hitch, G. J. (1999). Memory for serial order: a network model of the phonological loop and its timing. *Psychological Review*, *106*, 581.

Burgess, N. & Hitch, G. J. (2005). Computational models of working memory: putting long-term memory into context. *Trends in Cognitive Sciences*, *9*, 535–541.

Burgess, N. & O'Keefe, J. (1996). Neuronal computations underlying the firing of place cells and their role in navigation. *Hippocampus*, *6*, 749–762.

Burgess, N., Recce, M., & O'Keefe J. (1994). A model of hippocampal function. *Neural Networks*, *7*, 1065–1081.

Burgess, N., Becker, S., King, J., & O'Keefe, J. (2001). Memory for events and their spatial context: models and experiments. *Philosophical Transaction of the Royal Society of London, B: Biological Sciences*, *356*, 1493–1503.

Burgess, P. W. (2000). Strategy application disorder: the role of the frontal lobes in human multitasking. *Psychological Research*, *63*, 279–288.

Burgess, P. W. & Alderman, N. (2004). Executive dysfunction. In L. H. Goldstein & J. E. McNeil (Eds), *Clinical Neuropsychology: A Practical Guide to Assessment and Management for Clinicians*. Chichester, UK: Wiley.

Burgess, P. W. & Shallice, T. (1996a). Bizarre responses, rule detection and frontal lobe lesions. *Cortex*, *32*, 241–259.

Burgess, P. W. & Shallice, T. (1996b). Confabulation and the control of recollection. *Memory*, *4*, 359–411.

Burgess, P. W. & Shallice, T. (1996c). Response suppression, initiation and strategy use following frontal lobe lesions. *Neuropsychologia*, *34*, 263–272.

Burgess, P. W., Veitch, E., de Lacy Costello, A., & Shallice, T. (2000). The cognitive and neuroanatomical correlates of multitasking. *Neuropsychologia*, *38*(6), 848–863.

Burgess, P. W., Quayle, A., & Frith, C. D. (2001). Brain regions involved in prospective memory as determined by positron emission tomography. *Neuropsychologia*, *39*, 545–555.

Burgess, P. W., Scott, S. K., & Frith, C. D. (2003). The role of the rostral frontal cortex (area 10) in prospective memory: a lateral versus medial dissociation. *Neuropsychologia*, *41*, 906–918.

Burgess, P. W., Dumontheil, I., & Gilbert, S. J. (2007). The gateway hypothesis of rostral prefrontal cortex (area 10) function. *Trends in Cognitive Sciences*, *11*, 290–298.

Bussey, T. J. & Saksida, L. M. (2002). The organization of visual object representations: a connectionist model of effects of lesions in perirhinal cortex. *European Journal of Neuroscience*, *15*, 355–364.

Butterworth, B., Shallice, T., & Watson, F. (1990). Short-term retention without short-term memory. In G.Vallar & T. Shallice (Eds), *Neuropsychological impairments of short-term memory* (pp. 187–213). Cambridge: CUP.

Buxbaum, L. J. (2001). Ideomotor apraxia: a call to action. *Neurocase, 7*, 445–458.

Buxbaum, L. J. & Coslett, H. (2001). Specialised structural descriptions for human body parts: evidence from autotopagnosia. *Cognitive Neuropsychology, 18*, 289–306.

Buxbaum, L. J., Schwartz, M., & Montgomery, M. (1998). Ideational apraxia and naturalistic action. *Cognitive Neuropsychology, 15*, 617–643.

Buxbaum, L. J., Giovannetti, T., & Libon, D. (2000). The role of the dynamic body schema in praxis: evidence from primary progressive apraxia. *Brain and Cognition, 44*, 166–191.

Buxbaum, L. J., Johnson-Frey, S. H., & Bartlett-Williams, M. (2005). Deficient internal models for planning hand-object interactions in apraxia. *Neuropsychologia, 43*, 917–929.

Bybee, J. & Slobin, D. (1982). Rules and schemas in the development and use of the English past tense. *Language, 58*, 265–289.

Byrne, M. & Anderson, J. (2001). Serial modules in parallel: the psychology refractory period and perfect time-sharing. *Psychological Review, 108*, 847–869.

Byrne, P., Becker, S., & Burgess, N. (2007). Remembering the past and imagining the future. *Psychological Review, 114*(2), 340–375.

Cabeza, R., Locantore, J. K., & Anderson, N. D. (2003). Lateralization of prefrontal activity during episodic memory retrieval: evidence for the production-monitoring hypothesis. *Journal of Cognitive Neuroscience, 15*, 249–259.

Caccappolo-van Vliet, E., Miozzo, M., & Stern, Y. (2004a). Phonological dyslexia without phonological impairment? *Cognitive Neuropsychology, 21*, 820–839.

Caccappolo-van Vliet, E., Miozzo, M., & Stern, Y. (2004b). Phonological dyslexia: a test case for reading models. *Psychological Science, 15*, 583–590.

Cain, M. (2002). *Fodor: language, mind and philosophy.* Cambridge, UK: Polity.

Call, J. & Tomasello, M. (2008). Does the chimpanzee have a theory of mind? 30 years later. *Trends in Cognitive Sciences, 12*, 187–192.

Campanella, F. & Shallice, T. (in press). Refractoriness and the healthy brain: a behavioural study on semantic access. *Cognition.*

Campanella, F., Mondani, M., Skrap, M., & Shallice, T. (2009). Semantic access dysphasia resulting from left temporal lobe tumours. *Brain, 132*, 87–102.

Campanella, F., D'Agostini, S., Skrap, M., & Shallice, T. (2010). Naming manipulable objects: anatomy of a category specific effect in left temporal tumours. *Neuropsychologia, 48*, 1583–1597.

Campbell, R. (1990). Lipreading, neuropsychology, and immediate memory. In C. Vallar & T. Shallice (Eds), *Neuropsychological impairments of short-term memory* (pp. 268–286). Cambridge: CUP.

Campbell, R. & Butterworth, B. (1985). Phonological dyslexia and dysgraphia in a highly literate subject: A developmental case with associated deficits of phonemic processing and awareness. *Quarterly Journal of Experimental Psychology, 37A*, 435–475.

Campbell, R. & Dodd, B. (1980). Hearing by eye. *Quarterly Journal of Experimental Psychology, 32*, 85–89.

Campion, J., Latto, R., & Smith, Y. (1983). Is blindsight an effect of scattered light, spared cortex, and near-threshold vision? *Behavioral and Brain Sciences, 6*, 423–486.

Canolty, R. T., Soltani, M., Dalal, S. S., Edwards, E., Dronkers, N. F., Nagarajan, S. S. et al. (2007). Spatiotemporal dynamics of word processing in the human brain. *Frontiers in Neurosciences, 1*, 185–196.

Cantagallo, A. & Bonazzi, S. (1996). Acquired dysgraphia with selective damage to the graphemic buffer: a single case report. *Italian Journal of Neurological Sciences, 17*, 249–254.

Capitani, E., Laiacona, M. & Barbarotto, R. (1993). Dissociazioni semantiche intercategoriali [Parte II] procedura automatica di analisi di una batteria standardizzata. *Archivio di Psicolologia, Neurologia e Psichiatria, 54*, 457–476.

Capitani, E., Laiacona, M., Mahon, B., & Caramazza, A. (2003). What are the facts of semantic category-specific deficits? A critical review of the clinical evidence. *Cognitive Neuropsychology, 20*, 213–261.

Caplan, D. & Hildebrandt, N. (1988). *Disorders of Syntactic Comprehension.* Cambridge, MA: MIT Press.

Caplan, D. & Waters, G. S. (1992). Issues arising regarding the nature and consequences of reproduction conduction aphasia. In S. Kohn (Ed.), *Conduction aphasia.* Hillsdale, NJ: Lawrence Erlbaum Associates, Inc.

Caplan, D. & Waters, G. S. (1999). Verbal working memory and sentence comprehension. *Behavioral and Brain Sciences, 22*, 77–94.

Caplan, D., Baker, C., & Dehaut, F. (1985). Syntactic determinants of sentence comprehension in aphasia. *Cognition, 21*, 117–175.

Caplan, D., Hildebrandt, N., & Makris, N. (1996). Location of lesions in stroke patients with deficits in syntactic processing in sentence comprehension. *Brain, 119* (3), 933–949.

Caplan, D., Alpert, N., & Waters, G. (1998). Effects of syntactic structure and propositional number on patterns of regional cerebral blood flow. *Journal of Cognitive Neuroscience, 10*, 541–552.

Cappa, S. F., Perani, D., Schnur, T., Tettamanti, M., & Fazio, F. (1998). The effects of semantic category and knowledge type on lexical-semantic access: a PET study. *Neuroimage*, 8, 350–359.

Cappa, S. F., Moro, A., Perani, D., & Piattelli-Palmarini, M. (2000). Broca's aphasia, Broca's area, and syntax: a complex relationship. *Behavioral and Brain Sciences*, 23(1), 27–28.

Cappelletti, M., Kopelman, M., & Butterworth, B. (2002). Why semantic dementia drives you to the dogs (but not to the horses): a theoretical account. *Cognitive Neuropsychology*, 19, 483–503.

Caramazza, A. (1986). On drawing inferences about the structure of normal cognitive systems from the analysis of patterns of impaired performance: the case for single-patient studies. *Brain and Cognition*, 5, 41–66.

Caramazza, A. (1997). How many levels of processing are there in lexical access? *Cognitive Neuropsychology*, 14, 177–208.

Caramazza, A. & Hillis, A. (1990). Where do semantic errors come from? *Cortex*, 26, 95–122.

Caramazza, A. & Mahon, B. (2006). The organisation of conceptual knowledge in the brain: the future's past and some future directions. *Cognitive Neuropsychology*, 23, 13–38.

Caramazza, A. & Miceli, G. (1990). The structure of graphemic representations. *Cognition*, 37, 243–297.

Caramazza, A. & Shelton, J. (1998). Domain specific knowledge systems in the brain: the animate-inanimate distinction. *Journal of Cognitive Neuroscience*, 10, 1–34.

Caramazza, A. & Zurif, E. B. (1976). Dissociation of algorithmic and heuristic processes in language comprehension: evidence from aphasia. *Brain and Language*, 3, 572–582.

Caramazza, A., Miceli, G., & Villa, G. (1986). The role of (output) phonology in reading writing and repetition. *Cognitive Neuropsychology*, 3, 37–76.

Caramazza, A., Miceli, G., Villa, G., & Romani, C. (1987). The role of the graphemic buffer in spelling: evidence from a case of acquired dysgraphia. *Cognition*, 26, 59–85.

Caramazza, A., Hillis, A., Rapp, B., & Romani, C. (1990). The multiple semantics hypothesis: multiple confusions? *Cognitive Neuropsychology*, 7, 161–189.

Caramazza, A., Capitani, E., Rey, A., & Berndt, R. S. (2001). Agrammatic Broca's aphasia is not associated with a single pattern of comprehension performance. *Brain and Language*, 76, 158–184.

Card, S., Moran, T., & Newell, A. (1983). *The psychology of human-computer interaction*. Hillsdale, NJ: Lawrence Erlbaum Associates.

Carlesimo, G. A., Fadda, L., Sabbadini, M., & Caltagirone, C. (1994). Visual repetition priming for words relies on access to the visual input lexicon: evidence from a dyslexic patient. *Neuropsychologia*, 32, 1089–1100.

Carlesimo, G. A., Fadda, L., Turriziani, P., Tomaiuolo, F., & Caltagirone, C. (2001a). Selective sparing of face learning in a global amnesic patient. *The Journal of Neurology, Neurosurgery, and Psychiatry*, 71, 340–346.

Carlesimo, G. A., Perri, R., Turriziani, P., Tomaiuolo, F., & Caltagirone, C. (2001b). Remembering what but not where: independence of spatial and visual working memory in the human brain. *Cortex*, 37, 519–534.

Carnap, R. (1947). On the application of inductive logic. *Philosophy and Phenomenological Research*, 8, 133–148.

Carpenter, P. A., Just, M. A., & Shell, P. (1990). What one intelligence test measures: a theoretical account of the processing in the Raven Progressive Matrices Test. *Psycholical Review*, 97, 404–431.

Carpenter, P. A., Just, M. A., Keller, T. A., Eddy, W., & Thulborn, K. (1999). Graded functional activation in the visuospatial system with the amount of task demand. *Journal of Cognitive Neuroscience*, 11, 9–24.

Carter, C. S., Braver, T. S., Barch, D. M., Botvinick, M. M., Noll, D., & Cohen, J. D. (1998). Anterior cingulate cortex, error detection, and the online monitoring of performance. *Science*, 280, 747–749.

Catani, M., Howard, R. J., Pajevic, S., & Jones, D. K. (2002). Virtual in vivo interactive dissection of white matter fasciculi in the human brain. *Neuroimage*, 17, 77–94.

Catani, M., Piccirilli, M., Cherubini, A., Tarducci, R., Sciarma, T., Gobbi, G., Pelliccioli, G., et al. (2003). Axonal injury within language network in primary progressive aphasia. *Annals of Neurology*, 53(2), 242–247.

Cavanna, A. E. & Trimble, M. R. (2006). The precuneus: a review of its functional anatomy and behavioural correlates. *Brain*, 129, 564–583.

Cave, C. B. (1997). Very long-lasting priming in picture naming. *Psychological Science*, 8(4), 322–325.

Cave, K. R. & Zimmerman, J. M. (1997). Flexibility in spatial attention before and after practice. *Psychological Science*, 8, 399–403.

Cecchetto, C. & Papagno, C. (in press). Bridging the gap between brain and syntax. A case for a role of the phonological loop. In A. M. Di Sciullo & C. Boeckx (Eds), *The biolinguistic enterprise: new perspectives on the evolution and nature of the human language faculty*. Oxford: Oxford University Press.

Cermak, L. S. & O'Connor, M. (1983). The anterograde and retrograde retrieval ability of a patient with amnesia due to encephalitis. *Neuropsychologia*, 21, 213–234.

Chalmers, D. (1996). *The conscious mind: in search of a fundamental theory*. Oxford: OUP.

Chan, D., Fox, N. C., Scahill, R. I., Crum, W. R., Whitwell, J. L., Leschziner, G. et al. (2001). Patterns of temporal lobe atrophy in semantic dementia and Alzheimer's disease. *Annal of Neurology*, 49, 433–442.

Chan, D., Revesz, T., & Rudge, P. (2002). Hippocampal, but not parahippocampal, damage in a case of dense retrograde amnesia: a pathological study. *Neuroscience Letters*, 329(1), 61–64.

Chao, L. L. & Martin, A. (2000). Representation of manipulable man-made objects in the dorsal stream. *Neuroimage*, 12, 478–484.

Chao, L. L., Haxby, J. V., & Martin, A. (1999). Attribute-based neural substrates in temporal cortex for perceiving and knowing about objects. *Nature Neuroscience*, 2, 913–919.

Chater, N., Tenenbaum, J. B., & Yuille, A. (2006). Probabilistic models of cognition: conceptual foundations. *Trends in Cognitive Sciences*, 10, 287–291.

Cherry, E. (1953). Some experiments on the recognition of speech, with one and with two ears. *The Journal of the Acoustical Society of America*, 25, 975–979.

Chertkow, H. & Bub, D. (1990). Semantic memory loss in dementia of Alzheimer's type. *Brain*, 113, 347–417.

Chialant, D. & Caramazza, A. (1998). Perceptual and lexical factors in a case of letter-byletter reading. *Cognitive Neuropsychology*, 15, 167–201.

Choi, S., Na, D., Kang, E., Lee, K., Lee, S., & Na, D. (2001). Functional magnetic resonance imaging during pantomiming tool-use gestures. *Experimental Brain Research*, 139(3), 311–317.

Chomsky, N. (1959a). A note on phrase structure grammars. *Information and Control*, 2, 393–395.

Chomsky, N. (1959b). Verbal behaviour. *Language*, 35, 26–58.

Chomsky, N. (1965). *Aspects of the theory of syntax.* Cambridge, MA: MIT Press.

Chomsky, N. (1968). *Language and mind.* New York: Harcourt Brace Jovanovich.

Chomsky, N. (1969). *American power and the new mandarins.* New York: Pantheon.

Chomsky, N. (1980). The linguistic approach. In M.Piattelli-Palmarini (Ed.), *Language and learning* (pp. 109–116). Cambridge, MA: Cambridge University Press.

Chomsky, N. (1981). *Lectures on government and binding.* Dordrecht: Foris Publications.

Chomsky, N. (1986). *Knowledge of language: its nature, origin, and use.* Praeger.

Chomsky, N. (1995). *The minimalist program.* Cambridge, MA: MIT Press.

Chomsky, N. & Lasnik, H. (1993). The theory of principles and parameters. In Jacobs J., A. von Stechow, Sternfield W, Vennemann T, & . (Eds), *Syntax: an international handbook of contemporary research, Vol. 1.* Berlin: Walter de Gruyter.

Chow, T., Miller, B., Hayashi, V., & Geshwind, D. (1999). Inheritance of frontotemporal dementia. *Archives of Neurology*, 56, 817–822.

Christoff, K. & Gabrieli, J. (2000). The frontopolar cortex and human cognition: evidence for a rostrocaudal hierarchical organisation within the human prefrontal cortex. *Psychobiology*, 28, 168–186.

Christoff, K., Prabhakaran, V., Dorfman, J., Zhao, Z., Kroger, J. K., Holyoak, K. J. et al. (2001). Rostrolateral prefrontal cortex involvement in relational integration during reasoning. *Neuroimage*, 14, 1136–1149.

Christoff, K., Ream, J. M., Geddes, L. P. T., & Gabrieli, J. D. E. (2003). Evaluating self-generated information: Anterior prefrontal contributions to human cognition. *Behavioral Neuroscience*, 117, 1161–1168.

Churchland, P. S. (1986). *Neurophilosophy: toward a unified science of the mind/brain.* Cambridge, MA: MIT Press.

Churchland, P. S. & Sejnowski, T. J. (1992). *The computational brain.* Cambridge, MA: MIT Press.

Ciaramelli, E., Grady, C., Levine, B., Ween, J., & Moscovitch, M. (2010). Top-down and bottom-up attention to memory are dissociated in posterior parietal cortex: neuroimagingand and neuropsychological evidence. *Journal of Neuroscience*, 30, 4943–4956.

Cipolotti, L. (2000). Sparing of country and nationality names in a case modality-specific oral output impairment: implications for theories of speech production. *Cognitive Neuropsychology*, 17, 709–729.

Cipolotti, L. & Warrington, E. K. (1995a). Semantic memory and reading abilities: a case report. *Journal of the International Neuropsychological Society*, 1, 104–110.

Cipolotti, L. & Warrington, E. K. (1995b). Towards a unitary account of access dysphasia: a single case study. *Memory*, 3, 309–332.

Cipolotti, L., Shallice, T., Chun, D., Fox, N., Scahill, R., Harrison, G. et al. (2001). Long-term retrograde amnesia: the crucial role of the hippocampus. *Neuropsychologia*, 39, 151–172.

Cipolotti, L., Bird, C. M., Glasspool, D. W., & Shallice, T. (2004). The impact of deep dysgraphia on graphemic buffer disorders. *Neurocase*, 10, 405–419.

Cipolotti, L., Bird, C. M., Good, T., Macmanus, D., Rudge, P., & Shallice, T. (2006). Recollection and familiarity in dense hippocampal amnesia: a case study. *Neuropsychologia*, 44, 489–506.

Clahsen, H. (1999). Lexical entries and rules of language: a multidisciplinary study of German inflection. *Behavioral and Brain Sciences*, 22, 991–1013.

Clarke, D.S. (ed.) (2004). *Panpsychism: past and recent selected readings.* State University of New York Press, Albany, NY

Clarke, R. & Morton, J. (1983). Cross-modality facilitation in tachistoscopic word recognition. *Quarterly Journal of Experimental Psychology*, 35A, 79–96.

Clements, G. & Keyser, S. (1983). *CV phonology: a generative theory of the syllable.* Cambridge, MA: MIT Press.

Clifton, C. & Odom, P. (1966). Similarity relations among certain English sentence constructions. *Psychological Monographs*, *80*, 1–35.

Cohen, D. (1972). Magnetoencephalography: detection of the brain's electrical activity with a superconducting magnetometer. *Science*, *175*(4022), 664–666.

Cohen, J. D. & Servan-Schreiber, D. (1992). Context, cortex, and dopamine: a connectionist approach to behavior and biology in schizophrenia. *Psychological Review*, *99*, 45–77.

Cohen, L. & Dehaene, S. (1996). Cerebral networks for number processing: evidence from a case of posterior callosal lesion. *Neurocase*, *2*, 155–174.

Cohen, L. & Dehaene, S. (1998). Competition between past and present. Assessment and interpretation of verbal perseverations. *Brain*, *121* (9), 1641–1659.

Cohen, L., Dehaene, S., Naccache, L., Lehericy, S., haene-Lambertz, G., Henaff, M. A. et al. (2000). The visual word form area: spatial and temporal characterization of an initial stage of reading in normal subjects and posterior split-brain patients. *Brain*, *123* (2), 291–307.

Cohen, L., Martinaud, O., Lemer, C., Lehericy, S., Samson, Y., Obadia, M. et al. (2003). Visual word recognition in the left and right hemispheres: anatomical and functional correlates of peripheral alexias. *Cerebral Cortex*, *13*, 1313–1333.

Cohen, N. J. & Squire, L. R. (1980). Preserved learning and retention of pattern-analyzing skill in amnesia: dissociation of knowing how and knowing that. *Science*, *210*, 207–210.

Colby, C., Duhamel, J., & Goldberg, M. (1993). Ventral intraparietal area of the macaque: anatomic location and visual response properties. *Journal of Neurophisiology*, *69*, 902–914.

Coleman, M. R., Davis, M. H., Rodd, J. M., Robson, T., Ali, A., Owen, A. M., & Pickard, J. D. (2009). Towards the routine use of brain imaging to aid the clinical diagnosis of disorders of consciousness. *Brain*, *132*(9), 2541–2552.

Collins, A. & Quillian, M. (1969). Retrieval from semantic memory. *Journal of Verbal Learning and Verbal Behavior*, *8*, 240–247.

Coltheart, M. (1978). Lexical access in simple reading tasks. In G. Underwood (Ed.), *Strategies of information processing.* London: Academic Press.

Coltheart, M. (1980a). Deep dyslexia: a review of the syndrome. In M. Coltheart, K. E. Patterson, & J. C. Marshall (Eds). *Deep dyslexia.* (chapter 2, pp. 22–47). London: Routledge.

Coltheart, M. (1980b). Deep dyslexia: a right-hemisphere hypothesis. In M. Coltheart, K. E. Patterson, & J. C. Marshall (Eds). *Deep dyslexia.* (chapter 16, pp. 326–380). London: Routledge.

Coltheart, M. (2000). Dual-routes from print to speech and dual routes from print to meaning: some theoretical issues. In A.Kennedy, R. Radach, J. Pynte, & D. Heller (Eds), *Reading as a perceptual process.* Oxford, UK: Elsevier.

Coltheart, M. (2001). Assumptions and methods in cognitive neuropsychology. In B. Rapp (Ed.), *A handbook of cognitive neuropsychology: what deficits reveal about the human mind.* Hove, UK: Psychology Press.

Coltheart, M. (2004). Brain imaging, connectionism, and cognitive neuropsychology. *Cognitive Neuropsychology*, *21*, 21–25.

Coltheart, M. (2006a). Acquired dyslexias and the computational modelling of reading. *Cognitive Neuropsychology*, *23*, 96–109.

Coltheart, M. (2006b). What has functional neuroimaging told us about the mind (so far)? *Cortex*, *42*, 323–331.

Coltheart, M. & Rastle, K. (1994). Serial processing in reading aloud: Evidence for dual-route models of reading. *Journal of Experimental Psychology Human Perception Performance*, *20*, 1197–1211.

Coltheart, M., Davelaar, E., Jonasson, J., & Besner, D. (1977). Access to the internal lexicon. In S. Dornick (Ed.), *Attention and Performance VI.* London: Academic Press.

Coltheart, M., Patterson, K., & Marshall, J. (1980). *Deep dyslexia.* London: Routledge & Kegan Paul.

Coltheart, M., Patterson, K., & Marshall, J. (1987). Deep dyslexia since 1980. In M. Coltheart, K. Patterson, & J. Marshall (Eds), *Deep dyslexia* (pp. 407–451). London: Routledge & Kegan Paul.

Coltheart, M., Curtis, B., Atkins, P., & Haller, M. (1993). Models of reading aloud: Dual-route and parallel-distributed processing approaches. *Psychological Review*, *100* (4), 589–608.

Coltheart, M., Langdon, R., & Haller, M. (1996). Computational cognitive neuropsychology and acquired dyslexia. In B. Dodd, R. Campbell, & L. Worral (Eds), *Evaluating theories of language: evidence from disordered communication* (pp. 3–36). London: Whurr.

Coltheart, M., Rastle, K., Perry, C., Langdon, R., & Ziegler, J. (2001). DRC: A dual-route cascaded model of visual word recognition and reading aloud. *Psychological Review*, *108*, 204–256.

Connolly, J., Andersen, R., & Goodale, M. (2003). FMRI evidence for a 'parietal reach region' in the human brain. *Experimental Brain Research*, *153*(2), 140–145.

Conrad, M., Carreiras, M., & Jacobs, A. M. (2008). Contrasting effects of token and type syllable frequency in lexical decision. *Language and Cognitive Processes*, *23*, 296–326.

Conrad, R. (1964). Acoustic confusion in immediate memory. *British Journal of Psychology, 55*, 75–84.

Conway, M. A. (1996). Autobiographical knowledge and autobiographical memories. In D. C. Rubin (Ed.). *Remembering our past: studies in autobiographical memory.* Cambridge: Cambridge University Press, pp. 67–93.

Conway, M. A. & Pleydell-Pearce, C. W. (2000). The construction of autobiographical memories in the self-memory system. *Psychological Review, 107*, 261–288.

Conway, M. A., Turk, D. J., Miller, S. L., Logan, J., Nebes, R. D., Meltzer, C. C. et al. (1999). A positron emission tomography (PET) study of autobiographical memory retrieval. *Memory, 7*, 679–702.

Cooper, R. P. (2002). *Modelling high-level cognitive processes.* Mahwah, NJ: Erlbaum.

Cooper, R. P. (2006). Cognitive architectures as Lakatosian research programmes: two case studies. *Philosophical Psychology, 19*, 1–22.

Cooper, R. P. (2007a). The role of falsification in the development of Cognitive Architectures: Insights from a Lakatosian analysis. *Cognitive Science, 31*, 509–533.

Cooper, R. P. (2007b). Tool use and related errors in ideational apraxia: the quantitative simulation of patient error profiles. *Cortex, 43*, 319–337.

Cooper, R. P. & Fox, J. (1998). COGENT: a visual design environment for cognitive modeling. *Behaviour Research Methods, Instruments Computers, 30*, 553–564.

Cooper, R. P., Fox, J., Farringdon, J., & Shallice, T. (1996). A systematic methodology for cognitive modelling. *Artificial Intelligence, 85*, 3–44.

Cooper, R. P. & Shallice, T. (1995). Soar and the case for unified theories of cognition. *Cognition, 55*, 115–149.

Cooper, R. P. & Shallice, T. (2000). Contention scheduling and the control of routine activities. *17*, 338.

Cooper, R. P. & Shallice, T. (2006a). Hierarchical schemas and goals in the control of sequential behavior. *Psychological Review, 113*, 887–916.

Cooper, R. P. & Shallice, T. (2006b). Structured representations in the control of behavior cannot be so easily dismissed: A reply to Botvinick and Plaut (2006). *Psychological Review, 113*, 929–931.

Cooper, R. P., Yule, P., & Fox, J. (2003). Cue selection in category learning: a systematic comparison of three theories. *Cognitive Science Quarterly, 3*, 143–182.

Cooper, R. P., Schwartz, M., Yule, P., & Shallice, T. (2005). The simulation of action disorganization in complex activities of daily living. *Cognitive Neuropsychology, 22*, 959–1004.

Corbetta, M. & Shulman, G. (2002). Control of goal-directed and stimulus-driven attention in the brain. *Nature Reviews of Neuroscience, 3*, 201–215.

Corbetta, M., Kincade, J. M., & Shulman, G. L. (2002). Neural systems for visual orienting and their relationships to spatial working memory. *Journal of Cognitive Neuroscience, 14*, 508–523.

Corsi, P. (1972). Human memory and the medial temporal region of the brain. *Dissertation Abstracts International, 34*, 819B.

Cortes, C. & Vapnik, V. (1995). Support-vector networks. *Machine Learning, 20*, 273–297.

Coslett, H. B. & Saffran, E. M. (1989). Evidence for preserved reading in 'pure alexia'. *Brain, 112* (2), 327–359.

Coslett, H. B., Saffran, E. M., Greenbaum, S., & Schwartz, H. (1993). Reading in pure alexia. The effect of strategy. *Brain, 116* (1), 21–37.

Cosmides, L. & Tooby, J. (1994). Beyond intuition and instinct blindness—toward an evolutionarily rigorous cognitive science. *Cognition, 50*, 41–77.

Costello, A., Fletcher, P. C., Dolan, R. J., Frith, C. D., & Shallice, T. (1998). The origins of forgetting in a case of isolated retrograde amnesia following a haemorrhage: evidence from functional imaging. *Neurocase, 4*, 437–446.

Coughlan, A. & Warrington, E. K. (1981). The impairment of verbal semantic memory: a single-case study. *Journal of Neurology, Neurosurgery and Psychiatry, 44*, 1079–1083.

Coulthard, E., Parton, A., & Husain, M. (2006). Action control in visual neglect. *Neuropsychologia, 44*, 2717–2733.

Courtney, S., Ungerleider, L. G., Keil, K., & Haxby, J. V. (1996). Object and spatial visual working memory activate separate neural systems in human cortex. *Cerebral Cortex, 6*, 39–49.

Courtney, S., Petit, L., Maisog, J., Ungerleider, L. G., & Haxby, J. V. (1998). An area specialized for spatial working memory in human frontal cortex. *Science, 279*, 1347–1351.

Courtney, S., Roth, J., & Sala, J. (2007). A hierarchical biasedcompetition model of domain-dependent working memory maintenance and executive control. In N.Osaka, R. Logie, & M. D'Esposito (Eds), *Working memory: behavioural and neural correlates* (pp. 369–383). Oxford: OUP.

Cowan, N. (1995). *Attention and memory: an integrated framework.* (Oxford Psychology Series.) Oxford: OUP.

Cowey, A. & Stoerig, P. (1995). Blindsight in monkeys. *Nature, 373*, 247–249.

Cox, R. W. (1996). AFNI software for analysis and visualisation of functional magneticc resonance images. *Computers and Biomedical Research, 29*, 162–173.

Craik, F. (1968). Two components in free recall. *Journal of Verbal Learning and Verbal Behavior, 7*, 996–1004.

Craik, F.I.M. (2002). Levels of processing: past, present and future? *Memory, 10*, 305–318.

Craik, F. & Lockhart, R. (1972). Levels of processing: a framework for memory research. *Journal of Verbal Learning and Verbal Behavior*, 11, 671–684.

Craik, F. & Masani, P. (1969). Age and intelligence differences in coding and retrieval of word lists. *British journal of Psychology*, 60, 315–319.

Craik, F. & Tulving, E. (1975). Depth of processing and retention of words in episodic memory. *Journal of Experimental Psychology: General*, 104, 268–294.

Craik, F., Govoni, R., Naveh-Benjamin, M., & Anderson, N. D. (1996). The Effects of Divided Attention on Encoding and Retrieval Processes in Human Memory. *Journal of Experimental Psychology: General*, 125, 159–180.

Craik, K. J. W. (1943). *The Nature of Explanation*. Cambridge, UK: Macmillan.

Craik, K. J. W. (1947). Theory of the human operator in control systems. *British Journal of Psychology*, 58, 56–61.

Crawford, J. R. & Garthwaite, P. H. (2005a). Evaluation of criteria for classical dissociations in single-case studies by Monte Carlo simulation. *Neuropsychology*, 19, 664–678.

Crawford, J. R. & Garthwaite, P. H. (2005b). Testing for suspected impairments and dissociations in single-case studies in neuropsychology: evaluation of alternatives using monte carlo simulations and revised tests for dissociations. *Neuropsychology*, 19, 318–331.

Crawford, J. R. & Howell, D. (1998). Comparing an individual's test score against norms derived from small samples. *The Clinical Neuropsychologist*, 12, 482–486.

Crescentini, C., Shallice, T., & Macaluso, E. (2010). Item retrieval and competition in noun and verb generation: an fMRI study. *Journal of Cognitive Neuroscience*, 22, 1140–1157.

Crick, F. (1989). The recent excitement about neural networks. *Nature*, 337, 129–132.

Crick, F. & Koch, C. (1995). Are we aware of neural activity in primary visual cortex? *Nature*, 375, 121–123.

Crick, F. & Koch, C. (1998). Consciousness and neuroscience. *Cerebral Cortex*, 8, 97–107.

Crick, F. & Mitchison, G. (1983). The function of dream sleep. *Nature*, 304, 111–114.

Crisp, J. & Lambon Ralph, M. (2006). Unlocking the nature of the phonological-deep dyslexia continuum: The keys to reading aloud are in phonology and semantics. *Journal of Cognitive Neuroscience*, 2006, 18–348.

Critchley, H. D., Melmed, R. N., Featherstone, E., Mathias, C. J., & Dolan, R. J. (2002). Volitional control of autonomic arousal: a functional magnetic resonance study. *Neuroimage*, 16, 909–919.

Critchley, M. (1953). *The parietal lobes*. New York: Hafner Press.

Crovitz, H. F., & Schiffman, H. (1974). Frequency of episodic memories as a function of their age. *Bulletin of the Psychonomic Society*, 4, 517–518.

Crowder, R. (1993). Short-term memory: Where do we stand? *Memory and Cognition*, 21, 145.

Crowder, R. & Morton, J. (1969). Precategorical acoustic storage. *Perception and Psychophysics*, 5, 365–373.

Crutch, S. J. & Warrington, E. K. (2001). Refractory dyslexia: evidence of multiple task-specific phonological output stores. *Brain*, 124, 1533–1543.

Crutch, S. J. & Warrington, E. K. (2005). Abstract and concrete concepts have structurally different representational frameworks. *Brain*, 128, 615–627.

Crutch, S. J. & Warrington, E. K. (2007). Contrasting effects of semantic priming and interference in processing abstract and concrete words. *Brain and Language*, 103, 88–89.

Culham, J. C. & Valyear, K. F. (2006). Human parietal cortex in action. *Current Opinion in Neurobiology*, 16, 205–212.

Culham, J. C., Danckert, S. L., DeSouza, J. F., Gati, J. S., Menon, R. S., & Goodale, M. A. (2003). Visually guided grasping produces fMRI activation in dorsal but not ventral stream brain areas. *Experimental Brain Research*, 153, 180–189.

Cummins, R. (1983). *The nature of psychological explanation*. Cambridge, AM: MIT Press.

Curtiss, S. & Yamada, J. (1988). *Curtiss-Yamada comprehensive language evaluation*. Unpublished test, UCLA.

Dagher, A., Owen, A. M., Boecker, H., & Brooks, D. J. (1999). Mapping the network for planning: a correlational PET activation study with the Tower of London task. *Brain*, 122(10), 1973–1987.

Dale, A. & Buckner, R. (1997). Selective averaging of rapidly presented individual trials using fMRI. *Human Brain Mapping*, 5, 329–340.

Damasio, A. R. (1996). The somatic marker hypothesis and the possible functions of the prefrontal cortex. *Philos.Trans.R.Soc.Lond B Biol.Sci.*, 351, 1413–1420.

Damasio, H. & Damasio, A. R. (1980). The anatomical basis of conduction aphasia. *Brain*, 103, 337–350.

Damasio, A. R. & Damasio, H. (1983). The anatomic basis of pure alexia. *Neurology*, 33, 1573–1583.

Damasio, A. R., Graff-Radford, N. R., Eslinger, P. J., Damasio, H., & Kassell, N. (1985). Amnesia following basal forebrain lesions. *Archives of Neurology*, 42, 263–271.

Damasio, H., Grabowski, T. J., Tranel, D., Hichwa, R. D., & Damasio, A. R. (1996). A neural basis for lexical retrieval. *Nature*, 380, 499–505.

Daneman, M. & Carpenter, P. (1980). Individual differences in working memory and reading. *Journal of Verbal Learning and Verbal Behavior*, 19, 450–466.

Darvas, F., Pantazis, D., Kucukaltun-Yildirim, E., & Leahy, R. M. (2004). Mapping human brain function with MEG and EEG: methods and validation. *Neuroimage*, *23*, Suppl 1, S289–S299.

Darwin, C. (1859). *On the origin of species by means of natural selection, or the preservation of favoured races in the struggle for life*. New York: D. Appleton.

Das, S. K., Fox, J., Elsdon, D., & hammond, P. (1997). A flexible architecture for autonomous agents. *Journal of Experimental and Theoretical Artificial Intelligence*, *9*, 407–440.

Daselaar, S. M., Fleck, M. S., Dobbins, I. G., Madden, D. J. & Cabeza, R. (2006a). Effects of healthy aging on hippocampal and rhinal memory functions: an event-related fMRI study. *Cerebral Cortex*, *16*, 1771–1782.

Daselaar, S. M., Fleck, M. S., & Cabeza, R. (2006b). Triple dissociation in the medial temporal lobes: recollection, familiarity, and novelty. *Journal of Neurophysiology*, *96*, 1902–1911.

Daselaar, S. M., Fleck, M. S., Prince, S. E., & Cabeza, R. (2006c). The medial temporal lobe distinguishes old from new independently of consciousness. *Journal of Neuroscience*, *26*, 5835–5839.

Daselaar, S. M., Rice, H. J., Greenberg, D. L., Cabeza, R., Labar, K. S., & Rubin, D. C. (2008). The spatiotemporal dynamics of autobiographical memory: Neural correlates of recall, emotional intensity, and reliving. *Cerebral Cortex*, *18*, 217–229.

Davidson, D. (1987). Knowing one's own mind. *Proceedings and Addresses of the American Philosophical Association*, *60*, 441–458.

Davies, R., Hodges, J., Krill, J., Patterson, K., Halliday, G., & Xuereb, J. (2005). The pathological basis of semantic dementia. *Brain*, *128*, 1984–1995.

Daw, N. D., Niv, Y., & Dayan, P. (2005). Uncertainty-based competition between prefrontal and dorsolateral striatal systems for behavioral control. *Nature Neuroscience*, *8*, 1704–1711.

Dawson, M. R. W. (1998). *Understanding cognitive science*. Maiden, MA: Blackwell.

Dayan, P. & Abbott, L. (2001). *Theoretical Neuroscience: Computational and Mathematical Modeling of Neural Systems*. Cambridge, MA: MIT Press.

Dayan, P. & Huys, Q. J. (2009). Serotonin in affective control. *Annual Reviews of Neuroscience*, *32*, 95–126.

Dayan, P., Hinton, G. E., Neal, R. M., & Zemel, R. S. (1995). The Helmholtz machine. *Neural Comput.*, *7*, 889–904.

Debner, J. A. & Jacoby, L. L. (1994). Unconscious perception: attention, awareness, and control. *J.Exp. Psychol.Learn.Mem.Cogn*, *20*, 304–317.

Decety, J., Perani, D., Jeannerod, M., Bettinardi, V., Tadary, B., Woods, R. et al. (1994). Mapping motor representations with positron emission tomography. *Nature*, *371*, 600–602.

Decety, J., Grezes, J., Costes, N., Perani, D., Jeannerod, M., Procyk, E. et al. (1997). Brain activity during observation of actions. Influence of action content and subject's strategy. *Brain*, *120*(10), 1763–1777.

Deco, G. & Lee, T. S. (2004). The role of early visual cortex in visual integration: a neural model of recurrent interaction. *European Journal of Neuroscience*, *20*, 1089–1100.

De Groot, A. (1965). *Thought and choice in chess*. The Hague: Mouton.

De Groot, A. (1966). Perception and memory versus thought: some old ideas and recent findings. In B.Keinmuntz (Ed.), *Problem solving: research, method and theory* (pp. 19–50). New York: Wiley.

De Haan, E., Young, A., & Newcombe, F. (1987). Face recognition without awareness. *Cognitive Neuropsychology*, *4*, 385–415.

Dehaene, S., & Changeux, J. (2005). Ongoing spontaneous activity controls access to consciousness: a neuronal model for inattentional blindness. *PLoS Biology*, *3*(5), e141.

Dehaene, S. & Naccache, L. (2001). Towards a cognitive neuroscience of consciousness: basic evidence and a workspace framework. *Cognition*, *79*, 1–37.

Dehaene, S., Kerszberg, M., & Changeux, J. P. (1998a). A neuronal model of a global workspace in effortful cognitive tasks. *Proceedings of the National Academy of Sciences, USA*, *95*, 14529–14534.

Dehaene, S., Naccache, L., Le, C. G., Koechlin, E., Mueller, M., Dehaene-Lambertz, G. et al. (1998b). Imaging unconscious semantic priming. *Nature*, *395*, 597–600.

Dehaene, S., Naccache, L., Cohen, L., Bihan, D. L., Mangin, J. F., Poline, J. B. et al. (2001). Cerebral mechanisms of word masking and unconscious repetition priming. *Nature Neuroscience*, *4*, 752–758.

Dehaene, S., Sergent, C., & Changeux, J. (2003). A neuronal network model linking subjective reports and objective physiological data during conscious perception. *Proceedings of the National Academy of Sciences of the United States of America*, *100*(14), 8520–8525.

Dehaene, S., Cohen, L., Sigman, M., & Vinckier, F. (2005). The neural code for written words: a proposal. *Trends in Cognitive Science*, *9*, 335–341.

Dehaene, S., Changeux, J., Naccache, L., Sackur, J., & Sergent, C. (2006). Conscious, preconscious, and subliminal processing: a testable taxonomy. *Trends in Cognitive Sciences*, *10*(5), 204–211.

Deiber, M. P., Ibanez, V., Sadato, N., & Hallett, M. (1996). Cerebral structures participating in motor preparation in humans: a positron emission tomography study. *Journal of Neurophysiology*, *75*(1), 233–247.

Dejerine, J. (1892). Contribution à l'étude anatomo-pathologique et clinique des différentes variétés de cécité verbale. *Mémoires de la Société de Biologie*, *4*, 61–90.

Delbecq-Derouesné, J., Beauvois, M. F., & Shallice, T. (1990). Preserved recall versus impaired recognition. A case study. *Brain, 113* (4), 1045–1074.

Delius, J. & Siemann, M. (1998). Transitive responding in animals and humans: exaptation rather than adaptation. *Behavioural Processes, 42,* 107–137.

Dell, G. (1986). A spreading-activation theory of retrieval in sentence production. *Psychological Review, 93,* 283–321.

Dell, G. (1988). The retrieval of phonological forms in production: Tests of predictions from a connectionist model. *Journal of Memory and Language, 27,* 124–142.

Dell, G. S., Burger, L. K., & Svec, W. R. (1997a). Language production and serial order: A functional analysis and a model. *Psychological Review, 104*(1), 123–147.

Dell, G., Schwartz, M., Martin, N., Saffran, E., & Gagnon, D. (1997b). Lexical access in aphasic and nonaphasic speakers. *Psychological Review, 104,* 801–838.

Della Malva, C. L., Stuss, D. T., D'Alton, J., & Willmer, J. (1993). Capture errors and sequencing after frontal brain lesions. *Neuropsychologia, 31,* 363–372.

Della Sala, S. & Logie, R. (2002). Neuropsychological impairments of visual and spatial working memory. In A.Miyake & P. Shah (Eds), *Handbook of Memory Disorders, 2nd edition,* (pp. 271–292). Wiley.

Della Sala, S., Marchetti, C., & Spinnler, H. (1991). Right-sided anarchic (alien) hand: a longitudinal study. *Neuropsychologia, 29,* 1113–1127.

Della Sala, S., Gray, C., Baddeley, A., Allamano, N., & Wilson, L. (1999). Pattern span: a tool for unwelding visuo-spatial memory. *Neuropsychologia, 37,* 1189–1199.

Dennett, D. C. (1969). *Content and Consciousness.* London: International Library of Philosophy and Scientific Method. Routledge and Kegan Paul.

Dennett, D. C. (1978). *Brainstorms: Philosophical essays on mind and psychology.* Montgomery VT: Bradford.

Dennett, D. C. (1991). *Consciousness explained.* Boston, MA: Little, Brown & Co.

Dennett, D.C. (1996). *Kinds of minds: towards an understanding of consciousness.* Basic Books, New York.

Dennett, D. C. (1998). Reflections on language and mind. In P. Carruthers & J. Boucher (Eds), *Language and thought: interdisciplinary themes* (pp. 284–295). Cambridge: CUP.

Dennett, D. C. (2001). Are we explaining consciousness yet? *Cognition, 79,* 221–237.

Dennett, D. C. (2005). *Sweet dreams.* MIT Press.

Dennett, D. C., & Kinsbourne, M. (1992). Time and the observer. *Behavioral and Brain Sciences, 15,* 183–247.

Dennis, M. (1976). Dissociated naming and locating of body parts after left anterior temporal lobe resection: an experimental case study. *Brain and Language, 3,* 147–163.

Derbyshire, N., Ellis, R., & Tucker, M. (2006). The potentiation of two components of the reach-to-grasp action during object categorisation in visual memory. *Acta Psychologia, 122,* 74–98.

De Renzi E. & Barbieri, C. (1992). The incidence of the grasp reflex following hemispheric lesion and its relation to frontal damage. *Brain, 115* Pt 1, 293–313.

De Renzi, E. & Lucchelli, F. (1988). Ideational apraxia. *Brain, 111*(5), 1173–1185.

De Renzi, E. & Lucchelli, F. (1994). Are semantic systems separately represented in the brain? The case of living category impairment. *Cortex, 30,* 3–25.

De Renzi, E. & Nichelli, P. (1975). Verbal and nonverbal short-term memory impairment following hemispheric damage. *Cortex, 11,* 341–354.

De Renzi, E., Pieczuro, A., & Vignolo, L. (1968). Ideational apraxia: a quantitative study. *Neuropsychologia, 6,* 41–52.

De Renzi, E., Scotti, G., & Spinnler, H. (1969). Perceptual and associative disorders of visual recognition. Relationship to the side of the cerebral lesion. *Neurology, 19,* 634–642.

De Renzi, E., Faglioni, P., & Previdi, P. (1977). Spatial memory and hemispheric locus of lesion. *Cortex, 13,* 424–433.

De Renzi, E., Faglioni, P., & Sorgato, P. (1982). Modality-specific and supramodal mechanisms of apraxia. *Brain, 105,* 301–312.

Derouesné, J. & Beauvois, M.-F. (1979). Phonological processing in reading: data from alexia. *The Journal of Neurology, Neurosurgery, and Psychiatry, 42,* 1125–1132.

Derouesné, J. & Beauvois, M.-F. (1985). The 'phonemic' stage in the non-lexical reading process: evidence from a case of phonological alexia. In K.E. Patterson, M. Coltheart, & J. C. Marshall (Eds), *Surface dyslexia.* London: Erlbaum.

Derrfuss, J., Brass, M., Neumann, J., & von Cramon, D. Y. (2005). Involvement of the inferior frontal junction in cognitive control: meta-analyses of switching and Stroop studies. *Human Brain Mapping, 25,* 22–34.

Desai, R., Conant, L. L., Waldron, E., & Binder, J. R. (2006). fMRI of Past Tense Processing: The Effects of Phonological Complexity and Task Difficulty. *Journal of Cognitive Neuroscience, 18*(2), 278–297.

Desimone, R. & Duncan, J. (1995). Neural mechanisms of selective visual attention. *Annual Review of Neuroscience, 18,* 193–222.

Desimone, R. & Ungerleider, L. (1989). Neural mechanisms of visual processing in monkeys. In H.Goodglass & A. Damasio (Eds), *Handbook of neuropsychology* (pp. 267–300). Amsterdam: Elsevier.

Desimone, R., Albright, T.D., Gross, C.G. & Bruce, C. (1984). Stimulus selective properties of inferior temporal neurons in the macaque. *Journal of Neuroscience, 4*, 2051–2062.

Desmurget, M., Epstein, C. M., Turner, R. S., Prablanc, C., Alexander, G. E., & Grafton, S. T. (1999). Role of the posterior parietal cortex in updating reaching movements to a visual target. *Nature Neuroscience, 2*, 563–567.

D'Esposito, M. & Postle, B. R. (1999). The dependence of span and delayed-response performance on prefrontal cortex. *Neuropsychologia, 37*, 1303–1315.

D'Esposito, M., Zarahn, E., Aguirre, G. K., Shin, R. K., Auerbach, P., & Detre, J. A. (1997). The effect of pacing of experimental stimuli on observed functional MRI activity. *Neuroimage, 6*, 113–121.

D'Esposito, M., Postle, B. R., Ballard, D., & Lease, J. (1999). Maintenance versus manipulation of information held in working memory: an event-related fMRI study. *Brain and Cognition, 41*, 66–86.

Deutsch, D. & Deutsch, D. (1963). Attention: some theoretical considerations. *Psychological Review, 70*, 80–90.

Devlin, J. T. & Poldrack, R. A. (2007). In praise of tedious anatomy. *Neuroimage, 37*, 1033–1041.

Devlin, J. T., Gonnerman, L. M., Andersen, E. S., & Seidenberg, M. S. (1998). Category-specific semantic deficits in focal and widespread brain damage: a computational account. *Journal of Cognitive Neuroscience, 10*, 77–94.

Devlin, J. T., Moore, C. J., Mummery, C. J., Gorno-Tempini, M. L., Phillips, J. A., Noppeney, U. et al. (2002). Anatomic constraints on cognitive theories of category specificity. *Neuroimage, 15*, 675–685.

Diana, R. A., Yonelinas, A. P., & Ranganath, C. (2007). Imaging recollection and familiarity in the medial temporal lobe: a three-component model. *Trends in Cognitive Sciences, 11*, 379–386.

Diaz, M. T. & McCarthy, G. (2007). Unconscious word processing engages a distributed network of brain regions. *Journal of Cognitive Neuroscience, 19*, 1768–1775.

Dobbins, I. G. & Wagner, A. D. (2005). Domain-general and domain-sensitive prefrontal mechanisms for recollecting events and detecting novelty. *Cerebral Cortex, 15*, 1768–1778.

Dobbins, I. G., Schnyer, D. M., Verfaellie, M., & Schacter, D. L. (2004). Cortical activity reductions during repetition priming can result from rapid response learning. *Nature, 428*, 316–319.

Doeller, C. F., Barry, C., & Burgess, N. (2010). Evidence for grid cells in a human memory network. *Nature, 463*, 657–661.

Donders, F. (1868). On the speed of mental processes. In W-G Koster Editor (Ed.), *Attention and performance*. Amsterdam: North-Holland Publishing Company.

Doricchi, F. & Tomaiuolo, F. (2003). The anatomy of neglect without hemianopia: a key role for parietal-frontal disconnection? *NeuroReport, 14*(17), 2239–2243.

Doricchi, F., Perani, D., Incoccia, C., Grassi, F., Cappa, S. F., Bettinardi, V. et al. (1997). Neural control of fast-regular saccades and antisaccades: an investigation using positron emission tomography. *Experimental Brain Research, 116*, 50–62.

Douglas, R. & Martin, K. (1991). A functional microcircuit for cat visual cortex. *Journal of Physiology, 440*, 735–769.

Doumas, L. A. A., & Hummel, J. E. (2005). Modeling human mental representations: What works, what doesn't, and why. In K. J. Holyoak & R. Morrison (Eds), *The Cambridge handbook of thinking and reasoning* (pp. 73–94). New York: Cambridge University Press.

Drazin, DH. (1961). Effects of foreperiod, foreperiod variability, and probability of stimulus occurrence on simple reaction time. *Journal of Experimental Psychology, 62*, 43–50.

Dretske, F. (1995). *Naturalizing the mind.* Cambridge, MA: MIT Press.

Drewe, E. A. (1975). Go-no go learning after frontal lobe lesions in humans. *Cortex: A Journal Devoted to the Study of the Nervous System and Behavior, 11*(1), 8–16.

Driver, J. & Baylis, G. (1998). Attention and visual object segmentation. In R.Parasuraman (Ed.), *The attentive brain* (pp. 299–325). Cambridge, MA: MIT Press.

Driver, J. & Mattingley, J. B. (1998). Parietal neglect and visual awareness. *Nature Neuroscience, 1*, 17–22.

Driver, J. & Vuilleumier, P. (2001). Perceptual awareness and its loss in unilateral neglect and extinction. *Cognition, 79*, 39–88.

Driver, J., Baylis, G. C., & Rafal, R. D. (1992). Preserved figure-ground segregation and symmetry perception in visual neglect. *Nature, 360*, 73–75.

Driver, J., Vuilleumier, P., & Husain, M. (2004). Spatial neglect and extinction. In M.Gazzaniga (Ed.), *The cognitive neurosciences III* (pp. 589–606). Cambridge, MA: MIT Press.

Dronkers, N. (1996). A new brain region for coordinating speech articulation. *Nature, 384*, 159–161.

Dronkers, N. F., Wilkins, D. P., Van, V. R., Jr., Redfern, B. B., & Jaeger, J. J. (2004). Lesion analysis of the brain areas involved in language comprehension. *Cognition, 92*, 145–177.

Dror, I. & Gallogy, D. (1999). Computational analyses in cognitive neuroscience: In defense of biological implausibility. *Psychonomic Bulletin and Review, 6*, 173–182.

Dubner, R. & Zeki, S. (1971). Response properties and receptive fields of cells in an anatomically defined region of the superior temporal sulcus. *Brain Research, 35*, 528–532.

Dubois, J., Hécaen, H., Angerlegues, R., du Catelier, A., & Marcie, P. (1964). Etude neurolinguistique de l'aphasie de conduction. *Neuropsychologia, 2*, 9–44.

Duchaine, B. & Garrido, L. (2008). We're getting warmer - characterizing the mechanisms of face recognition with acquired prosopagnosia: a comment on Riddoch et al. (2008). *Cognitive Neuropsychology*, 25, 765–768.

Duchaine, B. C., Yovel, G., Butterworth, E. J., & Nakayama, K. (2006). Prosopagnosia as an impairment to face-specific mechanisms: Elimination of the alternative hypotheses in a developmental case. *Cognitive Neuropsychology*, 23, 714–747.

Duncan, J. (1980). The locus of interference in the perception of simultaneous stimuli. *Psychological Review*, 87, 272–300.

Duncan, J. (1984). Selective attention and the organization of visual information. *Journal of Experimental Psychology: General.*, 113, 501–517.

Duncan, J. (2001). An adaptive coding model of neural function in prefrontal cortex. *Nature Reviews Neuroscience*, 2, 820–829.

Duncan, J. (2010). The multiple-demand (MD) system of the primate brain: mental programs for intelligent behaviour. *Trends in Cognitive Sciences*, 14, 172–179.

Duncan, J. & Owen, A. M. (2000). Common regions of the human frontal lobe recruited by diverse cognitive demands. *Trends in Neurosciences*, 23, 475–483.

Duncan, J., Burgess, P., & Emslie, H. (1995). Fluid intelligence after frontal lobe lesions. *Neuropsychologia*, 33, 261–268.

Duncan, J., Seitz, R. J., Kolodny, J., Bor, D., Herzog, H., Ahmed, A. et al. (2000). A neural basis for general intelligence. *Science*, 289(5478), 457–460.

Duncker, K. (1945). On problem solving. *Psychological Monographs*, 58.

Dunn, J. C. & Kirsner, K. (1988). Discovering functionally independent mental processes: the principle of reversed association. *Psychol.Rev.*, 95, 91–101.

Duzel, E., Cabeza, R., Picton, T. W., Yonelinas, A. P., Scheich, H., Heinze, H. J. et al. (1999). Task-related and item-related brain processes of memory retrieval. *Proceedings of the National Academy of Sciences, USA*, 96, 1794–1799.

Dyson, F., Eddington, A., & Davidson, C. (1920). A determination of the deflection of light by the sun's gravitaional field made during the total eclipse of May 29th, 1919. *Philosophical Transaction of the Royal Society of London*, 220A, 291.

Eger, E., Sterzer, P., Russ, M. O., Giraud, A. L., & Kleinschmidt, A. (2003). A supramodal number representation in human intraparietal cortex. *Neuron*, 37, 719–725.

Egly, R., Driver, J., & Rafal, R. (1994). Shifting visual attention between objects and locations: evidence for normal and parietal lesion subjects. *Journal of Experimental Psychology: General*, 123, 161–177.

Eichenbaum, H. & Cohen, N. (2001). *From conditioning to conscious recollection*. New York: OUP.

Eichenbaum, H., Yonelinas, A. P., & Ranganath, C. (2007). The medial temporal lobe and recognition memory. *Annual Reviews of Neuroscience*, 30, 123–152.

Eimer, M. (1998). The lateralized readiness potential as an on-line measure of central response activation processes. *Behavior Research Methods, Instruments, & Computers*, 30(1), 146–156.

Eimer, M. & Schlaghecken, F. (1998). Effects of masked stimuli on motor activation: Behavioral and electrophysiological evidence. *Journal of Experimental Psychology: Human Perception and Performance*, 24, 1737–1747.

Eldridge, L., Knowlton, B., Furmanski, C., Bookheimer, S., & Engel, S. (2000). Remembering episodes: A selective role for the hippocampus during retrieval. *Nature Neuroscience*, 3, 1149–1152.

Elliott, R., Rees, G., & Dolan, R. J. (1999). Ventromedial prefrontal cortex mediates guessing. *Neuropsychologia*, 37, 403–411.

Ellis, A. (1979). Speech production and short-term memory. In J. Morton & J. Marshall (Eds), *Psycholinguistic series: structures and processes* (pp. 157–187). London: Paul Elek.

Ellis, A. (1982). Spelling and writing (and reading and speaking). In A. Ellis (Ed.), *Normality and pathology in cognitive functions* (pp. 113–146). London: Academic Press.

Ellis, R. & Tucker, M. (2000). Micro-affordance: the potentiation of components of action by seen objects. *British Journal of Psychology*, 91 (4), 451–471.

Ellis, A. & Young, A. W. (1988). *Human cognitive neuropsychology*. Hillsdale, NJ: Lawrence Erlbaum.

Elman, J. L. (1990). Finding structure in time. *Cognitive Science*, 14, 179–211.

Elsaesser, C. & Slack, M. (1994). Integrating deliberative planning in a robot architecture. In *Proceedings of the AIAA/NASA Conference on Intelligent Robots in Field, Factory, Service, and Space (CIRFFSS '94)* (pp. 782–787). Houston, TX.

Engel, A. K. & Singer, W. (2001). Temporal binding and the neural correlates of sensory awareness. *Trends in Cognitive Sciences*, 5, 16–25.

Enns, J. & Oriet, C. (2007). Visual similarity in masking and priming: the critical role of task relevance. *Advances in Cognitive Psychology*, 3, 211–240.

Ericsson, K. & Simon, H. (1993). *Protocol analysis: verbal reports as data*. Cambridge, MA: MIT Press.

Eriksen, C. W. (1960). Discrimination and learning without awareness: A methodological survey and evaluation. *Psychological Review*, 67(5), 279–300.

Erivn, S. (1964). Language and TAT content in bilinguals. *Journal of abnormal and social psychology*, *68*, 500–507.

Erman, L. D., Hayes-Roth, F., Lesser, V. R., & Reddy, D. R. (1980). The hearsay-II speech-understanding system: integrating knowledge to resolve uncertainty. *ACM Comput. Surv.*, *12*(2), 213–253.

Eslinger, P. J. (2002). The anatomic basis of utilisation behaviour: a shift from frontal-parietal to intra-frontal mechanisms. *Cortex*, *38*, 273–276.

Eslinger, P. J. & Damasio, A. R. (1985). Severe disturbance of higher cognition after bilateral frontal lobe ablation: patient EVR. *Neurology*, *35*, 1731–1741.

Evans, B. & Waites, B. (1981). *IQ and mental testing: an unnatural science and its social history*. London: Macmillan.

Evans, C. O. (1970). *The subject of consciousness*. George Allen & Unwin Ltd.

Evans, J. S. (2006). The heuristic-analytic theory of reasoning: extension and evaluation. *Psychonomic Bulletin & Review*, *13*, 378–395.

Evans, J. S. & Over, D. (1996). *Rationality and reasoning*. Hove, England: Psychology Press.

Evans, J. S., Barston, J. L., & Pollard, P. (1983). On the conflict between logic and belief in syllogistic reasoning. *Memory and Cognition*, *11*, 295–306.

Evans, N. & Levinson, S. C. (2009). The myth of language universals: language diversity and its importance for cognitive science. *Behavioral and Brain Sciences.*, *32*, 429–448.

Fabbri, A. & Navarro-Salas, J. (2005). *Modeling black hole evaporation*. Imperial College Press.

Faglioni, P. & Botti, C. (1993). How to differentiate retrieval from storage deficit: a stochastic approach to semantic memory modeling. *Cortex*, *29*, 518.

Fahlman, S. E. (1974). Planning system for robot construction tasks. *Artificial Intelligence*, *5*, 1–49.

Fan, J., McCandliss, B. D., Sommer, T., Raz, A., & Posner, M. I. (2002). Testing the efficiency and independence of attentional networks. *Journal of Cognitive Neuroscience*, *14*, 340–347.

Fan, J., McCandliss, B. D., Fossella, J., Flombaum, J. I., & Posner, M. I. (2005). The activation of attentional networks. *Neuroimage*, *26*, 471–479.

Farah, M. J. (1990). *Visual agnosia*. Cambridge, MA: MIT Press.

Farah, M. J. (1994). Perception and awareness after brain damage. *Current Opinion in Neurobiology*, *4*(2), 252–255.

Farah, M. J. & McClelland, J. (1991). A computational model of semantic memory impairment: modality-specificity and emergent category-specificity. *Journal of Experimental Psychology: General*, *120*, 339–357.

Farah, M. J., O'Reilly, R., & Vecera, S. (1993). Dissociated overt and covert recognition as on emergent

property of lesioned neural networks. *Psychological Review*, *100*, 571–588.

Farah, M. J., Meyer, M., & McMullen, P. (1996). The living/nonliving dissociation is not an artifact: giving an a priori implausible hypothesis a strong test. *Cognitive Neuropsychology*, *13*, 154.

Faroqi-Shah, Y. (2007). Are regular and irregular verbs dissociated in non-fluent aphasia? A meta-analysis. *Brain Research Bulletin*, *74*, 1–13.

Feigenbaum, J. D., Polkey, C. E., & Morris, R. G. (1996). Deficits in spatial working memory after unilateral temporal lobectomy in man. *Neuropsychologia*, *34*, 163–176.

Feigenson, L. & Carey, S. (2003). Tracking individuals via object-files: evidence from infant's manual search. *Developmental Psychology*, *6*, 568–584.

Fellows, L. K. & Farah, M. J. (2005). Different underlying impairments in decision-making following ventromedial and dorsolateral frontal lobe damage in humans. *Cerebral Cortex*, *15*, 58–63.

Fendrich, R., Wessinger, C., & Gazzaniga, M. (1992). Residual vision in a scotoma: implications for blindsight. *Science*, *258*(5087), 1489–1491.

Fernandez-Duque, D. & Posner, M. I. (2001). Brain imaging of attentional networks in normal and pathological states. *Journal of Clinical and Experimental Neuropsychology*, *23*, 74–93.

ffytche, D. H. & Howard, R. J. (1999). The perceptual consequences of visual loss: 'positive' pathologies of vision. *Brain*, *122* (7), 1247–1260.

Fias, W. & Fischer, M. (2005). Spatial representation of numbers. In J. Campbell (Ed.), *Handbook of mathematical cognition* (pp. 43–54). New York: Psychology Press.

Fiez, J. A. & Petersen, S. E. (1998). Neuroimaging studies of word reading. *Proceedings of the National Academy of Sciences, USA*, *95*, 914–921.

Fiez, J. A., Balota, D. A., Raichle, M. E., & Petersen, S. E. (1999). Effects of lexicality, frequency, and spelling-to-sound consistency on the functional anatomy of reading. *Neuron*, *24*, 205–218.

Fikes, R., Hart, P., & Nilsson, N. (1972). *Some new directions in robot problem solving*. (Stanford Research Institute Artificial Intelligence Center TN-68 ed.).

Fincham, J., VanVeen, V., Carter, C., Stenger, V., & Anderson, J. (2002). Integrating computational cognitive modeling and neuroimaging: an event-related fMRI study of the Tower of Hanoi task. *Proceedings of the National Academy of Sciences, USA*, *99*, 3346–3351.

Fink, G. R., Markowitsch, H. J., Reinkemeier, M., Bruckbauer, T., Kessler, J., & Heiss, W. D. (1996). Cerebral representation of one's own past: neural networks involved in autobiographical memory. *Journal of Neuroscience*, *16*, 4275–4282.

Finlay, A. L., Jones, S. R., Morland, A. B., Ogilvie, J. A., & Ruddock, K. H. (1997). Movement in the normal visual hemifield induces a percept in the 'blind' hemifield of a human hemianope. *Proceedings: Biological Sciences*, *264*, 267–275.

Finlayson, P. & Cynader, M. (1995). Synaptic depression in visual cortex tissue slices: an in vitro model for cortical neuron adaptation. *Experimental Brain Research*, *106*, 145–155.

Fischer, K. W. (1980). A theory of cognitive development: The control and construction of hierarchies of skills. *Psychological Review*, *87*(6), 477–531.

Flash, T. & Hogan, N. (1985). The coordination of arm movements: an experimentally confirmed mathematical model. *Journal of Neuroscience*, *5*, 1688–1703.

Fletcher, P. & Henson, R. (2001). Frontal lobes and human memory: Insights from functional neuroimaging. *Brain*, *124*, 849–881.

Fletcher, P. C., Frith, C. D., Grasby, P. M., Shallice, T., Frackowiak, R. S., & Dolan, R. J. (1995). Brain systems for encoding and retrieval of auditory-verbal memory. An in vivo study in humans. *Brain*, *118* (2), 401–416.

Fletcher, P. C., Shallice, T., Frith, C. D., Frackowiak, R. S., & Dolan, R. J. (1996). Brain activity during memory retrieval. The influence of imagery and semantic cueing. *Brain*, *119* (5), 1587–1596.

Fletcher, P. C., Frith, C. D., & Rugg, M. D. (1997). The functional neuroanatomy of episodic memory. *Trends in Neurosciences*, *20*(5), 213–218.

Fletcher, P. C., Shallice, T., & Dolan, R. J. (1998a). The functional roles of prefrontal cortex in episodic memory. I. Encoding. *Brain*, *121* (7), 1239–1248.

Fletcher, P. C., Shallice, T., Frith, C. D., Frackowiak, R. S., & Dolan, R. J. (1998b). The functional roles of prefrontal cortex in episodic memory. II. Retrieval. *Brain*, *121* (7), 1249–1256.

Fodor, J. (1975). *The language of thought*. New York: Crowell.

Fodor, J. (1983). *Modularity of mind*. Cambridge, MA: MIT Press.

Fodor, J. (1999). Diary (September 30). *London Review of Books*.

Fodor, J. (2000). *The mind doesn't work that way: The scope and limits of computational psychology*. Cambridge, MA: MIT Press.

Fodor, J. & Pylyshyn, Z. (1988). Connectionism and cognitive architecture: a critical analysis. *Cognition*, *28*, 3–71.

Fodor, J., Bever, T., & Garrett, M. (1974). *The psychology of language: an introduction to psycholinguistics and generative grammar*. New York: McGraw-Hill.

Fodor, J. D., Fodor, J. A., & Garrett, M. F. (1975). The psychological unreality of semantic representations. *Linguistic Inquiry*, *6*(4), 515–531.

Fogassi, L. & Luppino, G. (2005). Motor functions of the parietal lobe. *Current Opinion in Neurobiology*, *15*, 626–631.

Fogassi, L., Ferrari, P. F., Gesierich, B., Rozzi, S., Chersi, F., & Rizzolatti, G. (2005). Parietal lobe: from action organization to intention understanding. *Science*, *308*, 662–667.

Forde, E. M. & Humphreys, G. W. (2007). Contrasting effects of repetition across tasks: implications for understanding the nature of refractory behavior and models of semantic memory. *Cognive, Affective and Behavioral Neuroscience*, *7*, 198–211.

Forde, E., Francis, D., Riddoch, M., Rumiati, R., & Humphreys, G. W. (1997). On the links between visual knowledge and naming: a single case study of a patients with a category-specific impairment for living things. *Cognitive Neuropsychology*, *14*, 403–458.

Fox, J. (2005). Images of Mind. In D. N. Davis (Ed.) *Visions of mind: architectures for cognition and affect* (pp. 125–148). Hershey, PA: IDEA Group.

Fox, J. (2009). Arguing about the evidence: A logical approach. In P. Dawid, W. Twining, & M. Vasilaki (Eds), *Evidence, inference and enquiry*. London: British Academy.

Fox, J. & Das, S. (2000). *Safe and sound: artificial intelligence in hazardous applications*. AAAI Press/MIT Press.

Fox, J., Krause, P. J., & Elvang-Goransson, M. (1993). Argumentation as a general framework for uncertain reasoning. In *Proceedings of the 9th Conference on Uncertainty in Artificial Intelligence*. (pp. 428–434). Washington: Morgan Kaufman.

Fox, J., Glasspool, D. W., Modgil, S., Tolchinsky, P., & Black, L. (2006). Towards a canonical framework for designing agents to support healthcare organisations. In *Proceedings of the European Conference on Artificial Intelligence (ECAI) Workshop Agents Applied in Healthcare*.

Fox, P. T., Laird, A. R., Fox, S. P., Fox, P. M., Uecker, A. M., Crank, M. et al. (2005). BrainMap taxonomy of experimental design: description and evaluation. *Human Brain Mapping*, *25*, 185–198.

Foygel, D. & Dell, G. S. (2000). Models of impaired lexical access in speech production. *Journal of Memory and Language*, *43*, 182–216.

Frankish, C. R. (1974). *Organisational factors in short-term memory*. Unpublished doctoral dissertation, University of Cambridge.

Frankish, C. (2008). Precategorical acoustic storage and the perception of speech. *Journal of Memory and Language*, *58*, 815–836.

Frankish, C. & Barnes, L. (2008). Lexical and sublexical processes in the perception of transposed-letter anagrams. *Quarterly Journal Experimental Psychology*, *61*, 381–391.

Frazier, L. (1987). Sentence processing: a tutorial review. In M.Coltheart (Ed.), *Attention and performance XII* (pp. 559–585). Hillsdale, NJ: Erlbaum.

Frazier, L. & Rayner, K. (1982). Making and correcting errors during sentence comprehension: Eye movements in the analysis of structurally ambiguous sentences. *Cognitive Psychology, 14*, 178–210.

French, R. M. (1999). Catastrophic forgetting in connectionist networks. *Trends in Cognitive Sciences*, *3*, 128–135.

Freuder, E. (1974). A computer vision system for visual recognition using active knowledge. *MIT A.I. Laboratory, Technical Report*, *345*.

Fried, I., Katz, A., McCarthy, G., Sass, K. J., Williamson, P., Spencer, S. S. et al. (1991). Functional-organization of human supplementary motor cortex studied by electrical-stimulation. *Journal of Neuroscience*, *11*, 3656–3666.

Friederici, A. D., Schoenle, P. W., & Goodglass, H. (1981). Mechanisms underlying writing and speech in aphasia. *Brain and Language*, *13*(2), 212–222.

Friedman, R. (1996). Recovery from deep alexia to phonological alexia. *Brain and Language*, *52*, 114–128.

Friedrich, F., Glenn, C., & Marin, O. (1984). Interruption of phonological coding in conduction aphasia. *Brain and Language*, *22*, 266–291.

Friston, K. (2007). Statistical parametric mapping. In K. J. Friston, J. Ashburner, S. Kiebel, T. Nichols, & W. D. Penny (Eds), *Statistical parametric mapping: an analysis of functional brain images* (pp. 10–31). Amsterdam: Elsevier.

Friston, K. J., Frith, C. D., Frackowiak, R. S. J., & Turner, R. (1995). Characterizing dynamic brain responses with fMRI—a multivariate approach. *Neuroimage*, *2*, 166–172.

Friston, K. J., Price, C. J., Fletcher, P., Moore, C., Frackowiak, R. S., & Dolan, R. J. (1996). The trouble with cognitive subtraction. *Neuroimage*, *4*, 97–104.

Friston, K. J., Holmes, A. P., Price, C. J., Buchel, C., & Worsley, K. J. (1999). Multisubject fMRI studies and conjunction analyses. *Neuroimage*, *10*, 385–396.

Friston, K. J., Harrison, L., & Penny, W. (2003). Dynamic causal modelling. *Neuroimage*, *19*, 1273–1302.

Friston, K. J., Penny, W. D., & Glaser, D. E. (2005). Conjunction revisited. *Neuroimage*, *25*, 661–667.

Friston, K. J., Ashburner, J., Kiebel, S., Nichols, T., & Penny, W. D. (2007). *Statistical parametric mapping: the analysis of functional brain images*. Academic Press.

Frith, C. D. (1992). *The Cognitive Neuropsychology of Schizophrenia*. Hove.: Lawrence Erlbaum Associates.

Frith, C. D. & Frith, U. (1999). Interacting minds—a biological basis. *Science*, *286*, 1692–1695.

Frith, C. D., Friston, K. J., Liddle, P., & Frackowiak, R. S. (1991). Willed action and the prefrontal cortex in man: A study with PET. *Proceedings of the Royal Society of London*, *244*, 241–246.

Frith, U. (2001). Mind blindness and the brain in autism. *Neuron*, *32*, 969–979.

Frith, U. & Frith, C. D. (2001). The biological basis of social interaction. *Current Directions in Psychological Science*, *10*, 151–155.

Frith, U., Morton, J., & Leslie, A. M. (1991). The cognitive basis of a biological disorder: autism. *Trends in Neurosciences*, *14*(10), 433–438.

Fromkin, V. (1973). *Speech errors as linguistic evidence*. The Hague: Mouton.

Frost, R. (1998). Toward a strong phonological theory of visual word recognition: true issues and false trails. *Psycholical Bullettin*, *123*, 71–99.

Fudge, E. (1969). Syllables. *Journal of Linguistics*, *5*, 193–320.

Funahashi, S. (2001). Neuronal mechanisms of executive control by the prefrontal cortex. *Neuroscience Research*, *39*, 147–165.

Funahashi, S. & Inoue, M. (2000). Neuronal interactions related to working memory processes in the primate prefrontal cortex revealed by cross-correlation analysis. *Cerebral Cortex*, *10*, 535–551.

Funahashi, S., Bruce, C. J. & Goldman-Rakic, P.S. (1989). Mnemonic coding of visual space in the monkey's dorsolateral prefrontal cortex. *Journal of Neurophysiology*, *61*, 331–349.

Funahashi, S., Chafee, M., & Goldman-Rakic, P. (1993). Prefrontal neuronal activity in rhesus monkeys performing a delayed anti-saccade task. *Nature*, *365*, 756.

Funnell, E. & De Mornay Davies, P. (1997). JBR: a reassessment of concept familiarity and a category-speci.c disorder for living things. *Neurocase*, *2*, 461–474.

Funnell, E. & Sheridan, J. (1992). Categories of knowledge? Unfamiliar aspects of living and non-living things. *Cognitive Neuropsychology*, *9*, 135–153.

Fuster, J. M. (1973). Unit activity of prefrontal cortex during delayedresponse performance: neuronal correlates of transient memory. *Journal of Neurophisiology*, *36*, 61–78.

Fuster, J. M. (1989). *The prefrontal cortex* (2nd edn). Raven Press, New York.

Fuster, J. M. & Alexander, G. E. (1971). Neuron activity related to short-term memory. *Science*, *173*, 652–654.

Fuster, J. M., Bauer, R., & Jervey, J. (1982). Cellular discharge in the dorsolateral prefrontal cortex of the monkey in cognitive tasks. *Experimental Neurology, 77,* 679–694.

Fuster, J. M., Bodner, M., & Kroger, J. K. (2000). Cross-modal and cross-temporal association in neurons of frontal cortex. *Nature*, *405*, 347–351.

Gabrieli, J. (2001). Functional imaging of episodic memory. In R. Cabeza & A. Kingstone (Eds), *Handbook of functional neuroimaging of cognition* (pp. 253–292). MIT Press.

Gabrieli, J., Keane, M., Stanger, B., Kjelgaard, M., Corkin, S., & Growdon, J. (1994). Dissociations among structural-perceptual, lexical-semantic, and even-fact memory systems in amnesic, Alzheimers, and normal subjects. *Cortex, 30,* 75–103.

Gabrieli, J., McGlinchey-Berroth, R., Gluck, M., Cermak, L., & Disterhoft, J. (1995). Intact delay-eyeblink conditioning in amnesia. *Behavioual Neuroscience, 109,* 819–827.

Gabrieli, J., Desmond, J., Demb, J., & Wagner, A. (1996). Functional magnetic resonance imaging of semantic memory processes in the frontal lobes. *Psychological Science, 7,* 278–283.

Gaffan, D. (2002). Against memory systems. *Philosophical Transactions of the Royal Society B: Biological Sciences, 357,* 1111–1121.

Gaffan, D. & Heywood, C. (1993). A spurious categoryspecic visual agnosia for living things in normal humans and nonhuman primates. *Journal of Cognitive Neuroscience, 5,* 118–128.

Gaffan, D., Parker, A., Easton, A. (2001). Dense amnesia in the monkey after transection of fornix, amygdala and anterior temporal stem. *Neuropsychologia, 39,* 51–70.

Gainotti, G. (2000). What the locus of brain lesion tells us about the nature of the cognitive defect underlying category-specific disorders: a review. *Cortex, 36,* 539–559.

Gainotti, G., Marra, C., Villa, G., Parlato, V., & Chiarotti, F. (1998). Sensitivity and specificity of some neuropsychological markers of Alzheimer dementia. *Alzheimer Dis.Assoc.Disord., 12,* 152–162.

Galletti, C., Fattori, P., Battaglini, P., Shipp, S., & Zeki, S. (1996). Functional demarcation of a border between areas V6 and V6A in the superior parietal gyrus of the macaque monkey. *European Journal of Neuroscience, 8,* 30–52.

Gamer, M., Klimecki, O., Bauermann, T., Stoeter, P., & Vossel, G. (2009). fMRI-activation patterns in the detection of concealed information rely on memory-related effects. *Social Cognitive and Affective Neuroscience*.

Gardner, H. (1993). *Frames of mind: the theory of multiple intelligences*. New York: Basic books.

Gardiner, J. M. (1988). Functional aspects of recollective experience. *Memory and Cognition, 16,* 309–313.

Gardiner, J. M. & Java, R. I. (1990). Recollective experience in word and nonword recognition. *Memory and Cognition, 18,* 23–30.

Garner, W. R., Hake, H. W., & Eriksen, C. W. (1956). Operationism and the concept of perception. *Psychological Review, 63*(3), 149–159.

Garrard, P., Patterson, K., Watson, P., & Hodges, J. (1998). Category specific semantic loss in dementia of Alzheimer's type. Functional-anatomical correlations from cross-sectional analyses. *Brain, 121,* 633–646.

Garrard, P., Lambon Ralph, M. A., Hodges, J. R., & Patterson, K. (2001). Prototypicality, distinctiveness, and intercorrelation: analyses of the semantic attributes of living and nonliving concepts. *Cognitive Neuropsychology, 18,* 125–174.

Garrard, P., Carroll, E., Vinson, D., & Vigliocco, G. (2004). Dissociation of lexical syntax and semantics: evidence from focal cortical degeneration. *Neurocase, 10,* 353–362.

Garrett, M. (1980). Levels of processing in sentence production. In B. Butterworth (Ed.), *Language production: Vol. I. Speech and talk*. Academic Press.

Garrett, M. (1988). Processes in language production. In F.Nieuwmeyer (Ed.), *Linguistics: The Cambridge survey. Vol. III. Biological and psychological aspects of language*. Harvard University Press.

Gat, E. (1991). *Reliable goal-directed reactive control of autonomous mobile robots*. PhD thesis, Virginia Polytechnic Institute and State University.

Gat, E. (1998). Three-layer architectures. In P.Kortenkamp, R. Bonasso, & R. Murphy (Eds), *Artificial intelligence and mobile robots: case studies of successful robot systems* (pp. 195–210). Menlo Park, CA: AAAI Press/ The MIT Press.

Gauthier, I. & Tarr, M. J. (1997). Becoming a 'Greeble' expert: exploring mechanisms for face recognition. *Vision Research, 37,* 1673–1682.

Gaymard, B., Rivaud, S., Cassarini, J. F., Dubard, T., Rancurel, G., Agid, Y. et al. (1998). Effects of anterior cingulate cortex lesions on ocular saccades in humans. *Experimental Brain Research, 120,* 173–183.

Gazdar, G., Kelin, E., Pullum, G., & Sag, I. (1985). *Generalized phrase structure grammar*. Oxford: Blackwell Publishing.

Gazzaniga, M.S. (1966). Visuomotor integration in split-brain monkeys with other cerebral lesions. *Experimental Neurology, 16,* 289–298.

Genovesio, A. & Wise, S. P. (2008). The neurophysiology of abstract response strategies. In S.A.Bunge & J. D. Wallis (Eds), *Neuroscience of rule-guided behavior*. Oxford.

Genovesio, A., Brasted, P., Mitz, A., & Wise, S. (2005). Prefrontal cortex activity related to abstract response strategies. *Neuron, 47,* 307–320.

Gentilini, M., Derenzi, E., & Crisi, G. (1987). Bilateral paramedian thalamic artery infarcts—report of 8 cases. *Journal of Neurology Neurosurgery and Psychiatry, 50,* 900–909.

Gentner, D. (2006). Why verbs are hard to learn. In K.Hirsh-Pasek & R. Golinkoff (Eds), *Action meets word: how children learn verbs* (pp. 544–564). Oxford: OUP.

Gentner, D. & Stevens, A. (1983). *Mental models.* Erlbaum.

Gerhand, S. (2001). Routes to reading: a report of a non-semantic reader with equivalent performance on regular and exception words. *Neuropsychologia, 39,* 1473–1484.

Gerschlager, W., Alesch, F., Cunnington, R., Deecke, L., Dirnberger, G., Endl, W., et al. (1999). Bilateral subthalamic nucleus stimulation improves frontal cortex function in Parkinson's disease. An electrophysiological study of the contingent negative variation. *Brain, 122,* 2365–2373.

Geschwind, N. (1965). Disconnexion syndromes in animals and man. I. *Brain, 88,* 237–294.

Geschwind, N., Quadfassel, F., & Segarra, J. (1968). Isolation of the speech area. *Neuropsychologia, 6,* 327–340.

Ghent, L., Mishkin, M., & Teuber, H. (1962). Short-term memory after frontal lobe injury in man. *Journal of Comparative and Physiological Psychology, 55,* 705–709.

Giese, M. A. & Poggio, T. (2003). Neural mechanisms for the recognition of biological movements. *Nature Reviews Neuroscience, 4,* 179–192.

Gigerenzer, G., Todd, P. & the ABC Research Group (1999). *Simple heuristics that make us smart.* New York: OUP.

Gilbert, S. J. & Shallice, T. (2002). Task switching: a PDP model. *Cognitive Psychology, 44,* 297–337.

Gilbert, S. J., Frith, C. D., & Burgess, P. W. (2005). Involvement of rostral prefrontal cortex in selection between stimulus-oriented and stimulus-independent thought. *European Journal of Neuroscience, 21,* 1423–1431.

Gilbert, S. J., Spengler, S., Simons, J. S., Steele, J. D., Lawrie, S. M., Frith, C. D. et al. (2006). Functional specialization within rostral prefrontal cortex (area 10): a meta-analysis. *Journal of Cognitive Neuroscience, 18,* 932–948.

Gilboa, A. (2004). Autobiographical and episodic memory—one and the same? Evidence from prefrontal activation in neuroimaging studies. *Neuropsychologia, 42,* 1336–1349.

Gilboa, A. & Moscovitch, M. (2002). The cognitive neuroscience of confabulation: a review and a model. In A.D.Baddeley, M. D. Kopelman, & B. A. Wilson (Eds), *Handbook of memory disorders* (pp. 315–342). London: Wiley.

Gilboa, A., Winocur, G., Grady, C. L., Hevenor, S. J., & Moscovitch, M. (2004). Remembering our past: functional neuroanatomy of recollection of recent and very remote personal events. *Cerebral Cortex, 14,* 1214–1225.

Gilboa, A., Alain, C., Stuss, D. T., Melo, B., Miller, S., & Moscovitch, M. (2006). Mechanisms of spontaneous confabulations: a strategic retrieval account. *Brain, 129,* 1399–1414.

Giocomo, L. M. & Hasselmo, M. E. (2007). Neuromodulation by glutamate and acetylcholine can change circuit dynamics by regulating the relative influence of afferent input and excitatory feedback. *Molecular Neurobiology, 36,* 184–200.

Gipson, P. (1986). The production of phonology and auditory priming. *British Journal of Psychology, 77,* 359–375.

Girard, J. (1987). Linear logic. *Theoretical Computational Science, 50,* 1–102.

Glanzer, M. & Cunitz, A. R. (1966). Two storage mechanisms in free recall. *Journal of Verbal Learning and Verbal Behavior, 5,* 351–360.

Glanzer, M., Dorfman, D., & Kaplan, B. (1981). Short-term storage in the processing of text. *Journal of Verbal Learning and Verbal Behavior, 20,* 656–670.

Glasspool, D. W. (2005). The integration and control of behaviour: Insights from neuroscience and AI. In D. N. Davis (Ed.), *Visions of mind: architectures for cognition and affect.* Hershey. Pa: Idea Group Inc.

Glasspool, D. W. & Houghton, G. (2005). Serial order and consonant-vowel structure in a graphemic output buffer model. *Brain and Language, 94,* 304–330.

Glasspool, D. W., Shallice, T., & Cipolotti, L. (2006). Towards a unified process model for graphemic buffer disorder and deep dysgraphia. *Cognitive Neuropsychology, 23,* 479–512.

Gleitman, L., Cassidy, K., Nappa, R., Papafragou, A., & Trueswell, J. (2005). Hard words. *Language Learning and Development, 1,* 23–64.

Glenberg, A. (1990). Common processes underlie enhanced recency effects for auditory and changing state stimuli. *Memory and Cognition, 18,* 638–650.

Gluck, M. & Myers, C. (1993). Hippocampal mediation of stimulus representation: a computational theory. *Hippocampus, 3,* 491–516.

Glymour, C. (1994). On the methods of cognitive neuropsychology. *British Journal of Philosophical Science, 45,* 815–835.

Gnadt, J. & Andersen, R. (1988). Memory related motor planning activity in posterior parietal cortex of macaque. *Experimental Brain Research, 70,* 216–220.

Gödel, K. (1931). Über formal unentscheidbare Sätze der Principia Mathematica und verwandter Systeme. *Monatshefte für Mathematik und Physik, 38,* 173–198.

Goel, V. (2007). Anatomy of deductive reasoning. *Trends in Cognitive Sciences, 11,* 435–441.

Goel, V. (2009). Cognitive Neuroscience of Thinking. In G.Berntson & J. Cacioppo (Eds), *Handbook of neuroscience for the behavioral sciences.* Wiley.

Goel, V. & Dolan, R. J. (2000). Anatomical segregation of component processes in an inductive inference task. *Journal of Cognitive Neuroscience*, *12*, 110–119.

Goel, V. & Dolan, R. J. (2003a). Explaining modulation of reasoning by belief. *Cognition*, *87*, B11–B22.

Goel, V. & Dolan, R. J. (2003b). Reciprocal neural response within lateral and ventral medial prefrontal cortex during hot and cold reasoning. *Neuroimage*, *20*, 2314–2321.

Goel, V. & Grafman, J. (1995). Are the frontal lobes implicated in 'planning' functions? Interpreting data from the Tower of Hanoi. *Neuropsychologia*, *33*, 623–642.

Goel, V. & Grafman, J. (2000). Role of the right prefrontal cortex in ill-structured planning. *Cognitive Neuropsychology*, *17*, 415–436.

Goel, V. & Vartanian, O. (2005). Dissociating the roles of right ventral lateral and dorsal lateral prefrontal cortex in generation and maintenance of hypotheses in set-shift problems. *Cerebral Cortex*, *15*, 1170–1177.

Goel, V., Gold, B., Kapur, S., & Houle, S. (1997). The seats of reason? An imaging study of deductive and inductive reasoning. *Neuroreport*, *8*, 1305–1310.

Goel, V., Gold, B., Kapur, S., & Houle, S. (1998). Neuroanatomical correlates of human reasoning. *Journal of Cognitive Neuroscience*, *10*, 293–302.

Goel, V., Buchel, C., Frith, C., & Dolan, R. J. (2000). Dissociation of mechanisms underlying syllogistic reasoning. *Neuroimage*, *12*, 504–514.

Goel, V., Pullara, S., & Grafman, J. (2001). A computational model of frontal lobe dysfunction: Working memory and the Tower of Hanoi task. *Cognitive Science*, *25*, 287–313.

Goel, V., Tierney, M., Sheesley, L., Bartolo, A., Vartanian, O., & Grafman, J. (2007). Hemispheric specialization in human prefrontal cortex for resolving certain and uncertain inferences. *Cerebral Cortex*, *17*, 2245–2250.

Goense, J. B. & Logothetis, N. K. (2008). Neurophysiology of the BOLD fMRI signal in awake monkeys. *Current Biology*, *18*, 631–640.

Goldberg, E. (1995). Rise and fall of modular orthodoxy. *Journal of Clinical and Experimental Neuropsychology*, *17*, 193–208.

Goldenberg, G. & Hagmann, S. (1997). The meaning of meaningless gestures: a study of visuo-imitative apraxia. *Neuropsychologia*, *35*, 333–341.

Goldenberg, G. & Hagmann, S. (1998). Tool use and mechanical problem solving in apraxia. *Neuropsychologia*, *36*, 581–589.

Goldenberg, G. & Karnath, H. O. (2006). The neural basis of imitation is body part specific. *Journal of Neuroscience*, *26*, 6282–6287.

Goldenberg, G. & Strauss, S. (2002). Hemisphere asymmetries for imitation of novel gestures. *Neurology*, *59*, 893–897.

Golding, E. (1981). The effect of unilateral brain lesion on reasoning. *Cortex*, *17*, 31–40.

Goldman-Rakic, P. (1987). Development of cortical circuitry and cognitive function. *Child Development*, *58*, 601–622.

Goldman-Rakic, P. (1988). Topography of cognition: Parallel distributed networks in primate association cortex. *Annual Review of Neuroscience*, *11*, 137–156.

Goldman-Rakic, P. (1996). Regional and cellular fractionation of working memory. *Proceedings of the National Academy of Sciences*, *93*, 13473–13480.

Gonnerman, L., Andersen, E., Devlin, J., Kempler, D., & Seidenberg, M. (1997). Double dissociation of semantic categories in Alzheimer's disease. *Brain and Language*, *57*, 254–279.

Gonsalves, B. D., Kahn, I., Curran, T., Norman, K. A., & Wagner, A. D. (2005). Memory strength and repetition suppression: multimodal imaging of medial temporal cortical contributions to recognition. *Neuron*, *47*, 751–761.

Goodall, J. (1986). *The chimpanzees of Gombe*. Belknap Press of Harvard University Press.

Goodglass, H., & Kaplan, E. (1972). *The Assessment of aphasia and related disorders*. Philadelphia: Lea and Febiger.

Goodglass, H., Quadfasel, F., & Timberlake, W. (1964). Phrase length and the type and severity of aphasia. *Cortex 1*, 133–153.

Goodglass, H., Klein, B., Carey, P., & Jones, K. (1966). Specific semantic word categories in aphasia. *Cortex*, *2*, 74–89.

Goodwin, G. P. & Johnson-Laird, P. N. (2005). Reasoning about relations. *Psychological Review*, *112*, 468–493.

Gorno-Tempini, M. L., Price, C. J., Josephs, O., Vandenberghe, R., Cappa, S. F., Kapur, N. et al. (1998). The neural systems sustaining face and proper-name processing. *Brain*, *121*(11), 2103–2118.

Gorno-Tempini, M., Dronkers, N., Rankin, K., Ogar, J., Phengrasamy, L., Rosen, H. et al. (2004). Cognition and anatomy in three variants of primary progressive aphasia. *Annals of Neurology*, *55*, 335–346.

Goswami, U. (1995). Transitive relational mappings in three- and four-year-olds: The analogy of Goldilocks and the three bears. *Child Development*, *66*, 877–892.

Goswami, U., & Brown, A. L. (1990a). Melting chocolate and melting snowmen: analogical reasoning and causal relations. *Cognition*, *35*(1), 69–95.

Goswami, U. & Brown, A. L. (1990b). Higher-order structure and relational reasoning: contrasting analogical and thematic relations. *Cognition*, *36*, 207–226.

Gotts, S. J. & Plaut, D. C. (2002). The impact of synaptic depression following brain damage: a connectionist account of 'access/refractory' and 'degraded-store' semantic impairments. *Cognitive, Affective and Behavioral Neuroscience, 2*, 187–213.

Gotts, S. J., la Rocchetta, A. I., & Cipolotti, L. (2002). Mechanisms underlying perseveration in aphasia: evidence from a single case study. *Neuropsychologia, 40*, 1930–1947.

Graf, P., Squire, L. R., & Mandler, G. (1984). The information that amnesic patients do not forget. *Journal of Experimental Psychology: Learning, Memory and Cognition, 10*, 164–178.

Grafton, S. T. & Hamilton, A. F. (2007). Evidence for a distributed hierarchy of action representation in the brain. *Human Movement Science, 26*, 590–616.

Grafton, S. T., Fadiga, L., Arbib, M. A., & Rizzolatti, G. (1997). Premotor cortex activation during observation and naming of familiar tools. *Neuroimage, 6*, 231–236.

Graham, K. S. (1999). Semantic dementia: A challenge to multple trace theory. *Trends in Cognitive Science, 3*, 85–87.

Graham, K. S. & Hodges, J. R. (1997). Differentiating the roles of the hippocampal complex and the neocortex in long-term memory storage: evidence from the study of semantic dementia and Alzheimer's disease. *Neuropsychology, 11*, 77–89.

Graham, K. S., Simons, J. S., Pratt, K. H., Patterson, K., & Hodges, J. R. (2000). Insights from semantic dementia on the relationship between episodic and semantic memory. *Neuropsychologia, 38*, 313–324.

Grainger, J. & Jacobs, A. (1996). Orthographic processing in visual word recognition: a multiple read-out model. *Psychological Review, 103*, 518–565.

Grant, D. & Berg, E. (1948). A behavioral analysis of degree of reinforcement and ease of shifting to new responses in a Weigl-type card-sorting problem. *Journal of Experimental Psychology., 38*, 404–411.

Grasby, P. M., Frith, C. D., Friston, K. J., Bench, C., Frackowiak, R. S., & Dolan, R. J. (1993). Functional mapping of brain areas implicated in auditory—verbal memory function. *Brain, 116* (1), 1–20.

Grea, H., Desmurget, M., & Prablanc, C. (2000). Postural invariance in three-dimensional reaching and grasping movements. *Experimental Brain Research, 134*, 155–162.

Green, A. E., Fugelsang, J. A., Kraemer, D. J., Shamosh, N. A., & Dunbar, K. N. (2006). Frontopolar cortex mediates abstract integration in analogy. *Brain Research, 1096*, 125–137.

Green, D. M. & Swets, J. A. (1966). *Signal detection theory and psychophysics*. New York: Wiley.

Greenberg, D. L. (2007). Comment on 'detecting awareness in the vegetative state'. *Science, 315*(5816), 1221b.

Greenfield, P. M. (1991). Language, tools and brain: The ontogeny and phylogeny of hierarchically organized sequential behavior. *Behavioral and Brain Sciences, 14*(4), 531–595.

Greenwald, A. & Draine, S. (1997). Do subliminal stimuli enter the mind unnoticed? Tests with a new method. In J. Cohen & J. Schuler (Eds), *Scientific approaches to consciousness: 25th Carnegie Symposium on Cognition* (pp. 83–108). Hillsdale, NJ: LEA.

Greenwood, R., Bhalla, A., Gordon, A., & Roberts, J. (1983). Behaviour disturbances during recovery from herpes simplex encephalitis. *The Journal of Neurology, Neurosurgery, and Psychiatry, 46*, 809–817.

Gregory, R. L. (1961). The brain as an engineering problem. In W. H. Thorpe & O. L. Zangwill (Eds). *Current problems in animal behaviour*. Cambridge, CUP.

Grèzes, J. & Decety, J. (2001). Functional anatomy of execution, mental simulation, observation, and verb generation of actions: a meta-analysis. *Human Brain Mapping, 12*, 1–19.

Grill-Spector, K., Knouf, N., & Kanwisher, N. (2004). The fusiform face area subserves face perception, not generic within-category identification. *Nature Neuroscience, 7*(5), 555–562.

Grodzinsky, Y. (1984). The syntactic characterization of agrammatism. *Cognition, 16*, 99–120.

Grodzinsky, Y. (2000). The neurology of syntax: language use without Broca's area. *Behavioral and Brain Sciences, 23*, 1–21.

Grodzinsky, Y. & Friederici, A. D. (2006). Neuroimaging of syntax and syntactic processing. *Current Opinion in Neurobiology, 16*, 240–246.

Grodzinsky, Y., Pinango, M. M., Zurif, E., & Drai, D. (1999). The critical role of group studies in neuropsychology: comprehension regularities in Broca's aphasia. *Brain and Language, 67*, 134–147.

Gross, C. G., Rocha-Miranda, C. E., & Bender, D. B. (1972). Visual properties of neurons in inferotemporal cortex of the Macaque. *Journal of Neurophysiology, 35*, 96–111.

Gross J, Schmitz F, Schnitzler I, Kessler K, Shapiro K, Hommel B, & Schnitzler A. (2004). Modulation of long-range neural synchrony reflects temporal limitations of visual attention in humans. *Proceedings of the National Academy of Sciences of the USA, 101*, 13050–13055.

Grossberg, S. (1987). Competitive learning: from interactive activation to adaptive resonance. *Cognitive Science, 11*, 23–63.

Grossi, D., Becker, J. T., Smith, C., & Trojano, L. (1993). Memory for visuospatial patterns in Alzheimer's disease. *Psychological Medicine, 23*, 65–70.

Gurney, K., Prescott, T. J., & Redgrave, P. (2001a). A computational model of action selection in the basal ganglia. I. A new functional anatomy. *Biological Cybernetics, 84*, 401–410.

Gurney, K., Prescott, T. J., & Redgrave, P. (2001b). A computational model of action selection in the basal ganglia. II. Analysis and simulation of behaviour. *Biological Cybernetics*, *84*, 411–423.

Haaland, K. Y., Harrington, D. L., & Knight, R. T. (2000). Neural representations of skilled movement. *Brain*, *123*(11), 2306–2313.

Haarmann, H. (1997). Aphasic sentence comprehension as a resource deficit: a computational approach. *Brain and Language*, *59*(1), 76–120.

Haarmann, H. & Usher, M. (2001). Maintenance of semantic information in capacity-limited item short-term memory. *Psychonomic Bulletin and Review*, *8*, 568–578.

Haarmann, H. J., Just, M. A., & Carpenter, P. A. (1997). Aphasic sentence comprehension as a resource deficit: a computational approach. *Brain and Language*, *59*, 76–120.

Haarmann, H. J., Cameron, K. A., & Ruchkin, D. S. (2003). Short-term semantic retention during on-line sentence comprehension. Brain potential evidence from filler-gap constructions. *Brain Res. Cogn Brain Res.*, *15*, 178–190.

Hadjikhani, N., Liu, A.K., Dale, A.M., Cavanagh, P. & Tootell, R.B.H. (1998). Retinotopy and color sensitivity in human visual cortical area VB. *Nature Neuroscience*, *3*, 235–241.

Hadley, R. (1997). Cognition, systematicity, and nomic necessity. *Mind and Language*, *12*, 137–153.

Hafting, T., Fyhn, M., Molden, S., Moser, M., & Moser, E. (2005). Microstructure of a spatial map in the entorhinal cortex. *Nature*, *436*, 801–806.

Haggard, P. (2008). Human volition: towards a neuroscience of will. *Nature Reviews Neuroscience*, *9*(12), 934–946.

Haggard, P., & Eimer, M. (1999). On the relation between brain potentials and the awareness of voluntary movements. *Experimental Brain Research*, *126*(1), 128–133.

Hagoort, P. (2003). How the brain solves the binding problem for language: a neurocomputational model of syntactic processing. *NeuroImage*, *20*, S18–S29.

Hagoort, P. (2005). On Broca, brain, and binding: a new framework. *Trends in Cognitive Sciences*, *9*, 416–423.

Hagoort, P., Brown, C., & Osterhout, L. (1999). The neurocognition of syntactic processing. In C.Brown & P. Hagoort (Eds), *Neurocognition of language*. Oxford: OUP.

Hagoort, P., Wassenaar, M., & Brown, C. (2003a). Real-time semantic compensation in patients with agrammatic comprehension: electrophysiological evidence for multiple-route plasticity. *Proceedings of the National Academy of Sciences, USA*, *100*, 4340–4345.

Hagoort, P., Wassenaar, M., & Brown, C. M. (2003b). Syntax-related ERP-effects in Dutch. *Cognitive Brain Research*, *16*(1), 38–50.

Hagoort, P., Hald, L., Bastiaansen, M., & Petersson, K. M. (2004). Integration of word meaning and world knowledge in language comprehension. *Science*, *304*, 438–441.

Hale, K. L. (1983). Warlpiri and the grammar of non-configurational languages. *Natural Language and Linguistic Theory*, *1*, 5–47.

Hameroff, S. & Penrose, R. (1996). Orchestrated reduction of quantum coherence in brain microtubules: a model for cosciousness? In S.Hameroff, A. Kaszniak, & A. Scott (Eds), *Toward a science of consciousness—the first tucson discussions and debates*. Cambridge, MA: MIT Press.

Hamilton, A. C. & Coslett, H. B. (2008). Refractory access disorders and the organization of concrete and abstract semantics: do they differ? *Neurocase*, *14*, 131–140.

Hamilton, A. F. & Grafton, S. T. (2006). Goal representation in human anterior intraparietal sulcus. *Journal of Neuroscience*, *26*, 1133–1137.

Hamilton, A. F. & Grafton, S. T. (2007). The motor hierarchy: from kinematics to goals and intentions. In P.Haggard, Y. Rossetti, & M. Kawato (Eds), *Sensorimotor foundations of higher cognition. Attention and performance XXII*. Oxford: OUP.

Hamilton, A. F. D. C., & Grafton, S. T. (2008). Action outcomes are represented in human inferior frontoparietal cortex. *Cerebral Cortex*, *18*(5), 1160–1168.

Hampshire, A. & Owen, A. M. (2006). Fractionating attentional control using event-related fMRI. *Cerebral Cortex*, *16*, 1679–1689.

Hanley, J. R. & Kay, J. (1996). Reading speed in pure alexia. *Neuropsychologia*, *34*, 1165–1174.

Hanley, J. R., Young, A. W., & Pearson, N. A. (1991). Impairment of the visuo-spatial sketch pad. *Quarterly Journal of Experimental Psychology A*, *43*, 101–125.

Hare, M. & Elman, J. L. (1995). Learning and morphological change. *Cognition*, *56*, 61–98.

Hare, M., Elman, J. L., & Daugherty, K. G. (1995). Default generalisation in connectionist networks. *Language and Cognitive Processes*, *10*(6), 601–630.

Harley, T. (1993). Phonological activation of semantic competitors during lexical access in speech production. *Language and Cognitive Processes*, *8*, 291–309.

Harley, T. (2004). Promises, promises. *Cognitive Neuropsychology*, *21*, 51–56.

Harley, T. A. (2008). *The psychology of language: from data to theory*. Hove: Psychology Press.

Harm, M. & Seidenberg, M. (2001). Are there orthographic impairments in phonological dyslexia? *Cognitive Neuropsychology*, *18*, 71–92.

Harris, I. M. & Miniussi, C. (2003). Parietal lobe contribution to mental rotation demonstrated with rTMS. *Journal of Cognitive Neuroscience*, *15*, 315-323.

Harris, C. M. & Wolpert, D. M. (1998). Signal-dependent noise determines motor planning. *Nature*, *394*, 780-784.

Harris, I. M., Egan, G. F., Sonkkila, C., Tochon-Danguy, H. J., Paxinos, G., & Watson, J. D. (2000). Selective right parietal lobe activation during mental rotation: a parametric PET study. *Brain*, *123* (1), 65-73.

Harrison, L., Stephen, K., & Friston., K. (2007). Effective connectivity. In K.J.Friston, J. Ashburner, S. Kiebel, T. Nichols, & W. D. Penny (Eds), *Statistical parametric mapping: an analysis of functional brain images* (pp. 508-521). Amsterdam: Elsevier.

Hartley, T., Burgess, N., Lever, C., Cacucci, F., & O'Keefe, J. (2000). Modeling place fields in terms of the cortical inputs to the hippocampus. *Hippocampus*, *10*, 369-379.

Hartley, T. & Houghton, G. (1996). A linguistically constrained model of short-term memory for nonwords. *Journal of Memory and Language*, *35*, 1-31.

Hartline, H. & Graham, C. (1932). Nerve impulses from single receptors in the eye. *Journal of Cellular and Comparative Physiology*, *1*, 277-295.

Hartmann, K., Goldenberg, G., Daumüller, M., & Hermsdörfer, J. (2005). It takes the whole brain to make a cup of coffee: the neuropsychology of naturalistic actions involving technical devices. *Neuropsychologia*, *43*, 625-637.

Hashimoto, R., Tanaka, Y., & Nakano, I. (2000). Amnesic confabulatory syndrome after focal basal forebrain damage. *Neurology*, *54*, 978-980.

Hasselmo, M. E. & Wyble, B. P. (1997). Free recall and recognition in a network model of the hippocampus: simulating effects of scopolamine on human memory function. *Behavioral Brain Research*, *89*, 1-34.

Hasselmo, M. E., Wyble, B. P., & Wallenstein, G. V. (1996). Encoding and retrieval of episodic memories: role of cholinergic and GABAergic modulation in the hippocampus. *Hippocampus*, *6*, 693-708.

Hauser, M., Chomsky, N., & Fitch, W. (2002). The faculty of language: what is it, who has it, and how did it evolve? *Science*, *298*, 1569-1579.

Haxby, J. V., Gobbini, M. I., Furey, M. L., Ishai, A., Schouten, J. L., & Pietrini, P. (2001). Distributed and overlapping representations of faces and objects in ventral temporal cortex. *Science*, *293*, 2425-2430.

Haxby, J., Hoffman, E., & Gobbini, M. (2000). The distributed human neural system for face perception. *Trends in Cognitive Science*, *4*, 223-233.

Haynes, J. D. & Rees, G. (2005). Predicting the stream of consciousness from activity in human visual cortex. *Current Biology*, *15*, 1301-1307.

Haynes, J. D. & Rees, G. (2006). Decoding mental states from brain activity in humans. *Nature Reviews Neuroscience*, *7*, 523-534.

Haynes, J. D., Sakai, K., Rees, G., Gilbert, S., Frith, C., & Passingham, R. E. (2007). Reading hidden intentions in the human brain. *Current Biology*, *17*, 323-328.

Hazy, T. E., Frank, M. J., & O'Reilly, R. C. (2006). Banishing the homunculus: making working memory work. *Neuroscience*, *139*, 105-118.

Hazy, T. E., Frank, M. J., & O'Reilly, R. C. (2007). Towards an executive without a homunculus: computational models of the prefrontal cortex/basal ganglia system. *Philosophical Transactions of the Royal Society B: Biological Sciences*, *362*, 1601-1613.

Head, H. (1926). *Aphasia and kindred disorders of speech.* Cambridge: CUP.

Head, H., & Holmes, G. (1911). Sensory disturbances from cerebral lesions. *Brain*, *34*(2-3), 102-254.

Hebb, D. O. (1945). Man's frontal lobes: A critical review. *Archives of Neurology & Psychiatry*, *54*, 10-24.

Hebb, D. O. (1949). *The organization of behavior: a neuropsychological theory.* New York: Wiley.

Hécaen, H. & Albert, M. (1978). *Human neuropsychology.* New York: Wiley.

Hécaen, H., & Angelergues, R. (1963). *La cécité psychique. [Psychic blindness.]* Oxford, England: Masson Cie.

Heilman, K. M. (1973). Ideational apraxia a re-definition. *Brain*, *96*, 861-864.

Heilman, K. & Rothi, L. (2003). Apraxia. In K. Heilman & E. Valenstein (Eds), *Clinical neurophysiology* (pp. 215-235). Oxford University Press: New York.

Heilman, K. M., & Valenstein, E. (2003). *Clinical neuropsychology.* Oxford: OUP.

Heilman, K. M., Tucker, D. M., & Valenstein, E. (1976). A case of mixed transcortical aphasia with intact naming. *Brain*, *99*, 415-426.

Heilman, K. M., Rothi, L. J., & Valenstein, E. (1982). Two forms of ideomotor apraxia. *Neurology*, *32*, 342-346.

Heilman, K. M., Rothi, L. G., Mack, L., Feinberg, T., & Watson, R. T. (1986). Apraxia after a superior parietal lesion. *Cortex*, *22*, 141-150.

Heilman, K. M., Maher, L., Greenwald, M., & Rothi, L. J. (1997). Conceptual apraxia from lateralized lesions. *Neurology*, *49*, 457-464.

Heim, S., Eickhoff, S. B., Ischebeck, A. K., Friederici, A. D., Stephan, K. E., & Amunts, K. (2009). Effective connectivity of the left BA 44, BA 45, and inferior temporal gyrus during lexical and phonological decisions identified with DCM. *Human Brain Mapping*, *30*, 392-402.

Held, B. (1996). *Dissociating Perception and Action in a Metacontrast Paradigm.* PhD thesis, University of London.

Henson, R. N. (1998). Short-term memory for serial order: the Start-End Model. *Cognitive Psychology, 36,* 73–137.

Henson, R. N. (1999). Positional information in short-term memory: relative or absolute? *Memory and Cognition, 27,* 915–927.

Henson, R. N. (2005). What can functional neuroimaging tell the experimental psychologist? *Quarterly Journal of Experimental Psychology: A, 58,* 193–233.

Henson, R. N. (2006). Forward inference using functional neuroimaging: dissociations versus associations. *Trends in Cognitive Sciences, 10,* 64–69.

Henson, R. N. (2007a). Analysis of fMRI time series. In K. J. Friston, J. Ashburner, S. Kiebel, T. Nichols, & W. Penny (Eds), *Statistical parametric mapping: an analysis of functional brain images.* Academic Press.

Henson, R. N. (2007b). Efficient experimental design for fMRI. In K.J.Friston, J. Ashburner, S. Kiebel, T. Nichols, & W. D. Penny (Eds), *Statistical parametric mapping: an analysis of functional brain images* (pp. 193–210). Academic Press.

Henson, R. N., Norris, D., Page, M. P., & Baddeley, A. (1996). Unchained memory: error patterns rule out chaining models of immediate serial recall. *Quarterly Journal of Experimental Psychology, 49A,* 80–115.

Henson, R. N., Rugg, M., Shallice, T., Josephs, O., & Dolan, R. (1999). Recollection and familiarity in recognition memory: an event-related functional magnetic resonance imaging study. *Journal of Neuroscience, 19,* 3962–3972.

Henson, R. N., Shallice, T., & Dolan, R. (2000a). Neuroimaging evidence for dissociable forms of repetition priming. *Science, 287,* 1269–1272.

Henson, R. N., Burgess, N., & Frith, C. D. (2000b). Recoding, storage, rehearsal and grouping in verbal short-term memory: an fMRI study. *Neuropsychologia, 38,* 426–440.

Henson, R. N. A., Shallice, T., Josephs, O., & Dolan, R. J. (2002). Functional magnetic resonance imaging of proactive interference during spoken cued recall. *NeuroImage, 17*(2), 543–558.

Henson, R. N., Hartley, T., Burgess, N., Hitch, G., & Flude, B. (2003). Selective interference with verbal short-term memory for serial order information: a new paradigm and tests of a timing-signal hypothesis. *Quarterly Journal of Experimental Psychology: A, 56,* 1307–1334.

Hepner, I. J., Mohamed, A., Fulham, M. J., & Miller, L. A. (2007). Topographical, autobiographical and semantic memory in a patient with bilateral mesial temporal and retrosplenial infarction. *Neurocase, 13,* 97–114.

Hermsdörfer, J., Terlinden, G., Mühlau, M., Goldenberg, G., & Wohlschläger, A. M. (2007). Neural representations of pantomimed and actual tool use: evidence from an event-related fMRI study. *Neuroimage, 36 Suppl 2,* T109–T118.

Hertz, K., Krogh, A., & Palmer, R. (1991). *Introduction to the theory of neural computation.* Reading, MA.: Addison-Wesley Longman Publ. Co., Inc..

Hess, R. F. & Pointer, J. S. (1989). Spatial and temporal contrast sensitivity in hemianopia. A comparative study of the sighted and blind hemifields. *Brain, 112* (4), 871–894.

Heywood, C. A. & Cowey, A. (1998). With color in mind. *Nature Neuroscience, 1,* 171–173.

Heywood, C. A., Gadotti, A., & Cowey, A. (1992). Cortical area V4 and its role in the perception of color. *Journal of Neuroscience, 12,* 4056–4065.

Hick, W. E. (1952). On the rate of gain of information. *Quarterly Journal of Experimental Psychology, 4,* 11–26.

Hickok, G. & Poeppel, D. (2004). Dorsal and ventral streams: a framework for understanding aspects of the functional anatomy of language. *Cognition, 92,* 67–99.

Hilgard, E. R. (1948). *Theories of Learning.* New York: Appleton-Century-Crofts. Hyland.

Hillis, A. E. & Caramazza, A. (1989). The graphemic buffer and attentional mechanisms. *Brain and Language, 36,* 208–235.

Hillis, A. E. & Caramazza, A. (1991). Category-specific naming and comprehension impairment: a double dissociation. *Brain, 114,* 2081–2094.

Hillis, A., Rapp, B., Romani, C., & Caramazza, A. (1990). Selective impairment of semantics in lexical processing. *Cognitive Neuropsychology, 7,* 191–243.

Hillis, A. E., Rapp, B. C., & Caramazza, A. (1999). When a rose is a rose in speech but a tulip in writing. *Cortex, 35,* 337–356.

Hillyard, S. & Picton, T. (1987). Electrophysiology of cognition. In E.Plum (Ed.), *Handbook of physiology: Section 1. The nervous system: Vol. 5. Higher functions of the brain, Pt. 2* (pp. 519–584). Bethesda, MD: Waverly Press.

Hillyard, S., Hink, R., Schwent, V., & Picton, T. (1973). Electrical signs of selective attention in the human brain. *Science, 182,* 177–179.

Hinton, G. E. (1989). Connectionist Learning Procedures. *Artificial Intelligence, 40,* 185–234.

Hinton, G.E. (2010). Learning to represent visual input. *Philosophical Transactions of the Royal Society, B, 365,* 177–184.

Hinton, G. & Sejnowski, T. J. (1983). Optimal perceptual inference. In *Proceedings of the IEEE conference on computer vision and pattern recognition.* Washington DC.

Hinton, G. & Sejnowski, T. (1986). Learning and relearning in Boltzmann Machines. In D.Rumelhart & J. McClelland (Eds), *Parallel distributed processing:*

explorations in the microstructure of cognition. Volume 1: Foundations (pp. 282-317). Cambridge, MA: MIT Press.

Hinton, G. & Shallice, T. (1991). Lesioning an attractor network: Iivestigations of acquired dyslexia. *Psychological Review, 98*, 74-95.

Hinton, G., Sejnowski, T., & Ackley, D. (1984). Boltzmann machines: costraint satisfaction systems that learn. *Technical Report CMU-CS-84-119*.

Hinton, G. E., Osindero, S., & Teh, Y. (2006). A fast learning algorithm for deep belief nets. *Neural Computation, 18*(7), 1527-1554.

Hirano, M., Noguchi, K., Hosokawa, T., & Takayama, T. (2002). I cannot remember, but I know my past events: remembering and knowing in a patient with amnesic syndrome. *Journal of Clinical and Experimental Neuropsychology, 24*, 548-555.

Hockey, G. (1993). Cognitive energetical control mechanism in the management of work demands and psychological health. In AD.Baddeley & L. Weiskrantz (Eds), *Attention: selection, awareness, and control: a tribute to Donald Broadbent* (pp. 328-345). Oxford, England: Clarendon Press/Oxford.

Hodges, A. (1983). *Alan Turing: the enigma*. New York: Simon & Shuster.

Hodges, J. R. & Graham, K. S. (2001). Episodic memory: insights from semantic dementia. *Philosophical Transactions of the Royal Society, B, 356*, 1423-1434.

Hodges, J. R. & Miller, B. (2001a). The classification, genetics and neuropathology of frontotemporal dementia. Introduction to the special topic papers: Part I. *Neurocase, 7*, 31-35.

Hodges, J. R. & Miller, B. (2001b). The neuropsychology of frontal variant frontotemporal dementia and semantic dementia. Introduction to the special topic papers: Part II. *Neurocase, 7*, 113-121.

Hodges, J. R., Patterson, K., Oxbury, S., & Funnel, E. (1992). Semantic dementia. Progressive fluent aphasia with temporal lobe atrophy. *Brain, 115*, 1783-1806.

Hodges, J. R., Patterson, K., & Tyler, L. K. (1994). Loss of semantic memory: implications for the modularity of mind. *Cognitive Neuropsychology, 11*(5), 505-542.

Hodges, J. R., Graham, N., & Patterson, K. (1995). Charting the progression in semantic dementia. *Memory, 3*, 463-495.

Holdstock, J. S., Parslow, D. M., Morris, R. G., Fleminger, S., Abrahams, S., Denby, C. et al. (2008). Two case studies illustrating how relatively selective hippocampal lesions in humans can have quite different effects on memory. *Hippocampus, 18*, 679-691.

Holender, D. (1986). Semantic activation without conscious identification in dichotic listening, parafoveal vision, and visual masking: A survey and reappraisal. *Behavioral and Brain Sciences, 9*, 1-23.

Hopfield, J. J. (1982). Neural Networks and Physical Systems with Emergent Collective Computational Abilities. *Proceedings of the National Academy of Sciences, USA, 79*, 2554-2558.

Horel, J. (1978). The neuroanatomy of amnesia: a critique of the hippocampal memory hypothesis. *Brain, 101*, 403-445.

Horner, A. J. & Henson, R. N. (2008). Priming, response learning and repetition suppression. *Neuropsychologia, 46*, 1979-1991.

Houghton, G. (1990). The problem of serial order: aneural model of sequence learning and recall. In R. Dale, C. Mellish, & M. Zock (Eds), *Current research in natural language generation.* London: Academic Press.

Houghton, G. & Tipper, S. P. (1996). Inhibitory mechanisms of neural and cognitive control: applications to selective attention and sequential action. *Brain and Cognition, 30*(1), 20-43.

Houghton, G., Glasspool, D. W., & Shallice, T. (1994). Spelling and serial recall: Insights from a competitive queuing model. In G.Brown & N. Ellis (Eds), *Handbook of spelling: theory, process and intervention* (pp. 367-404). Chichester: John Wiley and Sons.

Howard, D. (1995). Lexical anomia: or the case of the missing lexical entries. *Quarterly Journal of Experimental Psychology, 48A*, 999-1023.

Howard, D. & Best, W. (1996). Developmental phonological dyslexia: real word reading can be completely normal. *Cognitive Neuropsychology, 13*, 887-934.

Howard, D. & Franklin, S. (1988). *Missing the meaning?* Cambridge, MA: MIT Press.

Howard, D. & Nickels, L. (2005). Separating input and output phonology: Semantic, phonological, and orthographic effects in short-term memory impairment. *Cognitive Neuropsychology, 22*, 42-77.

Howard, D. & Patterson, K. (1992). *Pyramids and palm trees: a test of semantic access from pictures and words.* Bury St Edmunds: Thames Valley.

Howes, A., Lewis, R. L., & Vera, A. (2009). Rational adaptation under task and processing constraints: implications for testing theories of cognition and action. *Psychological Review, 116*, 717-751.

Hubel, D. H. & Wiesel, T. N. (1961). Integrative action in the cat's lateral geniculate body. *Journal of Physiology, 155*, 385-398.

Hubel, D. H. & Wiesel, T. N. (1962). Receptive fields, binocular interaction and functional architecture in the cat's visual cortex. *Journal of Physiology, 160*, 106-154.

Huettel, S. A. & McCarthy, G. (2000). Evidence for a refractory period in the hemodynamic response to visual stimuli as measured by MRI. *Neuroimage, 11*, 547-553.

Huettel, S. A., Song, A. W., & McCarthy, G. (2009). *Functional magnetic resonance imaging* (2nd edn). Sunderland, MA: Sinauer Associates.

Hull, C. L. (1920). Quantitative aspects of the evolution of concepts. *Psychological Monographs, 28,* 1–86.

Hull, C. L. (1943). *Principles of behavior, an introduction of behavior theory.* New York: D. Appleton-Century.

Humphrey, G. (1951). *Thinking: an introduction to its experimental psychology.* London: Methuen.

Humphrey, N. K. (1970). What the frog's eye tells the monkey's brain. *Brain, Behavior Evolution, 3,* 324–337.

Humphreys, G. W. & Forde, E. M. (1998). Disordered action schemas and action disorganisation syndrome. *Cognitive Neuropsychology, 15,* 771–811.

Humphreys, G. W. & Forde, E. M. (2001). Hierarchies, similarity, and interactivity in object recognition: 'category-specific' neuropsychological deficits. *Behavioral and Brain Sciences, 24,* 453–476.

Humphries, C., Willard, K., Buchsbaum, B., & Hickok, G. (2001). Role of anterior temporal cortex in auditory sentence comprehension: an fMRI study. *Neuroreport, 12,* 1749–1752.

Huttenlocher, J. (1968). Constracting spatial images: a strategy in reasoning. *Psychological Review, 4,* 277–299.

Hyman, R. (1953). Stimulus information as a determinant of reaction time. *Journal of Experimental Psychology, 45,* 188–196.

Imamizu, H., Kuroda, T., Miyauchi, S., Yoshioka, T., & Kawato, M. (2003). Modular organization of internal models of tools in the human cerebellum. *Proceedings of the National Academy of Sciences, U.S.A, 100,* 5461–5466.

Incisa della Rocchetta, A., Cipolotti, L., & Warrington, E. K. (1998). Countries: their selective impairment and selective preservation. *Neurocase, 4,* 99–109.

Indefrey, P. & Levelt, W. (2004). The neural correlates of language production. In M.Gazzaniga (Ed.), *The cognitive neurosciences* (2nd edn). Cambridge, MA.

Iriki, A., Tanaka, M., & Iwamura, Y. (1996). Coding of modified body schema during tool use by macaque postcentral neurones. *Neuroreport, 7,* 2325–2330.

Irle, E., Wowra, B., Kunert, H. J., Hampl, J., & Kunze, S. (1992). Memory disturbances following anterior communicating artery rupture. *Annals of Neurology, 31,* 473–480.

Jack, A. I. (1998). *Perceptual awareness in visual masking.* Unpublished doctoral dissertation, University College London.

Jack, A. I. & Shallice, T. (2001). Introspective physicalism as an approach to the science of consciousness. *Cognition, 79,* 161–196.

Jackendoff, R. (1987). *Consciousness and the computational mind.* Cambridge, MA: MIT Press.

Jackendoff, R. (2002). *Foundations of language.* New York: OUP.

Jackendoff, R. & Pinker, S. (2005). The nature of the language faculty and its implications for evolution of language (Reply to Fitch, Hauser, and Chomsky). *Cognition, 97,* 221–225.

Jackson, F. (1986). What Mary didn't know. *Journal of Philosophy, 83,* 291–295.

Jacobs, A. & Grainger, J. (1994). Models of visual word recognition—sampling the state of the art. *Journal of Experimental Psychology: Human Perception Performance, 20,* 1311–1334.

Jacobs, B., Schall, M., Prather, M., Kapler, E., Driscoll, L., Baca, S. et al. (2001). Regional dendritic and spine variation in human cerebral cortex: a quantitative golgi study. *Cerebral Cortex, 11,* 558–571.

Jacobsen, C. F. (1935). Functions of frontal association area in primates. *Archives of Neurology and Psychiatry, 33,* 558–569.

Jacobsen, C. F., Wolfe, J. B., & Jackson, T. A. (1935). An experimental analysis of the frontal association areas in primates. *Journal of Nervous and Mental Disease, 82,* 1–14.

Jacoby, L. L. (1991). A process dissociation framework: separating automatic from intentional uses of memory. *Journal of Memory and Language, 30,* 513–541.

Jaeger, J. J., Lockwood, A. H., Kemmerer, D. L., Valin, R. D. V., Murphy, B. W., & Khalak, H. G. (1996). A positron emission tomographic study of regular and irregular verb morphology in English. *Language, 72*(3), 451–497.

Jahanshahi, M., Profice, P., Brown, R. G., Ridding, M. C., Dirnberger, G., & Rothwell, J. C. (1998). The effects of transcranial magnetic stimulation over the dorsolateral prefrontal cortex on suppression of habitual counting during random number generation. *Brain, 121* (8), 1533–1544.

Jahanshahi, M., Dirnberger, G., Fuller, R., & Frith, C. D. (2000). The role of the dorsolateral prefrontal cortex in random number generation: a study with positron emission tomography. *Neuroimage, 12,* 713–725.

James, W. (1890). *Principles of pychology.* New York: Holt.

Janowsky, J. S., Shimamura, A. P., Kritchevsky, M., & Squire, L. R. (1989). Cognitive impairment following frontal-lobe damage and its relevance to human amnesia. *Behavioral Neuroscience, 103,* 548–560.

Jarvella, R. (1971). Syntactic processing of connected speech. *Journal of Verbal Learning and Verbal Behavior, 10,* 409–416.

Jeannerod, M., & Frak, V. (1999). Mental imaging of motor activity in humans. *Current Opinion in Neurobiology, 9*(6), 735–739.

Jefferies, E., Lambon Ralph, M. A., Jones, R., Bateman, D., & Patterson, K. (2004). Surface dyslexia in semantic dementia: a comparison of the influence of consistency and regularity. *Neurocase, 10,* 290–299.

Jefferies, E. & Lambon Ralph, M. A. (2006). Semantic impairment in stroke aphasia versus semantic dementia: a case-series comparison. *Brain*, *129*, 2132–2147.

Jefferies, E., Patterson, K., & Lambon Ralph, M. A. (2008). Deficits of knowledge versus executive control in semantic cognition: insights from cued naming. *Neuropsychologia*, *46*, 649–658.

Jeffreys, H. (1961). *Theory of probability* (3rd edn). Oxford, UK: OUP.

Jenkins, I. H., Brooks, D. J., Nixon, P. D., Frackowiak, R. S., & Passingham, R. E. (1994). Motor sequence learning: a study with positron emission tomography. *Journal of Neuroscience*, *14*, 3775–3790.

Jetter, W., Poser, U., Freeman, R. B., & Markowitsch, H. J. (1986). A verbal long-term-memory deficit in frontal-lobe damaged patients. *Cortex*, *22*, 229–242.

Jezzard, P. & Clare, S. (1999). Sources of distortion in functional MRI data. *Human Brain Mapping*, *8*, 80–85.

Joanisse, M. F. & Seidenberg, M. S. (1999). Impairments in verb morphology following brain injury: a connectionist model. *Proceedings of the National Academy of Sciences, USA*, *96*, 7592–7597.

Joanisse, M. F. & Seidenberg, M. S. (2005). Imaging the past: neural activation in frontal and temporal regions during regular and irregular past-tense processing. *Cognitive Affective and Behavioral Neurosciences*, *5*, 282–296.

John, B. (1988). *Contributions to engineering models of human-computer interaction (vol. i and ii)*. Unpublished PhD Thesis. Department of Psychology, CMU.

John, B. E. & Newell, A. (1987) Predicting the time to recall computer command abbreviations. In *proceedings of CHI+GI, 1987* (Toronto, April 5-9, 1987) ACM, New York, 33–40.

Johnson-Frey, S. H. (2003a). Cortical representations of human tool use. In S. H. Johnson-Frey (Ed.), *Taking action: cognitive neuroscience perspectives on intential acts* (pp. 185–217). MIT Press.

Johnson-Frey, S. H. (2003b). What's so special about human tool use? *Neuron*, *39*, 201–204.

Johnson-Frey, S. H., Newman-Norlund, R., & Grafton, S. T. (2005). A distributed left hemisphere network active during planning of everyday tool use skills. *Cerebral Cortex*, *15*, 681–695.

Johnson-Laird, P. N. (1983). *Mental models: towards a cognitive science of language, inference and consciousness*. Cambridge, England: Cambridge University Press.

Johnson-Laird, P. N. (2006). *How we reason*. Oxford, England: Oxford University Press.

Johnson-Laird, P. N., & Steedman, M. (1978). The psychology of syllogisms. *Cognitive Psychology*, *10*(1), 64–99.

Johnson-Laird, P. N., Legrenzi, P., & Legrenzi, M. (1972). Reasoning and a sense of reality. *British Journal of Psychology*, *63*, 395–400.

Jones, C. R., Rosenkranz, K., Rothwell, J. C., & Jahanshahi, M. (2004). The right dorsolateral prefrontal cortex is essential in time reproduction: an investigation with repetitive transcranial magnetic stimulation. *Experimental Brain Research*, *158*, 366–372.

Jones, G. (1985). Deep dyslexia, imageability, and ease of predication. *Brain and Language*, *24*, 1–19.

Jones, T., Chesler, D. A., & Ter-Pogossian, M. M. (1976). The continuous inhalation of oxygen-15 for assessing regional oxygen extraction in the brain of man. *British Journal of Radiology*, *49*, 339–343.

Jones, W. H. S. (1923). *Hippocrates*, vol 2. New York, Putnam.

Jonides, J., Schumacher, E. H., Smith, E. E., Koeppe, R. A., Awh, E., Reuter-Lorenz, P. A. et al. (1998). The role of parietal cortex in verbal working memory. *Journal of Neuroscience*, *18*, 5026–5034.

Jonides, J., Smith, E. E., Koeppe, R. A., Awh, E., Minoshima, S., & Mintun, M. A. (1993). Spatial working memory in humans as revealed by PET. *Nature*, *363*, 623–625.

Jónsdóttir, M. K., Shallice, T., & Wise, R. (1996). Phonological mediation and the graphemic buffer disorder in spelling: cross-language differences? *Cognition*, *59*, 169–197.

Joshi, A.K. & Schabes, Y. (1997). Tree-adjoining grammars. In G. Rosenberg & A. Salomaa (Eds), *Handbook of formal languages, vol. 3: beyond words* (pp. 69–121). Berlin: Springer-Verlag.

Jung-Beeman, M., Bowden, E. M., Haberman, J., Frymiare, J. L., rambel-Liu, S., Greenblatt, R. et al. (2004). Neural activity when people solve verbal problems with insight. *PLoS.Biol.*, *2*, E97.

Just, M.A. & Carpenter, P. (1987). *The psychology of reading and language comprehension*. Newton, MA: Allyn & Bacon.

Just, M. A. & Carpenter, P. A. (1992). A capacity theory of comprehension: individual differences in working memory. *Psychological Review*, *99*, 122–149.

Just, M. A. & Varma, S. (2007). The organization of thinking: what functional brain imaging reveals about the neuroarchitecture of complex cognition. *Cognitive, Affective and Behavioral Neuroscience*, *7*, 153–191.

Just, M. A., Carpenter, P. A., Keller, T. A., Eddy, W. F., & Thulborn, K. R. (1996). Brain activation modulated by sentence comprehension. *Science*, *274*, 114.

Just, M. A., Carpenter, P. A., Keller, T. A., Emery, L., Zajac, H., & Thulborn, K. R. (2001). Interdependence of nonoverlapping cortical systems in dual cognitive tasks. *Neuroimage*, *14*, 417–426.

Kahneman, D. & Tversky, A. (1973). On the psychology of prediction. *Psychological Review*, *80*, 237–251.

Kanai, R., Tsuchiya, N., & Verstraten, F. A. (2006). The scope and limits of top-down attention in unconscious visual processing. *Current Biology*, *16*, 2332–2336.

Kane, M. J., Conway, A. R. A., Miura, T. K., & Colflesh, G. J. H. (2007). Working memory, attention control, and the N-back task: a question of construct validity. *Journal of Experimental Psychology: Learning Memory and Cognition*, *33*, 615–622.

Kanerva, P. (1989). *Sparse distributed memory*. Cambridge, MA: MIT Press.

Kanwisher, N. (2001). Neural events and perceptual awareness. *Cognition*, *79*, 89–113.

Kanwisher, N., McDermott, J., & Chun, M. M. (1997). The fusiform face area: a module in human extrastriate cortex specialized for face perception. *Journal of Neuroscience*, *17*, 4302–4311.

Kapur, N. (1993). Focal retrograde amnesia in neurological disease: a critical review. *Cortex*, *29*, 217–234.

Kapur, N. (1996). The 'Petites Madeleines' phenomenon in two amnesic patients: sudden recovery of forgotten memories [Letter]. *Brain*, *119*, 1401–1403.

Kapur, N. (1999). Syndromes of retrograde amnesia: a conceptual and empirical synthesis. *Psychological Bulletin*, *125*, 800–825.

Kapur, S., Craik, F. I., Tulving, E., Wilson, A. A., Houle, S., & Brown, G. M. (1994). Neuroanatomical correlates of encoding in episodic memory: levels of processing effect. *Proceedings of the National Academy of Sciences, USA*, *91*, 2008–2011.

Karlin, L. (1959). Reaction time as a function of foreperiod duration and variability. *Journal of Experimental Psychology*, *58*, 185–191.

Karnath, H. O. & Perenin, M. T. (2005). Cortical control of visually guided reaching: evidence from patients with optic ataxia. *Cerebral Cortex*, *15*, 1561–1569.

Karnath, H. O., Ferber, S., & Himmelbach, M. (2001). Spatial awareness is a function of the temporal not the posterior parietal lobe. *Nature*, *411*, 950–953.

Kartsounis, L., Rudge, P., & Stevens, J. (1995). Bilateral lesions of CA1 and CA2 fields of the hippocampus are sufficient to cause a severe amnesic syndrome in humans. *Journal of Neurology, Neurosurgery and Psychiatry*, *59*, 95–98.

Katona, G. (1940). *Organizing and memorizing*. New York: Columbia University Press.

Katz, B. (1980). A three-step procedure for language generation. *MIT Artificial Intelligence Laboratory Memo*, *599*.

Katz, J. & Fodor, J. (1963). The structure of a semantic theory. *Language*, *39*, 170–210.

Katz, R. B. (1991). Limited retention of information in the graphemic buffer. *Cortex*, *27*, 111–119.

Kavé, G., Ze'ev, H. B., & Lev, A. (2007). Morphological processing with deficient phonological short-term memory. *Cognitive Neuropsychology*, *24*, 516–534.

Kawato, M. (1999). Internal models for motor control and trajectory planning. *Current Opinion in Neurobiology*, *9*, 718–727.

Kay, P. (2000). Comprehension deficits of Broca's aphasics provide no evidence for traces. *Behavioral and Brain Sciences*, *23*(1), 37–38.

Kay, J. and Hanley, R. (1991). Simultaneous form perception and serial letter recognition in a case of letter-by-letter reading. *Cognitive Neuropsychology*, *8*, 249–273.

Kay, J. & Hanley, R. (1994). Peripheral disorders of spelling: The role of the graphemic buffer. In G. Brown & N. Ellis (Eds), *Handbook of Spelling: Theory, Process and Intervention* (pp. 295–315). Chichester: Wiley.

Kayser, C. & Logothetis, N.K. (2010). The electrophysiological background of the fMRI signal. In S. Ulmer & O. Jansen (Eds), *fMRI: basic and clinical applications* (pp. 23–33). Berlin: Springer.

Kellenbach, M., Brett, M., & Patterson, K. (2003). Actions speak louder than functions: the importance of manipulability and action in tool representation. *Journal of Cognitive Neuroscience*, *15*, 30–46.

Kello, C. (2003). The emergence of a double dissociation in the modulation of a single control parameter in a nonlinear dynamical system. *Cortex*, *39*, 132–134.

Kello, C. & Plaut, D. (2003). Strategic control over rate of processing in word reading: A computational investigation. *Journal of Memory and Language*, *48*, 207–232.

Kello, C., Sibley, D., & Plaut, D. (2005). Dissociations in performance on novel versus irregular items: Single-route demonstrations with input gain in localist and distributed models. *Cognitive Science*, *29*, 627–654.

Kennedy, D. N., Lange, N., Makris, N., Bates, J., Meyer, J., & Caviness, V. S., Jr. (1998). Gyri of the human neocortex: an MRI-based analysis of volume and variance. *Cerebral Cortex*, *8*, 372–384.

Kennerley, S. W., Sakai, K., & Rushworth, M. (2004). Organization of action sequences and the role of the pre-SMA. *Journal of Neurophysiology*, *91*(2), 978–993.

Kentridge, R., Heywood, C., & Weiskrantz, L. (1997). Residual vision in multiple retinal locations within a scotoma: implications for blindsight. *Journal of Cognitive Neuroscience*, *9*, 191–202.

Kerns, J. G., Cohen, J. D., MacDonald, A. W., III, Cho, R. Y., Stenger, V. A., & Carter, C. S. (2004). Anterior cingulate conflict monitoring and adjustments in control. *Science*, *303*, 1023–1026.

Kersten, D., Mamassian, P., & Yuille, A. (2004). Object perception as Bayesian inference. *Annual Review of Psychology*, *55*, 271–304.

Kertesz, A., Davidson, W., & McCabe, P. (1998). Primary progressive semantic aphasia: a case study. *Jounral of the International Neuropsychological Society*, 4, 388–398.

Kesner, R. P., Gilbert, P. E., & Barua, L. A. (2002). The role of the hippocampus in memory for the temporal order of a sequence of odors. *Behavioral Neuroscience*, 116, 286–290.

Kilpatrick, C., Murrie, V., Cook, M., Andrewes, D., Desmond, P. & Hopper, J. (1997). Degree of hippocampal atrophy correlates with severity of neuropsychological deficits. *Seizure*, 6, 213–218.

Kim, H., Na, D. L., & Park, E. S. (2007). Intransigent vowel-consonant position in Korean dysgraphia: evidence of spatial-constructive representation. *Behavioural Neurology*, 18, 91–97.

Kim, J. J. & Fanselow, M. S. (1992). Modality-specific retrograde amnesia of fear. *Science*, 256, 675–677.

Kimberg, D. & Farah, M. (1993). A unified account of cognitive impairments following frontal lobe damage: The role of working memory in complex, organized behaviour. *Journal of Experimental Psychology: General*, 122, 411–428.

Kinder, A. & Shanks, D. R. (2003). Neuropsychological dissociations between priming and recognition: a single-system connectionist account. *Psychological Review*, 110, 728–744.

Kinsbourne, M. (1988). Integrated field theory of consciousness. In *Consciousness in contemporary science.* (pp. 239–256). New York, NY: Clarendon Press/OUP.

Kinsbourne, M. & Warrington, E. (1962). A variety of reading disability associated with right hemisphere lesions. *Journal of Neurology, Neurosurgery and Psychiatry*, 25, 339–344.

Kinsbourne, M. & Wood, F. (1975). Short-term memory and the amnesic syndrome. In D.Deutsch & J. Deutsch (Eds), *Short-term memory.* (pp. 257–291). New York: Academic Press.

Kintsch, W., Healy, A., Hegarty, M., Pennington, B., & Salthouse, T. (1999). Eight questions and some general issues. In A. Miyake & P. Shah (Eds), *Models of working memory: mechanisms of active maintenance and executive control* (pp. 62–101). Cambridge: CUP.

Kitazawa, S., Kimura, T., & Yin, P. B. (1998). Cerebellar complex spikes encode both destinations and errors in arm movements. *Nature*, 392, 494–497.

Klauer, K. C. & Zhao, Z. (2004). Double dissociations in visual and spatial short-term memory. *Journal of Experimental Psychology: General*, 133, 355–381.

Kleinschmidt, A., Büchel, C., Hutton, C., Friston, K. J., & Frackowiak, R. S. (2002). The neural structures expressing perceptual hysteresis in visual letter recognition. *Neuron*, 34(4), 659–666.

Knoblich, G., Ohlsson, S., Haider, H., & Rhenius, D. (1999). Constraint relaxation and chunk decomposition in insight problem solving. *Journal of Experimental Psychology: Learning, Memory and Cognition*, 25, 1534–1556.

Koch, G., Oliveri, M., Torriero, S., & Caltagirone, C. (2003). Underestimation of time perception after repetitive transcranial magnetic stimulation. *Neurology*, 60, 1844–1846.

Koechlin, E. & Jubault, T. (2006). Broca's area and the hierarchical organization of human behavior. *Neuron*, 50, 963–974.

Koechlin, E. & Summerfield, C. (2007). An information theoretical approach to prefrontal executive function. *Trends in Cognitive Sciences*, 11, 229–235.

Koechlin, E., Basso, G., Pietrini, P., Panzer, S., & Grafman, J. (1999). The role of the anterior prefrontal cortex in human cognition. *Nature*, 399, 148–151.

Koechlin, E., Ody, C., & Kouneiher, F. (2003). The architecture of cognitive control in the human prefrontal cortex. *Science*, 302, 1181–1185.

Koffka, K. (1935). *The principles of gestal psychology.* New York: Harcourt, Brace.

Kolodner, J. (1985). Memory for experience. *The Psychology of Learning and Motivation*, 19, 1–57.

Konorski, J. & Lawicka, W. (1964). Analysis of errors by prefrontal animals on the delayed response test. In J. M. Warren & K. Akert (Eds), *The frontal granular cortex and behavior* (pp. 271–294). New York: McGraw-Hill.

Koriat, A., & Goldsmith, M. (1996). Monitoring and control processes in the strategic regulation of memory accuracy. *Psychological Review*, 103(3), 490–517.

Kornhuber, H. H. & Deecke, L. (1965). Hirnpotentialanderungen bei Willkurbewegungen und Passiven Bewegungen des Menschen - Bereitschaftspotential und Reafferente Potentiale. *Pflugers Archiv fur Die Gesamte Physiologie des Menschen und der Tiere*, 284, 1–17.

Kosslyn, S.M. & Intriligator, J.M. (1992). Is cognitive neuropsychology plausible? The perils of sitting on a one-legged stool. *Journal of Cognitive Neuroscience*, 4, 96–107.

Kosslyn, S. M., Koenig, O., Barrett, A., Cave, C. B., Tang, J., & Gabrieli, J. D. (1989). Evidence for two types of spatial representations: hemispheric specialization for categorical and coordinate relations. *Journal of Experimental Psychology: Human Perception and Performance*, 15, 723–735.

Kosslyn, S. M., Chabris, C. F., Marsolek, C. J., & Koenig, O. (1992). Categorical versus coordinate spatial relations: computational analyses and computer simulations. *Journal of Experimental Psychology: Human Perception and Performance*, 18, 562–577.

Kosslyn, S. M., Thompson, W. L., & Alpert, N. M. (1997). Neural systems shared by visual imagery and visual perception: a positron emission tomography study. *Neuroimage*, 6, 320–334.

Kouider, S. & Dehaene, S. (2007). Levels of processing during non-conscious perception: a critical review of visual masking. *Philosophical Transactions of the Royal Society B: Biological Sciences*, *362*, 857–875.

Kouider, S., Dehaene, S., Jobert, A., & Le Bihan, D. (2007). Cerebral bases of subliminal and supraliminal priming during reading. *Cerebral Cortex*, *17*(9), 2019-2029.

Kouneiher, F., Charron, S., & Koechlin, E. (2009). Motivation and cognitive control in the human prefrontal cortex. *Nature Neuroscience*, *12*, 939-945.

Kounios, J., Frymiare, J. L., Bowden, E. M., Fleck, J. I., Subramaniam, K., Parrish, T. B. et al. (2006). The prepared mind: neural activity prior to problem presentation predicts subsequent solution by sudden insight. *Psychological Science*, *17*, 882–890.

Kozel, F. A., Johnson, K. A., Mu, Q., Grenesko, E. L., Laken, S. J., & George, M. S. (2005). Detecting deception using functional magnetic resonance imaging. *Biological Psychiatry*, *58*, 605–613.

Kraeplin, E. (1910). *Ein Lehrbuch fur Studirende und Aerzte*. Leipzig: Barth.

Kremin, H. (1982). Alexia: Theory and research. In R.Malatesha & P. Aaron (Eds), *Reading disorders: varieties and treatments.* New York: Academic Press.

Kristjansson, A., Vuilleumier, P., Schwartz, S., Macaluso, E., & Driver, J. (2007). Neural basis for priming of pop-out during visual search revealed with fMRI. *Cerebral Cortex*, *17*, 1612–1624.

Kropff, E. & Treves, A. (2008). Semantic cognition: Distributed, but then attractive. *Behavioral and Brain Sciences*, *31*, 718–719.

Kuffler, S. W. (1953). Discharge patterns and functional organization of mammalian retina. *Journal of Neurophysiology*, *16*, 37–68.

Kurbat, M. & Farah, M. (1998). Is the category-specific deficit for living things spurious? *Journal of Cognitive Neuroscience*, *10*, 355–361.

Kwong, K. K., Belliveau, J. W., Chesler, D. A., Goldberg, I. E., Weisskoff, R. M., Poncelet, B. P. et al. (1992). Dynamic magnetic resonance imaging of human brain activity during primary sensory stimulation. *Proceedings of the National Academy of Sciences, USA*, *89*, 5675–5679.

Làdavas, E., Shallice, T., & Zanella, M. T. (1997a). Preserved semantic access in neglect dyslexia. *Neuropsychologia*, *35*, 257–270.

Làdavas, E., Umiltà, C., & Mapelli, D. (1997b). Lexical and semantic processing in the absence of word reading: evidence from neglect dyslexia. *Neuropsychologia*, *35*, 1075–1085.

Laiacona, M., Barbarotto, R., & Capitani, E. (1993). Perceptual and associative knowledge in category specific impairment of semantic memory: a study of two cases. *Cortex*, *29*, 727–740.

Laiacona, M., Capitani, E., & Barbarotto, R. (1997). Semantic category dissociations: a longitudinal study of two cases. *Cortex*, *33*, 441–461.

Laine, M., Rinne, J. O., Krause, B. J., Teras, M., & Sipila, H. (1999). Left hemisphere activation during processing of morphologically complex word forms in adults. *Neuroscience Letters*, *271*, 85–88.

Laird J. (2008). Extending the Soar cognitive architecture. In P. Wang & S. Franklin (Eds), *Artificial general intelligence, 2008: proceedings of the First AGI Conference.* IOS Press.

Laird, J., Newell, A., & Rosenbloom, P. (1987). SOAR: an architecture for general intelligence. *Artificial Intelligence*, *33*, 1–64.

Lakatos, I. (1970). Falsification and the methodology of scientific research programmes. In I. Lakatos & A. Musgrave (Eds), *Criticism and the growth of knowledge.* Cambridge: CUP.

Lambie, J. A. (2009). Emotion experience, rational action, and self-knowledge. *Emotion Review*, *1*(3), 272–280.

Lambie, J. A., & Marcel, A. J. (2002). Consciousness and the varieties of emotion experience: a theoretical framework. *Psychological Review*, *109*(2), 219–259.

Lambon Ralph, M. A. (1998). Distributed versus localist representations: evidence from a study of item consistency in a case of classical anomia. *Brain and Language*, *64*, 339–360.

Lambon Ralph, M. A. (2004). Reconnecting cognitive neuropsychology: commentary on Harley's does cognitive neuropsychology have a future? *Cognitive Neuropsychology*, *21*, 31–35.

Lambon Ralph, M. A., Ellis, A., & Franklin, S. (1995). Semantic loss without surface dyslexia. *Neurocase*, *1*, 363–369.

Lambon Ralph, M. A., Ellis, A., & Sage, K. (1998). Word meaning blindness revisited. *Cognitive Neuropsychology*, *15*, 389–400.

Lambon Ralph, M. A., McClelland, J. L., Patterson, K., Galton, C. J., & Hodges, J. R. (2001). No right to speak? The relationship between object naming and semantic impairment: neuropsychological evidence and a computational model. *Journal of Cognitive Neuroscience*, *13*, 341–356.

Lambon Ralph, M. A., Patterson, K., Garrard, P., & Hodges, J. (2003). Semantic dementia with category-specificity: a comparative case-series study. *Cognitive Neuropsychology*, *20*, 307–326.

Lambon Ralph, M. A., Lowe, C., & Rogers, T. T. (2007). Neural basis of category-specific semantic deficits for living things: evidence from semantic dementia, HSVE and a neural network model. *Brain*, *130*, 1127–1137.

Laming, D. (1997). *The measurement of sensation*. Oxford.: Oxford University Press.

Lamme, V. A. F. (2006). Towards a true neural stance on consciousness. *Trends in Cognitive Sciences*, *10*, 494–501.

Lamme, V. A. F. & Roelfsema, P. R. (2000). The distinct modes of vision offered by feedforward and recurrent processing. *Trends in Neurosciences*, *23*(11), 571–579.

Land, M., Mennie, N., & Rustead, J. (1999). The roles of vision and eye movements in the control of activities of daily living. *Perception*, *28*, 1311–1328. 564–574.

Lappin, S., Levine, R. D., & Johnson, D. E. (2000). The structure of unscientific revolutions. *Natural Language & Linguistic Theory*, *18*, 665–671.

LaRock, E. (2006). Why neural synchrony fails to explain the unity of visual consciousness. *Behavior and Philosophy*, *34*, 39–58.

LaRock, E. (2007). Disambiguation, binding, and the unity of visual consciousness. *Theory & Psychology*, *17*(6), 747–777.

Lassalle, J. M., Bataille, T., & Halley, H. (2000). Reversible inactivation of the hippocampal mossy fiber synapses in mice impairs spatial learning, but neither consolidation nor memory retrieval, in the Morris navigation task. *Neurobiology of Learning and Memory*, *73*, 243–257.

Lau, H. C. & Passingham, R. E. (2006). Relative blindsight in normal observers and the neural correlate of visual consciousness. *Proceedings of the National Academy of Sciences, USA*, *49*, 18763–18768.

Lau, H. C., & Passingham, R. E. (2007). Unconscious activation of the cognitive control system in the human prefrontal cortex. *Journal of Neuroscience*, *27*(21), 5805–5811.

Lauro-Grotto, R., Piccini, C., & Shallice, T. (1997). Modality-specific operations in semantic dementia. *Cortex*, *33*, 593–622.

Lavie, N. (1995). Perceptual load as a necessary condition for selective attention. *Journal of Experimental Psychology Human Perception Performance*, *21*, 380–391.

Laws, K. R. (2005). 'Illusions of normality': a methodological critique of category-specific naming. *Cortex*, *41*, 842–851.

Laws, K. & Neve, C. (1999). A 'normal' category-specific advantage for naming living things. *Neuropsychologia*, *37*, 1263–1269.

Laws, K. R. & Sartori, G. (2005). Category deficits and paradoxical dissociations in Alzheimer's disease and Herpes Simplex Encephalitis. *Journal of Cognitive Neuroscience*, *17*, 1453–1459.

Laws, K. R., Evans, J., Hodges, J., & McCarthy, R. (1995). Naming without knowing and appearance without associations: evidence for constructive processes in semantic memory? *Memory*, *3*, 409–433.

Laws, K. R., Gale, T. M., Leeson, V. C., & Crawford, J. R. (2005). When is category-specific in Alzheimer's disease. *Cortex*, *41*, 452–463.

Lebière, C., & Anderson, J. R. (1993). A connectionist implementation of the ACT-R production system. In *Proceedings of the Fifteenth Annual Meeting of the Cognitive Science Society*, pp. 635–640. Hillsdale, NJ: Erlbaum.

Lee, C. & Estes, W. (1981). Item and order information in short-term memory: evidence for multilevel perturbation processes. *Journal of Experimental Psychology: Learning, Memory and Cognition*, *7*, 149–169.

Lee, F. & Anderson, J. R. (2001). Does learning of a complex task have to be complex? A study in learning decomposition. *Cognitive Psychology*, *42*, 267–316.

Lee, I. & Kesner, R. P. (2004). Encoding versus retrieval of spatial memory: double dissociation between the dentate gyrus and the perforant path inputs into CA3 in the dorsal hippocampus. *Hippocampus*, *14*, 66–76.

Leech, R., Mareschal, D., & Cooper, R. P. (2008). Analogy as relational priming: a developmental and computational perspective on the origins of a complex cognitive skill. *Behavioral and Brain Sciences*, *31*, 357–378.

Legate, J. A. (2002). *Warlpiri: theoretical implications*. PhD thesis. MIT.

Lehmkuhl, G. & Poeck, K. (1981). A disturbance in the conceptual organization of actions in patients with ideational apraxia. *Cortex*, *17*, 153–158.

Leng, N. R. & Parkin, A. J. (1988). Double dissociation of frontal dysfunction in organic amnesia. *British Journal of Clinical Psychology*, *27* (4), 359–362.

Lengyel. M. & Dayan, P. (2008). Hippocampal contributions to control: the third way. *Advances in Neural Information Processing*, *20*, 889–896.

Leonard, J. (1959). Tactual choice reactions: Part I. *Quarterly Journal of Experimental Psychology*, *11*, 76–83.

Leopold, D. A. & Logothetis, N. K. (1996). Activity changes in early visual cortex reflect monkeys' percepts during binocular rivalry. *Nature*, *379*, 549–553.

Lepage, M., Habib, R., & Tulving, E. (1998). Hippocampal PET activations of memory encoding and retrieval: the HIPER model. *Hippocampus*, *8*, 313–322.

Lepage, M., Ghaffar, O., Nyberg, L., & Tulving, E. (2000). Prefrontal cortex and episodic memory retrieval mode. *Proceedngs of the National Academy of Sciences, USA*, *97*, 506–511.

Leslie, A. M. & Frith, U. (1988). Autistic childrens understanding of seeing, knowing and believing. *British Journal of Developmental Psychology*, *6*, 315–324.

Lettvin, J., Maturana, H., McCulloch, W., & Pitts, W. (1959). What the frog's eye tells the frog's brain. *Proceedings of the Institute of Radio Engineers*, *47*, 1950–1961.

Levelt, W. (1989). *Speaking: From intention to articulation*. Cambridge, MA: MIT Press.

Levelt, W., Roelofs, A., & Meyer, A. (1999). A theory of lexical access in speech production. *Behavioral and Brain Sciences*, *22*, 1–38.

Levin, E. D. (2006). *Neurotransmitter interactions and cognitive function*. Birkhauser-Verlag / Springer.

Levine, B., Svoboda, E., Hay, J. F., Winocur, G., & Moscovitch, M. (2002). Aging and autobiographicla memory: dissociating episodic from semantic retrieval. *Psychology and Aging*, *17*, 677–689.

Levy, B. A. (1971). Role of articulation in auditory and visual short-term memory. *Journal of Verbal Learning and Verbal Behavior*, *10*, 123–132.

Lewandowsky, S. & Murdock, B. (1989). Memory for serial order. *Psychological Review*, *96*, 25–57.

Lewin, K. (1935). *A dynamic theory of personality*. New York: McGraw-Hill.

Lewis, R. L. & Vasishth, S. (2005). An activation-based model of sentence processing as skilled memory retrieval. *Cognitive Science*, *2*, 375–419.

Lewis, R. L., Vasishth, S., & Van Dyke, J. A. (2006). Computational principles of working memory in sentence comprehension. *Trends in Cognitive Sciences*, *10*(10), 447–454.

Lhermitte, F. (1983). 'Utilization behaviour' and its relation to lesions of the frontal lobes. *Brain*, *106* (2), 237–255.

Libet, B. (1985). Subjective antedating of a sensory experience and mind–brain theories: reply to Honderich (1984). *Journal of Theoretical Biology*, *114*(4), 563–570.

Lichtheim, L. (1885). On aphasia. *Brain*, *7*, 433–484.

Liepmann, H. (1900). Das Krankheitsbild der Apraxie (motorischen Asymbolie) auf Grund eines Falles von einseitiger Apraxie. *Monatsschrift für Psychiatrie und Neurologie*, *8*.

Liepmann, H. (1908). *Die linke Hemisphäre und das Handeln—Drei Aufsätze aus dem Apraxiegebiet*. Berlin: Springer-Verlag.

Liepmann, H. (1920). Apraxia. *Ergebnisse der Gesamten Medizin*, *1*, 516–543.

Lindsay, P. & Norman, D. A. (1977). *Human information processing: an introduction to psychology*. New York: Academic Press.

Linebarger, M. C., Schwartz, M. F., & Saffran, E. M. (1983). Sensitivity to grammatical structure in so-called agrammatic aphasics. *Cognition*, *13*(3), 361–392.

Lingnau, A., Gesierich, B., & Caramazza, A. (2009). Asymmetric fMRI adaptation reveals no evidence for mirror neurons in humans. *Proceedings of the National Academy of Sciences, USA*, *106*(24), 9925–9930.

Locke, J. (1690). *An essay concerning human understanding*. London: Basset.

Lockhart, R. S., Craik, F. I. M., & Jacoby, L. L. (1976). Depth of processing, recognition and recall. In

J. Brown (Ed.), *Recall and recognition* (pp. 75–102). New York: Wiley.

Logan, G. D. (1988). Toward an instance theory of automatization. *Psychological Review*, *95*(4), 492–527.

Logan, G. D. (1990). Repetition priming and automaticity: Common underlying mechanisms? *Cognitive Psychology*, *22*, 1–35.

Logie, R. (1995). *Visuo-Spatial Working Memory*. Hove: LEA.

Logothetis, N. K. (1998). Single units and conscious vision. *Philosophical Transactions of the Royal Society B: Biological Sciences*, *353*(1377), 1801–1818.

Logothetis, N. K. & Schall, J. D. (1989). Neuronal correlates of subjective visual perception. *Science*, *245*, 761–763.

Logothetis, N. K. & Wandell, B. A. (2004). Interpreting the BOLD signal. *Annual Review of Physiology*, *66*, 735–769.

Lombardi, L. & Sartori, G. (2007). Models of relevant cue integration in name retrieval. *Journal of Memory and Language*, *57*, 101–125.

Longworth, C. E., Marslen-Wilson, W. D., Randall, B., & Tyler, L. K. (2005). Getting to the meaning of the regular past tense: evidence from neuropsychology. *Journal of Cognitive Neuroscience*, *17*, 1087–1097.

Los, S. A., Knol, D. L., & Boers, R. M. (2001). The foreperiod effect revisited: conditioning as a basis for nonspecific preparation. *Acta Psychologica*, *106*, 121–145.

Lovett, M. (2002). Modeling selective attention: not just another model of Stroop. *Cognitive Systems Research*, *3*, 67–76.

Lovett, M. (2005). A strategy-based interpretation of Stroop. *Cognitive Science*, *29*, 493–524.

Luce, D. (1959). *Individual choice behavior*. New York: John Wiley and Sons.

Luck, S. J. & Vogel, E. K. (1997). The capacity of visual working memory for features and conjunctions. *Nature*, *390*, 279–281.

Luck, S. J., & Vogel, E. K. (2001). Multiple sources of interference in dual-task performance: The cases of the attentional blink and the psychological refractory period. In *The limits of attention: Temporal constraints in human information processing.* (pp. 124–140). New York, NY, US: Oxford University Press.

Luck, S. J., Vogel, E. K., & Shapiro, K. L. (1996). Word meanings can be accessed but not reported during the attentional blink. *Nature*, *383*, 616–618.

Lück, M., Hahne, A., & Clahsen, H. (2006). Brain potentials to morphologically complex words during listening. *Brain Res.*, *1077*, 144–152.

Lueck, C. J., Zeki, S., Friston, K. J., Deiber, M. P., Cope, P., Cunningham, V. J. et al. (1989). The color center in the cerebral cortex of man. *Nature*, *340*, 386–389.

Lumer, E. D. & Rees, G. (1999). Covariation of activity in visual and prefrontal cortex associated with subjective visual perception. *Proceedings of the National Academy of Sciences, USA, 96*, 1669–1673.

Lumer, E. D., Friston, K. J., & Rees, G. (1998). Neural correlates of perceptual rivalry in the human brain. *Science, 280*, 1930–1934.

Luo, J. & Knoblich, G. (2007). Studying insight problem solving with neuroscientific methods. *Methods, 42*, 77–86.

Luo, J. & Niki, K. (2003). Function of hippocampus in 'insight' of problem solving. *Hippocampus, 13*, 316–323.

Luo, J., Niki, K., & Phillips, S. (2004). Neural correlates of the 'Aha! reaction'. *Neuroreport, 15*, 2013–2017.

Luo, J., Niki, K., & Knoblich, G. (2006). Perceptual contributions to problem solving: chunk decomposition of Chinese characters. *Brain Res.Bull., 70*, 430–443.

Luria, A. (1966). *Higher cortical functions in man*. London: Tavistock.

Luzzatti, C. & Davidoff, J. (1994). Impaired retrieval of object-colour knowledge with preserved colour naming. *Neuropsychologia, 32*, 933–950.

Luzzatti, C., Mondini, S., & Semenza, C. (2001). Lexical representation and processing of morphologically complex words: evidence from the reading performance of an Italian agrammatic patient. *Brain and Language, 79*, 345–359.

Macaluso, E. & Driver, J. (2005). Multisensory spatial interactions: a window onto functional integration in the human brain. *Trends Neurosci., 28*, 264–271.

MacDonald, A. W., III, Cohen, J. D., Stenger, V. A., & Carter, C. S. (2000). Dissociating the role of the dorsolateral prefrontal and anterior cingulate cortex in cognitive control. *Science, 288*, 1835–1838.

MacDonald, M. C., Pearlmutter, N. J., & Seidenberg, M. S. (1994). The lexical nature of syntactic ambiguity resolution. *Psychological Review, 101*, 676–703.

MacGregor, J. N., Ormerod, T. C., & Chronicle, E. P. (2001). Information processing and insight: a process model of performance on the nine-dot and related problems. *Journal of Experimental Psychology: Learning, Memory and Cognition, 27*, 176–201.

Machtynger, J. (2006). *Modelling graphemic buffer disorder: a connectionist approach*. PhD Thesis. Institute of Cognitive Neuroscience, University College London.

MacKay, D. (1970). Spoonerisms: the structure of errors in the serial order of speech. *Neuropsychologia, 8*, 323–350.

MacWhinney, B. & Leinbach, J. (1991). Implementations are not conceptualizations: revising the verb learning model. *Cognition, 40*, 121–157.

Maguire, E. A. (2001). Neuroimaging studies of autobiographical event memory. *Philos.Trans.R.Soc. Lond B Biol.Sci., 356*, 1441–1451.

Maguire, E. A. & Frith, C. D. (2003). Lateral asymmetry in the hippocampal response to the remoteness of autobiographical memories. *Journal of Neuroscience, 23*, 5302–5307.

Maguire, E. A. & Mummery, C. J. (1999). Differential modulation of a common memory retrieval network revealed by positron emission tomography. *Hippocampus, 9*, 54–61.

Maguire, A. & Ogden, J. (2002). MRI brain scan analyses and neuropsychological profiles of nine patients with persistent unilateral neglect. *Neuropsychologia, 40*, 879–887.

Maguire, E. A., Burgess, N., Donnett, J. G., Frackowiak, R. S., Frith, C. D., & O'Keefe, J. (1998). Knowing where and getting there: a human navigation network. *Science, 280*, 921–924.

Maguire, E. A., Gadian, D. G., Johnsrude, I. S., Good, C. D., Ashburner, J., Frackowiak, R. S. et al. (2000). Navigation-related structural change in the hippocampi of taxi drivers. *Proceedings of the National Academy of Sciences, USA, 97*, 4398–4403.

Maguire, E. A., Henson, R. N. A., Mummery, C. J., & Frith, C. D. (2001). Activity in prefrontal cortex, not hippocampus, varies parametrically with the increasing remoteness of memories. *NeuroReport, 12(3)*, 441–444.

Maguire, E. A., Spiers, H. J., Good, C. D., Hartley, T., Frackowiak, R. S., & Burgess, N. (2003). Navigation expertise and the human hippocampus: a structural brain imaging analysis. *Hippocampus, 13*, 250–259.

Maguire, E. A., Nannery, R., & Spiers, H. J. (2006a). Navigation around London by a taxi driver with bilateral hippocampal lesions. *Brain, 129*, 2894–2907.

Maguire, E. A., Woollett, K., & Spiers, H. J. (2006b). London taxi drivers and bus drivers: A structural MRI and neuropsychological analysis. *Hippocampus, 16*, 1091–1101.

Mahon, B. & Caramazza, A. (2005). The orchestration of the sensory-motor systems: clues from neuropsychology. *Cognitive Neuropsychology, 22*, 480–494.

Mai, X. Q., Luo, J., Wu, J. H., & Luo, Y. J. (2004). 'Aha!' effects in a guessing riddle task: an event-related potential study. *Human Brain Mapping, 22*, 261–270.

Maia, T. V. & McClelland, J. L. (2004). A reexamination of the evidence for the somatic marker hypothesis: what participants really know in the Iowa gambling task. *Proceedings of the National Academy of Sciences, USA, 101*, 16075–16080.

Maier, A., Wilke, M., Aura, C., Zhu, C., Ye, F. Q., & Leopold, D. A. (2008). Divergence of fMRI and neural signals in V1 during perceptual suppression in the awake monkey. *Nature Neuroscience, 11*, 1193–1200.

Mair, W. G., Warrington, E. K., & Weiskrantz, L. (1979). Memory disorder in Korsakoff's psychosis: a neuropathological and neuropsychological investigation of two cases. *Brain, 102*, 749–783.

Malt, B. C., Sloman, S. A., Gennari, S., Shi, M. Y., & Wang, Y. (1999). Knowing versus naming: Similarity and the linguistic categorization of artifacts. *Journal of Memory and Language, 40*, 230–262.

Mandler, G. (1967). Organisation and memory. In K. W. Spence & J. T. Spence (Eds), *The psychology of learning and motivation. Vol. 1.* New York: Academic.

Mandler, G. (1975). Memory storage and retrieval: Some limits on the reach of attention and consciousness. In P. M. A. Rabbitt & S. Dornic (Eds), *Attention and performance* (pp. 499–516). New York: Academic Press.

Mandler, G. (1980). Recognizing: The judgment of previous occurrence. *Psychological Review, 87*, 252–271.

Mandler, G. & Shebo, B. J. (1982). Subitizing: an analysis of its component processes. *Journal of Experimental Psychology: General, 111*, 1–22.

Mandler, J. M. (2004). The foundations *of mind: origins of conceptual thought.* New York: OUP.

Mandler, J. M. & Mandler, G. (1969). *The diaspora of experimental psychology. the gestaltists and others.* Cambridge, MA: Harvard University Press.

Manes, F., Sahakian, B., Clark, L., Rogers, R., Antoun, N., Aitken, M. et al. (2002). Decision-making processes following damage to the prefrontal cortex. *Brain, 125*, 624–639.

Mangels, J. A., Ivry, R. B., & Shimizu, N. (1998). Dissociable contributions of the prefrontal and neocerebellar cortex to time perception. *Cognitive Brain Research, 7*, 15–39.

Manns, J. R. & Squire, L. R. (1999). Impaired recognition memory on the Doors and People Test after damage limited to the hippocampal region. *Hippocampus, 9*, 495–499.

Maravita, A. & Iriki, A. (2004). Tools for the body (schema). *Trends in Cognitive Science, 8*, 79–86.

Marcar, V. & Cowey, A. (1992). The effect of removing superior temporal cortical motion areas in the macaque monkey. II. Motion discrimination using random dot displays. *European Journal of Neuroscience, 4*, 1228–1238.

Marcel, A. (1983a). Conscious and unconscious perception: an approach to the relations between phenomenal experience and perceptual processes. *Cognitive Psychology, 15*, 238–300.

Marcel, A. (1983b). Conscious and unconscious perception: experiments on visual masking and word recognition. *Cognitive Psychology, 15*, 197–237.

Marconi, B., Genovesio, A., Battaglia-Mayer, A., Ferraina, S., Squatrito, S., Molinari, M. et al. (2001). Eye-hand coordination during reaching. I. Anatomical relationships between parietal and frontal cortex. *Cerebral Cortex, 11*, 513–527.

Marcus, G. F., Brinkmann, U., Clahsen, H., Wiese, R., & Pinker, S. (1995). German inflection: the exception that proves the rule. *Cognitive Psychology, 29*(3), 189–256.

Marois, R., & Ivanoff, J. (2005). Capacity limits of information processing in the brain. *Trends in Cognitive Sciences, 9*(6), 296–305.

Marques, J. F., Canessa, N., Siri, S., Catricala, E., & Cappa, S. (2008). Conceptual knowledge in the brain: fMRI evidence for a featural organization. *Brain Research, 1194*, 90–99.

Marr, D. (1971). Simple memory: a theory for archicortex. *The Philosophical Transactions of the Royal Society of London: B, 262*, 23–81.

Marr, D. (1982). *Vision: A computational investigation into the human representation and processing of visual information.* W. H. Freeman.

Marr, D. & Poggio, T. (1976). *From understanding computation to understanding neural circuitry.* Massachusetts Institute of Technology. AI Memo 357. May 1976.

Marshall, J. & Newcombe, F. (1966). Syntactic and semantic errors in paralexia. *Neuropsychologia, 4*, 169–176.

Marshall, J. & Newcombe, F. (1973). Patterns of paralexia: a psycholinguistic approach. *Journal of Psycholinguistic Research, 2*, 175–199.

Marslen-Wilson, W. & Tyler, L. K. (1980). The temporal structure of spoken language understanding. *Cognition, 8*, 1–71.

Marslen-Wilson, W. & Tyler, L. K. (1997). Dissociating types of mental computation. *Nature, 387*, 592–594.

Marslen-Wilson, W. D. & Tyler, L. K. (2007). Morphology, language and the brain: the decompositional substrate for language comprehension. *Philosophical Transactions Royal Society London B Biological Sciences, 362*, 823–836.

Martin, A. (2007). The representation of object concepts in the brain. *Annual Review of Psychology, 58*, 25–45.

Martin, A. & Fedio, P. (1983). Word production and comprehension in Alzheimer's disease: the breakdown of semantic knowledge. *Brain and Language, 19*, 124–141.

Martin, A., Wiggs, C. L., Ungerleider, L. G., & Haxby, J. V. (1996). Neural correlates of category-specific knowledge. *Nature, 379*, 649–652.

Martin, N. & Saffran, E. M. (1992). A computational account of deep dysphasia: evidence from a single case study. *Brain and Language, 43*, 240–274.

Martin, R. C. (2005). Components of short-term memory and their relation to language processing: evidence from neuropsychology and neuroimaging. *Current Directions in Psychological Science, 14*(4), 204–208.

Martin, R. C. & Breedin, S. (1992). Dissociations between speech perception and phonological short-term memory deficits. *Cognitive Neuropsychology, 9*, 509–534.

Martin, R. C. & Cheng, Y. (2006). Selection demands versus association strength in the verb generation task. *Psychonomic Bulletin and Review, 13,* 396–401.

Martin, R. C. & Freedman, M. L. (2001). Short-term retention of lexical-semantic representations: Implications for speech production. *Memory, 9,* 261–280.

Martin, R. C. & He, T. (2004). Semantic short-term memory and its role in sentence processing: a replication. *Brain and Language, 89,* 76–82.

Martin, R. C. & Romani, C. (1994). Verbal working memory and sentence comprehension: A multiple-components view. *Neuropsychology, 8,* 506–523.

Martin, R. C., Shelton, J. R. & Yaffee, L. S. (1994). Language processing and working memory: Neuropsychological evidence for separate phonological and semantic capacities. *Journal of Memory and Language, 33,* 83–111.

Matelli, M., Luppino, G., & Rizzolatti, G. (1985). Patterns of cytochrome oxidase activity in the frontal agranular cortex of the macaque monkey. *Behavioural Brain Research, 18*(2), 125–136.

Mathis, W. & Mozer, M. (1996). Conscious and unconscious perception: a computational theory. In *Proceedings of the 18th Annual Conference of the Cognitive Science Society,* (pp. 324–328). Lawrence Erlbaum.

Matthews, G., Warm, J., & Reinerman, L. L. L. S. D. (2010). Task engagement, attention and cognitive control. In A. Gruszka, G. Matthews, & B. Szymura (Eds), *Handbook of individual differences in cognition: Attention, memory and cognitive control.* New York: Springer.

Mattingley, J., Davis, G., & Driver, J. (1997). Preattentive filling-in of visual surfaces in parietal extinction. *Science, 275,* 671–674.

Mayer, N., Schwartz, M. F., Montgomery, M. W., Buxbaum, L. J., Lee, S. S., Carew, T. G., Coslett, H. B., et al. (1998). Naturalistic action impairment in closed head injury. *Neuropsychology, 12*(1), 13–28.

Mayes, A. R., Meudell, P. R., Mann, D., & Pickering, A. (1988). Location of lesions in Korsakoffs syndrome—neuropsychological and neuropathological data on 2 patients. *Cortex, 24,* 367–388.

Mayes, A. R., Holdstock, J. S., Isaac, C. L., Hunkin, N. M., & Roberts, N. (2002). Relative sparing of item recognition memory in a patient with adult-onset damage limited to the hippocampus. *Hippocampus, 12,* 325–340.

McCandliss, B. D., Cohen, L., & Dehaene, S. (2003). The visual word form area: expertise for reading in the fusiform gyrus. *Trends in Cognitive Sciences, 7,* 293–299.

McCarthy, R. & Warrington, E. K. (1984). A two-route model of speech production: evidence from aphasia. *Brain, 107,* 463–485.

McCarthy, R., & Warrington, E. K. (1985). Category specificity in an agrammatic patient: the relative impairment of verb retrieval and comprehension. *Neuropsychologia, 23*(6), 709–727.

McCarthy, R. & Warrington, E. K. (1986a). Phonological reading: phenomena and paradoxes. *Cortex, 22,* 359–380.

McCarthy, R. & Warrington, E. K. (1986b). Visual associative agnosia: a clinicoanatomical study of a single case. *Journal of Neurology, Neurosurgery and Psychiatry, 49,* 1233–1240.

McCarthy, R. & Warrington, E. K. (1988). Evidence for modality-specific meaning systems in the brain. *Nature, 334,* 428–430.

McCarthy, R. & Warrington, E. K. (1990a). *Cognitive neuropsychology: a clinical introduction.* San Diego: Academic Press.

McCarthy, R. & Warrington, E. K. (1990b). The dissolution of semantics. *Nature, 343,* 599.

McClelland, J. L. (1979). On the time relations of mental processes: an examination of systems of processing in cascade. *Psychological Review, 86,* 287–330.

McClelland, J. L. & Elman, J. L. (1986). The trace model of speech-perception. *Cognitive Psychology, 18,* 1–86.

McClelland, J. L. & Patterson, K. (2002). Rules or connections in past-tense inflections: what does the evidence rule out? *Trends in Cognitive Sciences, 6,* 465–472.

McClelland, J. L. & Rumelhart, D. E. (1981). An interactive activation model of context effects in letter perception: Part 1. An account of basic findings. *Psychological Review, 88,* 375–407.

McClelland, J. L., St John, M., & Taraban, R. (1989). Sentence comprehension: a parallel distributed processing approach. *Language and Cognitive Processes, 4,* 287–335.

McClelland, J., MacNaughton, B., & O'Reilly, R. (1995). Why are there complementary learning systems in the hippocampus and neocortex: insights from the successes and failures of connectionist models of learning and memory. *Psychological Review, 102,* 419–457.

McCloskey, M. & Caramazza, A. (1991). On crude data and impoverished theory. *Behavioral and Brain Sciences, 14,* 453–455.

McCloskey, M. & Cohen, N. (1989). Catastrophic interference in connectionist networks: The sequential learning problem. In G.Bower (Ed.), *The psychology of learning and motivation* (pp. 109–165). New York: Academic Press.

McCulloch, W. & Pitts, W. (1943). A logical calculus of the ideas immanent in neural nets. *Bulletin of Mathematical Biophysics, 5,* 115–133.

McDermott, J. & Forgy, C (1978). Production system conflict resolution strategies. In D.Waterman &

F. Hayes-Roth (Eds), *Pattern-directed inference systems*. New York: Academic Press.

McGlinchey-Berroth, R., Milberg, W., Verfaellie, M., Alexander, M., & Kilduff, P. (1993). Semantic processing in the neglected visual field: evidence from a lexical decision task. *Cognitive Neuropsychology*, *10*, 79–108.

McGonigle, B. & Chalmers, M. (1992). Monkeys are rational!. *Quarterly Journal of Experimental Psychology*, *45*, 189–228.

McGrew, W. (1993). The intelligent use of tools: twenty propositions. In K. Gibson & T. Ingold (Eds), *Tools, language and cognition in human evolution* (pp. 151–170). Cambridge: CUP.

McKeeff, T. J. & Behrmann, M. (2004). Pure alexia and covert reading. *Cognitive Neuropsychology*, *21*, 443–458.

McKone, E. (1995). Short-term implicit memory for words and nonwords. *Journal of Experimental Psychology: Learning, Memory and Cognition*, *21*, 1108–1126.

McMullin, E. (1985). Galilean idealization. *Studies in History and Philosophy of Science*, *16*, 247–273.

McNaughton, B. L. (1989) Neural mechanisms for spatial computation and information storage. In L. A. Nadel, P. Cooper, P. Culicover amd R. Harnish (Eds). *Neural connections and mental computations*, pp. 285–349. Cambridge, MA: MIT Press.

McRae, K. & Cree, G. (2002). Factors underlying category-specific semantic deficits. In E. Forde & G. W. Humphreys (Eds), *Category-specificity in brain and mind* (pp. 291–314). Hove: Psychology Press.

Mecklinger, A. D., von Cramon, D. Y., Springer, A., & Matthes-von, C. G. (1999). Executive control functions in task switching: evidence from brain injured patients. *Journal of Clinical and Experimental Neuropsychology*, *21*, 606–619.

Meeter, M. & Murre, J. M. J. (2005). TraceLink: a model of consolidation and amnesia. *Cognitive Neuropsychology*, *22*, 559–587.

Mehler, J. & Miller, G. A. (1964). Retroactive interference in the recall of simple sentences. *British Journal of Psychology*, *55*, 295–301.

Meiran, N. (1996). Reconfiguration of processing mode prior to task performance. *Journal of Experimental Psychology: Learning, Memory, and Cognition*, *22*(6), 1423–1442.

Mendez, M. & Perryman, K. (2002). Neuropsychiatric features of frontotemporal dementia. Evaluation of consensus criteria and review. *Journal of Neurospsychiatry and Clinical Neuroscience*, *14*, 424–429.

Mercer, B., Wapner, W., Gardner, H., & Benson, D. F. (1977). A study of confabulation. *Archives of Neurology*, *34*, 429–433.

Merikle, P. M., Smilek, D., & Eastwood, J. D. (2001). Perception without awareness: perspectives from cognitive psychology. *Cognition*, *79*, 115–134.

Mesulam, M. (1982). Slowly progressive aphasia without generalised dementia. *Annals of Neurology*, *11*, 592–598.

Meunier, M., Bachevalier, J., Mishkin, M., & Murray, E. (1993). Effects on visual recognition of combined and separate ablations of the entorhinal and perirhinal cortex in rhesus monkeys. *Journal of Neuroscience*, *13*, 5418–5432.

Mewhort, D. & Beal, A. (1977). Mechanisms of word identification. *Journal of Experimental Psychology: Human Perception Performance*, *3*, 629–640.

Meyer A., Beck E., McLardy T. (1947). *Prefrontal leucotomy: a neuroanatomical report*. Brain, *70*, 18–49.

Meyer, A. M. & Peterson, R. R. (2000). Structural influences on the resolution of lexical ambiguity: an analysis of hemispheric asymmetries. *Brain and Cognition*, *43*, 341–345.

Meyer, D. E. & Kieras, D. E. (1997a). A computational theory of executive cognitive processes and multiple-task performance. 1. Basic mechanisms. *Psychological Review*, *104*, 3–65.

Meyer, D. E. & Kieras, D. E. (1997b). A computational theory of executive cognitive processes and multiple-task performance. 2. Accounts of psychological refractory-period phenomena. *Psychological Review*, *104*, 749–791.

Meyer, M., Friederici, A. D., & von Cramon, D. Y. (2000). Neurocognition of auditory sentence comprehension: event related fMRI reveals sensitivity to syntactic violations and task demands. *Cognitive Brain Research*, *9*(1), 19–33.

Miceli, G., Mazzucchi, A., Menn, L., & Goodglass, H. (1983). Contrasting cases of Italian agrammatic aphasia without comprehension disorder. *Brain and Language*, *19*, 65–97.

Miceli, G., Silveri, M. C., Villa, G., & Caramazza, A. (1984). On the basis for the agrammatic's difficulty in producing main verbs. *Cortex*, *20*, 207–220.

Miceli, G., Silveri, M. C., & Caramazza, A. (1985). Cognitive analysis of a case of pure dysgraphia. *Brain and Language*, *25*, 187–212.

Miceli, G., Benvegnu, B., Capasso, R., & Caramazza, A. (1995). Selective deficit in processing double letters. *Cortex*, *31*, 161–171.

Miceli, G., Fouch, E., Capasso, R., Shelton, J. R., Tomaiuolo, F., & Caramazza, A. (2001). The dissociation of color from form and function knowledge. *Nature Neuroscience*, *4*, 662–667.

Michel, F., Henaff, M. A., & Intriligator, J. (1996). Two different readers in the same brain after a posterior callosal lesion. *Neuroreport*, *7*, 786–788.

Milea, D., Lehericy, S., Rivaud-Pechoux, S., Duffau, H., Lobel, E., Capelle, L. et al. (2003). Antisaccade deficit after anterior cingulate cortex resection. *Neuroreport*, *14*, 283–287.

Milgram, S. (1974). *Obedience to authority: An experimental view*. New York: Harper & Row.

Miller, E. K. & Cohen, J. D. (2001). An integrative theory of prefrontal cortex function. *Annual Review of Neuroscience, 24*, 167–202.

Miller, G. A. (1956). The magical number seven plus or minus two: some limits on our capacity for processing information. *Psychological Review, 63*, 81–97.

Miller, G. & Selfridge, J. (1950). Verbal context and the recall of meaningful material. *American Journal of Psychology, 63*, 176–185.

Miller, G., Galanter, E., & Pribram, K. (1960). *Plans and the structures of behavior*. New York: Holt.

Miller, J., van der Ham, F., & Sanders, A. F. (1995). Overlapping stage models and reaction-time additivity—Effects of the activation equation. *Acta Psychologica, 90*, 11–28.

Miller, L. A. & Tippett, L. J. (1996). Effects of focal brain lesions on visual problem-solving. *Neuropsychologia, 34*, 387–398.

Milner, A. & Goodale, M. (1995). *The visual brain in action*. Oxford: OUP.

Milner, B. (1963). Effects of different lesions on card sorting. *Archives of Neurology, 9*, 101–110.

Milner, B. (1966). Amnesia following operation on the temporal lobes. In C. W. M. Whitty & O. I. Zangwill (Eds), *Amnesia*, Butterworths, London.

Milner, B. (1971). Interhemispheric differences in the localization of psychological processes in man. *British Medical Bulletin, 27*, 272–277.

Milner, B. (1972). Disorders of learning and memory after temporal lobe lesions in man. *Clinical Neurosurgery, 19*, 421–446.

Milner, B. & Teuber, H-L. (1968). Alteration of perception and memory in man: reflections on methods. In L. Weiskrantz (Ed.), *Analysis of behavioural change.* (pp. 268–375). New York: Harper & Row.

Milner, P. M. (1957). The cell assembly. Mark II. *Psychological Review, 64*, 242–252.

Miniussi, C., Ruzzoli, M. & Walsh, V. (2010). The mechanism of transcranial magnetic stimulation in cognition. *Cortex, 46*, 128–130.

Minsky, M. & Papert, S. (1968). *Perceptrons: an introduction to computational geometry*. Cambridge, MA: MIT Press.

Miozzo, M. (2003). On the processing of regular and irregular forms of verbs and nouns: evidence from neuropsychology. *Cognition, 87*, 101–127.

Miozzo, M. & Caramazza, A. (1998). Varieties of pure alexia: the case of failure to access graphemic representations. *Cognitive Neuropsychology, 15*, 203–238.

Mishkin, M. & Pribram, K. (1954). Visual discrimination performance following partial ablations of the temporal lobe. I. Ventral vs. lateral. *Journal of Comparative Physiology and Psychology, 47*, 14–20.

Mitchell, D. C. (1972). Short-term visual memory and pattern masking. *Quarterly Journal of Experimental Psychology, 24*, 394–405.

Miyake, A. & Shah, P. (1999a). *Models of working memory: mechanisms of active maintenance and executive control*. Cambridge: CUP.

Miyake, A., & Shah, P. (1999b). Toward unified theories of working memory: emerging general consensus, unresolved theoretical issues, and future research directions. In A. Miyake & P. Shah (Eds), *Models of working memory: mechanisms of active maintenance and executive control* (pp. 442–481). New York: Cambridge University Press.

Miyake, A., Friedman, N. P., Emerson, M. J., Witzki, A. H., Howerter, A., & Wager, T. D. (2000). The unity and diversity of executive functions and their contributions to complex 'Frontal Lobe' tasks: a latent variable analysis. *Cognitive Psychology, 41*, 49–100.

Mohr, J. P., Pessin, M. S., Finkelstein, S., Funkenstein, H. H., Duncan, G. W., & Davis, K. R. (1978). Broca aphasia: pathologic and clinical. *Neurology, 28*, 311–324.

Moll, J., de Oliveira-Souza, R., Passman, L. J., Cunha, F. C., Souza-Lima, F., & Andreiuolo, P. A. (2000). Functional MRI correlates of real and imagined tool-use pantomimes. *Neurology, 54*, 1331–1336.

Monsell, S. (1978). Recency, immediate recognition memory, and reaction time. *Cognitive Psychology, 10*, 465–501.

Monsell, S. (1984). Components of working memory underlying verbal skills: a 'distributed capacities' view. In H. Bouma & D. Bouwhuis (Eds), *Attention and performance X. Control of language processes* (pp. 327–350). Hove, UK: LEA.

Monsell, S. (2003). Task switching. *Trends in Cognitive Sciences, 7*, 134–140.

Monsell, S., Patterson, K.E., Graham, A. Hughes, C.H. & Milroy, R (1992). Lexical and sublexical translation of spelling to sound: Strategic anticipation of lexical status. *Journal of Experimental Psychology; Learning, Memory, and Cognition, 18*, 452–467.

Montaldi, D., Spencer, T. J., Roberts, N., & Mayes, A. R. (2006). The neural system that mediates familiarity memory. *Hippocampus, 16*(5), 504–520.

Monti, M. M., Osherson, D. N., Martinez, M. J., & Parsons, L. M. (2007). Functional neuroanatomy of deductive inference: a language-independent distributed network. *Neuroimage, 37*, 1005–1016.

Monti, M. M., Parsons, L. M., & Osherson, D. N. (2009). The boundaries of language and thought in deductive inference. *Proceedings of the National Academy of Sciences, USA, 106*(30), 12554–12559.

Moran, J. & Desimone, R. (1985). Selective attention gates visual processing in extrastriate cortex. *Science*, *229*, 782–784.

Moray, N. (1959). Attention in dichotic listening: affective cues and the influence of instructions. *Quarterly Journal of Experimental Psychology*, *11*, 56–60.

Morel, A. & Bullier, J. (1990). Anatomical segregation of two cortical visual pathways in the macaque monkey. *Visual Neuroscience*, *4*, 555–578.

Morlaas, J. (1928). *Contribution à l'étude de l'apraxie*. Paris: Amédée, Legrand.

Morris, C., Bransford, J., & Franks, J. (1977). Levels of processing versus test-appropriate strategies. *Journal of Verbal Learning and Verbal Behavior*, *16*, 519–533.

Morris, J. S., Ohman, A., & Dolan, R. J. (1998). Conscious and unconscious emotional learning in the human amygdala. *Nature*, *393*, 467–470.

Morris, M. K., Bowers, D., Chatterjee, A., & Heilman, K. M. (1992). Amnesia following a discrete basal forebrain lesion. *Brain*, *115* (6), 1827–1847.

Morris, R. (1984). Developments of a water-maze procedure for studying spatial learning in the rat. *Journal of Neuroscience Methods*, *11*, 47–60.

Morris, R. G., Ahmed, S., Syed, G. M., & Toone, B. K. (1993). Neural correlates of planning ability: frontal lobe activation during the Tower of London test. *Neuropsychologia*, *31*, 1367–1378.

Morris, R. G., Miotto, E. C., Feigenbaum, J. D., Bullock, P., & Polkey, C. E. (1997). The effect of goal-subgoal conflict on planning ability after frontal- and temporal-lobe lesions in humans. *Neuropsychologia*, *35*, 1147–1157.

Morsella, E. & Miozzo, M. (2002). Evidence for a cascade model of lexical access in speech production. *Journal of Experimental Psychology: Learning, Memory and Cognition*, *28*, 555–563.

Mort, D. J., Malhotra, P., Mannan, S. K., Rorden, C., Pambakian, A., Kennard, C. et al. (2003). The anatomy of visual neglect. *Brain*, *126*, 1986–1997.

Morton, J. (1969). Interaction of information in word recognition. *Psychological Review*, *76*, 165–178.

Morton, J. (1970). A functional model for memory. In D. A. Norman (Ed.), *Models of human memory* (pp. 203–254). New York: Academinc Press.

Morton, J. (1979). Word recognition. In J. Morton & J. Marshall (Eds), *Psycholinguistics, Ser. 2. Structures and processes*. Elek, London.

Morton, J. (1981). The status of information processing models of language. *Philosophical Transaction of the Royal Society of London: B: Biological Sciences*, *295*, 387–396.

Morton, J. (2004). *Understanding developmental disorders*. Oxford: Blackwell.

Morton, J. & Bekerian, D. A. (1986). Three ways of looking at memory. In N. E. Sharkey (Ed.), *Advances in cognitive science, vol 1.* (pp. 44–71). Chichester: Ellis Horwood.

Morton, J. & Patterson, K. (1980). A new attempt at an interpretation, or, an attempt at a new interpretation. In M. Coltheart, K. Patterson, & J. C. Marshall (Eds.), *Deep dyslexia*. London: Routledge & Kegan Paul.

Morton, J., Hammersley, R. H., & Bekerian, D. A. (1985). Headed records: a model for memory and its failures. *Cognition*, *20*, 1–23.

Morton, N. & Morris, R. (1995). Image transformation dissociated from visuospatial working memory. *Cognitive Neuropsychology*, *12*, 767–791.

Moscovitch, M. (1995). Confabulation. In D. L.Schacter, J. T. Coyle, G. D. Fischbach, Mesulam, M. M., & E. D. Sullivan (Eds), *Memory distortion: how minds, brains and societies reconstruct the past.* (pp. 226–254). Cambridge, MA: Harvard.

Moscovitch, M. & Nadel, L. (1999). Multiple-trace theory and semantic dementia: response to K. S. Graham (1999). *Trends in Cognitive Sciences*, *3*, 87–89.

Moscovitch, M. & Umiltà, C. (1990). Modularity and neuropsychology: modules and central processes in attention and memory. In M. Schwartz (Ed.), *Modular deficits in Alzheimertype dementia*. Cambridge, MA: MIT Press.

Moscovitch, M., Vriezen, E., & Gottstein, G. (1993). Implicit tests of memory in patients with focal lesions or degenerative brain disorders. In F. Boller & J. Grafman (Eds), *Handbook of neuropsychology* (pp. 133–173). Amsterdam: Elsevier.

Moscovitch, M., Winocur, G., & Behrmann, M. (1997). What is special about face recognition? Nineteen experiments on a person with visual object agnosia and dyslexia but normal face recognition. *Journal of Cognitive Neuroscience*, *9*, 555–604.

Moscovitch, M., Yaschyshyn, T., Ziegler, M., & Nadel, L. (1999). Remote episodic memory and amnesia: Was Endel Tulving right all along? In E.Tulving (Ed.), *Memory, consciousness and the brain: the Talinn conference.* New York: Psychology Press.

Moscovitch, M., Rosenbaum, R. S., Gilboa, A., Addis, D. R., Westmacott, R., Grady, C. et al. (2005). Functional neuroanatomy of remote episodic, semantic and spatial memory: a unified account based on multiple trace theory. *Journal of Anatomy*, *207*, 35–66.

Moscovitch, M., Nadel, L., Winocur, G., Gilboa, A., & Rosenbaum, R. S. (2006). The cognitive neuroscience of remote episodic, semantic and spatial memory. *Current Opinion in Neurobiology*, *16*, 179–190.

Moss, H. E., Tyler, L. K., & Jennings, F. (1997). When leopards lose their spots: Knowledge of visual properties in category-specific deficits for living things. *Cognitive Neuropsychology*, *14*, 901–950.

Motomura, N. & Yamadori, A. (1994). A case of ideational apraxia with impairment of object use and preservation of object pantomime. *Cortex*, *30*, 167–170.

Mottaghy, F. M., Willmes, K., Horwitz, B., Muller, H. W., Krause, B. J., & Sturm, W. (2006). Systems level modeling of a neuronal network subserving intrinsic alertness. *Neuroimage*, *29*, 225–233.

Moutoussis, K. & Zeki, S. (2002). The relationship between cortical activation and perception investigated with invisible stimuli. *Proceedings of the National Academy of Sciences, USA*, *99*, 9527–9532.

Mozer, M. & Behrmann, M. (1990). On the interaction of selective attention and lexical knowledge: a connectionist account of neglect dyslexia. *Journal of Cognitive Neuroscience*, *2*, 96–123.

Mumford, D. (1994). Neuronal architectures for pattern-theoretic problems. In Koch, C. & Davis, J. L. (Eds), *Large scale neuronal theories of the brain* (pp. 125–152). Cambridge, MA: MIT Press.

Mummery, C. J., Patterson, K., Hodges, J. R., & Wise, R. J. (1996). Generating 'tiger' as an animal name or a word beginning with T: differences in brain activation. *Proceedings. Biological Sciences*, *263*, 989–995.

Mummery, C. J., Patterson, K., Wise, R. J., Vandenberghe, R., Price, C. J., & Hodges, J. R. (1999). Disrupted temporal lobe connections in semantic dementia. *Brain*, *122* (1), 61–73.

Mummery, C. J., Patterson, K., Price, C. J., Ashburner, J., Frackowiak, R. S., & Hodges, J. R. (2000). A voxel-based morphometry study of semantic dementia: relationship between temporal lobe atrophy and semantic memory. *Annals of Neurology*, *47*, 36–45.

Murata, A., Gallese, V., Luppino, G., Kaseda, M., & Sakata, H. (2000). Selectivity for the shape, size, and orientation of objects for grasping in neurons of monkey parietal area AIP. *Journal of Neurophysiology*, *83*, 2580–2601.

Murdock, B. (1974). *Human memory: theory and data*. Hillsdale, New Jersey: Erlbaum.

Murre, J. M. (1996). TraceLink: a model of amnesia and consolidation of memory. *Hippocampus*, *6*, 675–684.

Murre, J. M. (1997). Implicit and explicit memory in amnesia: some explanations and predictions by the TraceLink model. *Memory*, *5*, 213–232.

Murre, J. M., Graham, K., & Hodges, J. (2001). Semantic dementia: relevance to connectionist models of long-term memory. *Brain*, *124*, 647–675.

Nachev, P., & Husain, M. (2007). Comment on 'detecting awareness in the vegetative state'. *Science*, *315*(5816), 1221–1221.

Nadel, L. & Moscovitch, M. (1997). Memory consolidation, retrograde amnesia and the hippocampal complex. *Current Opinion in Neurobiology*, *7*, 217–227.

Nagahama, Y., Fukuyama, H., Yamauchi, H., Matsuzaki, S., Konishi, J., Shibasaki, H. et al. (1996). Cerebral activation during performance of a card sorting test. *Brain*, *119* (5), 1667–1675.

Nagel, T. (1974). What is it like to be a bat? *Philosophical Review*, *83*, 435–450.

Nakamura, R. K. & Mishkin, M. (1986). Chronic 'blindness' following lesions of nonvisual cortex in the monkey. *Experimental Brain Research*, *63*, 173–184.

Navon, D. & Gopher, D. (1979). On the economy of the human processing system. *Psychological Review*, *86*, 214–225.

Neath, I. (1993). Distinctiveness and serial position effects in recognition. *Memory and Cognition*, *21*, 689–698.

Neisser, U. (1967). *Cognitive psychology*. Prentice-Hall.

Neisser, U. (1976). *Cognition and reality: principles and implications of cognitive psychology*. San Francisco: Freeman.

Nelson, H. E. (1976). A modified card sorting test sensitive to frontal lobe defects. *Cortex*, *12*, 313–324.

Nestor, P. J., Fryer, T. D., & Hodges, J. R. (2006). Declarative memory impairments in Alzheimer's disease and semantic dementia. *Neuroimage*, *30*, 1010–1020.

Neumann, O. & Klotz, W. (1994). Motor responses to non-reportable, masked stimuli: where is the limit of direct motor specification. In C. Umiltà & M. Moscovitch (Eds), *Conscious and non-conscious information processing. Attention and performance (Vol. XV)* (pp. 123–150). Cambridge, MA: MIT Press.

Newell, A. (1990). *Unified theories of cognition*. Harvard University Press.

Newell, A. & Simon, H. (1961). Computer simulation of human thinking. *Science*, *134*, 2011–2017.

Newell, A. & Simon, H. (1972). *Human problem solving*. Prentice-Hall.

Newell, A. & Simon, H. (1976). Computer science as an empirical inquiry: Symbols and search. (1975 ACM Turing Award Lecture). *Communications of the ACM*, *19*, 113–126.

Newell, A., Shaw, J. C., & Simon, H. (1958). Elements of a theory of human problem solving. *Psychological Review*, *65*, 151–166.

Newell, B. R. & Dunn, J. C. (2008). Dimensions in data: testing psychological models using state-trace analysis. *Trends in Cognitive Sciences*, *12*, 285–290.

Newman, A. J., Ullman, M. T., Pancheva, R., Waligura, D. L., & Neville, H. J. (2007). An ERP study of regular and irregular English past tense inflection. *Neuroimage*, *34*, 435–445.

Newman, S. D., Carpenter, P. A., Varma, S., & Just, M. A. (2003). Frontal and parietal participation in problem solving in the Tower of London: fMRI and computational modeling of planning and high-level perception. *Neuropsychologia, 41*, 1668-1682.

Newsome, W. & Paré, E. (1988). A selective impairment of motion perception following lesions of the middle temporal visual area (MT). *Journal of Neuroscience, 8*, 2201-2211.

Nicholls, J., Martin, A., Wallace, B., & Fuchs PA (2001). *From neuron to brain* (4th edn). Sunderland, MA: Sinauer.

Nichols, T., Brett, M., Andersson, J., Wager, T., & Poline, J. B. (2005). Valid conjunction inference with the minimum statistic. *Neuroimage, 25*, 653-660.

Nickels, L. (2001). Producing spoken words. In B.Rapp (Ed.), *A handbook of cognitive neuropsychology*. New York: Psychology Press.

Nielsen, J. (1946). *Agnosia, apraxia, aphasi*a: their value in cerebral localisation (2nd edn). New York: Harper.

Nisbett, R. E. & Wilson, T. D. (1977). The halo effect: evidence for unconscious alteration of judgments. *Journal of Personality and Social Psychology, 35*(4), 250-256.

Niv, Y., Daw, N. D., Joel, D., & Dayan, P. (2007). Tonic dopamine: opportunity costs and the control of response vigor. *Psychopharmacology, 191*, 507-520.

Nolde, S. F., Johnson, M. K., & Raye, C. L. (1998). The role of prefrontal cortex during tests of episodic memory. *Trends in Cognitive Sciences, 2*, 399-406.

Noppeney, U., Patterson, K., Tyler, L. K., Moss, H., Stamatakis, E. A., Bright, P. et al. (2007). Temporal lobe lesions and semantic impairment: a comparison of herpes simplex virus encephalitis and semantic dementia. *Brain, 130*, 1138-1147.

Norman, D. A. (1968). Toward a theory of memory and attention. *Psychological Review, 75*, 522-536.

Norman, D. A. & Bobrow, D. (1975). On data-limited and resource-limited processes. *Cognitive Psychology, 7*, 44-64.

Norman, D. A., & Bobrow, D. G. (1979). Descriptions: an intermediate stage in memory retrieval. *Cognitive Psychology, 11*(1), 107-123.

Norman, D. A. & Shallice, T. (1980). *Attention to action: willed and automatic control of behavior*. Chip report 99, University of California, San Diego.

Norman, D. A. & Shallice, T. (1986). Attention to action: willed and automatic control of behaviour. In R.Davidson, G. Schwartz, & D. Shapiro (Eds), *Consciousness and self regulation: advances in research vol. 4* (pp. 1-18). New York: Plenum.

Norris, D. (1994). A quantitative multiple-levels model of reading aloud. *Journal of Experimental Psychology Human Perception Performance, 20,* 1212-1232.

Novick, L. R. & Sherman, S. J. (2003). On the nature of insight solutions: evidence from skill differences in anagram solution. *Quarterly Journal of Experimental Psychology, A, 56*, 351-382.

Oaksford, M. & Chater, N. (1994). A rational analysis of the selection task as optimal data selection. *Psychological Review, 101*.

Oaksford, M. & Chater, N. (2007). *Bayesian rationality: the probabilistic approach to human reasoning*. Oxford: OUP.

Ochipa, C., Rothi, L. J., & Heilman, K. M. (1989). Ideational apraxia: a deficit in tool selection and use. *Annals of Neurology, 25*, 190-193.

Ochipa, C., Rothi, L. J., & Heilman, K. M. (1994). Conduction apraxia. *Journal of Neurology, Neurosurgery and Psychiatry, 57*, 1241-1244.

Ochsner, K. & Kosslyn, S. (1999). The cognitive neuroscience approach. In D. Rumelhart & B. Martin (Eds), *Handbook of cognition and perception, vol. x, cognitive science* (pp. 319-365). San Diego, CA: Academic Press.

O'Doherty, J., Dayan, P., Schultz, J., Deichmann, R., Friston, K., & Dolan, R. J. (2004). Dissociable roles of ventral and dorsal striatum in instrumental conditioning. *Science, 304*, 452-454.

Ogawa, S., Lee, T., Kay, A., & Tank, D. (1990). Brain magnetic resonance imaging with contrast dependent blood oxygenation. *Proceedings of the National Academy of Sciences, USA, 87*, 8868-8872.

Ohlsson, S. (1992). Information-processing explanations of insight and related phenomena. In M. Keane & K. Gilhooley (Eds), *Advances in the psychology of thinking*. Harvester-Wheatsheaf.

Okada, T., Tanaka, S., Nakai, T., Nishizawa, S., Inui, T., Sadato, N. et al. (2000). Naming of animals and tools: a functional magnetic resonance imaging study of categorical differences in the human brain areas commonly used for naming visually presented objects. *Neuroscience Letters, 296, 33-36.

O'Keefe, J. (1979). A review of the hippocampal place cells. *Progress in neurobiology, 13*, 419-439.

O'Keefe, J. (2007). Hippocampal neurophysiology in the behaving animal. In P.Anderson, R. Morris, Amaral D, T. Bliss, & J. O'Keefe (Eds), *The hippocampus book* (pp. 475-548). Oxford: OUP.

O'Keefe, J. & Burgess, N. (1996). Geometric determinants of the place fields of hippocampal neurones. *Nature, 381*, 425-428.

O'Keefe, J. & Dostrovsky, J. (1971). The hippocampus as a spatial map. Preliminary evidence from unit activity in the freely-moving rat. *Brain Research, 34*, 171-175.

O'Keefe, J. & Nadel, L. (1978). *The hippocampus as a cognitive map*. Oxford: Clarendon.

Okuda, J., Fujii, T., Yamadori, A., Kawashima, R., Tsukiura, T., Fukatsu, R. et al. (1998). Participation of the prefrontal cortices in prospective memory: evidence from a PET study in humans. *Neuroscience Letters, 253,* 127–130.

Oppenheimer, J. & Snyder, H. (1939). On continued gravitational contraction. *Physical Review, 56,* 455–459.

O'Regan, J. K. & Noë, A. (2001). A sensorimotor account of vision and visual consciousness. *Behavioral and Brain Sciences, 24,* 939–973.

O'Reilly, R. C. (1996). Biologically plausible error-driven learning using local activation differences: the generalized recirculation algorithm. *Neural Computation, 8,* 895–938.

O'Reilly, R. C. & Frank, M. J. (2006). Making working memory work: a computational model of learning in the prefrontal cortex and basal ganglia. *Neural Comput., 18,* 283–328.

O'Reilly, R. C. & Munakata, Y. (2000). *Computational explorations in cognitive neuroscience: understanding the mind by simulating the brain.* Cambridge, MA: MIT Press.

O'Reilly, R. C., Noelle, D. C., Braver, T. S., & Cohen, J. D. (2002). Prefrontal cortex and dynamic categorization tasks: representational organization and neuromodulatory control. *Cerebral Cortex, 12,* 246–257.

O'Reilly, R. C., Busby, R. S., Soto, R. (2003). Three forms of binding and their neural substrates: alternatives to temporal synchrony. In A. Cleeremans, (Ed.) *The unity of consciousness: binding, integration, and dissociation.* Oxford University Press.

Orpwood, L. & Warrington, E. K. (1995). Word specific impairments in naming and spelling but not reading. *Cortex, 31,* 239–265.

Osgood, C. (1953). *Method and theory in experimental psychology.* New York: OUP.

O'Shaughnessy, B. (2000). *Consciousness and the world.* Oxford: OUP.

Osherson, D., Perani, D., Cappa, S., Schnur, T., Grassi, F., & Fazio, F. (1998). Distinct brain loci in deductive versus probabilistic reasoning. *Neuropsychologia, 36,* 369–376.

Otten, L. J. & Rugg, M. D. (2001). Task-dependency of the neural correlates of episodic encoding as measured by fMRI. *Cerebral Cortex, 11,* 1150–1160.

Owen, A. M., & Coleman, M. R. (2008). Functional neuroimaging of the vegetative state. *Nature Reviews Neuroscience, 9*(3), 235–243.

Owen, A. M., Downes, J. J., Sahakian, B. J., Polkey, C. E., & Robbins, T. W. (1990). Planning and spatial working memory following frontal lobe lesions in man. *Neuropsychologia, 28,* 1021–1034.

Owen, A. M., Coleman, M. R., Boly, M., Davis, M. H., Laureys, S., & Pickard, J. D. (2006). Detecting awareness in the vegetative state. *Science, 313* (5792), 1402.

Page, M. P. (2000). Connectionist modelling in psychology: A localist manifesto. *Behavioral and Brain Sciences, 23,* 443–467.

Page, M. P. (2006). What can't functional neuroimaging tell the cognitive psychologist? *Cortex, 42,* 428–443.

Page, M. P. & Norris, D. G. (1998). The primacy model: a new model of immediate serial recall. *Psychological Review, 105,* 761–781.

Page, M. P., Madge, A., Cumming, N., & Norris, D. G. (2007). Speech errors and the phonological similarity effect in short-term memory: evidence suggesting a common locus. *Journal of Memory and Language, 56,* 49–64.

Paivio, A. (1969). Mental imagery in associative learning and memory. *Psychological Review, 76,* 241–263.

Paivio, A. (1971). *Imagery and verbal processes.* New York: Holt, Rinehart and Winston.

Paivio, A. (1986). *Mental representation: a dual coding approach.* New York: OUP.

Papagno, C. & Vallar, G. (1995). Verbal short-term memory and vocabulary learning in polyglots. *Quarterly Journal of Experimental Psychology 38A,* 98–107.

Papagno, C., Della Salla, S., & Basso, A. (1993). Ideomotor apraxia without aphasia and aphasia without apraxia: the anatomical support for a double dissociation. *Journal of Neurology, Neurosurgery and Psychiatry, 56,* 286–289.

Papagno, C., Cecchetto, C., Reati, F., & Bello, L. (2007). Processing of syntactically complex sentences relies on verbal short-term memory: evidence from a short-term memory patient. *Cognitive Neuropsychology, 24,* 292–311.

Papagno, C., Capasso, R., & Miceli, G. (2009). Reversed concreteness effect for nouns in a subject with semantic dementia. *Neuropsychologia, 47,* 1138–1148.

Papagno, C., Valentine, T., & Baddeley, A. D. (1991). Phonological short-term memory and foreign language vocabulary learning. *Journal of Memory and Language, 30,* 331–347.

Papeo, L., Vallesi, A., Isaja, A., & Rumiati, R. I. (2009). Effects of TMS on different stages of motor and non-motor verb processing in the primary motor cortex. *PLoS One, 4,* e4508.

Papineau, D. (2002). *Thinking about consciousness.* Oxford: OUP.

Pardo, J., Fox, P., & Raichle, M. (1991). Localization of a human system for sustained attention by positron emission tomography. *Nature, 3,* 61–64.

Parkin, A. J. (1997). *Memory and amnesia: an introduction* (2nd edn). Oxford: Blackwell.

Parkin, A. J. &, Leng, N. R. C. (1988). Aetiological variation in the amnestic syndrome. In: M. M. Gruneberg, P. E. Morris and R. N. Sykes (Eds). *Practical aspects of memory: current research and issues,* vol. 2. (pp. 16–21). Chichester: John Wiley.

Parsons, L. M. & Osherson, D. (2001). New evidence for distinct right and left brain systems for deductive versus probabilistic reasoning. *Cerebral Cortex, 11,* 954–965.

Pashler, H. (1998). *Attention.* Hove, UK: Psychology Press.

Passingham, R. (1997). The organization of the motor system. In R. S. J. Frackowiak (Ed.), *Human brain function* (pp. 243–274). New York: Academic Press.

Patsenko, E. G., & Altmann, E. M. (2010). How planful is routine behavior? A selective-attention model of performance in the Tower of Hanoi. *Journal of Experimental Psychology: General, 139*(1), 95–116.

Patterson, K. (1990). Alexia and neural nets. *Japanese Journal of Neuropsychology, 6,* 90–99.

Patterson, K. (2000). Phonological alexia: the case of the singing detective. In E.Funnell (Ed.), *Case Studies in the Neuropsychology of Reading* (pp. 57). Hove: Psychology Press.

Patterson, K. (2007). The reign of typicality in semantic memory. *Philosophical Transaction of the Royal Society of LondonB: Biological Sciences, 362,* 813–821.

Patterson, K. & Kay, J. (1982). Letter-by-letter reading: psychological descriptions of a neurological syndrome. *Quarterly Journal of Experimental Psychology, 34A,* 411–441.

Patterson, K. & Marcel, A. J. (1977). Aphasia, dyslexia and phonological coding of written words. *Quarterly Journal of Experimental Psychology, 29,* 307–318.

Patterson, K. & Marcel, A. J. (1992). Phonological ALEXIA or PHONOLOGICAL alexia? In D.Alegria, D. Holender, J. Junca de Morais, & M. Radeau (Eds), *Analytic approaches to human cognition* (pp. 259–274). New York: Elsevier.

Patterson, K., & Plaut, D. C. (2009). 'Shallow draughts intoxicate the brain': lessons from cognitive science for cognitive neuropsychology. *Topics in Cognitive Science, 1*(1), 39–58.

Patterson, K., Coltheart, M., & Marshall, J. (1985). *Surface Dyslexia.* Hillsdale, NJ: LEA.

Patterson, K., Vargha-Khadem, F., & Polkey, C. (1989). Reading with one hemisphere. *Brain, 112,* 39–63.

Patterson, K., Plaut, D., McClelland, J., Seidenberg, M., Behrmann, M., & Hodges, J. (1996). Connections and disconnections: a connectionist account of surface dyslexia. In J.Reggia, E. Ruppin, & R. Berndt (Eds), *Neural modeling of brain and cognitive disorders.* World Scientific.

Patterson, K., Lambon Ralph, M. A., Jefferies, E., Woollams, A., Jones, R., Hodges, J. R. et al. (2006). 'Presemantic' cognition in semantic dementia: six deficits in search of an explanation. *Journal of Cognitive Neuroscience, 18,* 169–183.

Patterson, K., Nestor, P. J., & Rogers, T. T. (2007). Where do you know what you know? The representation of semantic knowledge in the human brain. *Nature Reviews Neuroscience, 8,* 976–987.

Paulesu, E., Frith, C. D., & Frackowiak, R. S. (1993). The neural correlates of the verbal component of working memory. *Nature, 362,* 342–345.

Paulesu, E. Shallice, T. Frackowiak, R. S. J. Frith, C. D. (1999). Anatomical modularity of verbal working memory revealed by a famous patient. *NeuroImage, 9*(6), S963.

Paulesu, E., McCrory, E., Fazio, F., Menoncello, L., Brunswick, N., Cappa, S. F. et al. (2000). A cultural effect on brain function. *Nature Neuroscience, 3,* 91–96.

Paus, T., Kalina, M., Patockova, L., Angerova, Y., Cerny, R., Mecir, P. et al. (1991). Medial vs lateral frontal lobe lesions and differential impairment of central-gaze fixation maintenance in man. *Brain, 114*(5), 2051–2067.

Paus, T., Petrides, M., Evans, A. C., & Meyer, E. (1993). Role of the human anterior cingulate cortex in the control of oculomotor, manual, and speech responses: a positron emission tomography study. *Journal of Neurophysiology, 70,* 453–469.

Paus, T., Jech, R., Thompson, C. J., Comeau, R., Peters, T., & Evans, A. C. (1997). Transcranial magnetic stimulation during positron emission tomography: a new method for studying connectivity of the human cerebral cortex. *Journal of Neuroscience, 17,* 3178–3184.

Paus, T., Koski, L., Caramanos, Z., & Westbury, C. (1998). Regional differences in the effects of task difficulty and motor output on blood flow response in the human anterior cingulate cortex: a review of 107 PET activation studies. *Neuroreport, 9,* R37–R47.

Peacocke, C. (1986). *Thoughts: an essay on content.* Oxford: Blackwell.

Peigneux, P., van der Linden, M., Andres-Benito, P., Sadzot, B., Franck, G., & Salmon, E. (2000). A neuropsychological and functional brain imaging study of visuo-imitative apraxia. *Revue neurologique, 156,* 459–472.

Peigneux, P., van der Linden, M., Garraux, G., Laureys, S., Degueldre, C., Aerts, J. et al. (2004). Imaging a cognitive model of apraxia: the neural substrate of gesture-specific cognitive processes. *Human Brain Mapping, 21,* 119–142.

Penney, C. (1989). Modality effects and the structure of short-term verbal memory. *Memory and Cognition, 17,* 398–422.

Penrose, L. S., & Raven, J. C. (1936). A new series of perceptual tests: preliminary communication. *British Journal of Medical Psychology, 16,* 97–104.

Penrose, R. (1989). *The emperor's new mind.* Oxford: OUP.

Perani, D. (1998). Brain imaging and memory systems in humans: the contribution of PET methods. *Comptes Rendus de l'Académie des Sciences - Series III - Sciences de la Vie, 321,* 199–205.

Perenin, M. & Vighetto, A. (1988). Optic ataxia: a specific disruption in visuomotor mechanisms. Different aspects of the deficit in reaching for objects. *Brain, 111,* 643–674.

Perrett, D., Rolls, E., & Caan, W. (1982). Visual neurones responsive to faces in the monkey temporal cortex. *Experimental Brain Research, 47,* 329–342.

Perry, C., Ziegler, J., & Zorzi, M. (2007). Nested incremental modelling in the development of computational theories: The CDP+ model or reading aloud. *Psychological Review, 114,* 273–315.

Perry, C., Ziegler, J. C. & Zorzi, M. (2010). Beyond single syllables: large-scale modeling of reading aloud with the Connectionist Dual Process (CDP++) model. *Cognitive Psychology, 61,* 106–151.

Pessoa, L., Japee, S., & Ungerleider, L. G. (2005). Visual awareness and the detection of fearful faces. *Emotion, 5,* 243–237.

Peterson, C. & Anderson, J. (1987). A mean field theory learning algorithm for neural networks. *Complex Systems, 1,* 995–1019.

Petersen, S., Fox, P., Posner, M., Mintun, M., & Raichle, M. (1988). Positron emission tomographic studies of the cortical anatomy of single word processing. *Nature, 331,* 585.

Petersen, S., Fox, P., Posner, M., Mintun, M., & Raichle, M. (1989). Positron emission tomographic studies of the processing of single words. *Journal of Cognitive Neuroscience, 1,* 153.

Petrides, M. (1994). Frontal lobes and behaviour. *Current Opinion in Neurobiology, 4,* 207–211.

Petrides, M. & Milner, B. (1982). Deficits on subject-ordered tasks after frontal- and temporal-lobe lesions in man. *Neuropsychologia, 20,* 249–262.

Petrides, M. & Pandya, D. (1994). Comparative architectonic analysis of the human and macaque frontal cortex. In F. Boller & J. Grafman (Eds), *Handbook of neuropsychology* (pp. 17). Amsterdam: Elsevier.

Phillips, C., Rugg, M. D., & Friston, K. J. (2002). Anatomically informed basis functions for EEG source localization: combining functional and anatomical constraints. *Neuroimage, 16,* 678–695.

Phillips, W. & Christie, D. (1977). Interference with visualization. *Quarterly Journal of Experimental Psychology, 29,* 637–650.

Picton, T. W., Stuss, D. T., Shallice, T., Alexander, M. P., & Gillingham, S. (2006). Keeping time: effects of focal frontal lesions. *Neuropsychologia, 44,* 1195–1209.

Picton, T. W., Stuss, D. T., Alexander, M. P., Shallice, T., Binns, M. A., & Gillingham, S. (2007). Effects of focal frontal lesions on response inhibition. *Cerebral Cortex, 17,* 826–838.

Pinker, S. (1984). *Language learnability and language development.* Cambridge, MA: Harvard University Press.

Pinker, S. (1997). *How the Mind Works.* New York: W.W. Norton.

Pinker, S. (1999). *Words and rules: the ingredients of language.* New York: Harper Collins.

Pinker, S. & Prince, A. (1988). On language and connectionism: analysis of a parallel distributed processing model of language acquisition. *Cognition, 28,* 73–193.

Pinker, S. & Ullman, M. T. (2002). The past and future of the past tense. *Trends in Cognitive Sciences, 6,* 456–463.

Pinker, S. & Ullman, M. T. (2003). Beyond one model per phenomenon. *Trends in Cognitive Sciences, 7,* 108–109.

Pisella, L., Grea, H., Tilikete, C., Vighetto, A., Desmurget, M., Rode, G., Boisson, D., et al. (2000). An 'automatic pilot' for the hand in human posterior parietal cortex: toward reinterpreting optic ataxia. *Nature Neuroscience, 3*(7), 729–736.

Pisella, L., Binkofski, F., Lasek, K., Toni, I., & Rossetti, Y. (2006). No double-dissociation between optic ataxia and visual agnosia: multiple sub-streams for multiple visuo-manual integrations. *Neuropsychologia, 44,* 2734–2748.

Pisella, L., Sergio, L., Blangero, A., Torchin, H., Vighetto, A., & Rossetti, Y. (2009). Optic ataxia and the function of the dorsal stream: contributions to perception and action. *Neuropsychologia, 47,* 3033–3044.

Place, U. (1956). Is consciousness a brain process? *British journal of Psychology, 47,* 44–50.

Plaut, D. C. (1996). Relearning after damage in connectionist networks: Toward a theory of rehabilitation. *Brain and Language, 52,* 25–82.

Plaut, D. C. (2002). Graded modality-specific specialization in semantics: a computational account of optic aphasia. *Cognitive Neuropsychology, 19,* 603–639.

Plaut, D. C. (2003). Connectionist modeling of language: Examples and implications. In M. Banich & M. Mack (Eds), *Mind, brain and language* (pp. 143–167). Mahwah, NJ: Lawrence Erlbaum Associates.

Plaut, D. C. & McClelland, J. L. (2000). Stipulating versus discovering representations. *Behavioral and Brain Sciences, 23,* 489–491.

Plaut, D. C. & McClelland, J. L. (2010). Locating object knowledge in the brain: comment on Bowers's (2009) attempt to revive the grandmother cell hypothesis. *Psychological Review, 117,* 284–290.

Plaut, D. C. & Shallice, T. (1993a). Deep dyslexia: a case study of connectionist neuropsychology. *Cognitive Neuropsychology, 10,* 377–500.

Plaut, D.C. & Shallice, T. (1993b). Perseverative and semantic influences on visual object naming errors in optic aphasia: a connectionist account. *Journal of Cognitive Neuroscience, 5,* 89–117.

Plaut, D. C., McClelland, J. L., Seidenberg, M., & Patterson, K. (1996). Understanding normal and impaired word reading: computational principles in quasi-regular domains. *Psychological Review, 103,* 56–115.

Plunkett, K. & Bandelow, S. (2006). Stochastic approaches to understanding dissociations in inflectional morphology. *Brain and Language*, 98(2), 194–209.

Plunkett, K. & Marchman, V. (1993). From rote learning to system building: acquiring verb morphology in children and connectionist nets. *Cognition, 48,* 21–69.

Poeck, K. & Lehmkuhl, G. (1980). The syndrome of ideational apraxia and its localisation. *Nervenarzt, 51,* 217–225.

Poizner, H. & Soechting, J. (1992). New strategies for studying higher level motor disorders. In D.Margolin (Ed.), *Cognitive neuropsychology in clinical practice* (pp. 435–464). New York: Oxford UP.

Poizner, H., Merians, A. S., Clark, M. A., Gonzalez Rothi, L. J., & Heilman, K. M. (1997). Kinematic approaches to the study of apraxic disorders. In L. J. G. Rothi & K. M. Heilman (Eds), *Apraxia* (pp. 93–110). Psychology Press.

Poldrack, R. A. (2006). Can cognitive processes be inferred from neuroimaging data? *Trends in Cognitive Sciences, 10,* 59–63.

Polk, T. & Newell, A. (1995). Deduction as verbal reasoning. *Psychological Review, 102,* 533–566.

Pollard, C. & Sag, I. (1987). Information-based syntax and semantics, c sli lecture notes # 13, CSLI. Chicago University Press.

Pollard, C. & Sag, I. (1994). *Head-driven phrase structure grammar.* Chicago: University of Chicago Press.

Pollen, D.A. *(*2008*)*. Fundamental requirements for primary visual perception. *Cerebral Cortex, 18,* 1991–1998.

Pöppel, E., Held, R., & Frost, D. (1973). Leter: residual visual function after brain wounds involving the central visual pathways in man. *Nature, 243,* 295–296.

Port, R. & van Gelder, T. (1995). *Mind as motion.* Cambridge, MA: MIT Press.

Posner, M. (1978). *Chronometric explorations of mind.* Englewood Heights, NJ: Erlbaum.

Posner, M. (1980). The orienting of attention. *Quarterly Journal of Experimental Psychology, 32,* 3–25.

Posner, M. & Cohen, Y. (1984). Components of visual orienting. In H.Bouma & D. Bouwhuis (Eds), *Attention and Performance vol 10* (pp. 531–556). Hillsdale, NJ: Erlbaum.

Posner, M. & Di Girolamo, G. (1998). Executive attention: Conflict, target detection, and cognitive control. In R. Parasuraman (Ed.), *The attentive brain* (pp. 401–423). Cambridge, MA: MIT Press.

Posner, M. & Petersen, S. (1990). The attention system of the human brain. *Annual Review of Neuroscience, 13,* 25–42.

Post, E. (1936). Finite combinatory processes: formulation I. *Journal of Symbolic Logic, 1,* 103–105.

Post, E. (1943). Formal reductions of the general combinatorial decision problem. *American Journal of Mathematics, 65,* 197–215.

Posteraro, L., Zinelli, P., & Mazzucchi, A. (1988). Selective impairment of the graphemic buffer in acquired dysgraphia: a case study. *Brain and Language, 35,* 274–286.

Postle, B. R. & Corkin, S. (1999). Manipulation of familiarity reveals a necessary lexical component of the word-stem completion priming effect. *Memory and Cognition, 27,* 12–25.

Postle, B. R., Berger, J. S., & D'Esposito, M. (1999). Functional neuroanatomical double dissociation of mnemonic and executive control processes contributing to working memory performance. *Proceedings of the Natlional Academy of Sciences, USA, 96,* 12959–12964.

Postma, A. (2000). Detection of errors during speech production: a review of speech monitoring models. *Cognition, 77,* 97–132.

Pouget, A. & Sejnowski, T. J. (1997). Spatial transformations in the parietal cortex using basis functions. *Journal of Cognitive Neuroscience, 9,* 222–237.

Pouget, A. & Sejnowski, T. J. (2001). Simulating a lesion in a basis function model of spatial representations: comparison with hemineglect. *Psychological Review, 108,* 653–673.

Poulton, E. C. (1973). Unwanted range effects from using within-subject experimental designs. *Psychological Bulletin, 80,* 113–121.

Poulton, E. C. (1979). Models for biases in judging sensory magnitude. *Psychological Bulletin,* 86(4), 777–803.

Prabhakaran, V., Narayanan, K., Zhao, Z., & Gabrieli, J. D. (2000). Integration of diverse information in working memory within the frontal lobe. *Nature Neuroscience, 3,* 85–90.

Premack, D. & Woodruff, G. (1978). Does the chimpanzee have a 'theory of mind'? *Behavioral and Brain Sciences, 4,* 515–526.

Price, C. J. (1997). Functional anatomy of reading. In R. S. J. Frackowiak et al, *Human brain function* (pp. 301–328) London: Academic Press.

Price, C. J. (2000). The anatomy of language: contributions from functional neuroimaging. *Journal of Anatomy, 197* (3), 335–359.

Price, C. J. & Devlin, J. T. (2003). The myth of the visual word form area. *Neuroimage, 19,* 473–481.

Price, C. J. & Devlin, J. T. (2004). The pro and cons of labelling a left occipitotemporal region: 'the visual word form area'. *Neuroimage, 22,* 477–479.

Price, C. J. & Friston, K. J. (1997). Cognitive conjunction: a new approach to brain activation experiments. *Neuroimage, 5,* 261–270.

Price, C. J. & Humphreys, G. W. (1995). Contrasting effects of letter-spacing in alexia: further evidence that different strategies generate word length effects in reading. *Quarterly Journal of Experimental Psychology, A, 48,* 573–597.

Price, C. J. & Mechelli, A. (2005). Reading and reading disturbance. *Current Opinion in Neurobiology, 15,* 231–238.

Price, C. J., Moore, C. J., & Friston, K. J. (1997a). Subtractions, conjunctions, and interactions in experimental design of activation studies. *Human Brain Mapping, 5,* 264–272.

Price, C. J., Moore, C., Humphreys, GW., & Wise, R. J. (1997b). Segregating semantic from phonological processes during reading. *Journal of Cognitive Neuroscience, 9,* 727–733.

Price, C. J., Howard, D., Patterson, K., Warburton, E. A., Friston, K. J., & Frackowiak, S. J. (1998). A functional neuroimaging description of two deep dyslexic patients. *Journal of Cognitive Neuroscience, 10,* 303–315.

Price, C. J., Mummery, C. J., Moore, C. J., Frakowiak, R. S., & Friston, K. J. (1999). Delineating necessary and sufficient neural systems with functional imaging studies of neuropsychological patients. *Journal of Cognitive Neuroscience, 11,* 371–382.

Price, C. J., McCrory, E., Noppeney, U., Mechelli, A., Moore, C. J., Biggio, N. et al. (2006). How reading differs from object naming at the neuronal level. *Neuroimage, 29,* 643–648.

Prinzmetal, W., Hoffman, H., & Vest, K. (1991). Automatic processes in word perception: An analysis from illusory conjunctions. *Journal of Experimental Psychology: Human Perception Performance, 17,* 902–923.

Pulvermuller, F., Shtyrov, Y., & Ilmoniemi, R. (2005). Brain signatures of meaning access in action word recognition. *Journal of Cognitive Neuroscience, 17,* 884–892.

Pylyshyn, Z. (1973). What the mind's eye tells the mind's brain: A critique of mental imagery. *Psychological Bullettin, 80,* 1–22.

Pylyshyn, Z. (1983). Information science: its roots and relation as viewed from the prespective of cognitive science. In F. Machlup & U. Mansfield (Eds), *The study of information: interdisciplinary messages.* (pp. 63–118). New York: Wiley.

Pylyshyn, Z. (1984). *Computation and Cognition: Toward a Foundation for Cognitive Science.* Cambridge, MA: Bradford Books.

Pylyshyn, Z. (2003). Mental imagery: In search of a theory. *Behavioral and Brain Sciences, 25,* 157–238.

Pylyshyn, Z. & Storm, R.W. (1988). Tracking multiple independent targets: Evidence for a parallel tracking mechanism. *Spatial Vision, 3,* 179–197.

Quillian, M. R. (1968). Semantic memory. In Minsky, M. (Ed). *Semantic Information Processing.* (pp. 227–270). Cambridge, MA: MIT Press.

Quiroga, R. Q., Reddy, L., Kreiman, G., Koch, C., & Fried, I. (2005). Invariant visual representation by single neurons in the human brain. *Nature, 435,* 1102–1107.

Rademacher, J., Morosan, P., Schormann, T., Schleicher, A., Werner, C., Freund, H. J. et al. (2001). Probabilistic mapping and volume measurement of human primary auditory cortex. *Neuroimage, 13,* 669–683.

Raichle, M. E., Martin, W. R., Herscovitch, P., Mintun, M. A., & Markham, J. (1983). Brain blood flow measured with intravenous H2(15)O. II. Implementation and validation. *Jounral of Nuclear Medicine, 24,* 790–798.

Raichle, M. E., Fiez, J. A., Videen, T. O., MacLeod, A. M., Pardo, J. V., Fox, P. T. et al. (1994). Practice-related changes in human brain functional anatomy during nonmotor learning. *Cerebral Cortex, 4,* 8–26.

Rajaram, S. (1993). Remembering and knowing: two means of access to the personal past. *Memory and Cognition, 21,* 89–102.

Ramnani, N. & Owen, A. M. (2004). Anterior prefrontal cortex: insights into function from anatomy and neuroimaging. *Nature Reviews Neuroscience, 5,* 184–194.

Ramscar, M. (2002). The role of meaning in inflection: why the past tense does not require a rule. *Cognitive Psychology, 45,* 45–94.

Ranganath, C., Yonelinas, A. P., Cohen, M. X., Dy, C. J., Tom, S. M., & D'Esposito, M. (2004). Dissociable correlates of recollection and familiarity in the medial temporal lobes. *Neuropscyhologia, 42,* 2–13.

Rao, A. & Georgeff, M. (1995). BDI Agents: from theory to practice. In *Proceedings of the 1st international conference on multi-agent systems* (pp. 312–319). San Francisco, CA.

Rao, S. M., Mayer, A. R., & Harrington, D. L. (2001). The evolution of brain activation during temporal processing. *Nature Neuroscience, 4,* 317–323.

Rapcsak, S. Z., Beeson, P. M., Henry, M. L., Leyden, A., Kim, E., Rising, K. et al. (2009). Phonological dyslexia and dysgraphia: cognitive mechanisms and neural substrates. *Cortex, 45,* 575–591.

Rapp, B. & Caramazza, A. (1993). On the distinction between deficits of access and deficits of storage: A question of theory. *Cognitive Neuropsychology, 10,* 113–141.

Ratcliff, G. (1979). Spatial thought, mental rotation and the right cerebral hemisphere. *Neuropsychologia, 17,* 49–54.

Ratcliff, G. & Davies-Jones, G. (1972). Defective visual localisation in focal brain wounds. *Brain, 95,* 49–60.

Rattermann, M. & Gentner, D. (1998). More evidence for a relational shift in the development of analogy:

children's performance on a causal-mapping task. *Cognitive Develpment, 13,* 453–478.

Ravizza, S. M., Delgado, M. R., Chein, J. M., Becker, J. T., & Fiez, J. A. (2004). Functional dissociations within the inferior parietal cortex in verbal working memory. *Neuroimage, 22,* 562–573.

Raymer, A. & Berndt, R. (1996). Models of word reading: evidence from Alzheimer's Disease. *Brain and Language, 47,* 479–482.

Raymond, J. E., Shapiro, K. L., & Arnell, K. M. (1992). Temporary suppression of visual processing in an RSVP task: an attentional blink? *Journal of Experimental Psychology: Human Perception and Performance, 18*(3), 849–860.

Reason, J. T. (1979). Actions not as planned: the price of automatization. In G. Underwood & R. Stevens (Eds), *Aspects of consciousness* (pp. 67–89). London: Academic Press.

Reason, J. T. (1984). Lapses of attention in everyday life. In R.Parasuraman & R. Davies (Eds), *Varieties of attention* (pp. 515–549). Orlando, FL: Academic Press.

Redish, A. D. (1999). *Beyond the cognitive map: from place cells to episodic memory.* Cambridge, MA: MIT Press.

Redish, A. D. & Touretzky, D. (1996). Modeling interactions of the rat's place and head direction systems. In D. Touretzky, M. Mozer, & M. Hasselmo (Eds), *Advances in neural information processing systems, 8.* (pp. 61–67). Cambridge, MA: MIT Press.

Redish, A. D. & Touretzky, D. S. (1998). The role of the hippocampus in solving the Morris water maze. *Neural Comput., 10,* 73–111.

Reed, J. M., & Squire, L. R. (1997). Impaired recognition memory in patients with lesions limited to the hippocampal formation. *Behavioral Neuroscience, 111*(4), 667–675.

Reed, J. M. & Squire, L. R. (1998). Retrograde amnesia for facts and events: findings from four new cases. *Journal of Neuroscience, 18,* 3943–3954.

Rees, G. (2007). Neural correlates of the contents of visual awareness in humans. *Philosophical Transactions of the Royal Society B: Biological Sciences, 362*(1481), 877–886.

Rees, G., Frith, C. D., & Lavie, N. (1997). Modulating irrelevant motion perception by varying attentional load in an unrelated task. *Science, 278,* 1616–1619.

Rees, G., Wojciulik, E., Clarke, K., Husain, M., Frith, C., & Driver, J. (2000). Unconscious activation of visual cortex in the damaged right hemisphere of a parietal patient with extinction. *Brain, 123* (8), 1624–1633.

Rempel-Clower, N. & Barbas, H. (2000). The laminar pattern of connections between prefrontal and anterior temporal cortices in the Rhesus monkey is related to cortical structure and function. *Cerebral Cortex, 10,* 851–865.

Rempel-Clower, N. L., Zola, S. M., Squire, L. R., & Amaral, D. G. (1996). Three cases of enduring memory impairment after bilateral damage limited to the hippocampal formation. *Journal of Neuroscience, 16,* 5233–5255.

Repovs, G. & Baddeley, A. D. (2006). The multi-component model of working memory: explorations in experimental cognitive psychology. *Neuroscience, 139,* 5–21.

Reverberi, C., D'Agostini, S., Skrap, M., & Shallice, T. (2005a). Generation and recognition of abstract rules in different frontal lobe subgroups. *Neuropsychologia, 43,* 1924–1937.

Reverberi, C., Lavaroni, A., Gigli, G. L., Skrap, M., & Shallice, T. (2005b). Specific impairments of rule induction in different frontal lobe subgroups. *Neuropsychologia, 43,* 460–472.

Reverberi, C., Toraldo, A., D'Agostini, S., & Skrap, M. (2005c). Better without (lateral) frontal cortex? Insight problems solved by frontal patients. *Brain, 128,* 2882–2890.

Reverberi, C., Cherubini, P., Rapisarda, A., Rigamonti, E., Caltagirone, C., Frackowiak, R. S. J. et al. (2007). Neural basis of generation of conclusions in elementary deduction. *Neuroimage, 38,* 752–762.

Ribot, T. (1882). *Diseases of memory: an essay in positive psychology.* London: Kegan Paul Trench.

Riddoch, M. J., Johnston, R. A., Bracewell, R. M., Boutsen, L., & Humphreys, G. W. (2008). Are faces special? A case of pure prosopagnosia. *Cognitive Neuropsychology, 25,* 3–26.

Rips, L. (1994). *The psychology of proof.* Cambridge, MA: MIT Press.

Rips, L., Shoben, E., & Smith, E. (1973). Semantic distance and the verification of semantic relations. *Journal of Verbal Learning and Verbal Behavior, 12,* 1–20.

Rizzo, A., Ferrante, D., & Bagnara, S. (1995). Handling human error. In J.Hoc, P. Cacciabue, & E. Hollnagel (Eds), *Expertise and technology. Cognition and humancomputer interaction.* Hillsdale, NJ: LEA.

Rizzolatti, G. & Arbib, M. A. (1998). Language within our grasp. *Trends in Neurosciences, 21,* 188–194.

Rizzolatti, G. & Matelli, M. (2003). Two different streams form the dorsal visual system: anatomy and functions. *Experimental Brain Research, 153,* 146–157.

Rizzolatti, G. & Sinigaglia, C. (2010). The functional role of the parieto-frontal mirror circuit: interpretations and misinterpretations. *Nature Reviews Neuroscience, 11,* 264–274.

Rizzolatti, G., Fadiga, L., Gallese, V., & Fogassi, L. (1996a). Premotor cortex and the recognition of motor actions. *Cognitive Brain Research, 3*(2), 131–141.

Rizzolatti, G., Fadiga, L., Matelli, M., Bettinardi, V., Paulesu, E., Perani, D. et al. (1996b). Localization of grasp representations in humans by PET: 1.

Observation versus execution. *Experimental Brain Research, 111,* 246–252.

Roberts, S. (1981). Isolation of an internal clock. *Journal of Experimental Psychology: Animal Behavior Processes, 7,* 242–268.

Roberts, S. & Pashler, H. (2000). How persuasive is a good fit? A comment on theory testing. *Psychological Review, 107,* 358–367.

Roberts, S. & Sternberg, S. (1993). The meaning of additive reaction-time effects: Tests of three alternatives. In S.Meyer & S. Kornblum (Eds), *Attention and performance XIV: synergies in experimental psychology, artificial intelligence, and cognitive neuroscience—a silver jubilee* (pp. 611–653). Cambridge, MA: MIT Press.

Robinson, J.A. (1976). Sampling autobiographical memory. *Cognitive Psychology, 8,* 578–595.

Robinson, G., Blair, J., & Cipolotti, L. (1998). Dynamic aphasia: an inability to select between competing verbal responses? *Brain, 121* (1), 77–89.

Robinson, G., Shallice, T. & Cipolotti, L. (2005). A failure of high level verbal response selection in progressive dynamic aphasia. *Cognitive Neuropsychology, 22,* 661–694.

Robinson, G., Shallice, T., & Cipolotti, L. (2006). Dynamic aphasia in progressive supranuclear palsy: a deficit in generating a fluent sequence of novel thought. *Neuropsychologia, 44,* 1344–1360.

Robinson, G., Shallice, T., Bozzali, M., & Cipolotti, L. (2010). Conceptual proposition selection and the LIFG: neuropsychological evidence from a focal frontal group. *Neuropsychologia, 48,* 1652–1663.

Roca, M., Parr, A., Thompson, R., Woolgar, A., Torralva, T., Antoun, N. et al. (2009). Executive function and fluid intelligence after frontal lobe lesions. *Brain, 133,* 234–247.

Rock, I., Linnett, C. M., Grant, P., & Mack, A. (1992). Perception without attention: results of a new method. *Cognitive Psychology, 24*(4), 502–534.

Rockel, A., Hiorns, R., & Powell, T. (1980). The basic uniformity in structure of the neocortex. *Brain, 103,* 221–244.

Rodd, J. M. (2004). The effect of semantic ambiguity on reading aloud: a twist in the tale. *Psychonomic Bulletin and Review, 11,* 440–445.

Rodd, J., Gaskell, M., & Marslen-Wilson, W. (2002). Making sense of semantic ambiguity: semantic competition in lexical access. *Journal of Memory and Language, 46,* 245–266.

Rodd, J., Gaskell, M., & Marslen-Wilson, W. (2004). Modelling the effects of semantic ambiguity in word recognition. *Cognitive Science, 28,* 89–104.

Rodd, J. M., Davis, M. H., & Johnsrude, I. S. (2005). The neural mechanisms of speech comprehension: fMRI studies of semantic ambiguity. *Cerebral Cortex, 15,* 1261–1269.

Roelfsema, P. R., Lamme, V. A. F., & Spekreijse, H. (1998). Object-based attention in the primary visual cortex of the macaque monkey. *Nature, 395,* 376–381.

Roelofs, A. (1997). The WEAVER model of word-form encoding in speech production. *Cognition, 64*(3), 249–284.

Roeltgen, D. P. (1987). Loss of deep dyslexic reading ability from a second left hemisphere lesion. *Archives of Neurology, 44,* 346–348.

Rogers, R. & Monsell, S. (1995). Costs of a predictable switch between simple cognitive tasks. *Journal of Experimental Psychology: General, 124,* 207–231.

Rogers, R. D., Sahakian, B. J., Hodges, J. R., Polkey, C. E., Kennard, C., & Robbins, T. W. (1998). Dissociating executive mechanisms of task control following frontal lobe damage and Parkinson's disease. *Brain, 121* (5), 815–842.

Rogers, T. T., Hodges, J. R., Ralph, M. A. L., & Patterson, K. (2003). Object recognition under semantic impairment: The effects of conceptual regularities on perceptual decisions. *Language and Cognitive Processes, 18,* 625–662.

Rogers, T. T., Lambon Ralph, M. A., Garrard, P., Bozeat, S., McClelland, J. L., Hodges, J. R., & Patterson, K. (2004). Structure and deterioration of semantic memory: a neuropsychological and computational investigation. *Psychological Review, 111,* 205–235.

Roland, P. E. & Gulyás, B. (1995). Visual memory, visual imagery, and visual recognition of large field patterns by the human brain: functional anatomy by positron emission tomography. *Cerebral Cortex, 5,* 79–93.

Roland, P. E., Skinhøj, E., & Lassen, N. A. (1981). Focal activations of human cerebral-cortex during auditory-discrimination. *Journal of Neurophysiology, 45,* 1139–1151.

Romani, C. (1992). Are there distinct input and output buffers? Evidence from an aphasic patient with an impaired output buffer. *Language and Cognitive Processes, 7,* 131–162.

Romero, L., Walsh, V., & Papagno, C. (2006). The neural correlates of phonological short-term memory: a repetitive transcranial magnetic stimulation study. *Journal of Cognitive Neuroscience, 18,* 1147–1155.

Rorden, C. & Karnath, H. O. (2004). Using human brain lesions to infer function: a relic from a past era in the fMRI age? *Nature Reviews Neuroscience, 5,* 813–819.

Rorden, C., Karnath, H. O., & Bonilha, L. (2007). Improving lesion-symptom mapping. *Journal of Cognitive Neuroscience, 19,* 1081–1088.

Rosazza, C. & Shallice, T. (2006). Patterns of peripheral paralexia: pure alexia and the forgotten visual dyslexia? *Cortex, 42,* 892–897.

Rosazza, C., Apollonio, I., Isella, V., & Shallice, T. (2007). Qualitatively different forms of pure alexia. *Cognitive Neuropsychology, 24,* 393–418.

Rosch, E., Mervis, C., Gray, W., Johnson, D., & Boyes-Braem, P. (1976). Basic objects in natural categorization. *Cognitive Psychology, 8,* 382–439.

Rosenbaum, R. S., McKinnon, M. C., Levine, B., & Moscovitch, M. (2004). Visual imagery deficits, impaired strategic retrieval, or memory loss: disentangling the nature of an amnesic person's autobiographical memory deficit. *Neuropsychologia, 42,* 1619–1635.

Rosenbaum, R. S., Moscovitch, M., Foster, J. K., Schnyer, D. M., Gao, F., Kovacevic, N. et al. (2008). Patterns of autobiographical memory loss in medial-temporal lobe amnesic patients. *Journal of Cognitive Neuroscience, 20,* 1490–1506.

Rosenblatt, F. (1958). The perceptron: A probabilistic model for information storage and organization in the brain. *Psychological Review, 65,* 407.

Rosenblatt, F. (1962). *Principles of Neurodynamics.* New York: Spartan Books.

Ross, E. D. & Monnot, M. (2008). Neurology of affective prosody and its functional-anatomic organization in right hemisphere. *Brain and Language, 104*(1), 51–74.

Rossi, S., Cappa, S. F., Babiloni, C., Pasqualetti, P., Miniussi, C., Carducci, F. et al. (2001). Prefrontal cortex in long-term memory: an 'interference' approach using magnetic stimulation. *Nature Neuroscience, 4,* 948–952.

Rossi, S., Pasqualetti, P., Zito, G., Vecchio, F., Cappa, S. F., Miniussi, C. et al. (2006). Prefrontal and parietal cortex in human episodic memory: an interference study by repetitive transcranial magnetic stimulation. *European Journal of Neuroscience, 23,* 793–800.

Rothi, L. J., Mack, L., & Heilman, K. M. (1986). Pantomime agnosia. *Journal of Neurology, Neurosurgery and Psychiatry,* 49, 451–454.

Rothi, L. J., Ochipa, C., & Heilman, K. M. (1991). A cognitive neuropsychological model of limb praxis. *Cognitive Neuropsychology, 8,* 443–458.

Rowe, J. B., Toni, I., Josephs, O., Frackowiak, R. S., & Passingham, R. E. (2000). The prefrontal cortex: response selection or maintenance within working memory? *Science, 288,* 1656–1660.

Rowe, J. B., Owen, A. M., Johnsrude, I. S., & Passingham, R. E. (2001). Imaging the mental components of a planning task. *Neuropsychologia, 39,* 315–327.

Roy, E. & Square, P. (1985). Common considerations in the study of limb, verbal, and oral apraxia. In E.Roy (Ed.), *Neuropsychological studies of apraxia and related disorders* (pp. 111–161). Amsterdam: North-Holland.

Rubin, D. C. & Schulkind, M. D. (1997). The distribution of autobiographical memories across the lifespan. *Memory and Cognition, 25,* 859–866.

Rudge, P. & Warrington, E. K. (1991). Selective impairment of memory and visual perception in splenial tumours. *Brain, 114 (1B),* 349–360.

Rueckert, L. & Grafman, J. (1996). Sustained attention deficits in patients with right frontal lesions. *Neuropsychologia, 34,* 953–963.

Ruff, C. C., Blankenburg, F., Bjoertomt, O., Bestmann, S., Freeman, E., Haynes, J. D. et al. (2006). Concurrent TMS-fMRI and psychophysics reveal frontal influences on human retinotopic visual cortex. *Current Biology, 16,* 1479–1488.

Ruge, H. & Braver, T. S. (2008). Neural mechanisms in cognitive control in cued task-switiching: rules, representations and preparation. In S.A.Bunge & J. D. Wallis (Eds), *Neuroscience of rule-guided behavior.* Oxford: OUP.

Rugg, M. D. (1998). Convergent approaches to electrophysiological and hemodynamic investigations of memory. *Human Brain Mapping, 6,* 394–398.

Rugg, M. D., Fletcher, P. C., Allan, K., Frith, C. D., Frackowiak, R. S. J., and Dolan, R. J. (1998). Neural correlates of memory retrieval during recognition memory and cued recall. *Neuroimage, 8,* 262–273.

Ruh, N., Cooper, R. P., & Mareschal, D. (submitted). The goal circuit model: a hierarchical multi-route model of the acquisition and control of routine sequential actions in humans.

Rumelhart, D. E. (1990). Brain style computation: Learning and generalization. In S. F. Zornetzer, J. L. Davis, & C. Lau (Eds), *An introduction to neural and electronic networks.* New York: Academic Press.

Rumelhart, D. & McClelland, J. (1982). An interactive activation model of context effects in letter perception: Part 2. The contextual enhancement effect and some tests and extensions of the model. *Psychological Review, 89,* 60–94.

Rumelhart, D. & Norman, D. A. (1982). Simulating a skilled typist: A study of skilled cognitive-motor performance. *Cognitive Science, 6,* 1–36.

Rumelhart, D., Hinton, G., & Williams, R. (1986). Learning representations by back-propagating errors. *Nature, 323,* 533–536.

Rumelhart, D. & McClelland, J. (1986). On learning the past tenses of English verbs. In J. L. McClelland & D. E. Rumelhart and the PDP Research Group (Eds) *Parallel distributed processing: explorations in the microstructures of cognition* (pp. 216–271). Cambridge, MA: MIT Press.

Rumiati, R., Zanini, S., Vorano, L., & Shallice, T. (2001). A form of ideational apraxia as a selective deficit of contention scheduling. *Cognitive Neuropsychology, 18,* 617–642.

Rumiati, R. I., Weiss, P. H., Shallice, T., Ottoboni, G., Noth, J., Zilles, K. et al. (2004). Neural basis of pantomiming the use of visually presented objects. *Neuroimage, 21,* 1224-1231.

Ruml, W., & Caramazza, A. (2000). An evaluation of a computational model of lexical access: comment on Dell et al. (1997). *Psychological Review, 107*(3), 609-634.

Rushworth, M. F., Behrens, T. E., & Johansen-Berg, H. (2006). Connection patterns distinguish 3 regions of human parietal cortex. *Cerebral Cortex, 16,* 1418-1430.

Russell, S. & Norvig, P. (1995). *Artificial intelligence: a modern approach.* Los Altos, CA.: Morgan-Kaufman.

Rust, N. C., Mante, V., Simoncelli, E. P., & Movshon, J. A. (2006). How MT cells analyze the motion of visual patterns. *Nature Neuroscience, 9,* 1421-1431.

Ryan, J. (1969). Grouping and short-term memory: different means and patterns of groups. *Quarterly Journal of Experimental Psychology, 21,* 137-147.

Ryan, L., Nadel, L., Keil, K., Putnam, K., Schnyer, D., Trouard, T. et al. (2001). Hippocampal complex and retrieval of recent and very remote autobiographicla memories. *Hippocampus, 11,* 707-714.

Rylander, G. (1939). Personality changes after operations on the frontal lobes. *Acta Psychiatrica et Neurologica Scandinavica, Supplementum. 20.*

Sacchett, C. & Humphreys, G. (1992). Calling a squirrel a squirrel but a canoe a wigwam: a category-specific deficit for artifactual objects and body parts. *Cognitive Neuropsychology, 9,* 73-86.

Sacerdoti, E. (1974). Planning in a hierarchy of abstract spaces. *Artificial Intelligence, 5,* 115-136.

Sach, M., Seitz, R. J., & Indefrey, P. (2004). Unified inflectional processing of regular and irregular verbs: a PET study. *Neuroreport, 15,* 533-537.

Saffran, E. & Marin, S. (1975). Immediate memory for word lists and sentences in a patient with deficient auditory short-term memory. *Brain and Language, 2,* 420-433.

Saffran, E., Bogyo, L., Schwartz, M., & Marin, O. (1980). Does deep dyslexia reflect right-hemisphere reading? In M.Coltheart, K. Patterson, & J. Marshall (Eds), *Deep dyslexia* (pp. 381-406). London: Routledge & Keegan Paul.

Sage, K. & Ellis, A. (2004). Lexical influences in graphemic buffer disorder. *Cognitive Neuropsychology, 21,* 400.

Sahraie, A., Weiskrantz, L., Barbur, J. L., Simmons, A., Williams, S. C., & Brammer, M. J. (1997). Pattern of neuronal activity associated with conscious and unconscious processing of visual signals. *Proceedings of the National Academy of Sciences, USA, 94,* 9406-9411.

Sakai, K. & Passingham, R. E. (2003). Prefrontal interactions reflect future task operations. *Nature Neuroscience, 6,* 75-81.

Salame, P. & Baddeley, AD. (1982). Disruption of short-term memory by unattended speech: implications for the structure of working memory. *Journal of Verbal Learning and Verbal Behavior, 21,* 150-164.

Samson, D. & Pillon, A. (2003). A case of impaired knowledge for fruit and vegetables. *Cognitive Neuropsychology, 20,* 373-400.

Sanders, A. (1998). *Elements of human performance: reaction processes and attention in human skill.* Mahway, NJ: Erlbaum.

Sanders, A. F., Wijnen, J. L. C., & van Arkel, A. E. (1982). An additive factor analysis of the effects of sleep loss on reaction processes. *Acta Psychologica, 51,* 41-59.

Sanders, H. I., & Warrington, E. K. (1971). Memory for remote events in amnesic patients. *Brain, 94*(4), 661-668.

Sandkühler, S. & Bhattacharya, J. (2008). Deconstructing insight: EEG correlates of insightful problem solving. *PLoS One, 3,* e1459.

Sargolini, F., Fyhn, M., Hafting, T., MacNaughton, B., Witter, M., Moser, M. et al. (2006). Conjunctive representation of position, direction, and velocity in entorhinal cortex. *Science, 312,* 762.

Sartori, G. & Job, R. (1988). The oyster with four legs: A neuropsychological study on the interaction of visual and semantic information. *Cognitive Neuropsychology, 5,* 105-132.

Sartori, G., Miozzo, M., & Job, R. (1993). Category-specific naming impairments? Yes. *Quarterly Journal of Experimental Psychology, 46A,* 489-504.

Sartori, G., Gnoato, F., Mariani, I., Prioni, S., & Lombardi, L. (2007). Semantic relevance, domain specificity and the sensory/functional theory of category-specificity. *Neuropsychologia, 45,* 966-976.

Schacter, D. L. & Buckner, R. L. (1998). Priming and the brain. *Neuron, 20,* 185-195.

Schacter, D. & Tulving, E. (1994). What are the memory systems of 1994? In D. Schacter & E. Tulving (Eds), *Memoery systems* (pp. 1-38). Cambridge, MA: MIT Press.

Schacter, D. L., Chiu, C. Y., & Ochsner, K. N. (1993). Implicit memory: a selective review. *Annual Review of Neuroscience, 16,* 159-182.

Schacter, D. L., Alpert, N. M., Savage, C. R., Rauch, S. L., & Albert, M. S. (1996). Conscious recollection and the human hippocampal formation: evidence from positron emission tomography. *Proceedings of the National Academy of Sciences, U S A, 93,* 321-325.

Schall, U., Johnston, P., Lagopoulos, J., Juptner, M., Jentzen, W., Thienel, R. et al. (2003). Functional brain maps of Tower of London performance: a positron emission tomography and functional magnetic resonance imaging study. *Neuroimage, 20,* 1154-1161.

Schank, R.C. (1982). *Dynamic memory.* Cambridge University Press, Cambridge.

Schank, R. C. & Abelson, R. P. (1977). *Scripts, plans, goals and understanding.* Oxford: Erlbaum.

Schein, S. & DeSimone, R. (1990). Spectral properties of V4 neurons in the macaque. *Journal of Neuroscience, 10,* 3369–3389.

Scherg, M. & Berg, P. (1991). Use of prior knowledge in brain electromagnetic source analysis. *Brain Topography, 4,* 143–150.

Schiller, N. O., Greenhall, J. A., Shelton, J. R., & Caramazza, A. (2001). Serial order effects in spelling errors: evidence from two dysgraphic patients. *Neurocase, 7,* 1–14.

Schlaghecken, F. & Eimer, M. (2006). Active masks and active inhibition: a comment on Lleras and Enns (2004) and on Verleger, Jaśkowski, Aydemir, van der Lubbe, and Groen (2004). *Journal of Experimental Psychology: General, 135*(3), 484–494.

Schmidt, R. A. (1975). A schema theory of discrete motor skill learning. *Psychological Review, 82*(4), 225–260.

Schnider, A. (2003). Spontaneous confabulation and the adaptation of thought to ongoing reality. *Nature Reviews Neuroscience,* 4(8), 662–671.

Schnider, A. (2008). *The confabulating mind: how the brain creates reality.* Oxford: OUP.

Schnider, A., Treyer, V., & Buck, A. (2000). Selection of currently relevant memories by the human posterior medial orbitofrontal cortex. *Journal of Neuroscience, 20,* 5880–5884.

Schnider, A., von Däniken C., & Gutbrod, K. (1996). The mechanisms of spontaneous and provoked confabulations. *Brain, 119* (4), 1365–1375.

Schnider, A., Valenza, N., Morand, S., & Michel, C. M. (2002). Early cortical distinction between memories that pertain to ongoing reality and memories that don't. *Cerebral Cortex, 12,* 54–61.

Schott, B. H., Henson, R. N., Richardson-Klavehn, A., Becker, C., Thoma, V., Heinze, H. J. et al. (2005). Redefining implicit and explicit memory: the functional neuroanatomy of priming, remembering, and control of retrieval. *Proceedings of the National Academy of Sciences, USA, 102,* 1257–1262.

Schuell, H. & Jenkins, J. J. (1959). The nature of language deficit in aphasia. *Psychological Review, 66,* 45–67.

Schvaneveldt, R. & Meyer, D. (1973). Retrieval and comparison processes in semantic memory. In S. Kornblum (Ed.), *Attention and performance IV* (pp. 421–452). New York: Academic Press.

Schwartz, M. F. (1995). Re-examining the role of executive functions in routine action production. In *Structure and functions of the human prefrontal cortex. Annals of the New York Academy of Sciences, Vol. 769.* (pp. 321–335). New York, NY, US: New York Academy of Sciences.

Schwartz, M. F., Saffran, E. M., & Marin, O. S. M. (1980a). Fractionating the reading process in dementia: Evidence for word-specific print-to-sound. In M. Coltheart, K. E. Patterson, & J. C. Marshall (Eds), *Deep dyslexia* (pp. 259–269). London: Routledge.

Schwartz, M., Saffran, E., & Marin, O. (1980b). The word-order problem in agrammatism: I. Comprehension. *Brain and Language, 10,* 249–262.

Schwartz, M. F., Reed, E. S., Montgomery, M., Palmer, C., & Mayer, N. H. (1991). The quantitative description of action disorganization after brain-damage: a case-study. *Cognitive Neuropsychology, 8,* 381–414.

Schwartz, M. F., Montgomery, M. W., Buxbaum, L. J., Lee, S. S., Carew, T. G., Coslett, H. B. et al. (1998). Naturalistic action impairment in closed head injury. *Neuropsychology, 12,* 13–28.

Scott, S. K. & Johnsrude, I. S. (2003). The neuroanatomical and functional organization of speech perception. *Trends in Neurosciences, 26,* 100–107.

Scoville, W. & Milner, B. (1957). Loss of recent memory after hippocampal lesions. *Journal of Neurology, Neurosurgery and Psychiatry, 20,* 11–21.

Searle, J. (1980). Minds, brains and programs. *Behavioral and Brain Sciences, 3,* 417–457.

Seger, C. A. & Cincotta, C. M. (2006). Dynamics of frontal, striatal, and hippocampal systems during rule learning. *Cerebral Cortex, 16,* 1546–1555.

Seidenberg, M. S. & Joanisse, M. F. (2003). Show us the model. *Trends in Cognitive Sciences, 7,* 106–107.

Seidenberg, M. S. & MacDonald, M. C. (1999). A probabilistic constraints approach to language acquisition and processing. *Cognitive Science, 23,* 567–588.

Seidenberg, M. S. & McClelland, J. L. (1989). A distributed, developmental model of word recognition and naming. *Psychological Review, 96,* 523–568.

Sejnowski, T. J. & Churchland, P. S. (1989). Brain and cognition. In M.Posner (Ed.), *Foundations of cognitive science* (pp. 315–356). Cambridge, MA: MIT Press.

Selkirk, E. (1984). On the major class features and syllable theory. In M.Aronoff & R. Orehrle (Eds), *Language sound structure: studies in phonology presented to Morris Halle by his teachers and students.* Cambridge, MA: MIT Press.

Selz, O. (1913). *Über die Gesetze des geordenten Denkverlaufes-Erster Teil [The laws of thinking-part 1].* Stuttgart: Spemann.

Selz, O. (1922). *The psychology of productive thinking and of error: an experimental study.* Bonn, Germany: Cohen.

Seok, B. (2006). Diversity and unity of modularity. *Cognitive Science, 30,* 347–380.

Shadlen, M. N. & Movshon, J. A. (1999). Synchrony unbound: a critical evaluation of the temporal binding hypothesis. *Neuron, 24,* 67–25.

Shadlen, M., Britten, K., Newsome, W., & Movshon, J. (1996). A computational analysis of the relationship between neuronal and behavioral responses to visual motion. *Journal of Neuroscience, 16,* 1486–1510.

Shafto, M. A., Burke, D. M., Stamatakis, E. A., Tam, P. P., & Tyler, L. K. (2007). On the Tip-of-the-Tongue: Neural Correlates of Increased Word-finding Failures in Normal Aging. *Journal of Cognitive Neuroscience, 19*(12), 2060–2070.

Shallice, T. (1975). On the contents of primary memory. In P. Rabbitt & S. Dornick (Eds), *Attention and performance* (pp. 269–280). London: Academic Press.

Shallice, T. (1979). Neuropsychological research and the fractionalization of memory systems. In L. Nilsson (Ed.), *Perspectives on memory research* (pp. 257–277). Hillsdale, NJ: Erlbaum.

Shallice, T. (1981). Phonological agraphia and the lexical route in writing. *Brain, 104,* 413–429.

Shallice, T. (1982). Specific impairments of planning. *Philosophical Transactions of the Royal Society of London B Biological Sciences, 298,* 199–209.

Shallice, T. (1987). Impairments of semantic processing: Multiple dissociations. In M.Coltheart, G. Sartori, & R. Job (Eds), *The Cognitive Neuropsychology of Language* (pp. 111–128). Hove, UK: Lawrence Erlbaum Associates Ltd.

Shallice, T. (1988). *From neuropsychology to mental structure.* Cambridge, UK: Cambridge University Press.

Shallice, T. (1993). Multiple semantics: whose confusions? *Cognitive Neuropsychology, 10,* 251–261.

Shallice, T. (2003). Functional imaging and neuropsychology findings: How can they be linked? *Neuroimage, 20 Suppl 1,* S146–S154.

Shallice, T. & Burgess, P. W. (1991). Deficits in strategy application following frontal lobe damage in man. *Brain, 11,* 727–741.

Shallice, T. & Burgess, P. W. (1996). The domain of supervisory processes and temporal organization of behaviour. *Philosophical Transactions of the Royal Society of London B Biological Sciences, 351,* 1405–1411.

Shallice, T. & Butterworth, B. (1977). Short-term memory impairment and spontaneous speech. *Neuropsychologia, 15,* 729–735.

Shallice, T. & McCarthy, R. (1985). Phonological reading: From patterns of impairment to possible procedures. In K.Patterson, M. Coltheart, & J. Marshall (Eds), *Surface Dyslexia* (pp. 361–398). Hillsdale, NJ: Lawrence Erlbaum Associates.

Shallice, T. & Saffran, E. (1986). Lexical processing in the absence of explicit word identification: Evidence from a letter by-letter reader. *Cognitive Neuropsychology, 3,* 429–458.

Shallice, T. & Vallar, G. (1990). The impairment of auditory-verbal short-term storage. In G.Vallar & T. Shallice (Eds), *Neuropsychological Impairments of Short-Term Memory* (pp. 11–53). Cambridge: CUP.

Shallice, T. & Warrington, E. K. (1970). Independent functioning of the verbal memory stores: A neuropsychological study. *Quarterly Journal of Experimental Psychology, 22,* 261–273.

Shallice, T. & Warrington, E. K. (1975). Word recognition in a phonemic dyslexic patient. *Quarterly Journal of Experimental Psychology, 27,* 187–199.

Shallice, T. & Warrington, E.K. (1977a). Auditory-verbal short-term memory impairment and spontaneous speech. *Brain and Language, 4,* 479–491.

Shallice, T. & Warrington, E. K. (1977b). The possible role of selective attention in acquired dyslexia. *Neuropsychologia, 15,* 31–41.

Shallice, T. & Warrington, E. K. (1980). Single and multiple component central dyslexic syndromes. In M.Coltheart, K. Patterson, & J. Marshall (Eds), *Deep Dyslexia.* London: Routledge & Kegan Paul.

Shallice, T., Warrington, E. K., & McCarthy, R. (1983). Reading without semantics. *Quarterly Journal of Experimental Psychology, 35A,* 111–138.

Shallice, T., McLeod, P., & Lewis, K. (1985). Isolating cognitive modules with the dual task paradigm: Are speech perception and production separate processes? *Quarterly Journal of Experimental Psychology, 37A,* 507–532.

Shallice, T., Burgess, P. W., Schon, F., & Baxter, D. M. (1989). The origins of utilization behaviour. *Brain, 112* (6), 1587–1598.

Shallice, T., Fletcher, P., Frith, C. D., Grasby, P., Frackowiak, R., & Dolan, R. (1994). Brain regions associated with acquisition and retrieval of verbal episodic memory. *Nature, 368,* 633–635.

Shallice, T., Glasspool, D. W., & Houghton, G. (1995). Can neuropsychological evidence inform connectionist modelling? Analyses of spelling. *Language and Cognitive Processes, 10,* 195–225.

Shallice, T., Rumiati, R., & Zadini, A. (2000). The selective impairment of the phonological output buffer. *Cognitive Neuropsychology, 17,* 517–546.

Shallice, T., Stuss, D. T., Picton, T. W., Alexander, M. P., & Gillingham, S. (2008a). Multiple effects of prefrontal lesions on task-switching. *Frontiers in Human Neuroscience, 1,* 2.

Shallice, T., Stuss, D. T., Alexander, M. P., Picton, T. W., & Derkzen, D. (2008b). The multiple dimensions of sustained attention. *Cortex, 44,* 794–805.

Shallice, T., Stuss, D. T., Picton, T. W., Alexander, M. P., & Gillingham, S. (2008c). Mapping task switching in frontal cortex through neuropsychological group studies. *Frontiers in Neuroscience, 2,* 79–85.

Shammi, P. & Stuss, D. T. (1999). Humour appreciation: a role of the right frontal lobe. *Brain, 122,* 657–666.

Shannon, C. E. (1948). A mathematical theory of communication. *Bell System Technical Journal, 27,* 379–423.

Shapiro, K. & Caramazza, A. (2003). Grammatical processing of nouns and verbs in left frontal cortex? *Neuropsychologia, 41,* 1189–1198.

Shapiro, K. A., Pascual-Leone, A., Mottaghy, F. M., Gangitano, M., & Caramazza, A. (2001). Grammatical distinctions in the left frontal cortex. *Journal of Cognitive Neuroscience, 13,* 713–720.

Shapiro, K. A., Moo, L. R., & Caramazza, A. (2006). Cortical signatures of noun and verb production. *Proceedings of the National Academy of Sciences, USA, 103,* 1644–1649.

Sharp, D. J., Scott, S. K., & Wise, R. J. (2004). Monitoring and the controlled processing of meaning: distinct prefrontal systems. *Cerebral Cortex, 14,* 1–10.

Sharp, P. E. (1991). Computer-simulation of hippocampal place cells. *Psychobiology, 19,* 103–115.

Shastri, L. (2002). Episodic memory and cortico-hippocampal interactions. *Trends in Cognitive Sciences, 6*(4), 162–168.

Sheinberg, D. L. & Logothetis, N. K. (1997). The role of temporal cortical areas in perceptual organization. *Proceedings of the National Academy of Sciences, USA, 94,* 3408–3413.

Shelton, J. R., Fouch, E., & Caramazza, A. (1998). The selective sparing of body part knowledge: a case study. *Neurocase, 4,* 339–351.

Shepard, R. N. & Metzler, J. (1971). Mental rotation of three-dimensional objects. *Science, 171,* 701–703.

Shibahara, N., Zorzi, M., Hill, M., Wydell, T., & Butterworth, B. (2003). Semantic effects in word naming: Evidence from English and Japanese Kanji. *Quarterly Journal of Experimental Psychology, 56A,* 263–286.

Shiffrin, R. M. & Schneider, W. (1977). Controlled and automatic human information processing: II Perceptual learning, automatic attending and a general theory. *Psychological Review, 84,* 127–190.

Silvanto, J., Lavie, N., & Walsh, V. (2005). Double dissociation of V1 and V5/MT activity in visual awareness. *Cerebral Cortex, 15,* 1736–1741.

Silveri, M. & Gainotti, G. (1988). Interaction between vision and language in category-specic impairment. *Cognitive Neuropsychology, 5,* 677–709.

Simner, J., Mulvenna, C., Sagiv, N., Tsakanikos, E., Witherby, S. A., Fraser, C., Scott, K., et al. (2006). Synaesthesia: The prevalence of atypical cross-modal experiences. *Perception, 35,* 1024–1033.

Simon, H. A. (1975). The functional equivalence of problem solving skills. *Cognitive Psychology, 7*(2), 268–288.

Simon, O., Mangin, J. F., Cohen, L., Le, B. D., & Dehaene, S. (2002). Topographical layout of hand, eye, calculation, and language-related areas in the human parietal lobe. *Neuron, 33,* 475–487.

Simoncelli, E. & Heeger, D. (1998). A model of neuronal responses in visual area MT. *Vision Research, 38,* 743–761.

Simons, J. S., Peers, P. V., Hwang, D. Y., Ally, B. A., Fletcher, P. C., & Budson, A. E. (2008). Is the parietal lobe necessary for recollection in humans? *Neuropsychologia, 46,* 1185–1191.

Sirigu, A., Duhamel, J. R., Cohen, L., Pillon, B., Dubois, B., & Agid, Y. (1996). The mental representation of hand movements after parietal cortex damage. *Science, 273,* 1564–1568.

Sirigu, A., Grafman, J., Bressler, K., & Sunderland, T. (1991). Multiple representations contribute to body knowledge processing. Evidence from a case of autotopagnosia. *Brain, 114 (1B),* 629–642.

Skinner, B. (1957). *Verbal Behavior.* New York: Appleton-Century-Crofts.

Skinner, E. I. & Fernandes, M. A. (2007). Neural correlates of recollection and familiarity: a review of neuroimaging and patient data. *Neuropsychologia, 45,* 2163–2179.

Sloman, A. (1978). *The Computer Revolution in Philosophy: Philosophy Science and Models of Mind.* Hassocks: Harvester Press.

Sloman, A. (2000). Introduction: models of models of mind. In *Proceedings of the DAM symposium: how to design a functioning mind.* Symposium held at AISB 2000 conference.

Sloman, S. A. (1996). The empirical case for two forms of reasoning. *Psychological Bulletin, 119,* 3–22.

Smart, J. J. C. (1959). Sensations and brain processes. *The Philosophical Review, 68*(2), 141–156.

Smart, J. (1963). Materialism. *Journal of Phylosophy, 60,* 651–662.

Smith, E. & Medin, D. (1981). *Categories and concepts.* Cambridge, MA: Harvard University Press.

Smith, E. E. & Jonides, J. (1999). Storage and executive processes in the frontal lobes. *Science, 283,* 1657–1661.

Smith, E., Jonides, J., & Koeppe, R. (1996). Dissociating verbal and spatial working memory using PET. *Cerebral Cortex, 6,* 11–20.

Smolensky, P. (1986). Information processing in dynamical systems: foundations of harmony theory. In D. Rumelhart, J. L. McClelland & the PDP Resarch Goup (Eds), *Parallel distributed processing: explorations in the microstructure of cognition, volume 1: foundations* (pp. 194–281). Cambridge, MA: MIT Press/Bradford Books.

Smolensky, P. (1988). The proper treatment of connectionism. *Behavioral and Brain Sciences, 11,* 1–74.

Smulders, F. T., Kok, A., Kenemans, J. L., & Bashore, T. R. (1995). The temporal selectivity of additive factor effects on the reaction process revealed in ERP component latencies. *Acta Psychologica, 90,* 97–109.

Smyth, M. M., Hay, D. C., Hitch, G. J., & Horton, N. J. (2005). Serial position memory in the visual-spatial domain: reconstructing sequences of unfamiliar faces. *Quarterly Journal of Experimental Psychology, 58A*, 909–930.

Snowden, J., Goulding, P., & Neary, D. (1989). Semantic dementia: a form of circumscribed cerebral atrophy. *Beahvioral Neurology, 2*, 167–182.

Snowden, J. S., Griffiths, H. L., & Neary, D. (1996). Semantic-episodic memory interactions in semantic dementia: Implications for retrograde memory function. *Cognitive Neuropsychology, 13*, 1101–1139.

Snyder, L. H., Batista, A. P., & Andersen, R. A. (1997). Coding of intention in the posterior parietal cortex. *Nature, 386*, 167–170.

Snyder, L. H., Batista, A. P., & Andersen, R. A. (2000). Intention-related activity in the posterior parietal cortex: a review. *Vision Research, 40*, 1433–1441.

Solstad, T., Moser, E. I., & Einevoll, G. T. (2006). From grid cells to place cells: a mathematical model. *Hippocampus, 16*, 1026–1031.

Solstad, T., Boccara, C. N., Kropff, E., Moser, M. B., & Moser, E. I. (2008). Representation of geometric borders in the entorhinal cortex. *Science, 322*, 1865–1868.

Soon, C. S., Brass, M., Heinze, H., & Haynes, J. (2008). Unconscious determinants of free decisions in the human brain. *Nature Neuroscience, 11*(5), 543–545.

Sparks, D. & Mays, L. (1980). Movement fields of saccade-related burst neurons in the monkey superior colliculus. *Brain Research, 190*, 39–50.

Spearman, C. (1904). General Intelligence objectively determined and measured. *American Journal of Psychology, 15*, 201–293.

Speekenbrink, M., Channon, S., & Shanks, D. R. (2008). Learning strategies in amnesia. *Neuroscience and Biobehavioral Reviews, 32*, 292–310.

Spence, S. A., Hunter, M. D., Farrow, T. F., Green, R. D., Leung, D. H., Hughes, C. J. et al. (2004). A cognitive neurobiological account of deception: evidence from functional neuroimaging. *Philosophical Transations of the Royal Society of London B Biological Sciences, 359*, 1755–1762.

Sperling, G. (1960). The information available in brief visual presentations. *Psychological Monographs, 74*.

Sperling, G. (1967). Successive approximations to a model for short-term memory. *Acta Psychologica, 27*, 285–292.

Sperry, R. W. (1984). Consciousness, personal identity and the divided brain. *Neuropsychologia, 22*(6), 661–673.

Spillantini, M. G., Bird, T. D., & Ghetti, B. (1998). Frontotemporal dementia and Parkinsonism linked to chromosome 17: a new group of tauopathies. *Brain Pathology, 8*, 387–402.

Squire, L. R. (1987). The organization and neural substrates of human memory. *International Journal of Neurology, 21-22*, 218–222.

Squire, L. R. & Alvarez, P. (1995). Retrograde amnesia and memory consolidation: a neurobiological perspective. *Current Opinion in Neurobiology, 5*, 169–177.

Squire, L. R. & Cohen, N. (1979). Memory and amnesia: resistance to disruption develops for years after learning. *Behavioral and Neural Biology, 25*, 115–125.

Squire, L. R. & Zola, S. M. (1996). Structure and function of declarative and nondeclarative memory systems. *Proceedings of the National Academy of Sciences, USA, 93*, 13515–13522.

Squire, L. R., Chace, P. M., & Slater, P. C. (1975). Assessment of memory for remote events. *Psychological Reports, 37*, 223–234.

Squire, L. R., Ojemann, J. G., Miezin, F. M., Petersen, S. E., Videen, T. O., & Raichle, M. E. (1992). Activation of the hippocampus in normal humans: a functional anatomical study of memory. *Proceedings of the National Academy of Sciences, USA, 89*, 1837–1841.

Squire, L. R., Wixted, J. T., & Clark, R. E. (2007). Recognition memory and the medial temporal lobe: a new perspective. *Nature Neuroscience Reviews, 8*(11), 872–883.

Staller, J., Buchanan, D., Singer, M., Lappin, J., & Webb, W. (1978). Alexia without agraphia: an experimental case study. *Brain and Language, 5*, 378–387.

Standing, L. (1973). Learning 10,000 pictures. *Quarterly Journal of Experimental Psychology, 25*, 207–222.

Stanovich, K. E. & West, R. F. (2000). Individual differences in reasoning: implications for the rationality debate? *Behavioral and Brain Sciences, 23*, 645–665.

Steedman, M. (1996). *Surface Structure and Interpretation*. Cambridge, MA: MIT Press.

Steedman, M. (2000). Information structure and the syntax-phonology interface. *Linguistic Inquiry, 34*, 649–689.

Steingrimsson, R., & Luce, R. D. (2006). Empirical evaluation of a model of global psychophysical judgments: III. A form for the psychophysical function and intensity filtering. *Journal of Mathematical Psychology, 50*(1), 15–29.

Steinvorth, S., Levine, B., & Corkin, S. (2005). Medial temporal lobe structures are needed to re-experience remote autobiographical memories: evidence from H. M. and W. R. *Neuropsychologia, 43*, 479–496.

Stemberger, J. (1985). An interactive activation model of language production. In A.Ellis (Ed.), *Progress in the psychology of language, vol. 1*. Erlbaum.

Stenning, K. & Oberlander, J. (1995). A cognitive theory of graphical and linguistic reasoning: logic and implementation. *Cognitive Science, 19*, 97–140.

Stenning, K. & Yule, P. (1997). Image and language in human reasoning: a syllogistic illustration. *Cognitive Psychology, 34,* 109–159.

Sternberg, S. (1966). High-speed scanning in human memory. *Science, 153,* 652–654.

Sternberg, S. (1969). The discovery of processing stages: extensions of Donders' method. *Acta Psychologica,* 276–315.

Sternberg, S. (2001). Separate modifiability, mental modules, and the use of pure and composite measures to reveal them. *Acta Psychologica, 106,* 147–246.

Sternberg, S., Monsell, S., Knoll, R. L., & Wright, C. E. (1978). The latency and duration of rapid movement sequences: Comparisons of speech and typewriting. In G. E. Stelmach (Ed.), *Information processing in motor control and learning* (pp. 118–152). New York: Academic Press.

Sternberg, S., Knoll, R. L., Monsell, S., & Wright, C. E. (1998). Motor programs and hierarchical organization in the control of rapid speech. *Phonetica, 45,* 175–197.

Stevens, S. S. (1957). On the psychophysical law. *Psychological Review, 64*(3), 153–181.

Stewart, F., Parkin, A. J., & Hunkin, N. M. (1992). Naming impairments following recovery from herpes simplex encephalitis: category-specific? *Quarterly Journal of Experimental Psychology, 44A,* 261–284.

Stich, S. (1983). *From folk psychology to cognitive science.* Cambridge, MA: MIT Press.

Stowe, L. A., Wijers, A., Willemsen, A., Reuland, E., Paans, A., & Vaalburg, W. (1994). PET studies of language: An assessment of the reliability of the technique. *Journal of Psycholinguistic Research, 23*(6), 499–527.

Stowe, L. A., Paans, A. M., Wijers, A. A., Zwarts, F., Mulder, G., & Vaalburg, W. (1999). Sentence comprehension and word repetition: a positron emission tomography investigation. *Psychophysiology, 36,* 786–801.

Strain, E., Patterson, K., & Seidenberg, M. (1995). Semantic effects in single-word naming. *Journal of Experimental Psychology: Learning, Memory and Cognition, 21,* 1140–1154.

Strange, B. A., Henson, R. N., Friston, K. J., & Dolan, R. J. (2001). Anterior prefrontal cortex mediates rule learning in humans. *Cerebral Cortex, 11,* 1040–1046.

Stromswold, K., Caplan, D., Alpert, N., & Rauch, S. (1996). Localization of syntactic comprehension by positron emission tomography. *Brain and Language, 52,* 452–473.

Sturm, W. & Willmes, K. (2001). On the functional neuroanatomy of intrinsic and phasic alertness. *Neuroimage, 14,* S76–S84.

Stuss, D. T. & Alexander, M. P. (2007). Is there a dysexecutive syndrome? *Philosophical Transactions of the Royal Society of London, B, Biological Sciences, 362,* 901–915.

Stuss, D. T., Alexander, M. P., Lieberman, A., & Levine, H. (1978). An extraordinary form of confabulation. *Neurology, 28*(11), 1166–1172.

Stuss, D. T., Alexander, M. P., Palumbo, C. L., Buckle, L., & et al. (1994). Organizational strategies with unilateral or bilateral frontal lobe injury in word learning tasks. *Neuropsychology, 8*(3), 355–373.

Stuss, D. T., Shallice, T., Alexander, M. P., & Picton, T. W. (1995). A multidisciplinary approach to anterior attentional functions. *Annals of the New York Academy of Sciences, 769,* 191–211.

Stuss, D. T., Alexander, M. P., Hamer, L., Palumbo, C., Dempster, R., Binns, M. et al. (1998). The effects of focal anterior and posterior brain lesions on verbal fluency. *Journal of the International Neuropsychological Society, 4,* 265–278.

Stuss, D. T., Levine, B., Alexander, M. P., Hong, J., Palumbo, C., Hamer, L. et al. (2000). Wisconsin Card Sorting Test performance in patients with focal frontal and posterior brain damage: effects of lesion location and test structure on separable cognitive processes. *Neuropsychologia, 38,* 388–402.

Stuss, D. T., Gallup, G. G., Jr., & Alexander, M. P. (2001). The frontal lobes are necessary for 'theory of mind'. *Brain, 124,* 279–286.

Stuss, D. T., Binns, M. A., Murphy, K. J., & Alexander, M. P. (2002). Dissociations within the anterior attentional system: effects of task complexity and irrelevant information on reaction time speed and accuracy. *Neuropsychology, 16,* 500–513.

Stuss, D. T., Alexander, M. P., Shallice, T., Picton, T. W., Binns, M. A., Macdonald, R. et al. (2005). Multiple frontal systems controlling response speed. *Neuropsychologia, 43,* 396–417.

Sumner, P., & Husain, M. (2008). At the edge of consciousness: automatic motor activation and voluntary control. *Neuroscientist, 14*(5), 474–486.

Sussman, G. (1975). *A computer model of skill acquisition.* New York: Elsevier.

Sutherland, S. (1989). *The international dictionary of psychology* (revised edn). New York: Continuum.

Sutton, R. S. & Barto, A. G. (1998). *Reinforcement learning.* Cambridge, MA: MIT Press.

Swartz, B. E. & Goldensohn, E. S. (1998). Timeline of the history of EEG and associated fields. *Electroencephalography and Clinical Neurophysiology, 106,* 173–176.

Symes, E., Ellis, R., & Tucker, M. (2007). Visual object affordances: object orientation. *Acta Psychologica, 124,* 238–255.

Tainturier, M. & Caramazza, A. (1996). The status of double letter representations. *Journal of Memory and Language, 35,* 53–75.

Takayama, Y., Kinomoto, K., & Nakamura, K. (2004). Selective impairment of the auditory-verbal short-term memory due to a lesion of the superior temporal gyrus. *European Neurology, 51,* 115–117.

Talairach, J. & Tournoux, P. (1988). *A co-planar sterotactic atlas of the human brain.* Stuttgart, Germany: Thieme.

Talmy, L. (1975). Semantics and syntax of motion. In J.Kimball (Ed.), *Syntax and semantics, vol. 4* (pp. 181–238). New York: Academic Press.

Talmy, L. (1983). How language structures space. In H. Pick & L. Acredolo (Eds), *Spatial orientation: theory, research, and application.* Plenum.

Tanenhaus, M. K., Spiveyknowlton, M. J., Eberhard, K. M., & Sedivy, J. C. (1995). Integration of visual and linguistic information in spoken language comprehension. *Science, 268,* 1632–1634.

Tarr, M. J., & Gauthier, I. (2000). FFA: a flexible fusiform area for subordinate-level visual processing automatized by expertise. *Nature Neuroscience, 3*(8), 764–769.

Taube, J., Muller, R., & Ranck, J. (1990). Head-direction cells recorded from the postsubiculum in freely moving rats. I. Description and quantitative analysis. *Journal of Neuroscience, 10,* 420–435.

Temple, C. & Marshall, J. (1983). A case study of developmental phonological dyslexia. *British Journal of Psychology., 74,* 517–533.

Tenenbaum, J.B. (1999) Bayesian modeling of human concept learning. In M. Kearns et al., (Eds) *Advances in neural information processing systems vol. 11* , pp. 59–68, MIT Press.

Tenenbaum, J. & Barrow, H. (1976). Experiments in interpretation-guided segmentation. *Stanford Research Institute, Technical Note, 123.*

Tenpenny, P. & Shoben, E. (1992). Component processes and the utility of the conceptually-driven/data-driven distinction. *Journal of Experimental Psychology: Learning, Memory and Cognition, 18,* 25–42.

Ter-Pogossian, M. M., Phelps, M. E., Hoffman, E. J., & Mullani, N. A. (1975). A positron-emission transaxial tomograph for nuclear imaging (PETT). *Radiology, 114,* 89–98.

Tettamanti, M., Buccino, G., Saccuman, M. C., Gallese, V., Danna, M., Scifo, P. et al. (2005). Listening to action-related sentences activates fronto-parietal motor circuits. *Journal of Cognitive Neuroscience, 17,* 273–281.

Teyler, T. J. & DiScenna, P. (1986). The hippocampal memory indexing theory. *Behavioral Neuroscience, 100,* 147–154.

Thomas, A. (2003). An adverbial theory of consciousness. *Phenomenology and the Cognitive Sciences, 2*(3), 161–185.

Thomas, M., & Karmiloff-Smith, A. (2002). Are developmental disorders like cases of adult brain damage? implications from connectionist modelling. *Behavioral and Brain Sciences, 25*(6), 727–750.

Thompson, K. G. & Schall, J. D. (1999). The detection of visual signals by macaque frontal eye field during masking. *Nature Neuroscience, 2,* 283–288.

Thompson, P. M., Schwartz, C., Lin, R. T., Khan, A. A., & Toga, A. W. (1996). Three-dimensional statistical analysis of sulcal variability in the human brain. *Journal of Neuroscience, 16,* 4261–4274.

Thompson-Schill, S. L., D'Esposito, M., Aguirre, G. K., & Farah, M. J. (1997). Role of left inferior prefrontal cortex in retrieval of semantic knowledge: a reevaluation. *Proceedings of the National Academy of Sciences, USA, 94,* 14792–14797.

Thompson-Schill, S. L., Swick, D., Farah, M. J., D'Esposito, M., Kan, I. P., & Knight, R. T. (1998). Verb generation in patients with focal frontal lesions: a neuropsychological test of neuroimaging findings. *Proceedings of the National Academy of Sciences, USA, 95,* 15855–15860.

Thomson, G. H. (1935). Defintion and measurement of general intelligence. *Nature, 135,* 509.

Todd, J. J. & Marois, R. (2004). Capacity limit of visual short-term memory in human posterior parietal cortex. *Nature, 428,* 751–754.

Todd, J. J. & Marois, R. (2005). Posterior parietal cortex activity predicts individual differences in visual short-term memory capacity. *Cognitive, Affective and Behavioral Neuroscience, 5,* 144–155.

Tolman, E. (1932). *Purposive behavior in animals and man.* New York: Appleton-Century-Crofts.

Tomasino, B., Toraldo, A., & Rumiati, R. I. (2003). Dissociation between the mental rotation of visual images and motor images in unilateral brain-damaged patients. *Brain and Cognition, 51,* 368–371.

Tong, F., Nakayama, K., Vaughan, J. T., & Kanwisher, N. (1998). Binocular rivalry and visual awareness in human extrastriate cortex. *Neuron, 21*(4), 753–759.

Tootell, R. & Hadjikhani, N. (2001). Where is dorsal V4 in human visual cortex? Retinotopic, topographic and functional evidence. *Cerebral Cortex, 11,* 298–311.

Toraldo, A. & Shallice, T. (2004). Error analysis at the level of single moves in block design. *Cognitive Neuropsychology, 21,* 645–659.

Touretzky, D. & Hinton, G. (1988). A distributed connectionist production system. *Cognitive Science, 12,* 423–466.

Tranel, D., Damasio, A. R., Damasio, H., & Brandt, J. P. (1994). Sensorimotor skill learning in amnesia: additional evidence for the neural basis of nondeclarative memory. *Learning and Memory, 1,* 165–179.

Treisman, A. M. (1964). Selective Attention in Man. *British Medical Bulletin, 20,* 12–&.

Treisman, A. M. (1998). Feature binding, attention and object perception. *Philosophical Transactions of the Royal Society B: Biological Sciences, 353*(1373), 1295–1306.

Treisman, A. M. & Davies, A. (1973). Divided attention to ear and eye. In S.Kornblum (Ed.), *Attention and performance IV.* London: Academic Press.

Treisman, A. M. & Gelade, G. (1980). Feature-integration theory of attention. *Cognitive Psychology, 12,* 97–136.

Treves, A. (2005). Frontal latching networks: a possible neural basis for infinite recursion. *Cognitive Neuropsychology, 21,* 276–291.

Treves, A. & Rolls, E. T. (1992). Computational constraints suggest the need for 2 distinct input systems to the hippocampal Ca3-network. *Hippocampus, 2,* 189–200.

Treves, A. & Rolls, E. T. (1994). Computational analysis of the role of the hippocampus in memory. *Hippocampus, 4,* 374–391.

Treves, A. & Samengo, I. (2002). Standing on the gateway to memory: shouldn't we step in? *Cognitive Neuropsychology, 12,* 557–575.

Trueswell, J. C. & Tanenhaus, M. K. (1994). Toward a lexicalist framework for constraint-based syntactic ambiguity resolution. In C. Clifton, L. Frazier & K Rayner (Eds). *Perspectives on sentence processing.* (chapter 7, pp. 155–179) LEA.

Trueswell, J. C., Tanenhaus, M. K., & Gamsey, S. (1994). Semantic influences on parsing: use of thematic role information in syntactic ambiguity resolution. *Journal of Memory and Language, 33,* 285–318.

Tucker, M. & Ellis, R. (1998). On the relations between seen objects and components of potential actions. *Journal of Experimental Psychology: Human Perception and Performance, 24,* 830–846.

Tucker, M. & Ellis, R. (2004). Action priming by briefly presented objects. *Acta Psychologica, 116,* 185–203.

Tulving, E. (1983). *Elements of episodic memory.* Oxford: Clarendon.

Tulving, E. (1985). Memory and consciousness. *Canadian Psychology, 26,* 1–12.

Tulving, E. & Donaldson, W. (1972). Episodic and semantic memory. In E.Tulving & W. Donaldson (Eds), *Organization of memory* (pp. 381–403). New York: Academic.

Tulving, E. & Madigan, S. (1970). Memory and verbal learning. *Annual Review of Psychology, 21,* 437–484.

Tulving, E. & Schacter, D. (1990). Priming and human memory systems. *Science, 247,* 301–306.

Tulving, E., Kapur, S., Craik, F. I., Moscovitch, M., & Houle, S. (1994a). Hemispheric encoding/retrieval asymmetry in episodic memory: positron emission tomography findings. *Proceedings of the National Academy of Sciences of the United States of America, 91*(6), 2016 –2020.

Tulving, E., Kapur, S., Markowitsch, H. J., Craik, F. I., Habib, R., & Houle, S. (1994b). Neuroanatomical correlates of retrieval in episodic memory: auditory sentence recognition. *Proceedings of the National Academy of Sciences of the United States of America, 91*(6), 2012 –2015.

Turing, A. (1936). On computable numbers, with an applcation to the Entscheidungsproblem. *Proceedings of the London Mathematical Society Set 2, 42,* 230–265.

Turner, M., Cipolotti, L., Yousry, T., & Shallice, T. (2007). Qualitatively different memory impairments across frontal lobe subgroup. *Neuropsychologia, 45,* 1540–1552.

Turner, M. S., Cipolotti, L., Yousry, T. A., & Shallice, T. (2008). Confabulation: damage to a specific inferior medial prefrontal system. *Cortex, 44*(6), 637–648.

Turner, M. S., Cipolotti, L., & Shallice, T. (in press). Spontaneous confabulation, temporal context confusion and reality monitoring: A study of three patients with anterior communicating aneurysms. *Journal of the International Neuropsychological Society.*

Turvey, M. (1973). On peripheral and central processes in vision: inferences from an information-processing analysis of masking with patterned stimuli. *Psychological Review, 81,* 1–52.

Turvey, M. (1974). Constructive Theory, Perceptual systems and tacit knowledge. In W. Weimer & D. Palermo (Eds), *Cognition and the symbolic processes* (pp. 165–180). Hillsdale, NJ: Erlbaum.

Tversky, A. & Kahneman, D. (1974). Judgment under uncertainty: heuristics and biases. *Science, 185,* 1124–1131.

Tyler, L. K. & Moss, H. E. (2001). Towards a distributed account of conceptual knowledge. *Trends in Cognitive Sciences, 5,* 244–252.

Tyler, L. K., & Marslen-Wilson, W. (2008). Fronto-temporal brain systems supporting spoken language comprehension. *Philosophical Transactions of the Royal Society B: Biological Sciences, 363*(1493), 1037–1054.

Tyler, L. K., Moss, H. E., Durrant-Peatfield, M. R., & Levy, J. P. (2000). Conceptual structure and the structure of concepts: a distributed account of category-specific deficits. *Brain and Language, 75,* 195–231.

Tyler, L. K., Mornay-Davies, P., Anokhina, R., Longworth, C., Randall, B., & Marslen-Wilson, W. D. (2002a). Dissociations in processing past tense morphology: neuropathology and behavioral studies. *Journal of Cognitive Neuroscience, 14,* 79–94.

Tyler, L. K., Randall, B., & Marslen-Wilson, W. D. (2002b). Phonology and neuropsychology of the English past tense. *Neuropsychologia, 40,* 1154–1166.

Tyler, L. K., Bright, P., Fletcher, P., & Stamatakis, E. A. (2004a). Neural processing of nouns and verbs: the role of inflectional morphology. *Neuropsychologia, 42*(4), 512–523.

Tyler, L. K., Stamatakis, E. A., Bright, P., Acres, K., Abdallah, S., Rodd, J. M. et al. (2004b). Processing objects at different levels of specificity. *Journal of Cognitive Neuroscience, 16,* 351–362.

Tyler, L. K., Marslen-Wilson, W. D., & Stamatakis, E. A. (2005a). Differentiating lexical form, meaning, and structure in the neural language system. *Proceedings of the National Academy of Sciences, USA, 102*(23), 8375–8380.

Tyler, L. K., Stamatakis, E. A., Post, B., Randall, B., & Marslen-Wilson, W. (2005b). Temporal and frontal systems in speech comprehension: an fMRI study of past tense processing. *Neuropsychologia, 43,* 1963–1974.

Tyler, L.K., Shafto, M.A., Randall, B., Wright, P., Marslen-Wilson, W. D. & Stamatakis, E.A. (2010). Preserving syntactic processing across the adult life span: the modulation of the frontotemporal language system in the context of age-related atrophy. *Cerebral Cortex, 20,* 352–364.

Tzeng, O. J. (1973). Positive recency effect in a delayed free recall. *Journal of Verbal Learning and Verbal Behavior, 12,* 436–439.

Uhl, F., Podreka, I., and Deecke, L. (1994). Anterior frontal cortex and the effect of proactive interference in word pair learning—results of brain-spect. *Neuropsychologia, 32,* 241–247.

Ullman, M. T., Corkin, S., Coppola, M., Hickok, G., Growdon, J. H., Koroshetz, W. J., & Pinker, S. (1997). A neural dissociation within language: evidence that the mental dictionary is part of declarative memory, and that grammatical rules are processed by the procedural system. *Journal of Cognitive Neuroscience, 9*(2), 266–276.

Umiltà, C. (1988). The control operations of consciousness. In *Consciousness in contemporary science.* (pp. 334–356). New York, NY, US: Clarendon Press/Oxford University Press.

Uncapher, M. R., & Rugg, M. D. (2008). Fractionation of the component processes underlying successful episodic encoding: a combined fMRI and divided-attention study. *Journal of Cognitive Neuroscience, 20*(2), 240–254.

Underwood, B. J. (1957). Interference and forgetting. *Psychological Review, 64,* 49–60.

Ungerleider, L. G. & Mishkin, M. (1982). Two cortical visual systems. In D. J. Ingle, M. A. Goodale, & F. J. W. Mansfield (Eds), *Analysis of Visual Behavior* (pp. 549–586). Cambridge, MA: MIT Press.

Uno, Y., Kawato, M., & Suzuki, R. (1989). Formation and control of optimal trajectory in human multijoint arm movement. Minimum torque-change model. *Biological Cybernetics, 61,* 89–101.

Uttal, W. (2001). *The new phrenology: the limits of localizing cognitive processes in the brain.* Cambridge, MA: MIT Press.

Valenstein, E., Bowers, D., Verfaellie, M., Heilman, K. M., Day, A., & Watson, R. T. (1987). Retrosplenial amnesia. *Brain, 110*(6), 1631–1646.

Vallar, G. (1993). The anatomical basis of spatial hemineglect in humans. In I. Robertson & J. Marshall (Eds), *Unilateral neglect: clinical and experimental studies.* (pp. 27–62). Hove (UK): LEA.

Vallar, G. (2000). The methodological foundations of human neuropsychology: studies in brain-damaged patients. In F.Boller, J. Grafman & G. Rizzolatti (Eds) *Handbook of neuropsychology* (2nd edn) *Vol 1* (pp. 305–352). Amsterdam: Elsevier.

Vallar, G. & Baddeley, A. D. (1984). Phonological short-term store: phonological processing and sentence comprehension. *Cognitive Neuropsychology, 1,* 121–141.

Vallar, G. & Papagno, C. (1986). Phonological short-term store and the nature of recency effect: evidence from Neuropsychology. *Brain and Cognition, 5,* 428–442.

Vallar, G. & Papagno, C. (2002). Neuropsychological impairments of verbal short-term memory. In A. D. Baddeley, M. Kopelman, & B. Wilson (Eds), *Handbook of memory disorders* (2nd edn), (pp. 249–270). Chichester: Wiley.

Vallar, G. & Shallice, T. (1990). *Neuropsychological Impairments of Short Term Memory.* Cambridge: CUP.

Vallar, G., Di Betta, A. M., & Silveri, M. C. (1997). The phonological short-term store-rehearsal system: patterns of impairment and neural correlates. *Neuropsychologia, 35,* 795–812.

Vallesi, A. & Shallice, T. (2007). Developmental dissociations of preparation over time: deconstructing the variable foreperiod phenomena. *Journal of Experimental Psychology: Human Perception and Performance, 33,* 1377–1388.

Vallesi, A., Mussoni, A., Mondani, M., Budai, R., Skrap, M., & Shallice, T. (2007a). The neural basis of temporal preparation: Insights from brain tumor patients. *Neuropsychologia, 45,* 2755–2763.

Vallesi, A., Shallice, T., & Walsh, V. (2007b). Role of the prefrontal cortex in the foreperiod effect: TMS evidence for dual mechanisms in temporal preparation. *Cerebral Cortex, 17,* 466–474.

Vallesi, A., McIntosh, A. R., Shallice, T., & Stuss, D. T. (2009). When time shapes behavior: fMRI evidence of brain correlates of temporal monitoring. *Journal of Cognitive Neuroscience, 21,* 1116–1126.

van Beers, R. J., Sittig, A. C., & Gon, J. J. V. D. (1999). Integration of proprioceptive and visual position-information: an experimentally supported model. *Journal of Neurophysiology, 81*(3), 1355–1364.

van Dalen, D. (1986). Intuitionistic logic. In *Handbook of philosophical logic, vol. 3,* pp. 225–339. D. Reidel Publishing Company, Dordrecht.

Vandenberghe, R., Price, C., Wise, R., Josephs, O., & Frackowiak, R. S. (1996). Functional anatomy of a common semantic system for words and pictures. *Nature, 383,* 254–256.

Vandenbulcke, M., Peeters, R., Fannes, K., & Vandenberghe, R. (2006). Knowledge of visual attributes in the right hemisphere. *Nature Neuroscience, 9,* 964–970.

van der Linden, M., Bredart, S., Depoorter, N., & Coyette, F. (1996). Semantic memory and amnesia: a case study. *Cognitive Neuropsychology, 13,* 391–413.

van der Linden, M., Cornil, V., Meulemans, T., Ivanoiu, A., Salmon, E., & Coyette, F. (2001). Acquisition of a novel vocabulary in an amnesic patient. *Neurocase, 7,* 283–293.

van Essen, D. & Deyoe E. A. (1995). Concurrent processing in the primate visual cortex. In M. Gazzaniga (Ed), *The cognitive neurosciences* (pp. 385–400). Boston, MA: MIT Press.

van Gaal, S., Ridderinkhof, K. R., Fahrenfort, J. J., Scholte, H. S., & Lamme, V. A. F. (2008). Frontal cortex mediates unconsciously triggered inhibitory control. *Journal of Neuroscience*, 28(32), 8053–8062.

van Gaal, S., Ridderinkhof, K. R., van den Wildenberg, W. P. M., & Lamme, V. A. F. (2009). Dissociating consciousness from inhibitory control: Evidence for unconsciously triggered response inhibition in the stop-signal task. *Journal of Experimental Psychology: Human Perception and Performance*, 35(4), 1129–1139.

van Gelder, T. (1998). The dynamical hypothesis in cognitive science. *Behavioral and Brain Sciences, 21,* 615–665.

van Gulick, R. (1994). Deficit studies and the function of phenomenal consciousness. In G.Graham & G. Stephens (Eds), *Philosophical psychopathology* (8th edn), pp. 1–34. Cambridge, MA: MIT Press.

Vanier, M., & Caplan, D. (1990). CT-scan correlates of agrammatism. In L. Menn, L. K. Obler, & G. Miceli (Eds), *Agrammatic aphasia* (pp. 97–114). John Benjamins Publishing Company.

van Orden, G., Johnston, J., & Hale, B. (1988). Word identification in reading proceeds from spelling to sound to meaning. *Journal of Experimental Psychology Human Perception Performance, 14,* 371–385.

van Orden, G., de Haar, M., & Bosman, A. (1997). Complex dynamic systems also predict dissociations, but they do not reduce to autonomous components. *Cognitive Neuropsychology, 14,* 131–165.

van Orden, G., Pennington, B., & Stone, G. (2001). What do double dissociations prove? *Cognitive Science, 25,* 111–172.

Varela, J., Song, S., Turrigiano, G., & Nelson, S. (1999). Differential depression at excitatory and inhibitory synapses in visual cortex. *Journal of Neuroscience, 19,* 4293–4304.

Vargha-Khadem, F., Gadian, D. G., Watkins, K. E., Connelly, A., Van, P. W., & Mishkin, M. (1997). Differential effects of early hippocampal pathology on episodic and semantic memory. *Science, 277,* 376–380.

Vartanian, O. & Goel, V. (2005). Task constraints modulate activation in right ventral lateral prefrontal cortex. *Neuroimage, 27,* 927–933.

Verbruggen, F., & Logan, G. D. (2008). Automatic and controlled response inhibition: Associative learning in the go/no-go and stop-signal paradigms. *Journal of Experimental Psychology: General*, 137(4), 649–672.

Verfaellie, M., Reiss, L., & Roth, H. L. (1995a). Knowledge of New English vocabulary in amnesia: an examination of premorbidly acquired semantic memory. *Journal of the International Neuropsychological Society, 1,* 443–453.

Verfaellie, M., Croce, P., & Milberg, W. (1995b). The role of episodic memory in semantic learning: an examination of vocabulary acquisition in a patient with amnesia due to encephalitis. *Neurocase, 1,* 291–304.

Verfaellie, M., Koseff, P., & Alexander, M. P. (2000). Acquisition of novel semantic information in amnesia: effects of lesion location. *Neuropsychologia, 38,* 484–492.

Verguts, T. & De Boeck, P. (2002). The induction of solution rules in Raven's progressive matrices. *European Journal of Cognitive Psychology, 14,* 521–547.

Vicari, S., Bellucci, S., & Carlesimo, G. A. (2003). Visual and spatial working memory dissociation: evidence from Williams syndrome. *Developmental Medicine and Child Neurology, 45,* 269–273.

Vicari, S., Bellucci, S., & Carlesimo, G. A. (2006). Evidence from two genetic syndromes for the independence of spatial and visual working memory. *Developmental Medicine and Child Neurology, 48,* 126–131.

Vidal, C. & Changeux, J. (1993). Nicotinic and muscarinic modulations of excitatory synaptic transmission in the rat prefrontal cortex in vitro. *Neuroscience, 56,* 23–32.

Vigliocco, G., Vinson, D. P., Lewis, W., & Garrett, M. F. (2004). Representing the meanings of object and action words: the featural and unitary semantic space hypothesis. *Cognitive Psychology, 48,* 422–488.

Vigneau, M., Beaucousin, V., Herve, P. Y., Duffau, H., Crivello, F., Houde, O. et al. (2006). Meta-analyzing left hemisphere language areas: phonology, semantics, and sentence processing. *Neuroimage, 30,* 1414–1432.

Vilberg, K. L., & Rugg, M. D. (2008). Memory retrieval and the parietal cortex: a review of evidence from a dual-process perspective. *Neuropsychologia, 46*(7), 1787–1799.

Vinckier, F., Dehaene, S., Jobert, A., Dubus, J. P., Sigman, M., & Cohen, L. (2007). Hierarchical coding of letter strings in the ventral stream: dissecting the inner organization of the visual word-form system. *Neuron, 55,* 143–156.

Viskontas, I. V., McAndrews, M. P., & Moscovitch, M. (2000). Remote episodic memory deficits in patients with unilateral temporal lobe epilepsy and excisions. *Journal of Neuroscience, 20*(15), 5853–5857.

Vogel, E. K., Luck, S. J., & Shapiro, K. L. (1998). Electrophysiological evidence for a postperceptual locus of suppression during the attentional blink. *Journal of Experimental Psychology: Human Perception and Performance, 24*(6), 1656–1674.

von der Malsburg, C. (1981). *The correlation theory of brain function (Internal report 81–2).* Department of Neurobiology, Max-Planck-Institute for Biophysical Chemistry, Gottingen, Germany.

von Neumann, J. (1945). *First draft of a report on the EDVAC.* Technical report, University of Pennsylvania.

von Neumann, J. (1958). *The computer and the Brain.* Yale University Press.

Vorberg, D., Mattler, U., Heinecke, A., Schmidt, T., & Schwarzbach, J. (2003). Different time courses for visual perception and action priming. *Proceedings of the National Academy of Sciences, USA, 100*(10), 6275–6280.

Vosse, T. & Kempen, G. (2000). Syntactic structure assembly in human parsing: a computational model based on competitive inhibition and a lexicalist grammar. *Cognition, 75,* 105–143.

Vuilleumier, P. & Rafal, R. (1999). 'Both' means more than 'two': localizing and counting in patients with visuospatial neglect. *Nature Neuroscience, 2,* 783–784.

Vuilleumier, P., Valenza, N., & Landis, T. (2001). Explicit and implicit perception of illusory contours in unilateral spatial neglect: behavioural and anatomical correlates of preattentive grouping mechanisms. *Neuropsychologia, 39,* 597–610.

Vuilleumier, P., Henson, R. N., Driver, J., & Dolan, R. J. (2002). Multiple levels of visual object constancy revealed by event-related fMRI of repetition priming. *Nature Neuroscience, 5,* 491–499.

Waddington, C. (1963). *The Nature of Life.* London: Allen & Unwin.

Wager, T. D. & Smith, E. E. (2003). Neuroimaging studies of working memory: a meta-analysis. *Cognitive, Affective and Behavioral Neuroscience, 3,* 255–274.

Wagner, A. D., Schacter, D. L., Rotte, M., Koutstaal, W., Maril, A., Dale, A. M., Rosen, B. R., & Buckner, R. L. (1998). Building memories: remembering and forgetting of verbal experiences as predicted by brain activity. *Science, 281*(5380), 1188–1191.

Wagner, A. D., Shannon, B. J., Kahn, I., & Buckner, R. L. (2005). Parietal lobe contributions to episodic memory retrieval. *Trends in Cognitive Sciences, 9*(9), 445–453.

Wais, P. E., Wixted, J. T., Hopkins, R. O., & Squire, L. R. (2006). The Hippocampus supports both the recollection and the familiarity components of recognition memory. *Neuron, 49*(3), 459–466.

Wallis, J. D. (2008). Single neuron activity underlying behavior-guiding rules. In S.A.Bunge & J. D. Wallis (Eds), *Neuroscience of rule-guided behavior.* New York: Oxford.

Wallis, J. D., Anderson, K., & Miller, E. (2000). Neuronal representation of abstract rules in the orbital and lateral prefrontal cortices (PFC). *Society of Neuroscience Abstracts.*

Wallis, J. D., Anderson, K. C., & Miller, E. K. (2001). Single neurons in prefrontal cortex encode abstract rules. *Nature, 411,* 953–956.

Walsh, V. & Pascual-Leone, A. (2003) *Transcranial magnetic stimulation: a neurochronometrics of mind.* Cambridge, MA: MIT Press.

Walter, W., Cooper, R., Aldridge, V., McCallum, W., & Winter, A. (1964). Contingent negative variation: an electric sign of sensorimotor association and expectancy in the human brain. *Nature, 203,* 380–384.

Waltz, J., Knowlton, B., Holyoak, K., Boone, K., Mishkin, F., Santos, M. et al. (1999). A system for relational reasoning in human prefrontal cortex. *Psychological Science, 10,* 119–125.

Wapner, W., Hamby, S., & Gardner, H. (1981). The role of the right hemisphere in the apprehension of complex linguistic materials. *Brain and Language, 14,* 15–33.

Ward, J., & Mattingley, J. B. (2006). Synaesthesia: an overview of contemporary findings and controversies. *Cortex, 42*(2), 129–136.

Ward, J. & Romani, C. (1998). Serial position effects and lexical activation in spelling: Evidence from a single case study. *Neurocase, 4,* 189–206.

Ware, W. H. (1963). *Digitial computer technology and design: circuits and machine design.* New York: Wiley.

Warren, J. D., Warren, J. E., Fox, N. C., & Warrington, E. K. (2003). Nothing to say, something to sing: primary progressive dynamic aphasia. *Neurocase, 9,* 140–155.

Warren, J. M. & Akert, K. (1964). *The frontal granular cortex and behavior.* New York.

Warrington, E. K. (1975). The selective impairment of semantic memory. *Quarterly Journal of Experimental Psychology, 27,* 635–657.

Warrington, E. K. (1981). Concrete word dyslexia. *British Journal of Psychology, 72,* 175–196.

Warrington, E. K. (1982). Neuropsychological studies of object recognition. *Philosophical Transaction of the Royal Society of London B: Biological Sciences, 298,* 15–33.

Warrington, P. (1984). *Recognition memory test.* Windsor (UK): NFER-Nelson.

Warrington, E. K. & Cipolotti, L. (1996). Word comprehension. The distinction between refractory and storage impairments. *Brain, 119* (2), 611–625.

Warrington, E. K. & Crutch, S. J. (2004). A circumscribed refractory access disorder: a verbal semantic impairment sparing visual semantics. *Cognitive Neuropsychology, 21,* 299–315.

Warrington, E. K. & Duchen, L. (1992). A re-appraisal of a case of persistent global amnesia following right temporal lobectomy: a clinico-pathological study. *Neuropsychologia, 30,* 450.

Warrington, E. K. & James, M. (1991). *VOSP: visual object and space perception battery.* Bury St. Edmunds, UK.: Thames Valley Test Company.

Warrington, E. K. & Langdon, D. (2002). Does the spelling dyslexic read by recognizing orally spelled words? An investigation of a letter-by-letter reader. *Neurocase, 8,* 210–218.

Warrington, E. K. & McCarthy, R. A. (1983). Category specific access dysphasia. *Brain, 106* (4), 859–878.

Warrington, E. K. & McCarthy, R. A. (1987). Categories of knowledge. Further fractionations and an attempted integration. *Brain, 110* (5), 1273–1296.

Warrington, E. K. & McCarthy, R. A. (1988). The fractionation of retrograde amnesia. *Brain and Cognition, 7,* 184–200.

Warrington, E. K. & Shallice, T. (1969). The selective impairment of auditory verbal short-term memory. *Brain, 92,* 885–896.

Warrington, E. K. & Shallice, T. (1979). Semantic access dyslexia. *Brain, 102,* 43–63.

Warrington, E. K. & Shallice, T. (1980). Word-form dyslexia. *Brain, 103,* 99–112.

Warrington, E. K. & Shallice, T. (1984). Category specific semantic impairments. *Brain, 107* (3), 829–854.

Warrington, E. K. & Taylor, A. (1973). The contribution of right parietal lobe to object recognition. *Cortex, 9,* 152–164.

Warrington, E. K. & Taylor, A. (1978). Two categorical stages of object recognition. *Perception, 7,* 695–705.

Warrington, E. K. & Weiskrantz, L. (1968). A new method of testing long-term retention with special reference to amnesic patients. *Nature, 217,* 972–974.

Warrington, E. K. & Weiskrantz, L. (1970). The amnesic syndrome: consolidation or retrieval? *Nature, 228,* 628–630.

Warrington, E. K. & Weiskrantz, L. (1978). Further analysis of the prior learning effect in amnesia patients. *Neuropsychologia, 16,* 169–177.

Warrington, E. K., Logue, V., & Pratt, R. (1971). The anatomical localisation of selective impairment of auditory verbal short-term memory. *Neuropsychologia, 9,* 377–387.

Wason, P. C. (1968). Reasoning about a rule. *Quarterly Journal of Experimental Psychology, 20*(3), 273.

Waugh, N. C. & Norman, D. A. (1965). Primary memory. *Psychological Review, 72,* 89–104.

Weekes, B. (1997). Differential effects of number of letters on word and nonword naming latency. *Quarterly Journal of Experimental Psychology, 50A,* 439–456.

Weekes, B. & Coltheart, M. (1996). Surface dyslexia and surface dysgraphia: treatment studies and their theoretical implications. *Cognitive Neuropsychology, 13,* 277–315.

Wegner, D. M. (1994). Ironic processes of mental control. *Psychological Review, 101,* 34–52.

Wegner, D. M. (2003). *The illusion of conscious will.* MIT Press.

Weiskrantz, L. (1986a). *Blindsight: a case history and implications.* Oxford: OUP.

Weiskrantz, L. (1986b). Some aspects of memory functions and the temporal lobes. *Acta Neurologica Scandinavica (Suppl. 109),* 69–74.

Weiskrantz, L. (1997). *Consciousness lost and found.* Oxford: OUP.

Weiskrantz, L. & Warrington, E. K. (1970). A study of forgetting in amnesic patients. *Neuropsychologia, 8,* 281–288.

Weiskrantz, L. & Warrington, E. K. (1979). Conditioning in amnesic patients. *Neuropsychologia, 17,* 187–194.

Weiskrantz, L., Warrington, E. K., Sanders, M. D., & Marshall, J. (1974). Visual capacity in the hemianopic field following a restricted occipital ablation. *Brain, 97,* 709–728.

Weiskrantz, L., Harlow, A., & Barbur, J. L. (1991). Factors affecting visual sensitivity in a hemianopic subject. *Brain, 114* (5), 2269–2282.

Weiskrantz, L., Barbur, J. L., & Sahraie, A. (1995). Parameters affecting conscious versus unconscious visual discrimination with damage to the visual cortex (V1). *Proceedings of the National Academy of Sciences, USA, 92,* 6122–6126.

Welford, A. T. (1952). The 'psychological refractory period' and the timing of high-speed performance—a review and a theory. *British Journal of Psychology, 43,* 2–19.

Welsh, M. C., Satterlee-Cartmell, T., & Stine, M. (1999). Towers of Hanoi and London: contribution of working memory and inhibition to performance. *Brain and Cognition, 41,* 231–242.

Wendelken, C., Nakhabenko, D., Donohue, S. E., Carter, C. S., & Bunge, S. A. (2008). 'Brain is to thought as stomach is to ??': investigating the role of rostrolateral prefrontal cortex in relational reasoning. *Journal of Cognitive Neuroscience, 20,* 682–693.

Wertheimer, M. (1920). *Über Schlussprozesse im produktiven Denken.* De Gruiter.

Westermann, G. & Goebel, R. (1995). Connectionist rules of language. In J.Moore & J. Lehmann (Eds), *Proceedings of the Seventeenth Annual Conference of the Cognitive Science Society.* LEA.

Westermann, G., Willshaw, D., & Penke, M. (1999). A constructivist neural network model of German verb inflection in agrammatic aphasia. *IEE conference publications*, (CP470), 916–921.

Wharton, C. M., Grafman, J., Flitman, S. S., Hansen, E. K., Brauner, J., Marks, A. et al. (2000). Toward neuroanatomical models of analogy: a positron emission tomography study of analogical mapping. *Cognitive Psychology, 40,* 173–197.

Wheatley, T., Weisberg, J., Beauchamp, M. S., & Martin, A. (2005). Automatic priming of semantically related words reduces activity in the fusiform gyrus. *Journal of Cognitive Neuroscience, 17,* 1871–1885.

White, H. (1989). Some asymptotic results for learning in single hidden-layer feedforward network models. *Journal of the American Statistical Association, 84*(408), 1003–1013.

Whittlesea, B. W. A. (1993). Illusions of familiarity. *Journal of Experimental Psychology: Learning, Memory, and Cognition, 19*(6), 1235–1253.

Whittlesea, B., Jacoby, L. L., & Girard, K. (1990). Illusions of immediate memory: Evidence of an attributional basis for feelings of familiarity and perceptual quality. *Journal of Memory and Language, 29,* 716–732.

Wickelgren, W. A. (1968). Sparing of short-term memory in an amnesic patient: implications for a strength theory of memory. *Neuropsychologia, 6,* 235–244.

Wickelgren, W. A. (1969). Auditory or articulatory coding in verbal short-term memory. *Psychological Review, 76*(2), 232–235.

Wickelgren, W. A. (1979). Chunking and consolidation: a theoretical synthesis of semantic networks, configuring in conditioning, S-R versus cognitive learning, normal forgetting, the amnesic syndrome, and the hippocampal arousal system. *Psychological Review, 86*(1), 44–60.

Wiener, N. (1948). *Cybernetics.* New York: Wiley and Sons.

Wilding, E. L., & Rugg, M. D. (1996). An event-related potential study of recognition memory with and without retrieval of source. *Brain, 119*(3), 889–905.

Wilkins, M. (1963). Molecular configuration of nucleic acids. *Science, 140,* 941–950.

Wilkins, M., Gosling, R., & Seeds, W. (1951). Nucleic acid: an extensible molecule? *Nature, 167,* 759–760.

Wills, T. J., Lever, C., Cacucci, F., Burgess, N., & O'Keefe, J. (2005). Attractor dynamics in the hippocampal representation of the local environment. *Science, 308,* 873–876.

Wilshire, C. & McCarthy, R. (1996). Experimental investigations of an impairment in phonological encoding. *Cognitive Neuropsychology, 13,* 1059–1098.

Wilson, B. & Baddeley, A. (1988). Semantic, episodic, and autobiographical memory in a postmeningitic amnesic patient. *Brain and Cognition, 8,* 31–46.

Wilson, S. M., Brambati, S. M., Henry, R. G., Handwerker, D. A., Agosta, F., Miller, B. L. et al. (2009). The neural basis of surface dyslexia in semantic dementia. *Brain, 132,* 71–86.

Wimmer, H. & Perner, J. (1983). Beliefs about beliefs: representation and constraining function of wrong beliefs in young children's understanding of deception. *Cognition, 13,* 103–128.

Wing, A. & Baddeley, A. (1980). Spelling errors in handwriting: A corpus and a distribution analysis. In U. Frith (Ed.), *Cognitive processes in spelling.* London: Academic Press.

Winocur, G. (1990). Anterograde and retrograde amnesia in rats with dorsal hippocampal or dorsomedial thalamic lesions. *Behavioral and Brain Research, 38,* 145–154.

Winograd, T. (1972). *Understanding natural language.* New York: Academic Press.

Winston, P. (1975). *Learning structural descriptions from examples. The psychology of computer vision.* New York: McGraw-Hill.

Wise, R. J. (2003). Language systems in normal and aphasic human subjects: functional imaging studies and inferences from animal studies. *British Medical Bulletin, 65,* 95–119.

Wise, S. P. & Mauritz, K. H. (1985). Set-related neuronal activity in the premotor cortex of rhesus monkeys: effects of changes in motor set. *Proceedings of the Royal Society of London B: Biological Sciences, 223,* 331–354.

Wise, S. P., Murray, E. A., & Gerfen, C. R. (1996). The frontal cortex-basal ganglia system in primates. *Critical Reviews in Neurobiology, 10,* 317–356.

Wittgenstein, L. (1953). *Philosophical Investigations,* (trans. G. E. M. Anscombe). Oxford: Blackwell.

Wixted, J. T. (2007). Dual-process theory and signal-detection theory of recognition memory. *Psychological Review, 114*(1), 152–176.

Wolf, M., Ferrari, M., & Quaresima, V. (2007). Progress of near-infrared spectroscopy and topography for brain and muscle clinical applications. *Journal of Biomedical Optics, 12,* 062104.

Wolford, G., Miller, M. B., & Gazzaniga, M. (2000). The left hemisphere's role in hypothesis formation. *Journal of Neuroscience, 20,* RC64.

Wolpert, D. M. & Ghahramani, Z. (2000). Computational principles of movement neuroscience. *Nature Neuroscience Supplement, 3,* 1212–1217.

Wolpert, D. M. & Kawato, M. (1998). Multiple paired forward and inverse models for motor control. *Neural Networks, 11,* 1317–1329.

Wolpert, D. M., Goodbody, S. J., & Husain, M. (1998). Maintaining internal representations: the role of the superior parietal lobe. *Nature Neuroscience, 1,* 529–533.

Woodrow, H. (1914). The measurement of attention. *Psychological Monographs, 17,* 1–158.

Woollams, A. M., Lambon Ralph, M. A., Plaut, D. C., & Patterson, K. (2007). SD-squared: on the association between semantic dementia and surface dyslexia. *Psychological Review, 114,* 316–339.

Woollams, A. M., Taylor, J. R., Karayanidis, F., & Henson, R. N. (2008). Event-related potentials associated with masked priming of test cues reveal multiple potential contributions to recognition memory. *Journal of Cognitive Neuroscience, 20,* 1114–1129.

Wright, I., McGuire, P., Poline, J., Travere, J., Murray, R., Frith, C. et al. (1995). A voxel-based method for the statistical analysis of gray and white matter density applied to schizophrenia. *Neuroimage, 2,* 244–252.

Xu, Y. (2007). The role of superior intraparietal sulcus in supporting visual short-term memory for multifeature objects. *The Journal of Neuroscience, 27*(43), 11676–11686.

Xu, Y. & Chun, M. M. (2006). Dissociable neural mechanisms supporting visual short-term memory for objects. *Nature, 440,* 91–95.

Xu, Y. & Chun, M. M. (2007). Visual grouping in human parietal cortex. *Proceedings of the National Academy of Sciences, USA, 104,* 18766–18771.

Yi, H. A., Moore, P., & Grossman, M. (2007). Reversal of the concreteness effect for verbs in patients with semantic dementia. *Neuropsychology, 21,* 9–19.

Yonelinas, A. P. (2002). The nature of recollection and familiarity: a review of 30 years of research. *Journal of Memory and Language, 46,* 441–517.

Yonelinas, A. P., Kroll, N. E. A., Dobbins, I., Lazzara, M., & Knight, R. T. (1998). Recollection and familiarity deficits in amnesia: Convergence of remember-know, process dissociation, and receiver operating characteristic data. *Neuropsychology, 12*(3), 323–339.

Young, A. W., Hellawell, D., & de Haan, E. H. (1988). Cross-domain semantic priming in normal subjects and a prosopagnosic patient. *Quarterly Journal of Experimental Psychology, 40A,* 561–580.

Young, R. & Lewis, R. L. (1999). The Soar cognitive architecture and human working memory. In A. Miyake & P. Shah (Eds), *Models of working memory: mechanisms of active maintenance and executive control* (pp. 224–256). New York: CUP.

Yu, A. J. & Dayan, P. (2005). Uncertainty, neuromodulation, and attention. *Neuron, 46,* 681–692.

Zaidel, E. & Peters, A. (1981). Phonological encoding and ideographic reading by the disconnected right hemisphere: two case studies. *Brain and Language, 14,* 205–234.

Zanini, S., Rumiati, R. I., & Shallice, T. (2002). Action sequencing deficit following frontal lobe lesion. *Neurocase, 8,* 88–99.

Zarahn, E., Aguirre, G. K., & D'Esposito, M. (1999). Temporal isolation of the neural correlates of spatial mnemonic processing with fMRI. *Cognitive Brain Research, 7,* 255–268.

Zeki, S. (1974). Functional organization of a visual area in the posterior bank of the superior temporal sulcus of the rhesus monkey. *Journal of Physiology, 236,* 549–573.

Zeki, S. (1990a). A theory of multi-stage integration in the visual cortex. In J. Eccles & O. Creutzfeldt (Eds), *The principles of design and operation of the brain.* Rome: Vatican City: Pontificial Academy.

Zeki, S. (1990b). Parallelism and functional specialization in human visual cortex. *Cold Spring Harbour Symposia on Quantitative Biology, 55,* 651–661.

Zeki, S. (2005). The Ferrier Lecture 1995. Behind the seen: the functional specialization of the brain in space and time. *Philosophical Transactions of the Royal Society of London B Biological Sciences, 360,* 1145–1183.

Zeki, S. & Bartels, A. (1999). Toward a theory of visual consciousness. *Consciousness and Cognition, 8*(2), 225–259.

Zeki, S., Watson, J. D., & Frackowiak, R. S. (1993). Going beyond the information given: the relation of illusory visual motion to brain activity. *Proceedings. Biological Sciences, 252,* 215–222.

Zhang, D., Zhang, X., Sun, X., Li, Z., Wang, Z., He, S. et al. (2004). Cross-modal temporal order memory for auditory digits and visual locations: an fMRI study. *Human Brain Mapping, 22,* 280–289.

Zihl, J., Von Cramon, D., & Mai, N. (1983). Selective disturbance of movement vision after bilateral brain damage. *Brain, 106* (2), 340.

Zimmer, K. (2005). Examining the validity of numerical ratios in loudness fractionation. *Perception & Psychophysics, 67*(4), 569–579.

Zingeser, L. B. & Berndt, R. S. (1990). Retrieval of nouns and verbs in agrammatism and anomia. *Brain and Language, 39*(1), 14–32.

Zipser, D. (1985). A computational model of hippocampal place fields. *Behavioral Neuroscience, 99,* 1006–1018.

Zipser, D., & Andersen, R. (1988). A back propagation programmed network that simulates response properties of a subset of posterior parietal neurons. *Nature, 331,* 679–684.

Zola-Morgan, S. M. & Squire, L. R. (1990). The primate hippocampal formation: evidence for a time-limited role in memory storage. *Science, 250,* 288–290.

Zola-Morgan, S. M., Squire, L. R., & Amaral, D. G. (1989). Lesions of the amygdala that spare adjacent cortical regions do not impair memory or exacerbate the impairment following lesions of the hippocampal formation. *Journal of Neuroscience, 9,* 1922–1936.

Zola-Morgan, S. M., Squire, L. R., Clower, R. P., & Rempel, N. L. (1993). Damage to the perirhinal cortex exacerbates memory impairment following lesions to the hippocampal formation. *Journal of Neuroscience, 13,* 251–265.

Zorzi, M. (2005). Computational models of reading. In G. Houghton (Ed.), *Connectionist models in cognitive psychology* (pp. 403–444). London: Psychology Press.

Zorzi, M., Houghton, G., & Butterworth, B. (1998). Two routes or one in reading aloud? A connectionist dual-process model. *Journal of Experimental Psychology: Human Perception and Performance, 24,* 1131–1161.

Index

Note: page numbers in *italics* refer to Figures and Tables, and those with the suffix 'n' refer to footnotes.